IMAGING
OF
DISEASES
OF THE
CHEST

PETER ARMSTRONG

Professor of Radiology
St. Bartholomew's Hospital
London, England
(Formerly Professor and Vice Chairman
Department of Radiology
University of Virginia Health Sciences Center
Charlottesville, Virginia)

ALAN G. WILSON

Consultant Radiologist, St. George's Hospital
London, England

PAUL DEE

Professor of Radiology
University of Virginia Health Sciences Center
Charlottesville, Virginia

DAVID M. HANSELL

Consultant Radiologist
Royal Brompton Hospital
London, England

SECOND EDITION
with 1690 ilustrations

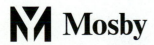 Mosby

St. Louis Baltimore Berlin Boston Carlsbad Chicago London Madrid
Naples New York Philadelphia Sydney Tokyo Toronto

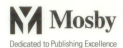

Mosby
Dedicated to Publishing Excellence

Executive Editor: Susan M. Gay
Developmental Editors: Maura K. Leib/Sandra Clark Brown
Project Manager: Patricia Tannian
Senior Book Designer: Gail Morey Hudson
Manufacturing Supervisors: John Babrick/Theresa Fuchs

SECOND EDITION

Printed in the United States of America
Composition by Clarinda Company
Printing/binding by Maple-Vail Book Mfg Group

Mosby–Year Book, Inc.
11830 Westline Industrial Drive
St. Louis, MO 63146

Library of Congress Cataloging in Publication Data
Imaging of diseases of the chest / Peter Armstrong . . . [et al.].—
  2nd ed.
    p. cm.
  Rev. ed. of: Imaging of diseases of the chest / Peter Armstrong,
Alan G. Wilson, Paul Dee. c1990.
  Includes bibliographical references and index.
  ISBN 0-8151-0011-6
  1. Chest — Imaging.   2. Chest — Diseases — Diagnosis.   I. Armstrong,
Peter, 1940- . II. Armstrong, Peter, 1940-   Imaging of diseases
of the chest.
  [DNLM: 1. Lung Diseases — diagnosis.   2. Diagnostic Imaging.
3. Thoracic Injuries — diagnosis.   WF 600 I31 1995]
RC941.A75   1995
617.5′40757 — dc20
DNLM/DLC
for Library of Congress   94-5302
                                            CIP

96 97 98 / 9 8 7 6 5 4 3

Contributors

PETER ARMSTRONG

Professor of Radiology
St. Bartholomew's Hospital
London, England
(Formerly Professor and Vice Chairman
Department of Radiology
University of Virginia Health Sciences Center
Charlottesville, Virginia)

PAUL DEE

Professor of Radiology
University of Virginia Health Sciences Center
Charlottesville, Virginia

DAVID M. HANSELL

Consultant Radiologist
Royal Brompton Hospital
London, England

THEODORE E. KEATS

Professor of Radiology
Department of Radiology
University of Virginia Health Sciences Center
Charlottesville, Virginia

A. MICHAEL PETERS

Reader in Nuclear Medicine
Department of Radiology
Royal Postgraduate Medical School
London, England

ALAN G. WILSON

Consultant Radiologist
St. George's Hospital
London, England

To
our families

Preface

This book has been written to provide radiologists, chest physicians, and thoracic surgeons with a one-volume account of chest imaging, primarily in the adult patient. An attempt has been made to present an integrated review of the appearances encountered in diseases of the lungs, pleura, and mediastinum using the various imaging modalities available in a modern radiology department. The plain chest radiograph is almost invariably the initial examination undertaken, and its interpretation continues to be a great challenge. Therefore the chest radiograph has been accorded the central position it deserves, but attention has also been directed to ultrasound, magnetic resonance imaging, radionuclide imaging, interventional procedures, and above all, computed tomography.

This second edition has been completely revised and updated. High-resolution computed tomography (HRCT) was in its relative infancy when the first edition was written. Now it forms a vital aspect of chest imaging. Therefore a whole new chapter is dedicated to this subject, written by our new coauthor Dr. David M. Hansell, and all the chapters on lung disease describe the HRCT appearances seen in specific disorders.

The magnitude of the AIDS epidemic has unfortunately become all too apparent since the previous edition was published, and a new chapter on AIDS has been added.

The clinical and pathologic aspects of conditions such as bronchial carcinoma, pulmonary embolism, and chest trauma are widely known, and detailed discussion of these aspects has been deliberately avoided. On the other hand, in less frequently encountered conditions, such as immunologic or systemic disorders and drug- or radiation-induced disease, we have chosen to deal with the clinicopathologic aspects in more detail. Our aim has been to provide answers to the many questions that in our experience arise in the day-to-day practice of chest imaging.

Peter Armstrong
Alan G. Wilson
Paul Dee
David M. Hansell

Acknowledgments

So many individuals contribute to a medical textbook that it is impossible to acknowledge all their help individually. We have had the assistance of many superb secretaries. In particular, Julie Jessop of St. Batholomew's Hospital, Sherry Deane, Pat West, Shirley Yowell, Geneva Shifflett, Diana Bowman, and Kelly Powell of the University of Virginia (UVa), Lisa Bolt of the Brompton Hospital, and Pat Vecchi, Hazel Bezodis, and Veronica King of St. George's Hospital have helped with typing manuscripts and making photocopies. Carol Chowdhry, our editorial assistant at UVa, was invaluable both for the many hours spent educating us on points of style and grammar and for checking and numbering the references in the first edition, and Natasha Armstrong spent many hours sorting images as well as checking and numbering references for both editions. The Medical Photography Departments of UVa, St. Bartholomew's, St. George's, and The Royal Marsden Hospitals were willing helpers in preparing photographs of an extremely high standard. Without good images a book such as this is of limited value. We therefore express our sincere gratitude to them for all their efforts.

Chest radiology is a team effort involving radiologists, chest surgeons, and pulmonary internists. It has been our great fortune to have worked with thoracic surgeons and physicians who were friendly, cooperative colleagues with a great interest in diagnostic imaging. They will recognize in these pages many of the patients that they have operated or consulted upon.

Thanks also to Mosby–Year Book Medical Publishers, notably Maura Leib and Patricia Tannian. This book would not have been possible without the support and resources of our own hospitals and medical schools. Finally, David Hansell would like to acknowledge his dog Baxter for enduring shorter walks.

Peter Armstrong
Alan G. Wilson
Paul Dee
David M. Hansell

Contents

IMAGING
OF
DISEASES
OF THE
CHEST

1 Technical Considerations

DAVID M. HANSELL

PLAIN CHEST RADIOGRAPHY

The standard views of the chest are the erect postero-anterior (PA) and lateral projections. With the greater availability of cross-sectional imaging, other views are less frequently required. The PA chest radiograph is taken at total lung capacity with the patient positioned so that the medial ends of the clavicle are equidistant from the spinous process of the thoracic vertebra at that level. The scapulae are held as far to the side of the chest as possible by rotating the patient's shoulders forward and placing the backs of the patient's wrists on the iliac crests. On a correctly exposed film most of the lungs should be visible (particularly the portions behind the heart), as well as the complex interfaces of the lung with the mediastinum. Many technical factors, notably the kilovoltage and film-screen combination used, determine how well the lungs are demonstrated.

The steep S-shaped dose/response curve of radiographic film (Figure 1-1) makes it impossible to obtain perfect exposure of the most radiolucent and radiodense parts of the chest in a single radiograph. Methods of overcoming this shortcoming of radiographic film include the use of high-kilovoltage (above 120 kV) techniques,[64] asymmetric screen-film combinations,[74] and sophisticated scanning equalization radiographic units.[79]

High-kilovoltage radiographs have several advantages over low-kilovoltage films. Because the coefficients of x-ray absorption of bone and soft tissue approach each other at high kilovoltage, the skeletal structures no longer obscure the lungs to the same degree as on low-kilovoltage radiographs. The high-kilovoltage radiograph thus demonstrates much more of the lung. Furthermore, the better penetration of the mediastinum with high-kilovoltage techniques allows greater detail of the airways to be seen. At high kilovoltage, exposure times are shorter and less scattered radiation reaches the intensifying screen, so that structures within the lung have a sharper

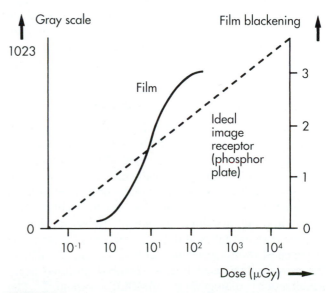

FIGURE 1-1
Radiation dose/response curve of conventional film-screen combination compared with the linear response (*dotted line*) of a phosphor plate image receptor.

outline. Although scattered radiation is greater with high kilovoltage, the use of a grid means that there is a net reduction of scattered radiation degrading the image compared with a low-kilovoltage, nongrid technique. An air gap of 15 cm in depth is often used, instead of a grid, with high-kilovoltage technique to disperse scattered radiation; this is as effective as a grid, and the radiation dose to the patient is similar for the two techniques.[78] To counteract the unwanted magnification and penumbra effects of interposing an air gap, the focus-film (or anode-to-image) distance is increased to approximately 4 m.

Although high-kilovoltage radiographs are preferable for routine examination of the lungs and mediastinum, low-kilovoltage radiographs provide excellent detail of unobscured lung because of the improved contrast between lung vessels and surrounding aerated lung. Moreover, calcified lesions, such as pleural plaques, and small pulmonary nodules[36] are particularly well demonstrated on low-kilovoltage films.

Film-screen combinations

The major advances in film-screen combinations over the last 20 years have been the introduction of "faster" rare earth phosphor screens and the development of wide-latitude film. The improved light emission from rare earth phosphors over traditional calcium tungstate crystal screens has resulted in shorter exposure times and thus sharper images. A significant advance in film-screen combinations for chest imaging has been the development of an asymmetric combination consisting of a thin front screen and high-contrast film emulsion and, on the reverse side of the film base, a thicker back screen and a low-contrast film emulsion. With this combination the two ends of the wide spectrum of transmission of x-rays through the thorax can be accommodated. In preliminary clinical trials, such a film-screen combination has shown significantly more detail in the mediastinum and lung obscured by the diaphragm and heart (Figure 1-2). A further benefit is that the radiation dose to the patient may be reduced by up to 30%.[74]

Scanning equalization radiography

Because attenuation of x-rays by the mediastinum is up to 10 times greater than that by the lungs, many attempts to produce a more uniformly exposed chest radiograph have been made. Exposure equalization may be achieved by using simple portal "trough" filters or by interposing a customized filter, unique to the patient, between the patient and the incident x-ray beam.[61] Newer techniques include devices that modulate the exposure for each part of the chest by an electronic feedback system.[25,82] One of the most widely used is the advanced multiple beam equalization radiography (AMBER) system.[79] The AMBER unit uses a horizontally oriented scanning slit beam that is effectively divided into 20 segments, each modulated by an electronic feedback loop from 20

corresponding detectors on the far side of the patient. Such a system is particularly good at demonstrating pathologic conditions of the lung that are obscured by the heart and diaphragm (Figure 1-2).[69] There does not appear to be any counterbalancing loss in observer performance in the detection of diffuse lung disease[28] or pulmonary consolidation[57] between scanning equalization radiography and conventional chest radiography.

Because of the dynamic exposure control of scanning equalization radiography, determining the exact radiation dose received by an individual patient is difficult. For an average-size patient the estimated effective dose for a PA and lateral projection with the AMBER technique is 0.14 mSv, compared with 0.085 mSv for conventional chest radiography.[18]

Extra radiographic views

The frontal and lateral projections suffice for most purposes in chest radiography. Other radiographic views are becoming less frequently requested as the availability of cross-sectional imaging increases. Nevertheless, they should not be overlooked, since they may solve a particular clinical problem quickly and cheaply.

The lateral decubitus view is not, as its name implies, a lateral view. It is a frontal view taken with a horizontal beam with the patient lying on his or her side. Its main purpose is to demonstrate the movement of fluid in the pleural space. If a pleural effusion is not loculated, it gravitates to the dependent part of the pleural cavity. If the patient lies on his or her side, the fluid layers between the chest wall and the lung edge. Because the ribs, unlike the diaphragm, are always identifiable, comparison of a standard frontal view with a lateral decubitus view is a reliable way of recognizing free pleural fluid.

A lordotic view is now rarely used and is virtually obsolete, but is included here for completeness. It is performed by angling the x-ray beam 15 degrees craniad either by positioning the patient upright and angling the beam up or by leaving the beam horizontal and leaning the patient backward. In this way the lung apices are better demonstrated, free from the superimposed clavicle and first rib. The lordotic view may be useful for distinguishing pulmonary shadows from incidental calcification of the costochondral junctions.

With the exception of identifying rib fractures and confirming the presence of a rib lesion, such as a lytic metastasis, oblique views of the thorax are rarely required.

Portable chest radiography

Portable or mobile chest radiography has the obvious advantage that the examination can be done without moving the patient to the radiology department. In many medical centers the proportion of portable to departmental chest radiographs has gradually increased over the years. However, the many disadvantages of portable radiography are often forgotten, particularly by request-

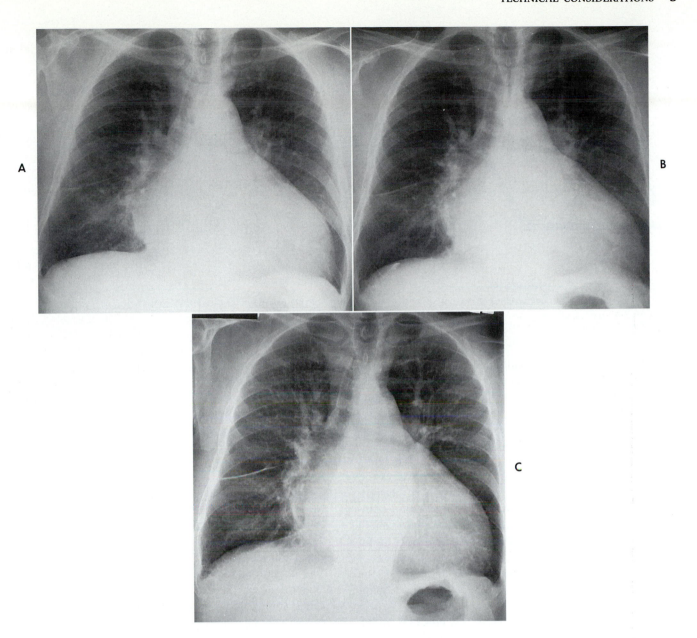

FIGURE 1-2
A patient with mitral valve disease. The three chest radiographs were taken at 140 kVp using, **A,** conventional film and rare earth screen combination, **B,** INSIGHT asymmetric film, and, **C,** AMBER scanning equalization unit. Note the differences in mediastinal detail between the radiographs produced with the three techniques.

ing clinicians. The shorter focus-film distance results in undesirable magnification. High-kilovoltage techniques cannot be used because portable machines are unable to deliver the high kilovoltage and because accurately aligning the x-ray beam with a grid is difficult. Furthermore, the maximum milliamperage is severely limited, necessitating long exposure times with the risk of significant blurring of the image. Portable lateral radiographs are even less likely to be successful because of the extremely long exposure times. Radiation exposure of nearby patients and staff is a further consideration.

Positioning of bed-bound patients is difficult, and the resulting radiographs are often of half-upright or rotated subjects. Even in the so-called erect position with the patient sitting up, the chest is rarely as vertical as it is in a standing patient. More important, the patient is unable to take a deep breath when propped up in bed.

Nevertheless, since many patients cannot be moved to the radiology department for a formal radiograph, any method of improving the quality of a portable chest radiograph represents a significant advance. In this area, digital chest radiography has proved valuable.

DIGITAL CHEST RADIOGRAPHY

Digital technology is an integral part of such techniques as computed tomography (CT), magnetic reso-

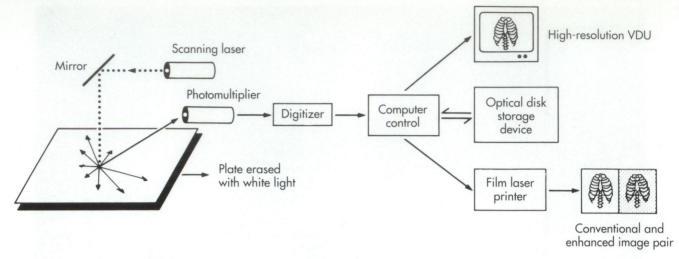

FIGURE 1-3
Components in a commercially available phosphor plate computed radiography system.

nance imaging (MRI), and ultrasonography. It has long been recognized that conventional film as a means of image capture, storage, and display represents something of a compromise,[24] and it has become apparent that digital image acquisition, transmission, display, and storage have advantages when applied to chest radiography.

Three fundamentally different methods of producing a digital chest radiography exist. The earliest work on digital chest radiography used digitization of conventional film radiographs by means of optical drum scanners or laser scanners. Although few indications remain for this approach in clinical practice, a great deal of useful information was derived from observer performance studies of digitized conventional film to establish the parameters for clinically acceptable digital radiographs.[23,39,42]

The second technique employed a dedicated digital chest unit that allowed digital acquisition of the image (rather than conversion of a conventional radiograph to a digital format). The prototype device was described more than 10 years ago and used a scanning slit beam and 1024 solid-state detectors.[76] The number of detectors limited the spatial resolution of this system and has precluded further development of this type of unit.

The third type of system employs conventional radiographic equipment but uses a reusable photostimulable phosphor plate (Europium-doped barium fluorohalide)[71] instead of a conventional film-screen combination. Phosphor plate computed, or digital, radiography has been adopted in many institutions, particularly as a substitute for portable film radiography. The phosphor plate is a large-area detector housed in a "filmless" cassette. The phosphor plate stores some of the energy of the incident x-ray photons as a latent image. When the plate is scanned with a focused laser beam, the stored energy is emitted as light that is detected by a photomultiplier and converted to a digital signal (Figure 1-3). The digital

information can then be manipulated, displayed, and stored in whatever format is desired (Figure 1-4). The phosphor plate can be reused once the latent image has been erased by exposure to white light. Most currently available computed radiography systems produce a digital radiograph with a 2 K × 2 K matrix (with a pixel size of 0.2 mm) and a gray scale of up to 1024 discrete levels. Because of the fundamental requirement of segmenting the image into a finite number of pixels, a great deal of work has been done to determine the relationship between pixel size, which affects spatial resolution, and lesion detectability.[14,39,43] Whether digital radiography can match conventional film radiography for the detection of extremely subtle pneumothoraces[12] and early interstitial lung disease[37] is still uncertain. Although an image composed of pixels of the smallest size possible would seem desirable, a direct inverse relationship exists between the pixel size and the cost and ease of data handling. Thus pixel size is ultimately a practical compromise between image fidelity and ease of data processing and storage.

Single-shot dual-energy imaging, a technique in which the bony thorax can be removed to reveal a "soft tissue image," can be performed relatively simply with phosphor plate computed radiography by separating two phosphor plates by a thin copper filter.[33] The resulting images, which separate the anatomic information into bone and soft tissue components, although remarkable, have not gained widespread clinical acceptance, probably because dual-energy imaging is competing with computed tomography to provide the same information.

An unequivocal advantage of phosphor plate computed radiography over conventional film radiography is the exactly linear photoluminescence-dose response, which is a full order of magnitude greater than that of conventional film (Figure 1-1). This extremely wide latitude, coupled with the facility for image processing, produces diagnos-

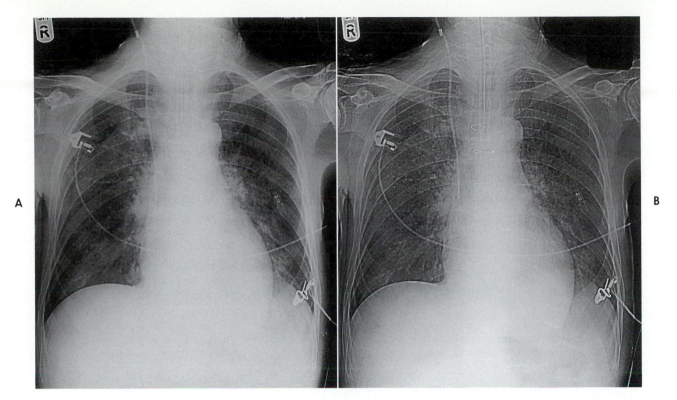

FIGURE 1-4
Portable computed radiograph pair that has been laser printed onto film. **A** is made to resemble analogue or conventional radiograph. **B** has been digitally processed to give an appearance of wider latitude and edge enhancement and wider latitude.

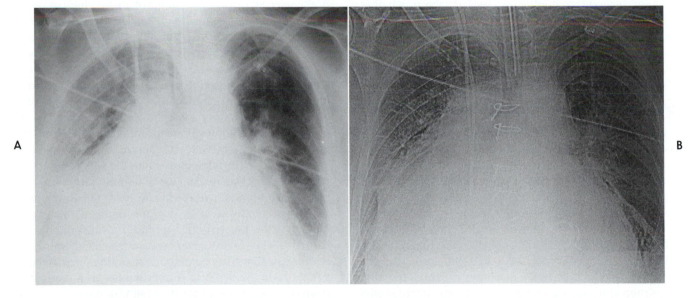

FIGURE 1-5
A, Portable postoperative conventional film radiograph of a patient after mitral valve replacement. Central venous lines and prosthetic valve are invisible. **B,** Phosphor plate computed radiograph showing considerably more detail despite adverse radiographic conditions.

tically acceptable images over a wide range of exposures. The ability to retrieve an image of diagnostic quality from a suboptimal exposure, which with conventional film would have resulted in an uninterpretable radiograph (Figure 1-5), has led to the increasing implementation of

such systems for portable chest radiography.

Numerous observer performance studies have shown that computed radiography can equal conventional film radiography in virtually any specific task.[66,67,77] For this, however, postprocessing of the digital image has to be

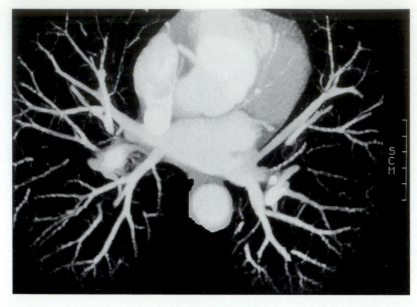

FIGURE 1-6
Three-dimensional reconstruction of the contrast-enhanced heart and pulmonary vasculature. Data acquired from continuous volume scanning using an electron beam ultrafast computed tomography scanner (Imatron Inc., San Francisco).

used to match the digital radiograph to the task. A problem inherent in all forms of digital manipulation is that enhancement of the image for one purpose degrades it for another.

There have been conflicting reports about whether digital chest radiographs can be satisfactorily interpreted on high-resolution television monitors, as distinct from laser-printed film. Recent studies suggest that 2 K × 2 K monitors may be adequate for making primary diagnoses of digital chest radiographs.[15,31,62]

COMPUTED TOMOGRAPHY

CT relies on the same physical principles as conventional radiography: the absorption of x-rays by tissues with constituents of differing atomic number. When multiple projections and computed calculations of radiographic density are used, slight differences in x-ray absorption can be displayed in a cross-sectional format.

The components of a conventional CT machine are an x-ray tube and an array of x-ray detectors opposite the tube; the number (up to 2400) and geometry of these detectors are variable. In CT machines in which both the x-ray tube and detectors rotate synchronously around the patient, the number of detectors is less (enough to be covered by the fan-shaped beam, but no more). The speed with which a mechanical CT scanner acquires a sectional image depends on the time the anode takes to rotate around the patient. Modern CT machines have scan times of below 2 seconds, and some scanners are capable of millisecond scan times. The signal from the x-ray detectors is reconstructed by a computer, displayed on the computer console, and usually laser printed onto film for interpretation.

A recent development in CT scanner technology is electron beam ultrafast CT scanning, which dispenses with a rotating mechanical anode: the patient is surrounded by a tungsten target ring, and a focused electron beam sweeps around the tungsten ring at high speed to produce an x-ray beam. Such machines are capable of acquiring an image in 100 msec or less, and thus "real-time" studies are possible with images acquired at 17 frames per second at a given level. Rapid acquisition studies allow the evaluation of normal and abnormal dynamic structural changes, for example, lung density during the respiratory cycle[87] or the excursion of the tracheal wall during respiratory maneuvers.[73] Spiral (also known as volume or helical) scanning entails continuous scanning while the table moves into the CT gantry.[35,80] In this way a continuous data set or "spiral" of information may be acquired in a single breath hold. The information is reconstructed into axial sections, perpendicular to the long axis of the patient, similar to conventional CT sections. The main advantage of so-called spiral CT scanning is that truly contiguous scanning, unaffected by variations in the depth of respiration between sections, is possible so that, for example, small pulmonary nodules are not missed.[63] Because a continuous data set is acquired with spiral scanning, exquisite three-dimensional reconstructions of complex anatomic areas can be produced (Figure 1-6).

Technical considerations

The CT image is composed of a matrix of picture element (pixels). There is a fixed number of pixels within the picture matrix so that the size of each pixel varies according to the diameter of the circle to be scanned. The smaller the scan circle size, the smaller the area represented by a pixel and the higher the spatial resolution of the final image. In practical terms the field of view size should be adjusted to the size of area of interest, usually the thoracic diameter of the patient. Depending on the field of view size, the pixel size varies between 0.3 and 1 mm across. By selecting a specific area of interest, the operator can achieve optimal spatial resolution (so-called targeted reconstruction of the raw data) for that region; extra information is available that is not displayed when the whole body section is viewed at once. Targeted reconstruction is used only when the finest morphologic detail is required, particularly in high-resolution CT examinations of the lung (see Chapter 5).

Sometimes a striking difference is apparent in the characteristics and "look" of the final CT image between different scanners. This is generally the result of differences in the software reconstruction algorithms that "smooth" the image to a greater or lesser extent by averaging the density of neighboring pixels. Smoothing is used to reduce the conspicuity of image noise and improve contrast, but it has the drawback of reducing the definition of fine structures. The lung is a high-contrast environment, and such smoothing is less necessary. Higher spatial resolution algorithms (which make image noise more conspicuous) are generally more desirable, and it has been recommended that their use not be confined to high-resolution CT but also be incorporated as routine contiguous 10 mm section scanning.[90]

SECTION THICKNESS. Although a CT section appears as a two-dimensional image, it has a third dimension of depth. Thus each pixel has a volume, and the three-dimensional element is referred to as a voxel. The computer calculates the average radiographic density of tissue within each voxel, and the final CT image consists of a representation of the numerous voxels in the section. Clearly, the single attenuation value of a voxel represents the average of the attenuation values of all the various structures within the voxel. The thicker the section, the greater the chance of different structures being included within the voxel and so the greater the averaging that occurs. The most obvious way to reduce this "partial volume" effect is to use thinner sections.

When the whole thorax is examined, contiguous 8 or 10 mm thick sections are usually employed. Thinner sections are occasionally required to clarify partial volume effects or to study areas of anatomy that are oriented obliquely to the plane of scanning. For example, contiguous 3 to 5 mm sections are sometimes preferable when examining the aortopulmonary window and subcarinal regions of the mediastinum. Another specific example of the use of narrow sections (less than 3 mm) to display differential densities (which would otherwise be lost because of the partial volume effect) is the small foci of fat or calcium that are sometimes seen within a hamartoma. Extremely fine sections of 1 to 2 mm thickness are used to study the fine morphologic detail of the lung parenchyma (high-resolution CT). This technique is discussed in more detail in Chapter 5. Apart from the evaluation of diffuse lung disease when sampling of a few parts of the lung (with sections taken at 20 or 30 mm intervals) is adequate, contiguous section scanning is necessary to allow accurate interpretation in most situations. Similarly, when pulmonary nodules are being sought, there is no alternative to contiguous scanning. There is a striking difference in the radiation dose to the patient between contiguous standard section and interspaced fine section scanning.[45] This difference is due largely to the imperfect beam collimation of most CT machines: because of the overlap between so-called contiguous sections, the effective dose to the patient is considerably greater than with interspaced scanning.

WINDOW SETTINGS. The average density of each voxel is measured in Hounsfield units (HU); these units have been arbitrarily chosen so that zero is water density and −1000 is air density. The range of Hounsfield units encountered in the thorax is wider than in any other part of the body, ranging from aerated lung (approximately −800 HU) to ribs (+700 HU). The operator uses two variables to select the range of densities to be viewed: window width and window center or level.

The window width determines the number of Hounsfield units to be displayed. Any densities greater than the upper limit of the window width are displayed as white, and any below the limit of the window are displayed as black. Between these two limits the densities are displayed in shades of gray. The median density of the window chosen is the center or level, and this center can be moved higher or lower at will, thus moving the window up or down through the range (Figure 1-7). The narrower the window width, the greater the contrast discrimination within the window. No single window setting can depict this wide range of densities on a single image. For this reason, thoracic work requires at least two sets of images, usually to demonstrate the lung parenchyma and the soft tissues of the mediastinum. Furthermore, it may be necessary for the operator to adjust the window settings to improve the demonstration of a particular abnormality. Standard window widths and centers for thoracic CT vary among institutions, but some generalizations can be made: for the soft tissues of the mediastinum and chest wall a window width of 400 to 600 HU and a center of +30 HU are appropriate. For the lungs a wide window of 1000 HU or more at a center of approximately −600 HU is usually satisfactory. For skeletal structures the widest possible window setting at a center of 30 HU is best.

The window settings have a profound influence on the visibility and apparent size of normal and abnormal structures. Nonetheless, precise window settings cannot be given because there is an element of observer preference and there are differences between machines. The most accurate representation of an object appears to be achieved if the value of the window level is halfway between the density of the structure to be measured and the density of the surrounding tissue.[3,38] For example, the

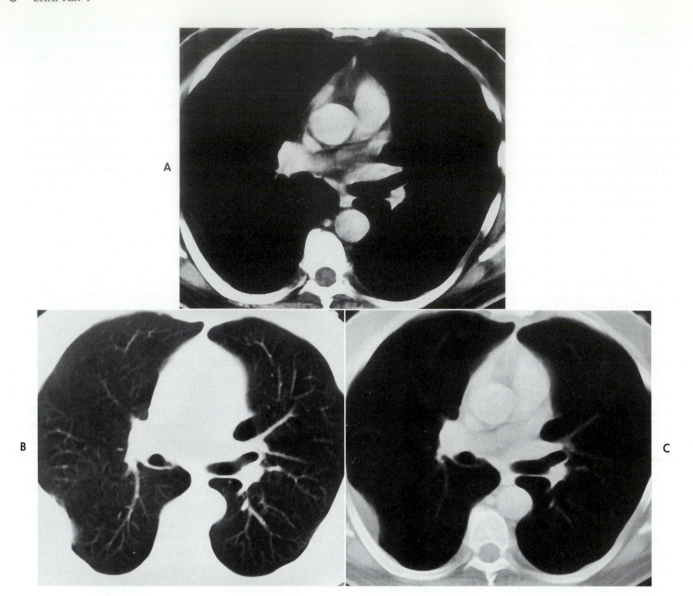

FIGURE 1-7
Computed tomography scans of the chest illustrating the effects of varying window levels and window widths. The section shows an extrapleural lipoma lying against the right chest wall. **A,** Window center 30 HU, window width 350 HU shows mediastinal soft tissue differences to advantage but does not show lung detail, nor is the lipoma easy to see. **B,** Window center 30 HU, window width 1500 HU shows the whole range of densities so that bone detail is well seen, the lipoma is recognizable as a soft tissue mass, and the mediastinal and lung structures are visible but subtle distinctions of contrast are invisible. **C,** Window center −600 HU, window width 1000 HU shows lung detail to advantage but provides no information about the mediastinum other than the outline.

diameter of a pulmonary nodule, measured on soft tissue settings appropriate for the mediastinum, will be grossly underestimated.[29] It is also important to remember that when inappropriate window settings are used, smaller structures (for example, peripheral pulmonary vessels) are proportionately much more affected than larger structures. A further factor that has a bearing on window settings is section thickness. Because pulmonary vessels imaged with thinner sections are less subject to partial volume effect, their density is greater and thus the window level should be correspondingly higher.[55]

Intravenous contrast enhancement

Because of the high contrast on CT between vessels and surrounding air in the lung, as well as between vessels and surrounding fat within the mediastinum, intravenous contrast enhancement is needed only in specific instances, for example, to aid the distinction between hilar vessels and lymph nodes. The exact timing of the injection of contrast media depends most on the time the CT scanner takes to scan the thorax. With faster and spiral scanners the circulation time of the patient becomes an important factor. However, general guidance about the time of arrival of contrast medium from the antecubital vein to various structures is possible[55]: in normal individuals arrival time in the superior vena cava is 4 seconds, pulmonary arteries 7 seconds, ascending aorta 11 seconds, descending aorta 12 seconds, and inferior vena cava 16 seconds.

The contrast medium rapidly diffuses out of the vascular space into the extravascular space, so that opacification of the vasculature following a bolus injection quickly declines and nonvascular structures such as lymph nodes steadily increase in density over time. Because of these dynamics, there is a time at which a solid structure may have exactly the same density as an adjacent vessel. The timing and duration of the contrast medium infusion must therefore be taken into account when interpreting a contrast-enhanced CT examination. Rapid scanning protocols with automated injectors tend to improve contrast enhancement of vascular structures at the expense of enhancement of solid lesions because of the rapidity of scanning. With rapid scanning and automated step-wise or continuous table movement, it is possible to achieve good opacification of all the thoracic vascular structures with a total dose of less than 120 ml of contrast (iodine content of 250 or 300 mg/ml) at a rate of about 1.5 ml/sec. For the examination of inflammatory lesions it may be necessary to delay scanning by 30 seconds to allow contrast to diffuse into the extravascular space. Each CT examination must be carefully tailored to the clinical problem; the protocol needed for a suspected aortic dissection with a fast scanner is clearly different from that required for the evaluation of an empyema with a conventional scanner.

Clinical indications for computed tomography

Despite continuing refinement of the indications for thoracic CT scanning, the radiologist should never forget that CT is a second-line study and should be used only when simpler tests, particularly chest radiography, have failed to resolve the clinical problem. Indications for CT can be broadly divided into situations in which CT elucidates an abnormality shown on a plain chest radiograph and those in which the chest radiograph appears normal but cryptic disease is suspected.

The indications for CT in a patient with a normal chest radiograph are rare. Specific instances include (1) the detection of pulmonary metastases in patients with extrathoracic malignancies that have a tendency to metastasize to the lung; (2) patients with endocrinologic or biochemical evidence of disease that might be related to a mediastinal or small pulmonary tumor, such as a thymoma, parathyroid adenoma, or bronchial carcinoid; and (3) a search for a peripheral lung tumor in patients with hemoptysis or abnormal findings on sputum cytology with no discoverable cause at bronchoscopy. High-resolution CT now has a major role in the evaluation of patients with abnormal lung function tests but a normal or near normal chest radiograph.

MAGNETIC RESONANCE IMAGING

The most significant advantages of MRI over other cross-sectional imaging are its excellent contrast resolution of soft tissues and its multiplanar imaging capability, which allows a truly three-dimensional appreciation of complex anatomic regions such as the hila and mediastinum. MRI has not replaced CT for the investigation of the majority of thoracic conditions that require cross-sectional imaging. However, there are specific instances in which MRI is superior to CT as a problem-solving technique; these include the identification of mediastinal or chest wall invasion by tumor,* the differentiation between solid and vascular hilar masses,[19,85] the evaluation of posterior and superior mediastinal masses,[41] the analysis of diaphragmatic disease, particularly after trauma,[51] and the assessment of mediastinal disease in patients with treated lymphoma.[21,34,58,59,84]

High spatial resolution imaging with MRI is technically possible, but there is a trade-off between resolution on one hand and signal-to-noise ratio and acquisition time on the other. This balance is particularly important for MRI of the lung parenchyma. The relatively poor spatial resolution of MRI remains a major obstacle to its more widespread use in thoracic imaging. For example, the spurious appearance of small clusters of lymph node in the mediastinum, which appear as a single mass, prevents the routine application of MRI to the staging of bronchogenic carcinoma. However, faster spin-echo techniques have improved contrast and spatial resolution by reducing motion artifact compared with standard T2-weighted images. Further developments in rapid breath hold imaging and improvements in cardiac and respiratory gating techniques and dedicated chest coils will improve image quality and lead to a wider role for MRI in the investigation of thoracic disease. More recently imaging sequences and protocols have been developed to evaluate the lung parenchyma.[5,7,47] Earlier studies showed the considerable difficulties in obtaining an adequate and reproducible signal from lung parenchyma.[46,48,54] The rapid development of MR angiography in other parts of the body has resulted in its increased use in the pulmonary circulation.[17,30,81]

Technical considerations

MRI of the thorax poses some unique challenges, particularly the consequences of cardiac and respiratory movement and the extremely low proton density of normal lung. The large tissue-air interface of the lung induces susceptibility artifacts that affect magnetic field homogeneity and lead to signal loss from intravoxel phase dispersion of spins in lung parenchyma,[4] although techniques have been devised to minimize this artifact.[10,53]

With the numerous imaging sequences, gating techniques, and planes of sections available to the radiologist, no single protocol can be prescribed for a thoracic MRI examination; more than any other imaging investigation

---

*References 2, 6, 9, 16, 27, 32, 49, 60, 89.

in the chest, the protocol needs to be tailored to the clinical question to be answered. For example, the MRI examination of a suspected thoracic aortic aneurysm will be different in virtually every respect from an examination of an area of pulmonary consolidation adjacent to the diaphragm. What follows therefore is an introduction to the factors affecting image quality.

SIGNAL-TO-NOISE RATIO. An appreciation of the factors that affect the signal-to-noise ratio (SNR) is crucial when considering the method of obtaining optimal MR images of the thorax. In MRI, signal intensity is proportional to the volume of tissue within a voxel. Because background noise is constant through the entire tissue volume, the voxel size in MRI needs to be larger than in CT to maintain a tolerable SNR. The same consideration applies to section thickness: section width is directly related to SNR. Sections less than 5 mm wide usually result in an unacceptably low SNR. The signal is further reduced with contiguous sections because of a phenomenon known as "cross-talk." For this reason most protocols include an interspace of approximately 25% of the section thickness between individual sections.[55]

In contrast to CT, in MRI a reduction in pixel size so that the finest matrix is used reduces the SNR by decreasing the voxel size. A further disadvantage is the increased scan time (which is proportional to the number of pixels in the phase encoding direction). Reducing the matrix size from 256×256 to 256×128 (the matrix most generally applicable to most thoracic work in which the highest resolution is not a priority) doubles the pixel size and consequently doubles the SNR.

The field of view has a profound effect on SNR. Although the field of view should be equivalent in size to the region of interest, SNR decreases dramatically below a field of view of 30 cm because of the reduction in pixel size inherent in decreasing the field of view (halving the field of view reduces the pixel size by fourfold and therefore the SNR by the same factor).

At high magnetic field strengths (1.5 Tesla or above), a higher SNR can be achieved in many parts of the body. However, in the thorax a high magnetic field induces a larger susceptibility artifact and movement artifacts leading to degradation of the image. A marked improvement in SNR can be achieved by using a smaller receiver coil: such a strategem is particularly effective in imaging infants, who may be imaged with head receiver coils. Dedicated thoracic surface coils are not widely available but increase both spatial resolution and SNR. However, the depth of penetration limits the clinical applicability of surface coils to the examination of chest wall lesions in adults.

The SNR can be increased by increasing the number of radiofrequency excitations and averaging the signal from each pixel. Doubling the number of radiofrequency excitations entails doubling the scanning time for what is only a modest increase in SNR; for this reason it is rarely employed.

MOVEMENT ARTIFACTS IN THORACIC MAGNETIC RESONANCE IMAGING. MR images are degraded by periodic respiratory and cardiovascular motion. The result is blurring of the image and superimposition of ghost images. At higher magnetic fields, degradation of the image by motion is more marked and the ghost images are more obvious because of the higher SNR. Artifacts from cardiovascular motion are minimized by synchronizing the acquisition of the images to a certain point in the cardiac cycle by electrocardiographic triggering. Such gating increases the scan time by approximately 15% while significantly improving image quality.[44]

The pulsatile flow of blood in major cardiovascular structures can generate variable amounts of signal and thus cause ghost artifacts in the phase direction of the image. The signal from flowing blood can be eliminated by saturating the incoming blood with repeated radiofrequency pulses, destroying its magnetization when it arrives in the volume being imaged.[13] The technique of presaturation is particularly valuable in high–field strength MRI machines.

Artifact from the movement of normal breathing cannot be countered by gating simply because the respiratory cycle is too long and a basic gating technique would require extremely long examination times.[40] Many data acquisition and processing techniques, including averaging, rephasing, and reordering of phase encoding (ROPE)[1] techniques, have been developed to overcome this problem. None is ideal, but fast scan techniques with single-section acquisition times of a few seconds can be used with breath holding. Rapid breath hold MRI has been successfully applied to cardiac studies.[11] For lung imaging, however, this technique suffers from the susceptibility artifacts encountered with gradient echo imaging. Further developments are needed to counteract this artifact. Echo planar techniques allow instantaneous real-time imaging.[65,72] In echo planar imaging a complete two-dimensional image is recovered from a single radiofrequency excitation using rapidly switched magnetic resonance field gradients to form an echo train. The data acquisition time can be reduced to tens of milliseconds and can be used after series of preparation pulses for anatomic, diffusion, or chemical shift imaging and velocity mapping. The echo planar technique makes severe demands on the hardware and software of currently available MRI systems.

Sometimes artifacts simulate or obscure the presence of thrombus in the major cardiovascular structures. In spin-echo imaging, increased signal intensity may be returned from slow-flowing blood because of the second echo of a symmetric double spin-echo sequence (known as even-echo rephasing). On the other hand, immobile thrombus often shows a reduction in signal intensity (with the caveat that the signal intensity of thrombus is affected by its age). Phase display images show either a high or a low signal intensity from moving objects, whereas static structures show constant signal inten-

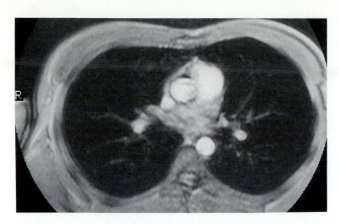

FIGURE 1-8
Gradient echo magnetic resonance image showing high signal from flowing blood, particularly in the great vessels running perpendicular to plane of section.

sity.[50,88] Perhaps the simplest technique for differentiating slow-flowing blood from a suspected thrombus is the use of gradient echo pulse sequences. The extremely high signal from even relatively slow-flowing blood usually allows the distinction to be made (Figure 1-8). However, if the vessel runs parallel to the plane of section, the contained blood receives multiple radiofrequency pulses and thus has a reduced signal, so that it potentially mimics thrombus. This can be resolved by imaging the vessel perpendicular to the scan plane.[26]

Tissue characteristics and paramagnetic contrast agents in magnetic resonance imaging

Differences in MR signal intensity among various tissues are due to a complex relationship between proton density and spin-lattice (T1) and spin-spin (T2) relaxation times.[68] Relaxation times are influenced by the size and freedom of molecules in tissues. After excitation by a radiofrequency pulse the nuclei return to their resting state. In the process an exchange of energy occurs; if the exchange is inefficient, the T1 time is long. T1 time is thus an index of the time taken for the spins to return or relax to their resting state. Fat has the shortest T1 relaxation time of all human tissues. In contrast, the large collagen macromolecules of fibrous (solid) tissue have much longer T1 relaxation times.

The T2 relaxation time is influenced mainly by interactions between molecules. In simple terms, large molecules that are restricted in motion have a very short T2 time, so that the MR signal is short lived and cannot be recorded within the echo time. Although the mobile molecules of water and fat generate the most signal, these molecules usually interact with the surrounding macromolecules that constitute the bulk of the soft tissue and thus their relaxation times are altered. It is this fundamental influence on water (and to a lesser extent fat)

molecules by the macromolecular components of different tissues that produces the striking contrast differences among various tissues on MRI. Thus an increase in the concentration of freely mobile water molecules and a decrease in the proportion of macromolecules (particularly protein) capable of interacting with water give long T1 and T2 relaxation times. Conversely, tissue with a high protein content shortens T1 relaxation times and at the same time has a less predictable effect on T2 relaxation times.

Paramagnetic agents, in the form of blood or gadolinium-complex contrast media, reduce T1 times; this phenomenon is the result of increasing the range of resonant frequency of protein protons by varying the magnetic field in the immediate vicinity of the paramagnetic material. In this way a wider range of proton-bearing molecules are recruited. The net result is a greater signal on T1 images with no substantial effect of T2 images at usual concentrations of gadolinium.

The MR signal intensity of a given tissue is an average of the contribution from each constituent of the tissue. In the same way, different pathologic processes produce different signal intensities depending on the proportions of, for example, fibrosis, edema, and necrosis. Because of the wide overlap in signal intensity resulting from the many components that contribute to the final signal, the signal intensity of a lesion cannot be regarded as specific; different pathologic conditions may produce similar signals. Any change in the various components of a tissue over time is reflected in the MR signal. For this reason, MRI, unlike CT, is more sensitive to serial change in a pathologic lesion; this characteristic has been exploited in monitoring some tumors.

The naturally occurring contrast agents in the thorax that provide the most clinically useful information on MRI are fat, flowing blood, and air. The high signal intensity of fat on T1-weighted images is of particular value because of its abundance in the mediastinum and in the extrapleural region around the chest wall: local invasion by a tumor relies largely on the striking contrast between its signal and the adjacent fat.

Certain pathologic conditions lend themselves to characterization by MRI because of their distinctive signals; hemorrhagic lesions or hematoma,[75] the proteinaceous contents of some foregut duplication cysts,[56] the high lipid content of lipoid pneumonia,[8] and to a lesser extent alveolar proteinosis, all result in a shortened T1 relaxation time. Differences in relaxation time between reactive mediastinal lymph nodes and those containing metastases are not large enough to be clinically useful.[20,83] Nevertheless, the differences in T2 relaxation time between tumor and established fibrosis are significant enough to allow clinically useful judgments about tumor recurrence versus postradiation fibrosis, particularly in patients with lymphoma.[22,58] There are some indications that the increased signal on T2-weighted images because of the edema associated with diffuse active alveolitis may

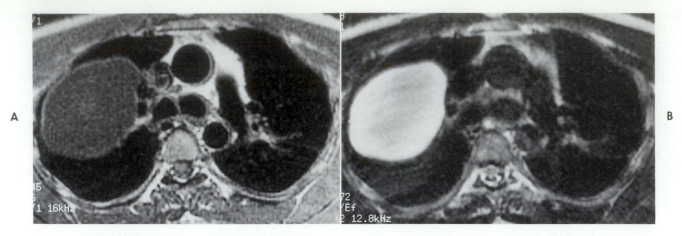

FIGURE 1-9
A, T1-weighted image of a patient with a hydatid cyst in the right lung (for accompanying chest radiograph and computed tomography images, see Figure 6-127). B, T2-weighted image showing increased contrast discrimination and increased noise associated with T2-weighted images.

be of clinical value in following patients with some forms of diffuse interstitial lung disease.[48,52]

Sequences for thoracic magnetic resonance imaging

Spin-echo sequences that have a short repetition time (TR) and a short echo time (TE), referred to as T1-weighted, increase the contrast between fat and surrounding tissues and reduce motion and susceptibility artifacts, respectively. T1-weighted images are therefore suited to anatomic studies. T2-weighted images have long TR and TE times and may allow further characterization of abnormalities detected on the T1-weighted images (Figure 1-9).[41,70] In general, if no abnormality is found on these T1-weighted sequences, further imaging with T2-weighted sequences is unlikely to reveal additional information that would otherwise be overlooked.[55] It has been recommended that the first part of a routine examination of the thorax should comprise coronal T1-weighted 10 mm wide sections with a 3 to 5 mm interspace between sections, a 256 × 192 matrix, and a 42 to 48 cm field of view.[86] A presaturation technique is desirable to suppress the flow-induced phase artifacts from flowing blood in the heart and great vessels.

Cardiac and respiratory gating considerably improve image quality by reducing motion artifact, particularly for the areas adjacent to the heart or diaphragm. Relatively static lesions, for example, at the lung apex, can be imaged satisfactorily without such gating. When cardiac gating is used, the TR time is equal to the R-R wave interval of the cardiac cycle. At a normal heart rate, cardiac gating produces pulse sequences with a TR of 800 to 1000 msec. The optimum echo time for lung studies depends on the magnetic field strength, but for most thoracic work the TE should be 20 msec or less. The long TR time of T2-weighted scans must be matched with the heart rate of the patient, and if necessary cardiac gating is adjusted to cover every third or fourth heartbeat. A

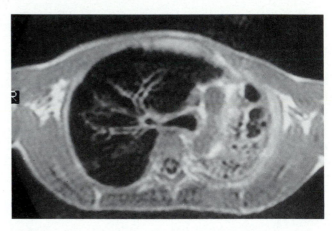

FIGURE 1-10
Short spin-echo (TE 8 msec) image of the lungs of a patient with cystic fibrosis, showing bronchiectatic airways in the right lung.

further consideration with T2-weighted images is that thicker sections are desirable; sections less than 8 mm make tissue characterization difficult because of poor signal-to-noise ratio.

In some circumstances suppressing the signal from fat may be useful; this can be done by choosing an appropriately short inversion time so that the signal from fat can be caught at its null time and thus be eliminated. The technique used for fat suppression is the so-called STIR (short T1 inversion recovery) sequence. It has the disadvantage that some signal loss from other tissues occurs.

The spin-echo sequence is not suited to very rapid imaging, so for this purpose gradient echo sequences (which have acronyms such as FEER, GRASS, FAST, and FLASH) have been developed. In these sequences magnetic field gradients are used to dephase and then rephase the protons following an excitation pulse, and an echo is produced much more rapidly than by the spin-echo sequence. Reduced flip angles are used for the initial exciting pulse to avoid saturation. An additional maneuver to maintain signal from moving blood is to make use of the "even echo rephasing" phenomenon and to acquire the second echo rather than the first. An extremely fast acquisition version of this sequence enables images to be acquired during a breath hold. The striking property of gradient echo images is the great contrast between the high signal from flowing blood and the surrounding structures. This type of sequence is particularly valuable for evaluating the patency or otherwise of major vessels.

The utility of MRI in the evaluation of parenchymal lung disease with extremely short spin-echo sequences has already been demonstrated (Figure 1-10).[47,52] Whether a T2-weighted sequence with an adequate SNR can be developed to characterize disease of the lung parenchyma remains to be seen.

REFERENCES

1. Bailes DR, Gilderdale DJ, Bydder GM, et al: Respiratory ordered phase-encoding (ROPE): a method for reducing respiratory motion artifacts in MR imaging, *J Comput Assist Tomogr* 9:835-838, 1985.
2. Barakos JA, Brown JJ, Brescia RJ, Higgins CB: High signal intensity lesions of the chest in MR imaging, *J Comput Assist Tomogr* 13:797-802, 1989.
3. Baxter BS, Sorenson JA: Factors affecting the measurements of size and CT number in computed tomography, *Invest Radiol* 16:337-341, 1981.
4. Bergin CJ, Glover GH, Pauly JM: Lung parenchyma: magnetic susceptibility in MR imaging, *Radiology* 180:845-848, 1991.
5. Bergin CJ, Glover GM, Pauly J: Magnetic resonance imaging of the lung parenchyma, *J Thorac Imag* 8:12-17, 1993.
6. Bergin CJ, Healy MV, Zincone GE, Castellino RA: MR evaluation of chest wall involvement in malignant lymphoma, *J Comput Assist Tomogr* 14:928-931, 1990.
7. Bergin CJ, Pauly JM, Macovski A: Lung parenchyma: projection reconstruction MR imaging, *Radiology* 179:777-781, 1991.
8. Brechot JM, Buy JN, Laaban JP, Rochemaure J: Computed tomography and magnetic resonance findings in lipoid pneumonia, *Thorax* 46:738-739, 1991.
9. Brown LR, Aughenbaugh GL: Masses of the anterior mediastinum: CT and MR imaging, *AJR* 157:1171-1180, 1991.
10. Cho ZH, Ro YM: Reduction of susceptibility artifact in gradient-echo imaging, *Magnet Reson Med* 23:193-200, 1992.
11. Edelman RR, Manning W, Burstein D, Paulin S: Coronary arteries: breath-hold MR angiography, *Radiology* 181:641-643, 1991.
12. Fajardo LL, Hillman BJ, Pond GD, et al: Detection of pneumothorax: comparison of digital and conventional chest imaging, *AJR* 152:475-480, 1989.
13. Felmlee JP, Ehman RL: Spatial presaturation: a method for suppressing flow artifacts and improving depiction of vascular anatomy in MR imaging, *Radiology* 164:559-564, 1987.
14. Foley WD, Wilson CR, Keyes GS, et al: The effect of varying spatial resolution on the detectability of diffuse pulmonary nodules, *Radiology* 141:25-31, 1981.
15. Frank MS, Jost RG, Molina PL, et al: High-resolution computer display of portable, digital, chest radiographs of adults: suitability for primary interpretation, *AJR* 160:473-477, 1993.
16. Gamsu G, Sostman D: Magnetic resonance imaging of the thorax, *Am Rev Respir Dis* 139:254-274, 1989.
17. Gefter WB, Hatabu H, Dinsmore BJ, et al: Pulmonary vascular cine MR imaging: a noninvasive approach to dynamic imaging of the pulmonary circulation, *Radiology* 176:761-770, 1990.
18. Geleijns J, Broerse JJ, Julius HW, et al: AMBER and conventional chest radiography: comparison of radiation dose and image quality, *Radiology* 185:719-723, 1992.
19. Glazer GM, Gross BH, Aisen AM, et al: Imaging of the pulmonary hilum: a prospective comparative study in patients with lung cancer, *AJR* 145:245-248, 1985.
20. Glazer GM, Orringer MB, Chenevert TL, et al: Mediastinal lymph nodes: relaxation time/pathologic correlation and implications in staging of lung cancer with MR imaging, *Radiology* 168:429-431, 1988.
21. Glazer HS, Lee JKT, Levitt RG, et al: Radiation fibrosis: differentiation from recurrent tumor by MR imaging; work in progress, *Radiology* 156:721-726, 1985.
22. Glazer HS, Lee JKT, Levitt RL, et al: Radiation fibrosis: differentiation from recurrent tumor by MR imaging, *Radiology* 156:721-726, 1985.
23. Goodman LR, Foley WD, Wilson CR, et al: Digital and conventional chest images: observer performance with film digital radiography system, *Radiology* 158:27-33, 1986.
24. Goodman LR, Wilson CR, Foley WD: Digital radiography of the chest: promises and problems, *AJR* 150:1241-1252, 1988.
25. Goodman LR, Wilson CR, Kim CS: Computed equalization radiography: preliminary clinical evaluation, *Radiology* 186:399-404, 1993.
26. Haase A, Frahm J, Matthaei D, et al: FLASH imaging: rapid NMR imaging using low flip angle pulses, *J Magnet Reson* 67:258-266, 1986.
27. Haggar AM, Pearlberg JL, Froelich JW, et al: Chest-wall invasion by carcinoma of the lung: detection by MR imaging, *AJR* 148:1075-1078, 1987.
28. Hansell DM, Coleman R, Du Bois RM, et al: Advanced multiple beam equalisation radiography (AMBER) in the detection of diffuse lung disease, *Clin Radiol* 44:227-231, 1991.
29. Harris KM, Adams H, Lloyd DCF, Harvey DJ: The effect on apparent size of simulated pulmonary nodules of using three standard CT window settings, *Clin Radiol* 47:241-244, 1993.
30. Hatabu H, Gefter WB, Listerud J, et al: Pulmonary MR angiography utilizing phased-array surface coils, *J Comput Assist Tomogr* 16:410-417, 1992.
31. Hayrapetian A, Aberle DR, Huang HK, et al: Comparison of 2048-line digital display formats and conventional radiographs: an ROC study, *AJR* 152:1113-1118, 1989.
32. Heelan RT, Demas BE, Caravelli JF, et al: Superior sulcus tumors: CT and MR imaging, *Radiology* 170:637-641, 1989.
33. Ishigaki T, Sakuma S, Horikawa Y, et al: One-shot dual-energy subtraction imaging, *Radiology* 161:271-273, 1986.
34. Jochelson M, Mauch P, Balikan J, et al: The significance of the residual mediastinal mass in treated Hodgkin's disease, *J Clin Oncol* 3:637-640, 1985.
35. Kalender WA, Seissler W, Klotz E, Vock P: Spiral volumetric CT with single-breath-hold technique, continuous transport, and continuous scanner rotation, *Radiology* 176:181-183, 1990.
36. Kelsey CA, Moseley RD, Mettler FA, et al: Comparison of nodule detection with 70-kVp and 120-kVp chest radiographs, *Radiology* 143:609-611, 1982.
37. Kido S, Ikezoe J, Takeuchi N, et al: Interpretation of subtle interstitial lung abnormalities: conventional versus storage phosphor radiography, *Radiology* 187:527-533, 1993.
38. Koehler PR, Anderson RE, Baxter B: The effect of computed tomography viewer controls on anatomical measurements, *Radiology* 130:189-194, 1979.
39. Lams PM, Cocklin ML: Spatial resolution requirements for digital chest radiographs: an ROC study of observer performance in selected cases, *Radiology* 158:11-19, 1986.
40. Lewis C, Prato FS, Drost DJ, Nicholson RL: Comparison of respiratory triggering and gating techniques for the removal of respiratory artifacts in MR imaging, *Radiology* 160:803-810, 1986.
41. Link KM, Samuels LJ, Reed JC, et al: Magnetic resonance imaging of the mediastinum, *J Thorac Imag* 8:34-53, 1993.
42. MacMahon H, Metz CE, Doi K, Digital chest radiography: effect on diagnostic accuracy of hard copy, conventional video, and

reversed gray scale video display formats, *Radiology* 168:669-674, 1988.

43. MacMahon H, Vyborny CJ, Metz CE, et al: Digital radiography of subtle pulmonary abnormalities: an ROC study of the effect of pixel size on observer performance, *Radiology* 158:21-26, 1986.

44. Mark AS, Winkler ML, Peltzer M, et al: Gated acquisition of MR images of the thorax: advantages for the study of the hila and mediastinum, *Magnet Reson Imag* 5:57-63, 1987.

45. Mayo JR, Jackson SA, Müller NL: High-resolution CT of the chest: radiation dose, *AJR* 160:479-481, 1993.

46. Mayo JR, MacKay A, Müller NL: T2 relaxation time in MR imaging of normal and abnormal lung parenchyma, *Radiology* 177(P):313, 1990.

47. Mayo JR, MacKay A, Müller NL: MR imaging of the lungs: value of short TE spin-echo pulse sequences, *AJR* 159:951-956, 1992.

48. McFadden RG, Carr TJ, Wood TE: Proton magnetic resonance imaging to stage activity of interstitial lung disease, *Chest* 92:31-39, 1987.

49. McLoud TC, Filion RB, Edelman RR, Shepard JO: MR imaging of superior sulcus carcinoma, *J Comput Assist Tomogr* 13:233-239, 1989.

50. Miller SW, Holmvang G: Differentiation of slow flow from thrombus in thoracic magnetic resonance imaging, emphasizing phase images, *J Thorac Imag* 8:98-107, 1993.

51. Mirvis SE, Keramati B, Buckman R, Rodriguez A: MR imaging of traumatic diaphragmatic rupture, *J Comput Assist Tomogr* 12:147-149, 1988.

52. Müller NL, Mayo JR, Zwirewich CV: Value of MR imaging in the evaluation of chronic infiltrative lung diseases: comparison with CT, *AJR* 158:1205-1209, 1992.

53. Munk PL, Morris DC, Nelems B: Left main bronchial-esophageal fistula: a complication of bronchial artery embolization, *Cardiovasc Intervent Radiol* 13:95-97, 1990.

54. Naidich DP, Weinreb JC, Schinella R: MR imaging of pulmonary parenchyma: comparison with CT in evaluating cadaveric lung specimens, *J Comput Assist Tomogr* 14:595-599, 1990.

55. Naidich DP, Zerhouni EA, Siegelman SS: Principles and techniques of thoracic CT and MR. In *Computed tomography and magnetic resonance of the thorax*, ed 2, New York, 1991, Raven Press, pp 13-15.

56. Nakata H, Egashira K, Watanabe H, et al: MRI of bronchogenic cysts, *J Comput Assist Tomogr* 17:267-270, 1993.

57. Nichols RD, Gurney JW, Jones KK, et al: Alveolar consolidation detection: advanced multiple beam equalization radiography versus conventional chest radiography, *Radiology* 187:65-69, 1993.

58. Nyman R, Rehn S, Glimelius B, et al: Magnetic resonance imaging for assessment of treatment effects in mediastinal Hodgkin's disease, *Acta Radiol* 28:145-151, 1987.

59. Nyman RS, Rehn SM, Glimelius BLG, et al: Residual mediastinal masses in Hodgkin disease: prediction of size with MR imaging, *Radiology* 170:435-440, 1989.

60. Padovani B, Mouroux J, Seksik L, et al: Chest wall invasion by bronchogenic carcinoma: evaluation with MR imaging, *Radiology* 187:33-38, 1993.

61. Peppler WW, Zink F, Naimuddin S, et al: Patient-specific beam attenuators. In *Proceedings of the chest imaging conference*, Madison, Wis, 1987, pp 64-78.

62. Razavi M, Sayre JM, Taira RK, et al: Receiver operating characteristic study of chest radiographs in children: digital hard-copy film vs 2K × 2K soft-copy images, *AJR* 158:443-448, 1992.

63. Remy-Jardin M, Remy J, Giraud F, Marquette CH: Pulmonary nodules: detection with thick-section spiral CT versus conventional CT, *Radiology* 187:513-520, 1993.

64. Revesz G, Shea FJ, Kundel HL: The effects of kilovoltage on diagnostic accuracy in chest radiography, *Radiology* 142:615-618, 1982.

65. Rzedzian RR, Pykett IL: Instant images of the human heart using a new, whole-body MR imaging system, *AJR* 149:245-250, 1987.

66. Schaefer CM, Greene R, Hall DA, et al: Mediastinal abnormalities: detection with storage phosphor digital radiography, *Radiology* 178:169-173, 1991.

67. Schaefer CM, Greene R, Oestmann JW, et al: Digital storage phosphor imaging versus conventional film radiography in CT-documented chest disease, *Radiology* 174:207-210, 1990.

68. Schmidt HC, Tscholakoff D, Hricak H, Higgins CB: MR image contrast and relaxation times of solid tumours in the chest, abdomen and pelvis, *J Comput Assist Tomogr* 9:738-748, 1985.

69. Schultze Kool LJ, Busscher DLT, Vlasbloem H, et al: Advanced multiple-beam equalization radiography in chest radiology: a simulated nodule detection study, *Radiology* 169:35-39, 1988.

70. Shioya S, Haida M, Ono Y, et al: Lung cancer: differentiation of tumor, necrosis and atelectasis by means of T1 and T2 values measured in vitro, *Radiology* 167:105-109, 1988.

71. Sonoda M, Takano M, Miyahara J, Kato H: Computed radiography utilizing scanning laser stimulated luminescence, *Radiology* 148:833-838, 1983.

72. Stehling MJ, Howseman AM, Ordidge RJ, et al: Whole-body echo planar MR imaging at 0.5T, *Radiology* 170:257-263, 1989.

73. Stern EJ, Graham CM, Webb WR, Gamsu G: Normal trachea during forced expiration: dynamic CT measurements, *Radiology* 187:27-31, 1993.

74. Swensen SJ, Gray JE, Brown LR, et al: A new asymmetric screen-film combination for conventional chest radiography: evaluation in 50 patients, *AJR* 160:483-486, 1993.

75. Swensen SJ, Keller PL, Berquist TH, et al: Magnetic resonance imaging of hemorrhage, *AJR* 145:921-927, 1985.

76. Tesic MM, Mattson RA, Barnes GT, et al: Digital radiography of the chest: design features and considerations for a prototype unit, *Radiology* 148:259-264, 1983.

77. Thompson MJ, Kubicka RA, Smith C: Evaluation of cardiopulmonary devices on chest radiographs: digital vs analog radiographs, *AJR* 153:1165-1168, 1989.

78. Trout ED, Kelley JP, Larson VL: A comparison of an air gap and a grid in roentgenography of the chest, *AJR* 124:404-411, 1975.

79. Vlasbloem H, Schultze Kool LJ: AMBER: a scanning multiple-beam equalization system for chest radiography, *Radiology* 169:29-34, 1988.

80. Vock P, Soucek M, Daepp M, Kalendar WA: Lung spiral volumetric CT with single breath-hold technique, *Radiology* 176:864-867, 1990.

81. von Schulthess GK, Fisher MR, Higgins CB: Pathologic blood flow in pulmonary vascular disease as shown by gated magnetic resonance imaging, *Ann Intern Med* 103:317-323, 1985.

82. Wandtke JC, Plewes DB: Comparison of scanning equalization and conventional chest radiography, *Radiology* 172:641-645, 1989.

83. Webb WR: Magnetic resonance imaging of the hila and mediastinum, *Cardiovasc Intervent Radiol* 8:306-313, 1986.

84. Webb WR: MR imaging of treated mediastinal Hodgkin disease, *Radiology* 170:315-316, 1989.

85. Webb WR, Gamsu G, Stark DD, Moore EH: Magnetic resonance imaging of the normal and abnormal pulmonary hila, *Radiology* 152:89-94, 1984.

86. Webb WR, Jensen BG, Gamsu G, et al: Coronal MRI of the chest: normal and abnormal, *Radiology* 153:729-735, 1984.

87. Webb WR, Stern EJ, Kanth N, Gamsu G: Dynamic pulmonary CT: findings in healthy adult men, *Radiology* 186:117-124, 1993.

88. White EM, Edelman RR, Wedeen VJ, et al: Intravascular signal in MR imaging: use of phase display for differentiation of blood-flow signal from intraluminal disease, *Radiology* 161:245-249, 1986.

89. Zerhouni EA, Scott WW, Baker RR, et al: Invasive thymomas: diagnosis and evaluation by computed tomography, *J Comput Assist Tomogr* 6:92-100, 1982.

90. Zwirewich CV, Terriff B, Müller NL: High-spatial-frequency (bone) algorithm improves quality of standard CT of the thorax, *AJR* 153:1169-1173, 1989.

2 Normal Chest

PETER ARMSTRONG

This chapter describes the normal anatomy of the lungs, mediastinum, and diaphragm as demonstrated on plain chest radiographs (Figure 2-1), computed tomography (CT), and magnetic resonance imaging (MRI).

LUNGS AND AIRWAYS
Central airways

The trachea is a straight tube that, in children and young adults, passes downward and backward in the midline; with unfolding and ectasia of the aorta, the trachea deviates to the right as it descends into the chest and may also bow forward. In cross section the trachea is usually round, oval, or oval with a flattened posterior margin; it occasionally shows other configurations such as square, inverted pear, or horseshoe.[22,36,37] The trachea enters the thorax 1 to 3 cm above the level of the suprasternal notch; the intrathoracic portion is 6 to 9 cm in length.[37] The upper limits of normal for coronal and sagittal diameters in adults on plain chest radiography are 21 and 23 mm, respectively, for women and 25 and 27 mm for men.[14] At CT, which allows precise assessment of diameters and cross-sectional areas without magnification, the mean transverse diameter is 15.2 mm (SD 1.4) for women and 18.2 mm (SD 1.2) for men, with the lower limit of normal 12.3 mm for women and 15.9 mm for men.[102] The diameters in growing children and young adults have been documented by Griscom and Wohl.[46]

Cross-sectional areas can also be measured: the mean is 194 mm^2 (SD 35) in women and 272 mm^2 (SD 33) in men. The normal cross-sectional area on forced expiration is considerably less than on full inspiration: Stern and co-workers[93] found that in 10 normal male volunteers the cross-sectional area dropped from a mean of 280 mm^2 (SD 50.5) at full inspiration to 178 mm^2 (SD 40.2) at end expiration. The major change is forward movement or invagination of the posterior wall of the trachea leading to a significant reduction in the anteroposterior diameter. Calcification of the cartilage rings of the trachea is a common normal finding after the age of 40 years, increasing in frequency with the age of the individual.[36,62]

The trachea divides into the two mainstem bronchi at the carina. In children the angles are symmetric, but in adults the right mainstem bronchus has a steeper angle than the left. The range of angles is wide, and alterations in angle can be diagnosed only by right-left comparisons, not by absolute measurement. The left main bronchus extends up to twice as far as the right main bronchus before giving off its upper lobe division.

The lobar and segmental branching pattern is shown in Figure 2-2. There are many variations of the segmental and subsegmental branches; these are of greater interest to the bronchoscopist and surgeon than to the radiologist now that bronchography is almost never performed. The central bronchi down to segmental level can be routinely identified with standard 10 mm sections. The interested

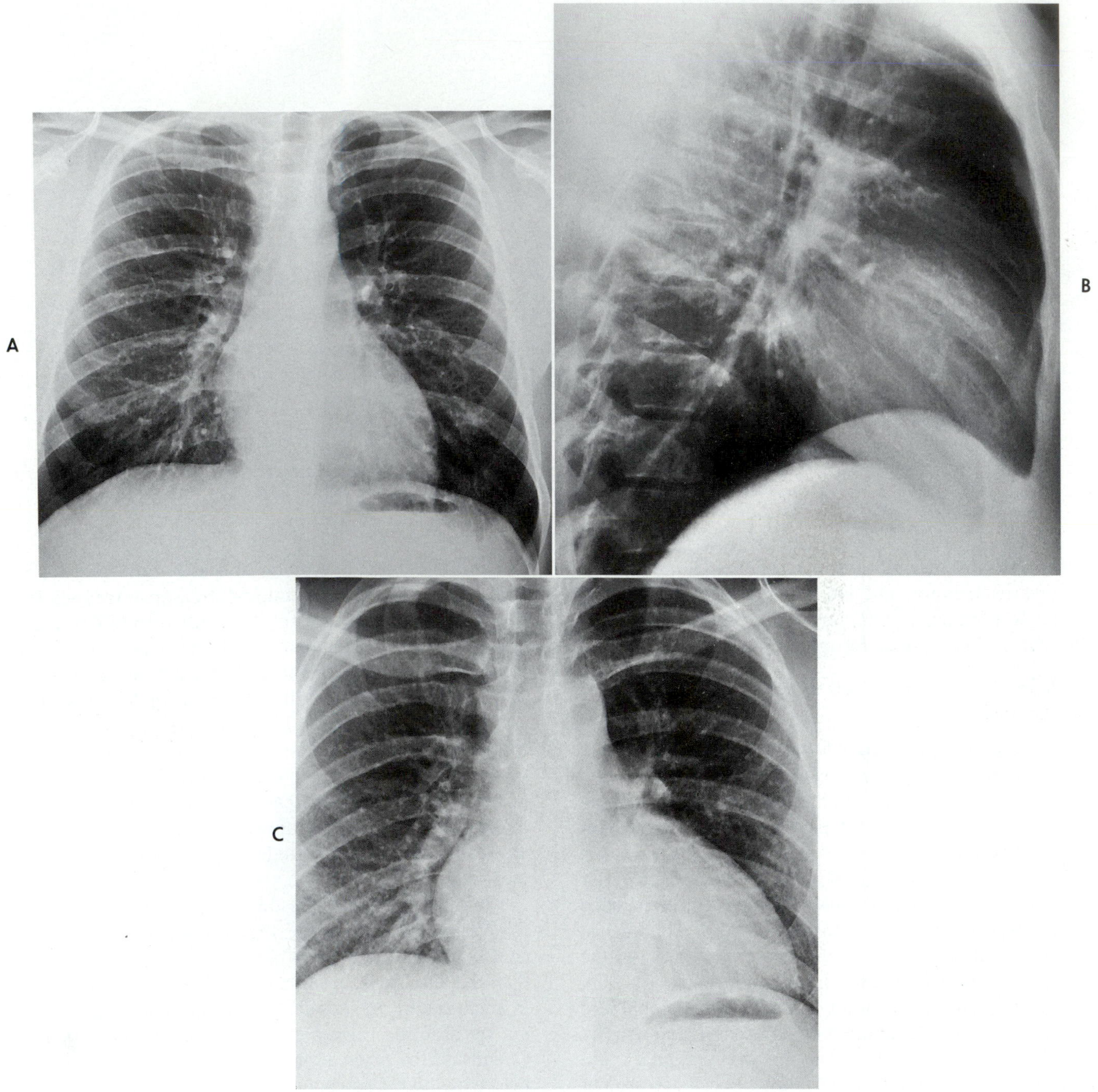

FIGURE 2-1
Radiograph of normal chest. **A**, Posteroanterior (PA) view. **B**, Lateral view. **C**, PA view on expiration (same patient). Note differences between appearances on inspiration and expiration, especially widening of heart and mediastinum on expiration.

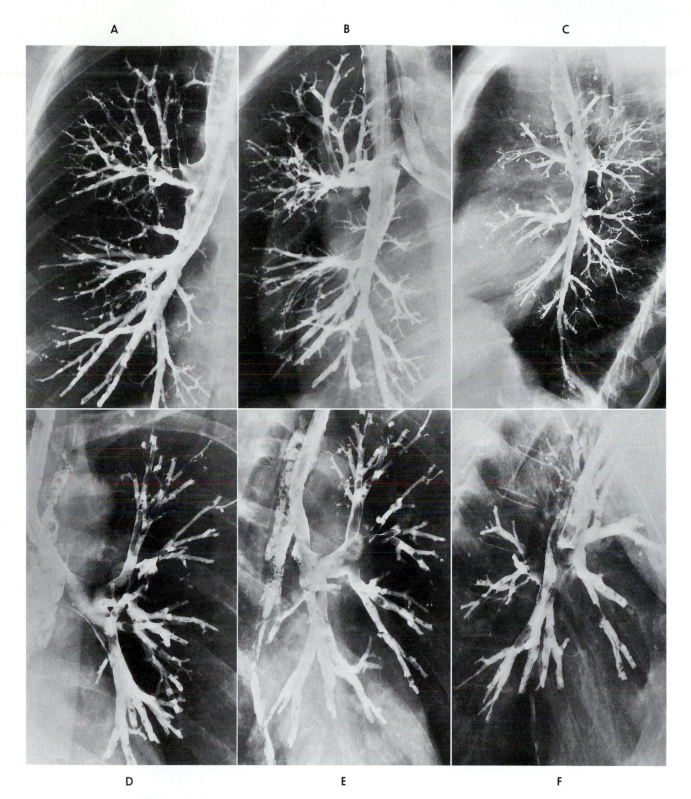

FIGURE 2-2

Divisions of bronchial tree shown by bronchography. **A,** Right bronchial tree, anteroposterior (AP) view. **B,** Right bronchial tree, right posterior oblique view. **C,** Right bronchial tree, lateral view. **D,** Left bronchial tree, AP view. **E,** Left bronchial tree, left posterior oblique view. **F,** Left bronchial tree, lateral view. *Continued.*

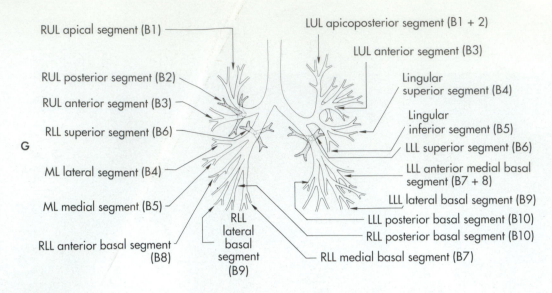

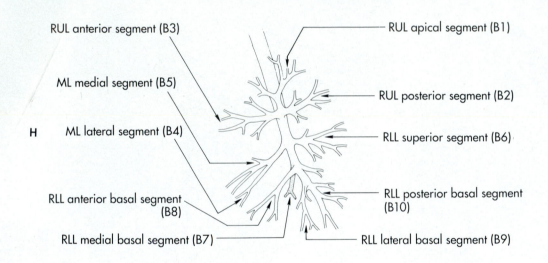

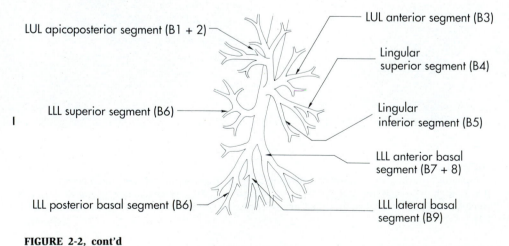

FIGURE 2-2, cont'd
G, Diagram of AP view. H, Diagram of lateral view of right bronchial tree. I, Diagram of lateral view of left bronchial tree.

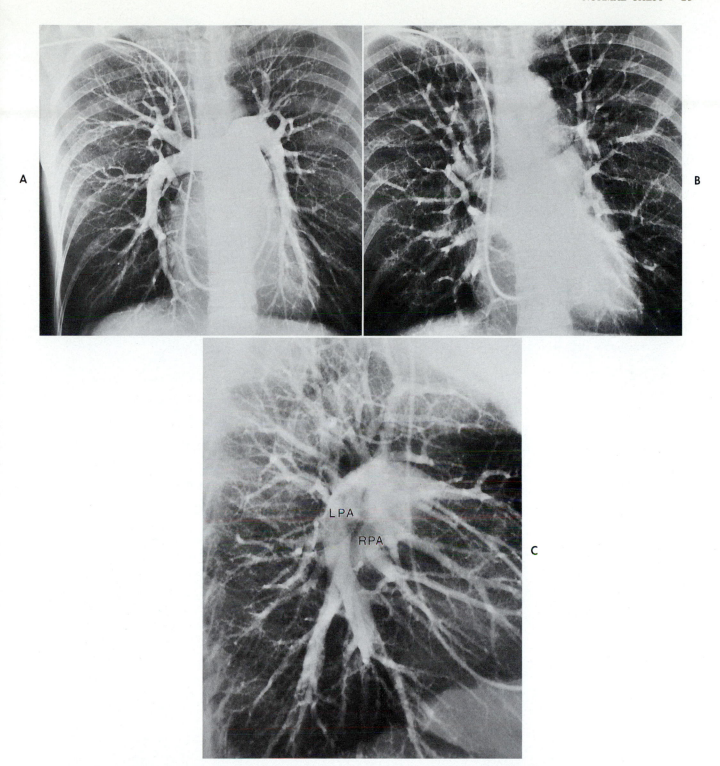

FIGURE 2-3
Pulmonary arteries and veins shown by pulmonary angiography. **A**, Anteroposterior (AP) view of pulmonary arteries. **B**, AP view of pulmonary veins in same patient. **C**, Lateral view of pulmonary arteries (different patient). *LPA*, Left pulmonary artery; *RPA*, right pulmonary artery.

reader is referred to several detailed descriptions of the CT anatomy of segmental bronchial anatomy.*

---

*Upper and middle lobe bronchi,[59,60,73] lower lobe bronchi,[53,71] whole lung.[108]

Pulmonary hila

Understanding the appearances of the normal hila requires an appreciation of the anatomy of the major bronchi (Figure 2-2) and hilar blood vessels (Figures 2-3 and 2-4)[38,70,101,104] because it is these structures that are

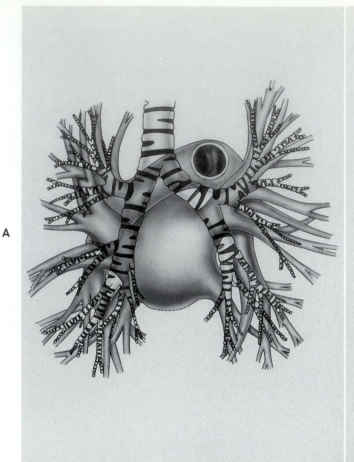

A

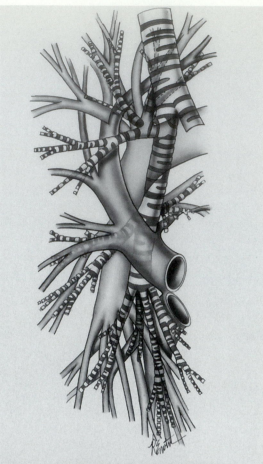

B

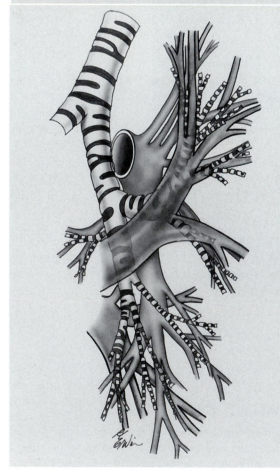

C

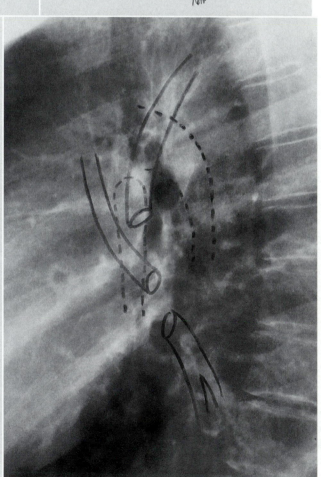

D

FIGURE 2-4
Diagram of hilar structures. A, Frontal view. B, Right hilum: oblique view. C, Left hilum: oblique view. D, Lateral radiograph with position of central pulmonary arteries and veins drawn in. Left and right pulmonary arteries are indicated by dotted lines (left lies posterior to right). Inferior pulmonary veins are similar on the two sides and are superimposed (only one is drawn in). Right superior pulmonary vein is on a more anterior plane than left superior pulmonary vein.

demonstrated with imaging (Figures 2-5 and 2-6). The normal lymph nodes, nerves, and connective tissue do not contribute significantly to the bulk of the hila, and the small amount of fat between the vessels is for practical purposes visible only at MRI.

The following points of anatomy should be remembered:

1. The right main bronchus has a more vertical course than the left main bronchus, and the right upper lobe bronchus arises more proximally than the left upper lobe bronchus.

2. The right main bronchus and its divisions into the right upper lobe bronchus and bronchus intermedius are outlined posteriorly by lung so that the posterior wall of these portions of the bronchial tree is seen as a thin stripe (Figures 2-6 and 2-7). This region is therefore a sensitive area in which to look for masses, such as lymphadenopathy. On the left side the lower lobe artery intervenes between the lung and the bronchial tree, and only a small tongue of lung can invaginate between the left lower lobe artery and the descending aorta to contact the posterior wall of the left mainstem bronchus (Figure 2-6).[103]

3. The right pulmonary artery passes anterior to the major bronchi to reach the lateral aspect of the bronchus intermedius and right lower lobe bronchus, whereas the left pulmonary artery arches over the left main bronchus and left upper lobe bronchus to descend posterolateral to the left lower lobe bronchus.

4. The pulmonary veins are similar on the two sides. The superior pulmonary veins are the anterior structures in the upper and middle hilum on both sides, and the inferior pulmonary veins run obliquely forward beneath the divisions of each lower lobe artery to enter the left atrium. Because the central portions of the pulmonary arteries are so differently organized on the two sides, the relationship between the major veins and arteries differs. On the right the superior pulmonary vein is separated from the central bronchi by the lower division of the right pulmonary artery, whereas on the left the superior pulmonary vein is separated from the lower division of the left pulmonary artery by the bronchial tree.

5. On plain chest radiographs the transverse diameter of the lower lobe arteries before their segmental divisions can be measured with reasonable accuracy. These arteries should normally be 9 to 16 mm in diameter (Figure 2-8). The large round shadow seen on lateral and oblique views of the right hilum is a combination of the right pulmonary artery and the superior pulmonary vein (Figure 2-5, *B*). The combined shadows of these two vessels may be sufficiently large to be confused with a mass.

6. Another feature of note with lateral or oblique plain chest radiographs is that normally no large vessels traverse the angle between the middle and the lower lobe bronchi on the right or the angle between the upper and lower lobe bronchi on the left (Figure 2-5). Therefore a rounded shadow larger than 1 cm in either of these angles is likely to be a mass rather than a normal vessel.[76]

Lungs beyond the hila

The segmental bronchi divide into progressively smaller airways until, after six to 20 divisions, they no longer contain cartilage in their walls and become bronchioles. The bronchioles divide, and the last of the purely conducting airways is known as the terminal bronchiole. Beyond the terminal bronchioles lie the acini, the gas exchange units of the lung. The walls of the segmental bronchi are invisible on chest radiographs except when seen end on as ring shadows. They are, however, clearly seen on CT.

The entire airway down to the terminal bronchiole can be demonstrated on a well-filled bronchogram (Figure 2-9). The acinus, which is 5 to 6 mm in diameter, comprises respiratory bronchioles, alveolar ducts, and alveoli. Up to 12 acini are grouped together in lobules 1 to 2 cm in diameter, which in the lung periphery are separated by interlobular septa. When thickened by disease, these septa form so-called septal lines (Kerley B lines). The anatomy of the secondary pulmonary lobule is discussed further in Chapter 5 (see p. 129).

The bronchopulmonary segments are based on the divisions of the bronchi (Figure 2-2). They can be identified with precision at bronchography and with reasonable accuracy at CT.[59,60,71,72,108] The boundaries between segments are complex in shape; the segments have been likened to the pieces of a three-dimensional jigsaw puzzle. With the rare exception of accessory fissures, the segments are not defined by septa. Although processes such as atelectasis, pneumonia, or edema may predominate in one segment or another, these processes never conform precisely to the whole of just one segment, since collateral air drift occurs across segmental boundaries. In other words, if these processes spread from segment to segment, there is no visible sign of the segmental boundary.

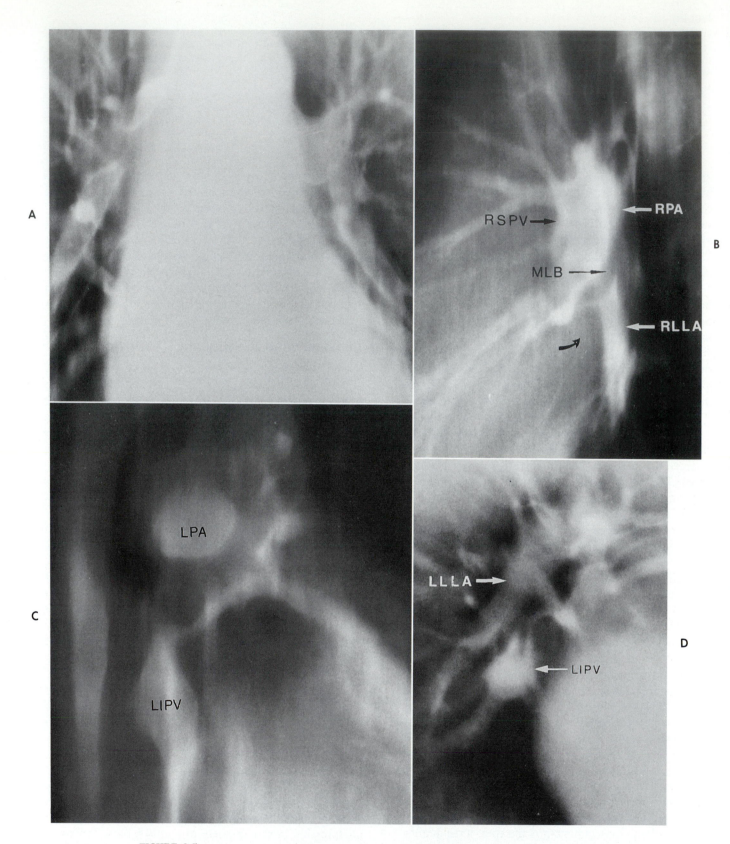

FIGURE 2-5
Conventional tomograms of hilar structures. **A,** Anteroposterior view. **B,** Lateral view of right hilum. **C,** Oblique view of left hilum. **D,** Lateral view of left hilum. *LIPV,* Left inferior pulmonary vein; *LLLA,* left lower lobe artery; *LPA,* left pulmonary artery; *MLB,* middle lobe bronchus; *RPA,* right pulmonary artery; *RLLA,* right lower lobe artery; *RSPV,* right superior pulmonary vein. Curved black arrow points to angle between middle and lower lobe bronchi, which is devoid of any normal rounded shadow.

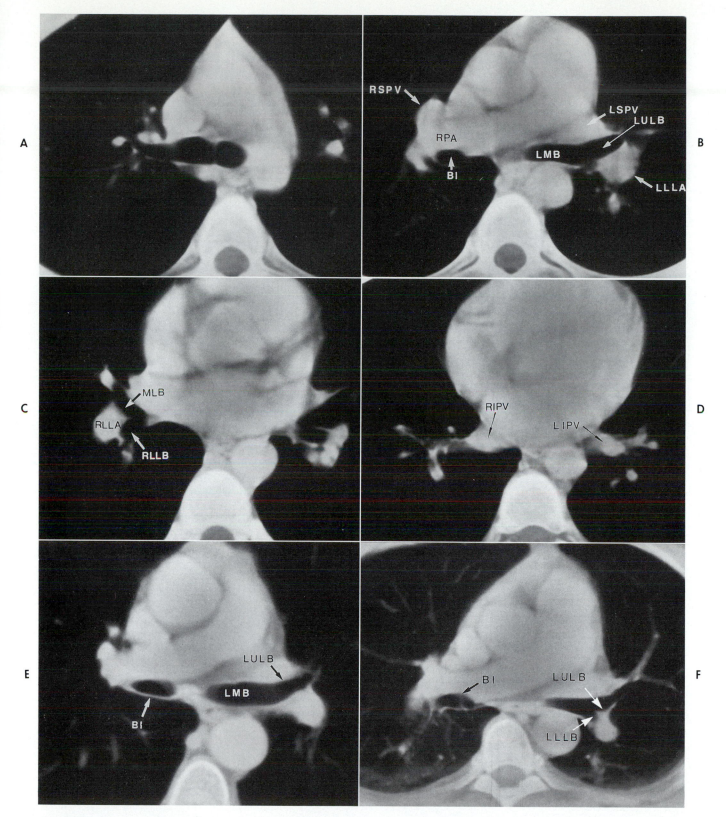

FIGURE 2-6

Computed tomography scans of pulmonary hila. **A,** At level of tracheal carina. Hilar vessels are segmental divisions. **B,** At level of bronchus intermedius. Note lack of major vessels behind bronchus intermedius and conglomerate density formed by right pulmonary artery and right superior pulmonary vein. **C,** At level of inferior (right) middle lobe bronchus. **D,** At level of inferior pulmonary veins. E illustrates posterior relationships of left and right bronchial tree. F also illustrates posterior relationships of left and right bronchial tree. Section shown in **E** is 1 cm higher than that in **F.** *BI,* Bronchus intermedius; *LIPV,* left inferior pulmonary vein; *LLLA,* left lower lobe artery; *LLLB,* left lower lobe bronchus; *LMB,* left main bronchus; *LSPV,* left superior pulmonary vein; *LULB,* left upper lobe bronchus; *MLB,* middle lobe bronchus; *RIPV,* right inferior pulmonary vein; *RLLB,* right lower lobe bronchus; *RPA,* right pulmonary artery; *RSPV,* right superior pulmonary vein.

FIGURE 2-7
A, Lateral radiograph of normal pulmonary hila. Arrow points to posterior wall of right main bronchus, and arrowheads point to posterior wall of bronchus intermedius. **B,** Lateral view in patient with lymphangitis carcinomatosa shows thickening of tissues posterior to bronchus intermedius *(arrows)*.

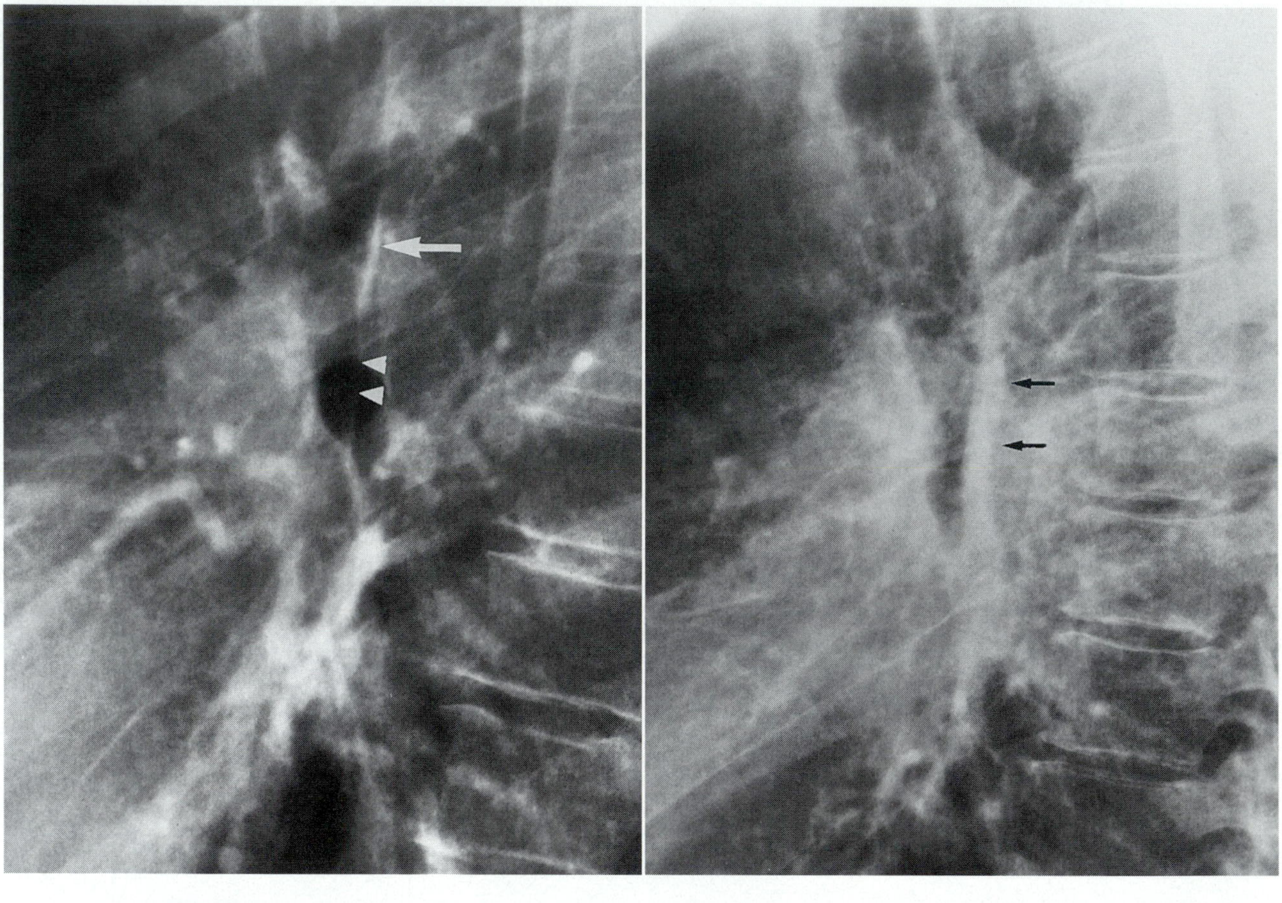

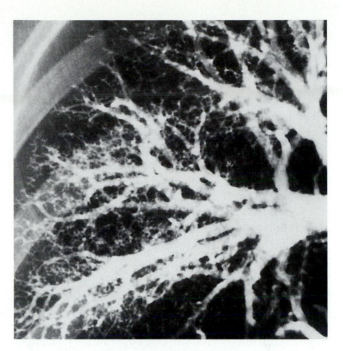

FIGURE 2-9
Terminal bronchiolar filling by bronchography.

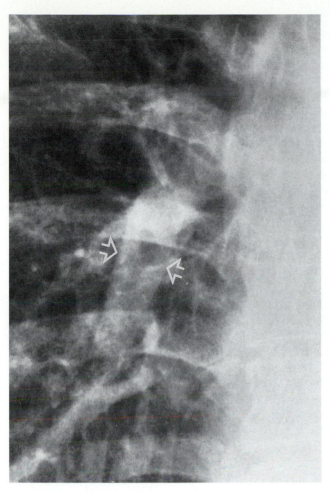

FIGURE 2-8
Right lower lobe artery. Diameter indicated by the arrows should be between 9 and 16 mm.

The pulmonary blood vessels (Figure 2-3) are responsible for the branching linear markings within the lungs both on conventional films and at CT scanning. In the outer two thirds of the lungs, arteries cannot be distinguished from veins except by angiography. More centrally the orientation of the arteries and veins differs: the inferior pulmonary veins draining the lower lobes run more horizontally, and the lower lobe arteries more vertically. In the upper lobes the arteries and veins show a similar gently curving vertical orientation, but the upper lobe veins (when not superimposed on the arteries) lie lateral to the arteries and can sometimes be traced to the main venous trunk, the superior pulmonary vein.

The diameter of the blood vessels beyond the hilum varies according to the patient's position. On plain chest films taken with the patient in the upright position, the diameter of both arteries and veins increases gradually from apex to base; for comparisons of diameter to be valid, the measurements must be made equidistant from the hilum. These changes in vessel size correlate with physiologic studies of perfusion, which show that in an erect subject the blood flow increases from apex to base, a difference that is less marked when supine. Although general statements regarding differences in regional blood vessel size can be made, meaningful measurements of individual peripheral pulmonary vessels are difficult to make on plain chest radiographs, since it is not possible to know whether the vessel being measured is an artery or a vein or what degree of magnification has been used. Certain measurements have been suggested for upright chest films:

1. The artery and bronchus of the anterior segment of either or both upper lobes are frequently seen end on. The diameter of the artery is usually much the same as the diameter of the bronchus (4 to 5 mm).
2. Woodring[107] measured the visible bronchi and immediately adjacent arteries in the upper and lower half of the chest in upright patients and found that the artery/bronchus ratio was 0.85 (SD 0.15) for the upper zone and 1.34 (SD 0.25) for the lower zone.
3. Vessels in the first anterior interspace should not exceed 3 mm in diameter.[54]

A rich network of lymphatics drains the lung and pleura. The subpleural lymphatic vessels are found just beneath the pleura, at the junction of the interlobular septa and pleura, where they interconnect with one another as well as with the lymphatic vessels in the interlobular septa. The lymph then flows to the hilum by way of lymphatic channels that run peribronchially and in the deep septa. The lymphatic network is radiographically invisible, but in certain conditions, such as when the lung is edematous or when the lymphatic channels are occluded by tumor, the thickened septa containing the dilated lymphatics may become visible.

There are a few intrapulmonary lymph nodes, which are small and not identifiable on plain chest radiographs. Very occasionally CT shows them as small, peripherally located nodules.

Fissures

The lobes of the lungs are separated by fissures that in the majority of people are incomplete. In other words, lung tissue, together with its bronchovascular bundles and draining veins, passes from one lobe to another through holes in the fissures.[7,41,73,108] These defects are important because they allow collateral air drift between lobes and also limit the accumulation of pleural fluid in the interlobar portions of the pleural cavity.[21]

The anatomy of the pleura and pleural fissures is described in detail in Chapter 15; only an outline of the fissures is given here. The major fissures on each side are similar. The left major (oblique) fissure divides the left lung into an upper and a lower lobe. The right lung has an additional fissure, the minor (horizontal) fissure, which separates the middle from the right upper lobe. The major fissures run obliquely forward and downward, passing through the hilum, commencing at approximately the level of the fifth thoracic vertebra to contact the diaphragm up to 3 cm behind the anterior chest wall. Portions of one or both major fissures are frequently seen on the lateral chest radiograph. It is, however, unusual to be able to trace both fissures in their entirety on plain films. Each major fissure follows a gently curving plane somewhat similar to that of a propeller blade, with the upper portion facing forward and laterally and the lower portion facing forward and medially. Below the hila the lateral portions of the major fissures lie farther forward than do the medial portions, whereas above the hila this relationship reverses. Because of these undulations the lateral aspect of the upper portion of the major fissures can sometimes be identified in the frontal view.[77,78] Although these undulations can be identified at CT,[78] they usually cannot be traced on the plain chest radiograph. Therefore on a lateral view the radiologist cannot be certain what portion of the fissure is being profiled, and it is easy to misinterpret a fissure as displaced when it is in fact in normal position. The inferior few centimeters of either or both major fissures are often wide as a result of fat or pleural thickening between the leaves of the pleura. This thickening may lead to loss of silhouette where the fissure contacts the diaphragm.

The minor fissure fans out forward and laterally in a horizontal direction from the right hilum. On a standard upright frontal chest radiograph the minor fissure contacts the lateral chest wall at or near the axillary portion of the right sixth rib. The fissure curves gently, usually downward in the anterior and lateral portions. Because of the undulations of the major fissure the minor fissure may be projected posterior to the right major fissure on a normal lateral view.

On standard 10 mm CT sections (Figure 2-10) the position of the major fissures can usually be predicted by noting the relatively avascular zone that forms the outer cortex of the lobe.[41,63,78] The region of the major fissures is seen as a band of avascularity, or a zone with much smaller vessels, traversing the lung. Because the major fissures run obliquely through the sections, the fissure itself may be invisible or may be seen as a poorly defined band of density. In early series[78] the fissure could not be appreciated as a line in a significant minority of cases, but with more modern CT equipment each oblique fissure is seen as a line in almost all instances.[41] With thin section CT the left major fissure is seen as a line throughout its course in almost all subjects (Figure 2-10, B), but the line may not be visible in upper and middle portions of the right major fissure in up to one fourth of patients, presumably because the right major fissure is more obliquely oriented to the scanning plane.[41]

The major fissures are seen as two parallel lines rather than a single line on thin section CT at least at one level in approximately one third of the population.[65] This so-called double fissure sign is an artifact related to cardiac and respiratory motion.[41,65]

The minor fissure is in the plane of section of the CT scanner, and therefore when in normal position it is not seen as a line on standard 10 mm sections. Its position can usually be inferred from the large, oval deficiency of vessels on one or more sections at the level of the bronchus intermedius (Figure 2-10, C).[45] With thin section CT a variety of normal patterns are encountered, depending on the precise shape of the minor fissure.[7] Because the fissure may assume the shape of an upward-arching dome, some portions may run sufficiently obliquely through the section to be seen as a line, an ill-defined band shadow, or even a rounded density (Figure 2-10).[7,32]

Occasionally, other fissures are present.[44] The most common, seen in up to 1% of the population, is the "azygos lobe fissure" (Figure 2-11), so called because it contains the azygos vein within its lower margin. The fissure is almost invariably on the right side, although left-sided "azygos" fissures have been described, in which case the vein at the base of the fissure is the superior intercostal vein.[96] The fissure results from failure of normal migration of the azygos vein from the chest wall through the upper lobe to its usual position in the tracheobronchial angle, so that the invaginated visceral and parietal pleurae persist to form a fissure in the lung. The altered course of the azygos vein together with the fissure is readily seen at CT.[92] Since there is no corresponding alteration in the segmental architecture of the lung, the term "lobe" is a misnomer: that portion of the lung is supplied by branches of the apical segment bronchus with or without a contribution from the posterior segmental airway.[13] The "azygos lobe" is not unduly susceptible to disease. A potential diagnostic pitfall is that the "azygos lobe" may occupy less volume than the equivalent normal lung and may therefore appear rela-

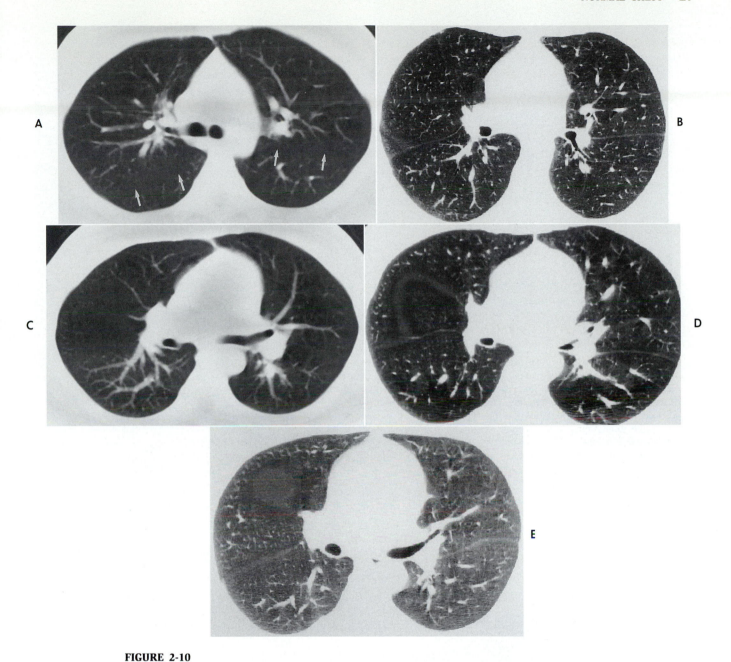

FIGURE 2-10
Pleural fissures at computed tomography. **A,** Major fissures *(arrows)* seen as a band of relative avascularity in upper zones. **B,** Thin section high-resolution scan showing region of major fissures in midzone. Smudgelike density close to right chest wall is minor fissure as it passes obliquely through section. **C,** Minor fissure seen as oval area of relative avascularity radiating from right hilum. **D,** Minor fissure seen as curvilinear bandlike density, because section is through dome of fissure. **E,** Minor fissure seen as faint homogeneous density because section is through apex of dome of fissure.

tively opaque,[16] even when no disease is present (Figure 2-11, *B*). The right brachiocephalic vein may on rare occasion course through the anterior portion of the azygos fissure.[64]

Fissures are very rarely seen at the boundaries between bronchopulmonary segments.[44] A minor fissure, similar to the minor fissure on the right, can occur on the left separating the lingular segments from the remainder of the upper lobe.[2] A horizontally oriented fissure, the superior accessory fissure, may be seen separating the

superior segment from the basal segments in either lower lobe. An inferior accessory fissure is common in one or the other lower lobe, particularly on the right, separating the medial basal segment from the remaining segments.[99] It runs obliquely upward and medially toward the hilum from the diaphragm (Figure 2-12).

The inferior pulmonary ligaments are pleural reflections, analogous in shape to the peritoneal reflections that form the broad ligaments of the uterus. These ligaments invest the hila and connect the mediastinal surface of

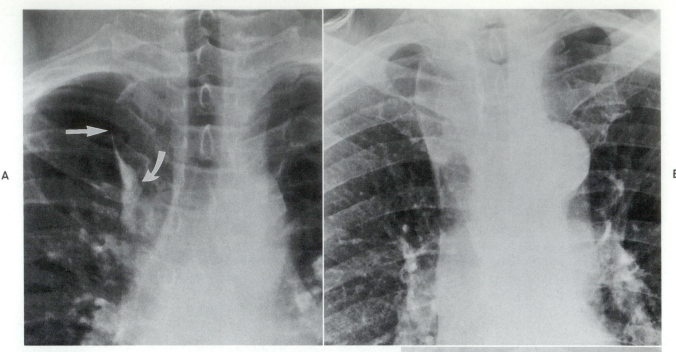

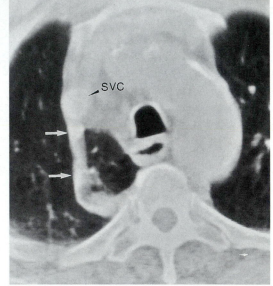

FIGURE 2-11
Azygos lobe fissure. **A,** Typical example. Horizontal arrow points to fissure. Curved arrow points to azygos vein running in lower margin of fissure. Note that the azygos vein is not in its usual position in the tracheobronchial angle. **B,** Example in which the lung lying medial to azygos fissure appears opaque. This opacity can be normal and does not represent disease, as is shown in **C,** computed tomography scan through azygos lobe in same patient. Band of azygos vein *(arrows)* crossing through the lung to join the superior vena cava *(SVC)* is clearly shown.

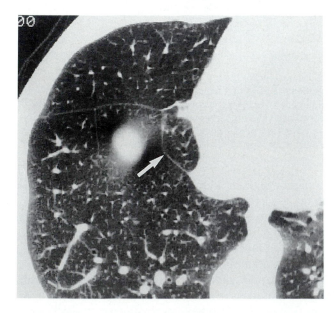

FIGURE 2-12
Inferior accessory fissure *(arrow)* separating medial basal segment from remainder of right lower lobe.

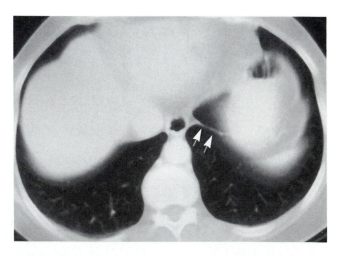

FIGURE 2-13
Inferior pulmonary ligament. Intersegmental septum *(arrows)* is shown on computed tomography scan.

each lower lobe to the mediastinum. They are discussed further in Chapter 15. A thin septum, known as the intersegmental (intersublobar) septum, extends inward into the lung between the attachment of the inferior pulmonary ligament and the inferior pulmonary vein. It is identifiable in the majority of normal chest CT scans (Figure 2-13).[9]

MEDIASTINUM

The mediastinum is divided by anatomists into superior, anterior, middle, and posterior divisions.* The exact anatomic boundaries between these divisions are unimportant to the radiologist because they do not provide a clear-cut guide to disease, nor do these boundaries form barriers to the spread of disease. Moreover, almost every writer on the subject seems to have a different definition.[25,29,49,109] The mediastinal structures and spaces as seen on CT and MRI are described before the appearances on plain film because the complex interfaces between the mediastinum and the lungs are best understood by careful correlation with cross-sectional images.

Normal mediastinum

The normal mediastinal structures always identified at CT and MRI (Figure 2-14) are the heart and blood vessels, which make up the bulk of the mediastinum; the major airways; and the esophagus. These structures are surrounded by a variable amount of connective tissue, largely fat, within which lie lymph nodes, the thymus, the thoracic duct, and the phrenic and laryngeal nerves.

MEDIASTINAL BLOOD VESSELS. On transaxial images the vertically oriented ascending and descending portions of the aorta appear round, whereas the arch is seen as a tapering oval that becomes narrower as it gives rise to the arteries to the neck, head, and arms. The average diameter of the ascending aorta is 3.5 cm, and that of the descending aorta is 2.5 cm.[47] Sections above the aortic arch show the three major aortic branches arranged in a curve lying anterior and to the left of the trachea. Their order from right to left is the brachiocephalic (innominate), left common carotid, and left subclavian arteries. The brachiocephalic artery is appreciably larger than the other two vessels. It varies slightly in position: in about half the population it is directly anterior to the trachea, and in the remainder, although still anterior to the trachea, it is either slightly to the right or left of the midline.[35] The left common carotid artery lies to the left of the trachea; the left subclavian artery also lies either to

the left of the trachea or posterior to it. It is the most lateral vessel of the three and often contacts the left lung.

In 0.5% of the population the right subclavian artery arises as a separate fourth major branch of the aorta, known as an aberrant right subclavian artery. Instead of arising from the brachiocephalic artery, it runs behind the esophagus from left to right, at or just above the level of the aortic arch, to lie against the right side of the vertebral bodies before entering the root of the neck. In individuals with an aberrant right subclavian artery the brachiocephalic artery (now the right common carotid artery) is smaller than usual and is similar in diameter to the left common carotid artery.

As the descending aorta travels through the chest, it gradually moves from a position to the left of the vertebral bodies to an almost midline position before exiting from the chest through the aortic hiatus in the diaphragm. The diameter should remain nearly constant, but dilation and tortuosity may develop with increasing age.

The mediastinal venous anatomy[43] is illustrated in Figure 2-15. The superior vena cava (SVC) has an oval or round configuration on transaxial section. Its diameter is one-third to two-thirds the diameter of the ascending aorta.[47] It can, however, be considerably smaller and may appear flattened.

In 0.3% to 0.5% of the healthy population, but in 4.4% to 12.9% of those with congenital heart disease,[15,18] a left SVC is present (Figure 2-16). This anomaly results from failure of obliteration of the left common cardinal vein during fetal development. A right SVC and an interconnecting brachiocephalic vein are also present in most persons with a left SVC. A left SVC arises from the junction of the left jugular and subclavian veins and travels vertically through the left mediastinum, passing anterior to the left main bronchus before joining the coronary sinus on the back of the heart. From this point the blood flows into the right atrium through the coronary sinus, which is significantly larger than normal because of the increased blood flow. A left SVC may be confused with lymphadenopathy if the full course of the vessel is not appreciated.

The left brachiocephalic vein forms a curved band anterior to the arteries arising from the arch of the aorta. Since it takes an oblique, downward course to join the SVC, its image on axial sections is usually oval rather than tubular. On rare occasion the left brachiocephalic vein descends vertically through the mediastinum before crossing the midline to join the right brachiocephalic vein,[33] and like left superior vena cava (which it resembles) may mimic lymphadenopathy.

The right brachiocephalic vein, which travels vertically, lies anterolateral to the trachea in line with the three major arteries. This vein is identifiable as the farthest right of the vessels; it is oval and larger than the arteries.

The azygos vein travels anterior to the spine, either behind or to the right of the esophagus, until at some variable point it arches forward to join the posterior wall of the SVC. Usually it remains within the mediastinum

---

*According to *Gray's Anatomy*,[106] the mediastinum is divided into superior and inferior compartments by an imaginary line from the lower border of the manubrium to the lower border of the fourth vertebra. The inferior compartment is divided into anterior, middle, and posterior. The anterior mediastinum lies anterior to the pericardium and the ascending aorta. The posterior mediastinum is bounded in front by the trachea, the pulmonary vessels, and the pericardium, and behind by the vertebral column. Its contents include the descending aorta, the esophagus, the azygos and hemiazygos veins, and the thoracic duct.

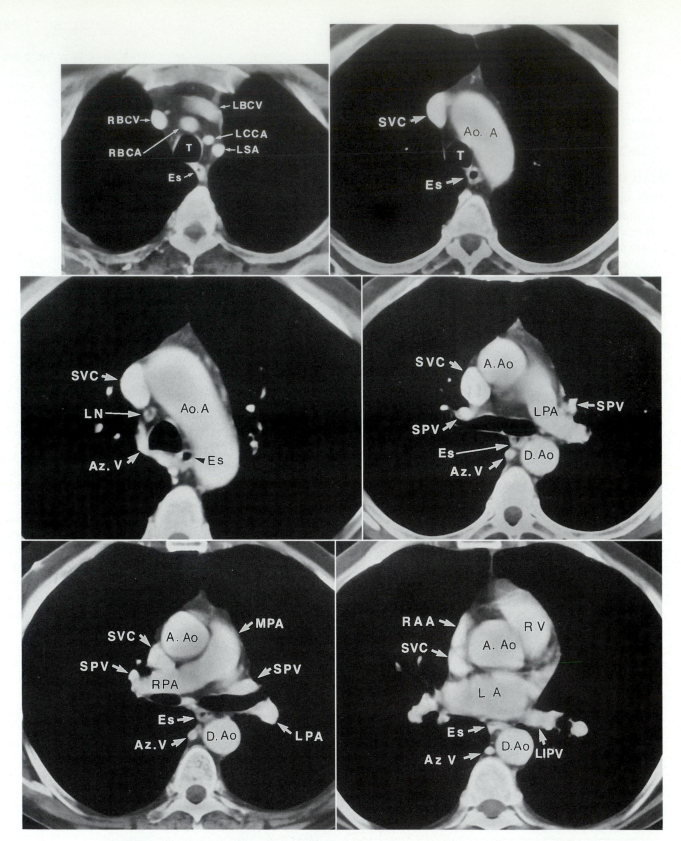

FIGURE 2-14

Anatomy of mediastinum on contrast-enhanced computed tomography and on magnetic resonance imaging (T1-weighted images). *A.Ao,* Ascending aorta; *Ao.A,* aortic arch; *Az.V,* azygos vein; *BI,* bronchus intermedius; *D.Ao,* descending aorta; *Es,* esophagus; *LBVC,* left brachiocephalic vein; *LCCA,* left common carotid artery; *LCCA,* left common carotid artery; *LA,* left atrium; *LMB,* left main bronchus; *LN,* lymph node; *LPA,* left pulmonary artery; *LIPV,* left inferior pulmonary vein; *LSA,* left subclavian artery; *LV,* left ventricle; *MPA,* main pulmonary artery; *RA,* right atrium; *RAA,* right atrial appendage; *RBCA,* right brachiocephalic artery; *RBCV,* right brachiocephalic vein; *RMB,* right middle lobe bronchus; *RPA,* right pulmonary artery; *RV,* right ventricle; *SPV,* superior pulmonary vein; *SVC,* superior vena cava; *T,* trachea.

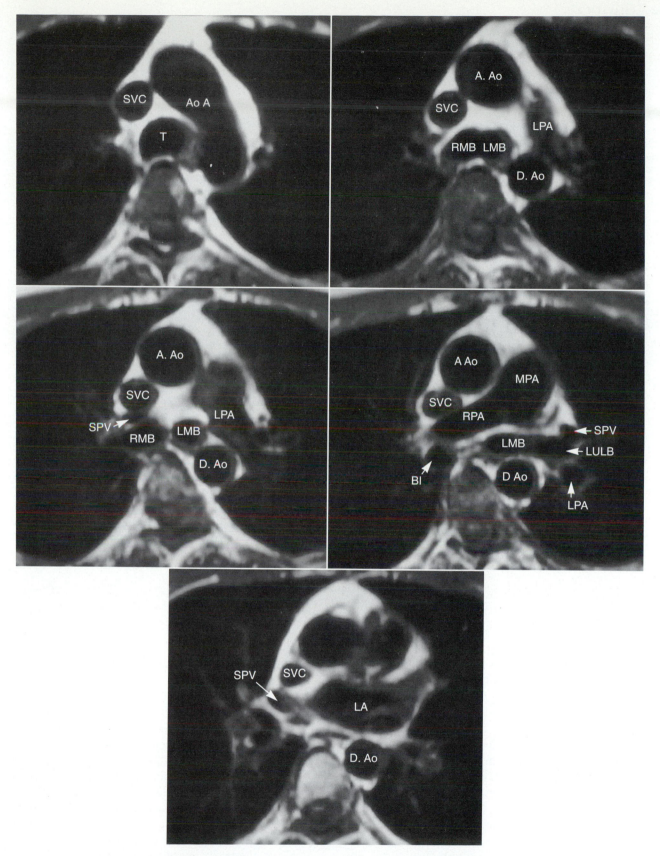

FIGURE 2-14, cont'd
For legend see opposite page.

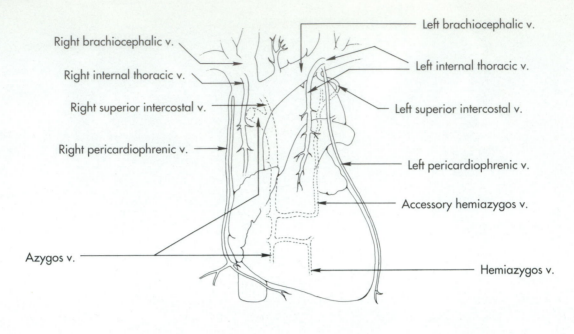

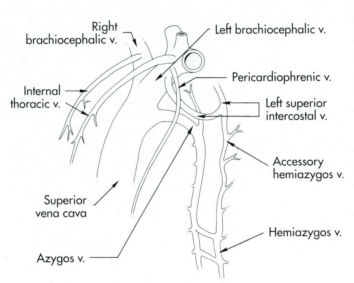

FIGURE 2-15
Diagrams illustrating mediastinal venous anatomy. (Redrawn from Godwin JD, Chen JTT: *AJR* 147:674-684, 1986.)

and occupies the right tracheobronchial angle. In the 1% of the population who have an azygos lobe, the azygos vein traverses the lung before entering the SVC, in which case the SVC may appear distorted both on plain film and CT.[92]

The hemiazygos and accessory hemiazygos veins also lie against the vertebral bodies but in a more posterior plane, usually just behind the descending aorta. The accessory hemiazygos vein may cross the midline in the midthoracic level to join the azygos vein, or it may drain into the left superior intercostal vein, which arches around the aorta more or less at the junction of the arch and the descending portion to join the left brachiocepha-

lic vein. The azygos and hemiazygos veins are routinely identifiable at CT, but they are generally not big enough to confuse with lymphadenopathy or other masses.[97] The left superior intercostal vein is much smaller than the azygos vein and is only occasionally identified on plain films or CT scans, although in 1% to 9.5% of normal patients it is seen on plain chest radiography as a small nipple on the lateral margin of the aortic arch.[5,30,66]

Occasionally the inferior vena cava (IVC) does not develop in the usual fashion and the azygos vein forms the venous conduit draining inferior vena caval blood back to the heart, an arrangement known as azygos continuation of the IVC. The hepatic veins in these cases

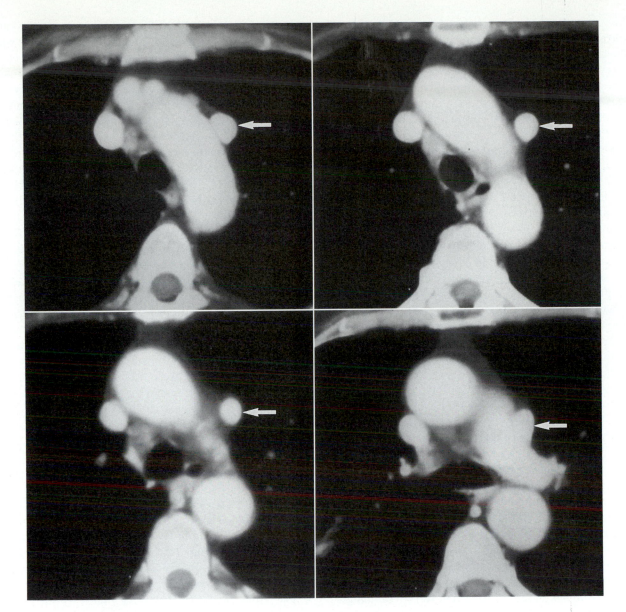

FIGURE 2-16
Persistent left superior vena cava *(arrows)*. Four adjacent sections showing the course of a left superior
vena cava.

drain into the right atrium, not into the IVC. The azygos
vein is therefore enlarged and is only slightly smaller than
the IVC. Its anatomy is otherwise unaltered. Azygos
continuation of the IVC may resemble a mediastinal mass
or lymphadenopathy.

The main pulmonary artery runs obliquely backward
and upward to the left of the ascending aorta. It divides
into right and left branches. The right branch travels more
or less horizontally through the mediastinum, between
the ascending aorta and SVC anteriorly and the major
bronchi posteriorly. The left pulmonary artery arches
higher than the right pulmonary artery and passes over
the left main bronchus to descend posterior to it. This
configuration leads to two important observations: the left
pulmonary artery is often seen on a higher CT section

than the right pulmonary artery, and the lung abuts the
posterior wall of the right airway but is partly or totally
excluded from contact with the left airway by the
descending limb of the left pulmonary artery. The
external diameter of the main pulmonary artery is slightly
smaller than that of the ascending aorta, averaging 2.8 cm
in the series by Guthaner et al.[47] The right pulmonary
artery is two-thirds the diameter of the main pulmonary
artery.

ESOPHAGUS. The esophagus is visible on all CT and
MRI axial sections from the root of the neck down to the
esophageal hiatus through the diaphragm. In approximately 80% of normal persons the esophagus contains
air, sometimes just a small amount. If there is sufficient
mediastinal fat, the entire circumference of the esophagus

can be identified. If air is present in the lumen, the uniform thickness of the wall can be appreciated. Without air the collapsed esophagus appears either circular or oval and is usually approximately 1 cm in its narrowest diameter. On MRI the signal intensity on T1-weighted images is similar to that of muscle, but on T2-weighted images the esophagus often shows a much higher signal intensity than muscle.

THYMUS. Microscopic examination of the thymus shows many lobules, each divided into a medulla, consisting predominantly of epithelial cells, and a cortex containing the major cell of the thymus, the T lymphocyte. Epithelioid cells form a general framework. Hassall's corpuscles are a characteristic feature of the medulla of the thymus; they consist of mature keratinized epithelial cells that layer on each other in concentric fashion. Myoid cells, similar to striated skeletal muscle, are found adjacent to Hassall's corpuscles; they are much more prevalent in children than in adults.

The thymus is anterior to the aorta and the right ventricular outflow tract or pulmonary artery. At CT scanning it is usually found inferior to the left brachiocephalic vein and superior to the level of the horizontal portion of the right pulmonary artery; it is often best appreciated on a section through the aortic arch (Figure 2-17).[69]

In childhood before puberty[48] the thymus occupies most of the mediastinum in front of the great vessels (Figure 2-17). The gland remains fairly constant in weight, enlarging slightly until puberty, after which the thymic follicles atrophy and fatty replacement occurs until eventually no residual thymic tissue can be seen. In children the gland varies so greatly in size that measurement is of little value in deciding normality. Shape is a more useful criterion: the thymus is soft and fills in the spaces between the great vessels and the anterior chest wall as if molded by these structures. The lateral margins may be concave, straight, or bulged outward, and approx-

imate symmetry is the rule. In children under 5 years of age the gland is usually quadrilateral in shape with a convex lateral margin.[90] A sharp angular border equivalent to the sail sign on plain films is occasionally visible at CT.[48] In young children the thymus may extend all the way into the posterior mediastinum[20,28] and may occasionally be confused with a posterior mediastinal mass.[3,67,85,89]

The thymus consists of two lobes, each enclosed in its own fibrous sheath.[86] Up to 30% of the population have a fat cleft visible by CT at the junction of the two lobes. The left lobe is usually larger[23] and slightly higher than the right.[87] But these asymmetries are moderate, and the two lobes cannot always be clearly defined.[69] A focal swelling, or a large lobe on one side with little or no thymic tissue visible on the other, suggests a mass. At CT the thymus is bilobed, triangular, or shaped like an arrowhead. The maximum width and thickness of each lobe decrease with advancing age. Between 20 and 50 years of age the average thickness measured by CT decreases from 8 or 9 mm to 5 or 6 mm, the maximum thickness of one lobe being up to 1.5 cm.[6,28] These diameters are greater at MRI, presumably because MRI demonstrates the thymic tissue even when it is partially replaced by fat.[23] At MRI sagittal images demonstrate that the gland is 5 to 7 cm in craniocaudad dimension.[23] It is impractical to measure the craniocaudad dimension at CT scanning, but the gland may be visible over a similar distance.[6,28]

In younger patients the CT density of the thymus is homogeneous and close to or slightly higher than muscle. The gland often enhances appreciably with intravenous contrast material.[48] After puberty the density gradually decreases owing to fatty replacement.[91] In patients older than 40 years of age the thymus may have an attenuation value identical to that of fat.[6] In some patients the whole gland shows fat density[6,24] and is therefore indistinguishable from mediastinal fat. In others residual thymic parenchyma is visible as a streaky or nodular density (Figure 2-18).[24,69]

On T1-weighted MR images the intensity of the normal thymic tissue is similar to or slightly higher than that of muscle.[12,90] As fatty replacement progresses, the thymus shows higher signal intensity to eventually blend in with the surrounding fat. On T2-weighted images the signal intensity is similar to or sometimes higher than fat[12,68,90] and does not change with age. Proton density images show significantly less signal than the surrounding fat.

"Mediastinal spaces"

The nomenclature of the connective tissue spaces within the mediastinum is not standard, and there are no exact definitions for the boundaries between them. Nevertheless, radiologists need to understand the terms in common use. Four named spaces surround the central airways (Figure 2-19): the pretracheal space, the aortopulmonary window, the subcarinal space, and the right paratracheal space. All four contain lymph nodes

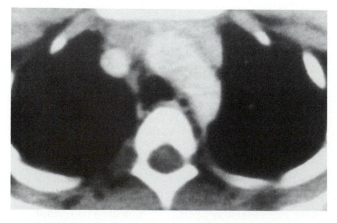

FIGURE 2-17
Normal thymus in a 12-year-old boy. The thymus fills in most of the mediastinum and molds to the aorta and superior vena cava.

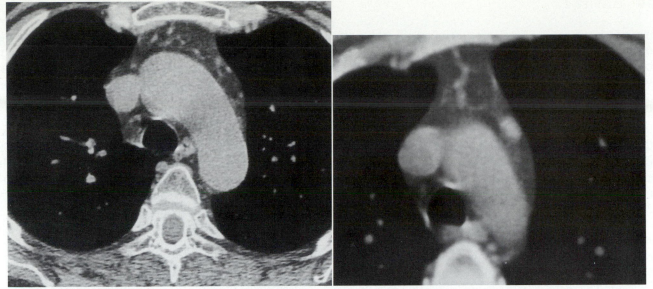

FIGURE 2-18
Normal thymic remnants. **A,** Typical small nodular and linear remnants. **B,** Large nodular and linear remnants in 36-year-old man.

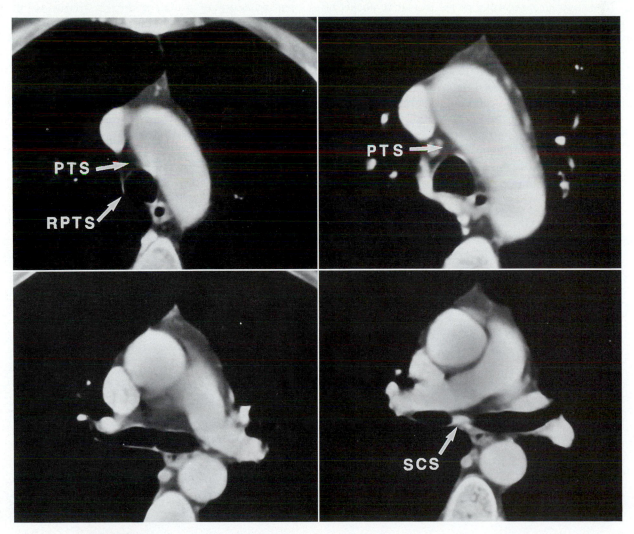

FIGURE 2-19
Mediastinal spaces. *PTS,* Paratracheal space; *RPTS,* right paratracheal space; *SCS,* subcarinal space. The four illustrations are adjacent sections.

that drain the lung and are therefore likely to be involved by bronchial carcinoma. In addition to these central spaces there are the junction areas, so called because in these areas the two lungs approximate each other. One lies anterior to the aorta and pulmonary artery and is variously known as the anterior junction[81] or the prevascular space[35]; the other lies posterior to the trachea and esophagus and is known as the posterior junction.[80] Finally, there are the paraspinal lines on either side of the spine and the junctional area between mediastinum and retroperitoneum known as the retrocrural space.

PRETRACHEAL SPACE. The pretracheal space[88] has no boundary with the lung and is therefore not imaged on plain chest radiographs. It is well known to surgeons because it is the space explored by transcervical mediastinoscopy. The space is triangular in axial cross section; the three boundaries are the trachea or carina posteriorly, either the superior vena cava or the right innominate vein anteriorly to the right, and the ascending aorta with its enveloping superior pericardial sinus anteriorly to the left.[1] The superior pericardial recess is a small pocket of pericardium investing the aorta. When distended the pericardial configuration is easy to recognize (Figure 2-20). In normal individuals, however, the small amount of pericardial fluid in the retroaortic extension of the superior pericardial recess (Figure 2-20) may mimic lymphadenopathy on CT scanning. At spin-echo MRI the signal characteristics of fluid permit differentiation from lymphadenopathy or other masses, but on gradient echo MRI the high signal intensity of fluid may resemble the signal from flowing blood and the superior pericardial recess may then mimic aortic dissection.[11]

The pretracheal space is continuous with the right paratracheal space, the aortopulmonary window, and the subcarinal space. Consequently, lymph nodes or other masses arising in any of these spaces may grow large enough to encroach on the pretracheal space and vice versa.

AORTOPULMONARY WINDOW. The aortopulmonary window is situated under the aortic arch above the left pulmonary artery. It is bounded medially by the trachea and esophagus and laterally by the lung. Its fatty density is not always appreciated at CT scanning because so often the sections include either the aortic arch or the left pulmonary artery, and volume averaging results in higher than fat density.

The ligamentum arteriosum and the recurrent laryngeal nerve traverse this space. How often they can be identified is not clear, but in any event they are not likely to be confused with lymphadenopathy or other masses. The ligamentum arteriosum may be calcified. It is easier to recognize as such in younger patients, in whom calcification was seen in 13% of 53 patients,[10] but none had evidence of a patent ductus arteriosus. In older patients calcification of the ligamentum is difficult to distinguish from atheromatous calcification of the adjacent aortic wall.

SUBCARINAL SPACE. The subcarinal space, lying beneath the tracheal carina, is bounded on either side by the major bronchi. The azygoesophageal recess of the right lung lies behind the subcarinal space, and distortion of the azygoesophageal recess is a sensitive method of detecting masses, usually lymphadenopathy, in this space. The posterior boundary is partly formed by the esophagus.

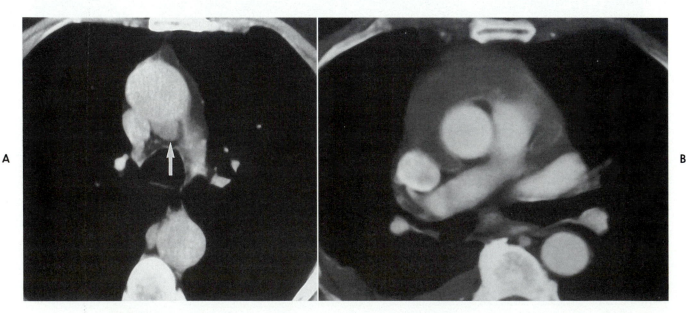

FIGURE 2-20
A, Normal superior pericardial recess (arrow). B, Patient with pericardial effusion showing marked distention of superior pericardial recess.

RIGHT PARATRACHEAL SPACE AND POSTERIOR TRACHEAL SPACE. These two adjacent spaces (they should more properly be called stripes) are best considered together. Normally the right lung is separated from the trachea only by a thin layer of fat (the only exception being at the tracheobronchial angle where the azygos vein lies between the lung and the airway). The degree to which the lung envelops the posterior wall of the trachea is variable. In up to half the population a substantial portion of the posterior tracheal wall is outlined by lung as it interposes between the spine and the trachea to contact the esophagus.

ANTERIOR JUNCTION. The anterior junction[81] (prevascular space) lies anterior to the pulmonary artery, the ascending aorta, and the three major branches of the aortic arch. It lies between the two lungs and is bounded anteriorly by the chest wall. If the two lungs approximate each other closely enough, the intervening mediastinum may consist of little more than four layers of pleura and is then sometimes known as the anterior junction line (see Figure 2-24). Coursing through the prevascular space superiorly is the left brachiocephalic vein. The internal mammary vascular bundles are to be found laterally and are visible at CT only if intravenous contrast material is administered. Embedded within the prevascular space are lymph nodes, the thymus, and the phrenic nerve.

POSTERIOR JUNCTION AND PARASPINAL AREAS. The term "posterior junction" describes the mediastinal region posterior to the trachea and the heart, where the two lungs lie close to each other.[80] The right lung always invaginates behind the right hilar structures and heart to contact the pleura overlying the azygos vein and esophagus, forming the so-called azygoesophageal recess. Displacement of the lung from the azygoesophageal recess is an important sign of a subcarinal mediastinal mass, particularly lymphadenopathy. Above the level of the azygos arch, the lung contacts the esophagus alone.

On the left the lung interface is with the aortic arch and descending aorta rather than with the esophagus, but in some individuals the lung below the aortic arch invaginates anterior to the descending aorta to almost reach the midline.

The paraspinal areas are contiguous with the posterior junction. Normally there is little or no discernible connective tissue between the lateral margins of the spine and the lungs. The only structures contained in these areas are intercostal vessels and small lymph nodes.

RETROCRURAL SPACE. The aorta exits the chest by passing through the aortic hiatus, which is bounded by the diaphragmatic crura and the spine (Figure 2-21). The diaphragmatic crura are ligaments that blend with the anterior longitudinal ligament of the spine. Apart from the aorta, the structures that pass through the aortic hiatus are the azygos and hemiazygos veins, intercostal arteries, and splanchnic nerves. All these structures are too small to be mistaken for lymphadenopathy.[17]

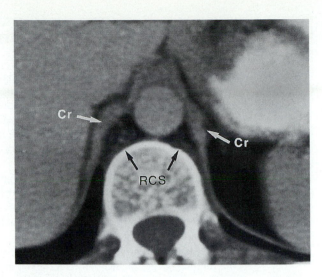

FIGURE 2-21
Retrocrural spaces (*RCS*). *Cr,* Diaphragmatic crura.

Mediastinal lymph nodes

Lymph nodes are widely distributed in the mediastinum. The nomenclature for these nodes is not standardized nor, unfortunately, does it correspond exactly with the terms used for the mediastinal spaces. The following description uses terms in keeping with the nomenclature of the American Thoracic Society (ATS) designed for the staging of carcinoma of the bronchus (see box on p. 38; Figure 2-22).[40,42,98]

Anterior mediastinal nodes lie anterior or anterolateral to the aorta and the innominate artery (station 6 in the ATS definitions).

Tracheobronchial nodes encircle the trachea and main bronchi except where the aorta, pulmonary artery, and esophagus are in direct contact with the airway. There is no clear division between the various nodes in this group, but they can be divided according to site:

1. Right and left paratracheal nodes, which can be further subdivided into upper and lower groups, depending on whether they lie above or below the level of the top of the aortic arch (stations 2R, 4R, 2L, and 4L). In the ATS-approved nomenclature this group includes the pretracheal nodes.
2. Aortopulmonary window nodes, which include nodes along the lateral surfaces of the aorta and left or main pulmonary arteries (station 5).
3. Subcarinal nodes, a group that comprises all the nodes found beneath the carina and main bronchi (station 7).
4. Tracheobronchial and hilar nodes. Tracheobronchial nodes (stations 10R and 10L) lie adjacent to right and left mainstem bronchi and according to the ATS definition are mediastinal in location. The lower tracheobronchial nodes may, however, be removed at standard pneumonectomy. (Friedman[31] has suggested that 10R nodes be considered hilar.)

AMERICAN THORACIC SOCIETY DEFINITIONS OF REGIONAL NODAL STATIONS

X   Supraclavicular nodes

2R   Right upper paratracheal nodes: nodes to the right of the midline of the trachea, between the intersection of the caudal margin of the innominate artery with the trachea and the apex of the lung

2L   Left upper paratracheal nodes: nodes to the left of the midline of the trachea, between the top of the aortic arch and the apex of the lung

4R   Right lower paratracheal nodes: nodes to the right of the midline of the trachea, between the cephalic border of the azygos vein and the intersection of the caudal margin of the brachiocephalic artery with the right side of the trachea

4L   Left lower paratracheal nodes: nodes to the left of the midline of the trachea, between the top of the aortic arch and the level of the carina, medial to the ligamentum arteriosum

5   Aortopulmonary nodes: subaortic and paraaortic nodes, lateral to the ligamentum arteriosum or the aorta or left pulmonary artery, proximal to the first branch of the left pulmonary artery

6   Anterior mediastinal nodes: nodes anterior to the ascending aorta or the innominate artery

7   Subcarinal nodes: nodes arising caudal to the carina of the trachea but not associated with the lower lobe bronchi or arteries within the lung

8   Paraesophageal nodes: nodes dorsal to the posterior wall of the trachea and to the right or left of the midline of the esophagus

9   Right or left pulmonary ligament nodes: nodes within the right or left pulmonary ligament

10R   Right tracheobronchial nodes: nodes to the right of the midline of the trachea, from the level of the cephalic border of the azygos vein to the origin of the right upper lobe bronchus

10L   Left peribronchial nodes: nodes to the left of the midline of the trachea, between the carina and the left upper lobe bronchus, medial to the ligamentum arteriosum

11   Intrapulmonary nodes: nodes removed in the right or left lung specimen, plus those distal to the mainstem bronchi or secondary carina

From Glazer GM, Gross BH, Quint LE, et al: *AJR* 144:261-265, 1985.

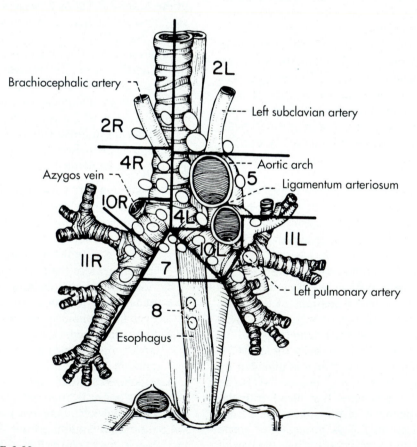

FIGURE 2-22
American Thoracic Society lymph node mapping scheme. See box above for definitions. (From Glazer GM, Gross BH, Quint LE, et al: *AJR* 144:261-265, 1985.)

The hilar nodes (stations 11R and 11L) are defined as nodes distal to the mainstem bronchi, and these are always part of standard pneumonectomy.

The posterior mediastinal nodes are divided into paraesophageal (station 8) and pulmonary ligament nodes (station 9). Glazer and associates[42] include nodes around the descending aorta with station 8 nodes. Nodes are also present in the retrocrural areas and in the anterior cardiophrenic angles.

NORMAL LYMPH NODE SIZE. The CT series documenting normal mediastinal lymph node size are in general agreement.[39,40,52,88] In these studies 95% of normal mediastinal lymph nodes were less than 10 mm in diameter, and the remainder, with few exceptions, were less than 15 mm in diameter. There is a significant variation in the number and size of lymph nodes seen in different locations within the mediastinum. Nodes in the region of the brachiocephalic veins are generally smaller, with over 90% measuring 5 mm or less, whereas nodes in the aortopulmonary window, the pretracheal and lower paratracheal spaces, and the subcarinal compartment are often 6 to 10 mm in diameter. Nodes in the paracardiac areas are rarely visible in normal subjects: their maximum size in a series of 50 persons was 3.5 mm.[94] Nodes in the retrocrural area do not normally exceed 6 mm in diameter.[17]

Normal mediastinal contours on plain chest radiographs

For descriptive convenience the frontal and lateral projections are treated separately, although in practice the information from these two views should be integrated. For further details of the normal appearances in the lateral projection, the reader is referred to the excellent accounts by Proto and Speckman.[82,83]

FRONTAL PROJECTION

Left mediastinal border. Above the aortic arch the mediastinal shadow to the left of the trachea is of low density and is caused by the left carotid and left subclavian arteries and the jugular veins. The usual appearance in the frontal projection is a gently curving border that fades out where the artery enters the neck. This border is formed by the left subclavian artery or more usually by the adjacent fat[79]; occasionally the interface is with the left carotid artery.[79] A separate interface may be discernible for the left carotid artery. The outer margin of the left tracheal wall is rarely outlined because the lung is almost invariably separated from the trachea by the aorta and great vessels.

Below the aortic arch the left mediastinal border is formed by the aortopulmonary pleural stripe,[55] the main pulmonary artery, and the heart. A small "nipple" may occasionally be seen projecting laterally from the aortic knob. This projection is caused by the left superior intercostal vein arching forward around the aorta just

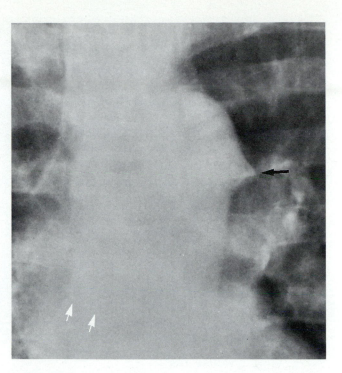

FIGURE 2-23
Left superior intercostal vein *(arrow)* seen as so-called aortic nipple.

beyond the origin of the left subclavian artery before entering the left brachiocephalic vein (Figure 2-23).[58] This vein should not be misinterpreted as lymphadenopathy projecting from the aortopulmonary window. Fat can sometimes be identified in the aortopulmonary window beneath the aortic arch.

The left border of the descending aorta can be traced through the shadow of the main pulmonary artery and heart as a continuous border from the aortic arch down to the aortic hiatus in the diaphragm. In patients with pectus excavatum a small portion of the left wall of the middle descending aorta may appear indistinct because it is in contact with the left atrium and left inferior pulmonary vein.[95]

Right mediastinal border. The right mediastinal border is normally formed by the right brachiocephalic (innominate) vein, the SVC, and the right atrium. The right paratracheal stripe can be seen through the right brachiocephalic vein and SVC because the lung contacts the right tracheal wall from the clavicles down to the arch of the azygos vein (Figure 2-24). This stripe, which should be of uniform thickness and no greater than 3 mm wide, is visible in approximately two thirds of healthy subjects. It consists of the wall of the trachea and adjacent mediastinal fat, but there should be no focal bulges caused by individual paratracheal lymph nodes. The azygos vein is outlined by air in the lung at the lower end of this stripe. The diameter of the azygos vein in the tracheobronchial angle is variable; it may be considered normal when 10 mm or less. The nodes immediately beneath the azygos vein, which are sometimes known as azygos nodes, are

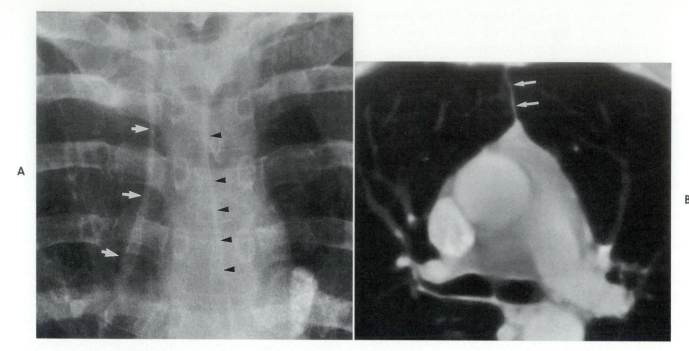

FIGURE 2-24
A, Anterior junction line *(black arrowheads)* and right paratracheal stripe *(white arrows)*. Lowest white arrow points to azygos vein. **B,** Computed tomography scan in another patient shows anterior junction line *(arrows)*.

not recognizable on normal chest radiographs. The right paratracheal stripe has diagnostic value because it excludes space-occupying processes in the area where the stripe is visible and appears normal.

Anterior junction. The two lungs approximate each other above the level of the heart and below the manubrium; the term "anterior junction" has therefore been applied to this area of the mediastinum.[81] When the two lungs are separated only by pleura, the anterior junction forms a visible line, known as the anterior junction line (Figure 2-24), which is usually straight and diverges to fade out superiorly as it reaches the clavicles. It descends for a variable distance, usually deviating to the left. The anterior junction line sometimes follows a vertical course or, very rarely, deviates to the right. It cannot extend below the point where the two lungs separate to envelop the right ventricle. Since the line is only occasionally seen, failure to identify it has no significance.

More often the two lungs are separated by fat and thymus, with the result that the borders of the anterior junction are invisible on plain film or that only one of the borders can be identified. Bulging of one or both borders indicates the presence of a mass. In young children the thymus can be a prominent structure and the sail shape is characteristic (Figure 2-25).

Proto, Simmons, and Zylak[81] used the terms "superior" and "inferior recesses" to describe the lung interfaces above and below the anterior junction region. The interfaces of the superior recesses are concave laterally.

They are formed by mediastinal fat anterior to the arteries that supply the head and neck. (The left and right brachiocephalic veins course through this fat but do not form visible borders on the frontal view). The inferior recesses are due to divergence of the lungs around fat in the lower mediastinum anterior to the heart.[81]

Posterior junction and azygoesophageal recess. In some patients the lungs almost touch each other behind the esophagus to form the posterior junction line, a structure that can be thought of as an esophageal mesentery (Figure 2-26).[49] This line, unlike the anterior junction line, diverges to envelop the aortic and azygos arches. Above the aortic arch the posterior junction line extends to the lung apices, where it diverges and disappears at the root of the neck, well above the level of the clavicles. The differences in the superior extent of the anterior and posterior junction lines are related to the sloping boundary between the thorax and the neck. Once again the width of the line depends on the amount of mediastinal fat. Whether both sides of the line are seen on plain chest radiograph depends on the tangent formed with the adjacent lung. Bulging of the borders of any portion of the posterior junction line or its superior recesses suggests a mass or other space-occupying process. The only normal convexities are those attributable to the azygos vein or aortic arch.

Whether or not there is a visible posterior junction line above the aortic arch, the interface between the lung and the right wall of the esophagus can often be seen as a shallow S extending from the lung apex down to the

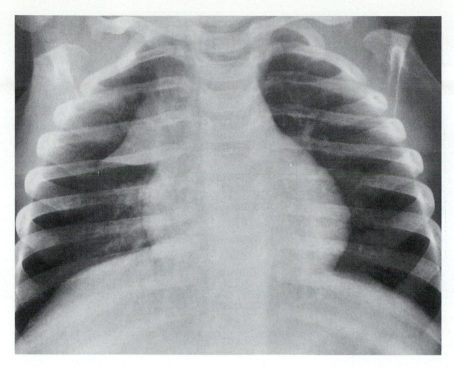

FIGURE 2-25
Normal thymus in a 3-year-old child. Sail shape projecting to the right of the mediastinum is characteristic.

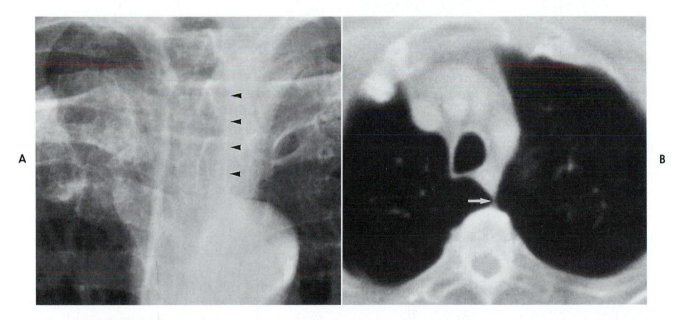

FIGURE 2-26
A, Posterior junction line *(arrowheads).* B, Computed tomography scan shows origin of line *(arrow)* in same patient.

azygos arch. If there is air in the esophagus, which there frequently is, the right wall of the esophagus is seen as a stripe, usually 3 to 5 mm thick.[19] This interface is known as the pleuroesophageal line or stripe (Figure 2-27).

Below the aortic arch the right lower lobe makes contact with the right wall of the esophagus and the

azygos vein as it ascends next to the esophagus. This portion of lung is known as the azygoesophageal recess, and the interface is known as the azygoesophageal line (Figure 2-28). The shape of the azygos arch varies considerably in different subjects, and therefore the shape of the upper portion of the azygoesophageal line varies

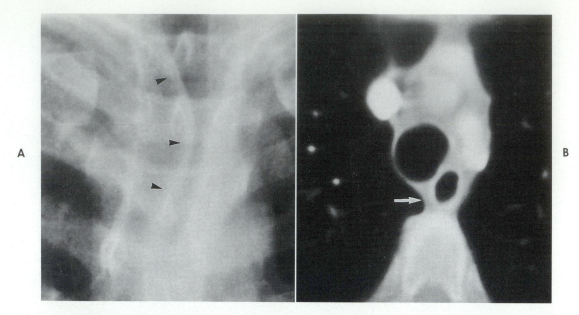

FIGURE 2-27
A, Pleuroesophageal line *(arrowheads)*. B, Computed tomography scan shows origin of line *(arrow)* in same patient.

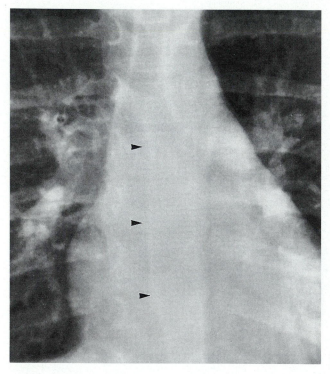

FIGURE 2-28
Azygoesophageal line *(arrowheads)*.

accordingly. In its upper few centimeters, however, the azygoesophageal line in adults is always straight or concave toward the lung, and a convex shape suggests a subcarinal mass. The azygoesophageal recess is somewhat different in children. Before 3 years of age the azygoesophageal line is usually convex, and various configurations are seen as the child becomes older.[27] The azygoesophageal line can be traced down into the posterior costophrenic angle in subjects with normal anatomy.

The near vertical border seen through the heart represents the left wall of the descending aorta. This border can be traced, with virtually no loss of continuity, upward to the aortic arch and downward to the diaphragm. In a few subjects a small segment of aortic outline may be invisible because of contact between the aorta and the descending division of the left pulmonary artery behind the left main bronchus.

Occasionally the lung contacts the left wall of the esophagus (Figure 2-29), and then the esophagus is outlined from both the right and the left. Because air is frequently present in the esophagus, identifying separately the thickness of the right and left walls may even be possible. The usual site for trapped air within the esophagus is just beneath the aortic arch (Figure 2-29).

Paraspinal lines. The term "paraspinal line" refers to a stripe of soft tissue density parallel to the left and right margins of the thoracic spine. Although lymph nodes and intercostal veins share this space with mediastinal fat and pleura, these structures cannot normally be recognized individually. With little fat the interface may closely follow the undulations of the lateral spinal ligaments, but with larger quantities of fat these undulations are smoothed out. The left paravertebral space is usually thicker than the right. The paravertebral stripes are usually less than 1 cm wide, although they can be wider in obese persons. Aortic unfolding contributes to the thickness of the left paraspinal line; as the aorta moves

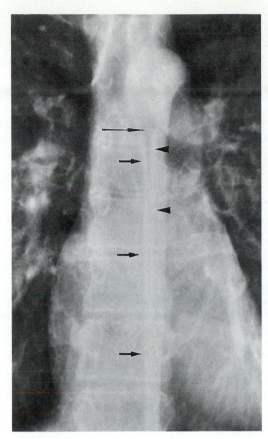

FIGURE 2-29
Right and left walls of esophagus. Arrowheads point to left wall. Arrows point to right wall (azygoesophageal line). Uppermost arrow points to air in the lumen of the esophagus trapped beneath the aortic arch.

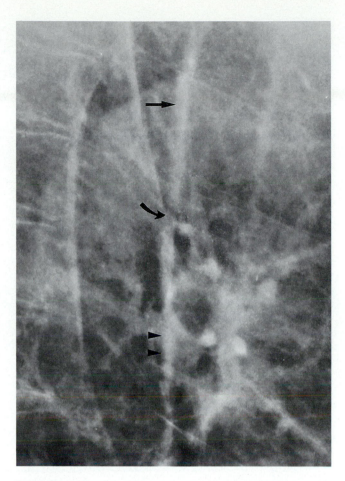

FIGURE 2-30
Posterior tracheal band *(straight arrow)*. Note that the posterior walls of the trachea, right main bronchus *(curved arrow),* and bronchus intermedius *(arrowheads)* are seen as a continuous thin band.

posteriorly, it strips the pleura from its otherwise close contact with the profiled portions of the spine.

LATERAL VIEW

Mediastinum above the aortic arch. A variable portion of the aortic arch and head and neck vessels is visible in the lateral view, depending on the degree of aortic unfolding. The brachiocephalic artery is the only artery recognized with frequency. It arises anterior to the tracheal air column. Unless involved by atheromatous calcification, the origin is usually invisible, but after a variable distance its posterior wall can be seen as a gentle S-shaped interface crossing the tracheal air column. The left and right brachiocephalic veins are also visible in the lateral view. The left brachiocephalic vein often forms an extrapleural bulge behind the manubrium. The posterior border of the right brachiocephalic vein and SVC can occasionally be identified curving downward in much the same position and direction as the brachiocephalic artery, but they are sometimes traceable below the upper margin of the aortic arch.

Trachea and retrotracheal area. The air column in the trachea can be seen throughout its length as it descends obliquely downward and posteriorly. The course of the trachea in the lateral view of adult subjects is straight, or bowed forward in patients with aortic unfolding, with no visible indentation by adjacent vessels. The carina is not visible on the lateral view. The anterior wall of the trachea is visible in only a minority of patients, but its posterior wall is usually visible because lung often passes behind the trachea, allowing the radiologist to see the "posterior tracheal stripe or band" (Figure 2-30).[4,36] This stripe is seen in 50% to 90% of healthy adults.[4,74] It is uniform in width and measures up to 3 mm (rarely, 4 mm). There is, however, a problem in applying this measurement. Because air is frequently present in the esophagus, the anterior wall of the esophagus may contribute to the thickness of the stripe in healthy persons.[74] Alternatively, the lung may be separated from the trachea by the full width of a collapsed esophagus, leading to a band of density 1 cm or more in thickness (Figure 2-31). Thus caution is needed in diagnosing abnormalities on the basis of an increase in thickness of the posterior tracheal stripe. CT study has shown that the visibility of the posterior tracheal stripe depends on the degree to which the lung passes behind the trachea.[57] Sometimes the

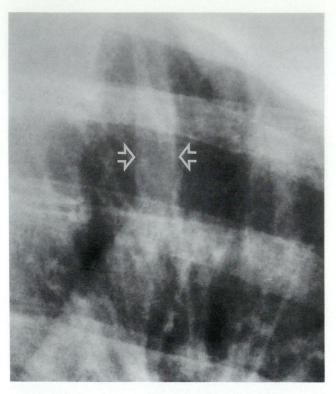

FIGURE 2-31
Normal collapsed esophagus appearing as a band shadow *(arrows)* posterior to the trachea.

airway is close to the spine and what little space is present is occupied by the esophagus and connective tissue. Clearly the quantity of mediastinal fat is an important factor in determining how much lung invaginates behind the trachea.

Retrosternal line. A bandlike opacity simulating pleural or extrapleural disease is often seen in healthy individuals along the lower half or lowest third of the anterior chest wall on the lateral view (Figure 2-32).[105] This density is due to the differing anterior extent of the left and right lungs. The left lung does not contact the most anterior portion of the left thoracic cavity at these levels because the heart with its epicardial fat occupies the space.

Inferior vena cava. In most healthy subjects the posterior wall of the inferior vena cava is visible just before it enters the right atrium. Even patients with azygos continuation of the inferior vena cava may show a similar vessel formed by the continuation of the hepatic veins as they drain into the right atrium. In approximately 5% of healthy people the posterior wall of the inferior vena cava is not visible on the lateral chest radiograph.

DIAPHRAGM

The diaphragm consists of a large, dome-shaped central tendon with a sheet of striated muscle radiating from the central tendon to attach to ribs 7 through 12 and to the xiphisternum.[34,50,56,75] The two crura arise from the upper three lumbar vertebrae and arch upward and forward to form the margins of the aortic and esophageal hiati. The median arcuate ligament connecting the two

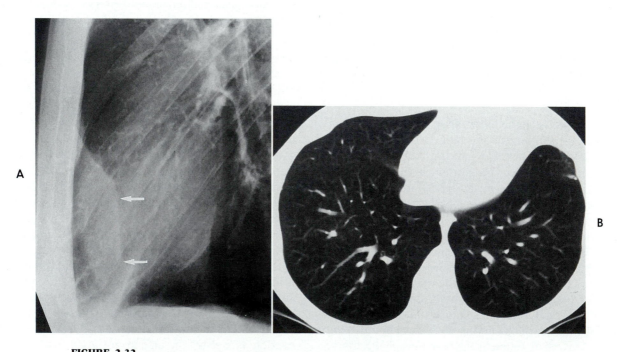

FIGURE 2-32
A, Retrosternal line *(arrows).* **B,** Computed tomography scan in same patient shows that the anterior margin of left lung lies more posterior than the anterior margin of right lung, in part because of the heart and in part because of epicardial fat.

crura forms the anterior margin of the aortic hiatus, and the crura themselves form the lateral boundary of the aortic hiatus. Accompanying the aorta through this opening are the azygos and hemiazygos veins and the thoracic duct. Anterior to the aortic hiatus lies the esophageal hiatus, through which run the esophagus, the vagus nerve, and the esophageal arteries. The most anterior of the three diaphragmatic hiati is the hiatus for the IVC, which is situated within the central tendon immediately beneath the right atrium. The diaphragm has a smooth dome shape in most individuals, but a scalloped outline is also common.

The position of the diaphragm in healthy subjects on upright plain chest radiographs taken at full inspiration was investigated by Lennon and Simon.[61] They used the anterior ribs to describe the position of each hemidiaphragm because the dome is closer to the anterior chest wall and both the domes and the anterior ribs are closer to the film in the PA projection. The normal right hemidiaphragm is found at about the level of the anterior sixth rib, being slightly higher in women and in individuals over 40 years of age. The range covers approximately one interspace above or below this level. In most people the right hemidiaphragm is 1.5 to 2.5 cm higher than the left, but the two hemidiaphragms are at the same level in about 9% of the population. In a few (3% in the series by Felson[26]) the left hemidiaphragm is higher than the right, but by less than 1 cm. The normal excursion of the domes of the diaphragm as measured by plain chest radiography is usually between 1.5 and 2.5 cm, although greater degrees of movement are sometimes seen. Transabdominal ultrasound, which allows more accurate real-time measurement of movement, shows that the normal range is considerable: between 2 and 8.6 cm, with the mean excursion of the right hemidiaphragm on deep inspiration 53 mm (SD 16.4) and that of the left side 46 mm (SD 12.4).[51]

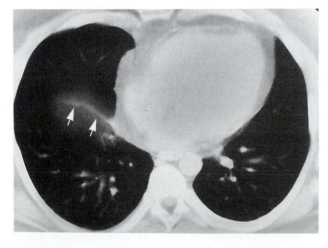

FIGURE 2-33
Phrenic nerve coursing over the surface of the right hemidiaphragm *(arrows).*

Incomplete muscularization, known as eventration, is also common. An eventration is composed of a thin membranous sheet replacing what should be muscle. Usually it is partial, involving one half to one third of the hemidiaphragm, frequently the anteromedial portion of the right hemidiaphragm. The lack of muscle manifests itself radiographically as elevation of the affected portion of the diaphragm, and the usual pattern is a smooth hump on the contour of the diaphragm. Total eventration of a hemidiaphragm, which is much more common on the left than the right, results in elevation of the whole hemidiaphragm; on fluoroscopy, hemidiaphragm movement is poor, absent, or paradoxic. In severe cases congenital eventration cannot be distinguished from acquired paralysis of the phrenic nerve.

A linear density arising from the lateral wall of the IVC (Figure 2-33) is often seen coursing over the superior surface of the right hemidiaphragm. This line represents an envelope of fat with investing pleura surrounding either the phrenic nerve, according to Berkmen and co-workers,[8] or the inferior phrenic artery and vein, according to Ujita and associates.[100]

REFERENCES

1. Aronberg DJ, Peterson RR, Glazer HS, et al: The superior sinus of the pericardium: CT appearance, *Radiology* 153:489-492, 1984.
2. Austin JHM: The left minor fissure, *Radiology* 161:433-436, 1986.
3. Bach AM, Hilfer CL, Holgerson LO: Left side posterior mediastinal thymus: MRI findings, *Pediatr Radiol* 21:440-441, 1991.
4. Bachman AL, Teixidor HS: The posterior tracheal band: a reflector of local mediastinal abnormality, *Br J Radiol* 48:352-359, 1975.
5. Ball JB, Proto AV: The variable appearance of the left superior intercostal vein, *Radiology* 144:445-452, 1982.
6. Baron RL, Lee JKT, Sagel SS, et al: Computed tomography of the normal thymus, *Radiology* 142:121-125, 1982.
7. Berkmen YM, Auh YH, Davis SD, et al: Anatomy of the minor fissure: evaluation with thin-section CT, *Radiology* 170:647-651, 1989.
8. Berkmen YM, Davis SD, Kazam E, et al: Right phrenic nerve: anatomy, CT appearance, and differentiation from the pulmonary ligament, *Radiology* 173:43-46, 1989.
9. Berkmen YM, Drossman SR, Marboe CC: Intersegmental (intersublobar) septum of the lower lobe in relation to the pulmonary ligament: anatomic, histologic, and CT correlations, *Radiology* 185:389-393, 1993.
10. Bisceglia M: Calcification of the ligamentum arteriosum in children: a normal finding on CT, *AJR* 156:351-352, 1991.
11. Black CM, Hedges LK, Javitt MC: The superior pericardial sinus: normal appearance on gradient-echo MR images, *AJR* 160:749-751, 1993.
12. Boothroyd AE, Hall-Craggs MA, Dicks-Mireaux CR, et al: The magnetic resonance appearances of the normal thymus in children, *Clin Radiol* 45:378-381, 1992.
13. Boyden EA: The distribution of bronchi in gross anomalies of the right upper lobe, particularly lobes subdivided by the azygos vein and those containing pre-eparterial bronchi, *Radiology* 58:797-807, 1952.
14. Breatnach E, Abbott GC, Fraser RE: Dimensions of the normal human trachea, *AJR* 142:903-906, 1984.

15. Buirski G, Jordan SC, Joffe HS, et al: Superior vena caval abnormalities: their occurrence rate, associated cardiac abnormalities and angiographic classification in a paediatric population with congenital heart disease, *Clin Radiol* 37:131-138, 1986.

16. Càceres J, Mata JM, Alegret X: Increased density of the azygos lobe on frontal radiographs simulating disease: CT findings in seven patients, *AJR* 160:245-248, 1993.

17. Callen PW, Korobkin M, Isherwood I: Computed tomographic evaluation of retrocrural prevertebral space, *AJR* 129:907-910, 1977.

18. Cha EM, Khoury GH: Persistent left superior vena cava: radiologic and clinical significance, *Radiology* 103:375-381, 1972.

19. Cimmino CV: The esophageal-pleural stripe: an update, *Radiology* 140:607-613, 1981.

20. Cohen MD, Weber TR, Sequeira FW, et al: The diagnostic dilemma of the posterior mediastinal thymus: CT manifestations, *Radiology* 146:691-693, 1983.

21. Dandy WE: Incomplete pulmonary interlobar fissure sign, *Radiology* 128:21-25, 1978.

22. Davis SD, Maldijian C, Perone RW, et al: CT of the airways, *Clin Imag* 14:280-300, 1990.

23. deGeer G, Webb WR, Gamsu G: Normal thymus: assessment with MR and CT, *Radiology* 158:313-317, 1986.

24. Dixon AK, Hilton CJ, Williams CT: Computed tomography and histological correlation of the thymic remnant, *Clin Radiol* 32:255-257, 1981.

25. Felson B: The mediastinum, *Semin Roentgenol* 4:41-58, 1969.

26. Felson B: *Chest roentgenology*, Philadelphia, 1973, WB Saunders.

27. Fitzgerald SW, Donaldson JS: Azygoesophageal recess: normal CT appearance in children, *AJR* 158:1101-1104, 1992.

28. Francis IR, Glazer GM, Bookstein FL, et al: The thymus: re-examination of age-related changes in size and shape, *AJR* 145:249-254, 1985.

29. Fraser RG, Pare JAP, Pare PD, et al: *Diagnosis of diseases of the chest*, vol 1, ed 3, Philadelphia, 1988, WB Saunders.

30. Friedman AC, Chambers E, Sprayregen S: The normal and abnormal left superior intercostal vein, *AJR* 131:599-602, 1978.

31. Friedman PJ: Lung cancer: update on staging classifications, *AJR* 150:261-264, 1988.

32. Frija J, Yan C, Laval-Jeantet M: Anatomy of the minor fissure: evaluation with thin-section CT (letter), *Radiology* 173:571-572, 1989.

33. Fujimoto K, Abe T, Kumabe T, et al: Anomalous left brachiocephalic (innominate) vein: MR demonstration, *AJR* 159:479-480, 1992.

34. Gale ME: Anterior diaphragm: variations in the CT appearance, *Radiology* 161:635-639, 1986.

35. Gamsu G: Computed tomography of the mediastinum. In Moss AA, Gamsu G, Genant HK, eds: *Computed tomography of the body*, Philadelphia, 1983, WB Saunders.

36. Gamsu G, Webb WR: Computed tomography of the trachea: normal and abnormal, *AJR* 139:321-326, 1982.

37. Gamsu G, Webb WR: Computed tomography of the trachea and main bronchi, *Semin Roentgenol* 18:51-60, 1983.

38. Genereux GP: Conventional tomographic hilar anatomy emphasizing the pulmonary veins, *AJR* 141:1241-1257, 1983.

39. Genereux GP, Howie JL: Normal mediastinal lymph node size and number: CT and anatomic study, *AJR* 142:1095-1100, 1984.

40. Glazer GM, Gross BH, Quint LE, et al: Normal mediastinal lymph nodes: number and size according to American Thoracic Society mapping, *AJR* 144:261-265, 1985.

41. Glazer HS, Anderson DJ, DiCroce JJ, et al: Anatomy of the major fissure: evaluation with standard and thin-section CT, *Radiology* 180:839-844, 1991.

42. Glazer HS, Aronberg DJ, Sagel SS, et al: CT demonstration of calcified mediastinal lymph nodes: a guide to the new ATS classification, *AJR* 147:17-20, 1986.

43. Godwin JD, Chen JTT: Thoracic venous anatomy, *AJR* 147:674-684, 1986.

44. Godwin JD, Tarver RD: Accessory fissures of the lung: pictorial essay, *AJR* 144:39-44, 1985.

45. Goodman LR, Golkow RS, Steiner RM, et al: The right mid-lung window, *Radiology* 143:135-138, 1982.

46. Griscom NT, Wohl ME: Dimensions of the growing trachea related to age and gender, *AJR* 146:233-237, 1986.

47. Guthaner DF, Wexler L, Harell G: CT demonstration of cardiac structures, *AJR* 133:75-81, 1979.

48. Heiberg E, Wolverson MK, Sundaram M, et al: Normal thymus: CT characteristics in subjects under age 20, *AJR* 138:491-494, 1982.

49. Heitzman ER: *The mediastinum: radiologic correlations with anatomy and pathology*, ed 2, Berlin, 1988, Springer-Verlag.

50. Heitzman ER: The diaphragm: radiologic correlations with anatomy and pathology, *Clin Radiol* 42:15-19, 1990.

51. Houston JG, Morris AD, Howie CA, et al: Quantitative assessment of diaphragmatic movement: a reproducible method using ultrasound, *Clin Radiol* 46:405-407, 1992.

52. Ingram CE, Belli AM, Lewars MD, et al: Normal lymph node size in the mediastinum: a retrospective study in two patient groups, *Clin Radiol* 40:35-39, 1989.

53. Jardin M, Remy J: Segmental bronchovascular anatomy of the lower lobes: CT analysis, *AJR* 147:457-468, 1986.

54. Jefferson K, Rees S: *Clinical cardiac radiology*, London, 1973, Butterworths.

55. Keats TE: The aortic-pulmonary mediastinal stripe, *AJR* 116:107-109, 1972.

56. Kleinman PK, Raptopoulos V: The anterior diaphragmatic attachments: an anatomic and radiologic study with clinical correlations, *Radiology* 155:289-293, 1985.

57. Kormano M, Yrjana J: The posterior tracheal band: correlation between computed tomography and chest radiography, *Radiology* 136:689-694, 1980.

58. Lane EJ, Heitzman ER, Dinn WM: The radiology of the superior intercostal veins, *Radiology* 120:263-267, 1976.

59. Lee KS, Bae WK, Lee BH, et al: Bronchovascular anatomy of the upper lobes: evaluation with thin section CT, *Radiology* 181:765-772, 1991.

60. Lee KS, Im JG, Bae WK, et al: CT anatomy of the lingular segmental bronchi, *J Comput Assist Tomogr* 15:86-91, 1991.

61. Lennon EA, Simon G: The height of the diaphragm in the chest radiograph of normal adults, *Br J Radiol* 38:937-943, 1965.

62. Lloyd DC, Taylor PM: Calcification of the intrathoracic trachea demonstrated by computed tomography, *Br J Radiol* 63:31-32, 1990.

63. Marks BW, Kuhns LR: Identification of the pleural fissures with computed tomography, *Radiology* 143:139-141, 1982.

64. Mata JM, Càceres J, Llauger J, et al: CT demonstration of intrapulmonary right brachiocephalic vein associated with an azygos lobe, *J Comput Assist Tomogr* 14:305-306, 1990.

65. Mayo JR, Müller NL, Henkelman RM: The double-fissure sign: a motion artifact on thin-section CT scans, *Radiology* 165:580-581, 1987.

66. McDonald CJ, Castellino RA, Blank N: The aortic "nipple": the left superior intercostal vein, *Radiology* 96:533-536, 1970.

67. Meaney JFM, Roberts DE, Carty H: Pseudo-tumour of the postero-superior mediastinum, *Br J Radiol* 66:741-742, 1993.

68. Molina PL, Siegel MJ, Glazer HS: Thymic masses on MR imaging: a pictorial essay, *AJR* 155:495-500, 1990.

69. Moore AV, Korobkin M, Olanow W, et al: Age-related changes in the thymus gland: CT-pathologic correlation, *AJR* 141:241-246, 1983.

70. Naidich DP, Khouri NF, Scott WW, et al: Computed tomogra-

phy of the pulmonary hila: normal anatomy, *J Comput Assist Tomogr* 5:459-467, 1981.

71. Naidich DP, Zinn WL, Ettinger NA, et al: Basilar segmental bronchi: thin-section CT evaluation, *Radiology* 169:11-16, 1988.

72. Osborne D, Vock P, Godwin JD, et al: CT identification of bronchopulmonary segments: 50 normal subjects, *AJR* 142:47-52, 1984.

73. Otsuji H, Uchida H, Maeda M, et al: Incomplete interlobar fissures: bronchovascular analysis with CT, *Radiology* 187:541-546, 1993.

74. Palajew MJ: The tracheo-esophageal stripe and the posterior tracheal band, *Radiology* 132:11-13, 1979.

75. Panicek DM, Benson CB, Gottlieb RH, et al: The diaphragm: anatomic, pathologic, and radiologic considerations, *Radiographics* 8:385-425, 1988.

76. Park C-K, Webb WR, Klein JS: Inferior hilar window, *Radiology* 178:163-168, 1991.

77. Proto AV, Ball JB: The superolateral major fissures, *AJR* 140:431-437, 1983.

78. Proto AV, Ball JB: Computed tomography of the major and minor fissures, *AJR* 140:439-448, 1983.

79. Proto AV, Corcoran HL, Ball JB: Left paratracheal reflection, *Radiology* 171:625-628, 1989.

80. Proto AV, Simmons JD, Zylak CJ: The posterior junction anatomy, *Crit Rev Diagn Imag* 20:121-173, 1983.

81. Proto AV, Simmons JD, Zylak CT: The anterior junction anatomy, *Crit Rev Diagn Imag* 19:111-173, 1983.

82. Proto AV, Speckman JM: The left lateral radiograph of the chest, Part 1, *Med Radiogr Photogr* 55:30-74, 1979.

83. Proto AV, Speckman JM: The left lateral radiograph of the chest, Part 2, *Med Radiogr Photogr* 56:36-64, 1980.

84. Raider L, Landry BA, Brogdon BG: The retrotracheal triangle, *Radiographics* 10:1055-1079, 1990.

85. Rollins NK, Currarino G: MR imaging of posterior mediastinal thymus, *J Comput Assist Tomogr* 12:518-520, 1988.

86. Rosai J, Levine GD: Normal thymus. In *Atlas of tumor pathology*, 2nd series, Fascicle 13, Washington, DC, 1976, Armed Forces Institute of Pathology.

87. Sagel SS, Aronberg DJ: Thoracic anatomy and mediastinum. In Lee JKT, Sagel SS, Stanley RJ, eds: *Computed body tomography*, New York, 1982, Raven Press.

88. Schnyder PA, Gamsu G: CT of the pretracheal retrocaval space, *AJR* 136:303-308, 1981.

89. Shackleford G, McAlister W: The aberrantly positioned thymus, *AJR* 120:291-296, 1974.

90. Siegel MJ, Glazer HS, Wiener JI, et al: Normal and abnormal thymus in childhood, *Radiology* 172:367-371, 1989.

91. Siegelman SS, Scott WW, Baker RR, et al: CT of the thymus. In Siegelman SS, ed: *Computed tomography of the chest*, New York, 1984, Churchill Livingstone.

92. Speckman JM, Gamsu G, Webb WR, et al: Alterations in CT mediastinal anatomy produced by an azygos lobe, *AJR* 137:47-50, 1981.

93. Stern EJ, Graham CM, Webb WR, et al: Normal trachea during forced expiration: dynamic CT measurements, *Radiology* 187:27-31, 1993.

94. Sussman SK, Halvorsen RA, Silverman PM, et al: Paracardiac adenopathy: CT evaluation, *AJR* 149:29-34, 1987.

95. Takahashi K, Sugimoto H, Ohsawa T: Obliteration of the descending aortic interface in pectus excavatum: correlation with clockwise rotation of the heart, *Radiology* 182:825-828, 1992.

96. Takasugi MD, Godwin JD: Left azygos lobe, *Radiology* 171:133-134, 1989.

97. Takasugi JE, Godwin JD: CT appearance of the retroaortic anastomoses of the azygos system, *AJR* 154:41-44, 1990.

98. Tisi GM, Friedman PJ, Peters RM, et al: Clinical staging of primary lung cancer, American Thoracic Society recommendations, *Am Rev Respir Dis* 127:659-663, 1983.

99. Trapnell DH: The differential diagnosis of linear shadows in chest radiographs, *Radiol Clin North Am* 11:77-92, 1973.

100. Ujita M, Ojiri H, Ariizumi M, et al: Appearance of the inferior phrenic artery and vein on CT scans of the chest: a CT and cadaveric study, *AJR* 160:745-747, 1993.

101. Vix VA, Klatte EC: The lateral chest radiograph in the diagnosis of hilar and mediastinal masses, *Radiology* 96:307-316, 1970.

102. Vock P, Spiegel, Fram EK, Effmann EL: CT assessment of the adult intrathoracic cross section of the trachea, *J Comput Assist Tomogr* 8:1076-1082, 1984.

103. Webb WR, Gamsu G: Computed tomography of the left retrobronchial stripe, *J Comput Assist Tomogr* 7:65-69, 1983.

104. Webb WR, Glazer G, Gamsu G: Computed tomography of the normal pulmonary hilum, *J Comput Assist Tomogr* 5:485-490, 1981.

105. Whalen JP, Meyers MA, Oliphant M, et al: The retrosternal line, *AJR* 117:861-872, 1973.

106. Williams PL, Warwick R, Dyson M, et al: *Gray's anatomy*, ed 37, Edinburgh, 1989, Churchill Livingstone.

107. Woodring JH: Pulmonary artery-bronchus ratios in patients with normal lungs, pulmonary vascular plethora, and congestive heart failure, *Radiology* 179:115-122, 1991.

108. Yamashita H: *Roentgenologic anatomy of the lung*, Tokyo, 1978, Igaku-Shoin.

109. Zylak CJ, Pallie W, Jackson R: Correlative anatomy and computed tomography: a module on the mediastinum, *Radiographics* 2:255-592, 1982.

3 Normal Variants That May Simulate Disease

THEODORE E. KEATS

Proper interpretation of chest films involves not only the detection of disease but also the avoidance of misinterpretations of normal anatomic variations or variations in appearance produced by operator technique. Errors of commission of this type may be an even greater error than the error of omission, for we may then subject a healthy patient to unwarranted investigation and treatment, with all its concomitant anxiety.

The illustrations that follow (Figures 3-1 through 3-31) demonstrate some of the normal entities that may confuse the observer if he or she is not familiar with them. Appropriate references are appended for those who wish to explore this subject further. The interested reader may also wish to consult a larger work on the same subject (Keats TE: *Atlas of normal roentgen variants that may simulate disease*, ed 5, St Louis, Mosby, 1992).

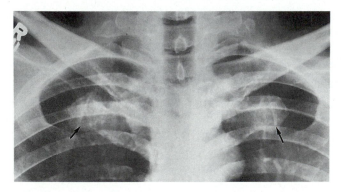

FIGURE 3-1
Developmental hypoplasia of first ribs bilaterally, but with presence of costal cartilage, which is calcified *(arrows)*.

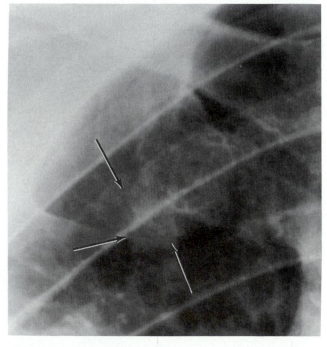

FIGURE 3-2
Hypertrophic calcified costal cartilage at anterior end of first rib *(arrows)* may simulate lesion in lung.

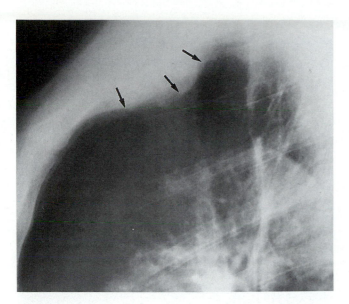

FIGURE 3-3
Anterior extrapleural line *(arrows)* represents deviation of pleura produced by innominate artery and vein and costal cartilage of first ribs. It should not be mistaken for lesion of sternum or mediastinal mass. (Reference: Whalen JP et al: Anterior extrapleural line: superior extension, *Radiology* 115:525, 1975.)

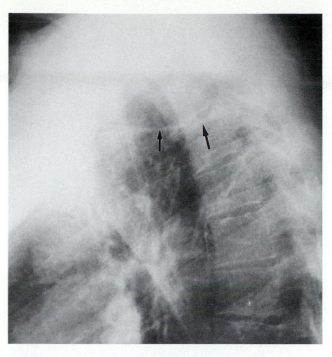

FIGURE 3-4
In improperly positioned chest study, spine of scapula may overlap lung and produce shadow *(arrows)* that may be mistaken for pneumothorax. (Reference: Harbin WP, Cimmino CV: The radiographic innominate lines of the scapular spine, *Va Med* 101:1050, 1974.)

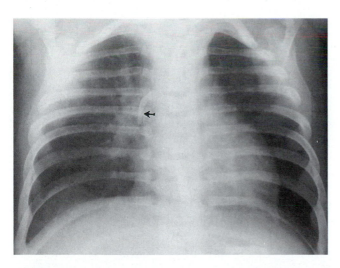

FIGURE 3-5
Intrathoracic rib *(arrow)* — anomaly of no clinical significance. (Reference: Weinstein AS, Mueller CF: Intrathoracic rib, *AJR* 94:587, 1965.)

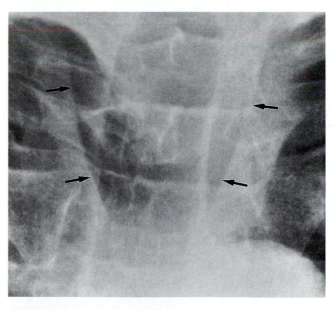

FIGURE 3-6
Suprasternal fossa *(arrows)* may be quite deep and cast radiolucency that might be mistaken for abnormal accumulation of air, such as esophageal diverticulum. (Reference: Ominsky S, Berinson HS: The suprasternal fossa, *Radiology* 122:311, 1977.)

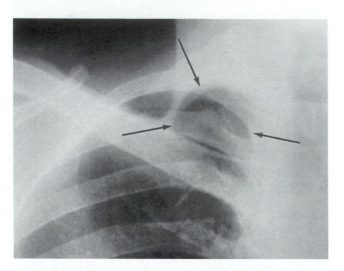

FIGURE 3-7
Confluence *(arrows)* of shadows of sternocleidomastoid muscle, first ribs, and clavicle may simulate bulla or cavity in apex of lung.

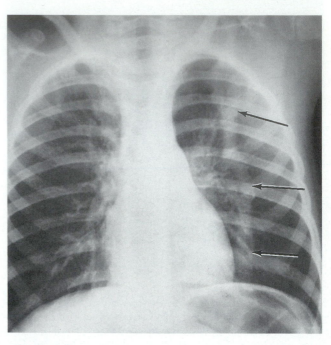

FIGURE 3-8
Hair braids *(arrows)* produced this unusual appearance of left lung.

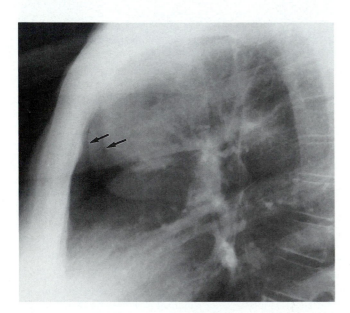

FIGURE 3-9
Redundant soft tissues of axilla produce rounded densities *(arrows)* projected into mediastinum.

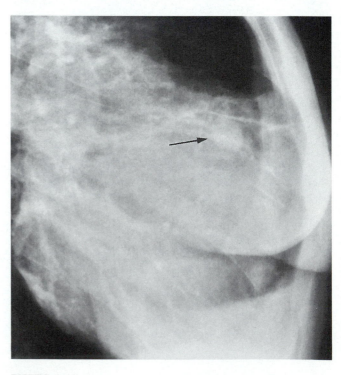

FIGURE 3-10
Nipple shadows *(arrow)* may cause confusing images in lateral projection in poorly positioned patients, in this case simulating nodular lesion in lung.

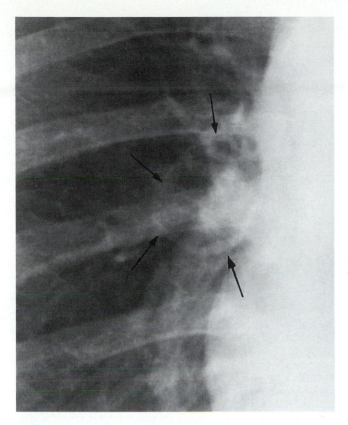

FIGURE 3-11
Superimposed shadows of vessels *(arrows)* may simulate cavitary lesion.

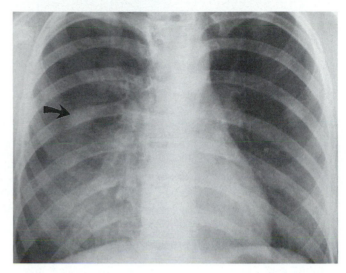

FIGURE 3-12
Opacity in right base in this 13-year-old patient is due to dense juvenile breast, accentuated by slight rotation of patient to left at time of filming. Linear shadow above *(arrow)* is due to hair braid.

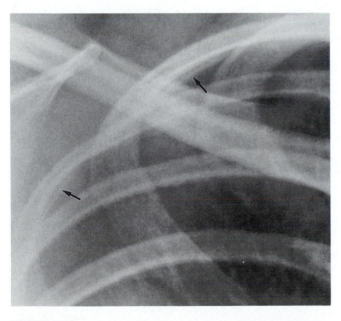

FIGURE 3-13
Companion soft tissue shadows of upper ribs and radiolucency laterally *(arrows)* should not be mistaken for pneumothorax.

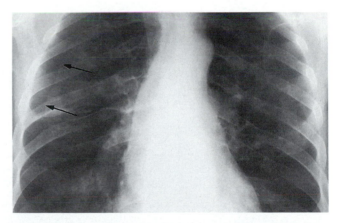

FIGURE 3-14
Skin folds in elderly *(arrows)* may simulate pneumothorax. Note that edge of fold has fading margin in contrast to sharp pleural line seen with true pneumothorax. (Reference: Fisher JK: Skin folds versus pneumothorax, *AJR* 130:791, 1978.)

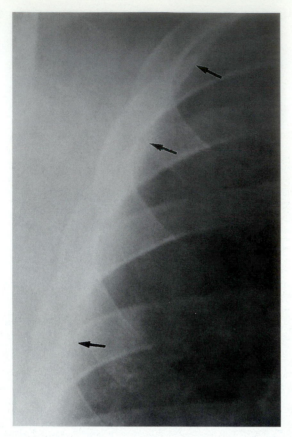

FIGURE 3-15
In obese individuals, extrapleural fat *(arrows)* may simulate pleural thickening. Absence of blunting of costophrenic angles is useful differential clue. (Reference: Vix VA: Extrapleural costal fat, *Radiology* 112:563, 1974.)

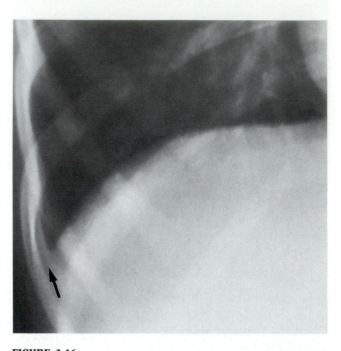

FIGURE 3-16
Blunted costophrenic angles *(arrow)* in young adults are often seen as apparently normal finding. This is apt to be misinterpreted as evidence of pleural effusion. It is possibly related to redundancy of pleura or possibly as reflection of presence of small amount of pleural fluid that is normally present in pleural space. (Reference: Ecklof O, Torngren A: Pleural fluid in healthy children, *Acta Radiol [Diagn] [Stockh]* 11:346, 1971.)

A

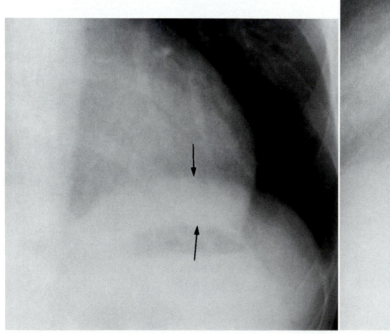 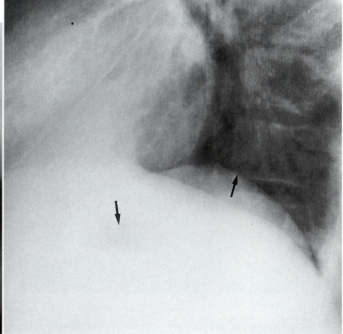

B

FIGURE 3-17
A, Increased distance between stomach gas bubble and diaphragm *(arrows)* suggests subpulmonic effusion. **B,** Lateral projection indicates that this appearance is due to fact that posterior portion of left diaphragm, seen posteriorly *(right arrow)*, is higher than anterior portion, which is adjacent to gas bubble *(left arrow)*.

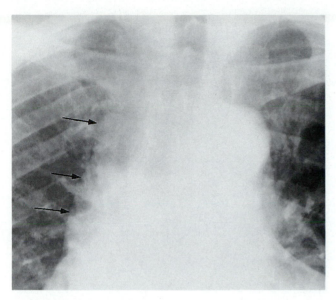

FIGURE 3-18
Mediastinal fat produces widening of mediastinal silhouette *(arrows)*. This may be seen in simple obesity, in Cushing's disease, and in patients receiving steroids. (Reference: Price JF, Rigler LG: Widening of the mediastinum resulting from fat accumulation, *Radiology* 96:497, 1970.)

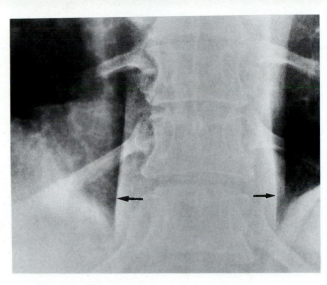

FIGURE 3-19
Paraspinous fat deposition *(arrows)* will displace paravertebral pleural reflections and may simulate disease process. (Reference: Streiter ML et al: Steroid induced thoracic lipomatosis: paraspinal involvement, *AJR* 139:679, 1982.)

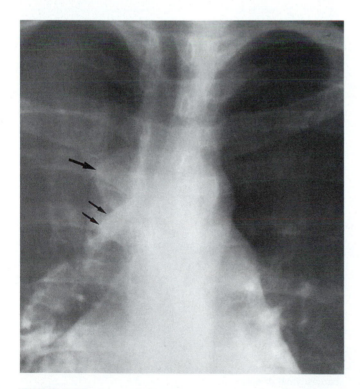

FIGURE 3-20
Manubrium presents laterally because of slight rotation and scoliosis and may simulate mediastinal mass *(top arrow)*. Azygous arch is seen below *(lower arrows)*.

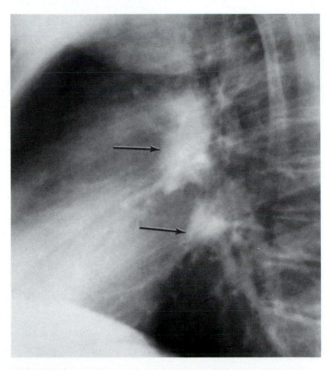

FIGURE 3-21
This normal lateral projection demonstrates pulmonary artery *(upper arrow)* and confluence of pulmonary veins *(lower arrow)*. Latter is sometimes mistaken for nodular lesion in lung.

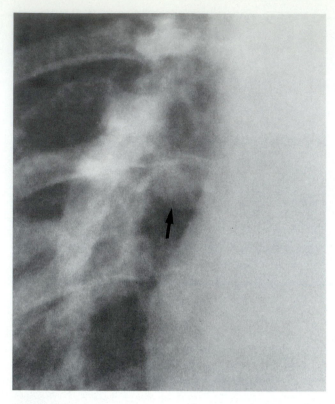

FIGURE 3-22
Large transverse process *(arrow)* may simulate nodular pulmonary lesion.

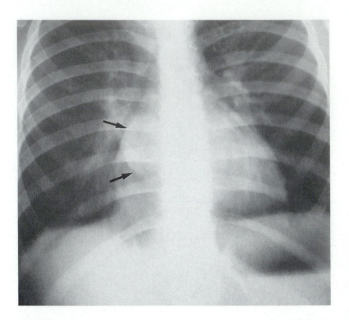

FIGURE 3-23
Right border of left atrium *(arrows)* may be seen in healthy individuals and should not be mistaken for chamber enlargement or mediastinal mass.

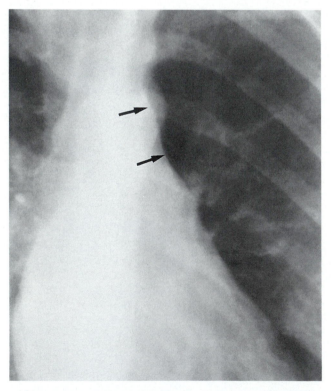

FIGURE 3-24
Aortic-pulmonary stripe is reflection of mediastinal pleura from aorta to pulmonary artery *(arrows)*. This should not be confused with displacement of mediastinal pleura resulting from adenopathy. (Reference: Keats TE: The aortic-pulmonary mediastinal stripe, *AJR* 116:107, 1972.)

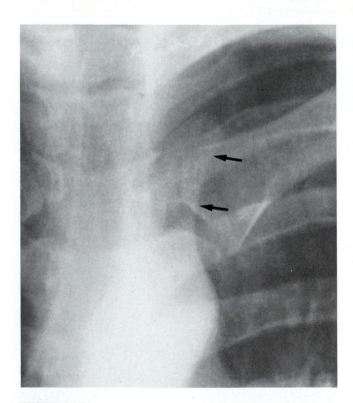

FIGURE 3-25
Shadow of left subclavian artery *(arrows)* may simulate pleural or parenchymal density.

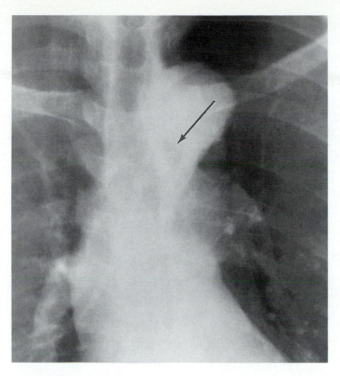

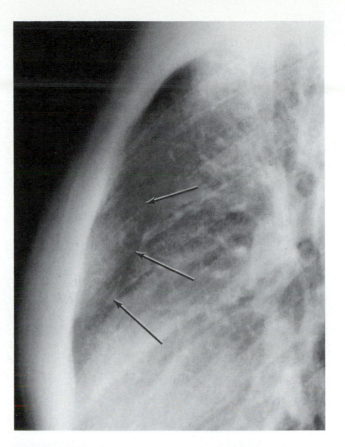

FIGURE 3-26

Air in esophagus may be confused with free air in mediastinum. In elderly people, esophagus follows ectatic descending aorta and air is trapped in knuckle of esophagus below arch *(arrow)*. (Reference: Proto AV: Air in the esophagus: a frequent radiologic finding, *AJR* 129:433, 1977.)

FIGURE 3-27

Mammary anterior mediastinal pseudotumor. Lateral aspects of dense, small breasts of young women *(arrows)* may project into anterior mediastinum in lateral projection and simulate mediastinal mass. (Reference: Keats TE: Mammary anterior mediastinal pseudotumor, *J Can Assoc Radiol* 27:262, 1976.)

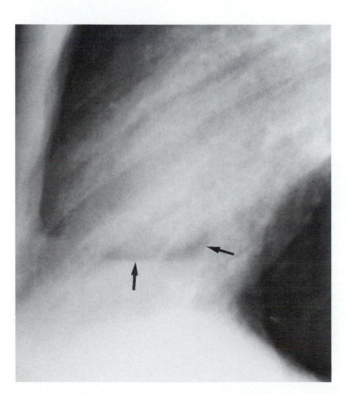

FIGURE 3-28

Confusing radiolucencies may be produced by inferior vena cava. With full inspiration, it is possible to clear portion of diaphragmatic surface of heart and expose anterior wall of inferior vena cava *(right arrow)*. This results in triangular area of radiolucency *(arrows)*. (Reference: Tonkin IL et al: Radiographic isolation of the inferior vena cava, *AJR* 129:657, 1977.)

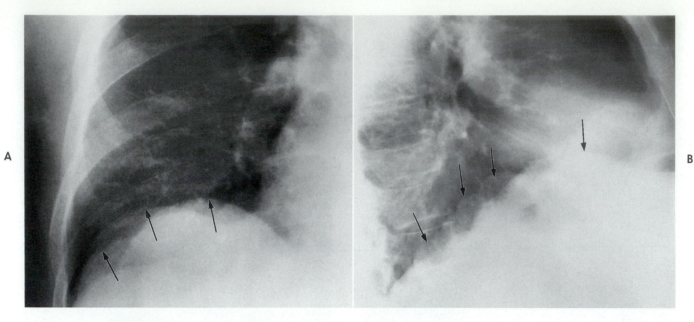

FIGURE 3-29
"Scalloping" of diaphragm *(arrows)* is normal variation in muscular architecture of diaphragm. **A,** Posterioranterior radiograph. **B,** Lateral radiograph.

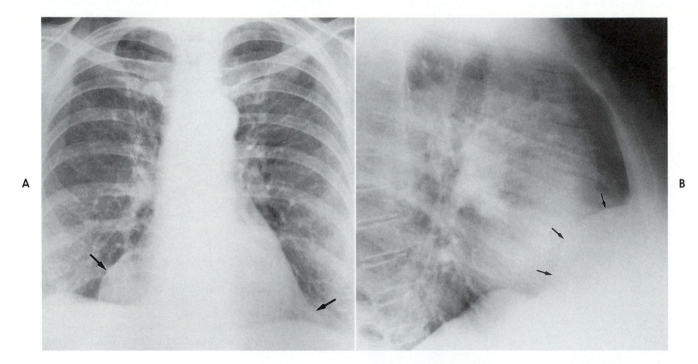

FIGURE 3-30
Epipericardial fat pads *(arrows)*. Note, **A,** their relative lucency in frontal film and, **B,** anterior position of fat pad in lateral projection. These fat collections may be confused with cysts and neoplasms. They vary in size with weight of patient. (Reference: Holt JF: Epipericardial fat shadows in differential diagnosis, *Radiology* 48:472, 1947.)

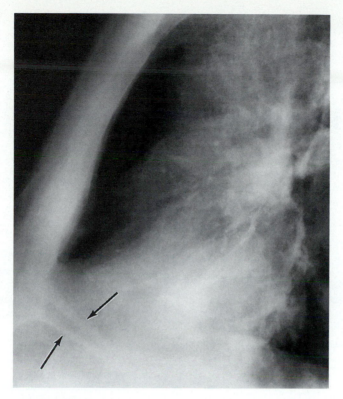

FIGURE 3-31
Sternal insertions of diaphragm *(arrows)* can be seen occasionally in healthy individuals.

4 Basic Patterns in Lung Disease

PETER ARMSTRONG

One of the most crucial decisions in diagnostic imaging is determining the location of any lesion, in particular whether the process is primarily in the lung, the hilum, the mediastinum, the pleura, the chest wall, or the diaphragm. Indeed the distinction is so important that most textbooks, including this one, are organized according to anatomic divisions. In this chapter we describe the signs of lung disease. The other sites are considered in their relevant chapters.

Although search patterns for chest disease by experienced viewers are far from orderly, it is wise for the inexperienced to adopt some sort of systematic scanning pattern in order to ensure that the search is complete. The apices, the hila, the retrocardiac regions, the lungs below the domes of the diaphragm, and the region just inside the chest wall should be specifically examined because experience has shown that opacities in these areas are easily overlooked.

Two interrelated signs — the silhouette sign and the air bronchogram sign — are considered first because these two signs have widespread applicability in the diagnosis of a variety of chest disorders.

SILHOUETTE SIGN

Felson and Felson[24] popularized the term "silhouette sign" to indicate an obliteration of the borders of the heart, mediastinum, or diaphragm by an adjacent opacity (Figure 4-1). They wrote, "An intrathoracic lesion touching a border of the heart, aorta, or diaphragm will obliterate that border on the roentgenogram. An intrathoracic lesion not anatomically contiguous with a border of one of the structures will not obliterate that border." The lesion responsible for obliterating a silhouette does not have to be large (Figure 4-2), nor does the opacity have to originate within the lung; pleural fluid, extrapleural fat, chest wall deformity, and mediastinal masses may all cause a loss of silhouette.

The mechanism responsible for the sign is debated. According to Felson and Felson,[24] the sign depends on direct contact, but another possible explanation is that the sign may be due simply to absorption of x-rays by whatever lies in the path of the beam, and the reason the border is lost only in cases of direct contact is that precise anatomic conformity of shape occurs only when intimate contact is present.

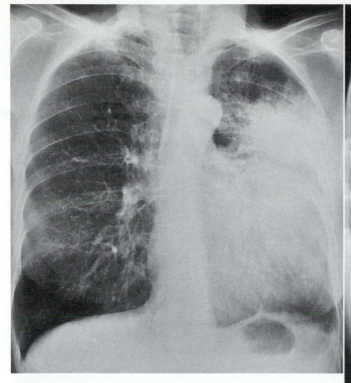

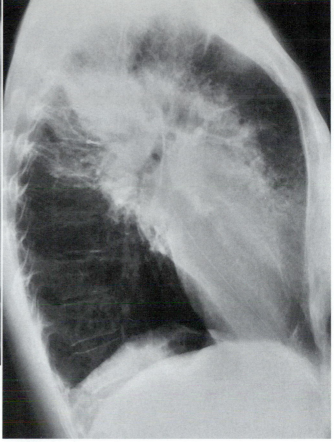

FIGURE 4-1
Silhouette sign. The left heart border is invisible because of consolidation in the adjacent left upper lobe. **A,** Posteroanterior view. **B,** Lateral view.

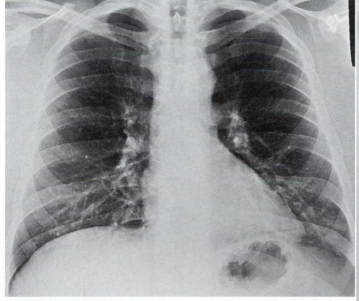

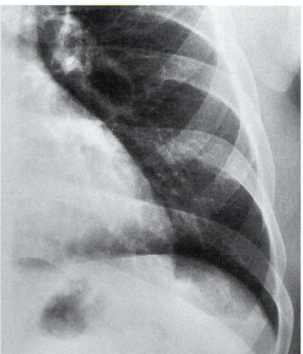

FIGURE 4-2
Silhouette sign. **A,** A small patch of pneumonia in the anterior segment of the left lower lobe has resulted in lack of visibility of the outer half of the left hemidiaphragm. (The lateral view in this patient is shown in Figure 4-14.) **B,** Normal diaphragm outline after the pneumonia has resolved.

A **B**

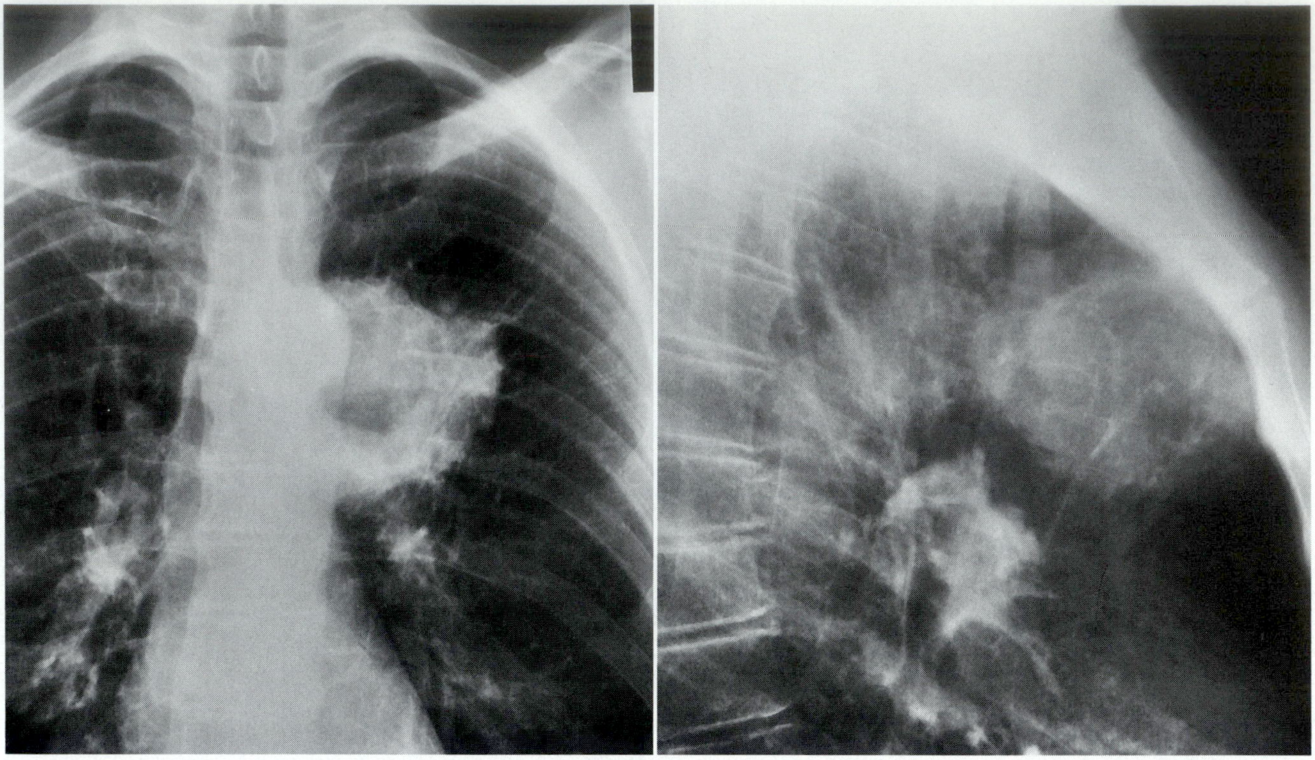

FIGURE 4-3
A, Preservation of the silhouette of the aortic knob and descending aorta in the posteroanterior view is good evidence that the pulmonary mass does not lie in the superior segment of the left lower lobe. **B,** The lateral view shows that the mass, in fact, lies well anteriorly. (It proved to be a squamous cell carcinoma.)

Regardless of the mechanism the silhouette sign can be used in two ways: (1) to localize a radiographic density (Figures 4-3 and 4-4) and (2) to detect lesions of low radiopacity when the shadow is less obvious than the loss of silhouette (Figure 4-2). The lesion must lie immediately adjacent to the structure in question to efface a silhouette. With a process that is remote from the interface and merely overlaps it on the radiograph, the radiographic boundary will still be visible, even though it may be more difficult to appreciate. Thus opacities in the right middle lobe or lingula may obliterate the right and left borders of the heart, respectively (Figures 4-1 and 4-5), whereas opacities in the lower lobes may partially obliterate the outline of the descending aorta and diaphragm, but leave the cardiac outline clearly visible (Figure 4-6). Similarly, the aortic knob will be rendered invisible if there is no air in the adjacent left upper lobe. The best example of detecting lesions of low radiopacity is collapse of the right middle lobe (Figure 4-5).

Felson and Felson[24] warned that mistakes will be made unless the following points are borne in mind:

1. The technical quality of the roentgenogram must be such that the diseased area is adequately penetrated. Underpenetration may result in loss of visibility of a normal border.

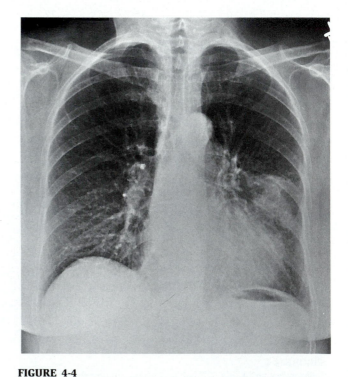

FIGURE 4-4
The loss of silhouette of the left cardiac border in the frontal view localizes the pulmonary consolidation to the lingula. It proved to be postobstructive pneumonia beyond a carcinoma in the lingular bronchus.

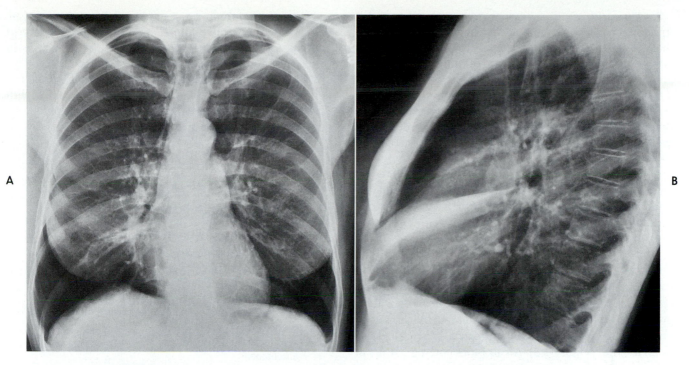

FIGURE 4-5
Right middle lobe collapse and consolidation obliterating the right heart border. **A,** Posteroanterior view. **B,** Lateral view.

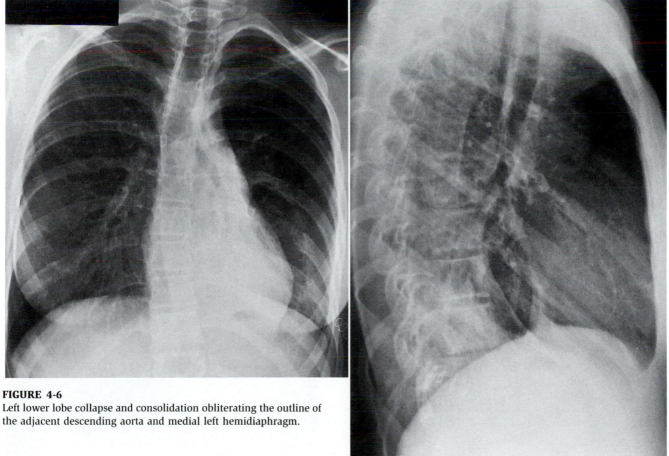

FIGURE 4-6
Left lower lobe collapse and consolidation obliterating the outline of the adjacent descending aorta and medial left hemidiaphragm.

2. The outline of a portion of the cardiovascular structure in question must be clearly visible beyond the shadow in the spine. In many healthy individuals the right border of the heart and ascending aorta do not project into the right side of the thorax. In these patients the silhouette sign cannot be applied on the right side.

3. In patients with pectus excavatum the right border of the heart is frequently obliterated because the depressed thoracic wall replaces aerated lung alongside the cardiac silhouette (Figure 4-7).

Felson and Felson also pointed out that there are patients in whom no disease and no satisfactory explanation for the loss of the right heart border will be found.[24] These cases are, however, few and far between and do little to reduce the general value of the sign.

AIR BRONCHOGRAM

Normal intrapulmonary airways are invisible unless end on to the x-ray beam, but air within bronchi or bronchioles passing through airless parenchyma may be visible as branching linear lucencies: a so-called air bronchogram (Figure 4-8). An air bronchogram within an opacity reliably indicates that the opacity is intrapulmonary, not pleural or mediastinal, in location. The sign is particularly well demonstrated with computed tomography (CT) (Figure 4-9).

The most common causes of an air bronchogram (see box below) are pneumonia and the various forms of pulmonary edema. Air bronchograms are also seen in atelectatic lobes provided the airway is patent. Examples of this condition include collapse caused by pleural effusion or pneumothorax, and collapse associated with bronchiectasis. Similarly, widespread air bronchograms are seen with hyaline membrane disease.

CAUSES OF AN AIR BRONCHOGRAM

Normal expiratory radiograph
Consolidation
Pulmonary edema
Nonobstructive pulmonary atelectasis
    Hyaline membrane disease
    Compression atelectasis (e.g., pleural effusion, pneumothorax)
    Fibrotic scarring (e.g., radiation fibrosis, bronchiectatic lobe)
Severe interstitial disease
    Sarcoidosis
    Fibrosing alveolitis
Certain neoplasms (notably bronchioloalveolar carcinoma, lymphoma, pseudolymphoma)

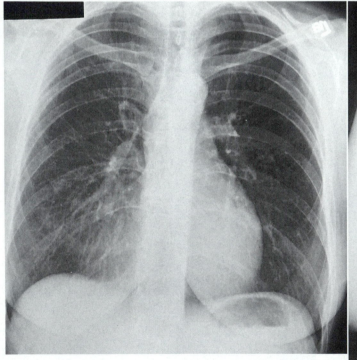
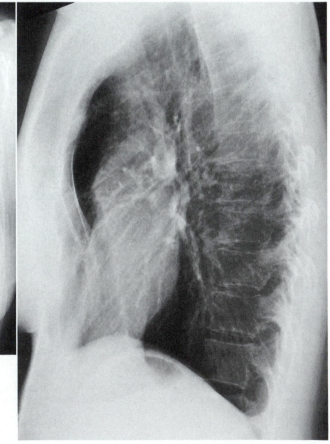

FIGURE 4-7
Pectus excavatum causing obliteration of the right border of the heart. **A,** Posteroanterior view. **B,** Lateral view.

There are four less predictable situations in which air bronchograms may be seen:

1. Bronchioloalveolar carcinoma (Figure 4-10), lymphoma, and pseudolymphoma grow around the airways without compressing them, and therefore air bronchograms may be visible on plain film radiography. Air bronchograms in lung cancers, other than bronchioloalveolar carcinoma, are visible only on high-resolution CT.[69]

2. Interstitial fibrosis may be so intense that it renders the lung parenchyma airless, producing an air bronchogram because the bronchi remain patent. Thus the nodular and consolidative lesions of sarcoidosis (Figure 4-11) may show an air bronchogram as may advanced fibrosing alveolitis and radiation fibrosis (Figure 4-12).[99]

3. Air bronchograms can sometimes be seen in postobstructive pneumonia, even though replacement of air by secretions beyond the obstruction might have been expected.

4. Air bronchograms can be normal at low lung volumes and in the segmental bronchi behind the heart in children.

PULMONARY OPACITY

Focal pulmonary opacities usually are readily detected in the frontal view by comparing one lung with the other. In the lateral view such right-left comparisons are not possible and therefore alternative signs are needed. In the normal lateral view, each thoracic vertebral body appears blacker than the one above it, as the eye travels down the spine, until the diaphragm is reached. Pulmonary opacity projected over the spine alters this continuum and allows

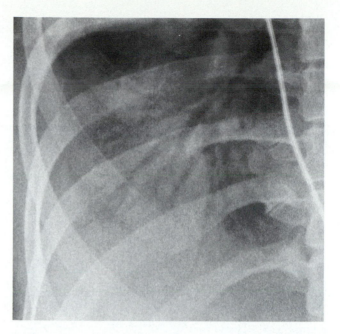

FIGURE 4-8
Air bronchogram. The branching linear lucencies within the consolidation in the right lower lobe are particularly well demonstrated in this example of staphylococcal pneumonia.

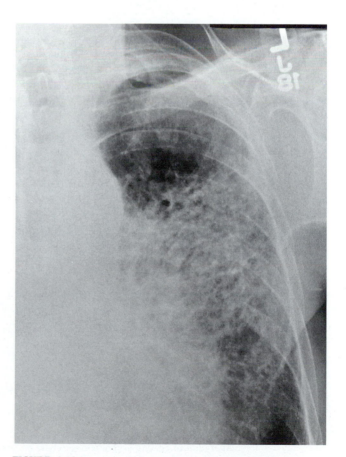

FIGURE 4-10
Air bronchogram in bronchioloalveloar cell carcinoma.

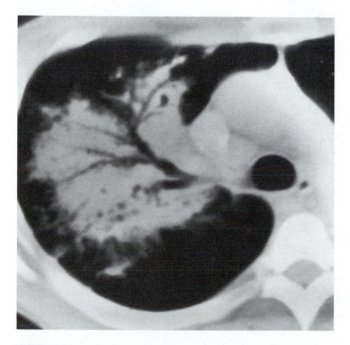

FIGURE 4-9
Air bronchogram shown by computed tomography in a patient with pneumonia.

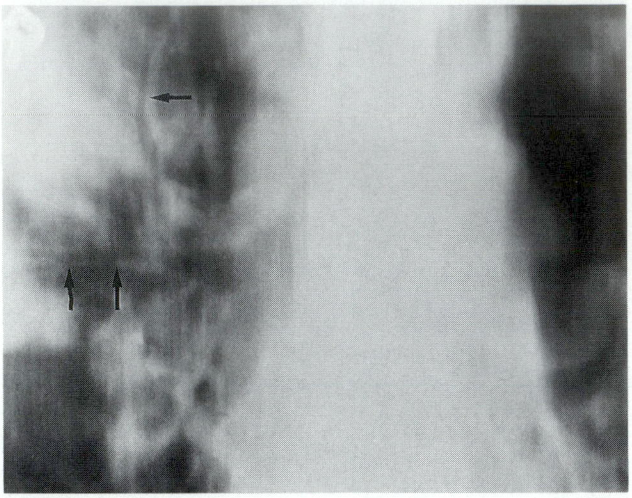

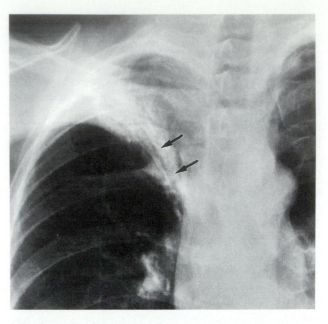

FIGURE 4-11
Sarcoidosis of the lung showing an air bronchogram *(arrows)* in an area of severe pulmonary involvement.

FIGURE 4-12
Air bronchogram *(arrows)* in radiation fibrosis of right upper lobe following treatment of carcinoma of breast.

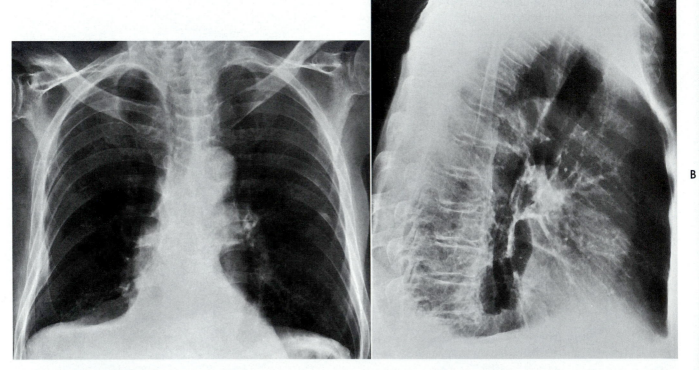

FIGURE 4-13
Alteration in opacity of thoracic vertebrae on lateral projection as a sign of lower lobe density. In this case, increasing opacity of vertebral bodies as eye travels down spine is one of the most obvious signs indicating presence of right lower lobe collapse. **A,** Posteroanterior view. **B,** Lateral view.

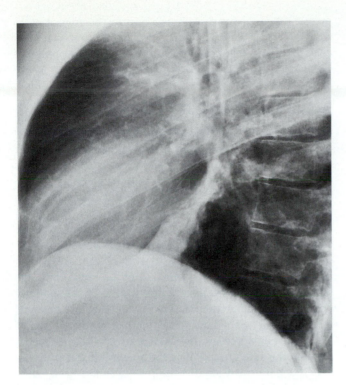

FIGURE 4-14
Abrupt change in density overlying cardiac shadow. Lateral view in patient with pneumonia in anterior segment of left lower lobe. (Posteroanterior view of this patient is shown in Figure 4-2.)

Beam   Object   Image

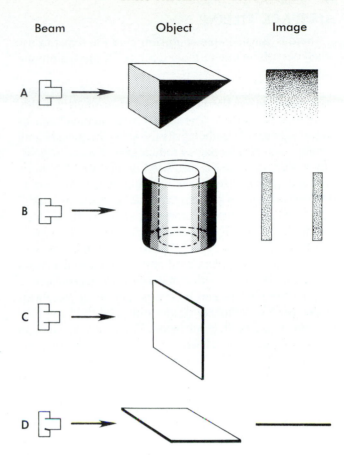

FIGURE 4-15
Density characteristics of pulmonary shadows. See text for explanation. (From Wilson AG: *Br J Hosp Med* 37:526, 1987.)

recognition of a shadow that might otherwise be over-looked (Figure 4-13). Another helpful point is that in a healthy subject there is no abrupt change in density across the heart shadow in the lateral projection (Figure 4-14). The rib shadows are of course an exception, and the radiologist must mentally subtract them from the image. Also, but less reliably, the high retrosternal area is usually more transradiant than all other areas on the lateral chest radiograph except the region immediately behind the heart.

The characteristics of a radiographic shadow depend on the absorptive capacity and geometry of the object. In order of increasing absorptive capacity, the major components of the chest are air, fat, fluid and soft tissues, and bone. For practical purposes, fluid and soft tissues, apart from fat, are isodense on plain film radiography. The following geometric features are worth noting (Figure 4-15)[132]:

1. Interfaces tangential to the x-ray beam are sharp and distinct, whereas interfaces oblique to the beam are not seen because the thin end of the wedge fades off and cannot be identified (Figure 4-15, *A*).

2. Hollow cylinders and hollow spheres are most absorptive at their edges because at the edge the beam has a longer path within the object and is therefore more attenuated. Also, the outside and inside marginal interfaces are sharp and distinct (Figure 4-15, *B*).

3. A thin sheet perpendicular to an x-ray beam usually causes no detectable opacity (Figure 4-15, *C*), whereas a thin sheet oriented in the direction of the beam casts a definite shadow (Figure 4-15, *D*).

There are innumerable patterns of pulmonary opacity, with no clear-cut divisions between them. Despite the imperfections, categorizing these patterns is worthwhile; the more certain the observer is of the description of an individual opacity, the shorter the differential diagnostic list will be. The diagnostic considerations for a particular pattern may be further reduced by reviewing serial images and by correlating the radiographic pattern with the clinical findings and laboratory data. The following classification of pulmonary shadows is suggested (pleural shadows are considered separately in Chapter 15):

1. Airspace filling
2. Collapse (atelectasis)
3. Pulmonary mass (nodule)
4. Line shadows and band shadows
5. Ring shadows, cysts, and bullae
6. Widespread nodular, reticulonodular, and honey-comb shadowing

More than one pattern may be present. The radiologist should look for calcification and cavitation, which will further limit the number of diagnostic possibilities.

AIRSPACE FILLING

There is considerable confusion over the terms to use when describing one or more discrete, ill-defined pulmonary densities.

The expressions "airspace filling" and "airspace shadows" seem to be the best because they imply a radiographic appearance.[26] The term "consolidation" can be confusing because pathologists use it synonymously with exudate, whereas its use by radiologists is more catholic. The word "infiltrate" is also used differently by radiologists and pathologists. Some radiologists use the term to describe almost any pulmonary shadow, whereas pathologists restrict its use to processes showing the specific histologic features of infiltration. This text uses the phrase "airspace filling/shadowing" for a radiographic appearance that implies replacement of air in the distal airways and alveoli by fluid or other material such as neoplasm or alveolar proteinosis, and no destruction or displacement of the gross morphology of the lung. The fluid can be a transudate, an exudate, or blood. Where it is possible to be certain that the shadow is caused by edema, the expression "pulmonary edema" is used instead. The term "consolidation" is restricted to shadows thought to be due to exudate, blood, or tumor. Thus edema and consolidation are subdivisions of airspace filling.

The features of airspace filling on plain chest radiography are one or more shadows with ill-defined margins, except where the shadow abuts the pleura. When multiple, the shadows typically coalesce. An air bronchogram may be visible, often as scattered branches or small twigs. On plain chest radiography the normal vascular markings within the shadow are invisible because of the silhouette sign. The lack of clarity of the edge of the shadows results, in part, from the piecemeal spread of the process through the bronchi and alveoli, the poorly defined margin being analogous to the edge of a three-dimensional jigsaw puzzle. Once the process abuts a fissure, the edge appears sharp. The ease with which it is possible to appreciate this edge on plain chest radiographs depends on how much of the fissure is tangential to the x-ray beam.

Many sublobar processes are vaguely conical, sometimes resembling the shape of a segment. Precise conformity to a segment almost never occurs because, with the rare exception of accessory fissures, there are no anatomic barriers to prevent the spread of fluid or other processes across segmental boundaries. Airspace filling is often peripheral in location, crossing segmental boundaries with impunity. Spherical consolidations are also seen but are unusual.

Ill-defined nodular shadows between 0.5 and 1 cm are sometimes seen within or adjacent to the larger opacities of airspace filling, particularly with pulmonary edema and pneumonia, notably varicella or tuberculous infection (Figure 4-16; see also Figure 4-19). These shadows have been called acinar shadows, since they are believed to be opaque acini contrasted against aerated lung.[139] They may coalesce as the disease progresses. The converse of the acinar shadow is the air alveologram (Figure 4-17), a pattern of small rounded lucencies seen when aerated acini are surrounded by opaque lung.

The term "ground glass" is sometimes applied to a homogeneous veiling opacity. Such opacity is seen in a large number of conditions, including airspace filling disorders and interstitial pulmonary diseases.

Cavitation may occur within areas of airspace filling.

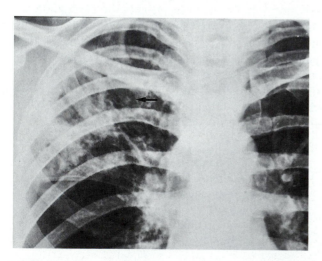

FIGURE 4-16
Acinar shadows in pulmonary tuberculosis *(arrow)*. In lateral portion of right upper lobe, acinar shadows have become confluent.

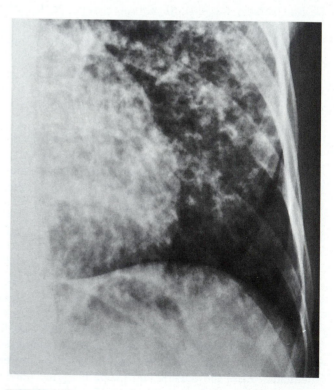

FIGURE 4-17
Air alveologram in bronchogenic spread of tuberculosis.

The term "cavitation" implies necrosis and liquefaction of lung tissue. If the necrotic center communicates with the bronchial tree, air enters the cavity (Figure 4-18) and is seen as a translucency within the shadow, often accompanied by an air-fluid level (Figure 4-18).

CT scanning (the topic of high-resolution CT is discussed in Chapter 5) may on occasion provide additional information about airspace filling.[86] It will show acinar filling to advantage (Figure 4-19). The excellent contrast discrimination of CT allows pneumonia in the immunocompromised host, for example, to be diagnosed when the plain chest radiographs still have a normal appearance. It can also demonstrate the size, shape, and precise position of any cavities (Figure 4-20).[42] Better definition of a cavity or the demonstration of more cavities may improve diagnostic accuracy, but if a cavity is clearly demonstrated on plain films, CT usually has little additional information to offer. Other morphologic features of airspace filling that are particularly well demonstrated by CT are air bronchograms (Figure 4-9), the satellite lesions of infectious granulomatous inflammation, and the conformity of radiation fibrosis to the radiation port (Figure 4-21).

It has been suggested that measuring CT numbers is sometimes helpful in diagnosing the nature of airspace shadowing. The CT density may be high in pulmonary hemorrhage, progressive massive fibrosis, and pulmonary calcinosis and may be low in lipoid pneumonia.[60] Great care must be taken in accepting a low CT number, however, because part of the volume being measured could be air in aerated alveoli or bronchi.

It is possible on occasion to recognize the so-called CT angiogram sign, a term that refers to the observation that contrast-enhanced blood vessels can be identified coursing through areas of homogeneous low-attenuation consolidation (Figure 4-22).[54] This sign has been described as reasonably specific for bronchioloalveolar carcinoma,[54] but while it is a common finding in lobar bronchioloalveolar carcinoma, it is also seen in pneumonia[54,82,126] and lymphoma.[106,125]

Another potential use of the CT angiogram sign is in the differential diagnosis of atelectatic lung resembling pleural effusion: the CT angiogram sign definitively indicates pulmonary pathology, since the sign cannot occur within pleural pathology.[4]

Differential diagnosis of airspace filling

The differential diagnosis of airspace shadows is long and covers diseases that require quite different forms of management.

Solitary airspace shadowing (Figure 4-23) is usually the result of pneumonia, atelectasis, infarction (Figure 4-24), or hemorrhage (Figure 4-25). Neoplasms, particularly bronchioloalveolar carcinoma (Figures 4-10 and 4-26), malignant lymphoma (Figure 4-27), and pseudolymphoma, may appear ill defined enough to be

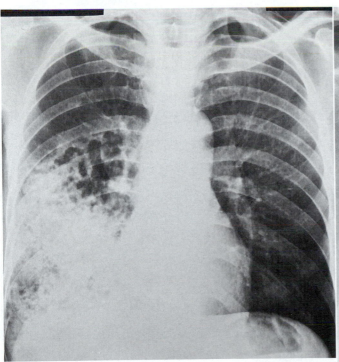

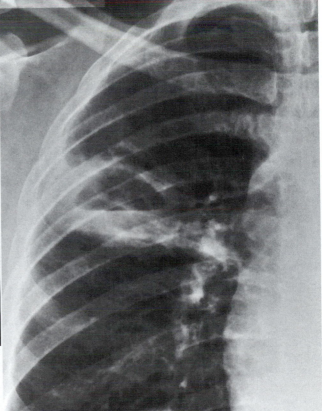

FIGURE 4-18
Cavitation. **A,** In this example of staphylococcal pneumonia, there are multiple transradiant areas within consolidation but no air-fluid levels. **B,** Another patient, illustrating air-fluid level in cavity within area of pneumonia.

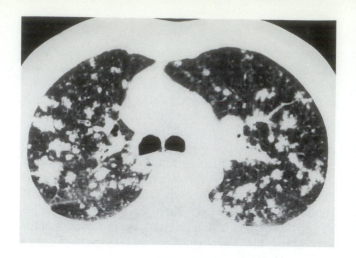

FIGURE 4-19
Acinar shadows, some of which have coalesced. Computed tomographic scan of bronchogenic spread in tuberculous pneumonia.

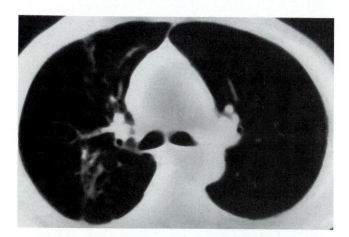

A

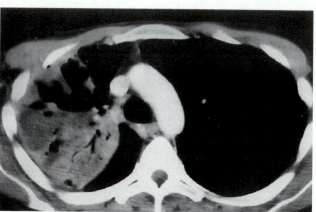

B

FIGURE 4-20
Computed tomographic scans showing, **A**, cavitation *(arrow)* in area of pneumonia and, **B**, complex cavitation with lower density fluid in dependent portion of a cavity.

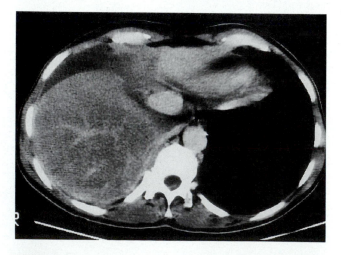

FIGURE 4-21
Computed tomographic scan showing conformity of radiation fibrosis to radiation port.

FIGURE 4-22
Computed tomographic angiogram sign. Branching contrast-enhanced pulmonary vessels are seen coursing through low-density pulmonary consolidation. In this instance, the diagnosis was lymphoma. (From Vincent JM, Ng YY, Norton AJ, et al: *J Comput Assist Tomogr* 16:829, 1992.)

A

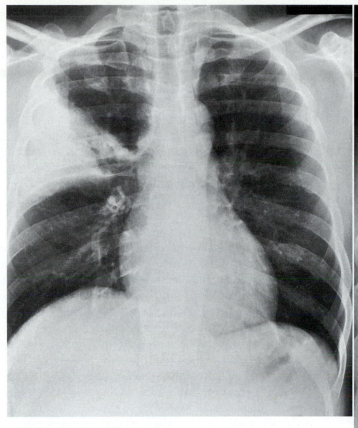

B

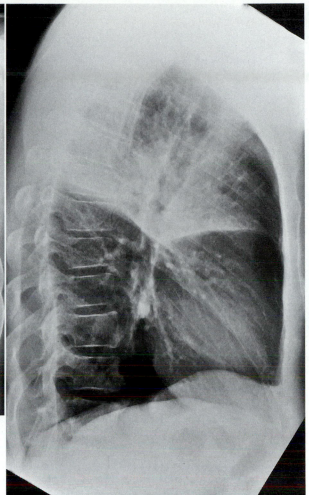

FIGURE 4-23
Solitary airspace shadow, in this case resulting from bacterial pneumonia. Note that the pneumonia occupies the gravitationally dependent portions of lobes, rather than being distributed according to segmental anatomy. A, Posteroanterior view. B, Lateral view.

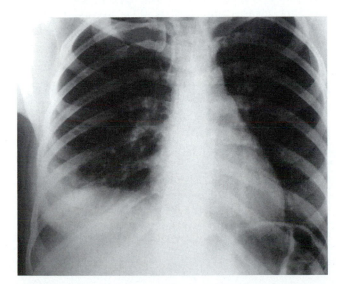

FIGURE 4-24
Pulmonary consolidation caused by pulmonary infarction lying peripherally in right lower lobe.

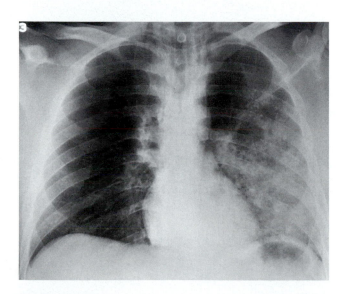

FIGURE 4-25
Solitary airspace shadow caused by pulmonary contusion following motor vehicle accident. (Pneumomediastinum is also present.)

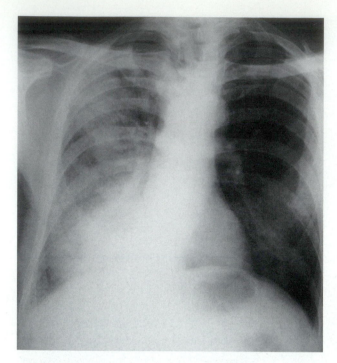

FIGURE 4-26
Consolidation of right lung caused by alveolar cell carcinoma.

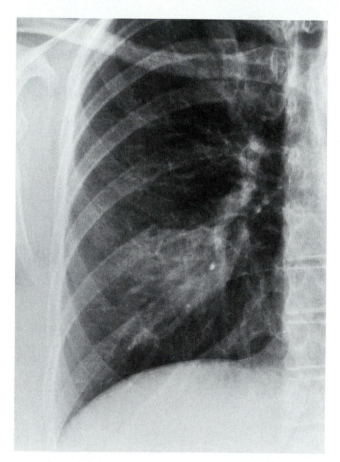

FIGURE 4-27
Solitary airspace shadow in Hodgkin's disease of lung parenchyma.

called consolidation. The full list of causes of solitary airspace shadows is given in Table 4-1.

Airspace filling is often multifocal and tends to coalesce as it progresses (Figure 4-28). The list of causes is given in the lefthand box on p. 72.

Certain generalizations may be helpful when considering airspace shadows:

1. Clinical correlation is essential and often decisive. A few examples suffice to emphasize this point: (a) In patients with noncardiogenic pulmonary edema, the chest film may not become abnormal until several hours after the onset of symptoms, whereas with cardiogenic pulmonary edema the pulmonary shadowing is almost always evident early on. (b) Widespread pneumonia is almost invariably accompanied by cough and fever. (c) Aspiration should be suspected as the cause of airspace shadowing in patients who have known predisposing factors such as alcoholism, a recent seizure, or a period of unconsciousness. (d) Immunocompromised patients are a special and complicated group. Widespread pulmonary shadows in such patients usually indicate infection, often from opportunistic organisms. (e) Substantial hemoptysis associated with widespread pulmonary consolidation usually indicates pulmonary hemorrhage.

2. Opacity of over half a lobe with no loss of volume is virtually diagnostic of pneumonia: this remains true even if a small portion of the lobe is spared (Figure 4-29). The common causes are pneumococcal or mycoplasma pneumonia and pneumonia distal to a bronchial neoplasm. Neoplastic obstruction of a lobar bronchus usually causes some degree of atelectasis, but consolidation without loss of volume is not uncommon. In these cases the tumor obstructs the drainage of secretions and bacterial pneumonia may supervene. Clinically, the condition may closely resemble simple pneumonia, but the consolidation, although it may improve with appropriate treatment, does not clear completely if it is secondary to an underlying tumor. Because the neoplasm involves a lobar

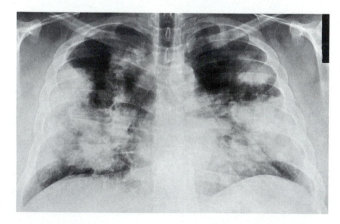

FIGURE 4-28
Multiple airspace shadows resulting from bacterial pneumonia.

Table 4-1   Differential diagnosis of a solitary airspace shadow

Diagnosis	Comment
Pneumonia	Pneumonia (bacterial [including tuberculous], viral, fungal, and parasitic) is the most common cause of solitary airspace filling. The opacity may be almost any shape from segmental/lobar to round or irregular. Cavitation and accompanying pleural effusion are both distinct features. In adults an associated hilar mass suggests a centrally located neoplasm causing postobstructive pneumonia, whereas in children an associated hilar mass suggests primary tuberculosis.
Atelectasis	The diagnosis of atelectasis is based on its characteristic shape. The appearances and causes are discussed in the section "Atelectasis and Collapse" later in this chapter. Discoid atelectasis results in a characteristic bandlike shape coursing through the lung, often in a horizontal orientation. Large areas of atelectasis that do not conform to either of these patterns may be indistinguishable from the other causes of airspace shadowing listed in this table.
Infarction or hemorrhage associated with pulmonary embolism	Infarcts are usually segmental in size, rarely larger. The shape is similar to a truncated cone with the base on the pleura. The apex of the cone, which may be rounded, points toward the hilum. The rounded medial margin, known as Hampton's hump (see Chapter 8), is a well known but infrequent sign suggestive, but not diagnostic, of the condition. Septic infarcts cavitate frequently, whereas bland infarcts rarely cavitate.
Pulmonary contusion	Contusions appear within hours of injury and clear within a few days. They are usually maximal in the general area of injury, although contrecoup damage may be seen at a distance. Pneumatocele formation is a distinct feature. Pulmonary contusion may surround a pulmonary hematoma. Hematomas resemble masses, may liquefy and cavitate, and take much longer to clear than contusions.
Collagen vascular disease, vasculitis	These conditions are infrequent causes of solitary airspace shadowing. They need to be considered in patients with appropriate clinical features. The opacity is usually sublobar in size and nonspecific in shape. Cavitation may be seen. Most solitary shadows in patients with collagen vascular disease or vasculitis represent pneumonia or infarction.
Drug reactions and allergic reactions	Airspace shadows in these conditions are rarely solitary. They may be almost any shape except lobar.
Hemorrhage	Solitary airspace shadows caused by hemorrhage are usually due to pulmonary emboli or to pulmonary contusion. When caused by systemic disease, pulmonary hemorrhage is usually multifocal. When single, the opacity can be any shape, even including lobar.
Neoplasm	Postobstructive pneumonia is a common cause of solitary airspace shadowing. Some neoplasms, particularly bronchioloalveolar carcinoma, malignant lymphoma, and pseudolymphoma, can closely resemble focal pneumonia and may even contain air bronchograms. The absence of clinical features of pneumonia and the lack of change of the shadow over many weeks point to one of these neoplasms. The longer the opacity persists, particularly if it grows slowly, the more likely it is to be a neoplasm.
Radiation pneumonitis, fibrosis	Airspace shadowing caused by radiation therapy conforms fairly precisely to the shape of the radiation port, a feature that is particularly evident in CT scans. The shape and the fact that radiation therapy was given usually permit a specific diagnosis to be made.
Eosinophilic pneumonia	Airspace shadowing in this condition is almost invariably multifocal; it is very rarely solitary. The opacity is likely to be noticeably peripheral in location.
Amyloidosis	Amyloidosis is an extremely rare cause of a solitary airspace shadow. When encountered, the opacity is nonspecific in appearance.

bronchus, it is always readily visible at bronchoscopy.

Bronchioloalveolar carcinoma (Figure 4-10) and malignant lymphoma may on occasion appear identical to lobar pneumonia radiologically. The lobar consolidation in these cases is due to neoplastic tissue spreading through the alveolar spaces without necessarily occluding the central bronchi.

3. Lobar consolidation with expansion of the lobe strongly suggests bacterial pneumonia (particularly *Strep-* *tococcus pneumoniae, Klebsiella pneumoniae, Pseudomonas aeruginosa,* and *Staphylococcus aureus* pneumonia) or obstructive pneumonia caused by a centrally positioned carcinoma of the bronchus.

4. A spherical consolidative process is likely to be due to pneumonia (Figure 4-30). The organisms most likely to cause round (spherical or nodular) pneumonia are *S. pneumoniae, S. aureus, K. pneumoniae, P. aeruginosa, Legionella pneumophila* or *L. micdadei, M. tuberculosis,*

CAUSES OF MULTIFOCAL AIRSPACE SHADOWS

EXUDATES AND TRANSUDATES

Pneumonia
Pulmonary emboli causing infarction (bland or septic)
Eosinophilic pneumonia
Collagen vascular disease and vasculitis
Pulmonary edema, both circulatory and noncirculatory (adult respiratory distress syndrome)
Inhalation of noxious gases or liquids
Hydrocarbon ingestion
Drug reactions
Allergic reactions
Alveolar proteinosis
Amyloidosis

HEMORRHAGE

Pulmonary contusion and hematoma
Hemorrhage due to pulmonary embolus
Aspiration of blood
Spontaneous hemorrhage, Goodpasture's syndrome, anticoagulant therapy, bleeding tendency

NEOPLASM

Bronchioloalveolar carcinoma
Lymphangitis carcinomatosa
Nonlymphangitic metastases
Malignant lymphoma
Pseudolymphoma

MISCELLANEOUS

Sarcoidosis
Silicosis, coal workers' pneumoconiosis
Alveolar microlithiasis
Diffuse pulmonary calcification

WIDESPREAD AIRSPACE SHADOWS: LIKELIHOOD OF BAT'S WING PATTERN

COMMON PATTERN FOR DISEASE

Pulmonary edema, both circulatory and noncirculatory (adult respiratory distress syndrome)
Pneumonia, notably that caused by aspiration or *Pneumocystis carinii*
Inhalation of noxious gases or liquids
Alveolar proteinosis
Pulmonary hemorrhage
    Spontaneous
    Goodpasture's syndrome
    Anticoagulant therapy
    Bleeding tendency

OCCASIONAL OR RARE PATTERN FOR DISEASE

Aspiration of blood
Bronchioloalveolar carcinoma
Lymphangitis carcinomatosa
Alveolar microlithiasis
Diffuse pulmonary calcification
Malignant lymphoma
Pulmonary emboli causing hemorrhage or infarction (bland or septic)
Collagen vascular disease, vasculitis
Drug reactions
Allergic reactions
Amyloidosis

EXTREMELY RARE PATTERN FOR DISEASE

Eosinophilic pneumonia
Nonlymphangitic metastases
Pseudolymphoma
Sarcoidosis
Silicosis, coal worker's pneumoconiosis

and several of the fungi. Clearly the major differential diagnosis is from neoplasm.

5. Air lucencies within consolidated lung may be due to (a) resolution of the process with intervening normal lung, (b) necrosis of tissue with cavitation, or (c) pneumatoceles.[98] The development of air-fluid levels within an area of consolidation that is known or presumed to be pneumonia strongly suggests necrotizing pneumonia (true abscess formation). Bacteria are the likely pathogens, notably *S. aureus,* gram-negative bacteria (especially *Klebsiella, Proteus,* and *Pseudomonas*), anaerobic bacteria, and tuberculosis. Those few cases of segmental or lobar consolidation with cavitation not caused by infection will be caused by vasculitis or, rarely, lymphoma. (Cavitation in pulmonary masses is a separate subject and is dealt with later in this chapter.) A meniscus of air within an area of segmental or lobar consolidation almost always represents resolving invasive aspergillosis or invasive mucormycosis.

6. The presence of rib or vertebral body destruction in the vicinity of a pulmonary shadow, whatever the shape of the shadow, is virtually diagnostic of invasion by primary carcinoma of the lung. With the rare exception of actinomycosis and the occasional case of pulmonary tuberculosis[55] or fungal disease, neither pulmonary infection nor any other nonneoplastic pulmonary process invades the adjacent bone.

7. Multiple airspace shadows that are clearly lobar or segmental in shape constitute another potentially useful subgroup (Figure 4-31; see box on p. 74).

It is useful to separate out those cases of multifocal airspace shadowing that show the so-called butterfly or bat's wing pattern because the presence of this pattern changes the likelihood of specific conditions (see box above). These fanciful terms are an attempt to describe bilateral shadowing that is perihilar in distribution; that is, the outer portion of each lobe is less involved than the perihilar area and is often normal (Figure 4-32). The shadowing consists of coalescent densities with ill-defined borders, sometimes with acinar shadows at the

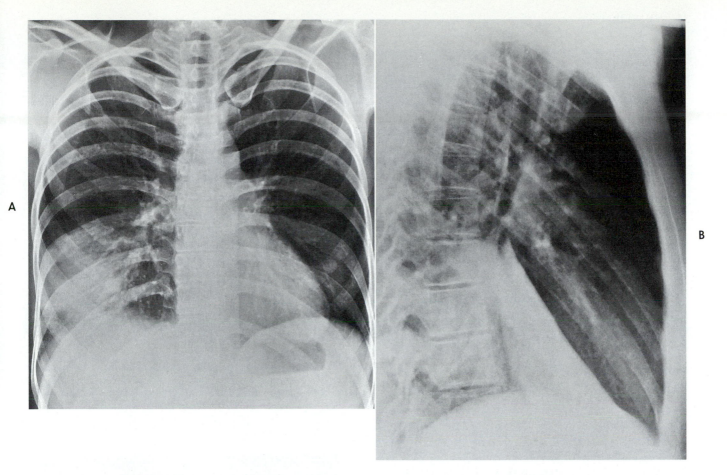

FIGURE 4-29
Lobar consolidation resulting from bacterial pneumonia. In this case, superior segment of right lower lobe is spared. **A,** Posteroanterior view. **B,** Lateral view.

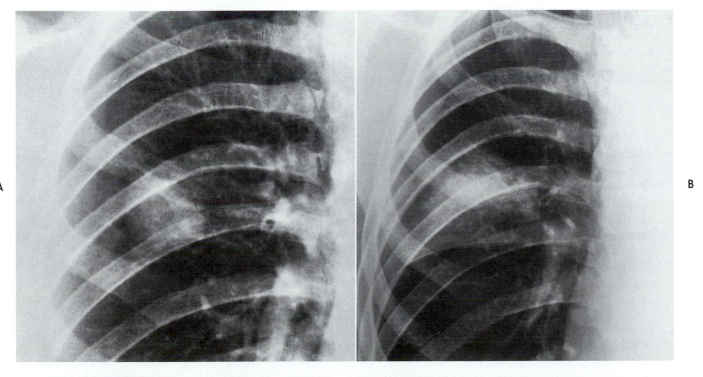

FIGURE 4-30
Round (spherical) pneumonia in patient with bacterial pneumonia. **A,** Radiograph on admission to hospital. **B,** One day later, pneumonia has spread through adjacent lung.

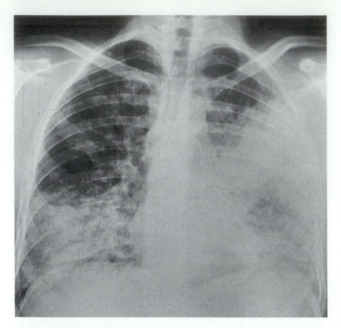

FIGURE 4-31
Multiple airspace shadows with lobar-segmental distribution, in this case of bacterial pneumonia.

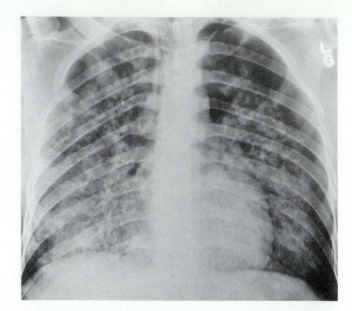

FIGURE 4-32
"Bat's wing" pattern caused by pulmonary edema. This example is typical in that it is bilateral, but asymmetric. Shadowing is maximal in the central (perihilar) portions of lung, and the outer portion of lungs is relatively clear.

DIFFERENTIAL DIAGNOSIS OF MULTIPLE AIRSPACE SHADOWS WHEN THEIR SHAPE IS CLEARLY LOBAR OR SEGMENTAL

Pneumonia
Infarction or hemorrhage caused by pulmonary emboli
Pulmonary edema*
Neoplasm (bronchioloalveolar carcinoma, lymphangitis carcinomatosa,* malignant lymphoma)

*Segmental or lobar shapes are a rare manifestation of the entity.

periphery. Bat's wing shadowing may be symmetric, but more often it is more severe on one side than the other. Air bronchograms and air alveolograms may be prominent features. By far the most common cause of the bat's wing pattern is pulmonary edema (Figure 4-32), particularly if air bronchograms, air alveolograms, or acinar shadows are present. The coexistence of Kerley B lines, for practical purposes, limits the diagnostic possibilities to edema, lymphangitis carcinomatosa, and alveolar proteinosis. Cases of bat's wing shadowing not caused by pulmonary edema or lymphangitis carcinomatosa are likely to be due to pneumonia, inhalation of noxious gases or liquids (including aspiration of gastric contents), multifocal pulmonary hemorrhage (Figure 4-33), vasculitis, or neoplasm. Multifocal pneumonia can be due to a vast array of organisms, but the bat's wing pattern in the immunocompetent patient should particularly suggest aspiration pneumonia, gram-negative bacterial pneumonia, and nonbacterial pneumonias such as mycoplasmal,

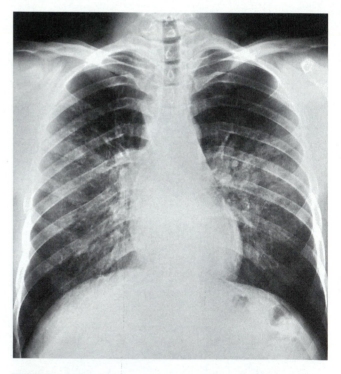

FIGURE 4-33
"Bat's wing" shadowing resulting from idiopathic pulmonary hemorrhage.

viral, and rickettsial pneumonia. Pneumonia in the immunocompromised host often results in the bat's wing pattern, most notably in infections with opportunistic organisms such as *Pneumocystis carinii* and various fungi.

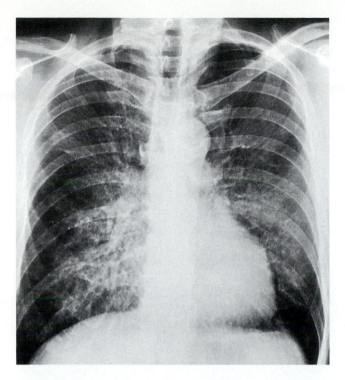

FIGURE 4-34
"Bat's wing" shadowing in alveolar proteinosis.

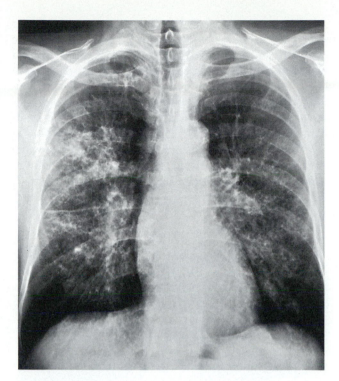

FIGURE 4-35
"Bat's wing" shadowing in lymphangitis carcinomatosa.

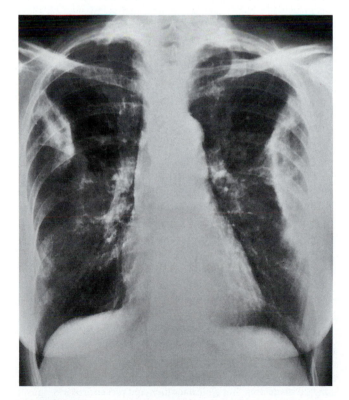

FIGURE 4-36
Chronic eosinophilic pneumonia showing nonsegmental strikingly peripheral distribution of airspace shadowing.

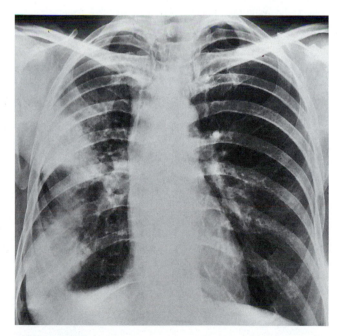

FIGURE 4-37
Chronic eosinophilic pneumonia with unilateral, nonsegmental, peripherally located airspace shadowing.

Bat's wing shadowing that remains unchanged over several weeks and is associated with nonspecific chronic symptoms suggests alveolar proteinosis (Figure 4-34) or a neoplasm, notably lymphangitis carcinomatosa (Figure 4-35), bronchioloalveolar carcinoma, or malignant lymphoma. Amyloidosis, sarcoidosis, and Wegener's granulomatosis are extremely rare possibilities for such shadowing.

9. Nonsegmental airspace shadows that are widespread, yet clearly peripheral in location (sometimes called ''the photographic negative of pulmonary edema'')

are highly indicative of chronic eosinophilic pneumonia (Figures 4-36 and 4-37).[29] The peripheral distribution may be more readily apparent on CT than on plain chest radiography.[75]

10. Many of the causes of multiple airspace shadows appear rapidly, but pulmonary edema is the only one that can clear within hours.

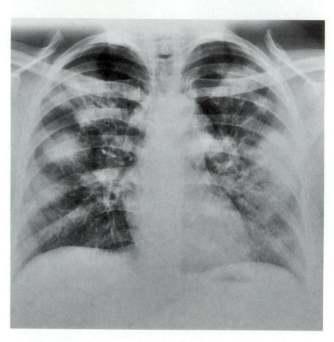

FIGURE 4-39
Sarcoidosis showing multiple, rounded, ill-defined areas of pulmonary shadowing. Note also bilateral hilar and mediastinal adenopathy.

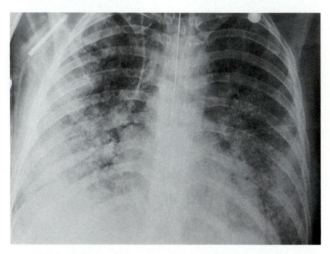

FIGURE 4-38
Widespread, uniform airspace shadowing in adult respiratory distress syndrome.

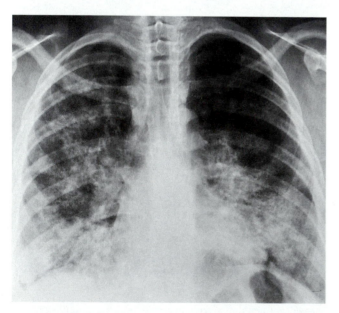

FIGURE 4-40
Sarcoidosis showing widespread nonspecific pulmonary shadowing closely resembling pneumonia.

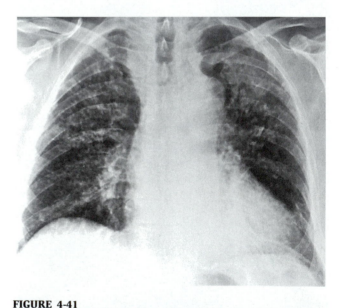

FIGURE 4-41
Progressive massive fibrosis (PMF) in a coal miner. Conglomerate PMF shadow in left upper lobe is ill defined enough to resemble airspace shadowing, but typical location and presence of widespread small nodules in lungs are characteristic of mineral dust pneumoconiosis.

11. Airspace shadowing that resolves only to reappear either in the same area or in some other part of either lung suggests pulmonary edema; eosinophilic pneumonia, either acute or chronic; or asthma, particularly when associated with bronchopulmonary aspergillosis.

12. Adult respiratory distress syndrome (ARDS) is the most likely diagnosis for uniform opacity of the whole of both lungs without pleural effusion in the immunocompetent patient (Figure 4-38). Air bronchograms are a noteworthy feature in these patients. The presence of associated pneumothorax or pneumomediastinum increases the likelihood of ARDS.

13. Sarcoidosis occasionally causes patchy shadows in the lungs that tend to be spherical, to contain air bronchograms, and to be associated with obvious hilar and mediastinal lymph node enlargement. Sometimes these opacities dominate the picture and, when irregular in shape, are radiologically indistinguishable from multifocal pneumonia (Figures 4-39 and 4-40).

14. Progressive massive fibrosis may rarely resemble airspace shadowing (Figure 4-41). It is seldom misdiagnosed, however, because the lesions are so characteristic in shape and position and because the other findings of pneumoconiosis are almost invariably visible.

ATELECTASIS (COLLAPSE)

The terms "atelectasis," "collapse," and "loss of lung volume" are used synonymously. They imply reduced inflation of the lung. There are several mechanisms for loss of volume, the most frequent being bronchial obstruction.

In adults, bronchial obstruction is usually the result of bronchial neoplasm, inhaled foreign body, or mucus plug. On occasion, it is due to inflammatory or posttraumatic bronchostenosis, a broncholith, or extrinsic compression by such phenomena as enlarged lymph nodes, aortic aneurysm, or left atrial enlargement.

Because bronchial tumors are uncommon in children, the probable causes of lobar atelectasis differ significantly from those in adults. In young children the airways are smaller and more vulnerable to mucus obstruction. Thus pneumonia is the most common cause of atelectasis in children, the inflammatory exudate and mucus causing significant airway obstruction. Other than pneumonia, the most likely causes of lobar collapse in children are mucus plug obstruction in conditions such as asthma or cystic fibrosis or inhaled foreign body. Less frequent causes of bronchial obstruction in children include inflammatory or posttraumatic bronchostenosis, compression of the bronchial tree by anomalous vessels, and, rarely, neoplastic obstruction.

The position of an obstructing lesion can be predicted by recognizing which lobes are collapsed. Obliteration or narrowing of the bronchial air column at the site of obstruction is often visible, even on plain film. Opaque foreign bodies or calcified broncholiths may be directly visible. All these findings are helpful in determining the need for bronchoscopy and in directing the procedure.

Although CT usually demonstrates the size and site of an obstructing lesion in a patient with a lobar collapse (Figures 4-42 and 4-43),[84] bronchoscopy is indicated to diagnose its nature and where possible, as with foreign body inhalation and mucus plug obstruction, to treat the cause.

The Golden S sign makes it possible to recognize that a lobe has collapsed around a large central mass (Figures 4-44 and 4-48). When the peripheral lung collapses and

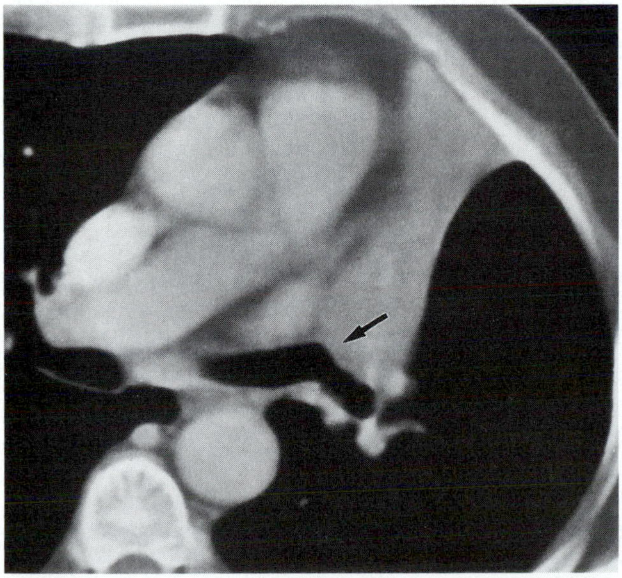

FIGURE 4-42
Carcinoma of bronchus obstructing left upper lobe bronchus and causing left upper lobe collapse. Bronchial occlusion by tumor (*arrow*) is well shown by computed tomography.

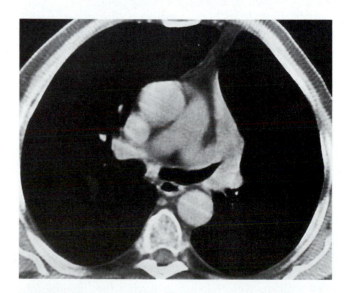

FIGURE 4-43
Carcinoma of bronchus causing "rat tail" narrowing of left upper lobe bronchus and collapse of left upper lobe.

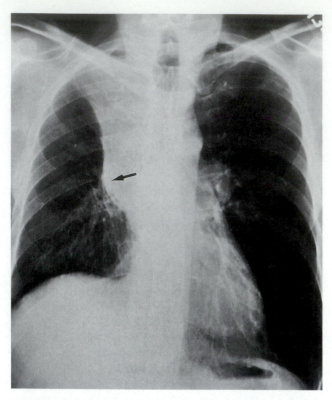

FIGURE 4-44
Right upper lobe collapse with Golden "S" sign. Outward bulge *(arrow)* of displaced minor fissure indicates underlying mass, which proved to be bronchial carcinoma.

the central portion is prevented from collapsing by the presence of a mass, the relevant fissures are concave peripherally but convex centrally; the shape of the fissure then resembles an S or a reverse S— hence the name Golden S sign, after Golden's description of cases of lobar collapse caused by carcinoma of the lung.[37]

Apart from bronchial obstruction, the major mechanisms for atelectasis are (1) retraction of the lung associated with pneumothorax or pleural effusion, (2) compression by adjacent masses or overinflated lung, (3) cicatrization of the lung, and (4) so-called adhesive atelectasis, which occurs when the alveolar walls adhere to one another, as for example in hyaline membrane disease of the newborn and in discoid atelectasis.

The middle lobe and lingula are particularly vulnerable to collapse, possibly because there are many lymph nodes surrounding their stem bronchi. In addition, in patients with complete minor and major fissures, the opportunity for collateral drift to the middle lobe is limited. In one series of 129 patients with chronic disease in the right middle lobe or lingula, 58 had no evidence of central obstruction, either by endobronchial or by exobronchial masses.[102] These patients, most of whom were middle-aged women, were labeled as having the "middle lobe syndrome" (Figure 4-56). The condition was originally thought to be due to tuberculous lymphadenopathy pressing on the lobar bronchus, but it is now believed that

the entity is due to chronic inflammatory disease, presumably a prior pneumonia, which clears very slowly because of poor collateral drift.[15]

Plain films are usually sufficient to diagnose the presence of a collapsed lobe. CT can be useful when the plain film findings are ambiguous, for example, when pleural fluid and pulmonary disease processes are both present. MRI has no particular value in the diagnosis of lobar collapse, although it may prove useful in distinguishing obstructive from nonobstructive collapse. Herold, Kuhlman, and Zerhouni[48] showed that the signal intensity on proton density and T2-weighted images was high in collapse because of a central obstruction but was low in nonobstructive collapse. They postulated that the high T2-dependent signal was related to trapped secretions, which were present only when the collapse was due to obstruction.

Signs of lobar collapse

The fundamental signs of lobar collapse are opacity of the lobe and evidence of loss of volume.[94] The signs can be divided into (1) direct signs, such as displacement of fissures, pulmonary blood vessels, and major bronchi, and (2) shift of other structures to compensate for the loss of volume. The compensatory shifts are in principle similar for each lobe, and therefore they are discussed first.

Compensatory overexpansion of the adjacent lobe may be recognizable because it results in spreading of the vessels so that there are fewer vessels per unit volume. This sign should not be relied on if it is an isolated finding, since previous lung damage, from infection for example, can lead to a similar appearance. Another sign of compensatory expansion is the shifting granuloma sign as illustrated in Figure 4-45.

The amount of mediastinal shift accompanying lobar collapse is variable. In general, it is greatest with lower lobe collapse and with chronic fibrotic upper lobe collapse, relatively mild with acute upper lobe collapse, and virtually nonexistent with collapse of the middle lobe. Its recognition depends on noting displacement of the trachea and mediastinum. Displacement of the trachea is a much more reliable sign. Normally, on a correctly centered frontal view, the trachea lies midway, or slightly to the right of the midpoint, between the medial ends of the clavicles. Minor obliquity of the chest radiograph does not make much difference because the trachea is only just behind the plane of the medial ends of the clavicles. Aortic unfolding, however, may move the trachea to the right.

The normal position of the mediastinum varies so greatly that displacement of the mediastinal contours is an insensitive sign of pulmonary collapse. Normally one fifth to one half of the cardiac shadow lies to the right of the midline. More than one half or less than one fifth of this suggests mediastinal shift.

Hemidiaphragm elevation is another form of compen-

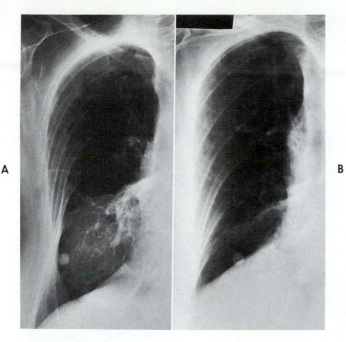

A **B**

FIGURE 4-45
Displacement of calcified granuloma secondary to right lower lobe collapse. **A,** At time when mild right lower lobe collapse is present. **B,** When complete collapse of right lower lobe is present.

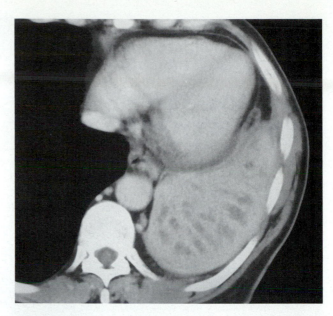

FIGURE 4-46
Fluid bronchogram at computed tomography. Fluid-filled bronchi beyond a carcinoma in this collapsed lower left lobe are clearly visible.

satory shift. It is usually unrecognizable in right middle lobe collapse and may be subtle in right upper lobe collapse. Collapse of either lower lobe or of the left upper lobe may lead to obvious elevation of the ipsilateral hemidiaphragm. The sign is, however, of limited value because the position of the normal diaphragm is highly variable, particularly in a hospital population. It depends on many factors, including the amount of gas in the stomach, and can vary from day to day in the same individual. Therefore great care must be taken when using this sign to support the diagnosis of lobar collapse.

Inward movement of the chest wall causes narrowing of the spaces between the affected ribs. This sign, which is seen only with a severely collapsed lobe, can be difficult to evaluate on chest films. It is much easier to recognize with CT where the volume of each hemithorax can be readily compared. Clearly, confusion with preexisting chest wall deformity, particularly when consequent to scoliosis, may cloud the issue.

Bronchial dilatation within collapsed lobes

Mucus-filled, dilated bronchi are frequently present beyond an obstructing lesion responsible for lobar collapse. This form of bronchiectasis is very familiar to pathologists. It cannot be recognized on plain films, although it is readily identified at CT as low-density branching structures (Figures 4-46 and 8-16).[33,108] The low density is due to trapped secretions. This so-called mucoid or fluid bronchogram should prompt a search for a central obstructing lesion.

Right upper lobe collapse

Right upper lobe collapse (Figures 4-44 and 4-47) is the easiest lobar collapse to recognize on plain chest radiographs. The major and minor fissures move upward toward each other rather like a half-closed book, the spine of which is represented by the hilum. At the same time these fissures rotate toward the mediastinum, with the result that the right upper lobe packs against the mediastinum and lung apex. The more the collapse, the greater the concavity of the minor fissure. Eventually, with extreme collapse, the minor fissure parallels the mediastinum and thoracic apex and resembles pleural thickening or mediastinal widening. The lobe is attached to the hilum by a conical wedge of collapsed lung, and therefore the curving inferior margin of the lobe always connects to the hilum. The intrinsic bulk of the central vessels and bronchi means that there is a limit to the loss of volume possible at the hilum; hence an outward bulge is discernible at the hilum in examples of extreme collapse even when no hilar mass is present. Because the collapsed right upper lobe has extensive contact with the mediastinum, the normal superior vena caval border is "silhouetted" out on the frontal chest film, as is the ascending aorta on the lateral view.

The middle and lower lobes expand to occupy the vacated space, leading to outward and upward displacement of the lower lobe artery. Because this displacement is easy to see on frontal radiographs, it is a good sign to look for. The corresponding upward angulation of the right mainstem and lower lobe bronchi is more difficult to recognize. Overexpansion of the opposite upper lobe is

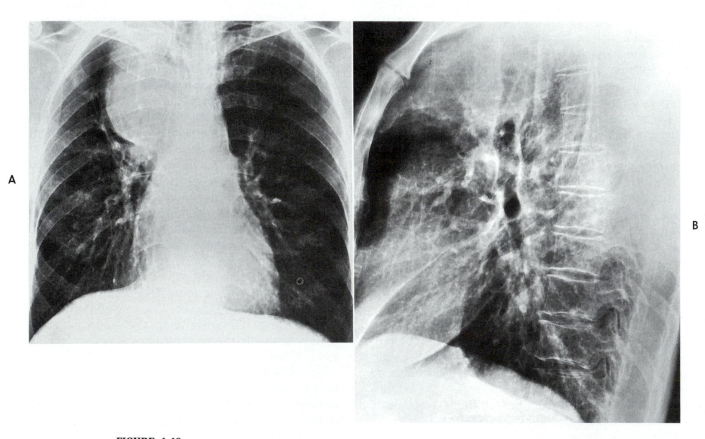

FIGURE 4-47
Right upper lobe collapse. Typical example. Also note juxtaphrenic peak *(arrow).* **A,** Posteroanterior view. **B,** Lateral view.

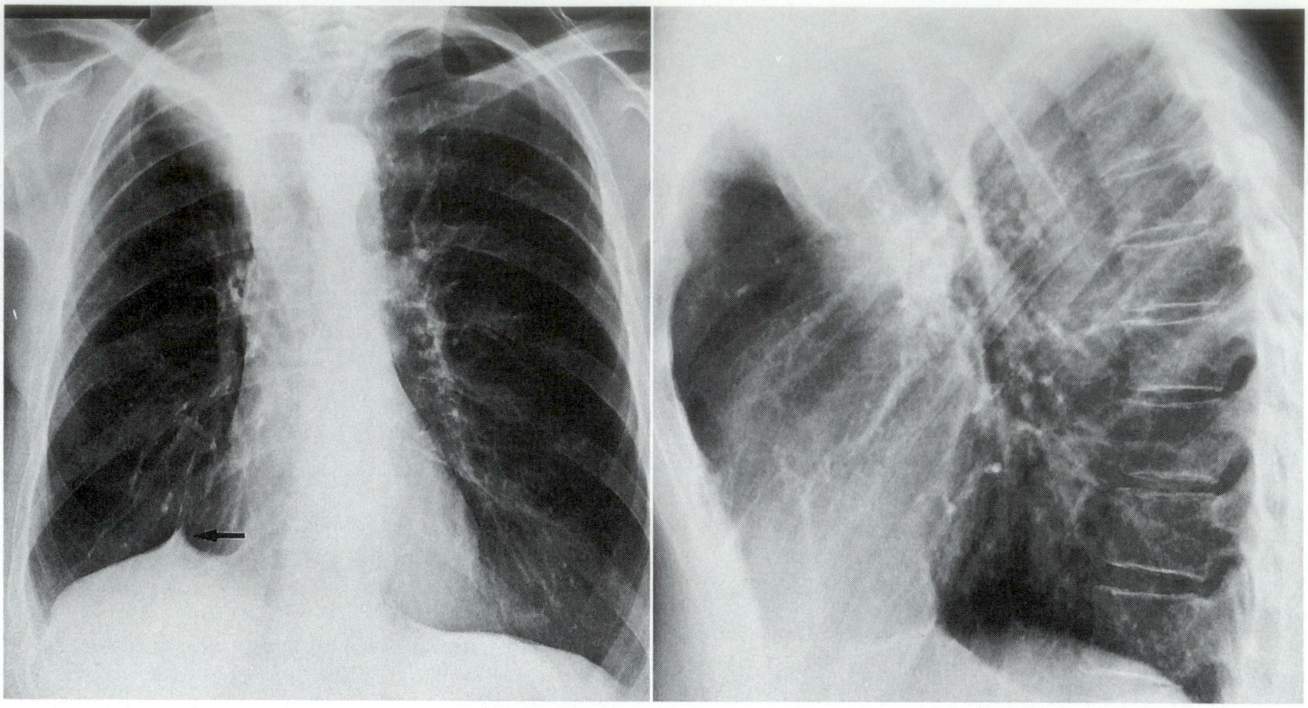

FIGURE 4-48
Right upper lobe collapse around large, centrally obstructing bronchial carcinoma (Golden "S" sign) resembling mediastinal mass. The best clue to correct interpretation is elevation of the right lower lobe artery. **A,** Posteroanterior view. **B,** Lateral view.

usually minor. For practical purposes it is visible only at CT scanning.

On the lateral view the upward displacement of the major and minor fissures is usually obvious. With severe loss of volume the wedge of collapsed lung radiating out from the hilum may be no more than an indistinct density on lateral views, since none of the fissures are tangential to the x-ray beam. The elevation of the right pulmonary trunk and the anterior displacement of the right bronchial tree can be identified on the lateral projection,[131] but only with great difficulty.

Occasionally, collapse of the right upper lobe around a large obstructing bronchial tumor closely mimics a mediastinal mass (Figure 4-48). An error in interpretation can be avoided by carefully analyzing the film for compensatory shift of other intrathoracic structures.

On rare occasions the normal chest wall contact is maintained even in severe collapse. This appearance (Figure 4-49) is most frequently reported in young children,[27] but it is also seen in adults.[18] It has been termed peripheral atelectasis because the collapsed lobe lies against the chest wall and the overexpanded lower lobe lies centrally.

A juxtaphrenic peak may be visible.[62] The term refers to a small triangular shadow based on the apex of the dome of the right hemidiaphragm with loss of silhouette of the adjacent hemidiaphragm (Figure 4-47), probably caused by traction on the lower end of the major fissure, the inferior accessory fissure, or the inferior pulmonary ligament.[35]

At CT scanning,[34,83-85,96] a collapsed right upper lobe appears as a triangular soft tissue density lying against the mediastinum and the anterior chest wall. The border formed by the major fissure posteriorly and the minor fissure laterally is sharp (Figure 4-50). In the absence of large intrapulmonary masses, each fissural boundary should be uniformly concave or convex, not a combination of the two. A severely collapsed right upper lobe assumes a bandlike configuration plastered against the mediastinum, an appearance that can be confused with mediastinal disease. Sometimes the hyperexpanded superior segment of the lower lobe insinuates itself between the mediastinum and the medial border of the collapsed lobe. Elevation of the right upper lobe bronchus may cause the bronchus intermedius to move laterally,[34] and the right middle lobe bronchus may be displaced anteriorly and reoriented in a more horizontal position.

Left upper lobe collapse

Because there is no minor fissure on the left, the appearance of collapse of the left upper lobe is significantly different from collapse of the right upper lobe

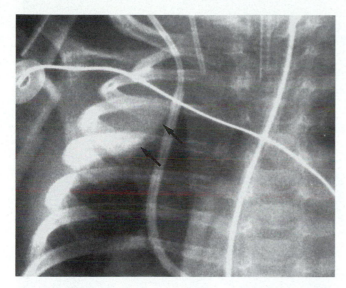

FIGURE 4-49
"Peripheral atelectasis" of right upper lobe *(arrows)* in infant following cardiac surgery. The lobe has collapsed against chest wall.

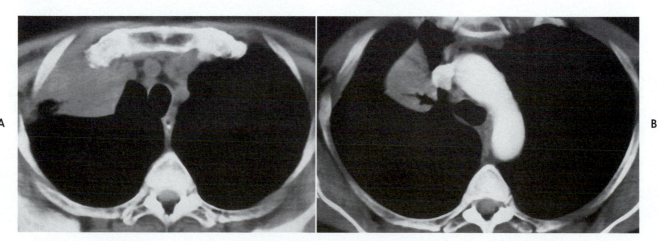

A

B

FIGURE 4-50
Computed tomographic scans of right upper lobe collapse showing characteristic wedge-shaped density radiating from right hilum with broad base against anterior chest wall.

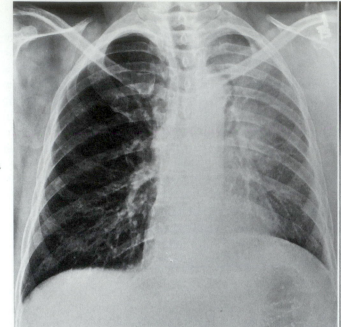
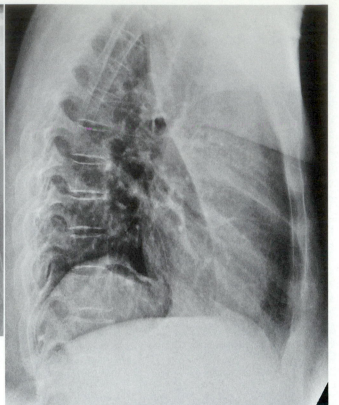

FIGURE 4-51
Left upper lobe collapse in patient with bronchial carcinoma.
A, Posteroanterior view. B, Lateral view.

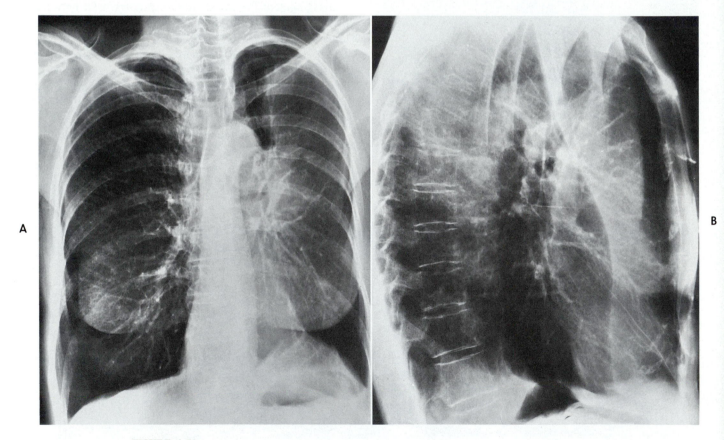

FIGURE 4-52
Left upper lobe collapse. In this example, the greatly expanded superior segment of left lower lobe occupies apex and consequently upper surface of aortic arch is visible. A, Posteroanterior view. B, Lateral view.

(Figure 4-51). The collapse is predominantly forward, pulling the expanding lower lobe behind it. Except at the edges the lobe in its collapsed state retains much of its original contact with the anterior chest wall and mediastinum.

Since the lobe thins as the fissure is pulled forward, the usual appearance on a frontal radiograph is a hazy density extending out from the left hilum, often reaching the lung apex, and fading laterally and inferiorly. The loss of the left cardiac and mediastinal silhouette is a striking feature on the frontal view. With mild loss of volume — provided the lobe is opaque — the entire cardiac and upper mediastinal border, together with the diaphragm outline adjacent to the cardiac apex, becomes invisible. With increasing loss of volume the upper margin of the aortic knob once again becomes visible because the superior segment of the lower lobe takes the place of the posterior segment of the upper lobe. With further loss of volume the upper border of the pulmonary opacity becomes hazy and its medial border becomes sharp because the apex is now occupied by the greatly overexpanded superior segment of lower lobe (Figure 4-52). The superior mediastinal and left hemidiaphragm contours then reappear, but with very few exceptions the left border of the heart remains indistinct even in the most severe cases of complete left upper lobe collapse.

The overexpansion of the left lower lobe results in elevation of the left hilum and outward angulation of the left lower lobe artery. The left bronchial tree assumes an S-shaped configuration, the left main bronchus assuming a near horizontal course and the lower lobe bronchus running more vertically than usual (Figure 4-53).

On the lateral view the lateral portion of the major fissure is usually seen as a clearly defined concave margin running approximately parallel to the anterior chest wall. The inevitable wedge of tissue radiating from the hilum is indistinct on the lateral projection unless there is a hilar mass to alter the tangents. The lingula segment, being thinner to start with, often appears to be no more than a sliver. The whole fissure may be so far forward that a collapsed upper lobe can be overlooked or misinterpreted as an anterior mediastinal density. Sometimes the fissure rotates, so that no part of it is tangential to the x-ray beam, and in these cases the edge of the shadow is ill defined in the lateral view also.

A striking feature of left upper lobe collapse is herniation of the opposite lung into the left hemithorax in front of the aorta (Figure 4-42), which leads to increased visibility of the ascending aorta on the lateral chest radiograph (Figure 4-52), a feature that should not be misinterpreted as the anterior edge of the collapsed lobe. In rare instances the edge of the herniated lung can be

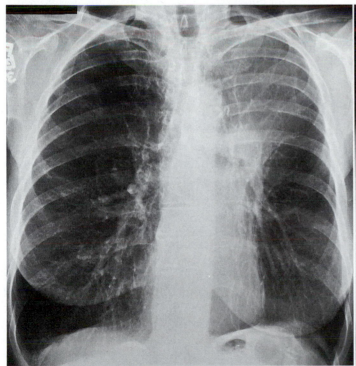

A

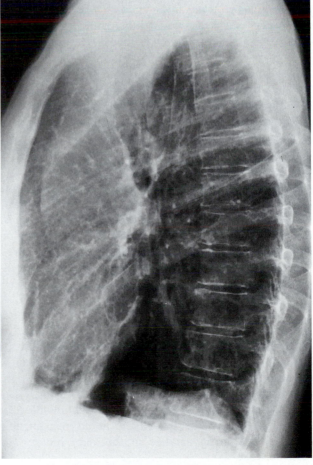

B

FIGURE 4-53
Left upper lobe collapse showing reorientation of left mainstem bronchus and left lower lobe bronchus. Note near horizontal alignment of mainstem bronchus and near vertical alignment of lower lobe bronchus. **A,** Posteroanterior view. **B,** Lateral view.

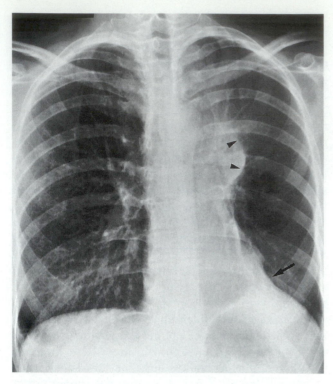

FIGURE 4-54
Left upper lobe collapse showing juxtaphrenic peak *(arrow)* and Golden "S" sign *(arrowheads)*. Collapse was due to a centrally obstructing bronchial carcinoma.

seen projected over the aortic knob on a frontal film. The more usual cause of aerated lung lying medial to the opacity of a collapsed left upper lobe is overexpansion of the left lower lobe invaginating between the collapsed lung and the mediastinum (Figure 4-52).

A juxtaphrenic peak on the hemidiaphragm (Figure 4-54) and the phenomenon of "peripheral" atelectasis may be seen on the left just as they may with collapse of the right upper lobe.

At CT (Figures 4-42, 4-43, 4-50, and 4-55)[34,38-85,96] collapsed left and right upper lobes appear similar, but with left upper lobe collapse the airless lingular segments are identified on sections below the carina as a narrow triangular density based on the heart and anterior chest wall extending almost to the diaphragm. The herniation of the right lung anterior to the aorta is particularly well demonstrated at CT scanning.

Right middle lobe collapse

The opacity of a collapsed middle lobe on the frontal chest radiograph may, in severe cases, be so minimal that middle lobe atelectasis is easy to overlook, because its depth in the plane of the beam may be no more than a few millimeters (Figure 4-56). Loss of silhouette of the right border of the heart is almost always a feature. The bronchial and vascular realignments in right middle lobe collapse are so slight that there is no recognizable alteration in the appearance of the right hilum. The

collapsed lobe is, however, easily and reliably recognized on the lateral chest radiograph. The major and minor fissures approximate one another, and if the collapse is pronounced, the lobe diminishes in volume and resembles a curved, elongated wedge. The wedge tapers in two directions: medial to lateral, and anterior to posterior. Because the wedge can be relatively thin, much of it is end on to the beam in the lateral projection. The image on the lateral chest radiograph is therefore a well-defined, curved triangular band of density, lying between the major and minor fissures, extending downward and forward from the hilum. The collapsed lobe may be so thin that it may be misinterpreted as a thickened fissure. Alternatively, there may occasionally be difficulty in distinguishing between collapse of the middle lobe and loculated fluid in the major fissure. With collapse the inferior margin of the opacity is concave, whereas with loculated fluid the fissure bulges downward. Also the fissures should not be separately visible in their normal positions, an important point in the differential diagnosis from fluid, fibrosis, or tumors lying within the fissures.

At CT (Figures 4-57 and 4-58),[34,83-85,96] right middle lobe collapse appears as a triangular density bounded posteriorly by the major fissure, medially by the mediastinum at the level of the right atrium, and anteriorly by the minor fissure. The posterior boundary should be well defined. Unless the minor fissure is pulled well down, the anterior margin may be poorly defined on the CT images. The right middle lobe bronchus enters the posteromedial corner of the opacity, an important point in the differential diagnosis from loculated pleural fluid. Because the collapsed middle lobe is effectively a sheet of tissue running obliquely through the chest, the axial sections of CT are not aligned with the lobe and only small portions of the collapsed lobe are seen on any one section.

Lower lobe collapse

The appearances of collapse of the lower lobes are sufficiently similar on the two sides that it is convenient to consider right and left lower collapse together. Collapse may affect the whole lobe, but the superior segment is frequently spared.

With collapse of either lower lobe (Figures 4-59 and 4-60), the major fissure rotates backward and medially and the upper half of the fissure swings downward. Thus collapsed lower lobes lie posteromedially in the lower thoracic cavity. The resulting triangular opacity is based on the diaphragm and mediastinum, with the fissure running obliquely through the thorax. On frontal projection the opacity of a collapsed lower lobe is easier to recognize on the right than on the left because on the left it is often hidden by the heart, especially if the film is underpenetrated. With severe loss of volume the lobe becomes notably thin and appears as a sliver lying against the mediastinum (Figure 4-61). Sometimes, presumably when the inferior pulmonary ligament does not attach to the diaphragm, the lobe is plastered against the mediasti-

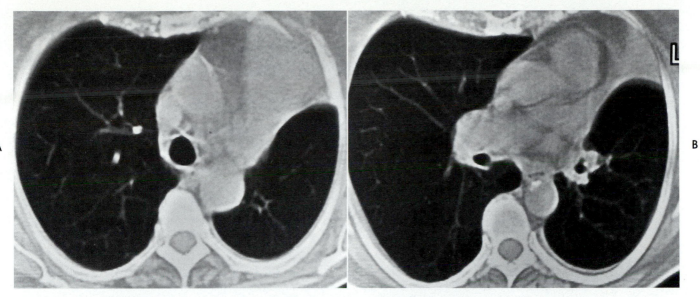

FIGURE 4-55
Computed tomographic scans showing left upper lobe collapse. Note forward displacement of major fissure and mediastinal shift to left. **A,** Section above level of left mainstem bronchus showing collapsed anterior, posterior, and apical segments. **B,** Section through collapsed lingular segments.

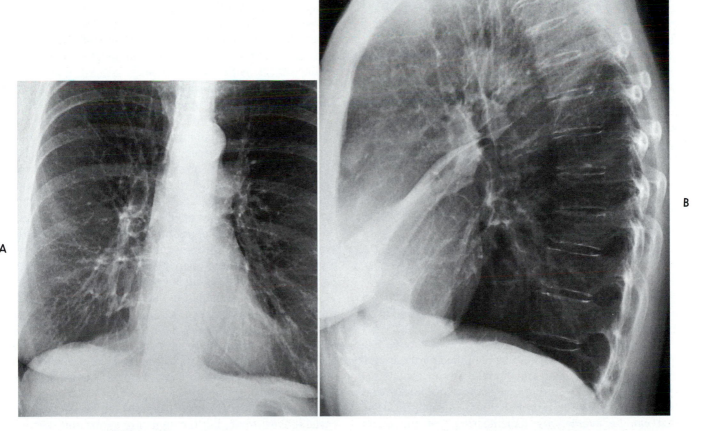

FIGURE 4-56
Right middle lobe collapse. **A,** Lobe is so severely atelectatic that the opacity in frontal view is difficult to see. There is, however, loss of right heart border owing to silhouette sign. **B,** Lateral view shows collapsed lobe to advantage. In this case, the collapse was chronic and the result of "middle lobe syndrome."

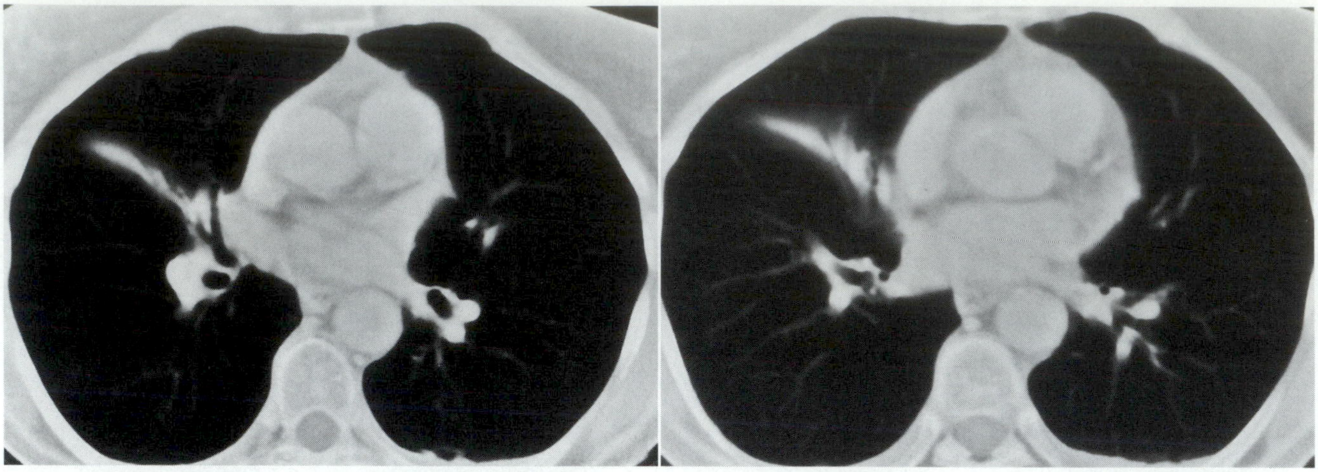

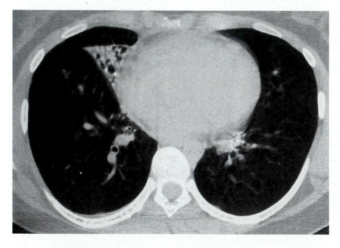

FIGURE 4-57
Computed tomographic scans of right middle lobe collapse in same patient as in Figure 4-56. Note patent middle lobe bronchus and air bronchogram. Two adjacent sections are shown: **A**, section at level of right middle lobe bronchus and, **B**, one section lower.

FIGURE 4-58
Computed tomographic scan of right middle lobe collapse showing dilated air-filled bronchi within collapsed lobe. This combination is typical of "right middle lobe syndrome."

num but has little if any contact with the diaphragm. In these cases the collapsed lobe assumes a rounded configuration and resembles a mediastinal mass (see Figure 15-24).

If the superior segment remains aerated, the upper half of the major fissure will often be identified on the frontal view as a line that may run horizontally to contact the spine (Figure 4-62). In these cases the major fissure may be confused with the minor fissure, a misinterpretation that can be avoided by remembering that the minor fissure does not cross medial to the hilum.

Lower lobe collapse is sometimes most obvious in the lateral view. With mild loss of volume the opaque lobe and the displaced major fissure are readily recognizable,

but with more severe loss of volume the fissure rotates and the triangular opacity in the lower posterior quadrant of the chest has an ill-defined anterior margin. Unless the collapse is severe, the outline of the posterior half of the right or left hemidiaphragm shadow is lost. With very severe collapse the outline of the ipsilateral hemidiaphragm once again becomes visible because compensatory expansion of the upper and middle lobe brings them into contact with the previously effaced diaphragm (Figure 4-61). The opacity of the collapsed lobe may be difficult to recognize unless the observer is careful to observe the density of the vertebrae. Normally, on lateral projection each vertebra appears blacker than the one above as the eye descends through the thorax to the diaphragm. In lower lobe collapse the lower vertebrae appear whiter than those higher up (Figures 4-59 and 4-60).

The major vascular trunks supplying the lobes are displaced, but more important, they are invisible because they are coursing through an opaque lobe. Therefore, with complete lower lobe collapse, the distal lobar and segmental divisions of the pulmonary artery are invisible. Careful analysis of the hilum may, however, be needed to recognize this difference because displaced middle or upper lobe trunks may resemble the lower lobe arteries. A similar analysis of the lobar bronchi may be even more revealing: in most cases air within the lobar bronchus can be identified coursing into the triangular density of the collapsed lobe.

Bronchial displacement can also be recognized on lateral chest films, but the signs are subtle and demand confident knowledge of the normal.[131] Normally the central bronchi run in the same direction as the trachea and course obliquely backward as they descend, so that the right and left major airways are virtually superim-

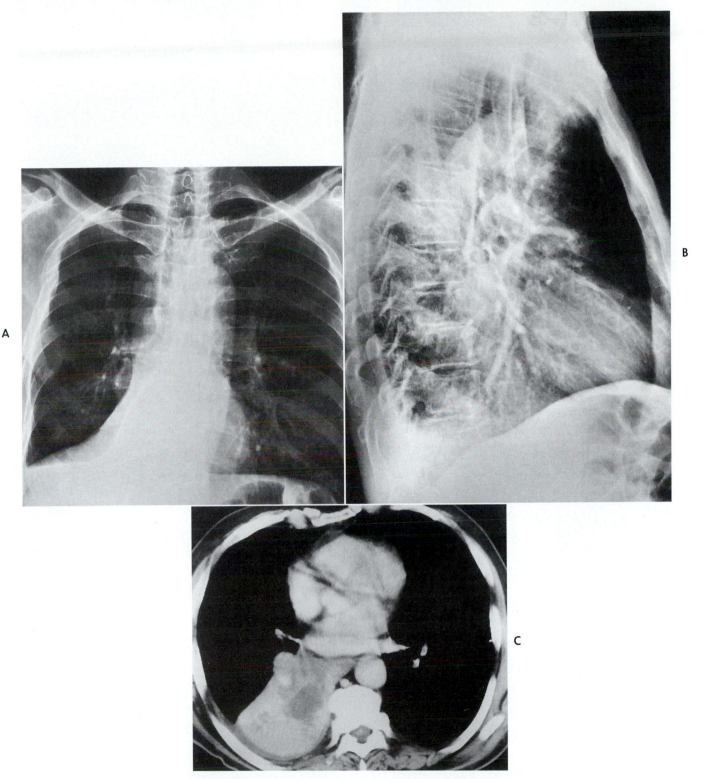

FIGURE 4-59
Right lower lobe collapse resulting from bronchial carcinoma. (Metastasis is present in right eighth rib, and there are multiple old fractures of right ribs.) **A,** Posteroanterior radiograph. **B,** Lateral radiograph. **C,** Computed tomographic scan in different patient.

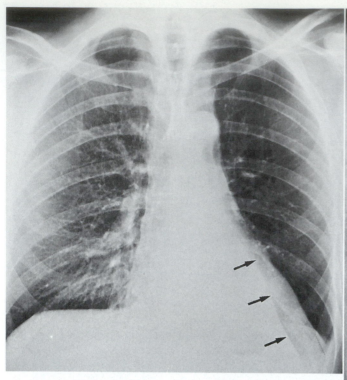

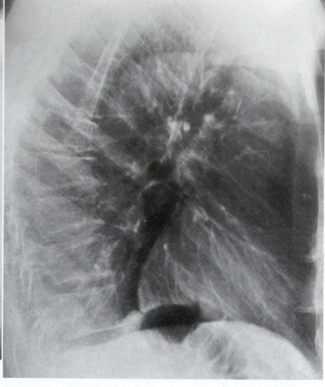

FIGURE 4-60
Left lower lobe collapse resulting from bronchial carcinoma. (Arrows point to displaced major fissure.) In this example, displacement of left hilar vessels is particularly well demonstrated. Left lower lobe artery is invisible because it is within collapsed lobe. Note also splaying of blood vessels in overexpanded left upper lobe. Flat waist sign is also present. **A,** Posteroanterior view. **B,** Lateral view.

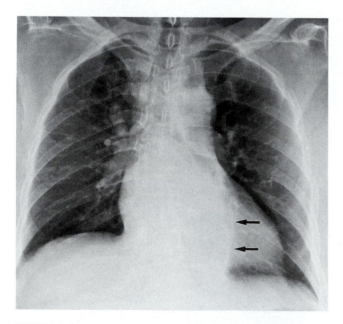

FIGURE 4-61
Very severe collapse of left lower lobe. Collapsed lobe *(arrows)* is no more than sliver against mediastinum. Altered configuration of left hilum is perhaps the most striking sign in this example.

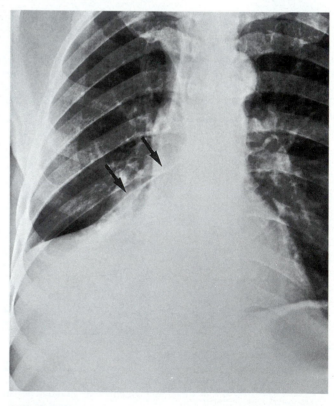

FIGURE 4-62
Right lower and right middle lobe collapse with partial aeration of superior segment of right lower lobe. Arrows point to displaced major fissure.

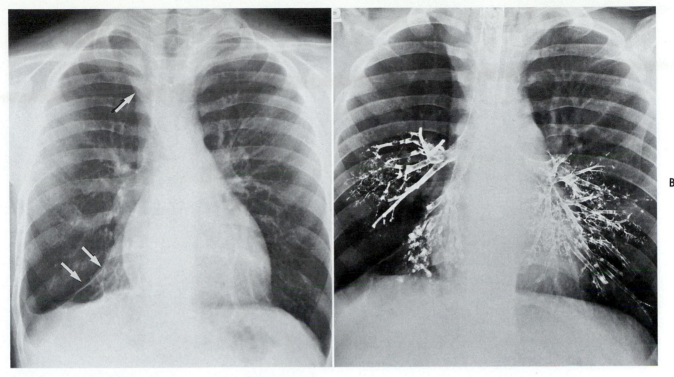

FIGURE 4-63
Right lower lobe collapse caused by bronchiectasis showing upper triangle sign *(upward-pointing arrow)*. Displaced major fissure *(downward-pointing arrows)* and right lower lobe artery entering collapsed lobe are well demonstrated. **A,** Posteroanterior radiograph. **B,** Bronchogram showing arrangement of bronchi.

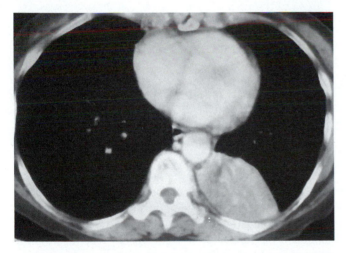

FIGURE 4-64
Contrast-enhanced computed tomographic scan of left lower lobe collapse.

posed on one another in a true lateral projection. The only difference is the higher origin of the right upper lobe bronchus and the differences inherent in the right lung having a middle lobe. Lower lobe collapse leads to backward displacement of the relevant airways. This displacement is useful in differentiating opacity caused primarily by pleural fluid from that caused by lower lobe collapse. With collapse the bronchi are pulled back,

whereas with pleural fluid the bronchi may be pushed forward.[91]

The appearance of the upper mediastinal contours may occasionally be helpful in drawing attention to, or confirming, the possibility of lower lobe collapse. Kattan[61] emphasized three signs:

1. The upper triangle sign[63] refers to a low-density, clearly marginated triangular shadow on frontal chest radiographs that resembles right-sided mediastinal widening. It is seen in right lower lobe collapse and is caused by rightward displacement of the anterior junctional tissues of the mediastinum (Figure 4-63). The appearance superficially resembles right upper lobe collapse but should not be confused with it, because the fissural, vascular, and bronchial realignments all point to overexpansion of the right upper lobe rather than to collapse.

2. The flat waist sign[64] refers to flattening of the contours of the aortic knob and adjacent main pulmonary artery (Figure 4-60). It is seen in severe collapse of the left lower lobe and is due to leftward displacement and rotation of the heart. The appearance therefore resembles a shallow right anterior oblique view of the normal mediastinum.

3. The outline of the top of the aortic knob may be obliterated in severe left lower lobe collapse.[61]

At CT scanning[34,83-85,96] a collapsed lower lobe produces a triangular opacity of soft tissue density in the posterior chest against the spine (Figures 4-59 and 4-64).

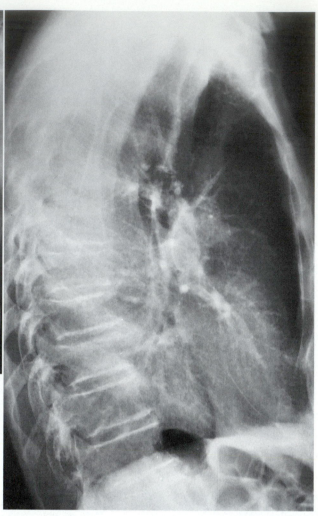

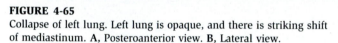

FIGURE 4-65
Collapse of left lung. Left lung is opaque, and there is striking shift of mediastinum. **A,** Posteroanterior view. **B,** Lateral view.

The major fissure rotates to lie obliquely across the thoracic cavity. The lobe is fixed at the hilum, and the medial basal segment cannot move further back than the attachment of the inferior pulmonary ligament to the mediastinum. In cases where the inferior pulmonary ligament is incomplete, collapse of the basal segments may simulate a mass on CT just as it may on the plain chest radiograph.[32]

Whole lung collapse

Whole lung collapse on either side leads to opacity of the whole hemithorax. The signs of compensatory shift are usually obvious. Mediastinal shift is invariably present, and herniation of the opposite lung is usually a striking feature (Figure 4-65).

Combined right upper and middle lobe collapse

Because there is no single bronchus to the right upper and middle lobes that does not also supply the right lower lobe, collapse of these two lobes with normal aeration of the lower lobe is unusual. The appearances are virtually identical to those seen with left upper lobe collapse (Figure 4-66). Occasionally collapse of the right upper lobe alone precisely mimics combined collapse of the right upper and middle lobes.[13]

Combined right lower and middle lobe collapse

The combination of right lower and middle lobe collapse is seen with obstruction to the bronchus intermedius. The appearances are similar to collapse of the right lower lobe alone in both the PA and lateral projections except that the abnormal density extends all the way to the lateral costophrenic angle (Figure 4-67).[94] Similarly, on the lateral view the opacity extends from the front to the back of the thorax.[94]

Diagnosing combined middle and lower lobe collapse is much easier at CT. Because the bronchi can be individually identified, it is possible to identify the middle lobe specifically and so diagnose or exclude the presence of combined middle and lower lobe collapse.

Distinguishing lower lobe collapse from pleural fluid

Lower lobe collapse can be difficult, and sometimes impossible, to distinguish from pleural effusion on conventional PA and lateral radiographs. This diagnostic dilemma is most frequent in postoperative or acutely ill

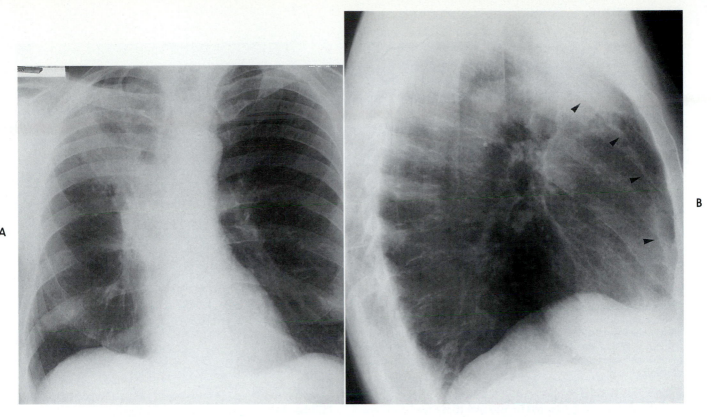

FIGURE 4-66
Combined right upper and middle lobe collapse. Note similarity to left upper lobe collapse. Arrowheads point to greatly displaced major fissure. **A,** Posteroanterior view. **B,** Lateral view. (Courtesy Dr. Michael Pearson, London.)

FIGURE 4-67
Combined right middle and lower lobe collapse. Note similarity to right lower lobe collapse alone, except that abnormal density extends all the way to costophrenic angle in frontal view and from front to back in lateral view. **A,** Posteroanterior view. **B,** Lateral view.

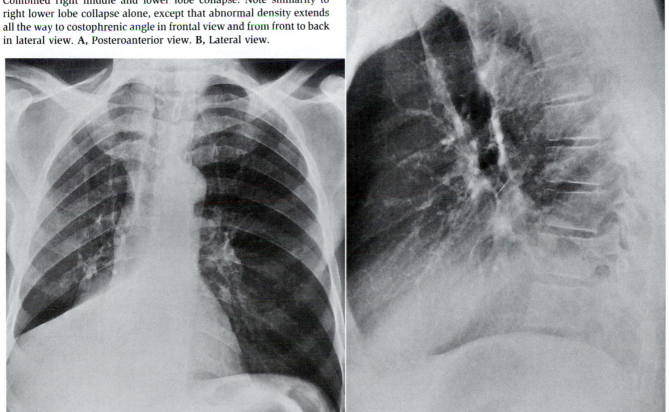

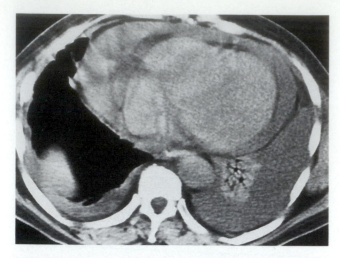

FIGURE 4-68
Computed tomographic scan of combined pleural effusion and left lower lobe collapse. Collapsed lobe with its air bronchogram is clearly distinguishable from adjacent left pleural effusion. (The patient, who had small cell carcinoma of lung, also has extensive mediastinal adenopathy, pericardial effusion, and right pleural effusion.)

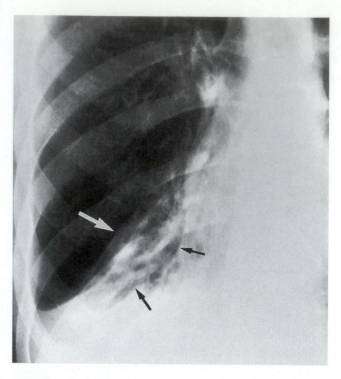

FIGURE 4-69
Right lower lobe collapse caused by bronchiectasis. Air in dilated bronchi (*black arrows*) is an important clue to the cause of the collapsed lobe. White arrow points to displaced major fissure.

patients and is compounded by the fact that these patients are frequently examined with portable equipment in frontal projection only.

The diagnosis of lobar collapse depends on recognizing shift of structures, particularly the fissures, the hilar blood vessels, and the major bronchi. If the position of the fissures can be confidently established, the diagnosis is easy. If not, attention should be turned to the hila, particularly the position of the lower lobe arteries and bronchi. Two questions should be addressed: (1) do these structures enter the opacity in question, and (2) are they displaced in a direction that suggests collapse? For example, in a patient with basal opacity, if the lower lobe artery is obscured and the lower lobe bronchus runs vertically through the opacity, lower lobe collapse should be diagnosed. If, on the other hand, the lower lobe artery is clearly seen lateral to the opacity and the bronchus is not surrounded by the density, the opacity is not the result of lower lobe collapse.

Lateral decubitus views may be necessary to distinguish between lower lobe collapse and pleural fluid. Provided fluid is free in the pleural cavity, it will layer against the lateral chest wall, whereas in lobar collapse there is little change in the shape or position of the density in question. If the pleural fluid is loculated, the decubitus view may not be helpful.

Distinguishing between pleural effusion and lobar collapse is easy at CT (Figure 4-68), but CT is only occasionally needed because the lateral decubitus view is a simpler method. At CT the density of the collapsed lobe is usually appreciably greater than that of the pleural effusion, particularly if intravenous contrast enhancement is used.[84,85] Also, blood vessels and bronchi can be traced into the compressed lung.

Cicatrization atelectasis

Pulmonary fibrosis leads to loss of lung volume owing to a combination of lung destruction and loss of compliance. There are many different patterns, the precise radiographic features depending on the distribution of the primary disease.

Following infection a lobe may lose volume because of destruction and fibrosis (Figure 4-69). Bronchial occlusion and dilatation may accompany the fibrosis, and if the disease affects the dependent portions of the lung, the patient may have the clinical features of bronchiectasis. Naidich and associates[85] have pointed out the following features of cicatrization atelectasis, all of which are best seen at CT, but which may be inferred from plain chest radiographs: no endobronchial mass; dilated, thick-walled bronchi within the atelectatic lobe; and associated extensive pleural thickening. The loss of volume can be severe and may be greater than is generally observed in lobar collapse caused by endobronchial obstruction.

Widespread interstitial pulmonary fibrosis causes generalized loss of lung volume. Reticulonodular shadowing of the lung is then the dominant radiographic feature (see the section "Widespread Nodular, Reticulonodular, and Honeycomb Shadowing" later in this chapter).

Round atelectasis

Round atelectasis, also known as folded lung,[3] is a form of chronic atelectasis that resembles a mass, which can be confused with bronchial carcinoma.[12,89,105] The process is frequently associated with asbestosis (see p. 441),[50,80,124] but it has been reported in other benign conditions.[113]

The mechanism that leads to the formation of round atelectasis is uncertain. One suggestion[45] is that a pleural exudate is the initial event and the resulting effusion causes passive atelectasis of the adjacent lung. The pleural surface of the atelectatic lung may then develop fibrinous adhesions to the adjacent parietal pleura and across any adjacent fissure. As the pleural effusion clears, the atelectatic lung is trapped and may even fold in on itself, leading to the condition of round atelectasis. This mechanism may occur with pleural effusion caused by asbestos exposure and with effusions caused by tuberculosis, other infections, therapeutic pneumothorax, uremic pleuritis,[135] or pulmonary infarction, as well as with idiopathic pleural exudates. An alternative explanation is that a sheet of pleural fibrosis alone is responsible: as the fibrosis matures, it contracts, causing atelectasis of the underlying lung.[17,50] Probably both mechanisms operate in different patients.[50]

The major feature on plain films and CT scans* is the peripheral location of the opacity based against the pleura. The pleura is thickened both over the lesion and sometimes in other parts of the pleural cavity (Figures

*References 7, 19, 31, 72, 77, 124.

4-70 to 4-72). The lesions, which may be single or multiple,[7] are most often encountered in the lower lobes.[50] However, in one large series the most common site was the lingula followed by the middle lobe.[50] Plaques of thickened or calcified pleura resulting from asbestos exposure may be seen in both thoracic cavities. Round atelectasis is usually oval in configuration and angled with respect to the pleural surface (Figure 4-70). The top, bottom, and lateral edges of the atelectatic mass are usually smooth, but the edge pointing to the hilum is often irregular or ill defined and blends with the bronchi and blood vessels that lead into the atelectatic mass. The feature of greatest diagnostic value, and one that is almost universally present,[7] is the distortion and displacement of the blood vessels and bronchi leading to, and immediately adjacent to, the area of round atelectasis. The vessels and bronchi appear pulled toward the lesion, are more numerous than normal for that portion of lung, and show

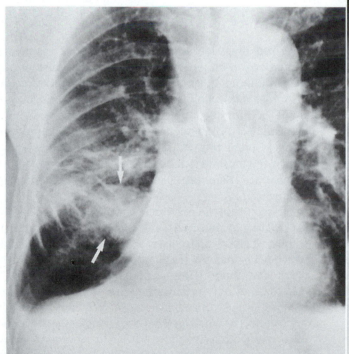

A

B

FIGURE 4-70
Round atelectasis (arrows) shows typical features of oval mass aligned obliquely in contact with pleural thickening along posterior chest wall. A, Posteroanterior radiograph. B, Lateral radiograph.

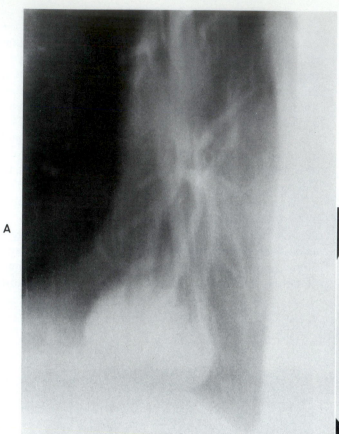

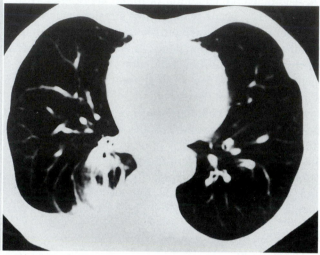

FIGURE 4-71
Round atelectasis showing distortion of blood vessels entering lesion. **A,** Lateral tomogram. **B,** Computed tomographic scan.

a characteristic curvilinear configuration (Figure 4-71), sometimes referred to as a comet tail sign. Air bronchograms are seen within the opacity at CT in the majority of cases; the thinner the CT section, the more frequently air bronchograms are identified. Calcifications may be seen within the area of rounded atelectasis, and the volume of the affected lobe is usually reduced. Round atelectasis, like lung cancer and many other pathologic conditions, enhances after intravenous injection of contrast agent; contrast enhancement is therefore of little diagnostic value.[120] Although usually static, round atelectasis may grow,[111] shrink,[45] or even resolve spontaneously.[50,135]

CT (Figures 4-71 and 4-72) shows all the features to advantage and may show that the pleural disease is more extensive than was previously appreciated. The CT findings may be definitive, so that further investigation to exclude carcinoma as the cause of the mass is unnecessary.

Discoid atelectasis

Discoid atelectasis (also known as plate or linear atelectasis) is a form of peripheral pulmonary collapse that is not secondary to bronchial obstruction. First described by Fleischner,[25] and therefore sometimes known as Fleischner lines, the atelectasis is disk or plate shaped (Figure 4-73). Sometimes the disk is so large that it crosses the whole lobe. Discoid atelectasis may be single or multiple. It usually abuts the pleura and is perpendicular to the pleural surface[130] with no predisposition to point toward the hilum. The thickness ranges from a few millimeters to a centimeter or more, and the lesions are therefore usually seen as line or band shadows.

Westcott and Cole[130] reviewed the mechanisms that lead to discoid atelectasis. The subject is complex, but put simply, discoid atelectasis is due to hypoventilation, which leads to alveolar collapse. Alveoli lying at the lung bases and those lying posteriorly are most likely to collapse, not only because they have the lowest volume but also because the physiologic mechanisms responsible for keeping the small airways and alveoli open are at their most vulnerable in these sites. In addition, discoid atelectasis may be seen in the lingula in patients with substantial collapse of the left lower lobe, possibly because of kinking of bronchi in the hyperexpanded lingula.[88,90]

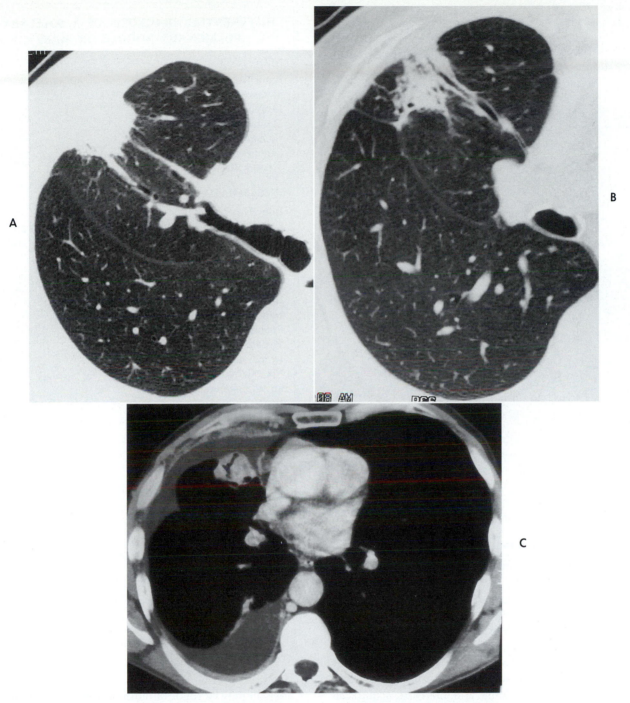

FIGURE 4-72
Round atelectasis. **A,** Computed tomographic (CT) scan showing pleura-based mass with crowding of vessels supplying lesion. **B,** Adjacent section showing air bronchogram within lesion. **C,** Contrast-enhanced CT scan in another patient showing contrast enhancement and air bronchograms.

Discoid atelectasis is common, particularly in hospitalized patients. Since it reflects hypoventilation, it is seen in a large variety of conditions, including general anesthesia, painful breathing (for example, pleurisy following surgery or trauma), pneumonia, pulmonary edema, pulmonary embolism, neoplasms, masses or fluid in the abdomen, or shallow breathing from any other cause.

Discoid atelectasis by itself is usually of little clinical importance, although the associated conditions may be of great significance. Occasionally, discoid atelectasis is of such magnitude and so widespread that it causes hypoxemia. It should be remembered that plain films may substantially underestimate the extent of the condition. Following general anesthesia, for example, widespread

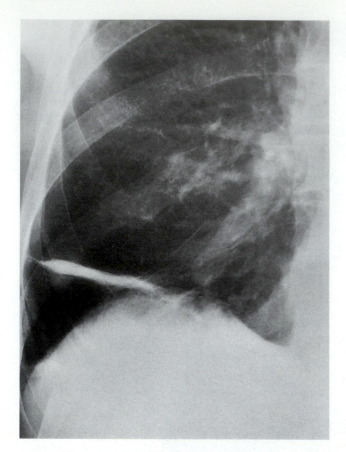

FIGURE 4-73
Discoid atelectasis showing typical bandlike shadow.

discoid atelectasis can be clinically significant, even in cases that show few signs on plain chest radiograph.

Compressive and passive atelectasis

The distinction between compressive and passive atelectasis is not clear cut. The lung is inherently elastic, and therefore any process that requires increased space within the thorax either compresses the lung or allows it to retract. For example, pleural effusion or pneumothorax allows retraction of the adjacent lung. With large pleural effusions the lobes surrounded by fluid may collapse completely. Large masses in any intrathoracic location frequently press on the lung and therefore acquire an ill-defined margin because of adjacent atelectatic lung. Similarly, emphysematous bullae are often surrounded by atelectatic lung. The shape of the collapsed lung in these cases reflects the cause.

PULMONARY MASS (NODULE)

The term "pulmonary mass" refers to an essentially spherical opacity with a well-defined edge. Although the Fleischner Society[26] and others use the word "nodule" for a lesion of up to 3 cm in diameter and "mass" for a lesion greater than 3 cm in diameter, the two terms are used interchangeably in this book.

DIFFERENTIAL DIAGNOSIS OF A SOLITARY PULMONARY NODULE OR MASS

NEOPLASTIC

Bronchial carcinoma*
Metastasis*
Lymphoma*
Carcinoid*
Hamartoma
Benign connective tissue and neural tumors, e.g., lipoma, fibroma, neurofibroma, mesothelioma

INFLAMMATORY

Infective
Granuloma,* e.g., tuberculosis, histoplasmosis, cryptococcosis, blastomycosis, coccidioidomycosis, nocardiosis, dirofilariasis
Round pneumonia, acute or chronic*
Lung abscess*
Hydatid cyst*
Noninfective
Rheumatoid arthritis*
Wegener's granulomatosis*
Lymphomatoid granulomatosis*
Necrotizing sarcoidal angiitis
Lipoid pneumonia
Behçet's disease*

CONGENITAL

Arteriovenous malformation
Sequestration*
Lung cyst*
Bronchial atresia with mucoid impaction

MISCELLANEOUS

Pulmonary infarct*
Round atelectasis
Intrapulmonary lymph node
Progressive massive fibrosis*
Mucoid impaction*
Hematoma*
Amyloidosis*

*May cavitate.

Masses may be single or multiple and range in diameter from a few millimeters to many centimeters. Sometimes it is impossible to distinguish between airspace shadowing and a mass. The multiple 2 to 5 mm nodules seen with widespread nodular or miliary shadowing are a separate category and are discussed in the section "Widespread Nodular, Reticulonodular, and Honeycomb Shadowing" later in this chapter.

Solitary pulmonary nodule

The solitary pulmonary nodule (SPN) is one of the most common diagnostic problems in pulmonary radiology. The possible diagnoses are numerous (see the box above

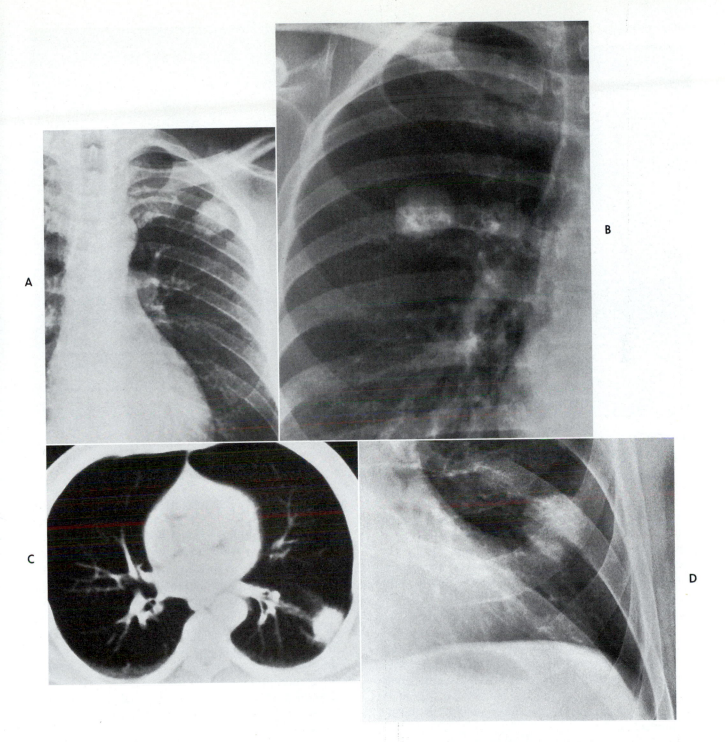

FIGURE 4-74
Examples of various causes of solitary pulmonary nodules. **A,** Bronchial carcinoma. **B,** Hamartoma.
C, Organizing pneumonia. **D,** Pulmonary infarct.

and Figure 4-74), but over 95% fall into one of three groups:

1. Malignant neoplasms, either primary or metastatic
2. Infectious granulomas, either tuberculous or fungal
3. Benign tumors, notably hamartomas

Nonradiologic factors are clearly vital when considering the differential diagnosis. For example, bronchogenic carcinoma is rare in patients under 30 years of age and is relatively rare in nonsmokers. Also, it is important to know whether the patient has an extrathoracic tumor of a type known to metastasize to the lungs. The chance that

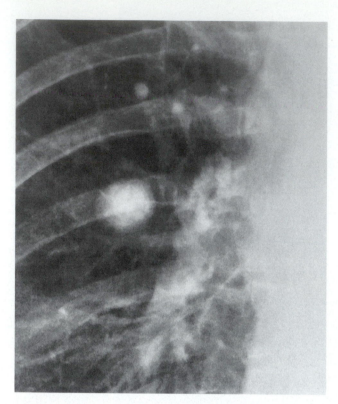

FIGURE 4-75
Concentric laminated calcification in histoplasmosis granuloma.

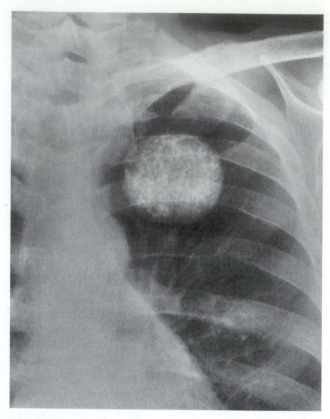

FIGURE 4-76
Popcorn calcification in pulmonary hamartoma.

an SPN is a metastasis is low if the patient does not have a known primary tumor and there are no clinical features to indicate the presence of such a tumor at the time of presentation. In the large multicenter series reported by Steele,[115] only 3 of 877 resected SPNs were metastases, and in a study of 705 patients without a known primary tumor,[40] only 1 nodule was a metastasis.*

Patients with SPN are generally divided into two groups: those in whom malignant neoplasm is either unlikely or impossible, and those in whom malignancy remains a serious consideration. If there is no known extrathoracic primary tumor, the problem usually centers on deciding whether or not the patient has a primary malignant neoplasm of the lung, notably bronchial carcinoma.

Morphologic features such as size, shape, and cavitation, which can help in making the distinction, are discussed later, but it must be emphasized that no radiologic features are entirely specific for lung carcinoma (or other primary malignant tumors). There are,

however, four imaging observations that exclude the diagnosis with reasonable certainty: (1) the detection of a benign pattern of calcification; (2) a rate of growth that is either too slow or too fast for the nodule to be primary lung cancer; (3) a specific shape, namely clear-cut identification of enlarged feeding and draining vessels, indicating that the nodule is an arteriovenous malformation, and the specific appearances of round atelectasis (see p. 93); and (4) unequivocal evidence on previous serial chest radiographs that the nodule is the end stage of a previous benign process, such as infarction or granulomatous infection.[70]

CALCIFICATION. Concentric (laminated) calcification is virtually specific to tuberculous or fungal granulomas (Figure 4-75).

Popcorn calcifications, which are randomly distributed, often overlapping, small rings of calcification, are seen only when cartilage is present in the nodule, a feature specific to hamartoma and cartilage tumors (Figure 4-76).

Punctate calcification occurs in a variety of benign and malignant lesions: granuloma, hamartoma, amyloidoma, carcinoid, and metastases, particularly osteosarcoma. Punctate calcification is rare in bronchial carcinoma unless the tumor engulfs a preexisting calcified granuloma (Figure 4-77), in which case the calcification is virtually never randomly distributed or at the center of the nodule. However, the presence of one or more focal

---

*There is an important practical point here. Imaging tests that search for an occult extrathoracic primary tumor to help in deciding whether an SPN is or is not a metastasis will inevitably be counterproductive. With such low probability of an extrathoracic primary tumor, the false-positive results of the various imaging procedures would swamp the true-positive findings, even with tests of high specificity.

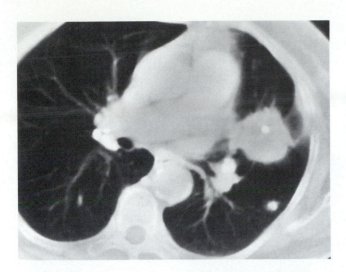

FIGURE 4-77
Bronchial adenocarcinoma. Computed tomographic scan shows focal calcification in granuloma engulfed by tumor. Note completely separate similar granuloma in lung behind tumor and widespread calcification in hilar lymph nodes.

calcifications arranged in an eccentric group, while reducing the probability of lung cancer, does not eliminate the possibility of carcinoma.

Widespread or uniform calcification of a nodule substantially reduces the probability of bronchial carcinoma, particularly if the calcification is present in sufficient quantities to be visible on plain chest radiographs, although, as discussed below, it does not exclude the diagnosis entirely. Calcification is better seen on plain chest radiographs taken with low kilovoltage than high kilovoltage. A few radiologists use fluoroscopic equipment because the patient can be maneuvered to project the nodule clear of overlying ribs or other structures and because fluoroscopic equipment can operate at low kilovoltage and often has x-ray tubes with fine focal spot sizes. Fluoroscopy in various oblique projections can be used to locate a nodule before tomography if the position is not certain from standard radiographs.

Conventional tomography provides better visualization of calcification within a nodule than plain chest radiography,[51] but it has largely been superseded by CT. Attempts to analyze the nodule using single- or dual-energy digital radiography remain experimental.[11]

CT, because of its superb density discrimination, is the most sensitive commercially available technique for the detection of calcification in an SPN (Figure 4-78). Siegelman and co-workers[110] were the first to use CT to identify nodules as benign by determining the CT density of the nodule. They measured the CT density of 91 nodules classed as uncalcified on conventional tomography and derived the "representative CT (RCT) number," a number representing the CT density of the 32 most dense contiguous voxels. On their scanner the average RCT number for bronchogenic carcinomas was 92 Hounsfield

units (HU); no carcinoma had an RCT number higher than 147 HU. Of the 33 benign lesions examined, 20 had an RCT number higher than 164 HU (164 HU was derived by adding 4 standard deviations to 92 HU). These authors concluded that CT densitometry of pulmonary nodules would be a clinically useful technique for determining that an SPN was benign, if it had an appropriately high RCT number. Proto and Thomas,[93] using a different scanner, confirmed these results but recommended 200 HU for the cutoff point above which the diagnosis of a benign lesion could be made.

The technical factors involved in measuring the attenuation values of intrathoracic nodules are complex.[137,138] The measurements can vary from scanner to scanner and may even vary from one examination to another with the same machine. Density measurements are also affected by the patient's anatomy and size, the diameter and position of the nodule within the chest, and the reconstruction algorithm being used.[53,137,138] Also, the CT density of the nodule is inversely related to the kilovoltage, a phenomenon that is more pronounced at high concentrations of calcium.[53] To overcome these problems, Zerhouni and associates.[136] designed a reference phantom that can simulate the shape, dimensions, and density of the thorax at multiple levels (Figure 4-79). Cylinders of various diameters made of resins containing radiopaque materials can be placed within the phantom. The CT density of the commercially available cylinders corresponds to 185 HU. The aim is to simulate the conditions under which an SPN is measured, so as to provide a meaningful measure of the density of the patient nodule regardless of equipment- or patient-related variations. The technique involves taking 1.5 to 2 mm sections of the patient's nodule. A reference cylinder with a diameter close to that of the patient's nodule is placed within the phantom in a position that corresponds to the nodule's position in the thorax. The chest wall thickness of the phantom is adjusted to correspond to the patient's body habitus, and the phantom is then scanned using the same table position and the identical technical factors used for the examination of the patient. The images of the patient's nodule and the simulated nodules are then compared. If more than 10% of the voxels in the patient nodule are higher in density than the density of the reference cylinder, the nodule is considered to be above the critical density level. If the high density either is uniformly distributed or clearly lies centrally within the nodule, the nodule is almost certainly not a bronchial carcinoma. As with plain film and conventional tomographic evaluation, however, CT scans may show eccentric calcification within a bronchial carcinoma if the tumor engulfs a preexisting calcified granulomatous lesion.[93,109] There are also well-documented reports of widespread or amorphous calcification in bronchial carcinoma (Figure 4-80).* Mahoney[73] and Zerhouni[138] and

---

*References 38, 59, 73, 74, 116, 118, 138.

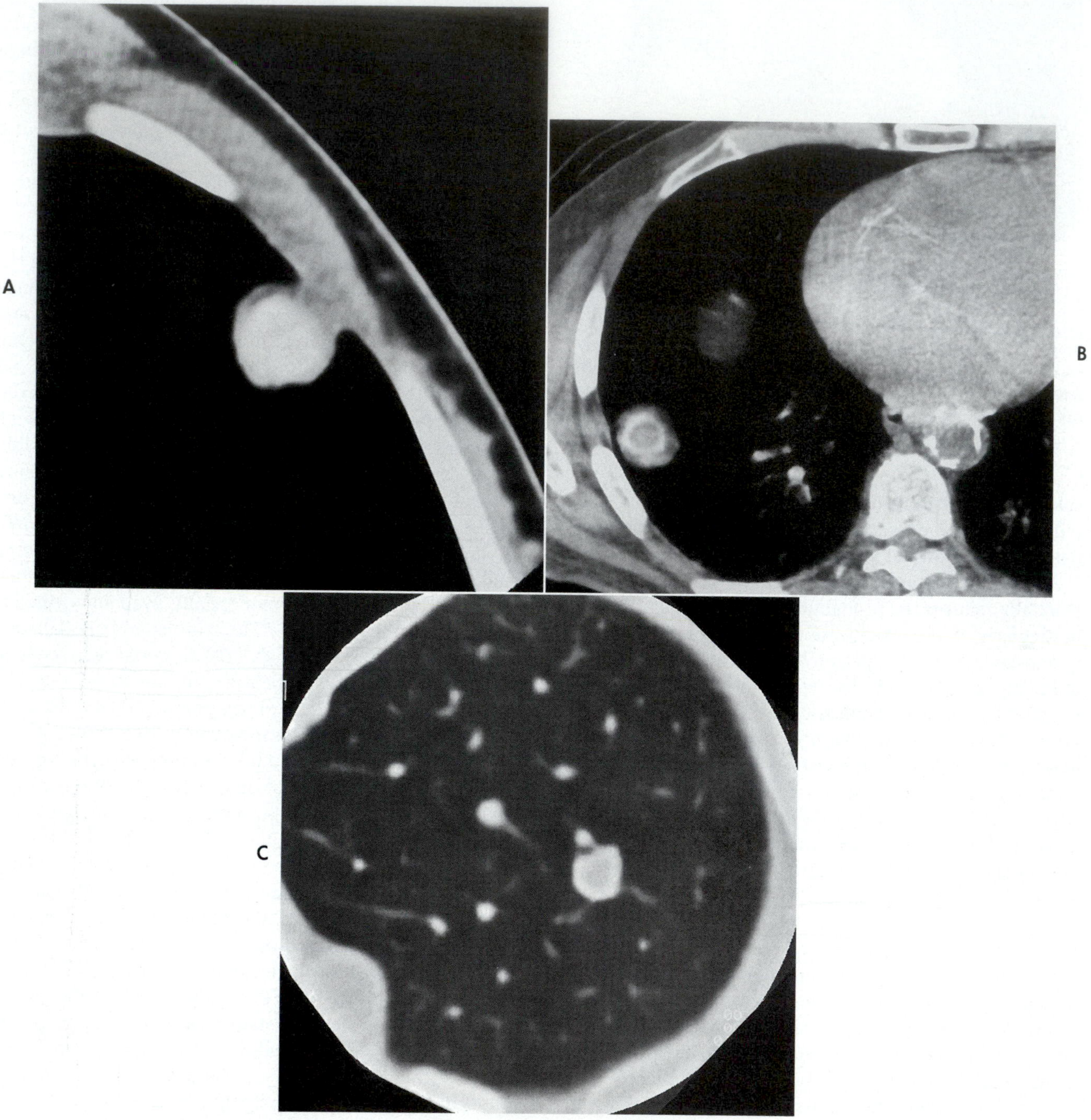

FIGURE 4-78
A, Computed tomographic (CT) scan of asymptomatic histoplasmoma showing that central portion of nodule is heavily calcified. It was not recognizably calcified on plain chest radiography. B, Another asymptomatic histoplasmoma that was not recognizably calcified on plain chest radiography, in which CT scanning shows concentric ring calcification within nodule. C, CT scan of another similar nodule that required comparison with a phantom. Over 90% of nodule was 100 HU denser than phantom nodule.

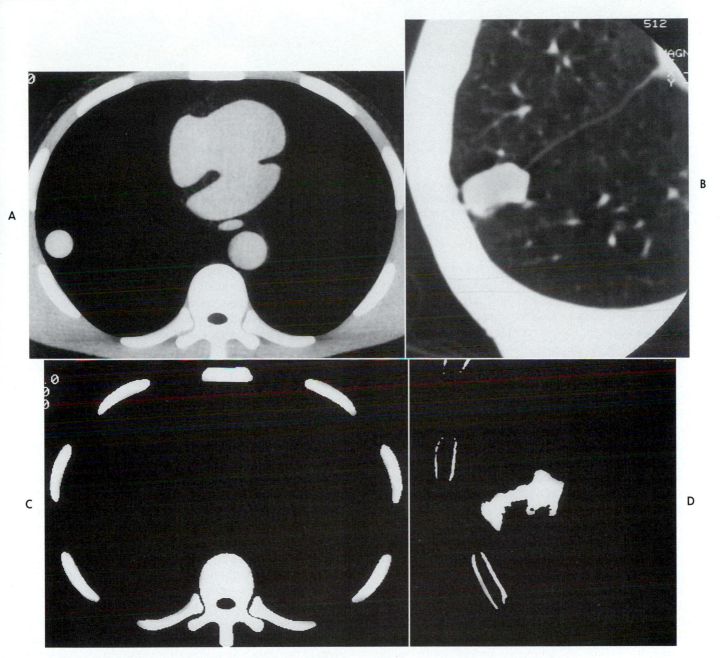

FIGURE 4-79
Computed tomography (CT) nodule densitometry. **A,** CT of phantom with phantom nodule placed in same position as patient nodule. **B,** Patient nodule at conventional window and level settings. **C,** Proportion of pixels above critical threshold is established by reducing window width to minimum possible and establishing the level at which phantom nodule is no longer visible. **D,** Patient nodule is then viewed at this critical level, and proportion of pixels still visible is compared with true size of the patient nodule.

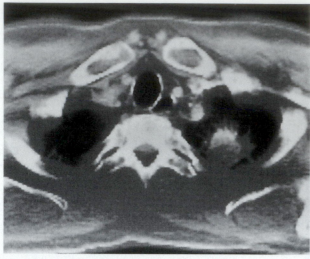
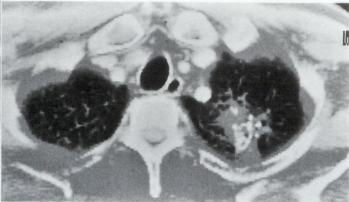

FIGURE 4-80
Adjacent computed tomographic sections showing primary adenocarcinoma of lung with widespread punctate, conglomerate calcification. On histologic examination, calcification proved to be necrotic foci of tumor. Further example of calcification in bronchogenic carcinoma can be seen in Figure 8-11. (Courtesy Dr. John Pitman, Williamsburg, Va.)

their co-workers found that 6% to 7% of patients with bronchial carcinoma showed calcification within the tumor mass at CT. To avoid misdiagnosing a benign lesion in the few cases of carcinoma that show calcification, the radiologist should consider a high-density lesion benign only if the edge of the nodule is smooth.[109,138] Also, evaluation of a nodule by CT scanning rarely yields a confident diagnosis of benign disease if the nodule is larger than 3 cm. CT densitometry is therefore not recommended for lesions greater than 3 cm in diameter or for nodules with irregular or spiculated borders,[138] nor is it recommended in patients with nodules that are known to be increasing in size at a rate compatible with bronchial carcinoma. Such nodules should not be automatically regarded as benign just because they show calcification.

Nodule densitometry is a useful diagnostic aid[52,127] and is more sensitive in detecting calcification than thin section CT alone[67] (just how necessary the reference phantom is with the newest scanners has, however, been questioned[16,103]). Even with good technique and awareness of the pitfalls, however, some malignant nodules will be misdiagnosed as benign: in the series of Swenson and associates at least 10 of the 85 nodules diagnosed as benign by nodule densitometry proved to be malignant.[118] Despite the introduction of nodule densitometry, in most cases the decision to perform surgery is still based on plain film characteristics, particularly the rate of growth of the nodule.[103]

RATE OF GROWTH. Bronchial carcinomas usually take between 1 and 18 months to double in volume, the average time being 4.2 to 7.3 months, depending on cell type.[30] A few take as long as 24 months, and a few double

their volume in under a month.* Therefore doubling times faster than 1 month or slower than 18 months make bronchial carcinoma unlikely but do not exclude the diagnosis completely (Figure 4-81).

Doubling times faster than 1 month suggest infection,[87] infarction,[87] histiocytic lymphoma,[20] or a fast-growing metastasis from tumors such as germ cell tumor and certain sarcomas.[14] Doubling times slower than 18 months suggest processes such as granuloma, hamartoma, bronchial carcinoid, and round atelectasis. One point to bear in mind is that primary lung tumors close to 1 cm are usually invisible on plain chest radiographs, so that it is not possible to calculate an accurate growth rate for small nodules developing in areas that were previously normal.

Patients who have an SPN with a rate of growth that is either indeterminate or in keeping with bronchial carcinoma, who do not have an extrathoracic primary tumor, and who do not have a benign pattern of calcification in the nodule form a discrete group. The proportion of SPNs that fall into this category varies greatly according to geography and the type of patients being seen. In the series reported by Good[39,40] this group formed 40% of patients with an SPN. In Europe the proportion is higher than in the United States because of the virtual absence of fungal granulomas. Figures from the large series of Steele,[115] Good and Wilson,[40] Bateson,[2] Toomes and associates,[121] and Huston and Muhm[51] suggest that between 25% and 50% of such cases in patients above 35 years of age will prove to be bronchial carcinoma, with

---

*References 10, 30, 79, 112, 117, 129.

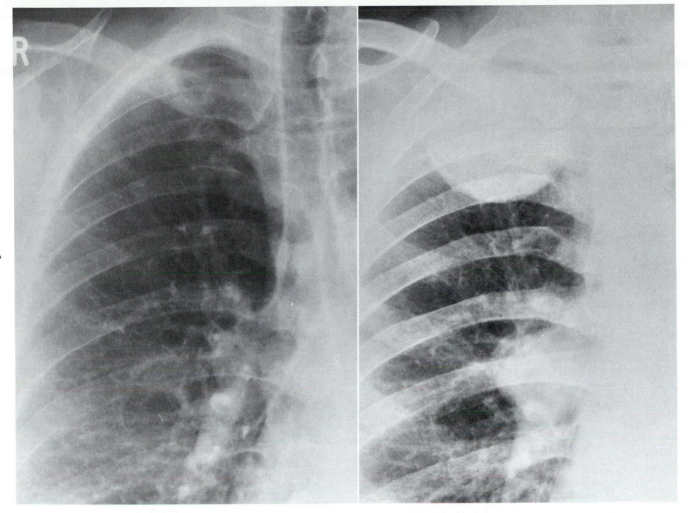

FIGURE 4-81
Unusually rapid growth of primary large cell carcinoma of lung. The two views (**A** and **B**) were taken
2 months apart.

the remainder composed of the various lesions listed in the box on p. 96.

SIZE, SHAPE, AND CAVITATION. An SPN resulting from lung cancer can be any size, but those less than 9 mm in diameter are virtually never visible on plain chest radiographs. Hence a well-defined nodule of smaller size that is clearly seen is likely to be calcified and is therefore likely to be benign. When the nodule is between 1 and 4 cm in diameter, there are no diagnoses in the box on p. 96 that can be excluded on the basis of size alone. Above 4 cm the probabilities begin to change dramatically. Most solitary nodules larger than 4 cm in diameter are bronchial carcinoma. With few exceptions, SPNs above this size that are not primary or metastatic carcinoma prove to be lung abscess, Wegener's granulomatosis, lymphoma or lymphomatoid granulomatosis, round pneumonia (see p. 70), round atelectasis (see p. 92), or hydatid cyst (see p. 218). The first three resemble one another and may be indistinguishable from bronchial

carcinoma. The latter three, however, may show characteristics that permit a specific diagnosis to be made.

There is substantial disagreement in the literature over how much attention should be paid to the shape of a nodule when trying to determine the nature of an SPN. Good[39] believed that calcification and lack of growth were the only important factors, and many subsequent authors have agreed. However, certain shapes do provide important diagnostic information and, in practice, shape is often used to make management decisions.[51]

A very irregular edge makes bronchial carcinoma highly probable,[140] and a corona radiata, the appearance of numerous strands radiating into the surrounding lung, is almost specific for bronchial carcinoma.[51] Exceptions do exist, however. For example, infectious granulomas and other chronic inflammatory lesions may have a very irregular edge (Figure 4-82) and may even show a corona radiata.

Lobulation and notching are seen with almost all the

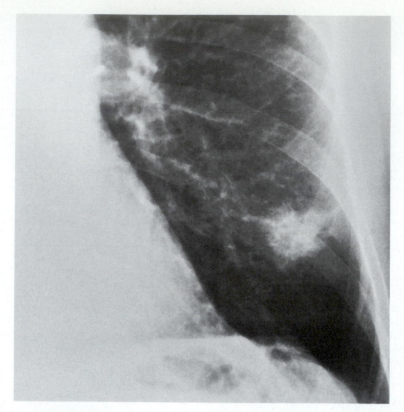

FIGURE 4-82
Organizing pneumonia, showing irregular edges and nodular shape. The lesion was removed because it was believed to be a bronchial carcinoma preoperatively.

diagnostic possibilities, but the more pronounced these signs are, the more likely it is that the lesion is a bronchogenic carcinoma. A well-defined, smooth, non-lobulated edge is most compatible with hamartoma, granuloma, and metastasis. It is rarely seen in patients with bronchial carcinoma.

If on high-quality tomography the opacity is composed of one or more narrow linear shadows without focal nodularity, the chances of bronchial carcinoma are so low that benignancy can be assumed and follow-up is the only recommendation.[51]

The presence of a pleuropulmonary tail in peripherally located nodules is not helpful in the differential diagnosis of an SPN. Much has been written about the "tail" sign because at one time it was believed to have potential diagnostic value. However, it turns out that the sign is seen with a variety of lesions, both malignant and benign, particularly granulomas.[5,49,107,140]

The precise relationship between an SPN and the adjacent pulmonary vessels may prove helpful in deciding the nature of the nodule, although at the moment this method of assessment has not been fully evaluated. Mori and associates,[81] using multiplanar CT reconstructions, found that involvement of a pulmonary vein was a feature of lung cancer and infrequent in nonneoplastic lesions.

Similarly, as discussed on p. 350, small pulmonary arteries can be shown by CT to lead directly to metastases.

AIR BRONCHOGRAM AND CAVITATION WITHIN A SOLITARY PULMONARY NODULE. The presence of air bronchograms visible on plain film radiography within an SPN makes lung carcinoma (other than bronchioloalveolar carcinoma) or metastasis an unlikely diagnosis. They may be seen in bronchioloalveolar carcinoma, lymphoma, and pseudolymphoma, as well as in round pneumonia and round atelectasis. Air bronchograms are, however, seen with some frequency in primary bronchial carcinoma on CT, particularly high-resolution CT.

CONTRAST ENHANCEMENT. SPNs caused by malignant neoplasm show a greater degree of contrast enhancement with iodinated contrast media than benign nodules. Littleton and co-workers[71] first demonstrated this phenomenon using very high-quality conventional tomography together with film densitometry, and Swensen and associates[119] subsequently showed that all 23 of the malignant nodules in their study enhanced by more than 20 HU whereas only one of seven benign nodules showed that degree of enhancement.

A preliminary report on the use of Gd-DTPA-enhanced MRI noted that tuberculoma showed ring enhancement of the capsule with no enhancement of the caseous center, whereas lung cancers did not show ring enhancement.[104]

ADJACENT BONE DESTRUCTION. Invasion of adjacent bone by a pulmonary mass is almost pathognomic of bronchogenic carcinoma. Actinomycosis and occasionally tuberculosis[55] or fungal disease are the alternative possibilities.

CAVITATION. A cavity is defined by the Fleischner Society[26] as a gas-filled space within a zone of pulmonary consolidation, a mass, or a nodule. There may or may not be an accompanying fluid level.

As can be seen from the box on p. 96, many of the causes of SPN may result in cavitation, so the presence or absence of cavitation is of limited diagnostic value. The morphology of the cavity may, however, be helpful. Lung abscess and benign lesions in general have a thinner, smoother wall than cavitating malignant neoplasms. Woodring and Fried[134] compared 126 patients with solitary cavities and found that when the maximum wall thickness was 16 mm or above only 4 cases were benign, whereas 35 cases were due to malignant neoplasm. Conversely, with a maximum wall thickness of 4 mm or less, only 2 cases were malignant neoplasm and 30 were benign. Between 4 and 16 mm the cases were almost equally divided, with 33 cases benign and 22 malignant.

In practice the diagnosis of acute lung abscesses usually depends on the clinical features together with the appearance of a cavity evolving in an area of undoubted pneumonia. The more difficult problem is distinguishing between cavitating neoplasm and chronic inflammatory processes. Fungal pneumonia, particularly cryptococcosis and blastomycosis, and various collagen vascular diseases, particularly Wegener's granulomatosis and rheumatoid arthritis, can appear identical to carcinoma of the lung and may even be indistinguishable clinically.

A cavity may contain a mass within it, the air within the cavity forming a peripheral halo or crescent of air between the intracavitary mass and the cavity wall, giving rise to the so-called air crescent or air meniscus sign. Intracavitary masses are most often due to fungal mycetomas. Other causes include complicated hydatid disease, blood clot (as a result of tuberculosis, laceration with hematoma, or infarct), abscess and necrotizing pneumonias (particularly caused by *Klebsiella* or *Aspergillus fumigatus*), and necrotic neoplasm.

CT is a useful modality for diagnosing the presence of a cavity within the lung but has little or no advantage over plain films in diagnosing the nature of the cavity because it rarely limits the differential diagnosis. CT can, however, distinguish with great reliability between lung abscess and empyema when this is a problem on plain chest radiograph (see Chapter 6).[1,114]

MANAGEMENT OF A SOLITARY PULMONARY NODULE. The management of a patient with an SPN depends heavily on radiologic factors.[8,9,43,44,128] The algorithm shown in Figure 4-83 is designed for patients in the cancer age group who have an SPN less than 3 cm in diameter with either no symptoms or symptoms compatible with lung cancer. The presence of visible calcification clearly conforming to a benign pattern or stability of size on retrospective review of chest radiographs (or CT scans) for 18 months is sufficient indication of a benign lesion to obviate surgical resection. Solitary masses larger than 3 cm, unless they show the specific features of round atelectasis or a congenital malformation such as an arteriovenous malformation, are so frequently lung cancers that benign entities should be diagnosed with caution.

If the nodule does not show any of the preceding features, thin section CT (CT densitometry) can be used to look for occult calcification. The presence of occult calcification must be interpreted with care and is not absolute proof of benignity, but because the probability of cancer becomes low when more than 10% of nodule shows calcification, it is prudent to institute a watch and wait program.[70] CT densitometry is not advised for nodules greater than 3 cm in diameter.

Nodules that are still indeterminate after all the preceding considerations have been taken into account may be benign, a solitary metastasis, or a bronchogenic carcinoma. Further distinction is difficult. Fine needle aspiration biopsy, as discussed on p. 894, can prove that a nodule is malignant but can only rarely exclude that possibility. Therefore resection of the nodule, with appropriate prior staging, is the recommended course of action.

RING SHADOWS AND CYSTS

Ring shadows are characterized by an annular shadow with a central transradiancy. There is no clear distinction between cavitating consolidation, cavitary masses, and ring shadows, but the term "ring shadow" is usually restricted to discrete round or oval spaces within the lung surrounded by a wall less than 2 mm thick.[36] Such ring shadows can be of any size and may be single or multiple, unilocular or multilocular. They may contain fluid, which is manifest as an air-fluid level. The term "cyst" is often reserved for cavitary lesions that are more than 1 cm in diameter and show a thin wall (less than 4 mm of uniform thickness). By common use the word "pneumatocele" is confined to air cysts that develop after lung trauma, infection, and hydrocarbon ingestion (Figure 4-84). CT may be useful in selected cases to define more accurately the shape, position, and contents of a ring shadow. CT is particularly helpful in distinguishing between loculated pneumothorax and an intrapulmonary cyst or bleb and in demonstrating any related pulmonary disease.[95] The causes of ring shadows and cysts are listed in the lefthand box on p. 107.

MULTIPLE PULMONARY NODULES

The differential diagnosis for multiple pulmonary nodules is given in the righthand box on p. 107. Once again the list is long, but well over 95% of multiple pulmonary

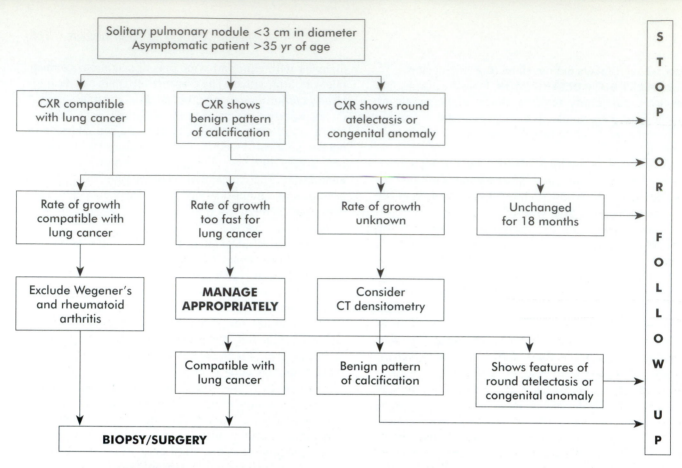

FIGURE 4-83
Algorithm for management of asymptomatic solitary pulmonary nodule less than 3 cm in diameter in patient in cancer age group.

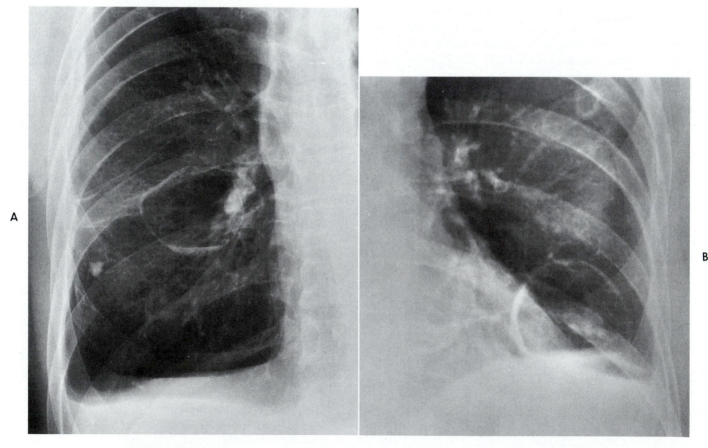

FIGURE 4-84
Pneumatoceles. **A,** Caused by previous trauma. Small amount of fluid is present in pneumatocele. **B,** Resulting from staphylococcal pneumonia. Second, smaller pneumatocele is seen in left middle zone.

PULMONARY RING SHADOWS AND CYSTS OF MORE THAN 1 CM

CONGENITAL

Sequestered segment
Bronchogenic cyst
Cystic adenomatoid malformation

INFECTION

Bacterial abscess, notably anaerobic bacteria, *Staphylococcus*, tuberculosis
Pneumocystis carinii pneumonia
Fungal abscess, notably coccidioidomycosis
Echinococcus cyst

COLLAGEN VASCULAR DISEASE

Rheumatoid necrobiotic nodule
Wegener's granulomatosis

NEOPLASM

Bronchial carcinoma, notably squamous cell
Metastases, notably squamous cell
Laryngeal papillomatosis with pulmonary spread
Malignant lymphoma

THROMBOEMBOLISM

Infarct, notably septic infarcts

AIRWAY DISEASE

Blebs and bullae
Bronchiectasis (individual ring shadows caused by dilated bronchi)

PNEUMATOCELES

Pulmonary laceration
Pulmonary infection, notably staphylococcal
Hydrocarbon ingestion

MIMICS

Bowel herniation
Empyema
Lucite plombage

DIFFERENTIAL DIAGNOSIS OF MULTIPLE PULMONARY NODULES AND MASSES

NEOPLASTIC

Malignant
Metastatic carcinoma or sarcoma*
Malignant lymphoma,* lymphomatoid granulomatosis*
Multifocal neoplasms, e.g., Kaposi's sarcoma and bronchioloalveolar carcinoma
Benign
Hamartomas, chondromas
Laryngeal papillomatosis*
Benign metastasizing leiomyoma

INFLAMMATORY

Infective
Granulomas,* e.g., tuberculosis, histoplasmosis, cryptococcosis, coccidioidomycosis, nocardiosis
Round pneumonias, particularly fungal and opportunistic infections*
Lung abscesses,* especially septicemic
Septic infarcts
Atypical measles
Hydatid cysts*
Paragonimiasis*
Noninfective
Rheumatoid arthritis,* Caplan's syndrome*
Wegener's granulomatosis*
Sarcoidosis
Drug-induced

CONGENITAL

Arteriovenous malformations

MISCELLANEOUS

Progressive massive fibrosis*
Hematomas*
Amyloidosis*
Pulmonary infarcts*
Mucoid impactions*

*May cavitate.

nodules are the result of either metastases or tuberculous or fungal granulomas. The great majority of patients who have multiple noncalcified nodules on plain chest radiographs have metastases, and the presence of an extrathoracic primary tumor is usually known or at least suspected because of clinical findings. The larger and more variable in size the nodules, the more likely they are to be neoplastic. The same statistic does not apply to nodules too small to be seen on plain chest radiographs and found only by CT; here the probability of multiple metastases is lower and the chance of multiple granulomas is higher.

The following points may help in limiting the diagnostic possibilities listed in the box above on the right:

1. Cavitation is seen in many of the disorders listed in the box. The major diagnostic value of cavitation is that it indicates an active disease process. It is not a feature of incidental lesions such as inactive granulomas or multiple hamartomas.

2. Metastases are usually spherical and have well-defined outlines (Figure 4-85), although metastases with irregular margins and poorly defined edges are occasionally encountered. Metastases vary considerably in size.

3. Nodules containing calcification are usually infectious granulomas, notably tuberculous or histoplasmal granulomas. On rare occasion, they are multiple hamartomas or even amyloidomas. Thus nodules that are extensively calcified can, with one important exception, be assumed to be benign. The one exception is in patients with osteosarcoma or chondrosarcoma, because metastases from these tumors frequently calcify (Figure 4-86). In the case of metastases from chondrosarcoma, the calcification may be the typical popcorn calcification of cartilage tumors. If calcified and noncalcified nodules coexist, the presence of the calcified nodules cannot be

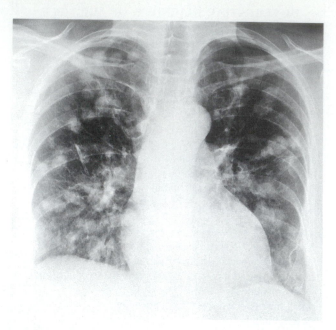

FIGURE 4-85
Multiple pulmonary nodules owing to metastases from squamous cell carcinoma of salivary gland.

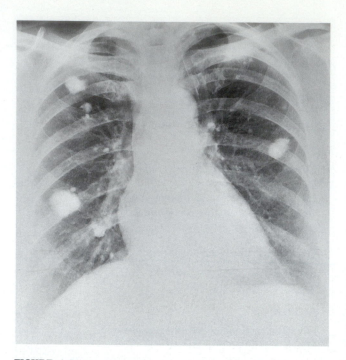

FIGURE 4-86
Multiple calcified pulmonary nodules caused by metastases from extrathoracic osteosarcoma.

taken as proof that the noncalcified nodules are also benign.

4. Growth rate can be a useful discriminator between granulomas and metastases. Strauss,[117] reviewing the literature on the doubling times of pulmonary metastases, found a wide range, much wider than for primary lung carcinoma: 11 to 745 days for breast carcinoma, 11 to 150 days for colorectal carcinomas, 10 to 205 days for testicular tumors, 17 to 253 days for soft tissue and bone sarcomas. Thus, to exclude the diagnosis of metastasis in the case of tumors with slow growth rates requires that the nodule in question remained the same size or grew very slowly over several years. Some tumors, for example, choriocarcinoma and osteosarcoma, may show explosive growth, doubling their volumes in less than a month.[56] Others, for example, thyroid carcinoma, can remain the same size for a very long time.[76]

5. Small pulmonary granulomas are common in the histoplasmosis belt of the United States. Elsewhere in the United States granulomas are less common. In parts of the world where fungal disease is uncommon, pulmonary granulomas are also uncommon and when encountered are usually caused by tuberculosis. Thus the likelihood of pulmonary nodules being granulomas is strongly influenced by where the patient has lived.

6. Multiple arteriovenous malformations can usually be diagnosed with certainty by noting large feeding arteries and draining veins. They are very rare and are usually part of the Osler-Weber-Rendu syndrome.

7. Sarcoidosis can produce multiple nodular shadows in the lung that may resemble metastases or lymphoma.

The uniform size, the slightly ill-defined edge, and the accompanying hilar and mediastinal adenopathy are important indicators of the diagnosis of sarcoidosis (Figure 4-87). Also, the age of the patient and the frequent lack of signs and symptoms of malignant neoplastic disease often help resolve the diagnostic difficulty.

8. Multiple nodules are a feature of coal worker's pneumoconiosis and chronic silicosis. When greater than 1 cm in diameter, they are known as progressive massive fibrosis. The presence of widespread nodulation in the rest of the lung and the characteristic shape and location of progressive massive fibrosis lead to a specific diagnosis in virtually every case (Figure 4-88). (The nodules of Caplan's syndrome may be more difficult to distinguish from metastases because the other signs of coal worker's pneumoconiosis are often absent.) The patient's work history is important in diagnosing progressive massive fibrosis because, on rare occasion, neoplasms (Figure 4-89) or inflammatory conditions such as Wegener's granulomatosis cause a similar appearance.

LINE SHADOWS AND BAND SHADOWS

The term "band shadow" is usually reserved for linear opacities more than 5 mm in diameter, whereas linear densities with a diameter less than 5 mm are simply referred to as line shadows. The causes of abnormal line and band shadows are given in the box on p. 110. A feature that may help in limiting the differential diagnosis is branching, a phenomenon seen only with vascular malformations and bronchiectatic or

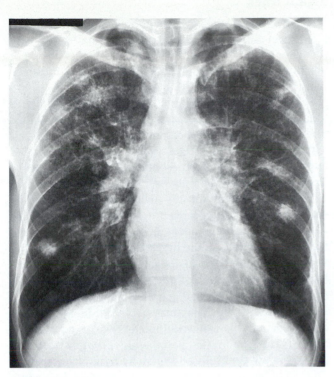

FIGURE 4-87
Multiple pulmonary nodules caused by sarcoidosis. Note that there is also hilar and mediastinal adenopathy. As is so often the case in sarcoidosis, the nodules are ill defined in outline and much the same size.

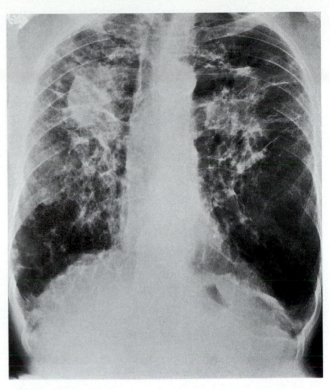

FIGURE 4-88
Multiple pulmonary nodules caused by progressive massive fibrosis *(PMF)*. Diagnosis here is easy because of characteristic location, shape of PMF shadows, background nodulation of lungs, and generalized emphysema.

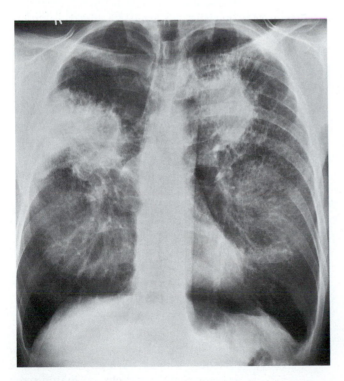

FIGURE 4-89
Bilateral primary bronchial carcinoma mimicking progressive massive fibrosis.

obstructed, secretion-filled airways (bronchoceles and mucoid impaction).

Of the items listed in the box on p. 110, only septal lines, mucoid impaction, and bronchial wall thickening are discussed further in this section. The other entities are described elsewhere in this book.

Mucoid impaction

With mucoid impaction (bronchocele, mucocele), a bandlike opacity is seen pointing to the hilum. The lesion is often very broad (1 cm or more) and is sharply marginated with branches that have been likened to fingers, the so-called gloved finger shadow. The presence of such shadows always implies bronchial obstruction.[22] Mucoid impactions are found typically in allergic bronchopulmonary aspergillosis (Figure 4-90) but may be seen with a variety of obstructing lesions provided collateral air drift maintains aeration to the affected segment, namely primary and metastatic carcinoma of the lung, bronchial carcinoid, tuberculous bronchostenosis, broncholithiasis, bronchial atresia (Figure 4-91), sequestration, pulmonary bronchogenic cyst, and foreign body aspiration.[22,133] If the surrounding lung collapses or consolidates, the shadow of the mucoid impaction becomes invisible because of the silhouette effect.

CAUSES OF LINE SHADOWS AND BAND SHADOWS

Skinfold
Clothing, tubes, etc.
Wall of a bleb or pneumatocele
Bronchial or peribronchial thickening, the causes of which are:
   Pulmonary edema
   Lymphangitis carcinomatosa
   Asthma
   Bronchiolitis
   Cystic fibrosis
   Bronchiectasis
Bronchocele (mucoid impaction)
Pleuroparenchymal scar
Discoid atelectasis
Anomalous blood vessels or feeding and draining vessels to arteriovenous malformation
Thickening of pleural fissures
Pleural tail associated with pleural nodule
Septal lines (Kerley lines), the causes of which are given in the box on p. 111.

Septal lines

The interstitial septa of normal lungs are not visible on plain chest radiographs except in a very small minority of thin patients and then only on very high-quality films. For practical purposes it is only when the septa are thickened that they become visible (Figure 4-92).[47,122]

Septal lines were first described by Kerley in patients with pulmonary edema.[65] He named them A, B, and C lines because he was not certain of their anatomic basis. "Septal lines" is a more descriptive and therefore better term because the lines represent thickening of connective tissue septa within the lung.[47,123]

The septa are anatomically divided into deep septa and peripheral interlobular septa.[101] Deep septal lines (Kerley A lines) are up to 4 cm in length, radiate from the hila into the central portions of the lungs, do not reach the pleura, and are most obvious in the middle and upper zones. Interlobular septal lines (Kerley B lines) are usually less than 1 cm in length and parallel one another at right angles to the pleura. They may be very thin and sharply defined or may be a few millimeters wide and fairly ill defined. They are located peripherally in contact with the pleura but are generally absent along fissural surfaces.[101] They may be seen in any zone but are most frequently observed at the lung bases.

The term "C lines" has been dropped because the crisscrossing lines that Kerley designated as C lines are actually due to superimposition of many B lines.[47]

Septal lines must be distinguished from blood vessels. Blood vessels are not seen in the outer centimeter of the lung, whereas interlobular septa, even though narrower in diameter, may be visible by virtue of having substantial

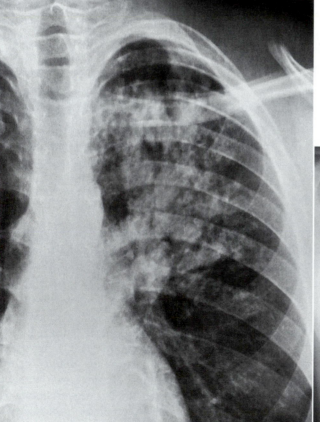

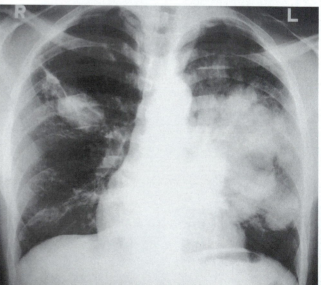

FIGURE 4-90
Mucoid impaction (mucocele) of bronchi in two patients with allergic bronchopulmonary aspergillosis. Branching tubular shadows, such as those illustrated in **A**, have been likened to "gloved finger." **B**, Dilated bronchi mimicking pulmonary mass lesions.

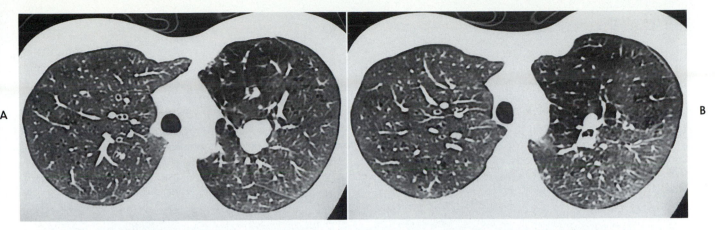

FIGURE 4-91
Bronchocele in the left upper lobe presumed to be secondary to congenital bronchial atresia. Adjacent computed tomographic sections showing branching pattern typical of bronchocele and emphysema distal to bronchocele.

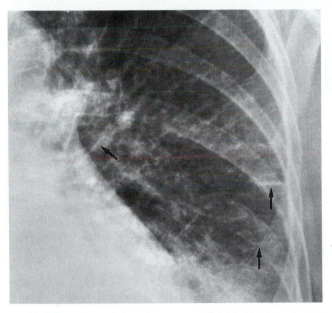

FIGURE 4-92
Septal lines caused by pulmonary edema. B lines are short horizontal lines at lung periphery *(vertical arrows)*. A lines are lines radiating from hila *(oblique arrow)*.

depth along the trajectory of the x-ray beam. Similarly, the deep septa are seen as narrow dense lines because they are thin sheets of tissue seen end on. Blood vessels of such a narrow diameter would be either invisible or of extremely low density. Another helpful feature is that deep septal lines, though they may interconnect or superimpose, do not branch in as uniform a manner as blood vessels.

The identification of septal lines is an extremely useful diagnostic feature, since thickened septal lines occur in few conditions (see the box at right above). If transient or

---

CAUSES OF SEPTAL LINES (KERLEY LINES)
Pulmonary edema
Lymphangitis carcinomatosa and malignant lymphoma
Congenital lymphangiectasia
Viral and mycoplasmal pneumonia
Interstitial pulmonary fibrosis from any cause
Pneumoconiosis
Sarcoidosis
Lymphocytic giant cell interstitial pneumonitis
Late-stage hemosiderosis
Lymphangiomyomatosis (tuberous sclerosis)

rapid in development, they are virtually diagnostic of interstitial pulmonary edema.

In addition to the classic septal lines described previously, Kreel and associates[68] described thick septal lines caused by pulmonary edema that resemble discoid atelectasis.

Bronchial wall (peribronchial) thickening

In normal chest radiographs the walls of the bronchi beyond the hila are invisible unless they are end on to the x-ray beam. The few that are seen end on have a thin, well-defined, ringlike wall. Portions of the walls of the lobar bronchi within the hila are also routinely visible in the healthy person. The posterior wall of the bronchus intermedius should measure less than 3 mm.[92] Since this portion of the bronchial tree is clearly seen in lateral chest radiographs and is even easier to identify on CT scans, it is a useful site at which to assess central bronchial wall thickening.

Intraparenchymal bronchial wall thickening on plain chest radiography (Figure 4-93) is seen in disorders of the bronchial wall such as recurrent asthma, allergic as-

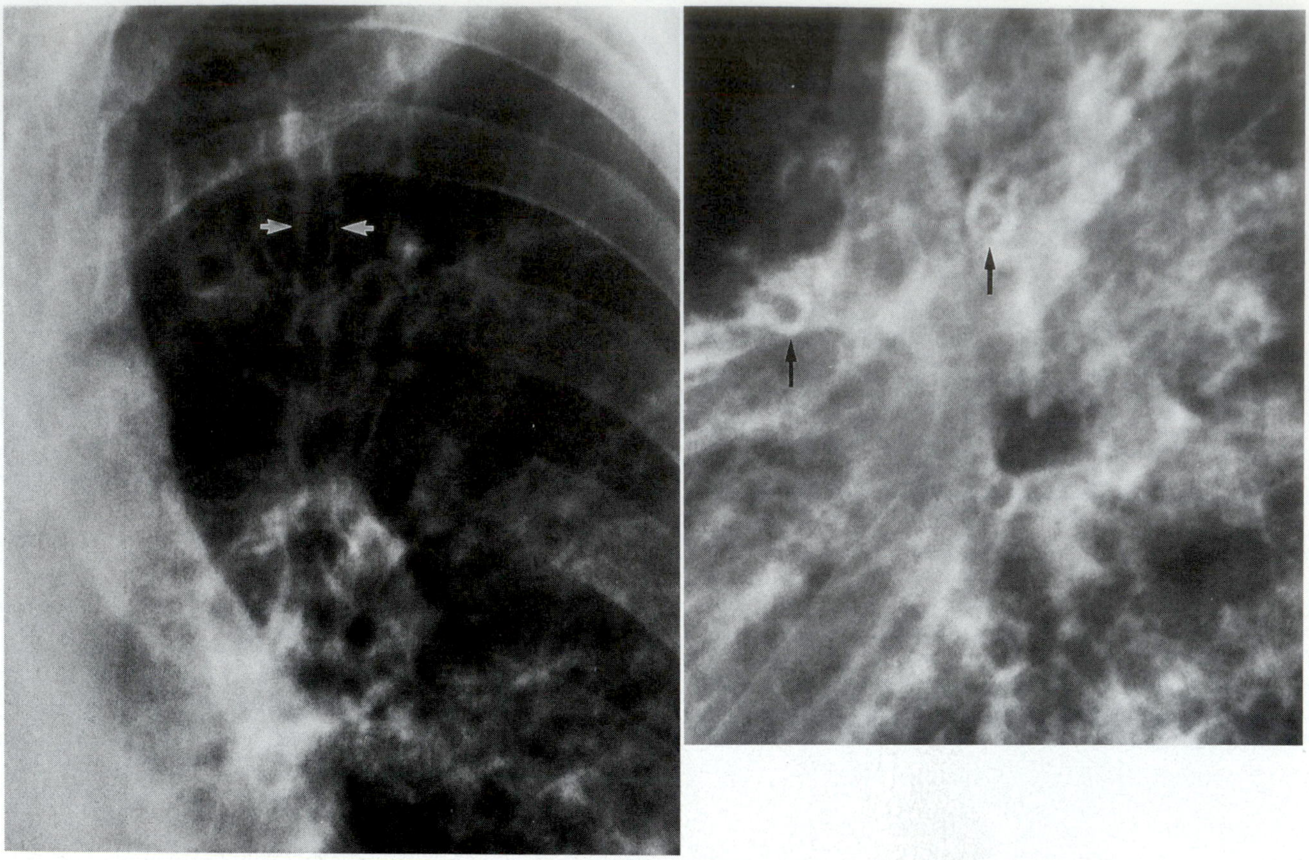

FIGURE 4-93
Bronchial wall thickening in patient with cystic fibrosis. **A,** Posteroanterior radiograph. Arrows point to parallel lines of thickened walls of representative moderately dilated bronchus. **B,** Lateral radiograph. Arrows point to two examples of ring shadows caused by thickened bronchial walls seen end on.

pergillosis, bronchiolitis, cystic fibrosis, and bronchiectasis. It is also seen with edema or neoplastic infiltration (lymphangitis carcinomatosa) of the peribronchial tissues. It is useful to note whether the bronchial wall thickening is associated with bronchial dilatation, a combination that would establish the diagnosis of bronchiectasis as the cause of the bronchial wall thickening.

If edema or inflammatory or neoplastic cells infiltrate the peribronchial interstitial space, the combination of the bronchial wall and the widened interstitium produces visible bronchial and peribronchial thickening. Not only do the bronchial walls appear thick, they are also usually less well defined. Although bronchial wall thickening may resemble two adjacent blood vessels, the distinction can be made by identifying the parallelism of the walls and by observing Y-shaped branching parallel walls where the bronchi divide.

WIDESPREAD NODULAR, RETICULONODULAR, AND HONEYCOMB SHADOWING

Many diseases cause widespread small pulmonary opacities. Occasionally the chest radiograph provides enough information for a specific diagnosis, but usually it is just one piece of information in a complex of clinical features and laboratory tests.

The numerous small opacities seen on chest radiographs probably do not represent the individual lesions seen by the pathologist: the pattern appears to be produced by summation. Carstairs[6] showed that when multiple superimposed sheets of small nodules are radiographed, the resulting image is a reticulonodular pattern. This observation is important because it suggests that the size and shape of the nodules and lines on the chest radiograph are not a precise reflection of the responsible lesion.

Many descriptive terms have been proposed for widespread small lung shadows on the plain chest radiograph; only a few are widely accepted. For diagnostic purposes the following are recommended[66]:

1. Nodular pattern. This pattern consists of clearly defined round or irregular opacities, ranging in diameter from 1 mm (Figure 4-94) to 1 cm. Such lesions may be partially or completely calcified. Above this size the nodules represent individual lesions, the differential diagnosis for which is discussed on p. 105.

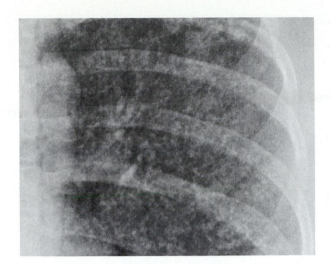

FIGURE 4-94
Nodular pattern in patient with miliary tuberculosis.

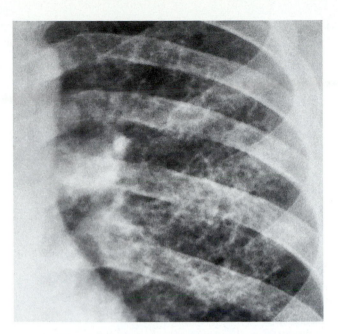

FIGURE 4-95
Reticular pattern in patient with histiocytosis X.

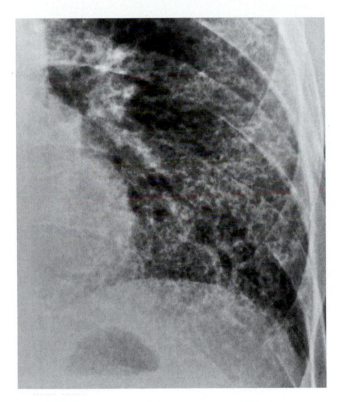

FIGURE 4-96
Reticulonodular pattern in patient with interstitial pulmonary fibrosis caused by scleroderma.

2. Reticular or linear pattern. This pattern consists of fine linear shadows, usually in an irregular netlike arrangement forming rings with thin walls surrounding spaces of air density (Figures 4-95 and 4-96). Kerley A and B lines (septal lines) are a specific form of linear shadowing of great diagnostic importance because their presence is reliable evidence of interstitial thickening.

3. Reticulonodular pattern. This pattern represents a mixture of nodular and reticular patterns. The nodules are usually irregular in shape. A reticulonodular appearance is much more common than a purely reticular or purely nodular pattern.

4. Honeycomb pattern. This term should be used to describe a coarse reticular or reticulonodular pattern in which the crisscrossing linear elements surround small cystic airspaces. This appearance corresponds to what the pathologist calls honeycomb lung when viewing the surface of a cut section of lung (Figure 4-96).

5. Cystic or ring pattern. Widespread ring shadows of 1 cm or more are diagnostic of cystic bronchiectasis (Figure 4-97).

6. Haze or ground-glass pattern. These terms refer to a diffuse increase in density that reduces the clarity of the pulmonary vessels but does not efface their outlines entirely. The diaphragmatic outlines may similarly be less clear cut. The abnormality is often subtle, and the sign can be highly subjective. It is a nonspecific sign of mild alveolar filling, interstitial thickening, or a combination of the two and is therefore seen in a large variety of conditions.

These six terms usually provide a reasonably accurate description of diffuse lung disease. They do not imply a specific disease process but are used to generate a differential diagnostic list.

Some authors have advocated two classes of diffuse lung disease, alveolar and interstitial, based on plain radiographic findings.[28,41] Alveolar disease is said to be manifest as opacities that are lobar, segmental, or "butterfly" in distribution.[21,46] The individual shadows have ill-defined margins (except when they contact a fissure), tend to coalesce, and may contain air bronchograms or air alveolograms. "Acinar" shadows, it is claimed, are distinctive enough to narrow the differential diagnosis of

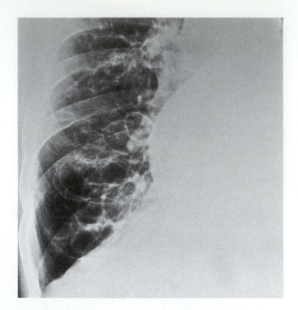

FIGURE 4-97
Cystic pattern in patient with cystic bronchiectasis.

DIFFUSE BILATERAL SMALL NODULAR OPACITIES OF THE LUNGS (MILIARY PATTERN)

Miliary tuberculosis
Nontuberculous infection, notably:
    Histoplasmosis
    Blastomycosis
    Coccidioidomycosis
    Cryptococcosis
    Nocardiosis
    Viral infection
Bronchiolitis obliterans
Pneumoconiosis, notably:
    Coal worker's pneumoconiosis
    Silicosis
    Siderosis
    Berylliosis
    Stannosis
Sarcoidosis
Metastases
Histiocytosis X
Amyloidosis
Alveolar microlithiasis

---

pulmonary opacities to diseases that cause filling of the alveolar airspaces. "Acinar" shadows are ill-defined coalescent nodular opacities, approximately the size of an acinus, that may initially appear as rosettes of small densities.[139] Interstitial disease, on the other hand, is manifest as a relatively well-defined linear, nodular, irregular, or honeycomb pattern together with septal lines, subpleural thickening, perivascular haze, or peribronchial cuffing.

The problem with this division is that widespread small shadows are often difficult to categorize into one or the other group on plain film findings. Many diseases that are classified by pathologists as alveolar show radiographic features of interstitial disease, and conversely there is an appreciable list of so-called interstitial diseases that show the radiographic signs ascribed to alveolar disease.[100] Even "acinar" shadows have been seen in interstitial processes.[57] Nevertheless, the division of diffuse lung disease into alveolar and interstitial patterns has its merits. The advent of high-resolution, thin section CT has refined the radiologist's ability to categorize diffuse lung disease into alveolar and interstitial patterns (see Chapter 5).

It is equally possible,[23] and in many instances preferable, to generate the differential diagnostic list according to the combination of radiographic signs without regard to an intermediate decision as to whether the process is predominantly alveolar or interstitial (see the lower box on the opposite page).

Other factors to note when deciding on differential diagnostic possibilities are zonal predominance, if any, and such signs as a reduction in lung volume, bronchial wall thickening, presence of airspace shadowing, masses, adenopathy, and pleural effusions. In some situations,

notably industrial lung disease, the problem is not diagnosis but quantification of the severity of disease. The International Labor Office and other groups have drawn up a classification based on reference radiographs to provide standardized descriptions (see Chapter 10).

The three boxes provide a general guide to the differential diagnosis of widespread nodular, reticular, reticulonodular, and honeycomb patterns on plain chest radiography. (The use of computed tomography for diagnosing diffuse lung disease is the principal topic of Chapter 5.) The boxes present a simplified approach, and it is important to realize that many exceptions exist. Certain generalizations can be applied with caution:

1. Acute conditions should be considered separately. If multiple linear markings appear acutely, that is, within hours or days, the most likely diagnosis is pulmonary edema, particularly cardiogenic edema, or pneumonia. In the immunocompetent patient with fever, viral or mycoplasmal pneumonia should be the major consideration. The line shadows indicate thickening of the interstitial septa of the lung, which may produce clear-cut septal lines or if numerous may appear as a reticular pattern owing to the superimposition of many thickened septa. In the case of cardiogenic edema the other signs of circulatory overload are often present.

2. The distribution of the shadows can be of help in differential diagnosis.

a. Reticulonodular shadows maximal at the bases or at the lung periphery, together with loss of lung volume but without pleural effusion or hilar adenopathy, are almost invariably due to one of the forms of interstitial pulmo-

CAUSES OF DIFFUSE BILATERAL RETICULONODULAR OPACITIES OF THE LUNGS

Idiopathic interstitial pulmonary fibrosis
Rheumatoid lung disease (interstitial fibrosis)
Scleroderma, dermatomyositis, systemic lupus erythematosus
Drug reaction/noxious gases (acute or fibrotic stages)
Extrinsic allergic alveolitis (acute or fibrotic stages)
Pneumoconiosis, notably:
    Coal worker's pneumoconiosis
    Silicosis
    Asbestosis
    Berylliosis
Extrinsic allergic alveolitis
    Acute stage
    Fibrotic stage
Sarcoidosis
Histiocytosis X
Interstitial pneumonia, notably:
    Fungi, particularly histoplasmosis
    Mycoplasma pneumoniae
    Viruses

Chronic aspiration
Bronchiolitis obliterans
Pulmonary edema
Lymphangitic spread of carcinoma or lymphoma
Lymphangiomyomatosis (tuberous sclerosis)
Lymphocytic interstitial pneumonitis, Waldenstrom's macroglobulinemia
Amyloidosis
Hemosiderosis
    Idiopathic, Goodpasture's syndrome
    Secondary to mitral valve disease
Talc granulomatosis
Alveolar microlithiasis
Gaucher's disease
Alveolar proteinosis
Neurofibromatosis

SIGNS THAT LIMIT THE DIFFERENTIAL DIAGNOSIS OF DIFFUSE BILATERAL RETICULONODULAR OPACITIES OF THE LUNGS

Acute appearance of shadows suggests:
    Pulmonary edema (both cardiac and noncardiac)
    Pneumonia, notably mycoplasma, viral, or opportunistic
Lower zone predominance of the opacities together with decrease in lung volume suggests:
    Idiopathic interstitial pulmonary fibrosis
    Rheumatoid lung disease (interstitial fibrosis)
    Scleroderma, dermatomyositis, systemic lupus erythematosus (interstitial fibrosis)
    Drug reaction, noxious gases (fibrotic stage)
    Extrinsic allergic alveolitis (fibrotic stage)
    Asbestosis
    Chronic aspiration
Mid or upper zone predominance of the opacities suggests:
    Chronic tuberculous and fungal disease
    Pneumoconiosis (coal worker's, silicosis, berylliosis)
    Sarcoidosis
    Histiocytosis X
    Extrinsic allergic alveolitis (fibrotic stage)
    Ankylosing spondylitis (fibrosis)
Associated increase in lung volume or bullae suggests:
    Underlying emphysema
    Cystic fibrosis
    Histiocytosis X
    Lymphangiomyomatosis (tuberous sclerosis)
    Neurofibromatosis
Associated septal (Kerley) lines suggest:
    Pulmonary edema
    Lymphangitic spread of carcinoma or lymphoma
    Viral or mycoplasmal pneumonia

    Sarcoidosis
    Extrinsic allergic alveolitis
    Interstitial pulmonary fibrosis (idiopathic, collagen vascular disease, etc.)
    Pneumoconiosis (notably silicosis)
Associated hilar lymphadenopathy suggests:
    Sarcoidosis
    Lymphangitis carcinomatosa
    Lymphoma
    Infections, notably:
        Tuberculosis
        Viral
    Pneumoconiosis, notably:
        Silicosis
        Berylliosis
Associated hilar node calcification suggests:
    Sarcoidosis
    Silicosis
    Chronic tuberculosis or histoplasmosis
    Treated lymphoma
Associated pleural effusion suggests:
    Pulmonary edema
    Lymphangitic spread of carcinoma or lymphoma
    Collagen vascular disease
    Lymphangiomyomatosis (particularly if effusion is chylous)
    NOTE: Pleural effusions are notably absent in idiopathic interstitial pulmonary fibrosis
Associated pleural thickening suggests:
    Asbestosis, particularly if pleural calcification is present.

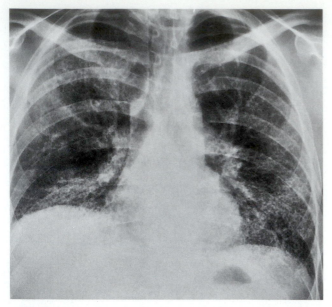

FIGURE 4-98
Interstitial pulmonary fibrosis in patient with scleroderma. Peripheral and basal predominance of shadowing, combined with small lung volumes, is typical of diffuse interstitial pulmonary fibrosis.

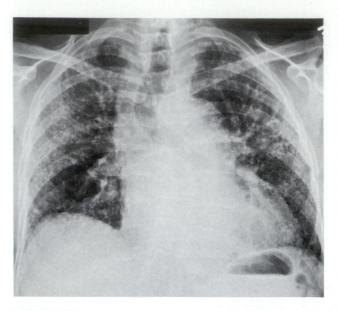

FIGURE 4-99
Idiopathic fibrosing alveolitis (interstitial fibrosis). This case demonstrates peripheral predominance of the shadowing. Note small volume of lungs.

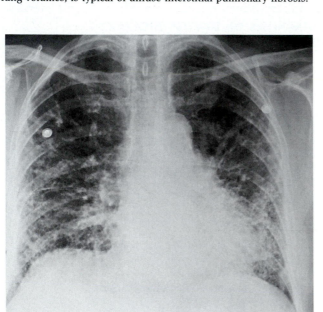

FIGURE 4-100
Diffuse interstitial pulmonary fibrosis in patient with rheumatoid arthritis. This example shows middle- and lower-zone predominance with only mild loss of volume.

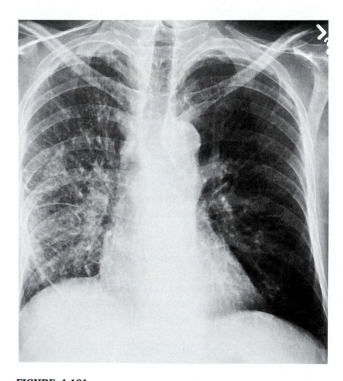

FIGURE 4-101
Lymphangitis carcinomatosa showing unilateral reticulonodular shadowing. Note fissural thickening and septal lines.

nary fibrosis (fibrosing alveolitis) (Figures 4-98 to 4-100). The major causes are idiopathic pulmonary fibrosis, asbestosis, rheumatoid lung disease, scleroderma, and dermatomyositis. Extrinsic allergic alveolitis and drug toxicity may also show this pattern. With chronic bilateral aspiration, bronchopneumonia may convert from consolidation to interstitial fibrosis and bronchiectasis, causing reticulonodular shadowing that may closely resemble late-stage idiopathic fibrosing alveolitis.

b. Unilateral reticulonodular shadowing without zonal or lobar predominance, particularly if septal lines are obvious and pleural effusions are present, is virtually diagnostic of lymphangitis carcinomatosa (Figure 4-101). Aspiration pneumonia may occasionally give this appearance, and sarcoidosis may rarely cause unilateral reticulonodular shadowing.

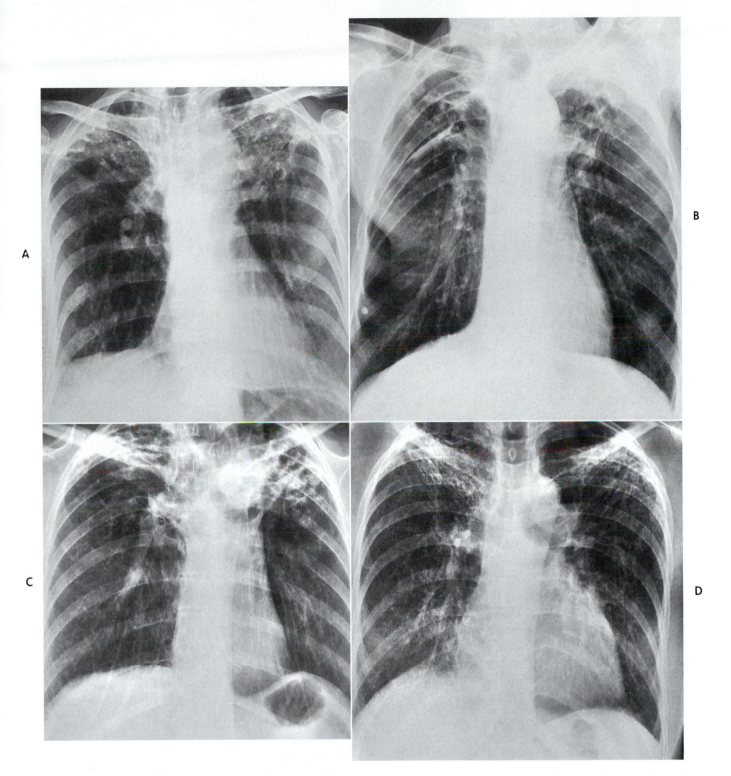

FIGURE 4-102
Coarse upper zone reticulonodular shadowing with fibrotic contraction of upper lobes. **A,** Tuberculosis. Note patchy small calcifications within fibrotic upper lobes. **B,** Histoplasmosis. **C,** Extrinsic allergic alveolitis: case of bird fancier's disease. **D,** Sarcoidosis.

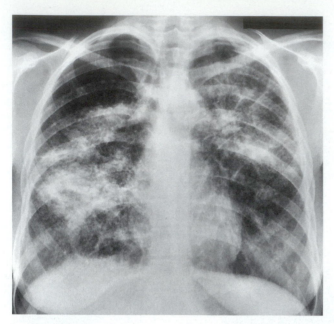

FIGURE 4-103
Pulmonary fibrosis caused by sarcoidosis. Midzone predominance radiating from hila with relative sparing of extreme apices and bases is typical of sarcoidosis.

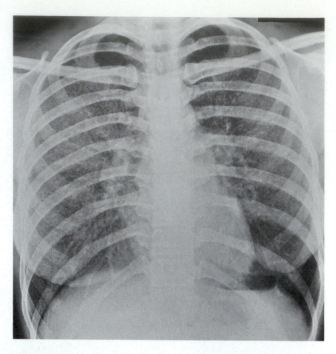

FIGURE 4-104
Uniformly distributed fine nodular shadowing in sarcoidosis. Note also bilateral hilar adenopathy.

c. Coarse reticulonodular shadowing maximal in the upper zones, particularly when associated with fibrotic contraction of the upper lobes, is seen particularly in chronic tuberculous (Figure 4-102, *A*) or fungal disease, notably histoplasmosis (Figure 4-102, *B*), the fibrotic end stage of extrinsic allergic alveolitis (Figure 4-102, *C*), sarcoidosis (Figure 4-102, *D*), ankylosing spondylitis, and radiation fibrosis.

d. Clear-cut reticular shadowing with pronounced upper zone predominance strongly suggests histiocytosis X, particularly if airspaces greater than 1 cm are seen.

e. Coarse shadowing radiating from the hila into the middle and upper zones, but sparing the extreme apices, is highly suggestive of sarcoidosis (Figure 4-103). The presence of hilar lymphadenopathy makes the diagnosis virtually certain.

f. Uniformly distributed, very small miliary nodules are virtually confined to miliary tuberculosis, sarcoidosis (Figure 4-104), or pneumoconiosis from coal, silica, or other inorganic dusts. The presence of bilateral lymphadenopathy makes sarcoidosis much the most likely, but does not exclude the other possibilities. Signs of mitral valve disease suggest the diagnosis of secondary hemosiderosis (Figure 4-105).

g. Miliary nodules maximal in the upper zones are strongly suggestive of coal worker's pneumoconiosis, silicosis, or other mineral dust pneumoconioses. The denser the nodules, the greater the likelihood of pneumoconiosis.

3. The components of the pattern itself may also be of help:

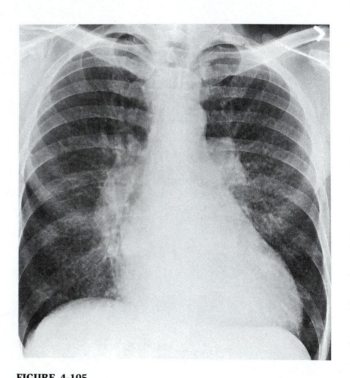

FIGURE 4-105
Uniformly distributed fine nodular shadowing caused by hemosiderosis in patient with mitral valve disease. Note other signs of mitral valve disease.

a. Obvious septal lines are seen only in the conditions listed in the box on p. 111. The most common cause by far is pulmonary edema; the next most frequent causes are lymphangitis carcinomatosa and interstitial pneumonia. Usually the other signs on the films, taken together with

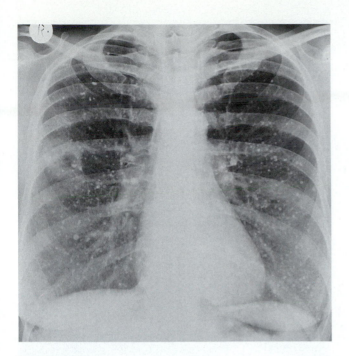

FIGURE 4-106
Multiple small calcifications in lungs caused by old healed varicella pneumonia. (Patient also has carcinoma of right upper lobe.)

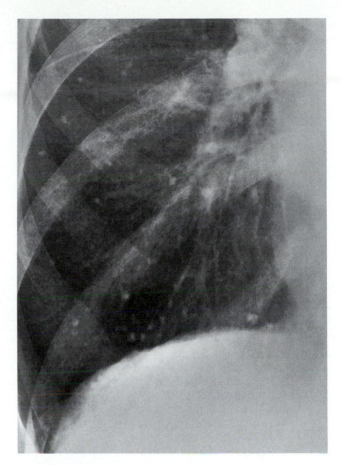

FIGURE 4-107
Multifocal ossification in lungs caused by long-standing mitral valve disease.

the knowledge of the patient's symptoms, permit one of the alternatives to be chosen, particularly if the chronicity or acuteness of the disease is known. For example, rapid appearance or disappearance of septal lines occurs only in pulmonary edema. Viral and mycoplasma pneumonia are associated with acute febrile illness, whereas relentless progression over weeks is virtually diagnostic of lymphangitis carcinomatosa.

b. True honeycomb pattern is virtually diagnostic of end-stage interstitial pulmonary fibrosis (fibrosing alveolitis) of many causes, histiocytosis X, or lymphangiomyomatosis. The honeycomb pattern is particularly well demonstrated at thin section high-resolution CT.

c. Multiple, partially, or totally calcified small nodular shadows are seen in only a few conditions. Most of the cases encountered are the result of calcification of widespread patchy pneumonia caused by disseminated histoplasmosis, tuberculosis, or varicella infection (Figure 4-106). Occasionally, pneumonia caused by coccidioidomycosis or blastomycosis calcifies. In each instance the responsible pneumonia will have occurred several years before. The presence of calcification indicates healing but, in the case of tuberculous and fungal infections, does not necessarily mean the disease is inactive.

Radiologically visible calcification in metastases is uncommon and for practical purposes is seen only with osteogenic sarcoma and chondrosarcoma.

d. High-density miliary nodulation may be seen with silicosis, stannosis, baritosis, or microlithiasis. The opacity of the nodules in baritosis may be even greater than calcific density.

e. Multifocal pulmonary ossification is occasionally seen in long-standing mitral valve disease (Figure 4-107). If the resulting small nodules clearly contain bony trabeculae, the diagnosis is easy. In most cases, however, only amorphous calcification can be recognized radiographically, and the distinction from postinfective calcification becomes impossible. Nowadays the entity is rare.

f. Cloudlike punctate calcification of the lung is seen only in alveolar microlithiasis (Figure 4-108) and hypercalcemia caused by conditions such as hyperparathyroidism, particularly secondary hyperparathyroidism resulting from renal failure (Figure 4-109).[58,78] In each instance the calcifications may be so minute that it is not possible to appreciate that the cloudlike shadows are in fact due to a myriad of calcifications. The appearance may then be confused with the other causes of multiple airspace shadows.

4. Certain combinations may make one diagnosis or a group of diagnoses more likely.

a. The combination of overinflation of the lung, widespread or basally predominant reticulonodular shadowing, and pleural effusion in a middle-aged woman is virtually diagnostic of the rare entity lymphangiomyomatosis (Figure 4-110).

b. The combination of small irregular shadows, maximal in the upper zone, with bronchial wall thickening

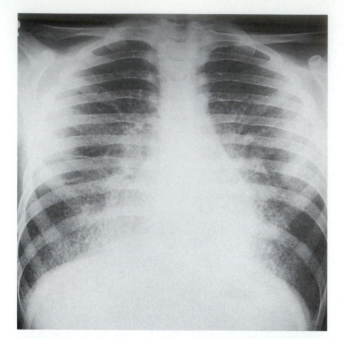

FIGURE 4-108
Alveolar microlithiasis. The innumerable fine pulmonary calcifications are so small that they appear cloudlike. (Courtesy Dr. Michael C. Pearson, London.)

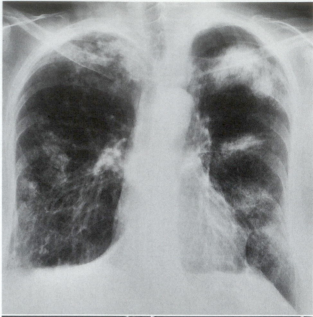

A

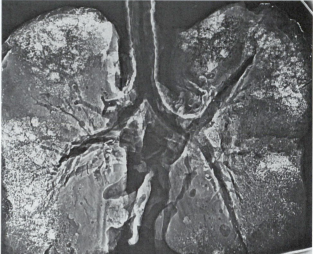

B

FIGURE 4-109
Pulmonary calcification caused by hyperparathyroidism. Fine calcifications are deposited in the lung in patchy fashion and produce coalescent cloudlike shadows. Patient died despite parathyroidectomy. **A,** Posteroanterior radiograph. **B,** Xerograph taken at autopsy shows pulmonary calcifications.

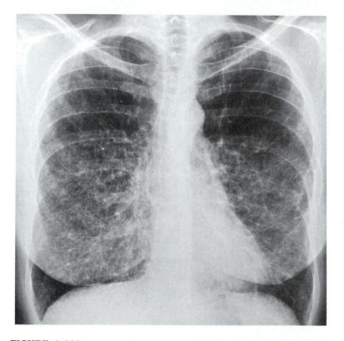

FIGURE 4-110
Lymphangiomyomatosis of lung. Typical example in middle-aged woman showing lower zone predominant reticulonodular shadowing and low, flat hemidiaphragms.

and overinflation of the lungs in a younger patient is virtually diagnostic of cystic fibrosis (Figure 4-111).

c. The presence of bilateral conglomerate shadows greater than 1 cm in diameter in the upper zones together with widespread or upper zone predominant

small nodules in the lungs makes pneumoconiosis virtually certain.

INCREASED TRANSRADIANCY OF THE LUNG

True increase in transradiancy of the lungs (that is, not due to technical factors) can be divided according to distribution into widespread, affecting both lungs; unilateral, affecting all or the majority of one lung; and focal, affecting a portion of one lobe only. (Increased transradiancy within a pulmonary opacity or contained within a cyst or cavity is a separate topic discussed earlier in this chapter.)

Widespread increase in transradiancy of both lungs is

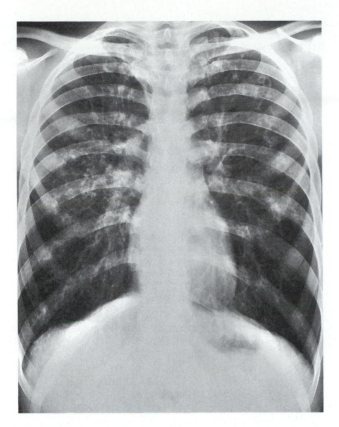

FIGURE 4-111
Cystic fibrosis. Note combination of small irregular shadows in upper lobe, bronchial wall thickening, and overinflation of lung in a 20-year-old man.

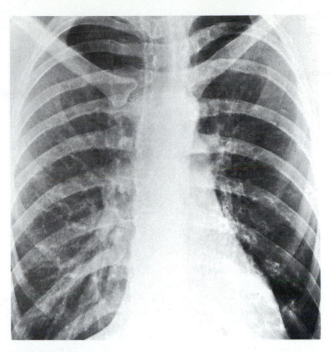

FIGURE 4-112
Swyer-James (McLeod's) syndrome. Note relative transradiancy of left hemithorax, reduction in size of hilar vessels, and small intrapulmonary vessels in left lung.

seen in two basic conditions: airway disease, notably emphysema, bronchiolitis, and asthma; and obstruction to blood flow from the right side of the heart, usually associated with right to left cardiac shunting, such as Fallot's tetralogy, Eisenmenger's physiology, or severe widespread peripheral pulmonary arterial stenoses. Massive pulmonary embolism is a theoretic possibility for widespread pulmonary oligemia but in practice is virtually never seen.

Focal increase in transradiancy is seen with emphysema and bullous disease and in some patients with pulmonary emboli.

Increased transradiancy of one lung (also known as unilateral hyperlucent lung) is a fairly commonly encountered radiographic finding. Basically, the causes may be subdivided as follows:

1. Radiographic artifact. Output of x-rays from the x-ray tube may not be uniform across the radiographic field. This so-called heel-toe effect is normally adjusted vertically so that output increases from the apices to the bases. If the heel-toe effect operates across the thorax, one hemithorax may appear more penetrated (that is, more transradiant) than the other. A similar appearance may result from slight rotation of the patient; the side to which the patient is rotated is the more penetrated, regardless of whether the film has been taken PA or AP. In both situations the relative exposures of the soft tissues,

especially around the shoulder girdles, should be compared. A clear-cut difference in penetration of these structures indicates that the explanation for increased transradiancy is technical rather than pathological.

2. Thoracic wall and soft tissue abnormalities. These are the most common cause of a unilateral hyperlucent lung (notably, a mastectomy on the ipsilateral side). Other causes include a congenital defect of the pectoral muscles (Poland syndrome).

3. Diminished vascular perfusion of the lung. A substantial reduction in vascular perfusion of one lung may cause that lung to be abnormally lucent. The causes may be either congenital (for example, aplasia of a pulmonary artery or hypoplasia of the lung) or acquired (for example, thromboembolic disease, fibrosing mediastinitis, tumor infiltration, or Swyer-James syndrome) (Figure 4-112).

4. Overexpansion of the lung. The lung as a whole may be relatively hyperexpanded when compared with the opposite lung. This state may result, for example, from foreign body impaction with obstructive emphysema. On occasion, emphysema, especially with bulla formation, may be asymmetric. Lobar collapse on one side with compensatory emphysema in the rest of the lung can superficially resemble a transradiant hemithorax, particularly if the collapse is chronic and extreme, since the collapsed lobe may be a relatively inconspicuous sliver of tissue wedged against the mediastinum. Careful study of the hilar airway and vascular anatomy should resolve this confusion. On occasion, a lobar resection may have been performed, leaving remarkably little radiographic evi-

dence of previous surgical intervention other than increased transradiancy.

5. Mild generalized increased opacity of one lung may be misinterpreted as increased transradiancy of the opposite normal lung. Examples are the filtering effect of a large pleural effusion layering out posteriorly in a supine patient and the occasional case of uniform loss of volume of a lung. The latter applies particularly to patients in intensive care who have mucus plugging. Some patchy pulmonary parenchymal density is likely to be present, indicating the true situation.

REFERENCES

1. Baber CE, Hedlund LW, Oddson TA, et al: Differentiating empyemas and peripheral pulmonary abscesses: the value of computed tomography, *Radiology* 135:755-758, 1980.
2. Bateson EM: An analysis of 155 solitary lung lesions illustrating the differential diagnosis of mixed tumors of the lung, *Clin Radiol* 16:51-65, 1965.
3. Blesovsky A: The folded lung, *Br J Dis Chest* 60:19-22, 1966.
4. Bressler EL, Francis IR, Glazer GM, et al: Bolus contrast medium enhancement for distinguishing pleural from parenchymal lung disease: CT features, *J Comput Assist Tomogr* 11:436-440, 1987.
5. Bryk D: Participating tail: new roentgenographic sign of pulmonary granuloma, *Am Rev Respir Dis* 100:406-408, 1969.
6. Carstairs LS: The interpretation of shadows in a restricted area of the lung field on a chest radiograph, *Proc R Soc Med* 54:978-980, 1961.
7. Carvalho PM, Carr DH: Computed tomography of folded lung, *Clin Radiol* 41:86-91, 1990.
8. Caskey CI, Templeton PA, Zerhouni EA: Current evaluation of the solitary pulmonary nodule, *Radiol Clin North Am* 28:511-520, 1990.
9. Caskey CI, Zerhouni EA: The solitary pulmonary nodule, *Semin Roentgenol* 25:85-95, 1989.
10. Chahinian P: Relationship between tumor doubling time and anatomoclinical features in 50 measurable pulmonary cancers, *Chest* 61:340-345, 1992.
11. Chiles C, Sherrier RH: Analysis of the solitary pulmonary nodule by means of digital techniques, *J Thorac Imag* 51:55-60, 1990.
12. Cho SR, Henry DA, Beachley MC, et al: Round (helical) atelectasis, *Br J Radiol* 54:643-650, 1981.
13. Chong BW, Weisbrod GL, Herman S: Atypical collapse of the upper lobe of the right lung simulating combined right upper and middle lobe collapse: report of two cases, *J Can Assoc Radiol* 41:358-362, 1990.
14. Collins VP, Loeffler RK, Tivey H: Observations on growth rates in human tumors, *AJR* 76:988-1000, 1956.
15. Culiner MM: The right middle lobe syndrome, a non-obstructive complex, *Dis Chest* 50:57-66, 1966.
16. de Geer G, Gamsu G, Cann C, et al: Evaluation of a chest phantom for CT nodule densitometry, *AJR* 147:21-25, 1986.
17. Dernevik L, Gatzinsky P: Long term results of operation for shrinking pleuritis with atelectasis, *Thorax* 40:448-452, 1985.
18. Don C, Desmarais R: Peripheral upper lobe collapse in adults, *Radiology* 170:657-659, 1989.
19. Doyle TC, Lawler GA: CT features of rounded atelectasis of the lung, *AJR* 143:225-228, 1984.
20. Dunnick NR, Parker BR, Castellino RA: Rapid onset of pulmonary infiltration due to histiocytic lymphoma, *Radiology* 118:281-285, 1976.
21. Felson B: The roentgen diagnosis of disseminated pulmonary alveolar diseases, *Semin Roentgenol* 2:3-21, 1967.
22. Felson B: Mucoid impaction (inspissated secretions) in segmental bronchial obstruction, *Radiology* 133:9-16, 1979.
23. Felson B: A new look at pattern recognition of diffuse pulmonary disease, *AJR* 133:183-189, 1979.
24. Felson B, Felson H: Localization of intrathoracic lesions by means of the postero-anterior roentgenogram: the silhouette sign, *Radiology* 55:363-374, 1950.
25. Fleischner F: Uber das Wesen der basalen horizontalen Schattenstreifen im Lungenfeld, *Wien Arch Intern Med* 28:461, 1936.
26. Fleischner Society: Glossary of terms for thoracic radiology: recommendation of the nomenclature committee of the Fleischner Society, *AJR* 143:509-517, 1984.
27. Franken EA, Klatte EC: Atypical (peripheral) upper lobe collapse, *Ann Radiol* 20:87-93, 1977.
28. Fraser RG, Pare JAP, Pare PD, et al: *Diagnosis of diseases of the chest*, ed 3, Philadelphia, 1988, WB Saunders.
29. Gaensler EA, Carrington CB: Peripheral opacities in chronic eosinophilic pneumonia: the photographic negative of pulmonary edema, *AJR* 128:1-13, 1977.
30. Garland LH, Coulson W, Wollin E: The rate of growth and apparent duration of untreated primary bronchial carcinoma, *Cancer* 16:694-707, 1963.
31. Glass TA, Armstrong P, Dyer RB, et al: Computed tomographic features of rounded atelectasis, *J Comput Tomogr* 7:183-185, 1980.
32. Glay J, Palayew MJ: Unusual patterns of left lower lobe atelectasis, *Radiology* 141:331-333, 1981.
33. Glazer HS, Anderson DJ, Sagel SS: Bronchial impaction in lobar collapse: CT demonstration and pathologic correlation, *AJR* 153:485-488, 1989.
34. Glazer HS, Aronberg DJ, Van Dyke JA, et al: CT manifestations of pulmonary collapse. In Siegelman SS, ed: *Computed tomography of the chest*, New York, 1984, Churchill Livingstone.
35. Godwin JD, Tarver RD: Accessory fissures of the lung, *AJR* 144:39-47, 1985.
36. Godwin JD, Webb WR, Savoca CJ, et al: Multiple, thin walled cystic lesions of the lung, *AJR* 135:593-604, 1980.
37. Golden R: The effect of bronchostenosis upon the roentgen-ray shadows in carcinoma of the bronchus, *AJR* 13:21-30, 1925.
38. Goldstein MS, Rush M, Johnson P, et al: A calcified adenocarcinoma of the lung with very high CT numbers, *Radiology* 150:785-786, 1984.
39. Good CA: The solitary pulmonary nodule: a problem of management, *Radiol Clin North Am* 1:429-438, 1963.
40. Good CA, Wilson TW: The solitary circumscribed pulmonary nodule: study of seven hundred five cases encountered roentgenologically in a period of three and one half years, *JAMA* 166:210-215, 1958.
41. Gould DM, Dalrymple GV: A radiological analysis of disseminated lung disease, *Am J Med Sci* 238:621-637, 1959.
42. Gross BH, Glazer GM, Wimbish KJ: CT of solitary cavitary infiltrates, *Semin Roentgenol* 19:236-242, 1984.
43. Gurney JW: Determining the likelihood of malignancy in solitary pulmonary nodules with Bayesian analysis. Part I. Theory, *Radiology* 186:405-413, 1993.
44. Gurney JW, Lyddon DM, McKay JA: Determining the likelihood of malignancy in solitary pulmonary nodules with Bayesian analysis. Part II. Application, *Radiology* 186:415-422, 1993.
45. Hanke R, Kretzschmar R: Round atelectasis, *Semin Roentgenol* 15:174-182, 1980.
46. Heitzman ER: *The lung — radiologic-pathologic correlations*, ed 2, St Louis, 1984, Mosby.
47. Heitzman ER, Ziter FM, Markarian B, et al: Kerley's interlobular septal lines: roentgen-pathologic correlation, *AJR* 100:578-582, 1967.
48. Herold CJ, Kuhlman JE, Zerhouni EA: Pulmonary atelectasis: signal patterns with MR imaging, *Radiology* 178:715-720, 1991.

49. Hill CA: "Tail" sign associated with pulmonary lesions: critical reappraisal, *AJR* 139:311-316, 1982.

50. Hillerdal G: Rounded atelectasis: clinical experience with 74 patients, *Chest* 95:836-841, 1989.

51. Huston J, Muhm JR: Solitary pulmonary opacities on plain tomography, *Radiology* 163:481-485, 1987.

52. Huston J, Muhm JR: Solitary pulmonary nodules: evaluation with a CT reference phantom, *Radiology* 170:653-656, 1989.

53. Im JG, Gamsu G, Gordon D, et al: CT densitometry of pulmonary nodules in a frozen human thorax, *AJR* 150:61-66, 1988.

54. Im JG, Han MC, Yu EJ: Lobar bronchioloalveolar carcinoma: "angiogram sign" on CT scans, *Radiology* 176:749-753, 1990.

55. Ip M, Chen NK, So SY, et al: Unusual rib destruction in pleuropulmonary tuberculosis, *Chest* 95:242-244, 1989.

56. Ishihara T, Kikuchi K, Ikeda T, et al: Metastatic pulmonary diseases: biologic factors and modes of treatment, *Chest* 63:227-232, 1973.

57. Itoh H, Tokunaga S, Asamoto H, et al: Radiologic-pathologic correlations of small lung nodules with special reference to peribronchiolar nodules, *AJR* 130:223-231, 1978.

58. Johkoh T, Ikezoe J, Nagaveda T, et al: Metastatic pulmonary calcification: early detection by high-resolution CT, *J Comput Assist Tomogr* 17:471-473, 1993.

59. Jones FA, Wiedemann HP, O'Donovan PB, et al: Computerized tomographic densitometry of the solitary pulmonary nodule using a nodule phantom, *Chest* 96:779-783, 1989.

60. Joshi RR, Cholankeril JV: Computed tomography in lipoid pneumonia, *J Comput Assist Tomogr* 9:211-213, 1985.

61. Kattan KR: Upper mediastinal changes in lower lobe collapse, *Semin Roentgenol* 15:183-186, 1980.

62. Kattan KR, Eyler WR, Felson B: The juxtaphrenic peak in upper lobe collapse, *Semin Roentgenol* 15:187-193, 1980.

63. Kattan KR, Felson B, Holder LE, et al: Superior mediastinal shift in right lower lobe collapse: the "upper triangle sign," *Radiology* 116:305-309, 1975.

64. Kattan KR, Wiot JF: Cardiac rotation in left lower lobe collapse: "the flat waist sign," *Radiology* 118:275-279, 1976.

65. Kerley P: Radiology in heart disease, *Br Med J* 2:594-597, 1933.

66. Kerr IH: Interstitial lung disease: the role of the radiologist, *Clin Radiol* 35:1-7, 1984.

67. Khan A, Herman PG, Vorwerk P, et al: Solitary pulmonary nodules: comparison of classification with standard, thin-section, and reference phantom CT, *Radiology* 179:477-481, 1991.

68. Kreel L, Slavin G, Herbert A, et al: Intralobar septal oedema: D lines, *Clin Radiol* 26:209-221, 1975.

69. Kuriyama K, Tateishi R, Doi O, et al: CT-pathologic correlation in small peripheral lung cancers, *AJR* 149:1139-1143, 1987.

70. Lillington GA, Caskey CI: Evaluation and management of solitary and multiple pulmonary nodules, *Clin Chest Med* 14:111-119, 1993.

71. Littleton JT, Durizch ML, Moeller G, et al: Pulmonary masses: contrast enhancement, *Radiology* 177:861-871, 1990.

72. Lynch DA, Gamsu G, Ray CS, et al: Asbestos-related focal lung masses: manifestations on conventional and high-resolution CT scans, *Radiology* 169:603-607, 1988.

73. Mahoney MC, Shipley RT, Corcoran HL, et al: CT demonstration of calcification in carcinoma of the lung, *AJR* 154:255-258, 1990.

74. Mallens WMS, Nijhuis-Heddes JMA, Bakker W: Calcified lymph node metastases in bronchioloalveolar carcinoma, *Radiology* 161:103-104, 1986.

75. Mayo JR, Müller NL, Road J, et al: Chronic eosinophilic pneumonia: CT findings in six cases, *AJR* 153:727-730, 1989.

76. McGee AR, Warren R: Carcinoma metastatic from the thyroid to the lungs: a twenty-four year follow up, *Radiology* 87:516-517, 1966.

77. McHugh K, Blaquiere RM: CT features of rounded atelectasis, *AJR* 153:257-260, 1989.

78. McLachlan MSF, Wallace DM, Seneriratne C: Pulmonary calcification in renal failure: report of three cases, *Br J Radiol* 41:99-106, 1968.

79. Meyer JA: Growth rate versus prognosis in resected primary bronchogenic carcinomas, *Cancer* 31:1468-1472, 1973.

80. Mintzer RA, Gore RM, Vogelzang RL, et al: Rounded atelectasis and its association with asbestosis-induced pleural disease, *Radiology* 139:567-570, 1981.

81. Mori K, Saitou Y, Tominaga K, et al: Small nodular lesions in the lung periphery: new approach to diagnosis with CT, *Radiology* 177:843-849, 1990.

82. Murayama S, Onitskua H, Murakami J, et al: "CT angiogram sign" in obstructive pneumonitis and pneumonia, *J Comput Assist Tomogr* 17:609-612, 1993.

83. Naidich DP, Ettinger N, Leitman BS, et al: CT of lobar collapse, *Semin Roentgenol* 19:222-235, 1984.

84. Naidich DP, McCauley DI, Khouri NF, et al: Computed tomography of lobar collapse. 1. Endobronchial obstruction, *J Comput Assist Tomogr* 7:745-757, 1983.

85. Naidich DP, McCauley DI, Khouri NF, et al: Computed tomography of lobar collapse. 2. Collapse in the absence of endobronchial obstruction, *J Comput Assist Tomogr* 7:758-767, 1983.

86. Naidich DP, Zerhouni EA, Hutchins GM, et al: Computed tomography of the pulmonary parenchyma. 1. Distal air space disease, *J Thorac Imag* 1:39-53, 1985.

87. Nathan MH, Collins VP, Adams RA: Differentiation of benign and malignant pulmonary nodules by growth rate, *Radiology* 79:221-232, 1962.

88. Nordenstrom B, Novek J: The atelectatic complex of the left lung, *Acta Radiol* 53:177-183, 1960.

89. Payne CR, Jacques PF, Kerr IH: Lung folding simulating peripheral pulmonary neoplasm (Blesovky's syndrome), *Thorax* 35:936-940, 1980.

90. Price J: Linear atelectasis in the lingula as a diagnostic feature of left lower lobe collapse: Nordenstrom's sign, *Australas Radiol* 35:56-60, 1991.

91. Proto AV, Merhar GL: Central bronchial displacement with large posterior pleural collections: findings on the lateral chest radiograph and CT scans, *J Can Assoc Radiol* 35:128-132, 1984.

92. Proto AV, Speckman JM: The left lateral radiograph of the chest, *Med Radiogr Photogr* 55:30-74, 1979.

93. Proto AV, Thomas SR: Pulmonary nodules studied by computed tomography, *Radiology* 156:149-153, 1985.

94. Proto AV, Tocino I: Radiographic manifestations of lobar collapse, *Semin Roentgenol* 15:117-173, 1980.

95. Putman CE, Godwin JD, Silverman PM, et al: CT of localized lucent lung lesions, *Semin Roentgenol* 19:173-188, 1984.

96. Raasch BN, Heitzman ER, Carsky EW, et al: A computed tomographic study of bronchopulmonary collapse, *Radiographics* 4:195-232, 1984.

97. Reed JC: Pathologic correlations of the air bronchogram: a reliable sign in chest radiology, *Crit Rev Diagn Imag* 10:235-255, 1977.

98. Reed JC: *Chest radiology: plain film patterns and differential diagnosis*, ed 2, Chicago, 1987, Year Book.

99. Reed JC, Madewell JE: The air bronchogram in interstitial disease of the lungs, *Radiology* 116:1-9, 1975.

100. Reeder MM, Felson B: *Gamuts in radiology: comprehensive lists of roentgen differential diagnosis*, Cincinnati, 1975, Audiovisual Radiology of Cincinnati.

101. Ried L: The connective tissue septa in the adult human lung, *Thorax* 14:138-145, 1959.

102. Rosenbloom SA, Ravin CE, Putman CE, et al: Peripheral middle lobe syndrome, *Radiology* 149:17-21, 1983.

103. Sagel SS: The solitary pulmonary nodule: role of CT, commentary, *AJR* 147:26-27, 1986.

104. Sakai F, Sone S, Murayama A, et al: Thin-rim enhancement in Gd-DTPA-enhanced magnetic resonance images of tubercu-

loma: a new finding of potential differential diagnostic importance, *J Thorac Imag* 7(4):64-69, 1992.

105. Schneider JH, Felson B, Gonzales LL: Rounded atelectasis, *AJR* 134:225-232, 1980.

106. Schuster MR, Scanlan KA: "CT angiogram sign": establishing the differential diagnosis (letter), *Radiology* 181:903, 1991.

107. Shapiro R, Wilson GL, Yesner R, et al: A useful roentgen sign in the diagnosis of localized bronchioloalveolar carcinoma, *AJR* 114:516-524, 1972.

108. Shin MS, Ho KJ: CT fluid bronchogram: observation in postobstructive pulmonary consolidation, *Clin Imag* 16:109-113, 1993.

109. Siegelman SS, Khouri NF, Leo FP, et al: Solitary pulmonary nodules: CT assessment, *Radiology* 160:307-312, 1986.

110. Siegelman SS, Zerhouni EA, Leo FP, et al: CT of the solitary pulmonary nodule, *AJR* 135:1-13, 1980.

111. Silverman SP, Marino PL: Unusual case of enlarging pulmonary mass, *Chest* 91:457-458, 1987.

112. Spratt JS, Spjut HJ, Roper CI: The frequency distribution of the rates of growth and the estimated duration of primary pulmonary carcinomas, *Cancer* 16:687-693, 1963.

113. Stancato-Pasik A, Mendelson DS, Marom Z: Rounded atelectasis caused by histoplasmosis, *AJR* 155:275-276, 1990.

114. Stark DD, Federle MP, Goodman PC, et al: Differentiating lung abscess and empyema: radiography and computed tomography, *AJR* 141:163-167, 1983.

115. Steele JD: The solitary pulmonary nodule — report of a cooperative study of resected asymptomatic solitary pulmonary nodules in males, *J Thorac Cardiovasc Surg* 46:21-39, 1963.

116. Stewart JG, MacMahon H, Vyborny CJ, et al: Dystrophic calcification in carcinoma of the lung: demonstration by CT, *AJR* 148:29-30, 1987.

117. Strauss MJ: The growth characteristic of lung cancer and its application to treatment design, *Semin Oncol* 1:167-174, 1974.

118. Swensen SJ, Harms GF, Morin RL, et al: CT evaluation of solitary pulmonary nodules: value of 185-H reference phantom, *AJR* 156:925-929, 1991.

119. Swensen SJ, Morin RL, Schueler BA, et al: Solitary pulmonary nodule: CT evaluation of enhancement with iodinated contrast material — a preliminary report, *Radiology* 182:343-347, 1992.

120. Taylor PM: Dynamic contrast enhancement of asbestos-related pulmonary pseudotumours, *Br J Radiol* 61:1070-1072, 1988.

121. Toomes H, Delphendahl A, Marike HG, et al: The coin lesion of the lung: a review of 955 resected coin lesions, *Cancer* 51:534-537, 1983.

122. Trapnell DH: The peripheral lymphatics of the lung, *Br J Radiol* 36:660-672, 1963.

123. Trapnell DH: The differential diagnosis of linear shadows in chest radiographs, *Radiol Clin North Am* 11:77-92.

124. Tylen V, Nilsson V: Computed tomography in pulmonary pseudotumors and their relation to asbestos exposure, *J Comput Assist Tomogr* 6:229-237, 1982.

125. Vincent JM, Ng YY, Norton AJ, et al: CT "angiogram sign" in primary pulmonary lymphoma, *J Comput Assist Tomogr* 16:829-831.

126. Walkey MM: And what is your sign? (letter), *Radiology* 178:894, 1991.

127. Ward HB, Pliego M, Diefenthal HC, et al: The impact of phantom CT scanning on surgery for the solitary pulmonary nodule, *Surgery* 106:734-739, 1989.

128. Webb WR: Radiologic evaluation of the solitary pulmonary nodule, *AJR* 154:701-708, 1990.

129. Weiss W: Tumor doubling time and survival of men with bronchogenic carcinoma, *Chest* 65:3-8, 1974.

130. Westcott JL, Cole S: Plate atelectasis, *Radiology* 155:1-9, 1985.

131. Whalen JP, Lane EJ: Bronchial rearrangements in pulmonary collapse as seen on the lateral radiograph, *Radiology* 93:285-288, 1969.

132. Wilson AG: The interpretation of shadows on the adult chest radiograph, *Br J Hosp Med* 37:526-534, 1987.

133. Woodring JH: Unusual radiographic manifestations of lung cancer, *Radiol Clin North Am* 28:588-618, 1990.

134. Woodring JH, Fried AM: Significance of wall thickness in solitary cavities of the lung: a follow-up study, *AJR* 140:473-474, 1983.

135. Yao L, Killam DA: Round atelectasis associated with end-stage renal disease, *Chest* 96:441-443, 1989.

136. Zerhouni EA, Boukadoum M, Siddiky MA, et al: A standard phantom for quantitative CT analysis of pulmonary nodules, *Radiology* 149:767-773, 1983.

137. Zerhouni EA, Spivey JF, Morgan RH, et al: Factors influencing quantitative CT measurements of solitary pulmonary nodules, *J Comput Assist Tomogr* 6:1075-1087, 1982.

138. Zerhouni EA, Stitik FP, Siegelman SS, et al: CT of the pulmonary nodule: a cooperative study, *Radiology* 160:319-327, 1986.

139. Ziskind MM, Weill H, Rayzant AR: The recognition and significance of acinus-filling processes of the lung, *Am Rev Respir Dis* 87:551-559, 1963.

140. Zwirewich CV, Vedal S, Miller RR, et al: Solitary pulmonary nodule: high-resolution CT and radiologic-pathologic correlation, *Radiology* 179:469-476, 1991.

High-Resolution Computed Tomography of the Lung

DAVID M. HANSELL

The limitations of chest radiography in diagnosing diffuse lung disease are well known.[19,38] The two-dimensional chest radiograph cannot clearly depict the alteration in morphology that occurs in diffuse lung disease. The radiographic pattern of diffuse lung disease is often nonspecific[55] and is subject to considerable interobserver variation.[25] Furthermore, the inability of chest radiography to resolve small differences in density makes it insensitive in the detection of early parenchymal disease.[17,24] In the last 10 years the development of high-resolution computed tomography (HRCT) has revolutionized the imaging of diffuse interstitial lung disease[59] and bronchiectasis.[27] HRCT images of the lung correlate closely with the macroscopic appearances of pathologic specimens,[15,35,37,117] so that in the context of diffuse lung disease, HRCT represents a substantial improvement over chest radiography in sensitivity, specificity, diagnostic accuracy, and assessment of disease activity.[31,63,64,83]

TECHNIQUE

Although no definition of "high-resolution" CT has been established, three factors significantly improve the spatial resolution of CT images of the lung: narrow scan collimation, a high spatial reconstruction algorithm, and a small field of view.[53] Other aspects that affect the final image, but that the user cannot control, include the x-ray focal spot size, the geometry and array of detectors, and the frequency of data sampling.[50]

Scan collimation

Narrow collimation of the x-ray beam reduces volume averaging within the section and so increases spatial resolution compared with standard 10 mm collimation.[71,72] No consensus has been reached on the optimum scan collimation for HRCT. A section thickness of more than 3 mm does not improve spatial resolution much over standard section widths. In contrast, reducing the section thickness to less than 1 mm does not yield any significant further improvement in spatial resolution and at the same time significantly reduces the signal-to-noise ratio of the image. Thus, for routine HRCT scanning, 1.5 mm collimation is generally regarded as optimal.[15,72,114] Narrow collimation has a marked effect on the appearance of the lungs, notably the vessels and bronchi: the branching vascular pattern seen particularly in the midzones on standard 10 mm sections has a more nodular appearance on narrow sections because shorter segments of the obliquely running vessels are included in the plane of section (Figure 5-1). The resulting "nodular" pattern of the normal lungs can be pronounced on some CT scanners, and the observer must take this into account when interpreting HRCT images from an unfamiliar machine. Another effect of narrow collimation is an apparent increase in the diameter of vessels that run parallel with the plane of section. This is due to the elimination of the partial volume effect of air surrounding the rounded surface of the vessel that occurs with standard width sections. The diameter of vessels or

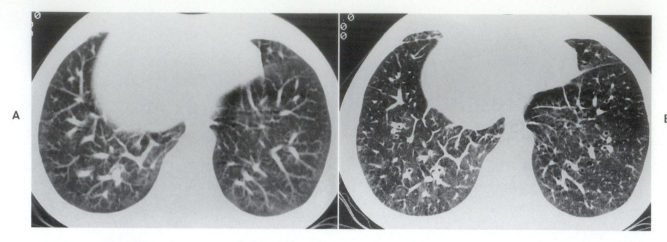

FIGURE 5-1
A, A 10 mm section with standard reconstruction algorithm through the lower lobes of a patient with lung cancer at the right hilum. Irregular polyhedral outline adjacent to the posterior surface of the right dome of the diaphragm represents interlobular septal thickening caused by lymphangitis carcinomatosa. B, A 1.5 mm section with high spatial resolution reconstruction algorithm at the same level. Note the increased clarity of the subsegmental bronchi, interlobular septa, and major fissures.

bronchi running perpendicular to the plane of section is the same irrespective of the scan collimation.

Reconstruction algorithm

The type and characteristics of the software algorithm used to reconstruct the CT image are at least as crucial as the chosen section width. In conventional body CT, images are reconstructed with a medium or relatively low spatial frequency algorithm that is designed to smooth the image and so reduce the visibility of image noise and improve contrast resolution. HRCT of the lung employs a high spatial frequency algorithm that takes advantage of the inherently high-contrast environment of the lung. The high spatial frequency algorithm (also known as the edge-enhancing, sharp, or formerly "bone" algorithm) reduces image smoothing and makes structures visibly sharper but at the same time makes image noise more conspicuous (Figure 5-1).[53,72] More than any other manipulation in HRCT technique, it is the combination of section thickness and the unique reconstruction algorithm that determines the final appearance of the lung image; in some instances the inconsistency of appearances obtained on different CT scanners makes comparisons between images difficult.

Targeted reconstruction

HRCT scanning is usually performed using a field of view that encompasses the whole patient in cross section (approximately 40 cm diameter). After the image data are acquired, it is possible to "target" the reconstruction to a single lung, thus reducing the image pixel size, and so increase spatial resolution. For example, with a matrix of 512 × 512 pixels and a 40 cm field of view the pixel size is 0.78 mm. If the image reconstruction is targeted to a 25

cm diameter field of view (large enough to encompass an average size single lung in cross section), the pixel size is reduced to 0.5 mm and the spatial resolution is correspondingly increased. For retrospective targeting of the image reconstruction, the raw scan data have to be saved and the process is laborious. In practice, of the three factors under operator control that contribute to the high spatial resolution of the image, adjusting the field of view is the least frequently employed: the greatest return is from the combination of narrow collimation and a high spatial frequency reconstruction algorithm.

Artifacts

Although several artifacts can be consistently identified on HRCT images, they do not usually degrade the diagnostic content. It is useful to be aware of the most common artifacts, which are caused by patient motion, quantum noise, and aliasing.

Probably the most frequently encountered artifact on HRCT images of the lung is a streaking appearance caused by patient motion. When scan acquisition time is less than 3 seconds, respiratory motion is rarely responsible for significant motion artifact. However, even with millisecond scan acquisition, movement of the lung resulting from cardiac motion sometimes degrades the image quality of the adjacent lingula and to a lesser extent the right middle lobe. Pulsation artifacts take the form of high-density linear streaks, usually arising from the heart border. Another manifestation of movement is a star pattern centered on pulmonary vessels,[43] and these vessels may show a superficial resemblance to bronchiectatic airways in cross section.[107] Sometimes the oblique fissure is seen as two fine lines in parallel.[52] This artifact is due to linear structures being scanned in different

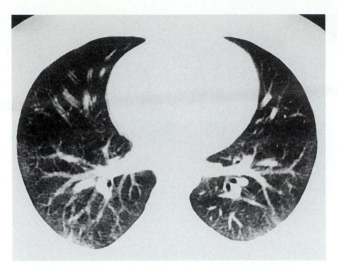

FIGURE 5-2
Artifact from cardiac pulsation, despite a scan time of 0.2 sec, causing double imaging of the pulmonary vessels in the right middle lobe that resembles bronchiectasis (6 mm section).

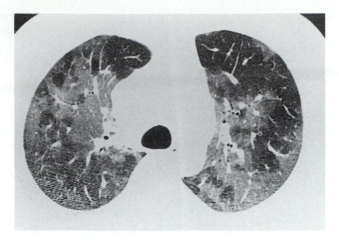

FIGURE 5-3
Considerable amount of artifact in paravertebral regions because of quantum mottle in a large patient. Ground-glass parenchymal opacification was due to cellular fibrosing alveolitis.

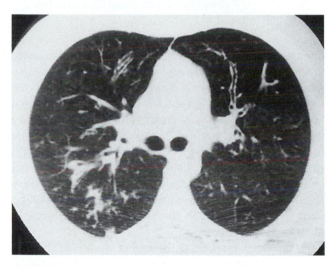

FIGURE 5-4
Another example of marked artifact from image noise. Nontapering of thickened anterior segmental bronchus of the left upper lobe indicating bronchiectasis (surrounding transradiancy of lung indicates underventilation and perfusion of this region). Similar, less severe changes are present in the right lung; some bronchi are plugged.

positions after the gantry has turned through 180 degrees. Although the double-fissure artifact is unlikely to cause misdiagnosis, "double vessels" may convincingly resemble bronchiectasis (Figure 5-2).[107]

The patient's size has a direct effect on the quality of the lung image: the larger the patient, the more conspicuous the noise because of increased x-ray absorption by the patient. Image noise or quantum mottle takes the form of granular streaks arising from high-attenuation structures and is particularly evident in the posterior lung adjacent to the vertebral column (Figures 5-3 and 5-4). Image noise rarely interferes with diagnosis, and while the problem can be counteracted by increasing the kilovoltage and milliamperage settings, the reduction in noise is barely perceptible except in the largest patients.

The phenomenon of aliasing results in a fine, streaklike pattern radiating from sharp, high-contrast interfaces. The severity of the aliasing artifact is related to the geometry of the CT scanner and particularly the spacing of the detectors and scan collimation; unlike quantum mottle, aliasing is independent of the radiation dose. Aliasing and quantum mottle are most prominent in the paravertebral regions and often parallel the pleural surface.[53] These artifacts are exaggerated by the non-smoothing high spatial resolution reconstruction algorithm but do not mimic normal anatomic structures and are rarely severe enough to obscure important detail in the lung parenchyma.

Scanning protocols

An HRCT examination can be varied in terms of the number of sections, the levels at which the sections are obtained, the position of the patient, the phase in which respiration is suspended, and the window settings at which the images are displayed. No single protocol can be recommended for every eventuality, since in some cases the examination would be prohibitively time consuming or require an excessive radiation dose. Early investigators recommended a conventional CT study of the lungs using contiguous 10 mm collimation scans, followed by as few as five HRCT sections at selected levels.[71] This approach provides conventional images that may help in the interpretation of HRCT for those unfamiliar with the technique. A further benefit is the improved detection of small nodules on the contiguous 10 mm collimation CT sections.[92] The disadvantage of this approach is that even with the widespread distribution of most interstitial lung

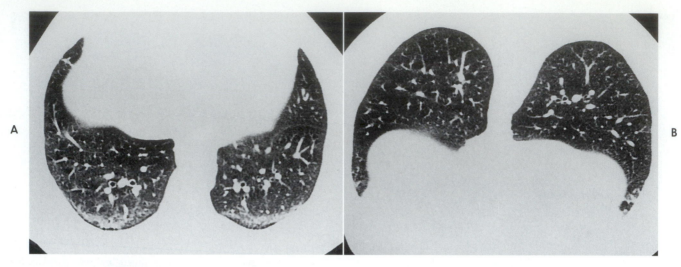

FIGURE 5-5
A, Increased parenchymal opacification in the dependent part of the lower lobes in a patient scanned while in the supine position. **B,** When the patient is turned over and scanned in the prone position, the density in the posterobasal segments disappears, confirming that this is a gravity-dependent phenomenon, rather than fixed pathology.

diseases, the usual indication for HRCT, the pathologic process is often patchy and so better assessed with a greater number of fine sections.[114] In many centers the most frequently used protocol is simply 1.5 mm collimation sections at 10 mm intervals from apex to lung bases with the patient supine. Clearly, any given scanning protocol may need to be modified: a patient referred with unexplained hemoptysis should ideally be scanned with contiguous standard sections through the main airways (to show a small endobronchial tumor) and interspaced narrow sections through the remainder of the lungs (to identify bronchiectasis).[76]

When early interstitial fibrosis is suspected, particularly in individuals exposed to asbestos, HRCT scans are often performed with the patient in the prone position. This prevents confusion with the increased opacification seen in the dependent posterobasal segments of many normal individuals scanned in the usual supine position. The increased density seen in the posterior dependent lung in the supine position disappears in normal individuals when the scan is repeated at the same level with the subject in the prone position (Figure 5-5). The poorly defined increased density in the dependent lung in normal individuals has been ascribed to "gravity-dependent perfusion," although it is more likely to result from relative atelectasis of the dependent lung.[58]

There are a number of conditions in which small airways disease may cause patchy air trapping because of a bronchiolitic component. A limited number of scans taken at full expiration may reveal evidence of air trapping not detectable on routine inspiratory scans: areas of air trapping range from a single secondary pulmonary lobule to a cluster of lobules giving a patchwork appearance of low-attenuation areas adjacent to

higher attenuation normal lung parenchyma (Figures 5-6 and 5-19).

The settings of window level and width (see Chapter 1) have a significant effect on both the HRCT appearances of the lung and the apparent dimensions of structures, notably the thickness of bronchial walls.[113] Alterations of the window settings may make detection of parenchymal abnormalities impossible if the attenuation of the lung parenchyma is subtly increased or decreased. Although no absolute window settings can be given because of machine variation and individual preferences, uniformity of window settings from patient to patient will make interpretation of the lung images more consistent. In general, a window level of −500 to −800 Hounsfield units (HU) and a width of between 900 and 1500 HU are satisfactory. Modifying the window settings for particular tasks is often desirable; for example, in looking for pleuroparenchymal abnormalities in asbestos-exposed individuals, a window of up to 2000 HU may be useful. Conversely, a narrower window width (approximately 600 HU) may emphasize the subtle density difference between areas of emphysema and normal lung parenchyma.

The relatively high radiation dose to the patient inherent in CT scanning needs constant consideration. The radiation burden to the patient is considerably less with interspaced finely collimated HRCT scans than with conventional contiguous CT scanning because the overlap between contiguous sections substantially increases the effective radiation dose.[18] The mean skin radiation dose delivered with HRCT using 1.5 mm sections at 20 mm intervals has been estimated to be 6% that of conventional 10 mm contiguous scanning protocols.[51] A further method of reducing the radiation burden to the patient is

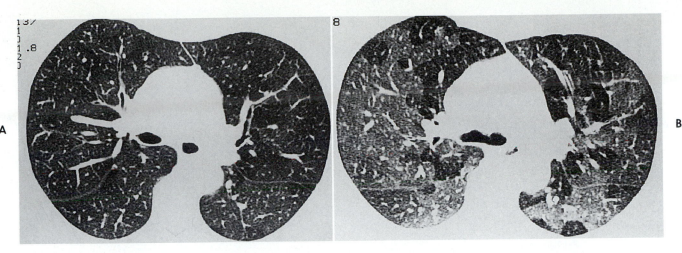

FIGURE 5-6
A, Section through the midzones of a patient with the rheumatoid arthritis (treated with penicillamine). There is minimal inhomogeneity of lung density in the left midzone; the lungs otherwise appear normal. **B,** Scan repeated with the patient breath holding at end expiration. Patchwork appearance of numerous well-defined transradiant areas represents air trapping at the level of the secondary pulmonary lobule. This phenomenon is pathognomonic of small airways disease, in this case an obliterative bronchiolitis. (Courtesy Dr. C.D.R. Flower, Cambridge, U.K.)

to decrease the milliamperage; it is possible to reduce the milliamperage by up to 10-fold and still obtain diagnostic images.[126] Such a low-dose technique considerably increases image noise (Figure 5-3), and subtle parenchymal abnormalities such as early emphysema or ground-glass opacification may be obscured. Nevertheless, this technique should be considered for young patients who are likely to be monitored with HRCT.

NORMAL LUNG ANATOMY ON HIGH-RESOLUTION COMPUTED TOMOGRAPHY

The limits of resolution determine the anatomy that can be identified on HRCT. The smallest objects that can be resolved on HRCT range from 100 to 400 μm and depend mainly on the geometry and orientation of the object in relation to the voxel.

Accurate interpretation of HRCT of the lung requires an appreciation of the normal appearances of the bronchi, blood vessels, and secondary pulmonary lobule. Throughout the lung the bronchi and pulmonary arteries run and branch together. Both the bronchi and pulmonary arteries taper slightly as they travel radially; this is most obvious in bronchi running within and parallel to the plane of section. At any given level the diameter of the bronchus is the same or marginally smaller than that of its accompanying pulmonary artery. The bronchovascular bundle is surrounded by a connective tissue sheath from its origin at the hilum to the respiratory bronchioles in the lung periphery. The concept of separate, but connected, components making up the lung interstitium, propounded by Weibel,[118] is important to the understanding of HRCT

findings in interstitial lung disease: the "peripheral" interstitium surrounds the surface of the lung beneath the visceral pleura and penetrates the lung to surround the secondary pulmonary lobules. Within the lobules a finer network of "septal" connective tissue fibers supports the alveoli. The "axial" fibers form a sheath around the bronchovascular bundles extending from the pulmonary hila to the lung periphery, as far out as the alveolar ducts and sacs. The connective tissue stroma of these three separate components is in continuity and thus forms a fibrous skeleton for the lungs.

The interface between the bronchovascular bundle and surrounding lung is normally sharp on HRCT. Any thickening of the connective tissue interstitium results in apparent bronchial wall thickening and blurs this interface. The size of the smallest subsegmental bronchi visible on HRCT is determined by the thickness of the bronchial wall rather than the bronchial diameter. In general, bronchi with a diameter of less than 3 mm and walls less than 300 μm thick are not identifiable on HRCT.[70,117] Airways reach this critical size about 3 cm from the pleural surface.

The secondary pulmonary lobule is the smallest anatomic unit of the lung surrounded by a connective tissue septum (Figure 5-7). Within the septa are lymphatic channels and venules. Thickening of the septa between the lobules is responsible for the Kerley B lines seen on chest radiography. The lobule contains up to 12 acini, each of which is approximately 6 to 10 mm in diameter. Each lobule is approximately 2 cm in diameter and is polyhedral, often resembling a misshapen or truncated cone.[8,104] In the lung periphery the bases of the cone-

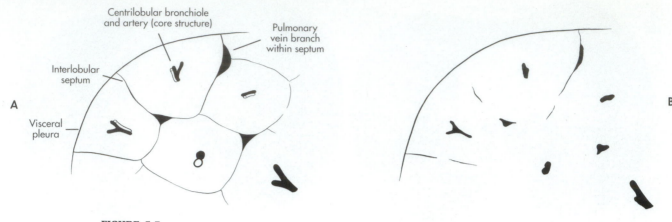

FIGURE 5-7
A, Anatomy of a group of secondary pulmonary lobules. B, Features of secondary pulmonary lobules identifiable on HRCT. Lumens of centrilobular bronchioles are not resolved on HRCT, and normal interlobular septa are rarely demonstrated in their entirety.

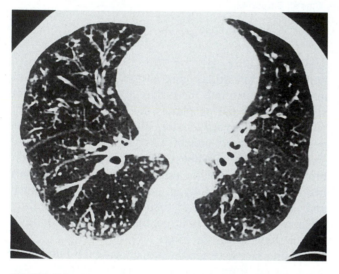

FIGURE 5-8
Widespread bronchial wall thickening and dilatation, most pronounced in right middle lobe, in a Japanese patient with panbronchiolitis. The numerous dot, V-like, and Y-like opacities in the lung periphery represent plugged and thickened centrilobular bronchioles.

shaped lobules lie on a visceral pleural surface and the centrilobular bronchiole and pulmonary artery enter through the apex of the lobule.

The connective tissue interlobular septa are well developed in the subpleural regions, particularly on the diaphragmatic surfaces and anterolateral regions of the lungs. In normal individuals these interlobular septa are approximately 100 μm thick. Because the lower limit of effective resolution of HRCT in vivo is approximately 200 μm, they are not often seen on HRCT. The few interlobular septa that are visible in normal individuals are usually inconspicuous and are seen as straight lines, 1 to 2 cm long, terminating at a visceral pleural surface.

Sometimes several septa joined end to end are seen as a nonbranching linear structure measuring up to 4 cm[117]; these are most common at the lung bases just above the diaphragmatic surface. Deep within the lung where the septa are less well developed, the interlobular septa are visible only when they are pathologically thickened.

The secondary pulmonary lobule is supplied by a centrilobular artery and bronchiole, which are approximately 1 mm in diameter as they enter the lobule.[70,117] In the normal state the core structures, effectively the 500 μm diameter centrilobular artery alone, are visible as dots 1 cm from the pleural surface. Only when the bronchioles become considerably thickened or dilated with an exudate do they become visible as V- or Y-shaped opacities (Figure 5-8). The lung parenchyma between the core structures and interlobular septa is usually of homogeneous low density, marginally greater than air.

PATTERNS OF LUNG DISEASE ON HIGH-RESOLUTION COMPUTED TOMOGRAPHY

The close correlation between HRCT appearances and macroscopic pathologic abnormalities often allows the use of accurate anatomic terms in describing patterns of diffuse lung disease. Inexact descriptive terms, so often used in the analysis of plain chest radiographs, can be replaced by precise morphologic terms derived from an understanding of normal HRCT anatomy. Nevertheless, there are a few nonspecific findings on HRCT that do not always have a definite counterpart at a pathologic level. Abnormal patterns on HRCT that denote pulmonary disease were initially given many names,[75,125] but there has been some convergence[116] and HRCT abnormalities can be broadly categorized into one of four patterns: (1) reticular and short linear opacities, (2) nodular opacities, (3) increased lung opacity ("ground-glass"), and (4) cystic airspaces and areas of decreased lung density.

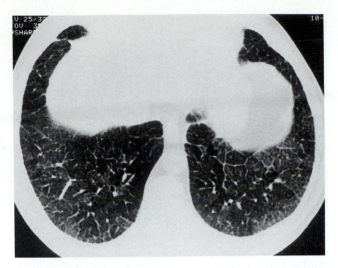

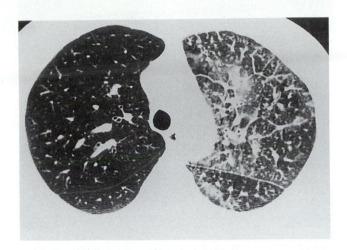

FIGURE 5-9
Widespread uniform thickening of interlobular septa and fine intralobular reticular pattern in a patient with interstitial fibrosis.

FIGURE 5-10
Unilateral irregular thickening of the interlobular septa and bronchovascular bundles caused by lymphangitis carcinomatosa.

Although these HRCT patterns have their corresponding patterns on chest radiography, they are seen with much greater clarity on the cross-sectional images of HRCT and the precise distribution of disease can be more readily appreciated.

Reticular pattern

Recognition of a reticular pattern on HRCT almost always indicates significant interstitial disease. A reticular pattern caused by thickening of interlobular septa is a common finding in many different interstitial lung diseases. Numerous interlobular septa that join to form polygonal outlines indicate an extensive interstitial abnormality caused by infiltration with fibrosis, abnormal cells, or fluid (for example, fibrosing alveolitis, lymphangitis carcinomatosa, and alveolar proteinosis, respectively) (Figure 5-9). At a pathologic level, interlobular septal thickening caused by fibrosis is often associated with bronchovascular thickening, intralobular interstitial thickening (beyond the resolution of HRCT), and finally the coarse reticular "honeycomb" of destroyed lung. Longer thickened interlobular septa, up to 4 cm in length and outlining part of more than one lobule, are occasionally seen, usually on a background of extensive interlobular septal thickening; distinguishing these linear opacities from a small area of subsegmental collapse or a dense fibrotic scar may be impossible.

Thickening of the interlobular septa may appear smooth or irregular on HRCT,[115] but this distinction is not always obvious: irregular septal thickening is a feature of lymphangitic spread of tumor (Figure 5-10),[68,95,104] whereas pulmonary edema and alveolar proteinosis cause smooth thickening.[73] Sarcoidosis may cause some nodular septal thickening.[62]

As a consequence of the continuity of the various parts of the lung interstitium,[118] widespread interstitial disease that causes thickening of the interlobular septa also results in bronchovascular interstitial thickening (typified by lymphangitis carcinomatosa) (Figures 5-1 and 5-10). The bronchovascular thickening depicted on HRCT is equivalent to the peribronchial "cuffing" seen around end-on bronchi on chest radiography. This HRCT finding may be obvious, particularly in regional or unilateral interstitial lung disease, but is sometimes subtle when it is minimal and diffuse. The HRCT finding of peribronchovascular thickening in isolation should be interpreted with caution, since it may be a manifestation of reversible airways disease such as asthma. In early bronchiectasis the thickened bronchi are generally, but not always, dilated. Thickening of the subsegmental and segmental bronchovascular bundles, such as that caused by lymphangitis carcinomatosa, sometimes gives the interface between the bronchial wall and surrounding lung an irregular and "feathery" appearance.[124,125]

At the level of the secondary pulmonary lobule, axial interstitial thickening of the centrilobular artery and bronchiole is seen as a prominent dot or Y-shaped opacity; often the interlobular septa are thickened. Such thickening is seen in a variety of interstitial lung diseases and is recognized as one of the earliest manifestations of asbestosis.[4,5] Diseases involving the smallest airways can produce apparent thickening of the core structures on HRCT; in these instances the abnormal core structure visible on HRCT is due to dilatation and thickening of the central bronchiole, which is filled with an exudate (Figure 5-8).[3,79] Perhaps surprisingly, confusion between axial interstitial disease and small airways disease, both of which give rise to prominent core structures, is rarely a problem: in the latter situation the larger subsegmental and segmental bronchi are usually abnormal.

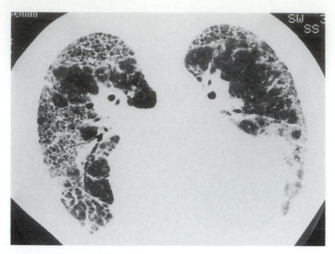

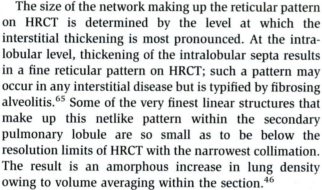

FIGURE 5-11
Characteristic peripheral basal distribution of disease in a patient (prone position) with established fibrosing alveolitis. The reticular pattern is made up of a myriad of small cystic airspaces surrounded by fibrotic walls.

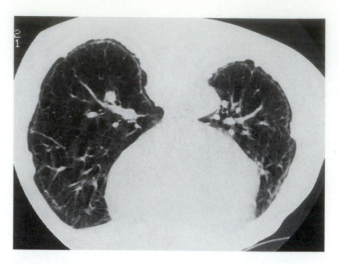

FIGURE 5-12
Fine dense curvilinear line parallel to chest wall in a patient (prone position) with pleural plaques. There was clinical and functional evidence of asbestosis.

The size of the network making up the reticular pattern on HRCT is determined by the level at which the interstitial thickening is most pronounced. At the intralobular level, thickening of the intralobular septa results in a fine reticular pattern on HRCT; such a pattern may occur in any interstitial disease but is typified by fibrosing alveolitis.[65] Some of the very finest linear structures that make up this netlike pattern within the secondary pulmonary lobule are so small as to be below the resolution limits of HRCT with the narrowest collimation. The result is an amorphous increase in lung density owing to volume averaging within the section.[46]

At the other end of the spectrum, extensive pulmonary fibrosis that destroys the architecture of the secondary pulmonary lobules results in a characteristic coarse reticular pattern made up of irregular linear opacities. The reticular pattern of end-stage fibrotic or honeycomb lung mirrors the appearances on chest radiography and is characterized by cystic spaces measuring a few millimeters to several centimeters across surrounded by thick irregular walls (Figure 5-11).[65,80,105,117] The distortion of normal lung morphology by extensive fibrosis may result in irregular dilatation of the segmental and subsegmental bronchi; in the lung periphery the dilated bronchi and bronchioles may be difficult to distinguish from the surrounding cystic airspaces of the honeycomb lung. This phenomenon has been termed traction bronchiectasis,[122] although these patients rarely have symptoms of bronchiectasis.

In a minority of patients with interstitial fibrosis an additional HRCT finding is a fine peripheral curvilinear line lying 1 cm from the visceral pleural surface. This dense line is extremely well defined and parallels the chest wall (Figure 5-12). The subpleural curvilinear line has caused confusion since it was first described in patients with asbestosis,[123] when such a line was thought to be virtually pathognomonic of asbestos-induced interstitial fibrosis. It is now recognized that this HRCT sign is seen in a minority of patients with interstitial fibrosis of various causes, including asbestosis,[4] and it should not be regarded as specific. An identical appearance has been reported in a patient treated for lymphoma,[41] in patients with cardiogenic pulmonary edema,[6] and in normal individuals.[1] In some cases the subpleural line is transient, and in others it disappears when the scans are repeated with the patient in a prone position. An anatomic explanation for the subpleural line remains elusive: one hypothesis implicates the rich leash of subpleural lymphatics at the site of the subpleural curvilinear line.[89] However, against this is the lack of a subpleural line in cases of lymphangitis carcinomatosa. A second possibility is the subpleural line represents focal atelectasis, which may or may not become fixed depending on the nature of the underlying pathologic condition.

Nodular pattern

A nodular pattern, defined on chest radiography as innumerable small discrete opacities ranging in diameter from 2 to 10 mm,[21] is a feature of both interstitial and airspace disease. The localization of nodules, as well as other characteristics such as their density, clarity of outline, and uniformity of size, may indicate whether the nodules are lying predominantly within the interstitium or within the airspaces. Since many lung diseases have both interstitial and airspace components, this distinction is not always helpful in refining the differential diagnosis. Whether pulmonary nodules can be detected on CT depends on their size, profusion, and density and the scanning technique. Although a standard section width has been advocated for the demonstration of nodular

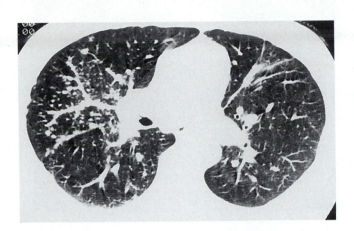

FIGURE 5-13
Typical beading of the bronchovascular bundles in pulmonary sarcoidosis (most obvious in right middle lobe). As well as discrete intrapulmonary nodules, there is thickening of the major fissures and irregularity of the pleural surface caused by conglomerates of subpleural granulomas.

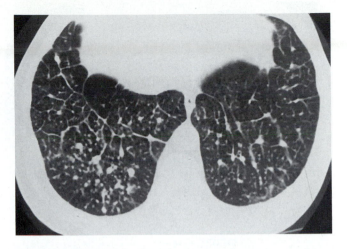

FIGURE 5-14
Marked thickening of the interlobular septa interspersed with uniformly small nodules in a patient with silicosis.

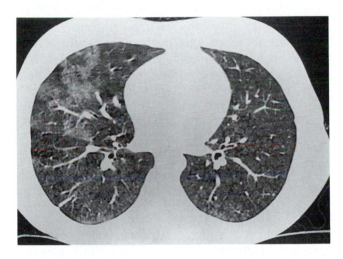

FIGURE 5-15
Profuse poorly defined nodules in the left lung of a patient with biopsy-proven idiopathic pulmonary hemorrhage. These indistinct nodules, 4 to 8 mm in diameter, were due to partial filling of the acini with hemosiderin-laden macrophages. Denser opacification in the right middle lobe was due to recent hemorrhage and subsequently resolved.

disease in sarcoidosis, where there is superimposition of the relatively large nodules,[62] narrow-collimation HRCT is generally superior for the detection of micronodular disease because HRCT has less partial volume effect, which can average out the attenuation of minute nodules.[92] Many pulmonary diseases, particularly the granulomatous disorders, are characterized by a fine nodular pattern. These include sarcoidosis, miliary tuberculosis, histiocytosis X, and extrinsic allergic alveolitis. Nongranulomatous diseases responsible for a nodular pattern include miliary metastases, pneumoconioses, and idiopathic pulmonary hemorrhage.

Nodules within the lung interstitium are seen in the interlobular septa, in subpleural regions (particularly in relation to the fissures), and in a peribronchovascular distribution. Nodular thickening of the bronchovascular interstitium results in an irregular interface between the margins of the bronchovascular bundles and the surrounding lung parenchyma. This irregularity, which has been called the interface sign,[124] may be seen in lymphangitis carcinomatosa[95,104] but is most obvious in cases of sarcoidosis when a coalescence of perilymphatic granulomas results in a beaded appearance of the thickened bronchovascular bundles.[47,62] The bronchovascular distribution of nodules, in conjunction with a perihilar concentration of disease, is virtually pathognomonic of sarcoidosis (Figure 5-13). In a few patients with histiocytosis X a centrilobular distribution of nodules has also been reported.[57] In practice, the size and character of the nodules and other CT features rarely cause confusion between these two diagnoses. The nodular pattern seen in coal worker's pneumoconiosis and silicosis is generally more uniform in distribution; the centrilobular nodules may be more upper zone and subpleural in distribution,

but overall they tend to be more evenly spread throughout the lung parenchyma than those in sarcoidosis. Thickening of the interlobular septa may be pronounced (Figure 5-14).[90,91]

When the airspaces are filled, or partially filled, with the products of disease, individual acini may become visible on HRCT as low-density poorly defined nodules approximately 8 mm in diameter. Acinar nodules may merge with areas of ground-glass opacification and are often seen around the periphery of areas of dense parenchymal consolidation. Acinar or airspace nodules are usually centrilobular, although this is not invariable and may not be appreciated if these nodules are profuse.

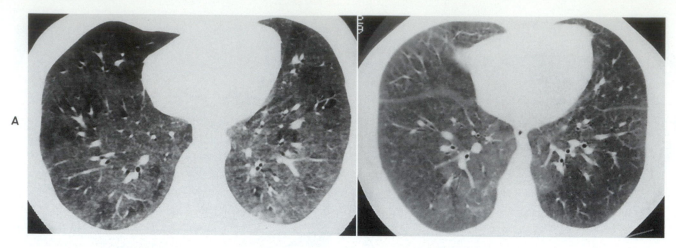

FIGURE 5-16
Nonspecific sign of ground-glass opacification of the lung parenchyma in patients with, **A,** subacute extrinsic allergic alveolitis and, **B,** idiopathic pulmonary hemorrhage. In both cases the pulmonary vasculature is not obscured and there is a considerable difference between the density of the lung parenchyma and air within bronchi.

Conditions in which this nonspecific pattern is seen include organizing pneumonia,[66] extrinsic allergic alveolitis,[32] endobronchial spread of tuberculosis,[70] idiopathic pulmonary hemorrhage (Figure 5-15),[12] pulmonary edema,[69,103] and some cases of bronchioloalveolar cell carcinoma.

Ground-glass pattern and increased lung density

A hazy increase in the density of the lung parenchyma on HRCT is often described as a "ground-glass" opacification. Unlike the analogous abnormality on chest radiography, in which the pulmonary vessels are often indistinct, a ground-glass pattern on HRCT does not obscure the pulmonary vasculature (Figure 5-16).[16,93] In cases in which the presence of a ground-glass pattern is equivocal, comparing the attenuation of the lung parenchyma with air in the bronchi may be helpful: in normal individuals the difference in density is marginal. Although this HRCT abnormality usually is easily recognizable, particularly when it is interspersed with areas of normal lung parenchyma, subtle degrees of increased parenchymal opacification may not be obvious and the conspicuity of this abnormality is susceptible to alterations in window settings. Furthermore, an increase in parenchymal density, indistinguishable from a widespread ground-glass pattern, is seen in patients breath holding at residual volume.

The morphologic changes responsible for a ground-glass pattern are complex and include partial filling of the airspaces, thickening of the interstitium, or a combination of the two.[46] Thickening of the intralobular interstitium by fluid or a cellular infiltrate is below the limits of resolution of HRCT, and volume averaging results in an amorphous increase in lung density. Conditions that are characterized by these pathologic changes and result in

the nonspecific pattern of ground-glass opacification include fibrosing alveolitis in the active inflammatory or cellular phase (Figure 5-3),[34,67,119] *Pneumocystis carinii* pneumonia,[9] subacute extrinsic allergic alveolitis (Figure 5-16, *A*),[32,100] sarcoidosis,[11,26,47] drug-induced lung damage,[82] diffuse pulmonary hemorrhage (Figure 5-16, *B*),[12] and acute lung injury including radiation pneumonitis.[36] In general, the amorphous ground-glass density seen on HRCT in these conditions represents a potentially reversible phase of the disease.[46] However, mild thickening of the intralobular interstitium by irreversible fibrosis may produce a ground-glass appearance in a minority of cases of fibrosing alveolitis[46] or asbestosis.[4] Similarly, a ground-glass pattern may be seen in areas of bronchioloalveolar cell carcinoma, usually in conjunction with patches of denser consolidated lung (Figure 5-17).

A pitfall in identifying a ground-glass pattern on HRCT is the patient with regions of either underperfused or underventilated lung. Regional alterations in pulmonary blood flow may result in striking differences in lung density; for example, in patients with pulmonary embolism the density difference between the oligemic lung and normal lung may give the appearance of a ground-glass density in the normal lung parenchyma. These areas of different density often have definable geographic margins, and the term "mosaic oligemia" has been used to describe this pattern on CT (Figure 5-18).[48] Similarly, in patients with patchy air trapping caused by small airways disease such as obliterative bronchiolitis, the relatively transradiant areas of underventilated and underperfused lung may make the normal lung parenchyma appear denser than usual and thus simulate a ground-glass infiltrate. This spurious appearance of ground-glass opacification can usually be recognized for what it is by the relative paucity of vessels in the underventilated parts

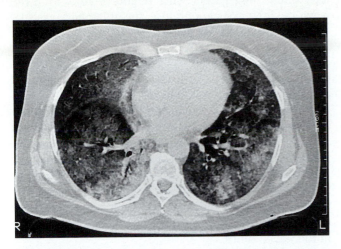

FIGURE 5-17
Areas of ground-glass opacification that merge with denser areas of consolidation in patient with bronchioloalveolar cell carcinoma.

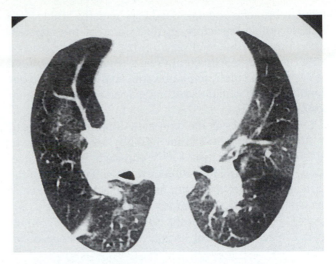

FIGURE 5-18
Mosaic oligemia in a patient with chronic thromboembolic disease (hence the dilated proximal pulmonary arteries). The abnormal areas of lung are the underperfused transradiant regions rather than the denser (ground-glass) areas to which blood is being shunted.

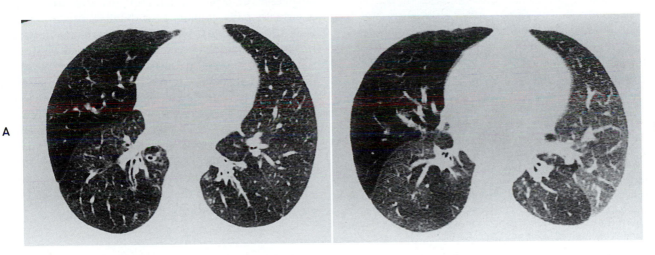

A   B

FIGURE 5-19
A, Regional inhomogeneity of lung density in patient with postviral obliterative bronchiolitis. B, Scan taken at end expiration confirms air trapping in the right middle lobe and emphasizes paucity of vessels in this underventilated region.

of the lungs owing to hypoxic vasoconstriction. By contrast the vessels in the relatively normal lung of higher density are engorged because of shunting of blood to these regions. If an obliterative bronchiolitis is suspected, additional scans should be performed in full expiration; the regional differences in lung density caused by the ventilatory imbalance will then be even more striking (Figure 5-19).

Cystic airspaces and decreased lung density

The terms "cystic airspace" and "lung cyst" are used to describe a clearly defined air-containing space with a definable wall between 1 and 3 mm thick. Innumerable cystic spaces may not be individually identifiable on chest radiography because of the superimposition of the thin walls, which results in a delicate reticular pattern. Several conditions are characterized by a profusion of cystic airspaces, and the size and distribution of these cysts on HRCT are often helpful in suggesting a diagnosis.

The abnormal airspaces of emphysema resulting from destruction of alveolar walls of the distal airspaces produce areas of low attenuation on HRCT that often merge imperceptibly and have no discernible interface with normal lung.[35] In patients with predominantly centrilobular emphysema there may be circular areas of lung destruction that resemble cysts; however, the centrilobular bronchovascular bundle is usually visible as a minute dotlike structure in the center of the apparent cyst. Although bullae of varying sizes are clearly seen on HRCT in patients with emphysema, usually a background of destructive emphysema prevents confusion with other conditions in which cystic airspaces are a prominent feature.

Cystic airspaces as the dominant abnormality are seen in only a few conditions, including lymphangioleiomyomatosis,[2,61] histiocytosis X,[10,57] end-stage fibrosing alveolitis,[65] and transient postinfective pneumatoceles. In the case of *Pneumocystis carinii* pneumonia a coalescence of bizarrely shaped, sometimes thick-walled, cystic airspaces is often superimposed on a background of ground-glass opacification or frank pulmonary consolidation.[20,30,42]

In lymphangioleiomyomatosis the cysts are usually uniformly scattered throughout the lungs with normal intervening lung parenchyma (Figure 5-20).[99,108] Even when the lung cysts are profuse, the pulmonary vasculature remains relatively normal with little distortion or attenuation. Paradoxically, as the disease progresses with coalescence of the larger cystic airspaces, the circumferential well-defined walls of the cysts become disrupted and the HRCT pattern of advanced lymphangioleiomyomatosis, and indeed histiocytosis X, may be practically indistinguishable from severe centrilobular emphysema (Figure 5-21). The distinction of this delicate lacelike pattern on HRCT from end-stage fibrosing alveolitis is usually straightforward because the cystic airspaces in honeycomb lung have thicker walls. Furthermore, the tendency for fibrosing alveolitis to have a peripheral distribution, even in its end stage, is often still discernible in the upper zones.

Similar confluent cystic airspaces giving a delicate pattern on HRCT are seen in patients with late histiocytosis X. However, in the earlier stages of the disease there is often a nodular component and some of the nodules cavitate.[10,57] The constellation of HRCT findings of cavitating nodules, some of which have odd shapes and cystic airspaces with a predominantly upper zone distribution, is virtually pathognomonic for the diagnosis of histiocytosis X (Figure 5-22). Serial HRCT scans show the natural history of nodules, which cavitate, become cystic airspaces, and finally coalesce. A curious feature of the disease is that some of the cavitating nodules and cystic airspaces may resolve, with the lung parenchyma reverting to a normal appearance. The strange shapes of some of the cavitating nodules in histiocytosis X sometimes resemble bronchiectatic airways. Distinguishing this pattern from bronchiectasis on HRCT is usually simple because there is a lack of continuity of these lesions on adjacent sections and the segmental bronchi do not have any of the HRCT features of bronchiectasis.

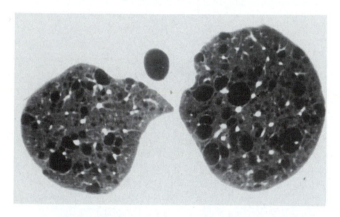

FIGURE 5-20
Numerous cystic airspaces with well-defined walls in a female patient with lymphangioleiomyomatosis. The cysts are uniformly distributed throughout the lung, and the intervening lung parenchyma appears normal. (Courtesy Dr. D.R. Aberle, Los Angeles.)

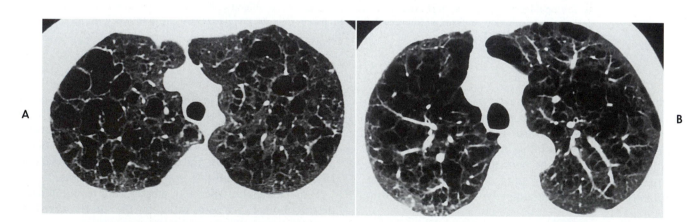

FIGURE 5-21
A, Advanced histiocytosis X with many of the cystic airspaces merging and causing widespread lung destruction. B, Severe centrilobular emphysema. The appearance of these two conditions is similar in advanced cases.

Distribution of disease

A frontal chest radiograph provides valuable information about the distribution of diffuse lung disease: an upper, middle or lower zonal predominance may help to narrow the differential diagnosis. Nevertheless, the radiographic pattern of distribution of diffuse lung disease may be more apparent than real. Some diseases that macroscopically have a truly uniform distribution throughout the lung parenchyma appear to have a middle and lower zone predominance on a frontal chest radiograph. In the subacute phase of extrinsic allergic alveolitis the poorly defined nodular or ground-glass pattern on a chest radiograph appears most pronounced in the middle and lower zones.[14] In contrast the distribution of the nodular or ground-glass pattern on CT in patients with subacute

extrinsic allergic alveolitis is usually uniform with no zonal predominance.[32] This misleading impression of a concentration of disease in the lower zones on chest radiography can be explained by the greater width of lung traversed by the x-ray beam in the lower zones, which results in summation of innumerable foci of disease and thus greater x-ray attenuation.[56] The cross-sectional nature of CT gives an accurate estimation of the uniformity of diffuse disease or the zonal distribution, in both transverse and longitudinal axes.

In established fibrosing alveolitis a lower zone and subpleural concentration of disease are typical, and this distribution is virtually pathognomonic of the disease.[65,105,110] Quite subtle regional variations in the distribution of disease may be a pointer to the diagnosis. For example, in the less common cellular form of fibrosing alveolitis the chest radiograph may show widespread ground-glass opacification with no obvious zonal distribution. In over half of patients with this form of fibrosing alveolitis, CT demonstrates a lower zone and peripheral predominance,[34] similar to the typical distribution in the more advanced fibrotic form of the disease. In the case of histiocytosis X the lower third of the lung is relatively unaffected. Although this distribution may be evident on a chest radiograph, in more widespread disease the sparing of the costophrenic recesses[57] or the anteromedial tips of the right middle lobe and lingula may be appreciated only on CT.

CT not only confirms the general distribution of disease that may be evident on chest radiography, it also gives important information about the distribution of disease in relation to the bronchovascular bundles, secondary pulmonary lobule, and visceral pleura. HRCT graphically shows peribronchial disease, particularly around bronchi that lie in the plane of section. The demonstration of a bronchocentric distribution has practical clinical use,

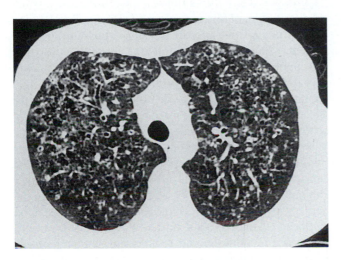

FIGURE 5-22
Histiocytosis X at a relatively early stage with numerous nodules, several of which are cavitating. In this patient, the disease was concentrated in the upper lobes.

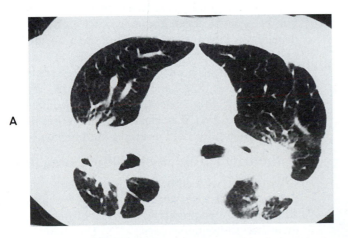
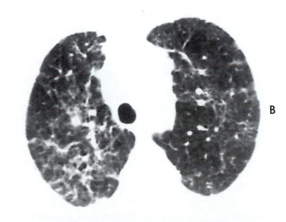

FIGURE 5-23
A, Dense confluent bronchocentric fibrosis radiating from the hila in a patient with long-standing sarcoidosis. **B,** Widespread reticular pattern in the upper lobes with distortion of the underlying pulmonary vasculature in a patient with chronic extrinsic allergic alveolitis. The distribution of fibrosis in an axial plane is quite different in these two conditions, both of which are characterized by upper zone fibrosis.

since it predicts that a transbronchial biopsy is likely to obtain diagnostic material.[49] Conditions that show a "bronchocentric" distribution are typified by sarcoidosis and lymphangitis carcinomatosa, and these diseases tend to have a more central distribution because of the confluence of the bronchovascular tree toward the hilum. Even in the advanced fibrotic stage of pulmonary sarcoidosis the peribronchial distribution remains evident (Figure 5-23, *A*). Such a striking predilection for the peribronchial regions is uncommon with other causes of upper zone fibrosis, such as chronic extrinsic allergic alveolitis (Figure 5-23, *B*).

CLINICAL APPLICATIONS

Clinical experience and the existing body of literature confirm that HRCT has become invaluable in the assessment of patients with suspected or clinically obvious diffuse lung disease. HRCT's superiority over plain chest radiography in identifying diffuse lung disease and suggesting a pathologic diagnosis is now discussed.

Sensitivity for the presence of diffuse lung disease

The frequency with which HRCT reveals pulmonary abnormalities when chest radiography is normal is difficult to gauge. Several studies have shown that HRCT scans were abnormal despite normal chest radiographs in 10% of cases of sarcoidosis,[62] 21% of cases of lymphangioleiomyomatosis.[61] 29% of cases of systemic sclerosis (Figure 5-24),[98] and approximately 30% of cases of asbestosis.[102] When these and other studies are taken into account, the prevalence of normal chest radiographs in patients with abnormalities on HRCT and confirmed diffuse lung disease is in the region of 20%. Although it is impossible to predict how often HRCT will reveal parenchymal abnormalities despite a normal chest radiograph,

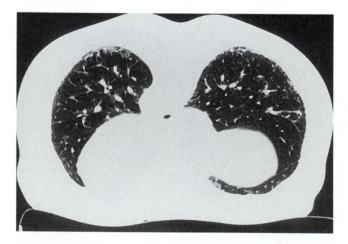

FIGURE 5-24
Subpleural linear and reticular opacities denoting fibrosing alveolitis in a patient (prone position) with systemic sclerosis. The patient had a normal chest radiograph and mildly reduced gas transfer on lung function testing.

HRCT clearly has an important role in patients with a questionably abnormal chest radiograph, particularly if clinical findings and lung function tests suggest disease.

Between 10% and 15% of patients with histologically proven interstitial lung disease have a normal chest radiograph.[17,23] In many studies describing the HRCT appearances of individual chronic diffuse lung diseases, a proportion of patients are reported to have had normal chest radiographs. The characteristics of HRCT abnormalities likely to be encountered in patients with diffuse lung disease and a normal chest radiograph can be summarized as (1) subtle differences in density of the lung parenchyma (for example, subacute extrinsic allergic alveolitis [Figure 5-16, *A*][32] and obliterative bronchiolitis [Figure 5-19, *A*][106]); (2) parenchymal abnormalities involving a small volume of the lung often obscured by superimposed structures (for example, the basal subpleural distribution of fibrosing alveolitis [Figure 5-24][98]), this is of particular relevance in asbestos-exposed individuals, who may have considerable pleural thickening obscuring the underlying lung parenchyma on chest radiography[1,22,102]; and (3) structural changes requiring high spatial resolution for their demonstration (for example, the thin-walled cystic airspaces of lymphangioleiomyomatosis[45] and the sometimes fine interstitial thickening in early lymphangitis carcinomatosa[104]). Patients with suspected diffuse lung disease on clinical grounds but normal chest radiographs are likely to have relatively limited changes on HRCT; the specificity and interobserver variation of such minimal changes on HRCT has not been evaluated. Some normal individuals have thickening of a few interlobular septa or parenchymal opacification mimicking early interstitial fibrosis.[1] Diffuse lung disease that is characterized by well-defined nodules or areas of frank pulmonary consolidation is not likely to result in HRCT abnormalities that are not also visible on chest radiography.

Chest radiography is similarly insensitive in the detection of bronchiectasis; the magnitude of this difference depends on the cause and extent of the bronchiectasis. In one study of adults with cystic fibrosis, 11% of patients had evidence of bronchiectasis on chest radiography, compared with 77% on HRCT.[97] Although the clinical utility of detecting evidence of very early emphysema is questionable, HRCT is clearly far more sensitive than chest radiography[7,39,40] or even lung function testing.[96]

Pathologic specificity in diffuse lung disease

In patients with clinical and lung function evidence of diffuse lung disease, several studies have confirmed that HRCT more often predicts the correct histologic diagnosis than chest radiography does.[29,49,84] The ability to narrow the differential diagnosis from the chest radiograph appearances alone in patients with diffuse lung disease is limited, and in one study the correct histologic diagnosis was included in the first two radiologic diagnoses offered by an experienced chest radiologist in only 50% of cases;

furthermore, interobserver agreement about the pattern of radiographic abnormality and the severity of disease was only 70%.[55]

In the first study to compare the diagnostic accuracy of chest radiography and CT in the prediction of specific histologic diagnoses in patients with diffuse lung disease, Mathieson and associates[49] showed that three observers could make a confident diagnosis in 23% of cases on the basis of chest radiographs and 49% using CT; the correct diagnoses were made in 77% and 93% of these readings, respectively. In this study approximately half of the patients had conventional CT sections only. In another study using HRCT exclusively in 140 consecutive patients with diffuse lung disease, Grenier and co-workers[29] showed that the high-confidence diagnoses of each of three observers that were correct on the basis of chest radiography findings alone were 29%, 34%, and 19%, whereas with HRCT the results were 57%, 55%, and 47%. Moreover, the intraobserver agreement for the proposed diagnosis was better with HRCT than with chest radiography.

A less striking difference in performance was found in a study by Padley and associates[84]: a confident diagnosis was offered in 41% of cases with chest radiography and 49% of cases with CT; of these readings, 69% and 82%, respectively, were correct. In this and similar studies, the degree of difference between the two techniques in the diagnosis of diffuse lung disease is likely to vary because of differences in case mixes, in the technical quality of the images, and in the observers' experience in interpreting chest radiographs and HRCT images. In the study by Padley and associates 14 normal subjects were included in the study group of 100 cases, which allowed an estimation of the ability of chest radiography and HRCT to identify normality correctly. Of patients thought to have normal chest radiographs, 42% had diffuse lung disease. In contrast, of patients thought to have normal lungs on CT, only 18% had diffuse lung disease. Normal subjects were correctly identified as such in 82% of cases with chest radiography and 96% of cases with CT.

The preceding studies show that HRCT is clearly useful for assessing patients with suspected diffuse lung disease when the clinical features and chest radiograph do not allow a confident diagnosis to be made. In some instances the HRCT appearances are virtually pathognomonic of a specific diffuse lung disease, and as experience increases, the need for lung biopsy to provide diagnostic confirmation may be reduced. The decision of whether to confirm a diagnosis of diffuse lung disease by biopsy is often complex, but HRCT has an increasingly influential role in such decision making.

Assessment of disease activity

Many attempts have been made to use noninvasive tests for assessing disease activity in interstitial lung diseases, particularly fibrosing alveolitis. Chest radiography, lung function tests, bronchoalveolar lavage, and

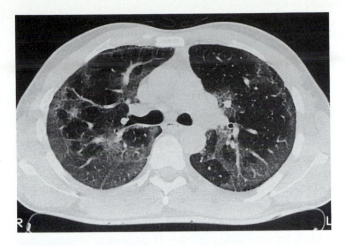

FIGURE 5-25
Ground-glass pattern in a patient with biopsy-proven cellular fibrosing alveolitis: there was no interstitial fibrosis. Nine months after treatment, the patient was symptom free.

radionuclide techniques all have limitations.[33,81,86,87] As a result, there has been great interest in defining the role of HRCT in staging disease activity. This is particularly true for fibrosing alveolitis, in which histologic findings indicating disease activity predict both response to treatment and prognosis.[111] Several studies have shown that a ground-glass pattern on CT in patients with fibrosing alveolitis corresponds histologically to active alveolitis (Figure 5-25).[46,67,93,119] Furthermore, a predominance of ground-glass opacification in fibrosing alveolitis predicts a good response to treatment[44,112] and longer actuarial survival[120] than in patients with a more reticular pattern, which denotes established fibrosis. The identification of these patterns on chest radiography is handicapped by significantly greater interobserver and intraobserver variation than with thin section CT.[13] Similar predictions about the potential reversibility of disease on HRCT can be made in patients with sarcoidosis in whom a ground-glass or a nodular pattern predominates.[11,47,74] In other conditions the identification of ground-glass opacification on HRCT, although nonspecific, almost invariably indicates a potentially reversible disease[46] such as extrinsic allergic alveolitis,[32] diffuse pulmonary hemorrhage,[12] or *Pneumocystis carinii* pneumonia.[9] An important exception is bronchioloalveolar cell carcinoma, in which there may be areas of ground-glass opacification that merge into areas of frank consolidation or a more nodular pattern (Figure 5-17).

Since the HRCT pattern of some diffuse lung diseases indicates disease activity and so predicts the subsequent behavior of the disease, HRCT may be used to follow up patients with these diseases.[94,109,121] Anatomically comparable sections are needed on follow-up studies. To achieve strictly comparable sections without imposing an excessive radiation burden on the patient, the protocol used should aim to achieve anatomically similar, if not identical, sections at two or three predetermined levels. In practice this may be difficult to achieve, so any judgment about change in extent or pattern of diffuse lung disease should take account of the comparability of sections on serial HRCT scans.

In patients who are to undergo lung biopsy, HRCT may be invaluable in indicating which biopsy procedure is likely to obtain useful diagnostic material. The broad distinction between peripheral disease and central and bronchocentric disease is easily made on HRCT; disease with a subpleural distribution such as fibrosing alveolitis is unlikely to be successfully sampled by transbronchial biopsy, whereas bronchocentric disease such as sarcoidosis and lymphangitis carcinomatosa is consistently accessible to transbronchial biopsy. If an open or thoracoscopic

lung biopsy is contemplated, HRCT will assist the surgeon in determining the optimal biopsy site and avoiding areas of end-stage interstitial fibrosis.[23]

BRONCHIECTASIS ON HIGH-RESOLUTION COMPUTED TOMOGRAPHY

The diagnosis of bronchiectasis on the basis of chest radiography alone is often uncertain unless the disease is extensive and severe. HRCT has rapidly supplanted bronchography as the imaging technique of choice for patients with suspected bronchiectasis. The opportunity for large-scale prospective studies to compare the accuracy of HRCT with the latter-day "gold standard" of bronchography has now passed. Most of the evidence suggesting that HRCT is at least as good as bronchography is based on small retrospective studies with different bronchographic and, more important, CT techniques. Nevertheless, with the demise of bronchography, no other imaging technique begins to compare to the sensitivity and specificity of a properly performed HRCT examination.*

HRCT has several advantages over bronchography in assessing patients with bronchiectasis: not only is bronchography unpleasant for the patient and sometimes hazardous, but also the quality of bronchographic images is variable and depends heavily on the operator's experience. Furthermore, the information on the bronchogram is limited to an assessment of the bronchial lumens; evaluation of the state of the bronchial wall is impossible. Although interpretation of the appearance of the bronchi on HRCT relies on some of the same criteria as bronchography, several supplementary signs help to confirm the diagnosis of bronchiectasis.

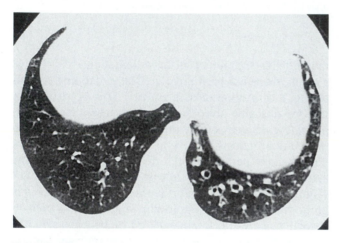

FIGURE 5-26
Signet ring sign: bronchiectasis confined to the subsegmental airways of the left lower lobe.

*References 28, 60, 77, 85, 88, 101.

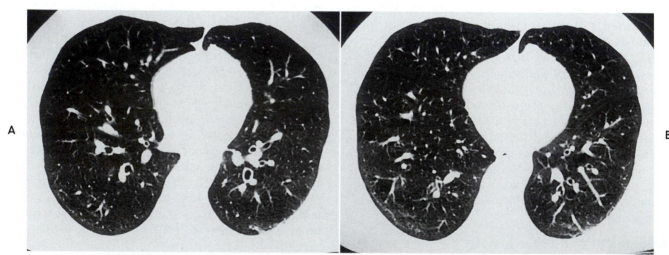

FIGURE 5-27
A, The posterobasal segmental bronchus of the left lower lobe has a larger diameter than its accompanying pulmonary artery, suggesting that it is bronchiectatic. **B,** Section 10 mm below this level shows that this is a spurious appearance caused by the confluence of two subsegmental bronchi.

Bronchiectasis is defined pathologically as damage to the bronchial wall that causes irreversible dilatation of the bronchi, whatever the cause. Thus the cardinal sign of bronchiectasis is dilatation of the bronchi with or without bronchial wall thickening.[27] Reversible bronchial dilatation does occur when there is adjacent pulmonary consolidation caused by acute infection.[78] For this reason, bronchiectasis should not be diagnosed when dilated bronchi are seen within densely consolidated lung. HRCT criteria for the identification of abnormally dilated bronchi depend on the orientation of the bronchi in relation to the plane of CT section.

Vertically oriented bronchi (in the lower lobes and apical segments of the upper lobes) are seen in transverse section, and reference can then be made to the accompanying pulmonary artery, which in normal individuals is of approximately the same caliber; any dilatation of the bronchus results in the so-called signet ring sign (Figure 5-26). Although this is generally a reliable sign of abnormal bronchial dilatation, conditions in which the pulmonary arteries are themselves of abnormal diameter must be considered. Furthermore, comparing the diameter of the bronchi and adjacent pulmonary arteries just below the division of the lower lobe bronchus may be misleading: at this level, pairs of segmental and sometimes subsegmental bronchi converge, and the fusion of the two bronchi may give the spurious impression of an abnormally dilated bronchus (Figure 5-27). Symmetry of the caliber of the bronchi between the right and left lungs is sometimes useful in establishing normality. However, a difference in the height of the two domes of the diaphragm may result in the two lower lobes being sectioned at different levels. The result is apparent prominence and dilatation of bronchi in the lobe that is being sectioned at a more proximal level. A false-positive diagnosis of bronchiectasis on HRCT is usually the result of scanning artifacts or another disease that superficially mimics bronchiectasis (such as histiocytosis X or cavitating bronchioloalveolar cell carcinoma [Figure 5-28])[54]; false-negative findings are more often due to a technically imperfect examination.

Bronchi that have a more horizontal course on CT, particularly the anterior segmental bronchi of the upper lobes and the segmental bronchi of the lingula and right middle lobe, are demonstrated along their length. Abnormal dilatation is seen as nontapering parallel walls or sometimes distinct flaring of the bronchi as they course distally (Figure 5-4). In more severe cases of bronchiectasis the bronchi are obviously dilated and have a concertina or varicose appearance. Because there is usually peribronchial fibrosis resulting in a thickened bronchial wall, the small airways can be identified more readily in the lung periphery, more than two thirds of the way out radially from the hilum. Although there is no exact level beyond which visualization of the bronchi can be regarded as abnormal on HRCT, normal bronchi should not be visible within 3 cm of the pleural surface (Figure 5-8).[70,117]

A supplementary HRCT sign of bronchiectasis is crowding of the affected bronchi with obvious volume loss of the lobe, as indicated by the position of the fissures. Patients with severe airway involvement by bronchiectasis may show definite regional differences in density of the lung parenchyma resulting from impaired ventilation partly because of bronchial obstruction by mucus plugging and bronchial wall thickening (Figure 5-29). The appearance of elliptic and circular opacities representing mucus- or pus-filled dilated bronchi is a sign of gross bronchiectasis and is almost invariably seen in the presence of other obviously dilated bronchi, some of which may contain air-fluid levels. When mucus plugging is present in the smaller airways, minute branching

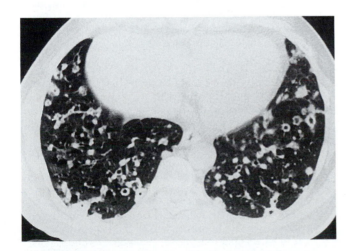

FIGURE 5-28
Unusual manifestation of bronchioloalveolar cell carcinoma: a profusion of cavitating nodules of approximately uniform size, which superficially resembles bronchiectasis.

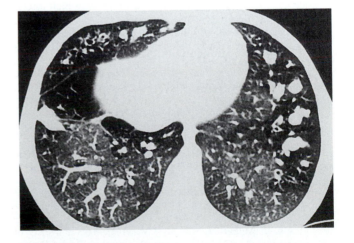

FIGURE 5-29
Plugging of the airways in severe bronchiectasis in a patient with cystic fibrosis. The surrounding lung is transradiant, reflecting reduced ventilation and perfusion.

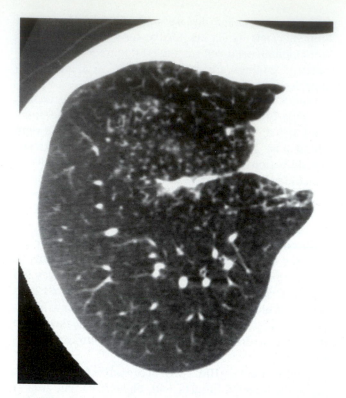

FIGURE 5-30
"Spotty" appearance in the anterior segment of the right lower lobe caused by plugging of the centrilobular bronchi. There were computed tomographic features of mild bronchiectasis in the subsegmental bronchi of the right lower lobe.

structures or dots in the lung periphery may be identifiable. In some cases plugging of the numerous centrilobular bronchioles gives a curious spotty appearance to the lungs, which may be confined to one bronchiectatic lobe (Figure 5-30).

REFERENCES

1. Aberle DR, Gamsu G, Ray CS, Feuerstein IM: Asbestos-related pleural and parenchymal fibrosis: detection with high resolution CT, *Radiology* 166:729-734, 1988.
2. Aberle DR, Hansell DM, Brown K, Tashkin DP: Lymphangiomyomatosis: CT, chest radiographic and functional correlations, *Radiology* 176:381-387, 1990.
3. Akira M, Kitatani F, Yong-Sik L, et al: Diffuse panbronchiolitis: evaluation with high-resolution CT, *Radiology* 168:433-438, 1988.
4. Akira M, Yamamoto S, Yokoyama K, et al: Asbestosis: high-resolution CT–pathologic correlation, *Radiology* 176:389-394, 1990.
5. Akira M, Yokoyama K, Yamamoto S, et al: Early asbestosis: evaluation with high-resolution CT, *Radiology* 178:409-416, 1991.
6. Arai K, Takashima T, Matsui O, et al: Transient subpleural curvilinear shadow caused by pulmonary congestion, *J Comput Assist Tomogr* 14:87-88, 1990.
7. Bergin C, Müller N, Nichols DM, et al: The diagnosis of emphysema: a computed tomographic–pathologic correlation, *Am Rev Respir Dis* 133:541-546, 1986.
8. Bergin CJ, Roggli V, Coblentz C, Chiles C: The secondary pulmonary lobule: normal and abnormal CT appearances, *AJR* 151:21-25, 1988.
9. Bergin CJ, Wirth RL, Berry GJ, Castellino RA: *Pneumocystis carinii* pneumonia: CT and HRCT observations, *J Comput Assist Tomogr* 14:756-759, 1990.
10. Brauner MW, Grenier P, Mouelhi MM, et al: Pulmonary histiocytosis X: evaluation with high-resolution CT, *Radiology* 172:255-258, 1989.
11. Brauner MW, Lenoir S, Grenier P, et al: Pulmonary sarcoidosis: CT assessment of lesion reversibility, *Radiology* 182:349-354, 1992.
12. Cheah FK, Sheppard MN, Hansell DM: Computed tomography of diffuse pulmonary haemorrhage with pathological correlation, *Clin Radiol* 48:89-93, 1993.
13. Collins CD, Wells AU, Hansell DM, et al: Observer variation in pattern type and extent of disease in fibrosing alveolitis on thin section computed tomography and chest radiography, *Clin Radiol* 49:236-240, 1994.
14. Cook PG, Wells IP, McGavin CR: The distribution of pulmonary shadowing in farmer's lung, *Clin Radiol* 39:21-27, 1988.
15. Corcoran HL, Renner WR, Milstein MJ: Review of high-resolution CT of the lung, *Radiographics* 12:917-939, 1992.
16. Engeler CE, Tashjian JH, Trenkner SW, Walsh JW: Ground-glass opacity of the lung parenchyma: a guide to analysis with high-resolution CT, *AJR* 160:249-251, 1993.
17. Epler GR, McLoud TC, Gaensler EA, et al: Normal chest roentgenograms in chronic diffuse infiltrative lung disease, *N Engl J Med* 298:935-939, 1978.
18. Evans SH, Cooke DJ, Anderson W: A comparison of radiation doses to the breast in computed tomographic chest examinations for two scanning protocols, *Clin Radiol* 40:45-46, 1989.
19. Felson B: A new look at pattern recognition of diffuse pulmonary disease, *AJR* 133:183-189, 1979.
20. Feuerstein IM, Archer A, Pluda JM, et al: Thin-walled cavities cysts and pneumothorax in *Pneumocystis carinii* pneumonia: further observations with histopathologic correlation, *Radiology* 174:697-702, 1990.
21. Fleischner Society: Glossary of terms for thoracic radiology: recommendations of the nomenclature committee of the Fleischner Society, *AJR* 143:509-517, 1984.
22. Friedman AC, Fiel SB, Fisher MS, et al: Asbestos-related pleural disease and asbestosis: a comparison of CT and chest radiography, *AJR* 150:269-275, 1988.
23. Gaensler EA, Carrington CB: Open lung biopsy for chronic diffuse infiltrative lung disease: clinical, roentgenographic and physiological correlations in 502 patients, *Ann Thorac Surg* 30:411-426, 1980.
24. Gaensler EA, Moister VB, Hamm J: Open lung biopsy in diffuse pulmonary disease, *N Engl J Med* 270:1319-1331, 1964.
25. Genereux GP: Pattern recognition in diffuse lung disease: a review of theory and practice, *Med Radiogr Photogr* 61:2-31, 1985.
26. Gilman MJ, Laurens RG, Jr, Somogyi JW, Honig EG: CT attenuation values of lung density in sarcoidosis, *J Comput Assist Tomogr* 7:407-410, 1983.
27. Grenier P, Cordeau MP, Beigelman C: High-resolution computed tomography of the airways, *J Thorac Imag* 8:213-229, 1993.
28. Grenier P, Maurice F, Musset D, et al: Bronchiectasis: assessment by thin-section CT, *Radiology* 161:95-99, 1986.
29. Grenier P, Valeyre D, Cluzel P, et al: Chronic diffuse interstitial lung disease: diagnostic value of chest radiography and high-resolution CT, *Radiology* 179:123-132, 1991.
30. Gurney JW, Bates FT: Pulmonary cystic disease: comparison of *Pneumocystis carinii* pneumatoceles and bullous emphysema due to intravenous drug abuse, *Radiology* 173:27-31, 1989.
31. Hansell DM, Kerr IH: The role of high resolution computed tomography in the diagnosis of interstitial lung disease, *Thorax* 46:77-84, 1991.
32. Hansell DM, Moskovic E: High-resolution computed tomography in extrinsic allergic alveolitis, *Clin Radiol* 43:8-12, 1991.

33. Harrison NK, Glanville AR, Strickland B, et al: Pulmonary involvement in systemic sclerosis: the detection of early changes by thin section CT scan bronchoalveolar lavage and 99mm Tc-DTPA clearance, *Respir Med* 83:1-12, 1989.

34. Hartman TE, Primack SL, Swensen SJ, et al: Desquamative interstitial pneumonia: thin-section CT findings in 22 patients, *Radiology* 187:787-790, 1993.

35. Hruban RH, Meziane MA, Zerhouni EA, et al: High resolution computed tomography of inflation-fixed lungs, *Am Rev Respir Dis* 136:935-940, 1987.

36. Ikezoe J, Takashima S, Morimoto S, et al: CT appearance of acute radiation-induced injury in the lung, *AJR* 150:765-770, 1988.

37. Itoh H, Murata K, Konishi J, et al: Diffuse lung disease: pathologic basis for the high-resolution computed tomography findings, *J Thorac Imag* 8:176-188, 1993.

38. Kerr IH: Interstitial lung disease: the role of the radiologist, *Clin Radiol* 35:1-7, 1984.

39. Klein JS, Gamsu G, Webb WR, et al: High-resolution CT diagnosis of emphysema in symptomatic patients with normal chest radiographs and isolated low diffusing capacity, *Radiology* 182:817-821, 1992.

40. Knudson RJ, Standen JR, Kaltenborn WT, et al: Expiratory computed tomography for assessment of suspected pulmonary emphysema, *Chest* 99:1357-1366, 1991.

41. Kubota H, Hosoya T, Kato M, et al: Plate-like atelectasis at the corticomedullary junction of the lung: CT observation and hypothesis, *Radiat Med* 1:305-310, 1983.

42. Kuhlman JE, Knowles MC, Fishman EK, Siegelman SS: Premature bullous pulmonary damage in AIDS: CT diagnosis, *Radiology* 173:23-26, 1989.

43. Kuhns LR, Borlaza G: The "twinkling star" sign: an aid in differentiating pulmonary vessels from pulmonary nodules on computed tomograms, *Radiology* 135:763-764, 1980.

44. Lee JS, Im JG, Ahn JM, et al: Fibrosing alveolitis: prognostic implication of ground-glass attenuation at high-resolution CT, *Radiology* 184:451-454, 1992.

45. Lenoir S, Grenier P, Brauner MW, et al: Pulmonary lymphangiomyomatosis and tuberous sclerosis: comparison of radiographic and thin-section CT findings, *Radiology* 175:329-334, 1990.

46. Leung AN, Miller RR, Müller NL: Parenchymal opacification in chronic infiltrative lung diseases: CT-pathologic correlation, *Radiology* 188:209-214, 1993.

47. Lynch DA, Webb WR, Gamsu G, et al: Computed tomography in pulmonary sarcoidosis, *J Comput Assist Tomogr* 13:405-410, 1989.

48. Martin KW, Sagel SS, Siegel BA: Mosaic oligemia simulating pulmonary infiltrates on CT, *AJR* 147:670-673, 1986.

49. Mathieson JR, Mayo JR, Staples CA, Müller NL: Chronic diffuse infiltrative lung disease: comparison of diagnostic accuracy of CT and chest radiography, *Radiology* 171:111-116, 1989.

50. Mayo JR: High resolution computed tomography: technical aspects, *Radiol Clin North Am* 29:1043-1049, 1991.

51. Mayo JR, Jackson SA, Müller NL: High-resolution CT of the chest: radiation dose, *AJR* 160:479-481, 1993.

52. Mayo JR, Müller NL, Henkelman RM: The double-fissure sign: a motion artifact on thin-section CT scans, *Radiology* 165:580-581, 1987.

53. Mayo JR, Webb WR, Gould R, et al: High-resolution CT of the lungs: an optimal approach, *Radiology* 163:507-510, 1987.

54. McGuinness G, Naidich DP, Leitman BS, McCauley DI: Bronchiectasis: CT evaluation, *AJR* 160:253-259, 1993.

55. McLoud TC, Carrington CB, Gaensler EA: Diffuse infiltrative lung disease: a new scheme for description, *Radiology* 149:353-363, 1983.

56. Mindell HJ: Roentgen findings in farmer's lung, *Radiology* 97:341-346, 1970.

57. Moore ADA, Godwin JD, Müller NL, et al: Pulmonary histiocytosis X: comparison of radiographic and CT findings, *Radiology* 172:249-254, 1989.

58. Morimoto S, Takeuchi N, Imanaka H, et al: Gravity-dependent atelectasis: radiologic, physiologic and pathologic correlation in rabbits on high-frequency oscillation ventilation, *Invest Radiol* 24:522-533, 1989.

59. Müller NL: Clinical value of high resolution CT in chronic diffuse lung disease, *AJR* 157:1163-1170, 1991.

60. Müller NL, Bergin CJ, Ostrow DN, Nichols DM: Role of computed tomography in the recognition of bronchiectasis, *AJR* 143:971-976, 1984.

61. Müller NL, Chiles C, Kullnig P: Pulmonary lymphangiomyomatosis: correlation of CT with radiographic and functional findings, *Radiology* 175:335-339, 1990.

62. Müller NL, Kullnig P, Miller RR: The CT findings of pulmonary sarcoidosis: analysis of 25 patients, *AJR* 152:1179-1182, 1989.

63. Müller NL, Miller RR: Computed tomography of chronic diffuse infiltrative lung disease (part 1), *Am Rev Respir Dis* 142:1206-1215, 1990.

64. Müller NL, Miller RR: Computed tomography of chronic diffuse infiltrative lung disease (part 2), *Am Rev Respir Dis* 142:1440-1448, 1990.

65. Müller NL, Miller RR, Webb WR, et al: Fibrosing alveolitis: CT pathologic correlation, *Radiology* 160:585-588, 1986.

66. Müller NL, Staples CA, Miller RR: Bronchiolitis obliterans organizing pneumonia: CT features in 14 patients, *AJR* 154:983-987, 1990.

67. Müller NL, Staples CA, Miller RR, et al: Disease activity in idiopathic pulmonary fibrosis: CT and pathologic correlation, *Radiology* 165:731-734, 1987.

68. Munk PL, Müller NL, Miller RR, Ostrow DN: Pulmonary lymphangitic carcinomatosis: CT and pathologic findings, *Radiology* 166:705-709, 1988.

69. Murata K, Herman PG, Khan A, et al: Intralobular distribution of oleic acid–induced pulmonary edema in the pig: evaluation by high-resolution CT, *Invest Radiol* 24:647-653, 1989.

70. Murata K, Itoh H, Todo G, et al: Centrilobular lesions of the lung: demonstration by high-resolution CT and pathologic correlation, *Radiology* 161:641-645, 1986.

71. Murata K, Khan A, Herman PG: Pulmonary parenchymal disease: evaluation with high-resolution CT, *Radiology* 170:629-635, 1989.

72. Murata K, Khan A, Rojas KA, Herman PG: Optimization of computed tomography technique to demonstrate the fine structure of the lung, *Invest Radiol* 23:170-175, 1988.

73. Murch CR, Carr DH: Computed tomography appearances of pulmonary alveolar proteinosis, *Clin Radiol* 40:240-243, 1989.

74. Murdoch J, Müller NL: Pulmonary sarcoidosis: changes on follow-up CT examination, *AJR* 159:473-477, 1992.

75. Naidich DP: Pulmonary parenchymal high-resolution CT: to be or not to be, *Radiology* 171:22-24, 1989.

76. Naidich DP, Funt S, Ettenger NA, Arranda C: Hemoptysis: CT-bronchoscopic correlations in 58 cases, *Radiology* 177:357-362, 1990.

77. Naidich DP, McCauley DI, Khouri NF, et al: Computed tomography of bronchiectasis, *J Comput Assist Tomogr* 6:437-444, 1982.

78. Nelson SW, Christoforidis A: Reversible bronchiectasis, *Radiology* 71:375-382, 1958.

79. Nishimura K, Kitaichi M, Izumi T, Itoh H: Diffuse panbronchiolitis: correlation of high-resolution CT and pathologic findings, *Radiology* 184:779-785, 1992.

80. Nishimura K, Kitaichi M, Izumi T, et al: Usual interstitial pneumonia: histologic correlation with high-resolution CT, *Radiology* 182:337-342, 1992.

81. Nugent KM, Peterson MW, Jolles H, et al: Correlation of chest roentgenograms with pulmonary function and bronchoalveolar lavage in interstitial lung disease, *Chest* 96:1224-1228, 1989.

82. Padley SPG, Adler B, Hansell DM, Müller NL: High resolution computed tomography of drug-induced lung disease, *Clin Radiol* 46:232-236, 1992.

83. Padley SPG, Adler B, Müller NL: High-resolution computed tomography of the chest: current indications, *J Thorac Imag* 8:189-199, 1993.

84. Padley SPG, Hansell DM, Flower CDR, Jennings P: Comparative accuracy of high resolution computed tomography and chest radiography in the diagnosis of chronic diffuse infiltrative lung disease, *Clin Radiol* 44:227-231, 1991.

85. Pang JA, Hamilton-Wood C, Metreweli C: Value of computed tomography in the diagnosis and management of bronchiectasis, *Clin Radiol* 40:40-44, 1989.

86. Panos RJ, Moretensen RL, Niccoli SA, King TE: Clinical deterioration in patients with idiopathic pulmonary fibrosis: causes and assessment, *Am J Med* 88:396-404, 1990.

87. Pantin CF, Valind SO, Sweatman M, et al: Measures of the inflammatory response in cryptogenic fibrosing alveolitis, *Am Rev Respir Dis* 138:1234-1241, 1990.

88. Philips MS, Williams MP, Flower CDR: How useful is computed tomography in the diagnosis and assessment of bronchiectasis? *Clin Radiol* 37:321-325, 1986.

89. Pilate I, Marcelis S, Timmerman H, et al: Pulmonary asbestosis: CT study of subpleural curvilinear shadow, *Radiology* 164:584, 1987.

90. Remy-Jardin M, Beuscart R, Sault MC, et al: Subpleural micronodules in diffuse infiltrative lung diseases: evaluation with thin-section CT scans, *Radiology* 177:133-139, 1990.

91. Remy-Jardin M, Degreef JM, Beuscart R, et al: Coal worker's pneumoconiosis: CT assessment in exposed workers and correlation with radiographic findings, *Radiology* 177:363-371, 1990.

92. Remy-Jardin M, Remy J, Deffontaines C, Duhamel A: Assessment of diffuse infiltrative lung disease: comparison of conventional CT and high-resolution CT, *Radiology* 181:157-162, 1991.

93. Remy-Jardin M, Remy J, Giraud F, et al: Computed tomography (CT) assessment of ground-glass opacity: semiology and significance, *J Thorac Imag* 8:249-264, 1993.

94. Remy-Jardin M, Remy J, Wallaert B, et al: Pulmonary involvement in progressive systemic sclerosis: sequential evaluation with CT, pulmonary function tests, and bronchoalveolar lavage, *Radiology* 188:499-506, 1993.

95. Ren H, Hruban RH, Kuhlman JE, et al: Computed tomography of inflation-fixed lungs: the beaded septum sign of pulmonary metastases, *J Comput Assist Tomogr* 13:411-416, 1989.

96. Sanders C, Nath PH, Bailey WC: Detection of emphysema with computed tomography: correlation with pulmonary function tests and chest radiography, *Invest Radiol* 23:262-266, 1988.

97. Santis G, Hodson ME, Strickland B: High resolution computed tomography in adult cystic fibrosis patients with mild lung disease, *Clin Radiol* 44:20-22, 1991.

98. Schurawitzki H, Stiglbauer R, Graninger W, et al: Interstitial lung disease in progressive systemic sclerosis: high resolution CT versus radiography, *Radiology* 176:755-759, 1990.

99. Sherrier RH, Chiles C, Roggli V: Pulmonary lymphangioleiomyomatosis: CT findings, *AJR* 153:937-940, 1989.

100. Silver SF, Müller NL, Miller RR, Lefcoe MS: Hypersensitivity pneumonitis: evaluation with CT, *Radiology* 173:441-445, 1989.

101. Silverman PM, Godwin JD: CT/bronchographic correlations in bronchiectasis, *J Comput Assist Tomogr* 11:52-56, 1987.

102. Staples CA, Gamsu G, Ray CS, Webb WR: High resolution computed tomography and lung function in asbestos-exposed workers with normal chest radiographs, *Am Rev Respir Dis* 139:1502-1508, 1989.

103. Stark P, Jasmine J: CT of pulmonary edema, *Crit Rev Diagn Imaging* 29:245-255, 1989.

104. Stein MG, Mayo J, Müller N, et al: Pulmonary lymphangitic spread of carcinoma: appearance on CT scans, *Radiology* 162:371-375, 1987.

105. Strickland B, Strickland NH: The value of high definition, narrow section computed tomography in fibrosing alveolitis, *Clin Radiol* 39:589-594, 1988.

106. Sweatman MC, Millar AB, Strickland B, Turner-Warwick M: Computed tomography in adult obliterative bronchiolitis, *Clin Radiol* 41:116-119, 1990.

107. Tarver RD, Conces DJ, Godwin JD: Motion artifacts on CT simulate bronchiectasis, *AJR* 151:1117-1119, 1988.

108. Templeton PA, McLoud TC, Müller NL, et al: Pulmonary lymphangioleiomyomatosis: CT and pathologic findings, *J Comput Assist Tomogr* 13:54-57, 1989.

109. Terriff BA, Kwan SY, Chan-Yeung MM, Müller NL: Fibrosing alveolitis: chest radiography and CT as predictors of clinical and functional impairment at follow-up in 26 patients, *Radiology* 184:445-449, 1992.

110. Tung KT, Wells AU, Rubens MB, et al: Accuracy of the typical computed tomographic appearances of fibrosing alveolitis, *Thorax* 48:334-338, 1993.

111. Turner-Warwick M, Burrows B, Johnson A: Cryptogenic fibrosing alveolitis: clinical features and their influence on survival, *Thorax* 35:171-180, 1980.

112. Vedal S, Welsh EV, Miller RR, Müller NL: Desquamative interstitial pneumonia: computed tomographic findings before and after treatment with corticosteroids, *Chest* 93:215-217, 1988.

113. Webb WR, Gamsu G, Wall SD, et al: CT of a bronchial phantom: factors affecting appearance and size measurements, *Invest Radiol* 19:394-398, 1984.

114. Webb WR, Müller NL, Naidich DP: High-resolution CT technique. In *High-resolution CT of the lung*, New York, 1992, Raven Press, pp 4-13.

115. Webb WR, Müller NL, Naidich DP: HRCT findings of lung disease. In *High-resolution CT of the lung*, New York, 1992, Raven Press, pp 24-50.

116. Webb WR, Müller NL, Naidich DP: Standardized terms for high resolution lung CT: a proposed glossary, *J Thorac Imag* 8:167-175, 1993.

117. Webb WR, Stein MG, Finkbeiner WE, et al: Normal and diseased isolated lungs: high-resolution CT, *Radiology* 166:81-87, 1988.

118. Weibel ER: Looking into the lung: what can it tell us? *AJR* 133:1021-1031, 1979.

119. Wells AU, Hansell DM, Corrin B, et al: High resolution computed tomography assessment of disease activity in the fibrosing alveolitis of systemic sclerosis: a histopathological correlation, *Thorax* 47:738-742, 1992.

120. Wells AU, Hansell DM, Rubens MB, et al: The predictive value of high resolution computed tomography in fibrosing alveolitis, *Am Rev Respir Dis* 148:1076-1082, 1993.

121. Wells AU, Rubens MB, Du Bois RM, Hansell DM: Serial computed tomography in fibrosing alveolitis: the prognostic significance of the initial pattern, *AJR* 162:473-478, 1993.

122. Westcott JL, Cole SR: Traction bronchiectasis in end-stage pulmonary fibrosis, *Radiology* 161:665-669, 1986.

123. Yoshimura H, Hatakeyama M, Otsuji H, et al: Pulmonary asbestosis: CT study of subpleural curvilinear shadow, *Radiology* 158:653-658, 1986.

124. Zerhouni EA: Computed tomography of the pulmonary parenchyma: an overview, *Chest* 95:901-907, 1989.

125. Zerhouni EA, Naidich DP, Stitik FP, et al: Computed tomography of the pulmonary parenchyma. II. Interstitial disease, *J Thorac Imag* 1:54-64, 1985.

126. Zwirewich CV, Mayo JR, Müller NL: Low dose high resolution CT of lung parenchyma, *Radiology* 180:413-417, 1991.

6 Infections of the Lungs and Pleura

PETER ARMSTRONG
PAUL DEE

Pneumonias are best classified according to the infecting organism because the cause dictates the treatment. Unfortunately, radiologic techniques are usually poor at predicting even the broad category of infectious agent, let alone the specific organism.[368] Imaging nevertheless has many important roles in patients with suspected pulmonary infection. The plain chest radiograph is the primary method of establishing the presence of pneumonia and of determining its location and extent. Predisposing conditions, notably bronchial carcinoma, may be visible, and complications, such as pleural effusion, empyema, and abscess formation, are readily demonstrated. Once pneumonia and its complications have been diagnosed, chest radiographs are an excellent method of following the response to treatment.

The essential radiographic feature of pneumonia is pulmonary consolidation, which may show cavitation and may be accompanied by pleural effusion. The appearance varies almost infinitely from one or more small, ill-defined shadows to large airspace shadows involving the whole of one or more lobes. The pattern depends not only on the infecting organism, but also on the integrity of the host defenses.

Pneumonias are sometimes divided according to their chest radiographic appearances into bronchopneumonia, lobar pneumonia, spherical (round or nodular) pneumonia, and interstitial pneumonia. Although widely used, these terms have limited value because the same organism may produce several patterns and because patterns often overlap in the individual patient. Also, pathologists and radiologists do not always agree in their use of these descriptive phrases.

Bronchopneumonia is the most common pattern. In bronchopneumonia the inflammatory exudate is multifocal and centered on large inflamed airways, involving some acini and sparing others. On radiologic examination, bronchopneumonia is characterized by patchy consolidation, loss of volume, and absence of air bronchograms (Figure 6-1). When affected areas coalesce, the shadowing may become more uniform and resemble lobar pneumonia. Although the term "segmental consolidation" is in common use, consolidation conforming precisely to segmental anatomy is rarely seen.

In lobar pneumonia (Figure 6-2) the inflammatory exudate begins in the distal airspaces and spreads via the pores of Kohn across segmental boundaries, giving rise to homogeneous nonsegmental consolidation. Eventually the pneumonia may involve a whole lobe, but usually symptoms develop before the entire lobe is consolidated and then antibiotic therapy halts the process. The consolidation is usually confined to one lobe, although multilobar involvement is not uncommon. Because the airways are not primarily affected, there is little or no volume loss and visible air bronchograms are common.

Some pneumonias present as spherical or nodular consolidations (Figure 6-3). The nodules are usually ill defined and may contain air bronchograms.

Interstitial pneumonia refers to a radiographic pattern comprising extensive peribronchial thickening and ill-defined reticulonodular shadowing of the lungs, which may be relatively localized or may be widespread (Figure 6-4). Associated patchy subsegmental or discoid atelectasis is common. This pattern, although it may show a lobar or segmental distribution, is frequently independent of the lobar architecture of the lung. The usual causes are viral and *Mycoplasma pneumoniae* infections.

DIAGNOSING THE CAUSE OF PNEUMONIA

Pneumonias caused by viruses or *M. pneumoniae* are usually self-limiting and resolve without treatment, whereas bacterial pneumonias require accurate diagnosis and therapy if serious complications, and even death, are to be avoided. It is bacterial pneumonia therefore that forms the bulk of cases seen in the hospital. The choice of which antibiotic to use may have to rest on a combination of clinical findings, radiographic features, and an initial Gram stain of the sputum[221] because the results of bacteriologic tests may be delayed and are sometimes uninformative.[46] Such guesses are based on many factors:

1. The age of the patient and any history of exposure to a specific organism. In infants viral infections are the dominant cause of pneumonia, and *Mycoplasma* infection becomes an important cause in young children.[70] Bacterial pneumonia is relatively rare at these ages. In adults with radiographically evident pulmonary consolidation the predominant cause is bacterial infection.[221]

2. The source of the infection, particularly whether it was acquired in the hospital or in the community. Pneumococcal, mycoplasmal, and viral pneumonias are the common community-acquired pneumonias in adults,[154] with *Staphylococcus aureus*, *Streptococcus pyogenes*, *Klebsiella*, *Chlamydia*, *Rickettsia*, and *Legionella pneumophila* as alternative agents, whereas gram-negative bacilli, *S. aureus*, anaerobic organisms, and pneumococci are the particularly prevalent causes in hospital-acquired infections.[27] Nearly half the cases of hospital-acquired pneumonia have more than one potential pathogen.[27]

3. The character of the illness. Bacterial pneumonia typically presents as an acute illness with chest pain, chills, high fever, and cough productive of purulent sputum. Neutrophilia is common. *Mycoplasma* and viral pneumonias, on the other hand, usually have prodromal symptoms, mild pyrexia, and less sputum; neutrophilia is absent and the white blood cell count is usually only slightly elevated.

4. Predisposing conditions. The list of predisposing conditions is long and complex. For example, aspiration pneumonia, which is most often due to anaerobic organisms, gram-negative bacteria, or *S. aureus*, is particularly prevalent in patients who are alcoholics, have had recent general anesthesia or a bout of unconsciousness, or have disturbances of swallowing.[131] Pneumococcal pneumonia is particularly likely in sickle cell disease and following

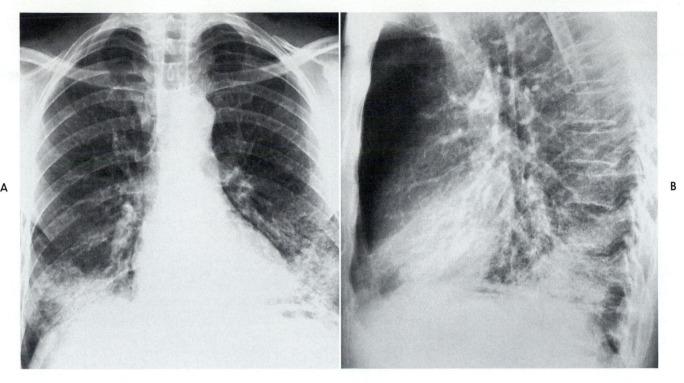

FIGURE 6-1
Bronchopneumonia. Bilateral lower zone predominant aspiration pneumonia in an alcoholic patient.
A, Posteroanterior view. B, Lateral view.

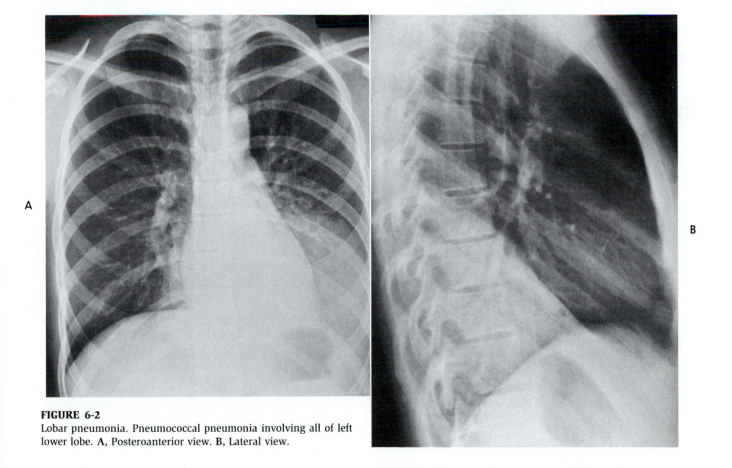

FIGURE 6-2
Lobar pneumonia. Pneumococcal pneumonia involving all of left
lower lobe. A, Posteroanterior view. B, Lateral view.

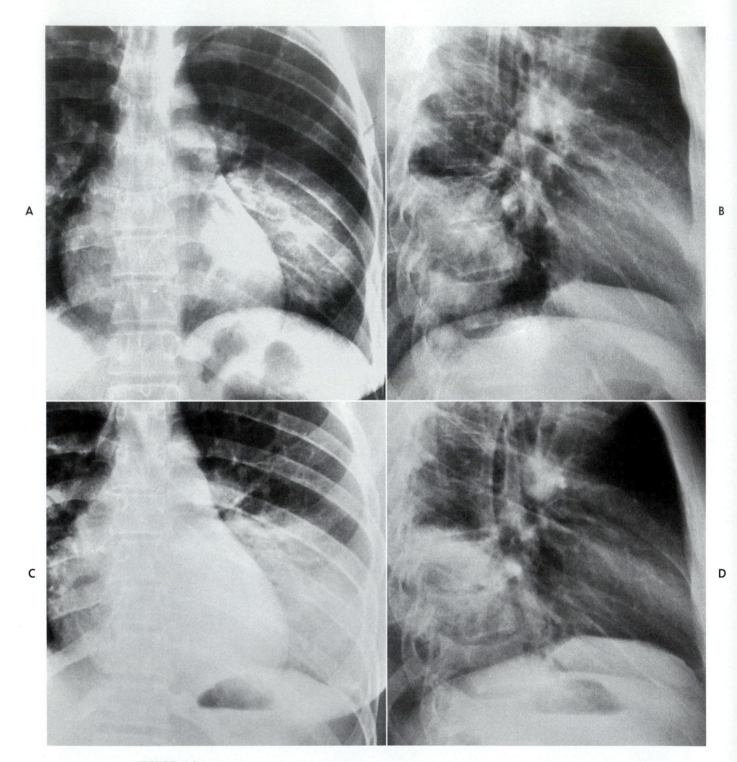

FIGURE 6-3
Round pneumonia in left lower lobe caused by pneumococcal pneumonia. **A,** Posteroanterior and, **B,** lateral radiographs on admission to hospital. **C** and **D,** Twelve hours later, round pneumonia has progressed to become lobar in shape.

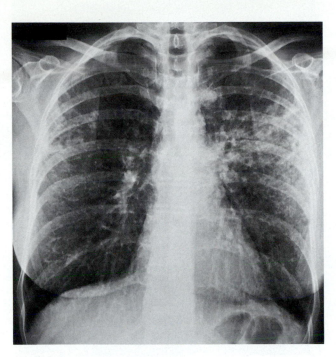

FIGURE 6-4
Interstitial viral pneumonia showing bilateral streaky shadowing radiating from both hila.

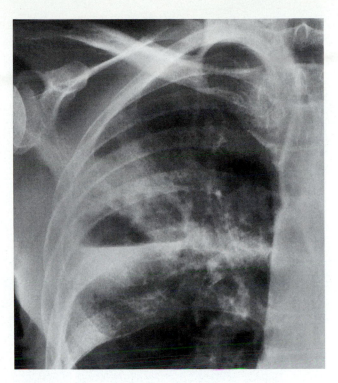

FIGURE 6-5
Consolidation with cavitation caused by gram-negative bacterial pneumonia.

splenectomy. *Pseudomonas aeruginosa* or *S. aureus* is the likely pathogen responsible for pneumonia in patients with cystic fibrosis.[87,207] Patients who are immunocompromised present a special category and are discussed in Chapter 7.

Before a discussion of individual pneumonias, it may be helpful to consider a few generalizations regarding pulmonary infection of the immunocompetent host:

1. Consolidation of all or most of a lobe is usually bacterial in origin (Figure 6-1), and postobstructive pneumonia should be strongly considered, particularly in patients who may have carcinoma of the bronchus. When lobar consolidation is due to a primary bacterial infection, the usual organism is *Streptococcus pneumoniae* (pneumococcus). Occasionally the infection is due to *Klebsiella, S. aureus, Mycobacterium tuberculosis,* or *L. pneumophila* or to aspiration of anaerobic or gram-negative bacteria from the upper respiratory tract or pharynx. Expansion of the lobe is a sign that suggests pneumococcal or *Klebsiella* pneumonia.

2. Aspiration pneumonia frequently causes patchy consolidation in the dependent portions of the lungs (Figure 6-1). The consolidations are usually multilobar and bilateral in distribution.

3. Consolidation with cavitation (Figure 6-5) suggests bacterial or fungal disease rather than viral or *Mycoplasma* infection. The bacteria that commonly cause cavitation are *S. aureus,* gram-negative bacteria (especially *Klebsiella, Proteus,* and *Pseudomonas*), anaerobic

bacteria, and *M. tuberculosis.* A large solitary abscess in a patient without underlying lung disease, the so-called primary lung abscess, is usually due to anaerobic bacteria. Such abscesses are usually due to aspiration of oropharyngeal secretions, alone or in combination with impairment of local or systemic host defense mechanisms.[144]

Pneumatocele formation (see p. 105) can be difficult to distinguish from cavitation (Figure 6-6). When pneumatoceles are due to pneumonia, the responsible organism is likely to be *S. aureus,* although pneumatoceles have also been described in infants with pneumonia caused by *S. pneumoniae.*[11]

Care needs to be taken to avoid misdiagnosing cavitation or pneumatocele formation when the focal transradiancies within consolidation are due to underlying emphysema. Emphysematous areas within the lung prevent homogeneous consolidation and may mimic cavitation.[413]

Pulmonary gangrene is a rare but interesting form of cavitation that produces sloughed lung within a large cavity secondary to thrombosis of the pulmonary vessels as they pass through the pneumonia (Figure 6-7).[305] *S. pneumoniae* and *Klebsiella*[78,195,271] are the most common responsible agents. The condition is unusual with other gram-negative pneumonias.[148] Pulmonary gangrene has also been described with *M. tuberculosis,*[195] possibly with anaerobic bacteria,[271] with *Aspergillus* infection,[350] and with mucormycosis in the immunocompromised host.[410]

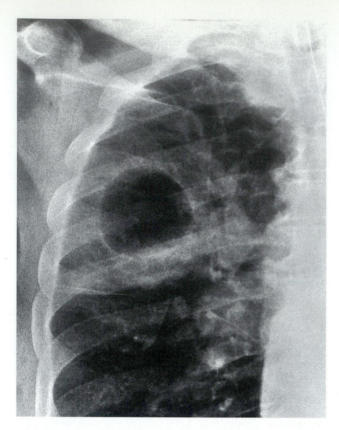

FIGURE 6-6
Pneumatocele formation in staphylococcal pneumonia.

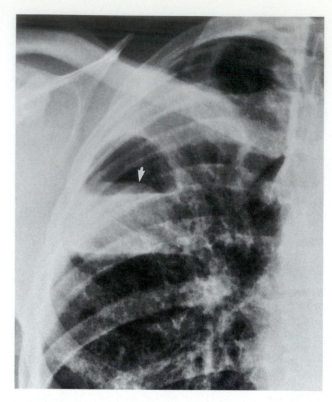

FIGURE 6-7
Pulmonary gangrene. Sloughed lung *(arrow)* can be seen projecting above air-fluid level in cavity. Organism in this case was *Pseudomonas.*

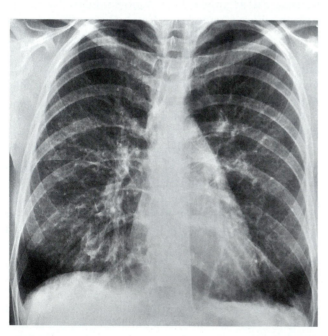

FIGURE 6-8
Mycoplasma pneumonia showing widespread reticulonodular shadowing in lung.

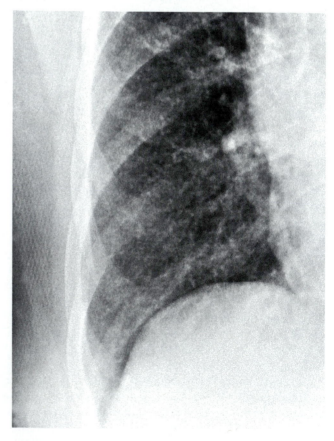

FIGURE 6-9
Miliary tuberculosis.

4. Nodular (spherical) pneumonia (Figure 6-3) is usually due to pneumococcal infection,[317] *L. pneumophila, Legionella micdadei,*[86,287] Q fever,[250] or fungal disease. It may also be due to hematogenous spread of bacteria, most commonly *S. aureus.* Although spherical pneumonia can be confused with lung carcinoma, the distinction is relatively straightforward when the pneumonia is bacterial in origin, since at least part of the border of a spherical pneumonia is ill defined in almost all instances. Spherical pneumonias expand to involve the adjacent lung over the next few hours or days, may contain air bronchograms, and are associated with obvious clinical features of acute bacterial infection. Also, they are common in childhood, an age at which lung carcinoma is nonexistent. Spherical pneumonias caused by fungal infections, however, are often chronic and may closely resemble carcinoma of the lung both clinically and radiographically.

5. Pneumonia that presents with focal or widespread, small, ill-defined reticulonodular shadows (Figure 6-8), whether or not lobar or segmental infiltrates are also present, is likely to be due to viral or mycoplasmal infection.[72,363] In exceptional cases fungal and streptococcal infection gives rise to this pattern.

6. Miliary nodulation of the lungs has many causes. When it is due to infection, the likely organisms are *M. tuberculosis* (Figure 6-9) and various fungi. The nodules are even in size, usually 2 to 4 mm in diameter, well defined, and uniformly distributed.

7. Patchy upper lobe consolidations (Figure 6-10) are very suggestive of tuberculous or fungal infection, notably histoplasmosis but occasionally North American blastomycosis, cryptococcosis, and coccidioidomycosis. Patchy lower lobe consolidations together with loss of volume suggests aspiration pneumonia.

8. Large pleural effusions are most commonly associated with pneumonia caused by anaerobic bacteria, gram-negative bacteria, *S. aureus,* or *S. pyogenes.* Empyemas can be radiologically indistinguishable from pleural effusions, but empyema should be considered if the effusion is large, delayed in appearance, or loculated, particularly if it loculates rapidly.

9. Most pneumonias resolve radiologically within a month, often within 10 to 21 days, and most of the remainder by 2 months. The most indolent shadowing is seen with infection caused by tuberculosis, anaerobes, *Coxiella burnetti, L. pneumophila,* or *Chlamydia psittaci* and with some cases of *M. pneumoniae* pneumonia. Consolidation persisting beyond 2 months represents delayed resolution, and an explanation should be sought. The most likely reasons are that the patient is old or has a systemic disease. Alternatively, the pneumonia may have been extensive or have been complicated by atelectasis, cavitation, or empyema. If none of these explanations appears satisfactory, a predisposing local cause such as obstructing neoplasm or bronchiectasis should be carefully sought.

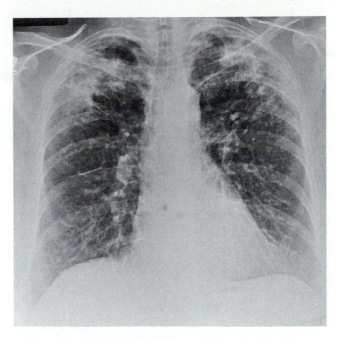

FIGURE 6-10
Patchy upper zone consolidations caused by histoplasmosis.

10. It has been suggested, but not substantiated, that symptomatic bacterial pneumonia may not be radiographically evident in severely dehydrated patients and that the consolidation caused by the pneumonia will become apparent only with rehydration of the patient. This widespread belief was refuted by animal experiments conducted by Caldwell and associates,[53] and only one possible clinical case has been reported in the literature.[150]

11. Diagnosing pneumonia in patients receiving mechanical ventilation can be difficult. Pneumonia, edema, adult respiratory distress syndrome (ARDS), infarction, and hemorrhage have overlapping signs, so that a confident diagnosis based on radiographic features alone is often not possible. Air bronchograms have the best predictive value for pneumonia, except in patients with ARDS in whom air bronchograms are part of the ARDS, but even air bronchograms have a predictive value for pneumonia of less than 70%.[405]

12. The distinction between normal and early pneumonia is often difficult, with relatively poor interobserver agreement.[248]

BACTERIAL PNEUMONIA
Streptococcus pneumoniae pneumonia

S. pneumoniae (pneumococcal) pneumonia occurs at any age, is the most common community-acquired bacterial pneumonia,[351] and is a leading cause of hospital-acquired infection. Dementia, seizure disorders, institutionalization, smoking, previous splenectomy, and various chronic illnesses are all predisposing factors. The initial symptoms of pneumococcal pneumonia typically

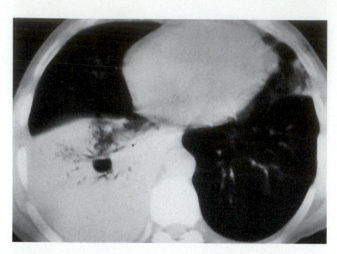

FIGURE 6-11
Computed tomographic scan of lobar consolidation caused by pneumococcal pneumonia. Note cavity and forward bowing of major fissure, indicating expansile consolidation.

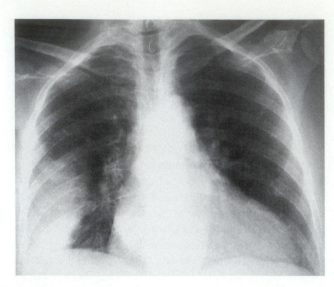

FIGURE 6-12
Pneumococcal pneumonia presenting as large peripheral consolidation in right lower lobe.

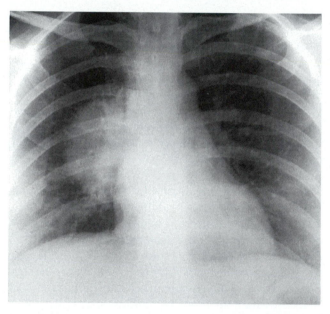

FIGURE 6-13
Round pneumonia caused by *Streptococcus pneumoniae* resembling a mediastinal mass.

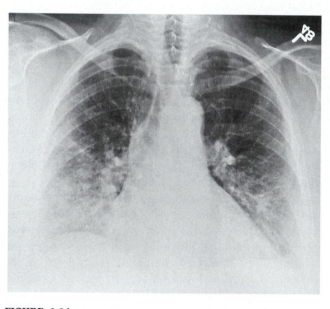

FIGURE 6-14
Pneumococcal pneumonia presenting as bilateral middle and lower zone patchy consolidations.

include sudden onset of high fever, shaking chills, pleuritic pain, and cough productive of sputum that is sometimes streaked with blood.

A variety of radiographic patterns are described. Pneumococcal pneumonia is the prototype pathologic condition for lobar consolidation (Figures 6-2 and 6-11). Bacteria are inhaled into the periphery of a lobe where they incite an intense inflammatory reaction, which is seen radiographically as an area of homogeneous nonsegmental shadowing (Figure 6-12).[115] Air bronchograms

may be evident. The exudate spreads rapidly across interalveolar connections rather than via the bronchial tree. It crosses segmental boundaries through the pores of Kohn and therefore does not show a segmental pattern. If untreated the pneumonia may involve the whole of the lobe, which may be expanded by the intense exudate. Frequently the gravitationally dependent portions of the lobes are the most densely opacified. Sometimes more than one lobe is involved. Early in its course, before any pleural boundaries have been reached, the pneumonia

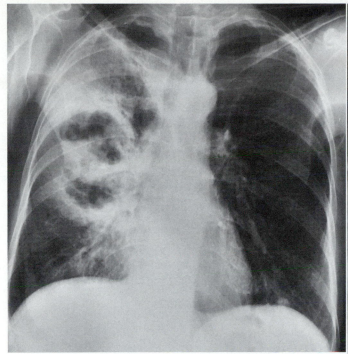

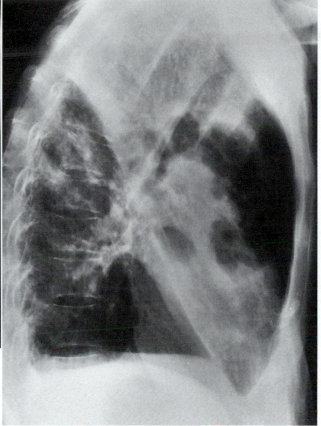

FIGURE 6-15
Pneumococcal pneumonia showing extensive cavitation in lobar consolidation of right upper and middle lobes. A, Posteroanterior view. B, Lateral view.

may be spherical (Figure 6-13), a phenomenon seen most frequently in children.

Nowadays this classic picture of lobar pneumonia is seen less often. Recent reports have emphasized that the more usual pattern is patchy or peribronchial consolidation (Figure 6-14), patterns that occurred in 57 (61%) of Ort's 94 patients[272] and in 28 (70%) of 40 patients in Kantor's series.[189] A widespread, small nodular and linear pattern resembling interstitial disease was seen in 22% of Kantor's patients; others do not emphasize this pattern, presumably regarding it as one of the bronchopneumonic varieties. With appropriate treatment the pneumonia usually clears within 14 days.

Pleural effusion is seen in up to 57% of patients,[227,366] and occasionally, particularly if treatment has been delayed, the effusion turns into an empyema. The presence of parapneumonic effusions correlates with the duration of symptoms before admission, with bacteremia, and with prolonged fever after commencement of therapy.[366]

Cavitation is distinctly unusual (Figure 6-15). A very rare complication is pulmonary gangrene.[78,271]

Streptococcus pyogenes pneumonia

S. pyogenes pneumonia is now much less common than pneumococcal pneumonia. In the early part of this century it was a major cause of pneumonia in both adults

and children. It may complicate viral infections or may follow streptococcal upper respiratory tract infections. On chest radiographs (Figure 6-16), *S. pyogenes* pneumonia appears as lower lobe–predominant, confluent or patchy consolidation. Large pleural effusions and empyema are common.[28]

Staphylococcal pneumonia

Pneumonia caused by *S. aureus* usually follows aspiration of organisms from the upper respiratory tract, occurring particularly in debilitated hospitalized patients. It may also be community acquired, particularly in infants and elderly individuals, often complicating influenza. Pneumonia caused by hematogenous spread may result from endocarditis, thrombophlebitis, or staphylococcal infection of indwelling catheters. Septicemic infection is also seen in drug addicts and immunocompromised patients.

Typically the plain chest radiograph (Figure 6-17)[395] shows patchy segmental consolidation, often with loss of volume. Air bronchograms are rare. The consolidation may spread rapidly and become confluent, resembling lobar pneumonia (Figure 6-18). Several lobes are frequently involved, and the disease may be bilateral. Abscess cavities may form within the pneumonia and are common at any age (Figure 6-18). Pneumatoceles (Figure 6-19) are much more common in childhood than adult

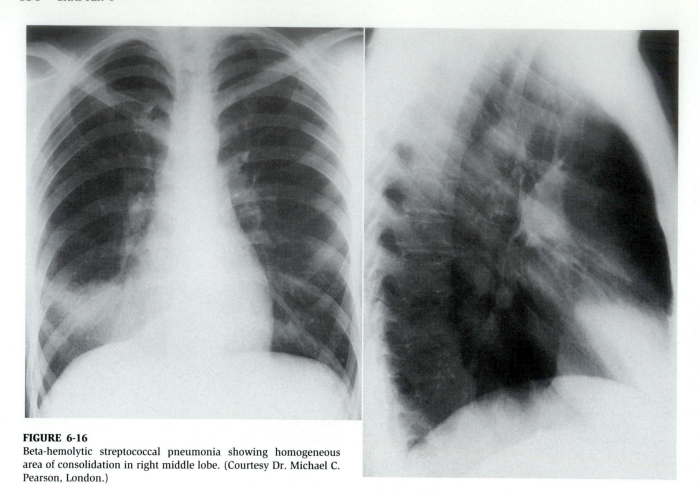

FIGURE 6-16
Beta-hemolytic streptococcal pneumonia showing homogeneous area of consolidation in right middle lobe. (Courtesy Dr. Michael C. Pearson, London.)

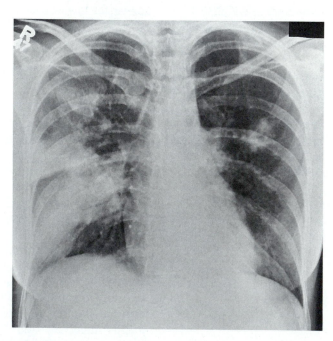

FIGURE 6-17
Staphylococcal pneumonia showing bilateral multifocal consolidation.

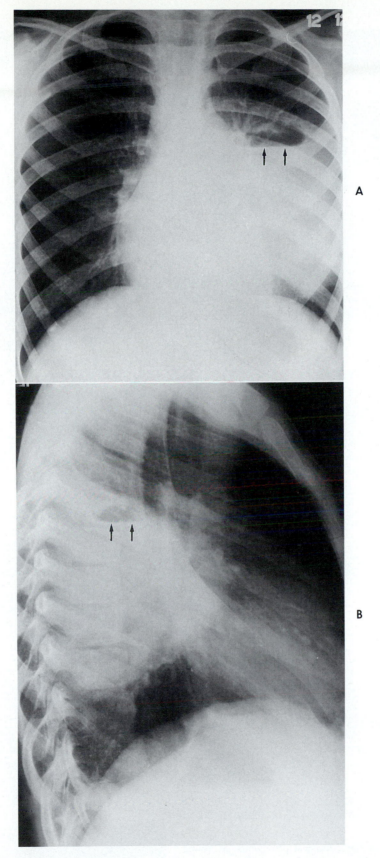

FIGURE 6-18
Staphylococcal pneumonia showing confluent lobar-type consolidations with cavitation (arrows point to air-fluid level in superior segment of left lower lobe). **A,** Posteroanterior view. **B,** Lateral view. (Courtesy Dr. Michael C. Pearson, London.)

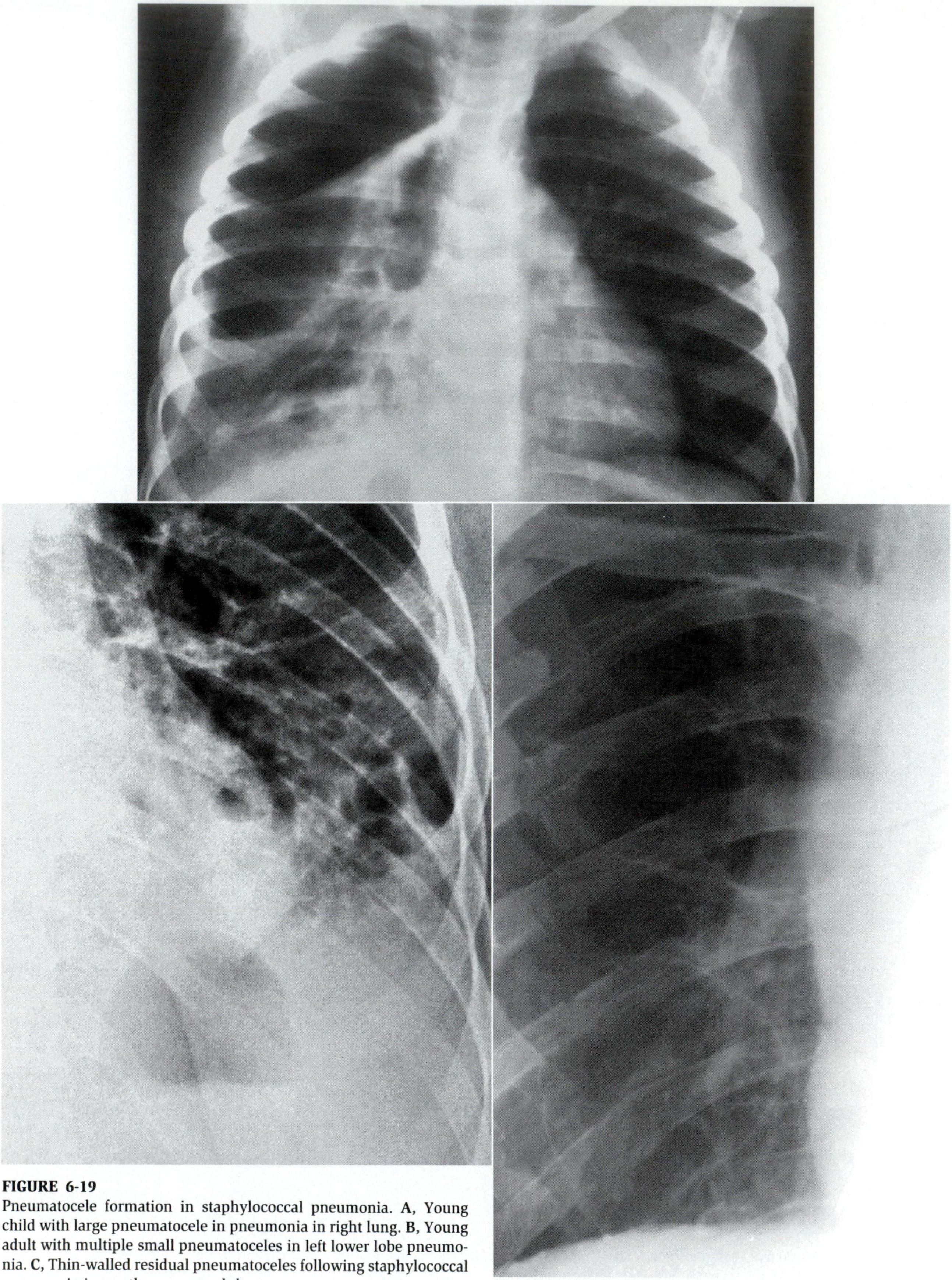

FIGURE 6-19
Pneumatocele formation in staphylococcal pneumonia. **A,** Young child with large pneumatocele in pneumonia in right lung. **B,** Young adult with multiple small pneumatoceles in left lower lobe pneumonia. **C,** Thin-walled residual pneumatoceles following staphylococcal pneumonia in another young adult.

infection and may lead to pneumothorax. Pleural effusions, which may develop rapidly, are common. In one large series of adults they were seen in just under 40% of cases.[395] Empyema formation is a common and serious complication, particularly in children. Septicemic staphylococcal infection, in contrast to infection following aspiration, causes multiple spherical (round) consolidations, which may cavitate.[263]

Anthrax

Anthrax, a major scourge before the introduction of vaccines originated by Louis Pasteur, is due to *Bacillus anthracis,* a gram-positive aerobic bacillus. Anthrax is now an extremely rare cause of pneumonia in the United States and United Kingdom. It is usually acquired from contact with infected goats or their products, particularly unfinished hides and wools imported from endemic areas in Asia, the Middle East, or Africa (Figure 6-20). The spores may be inhaled directly into the lungs, but cutaneous anthrax is the usual clinical presentation. The spores are carried to regional lymph nodes, from which they may disseminate to the lungs and cause hemorrhagic pneumonia. Mediastinal widening caused by lymphadenopathy appears to be a common radiographic feature.[377] The lungs may also show patchy consolidation, particularly at the bases, and pleural effusions.

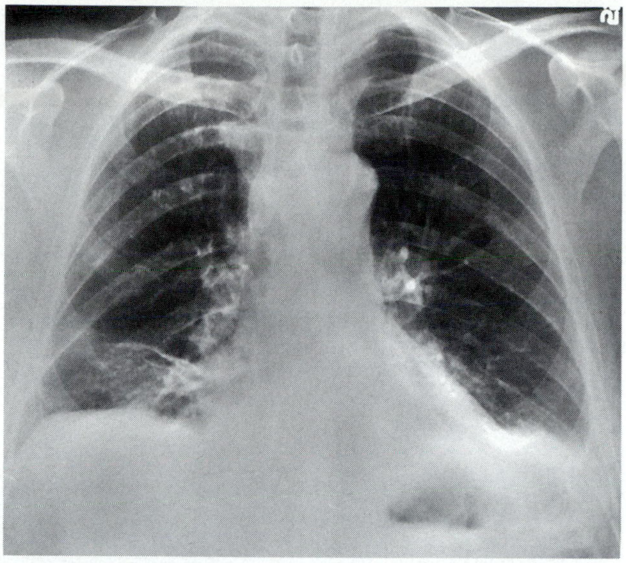

Gram-negative bacterial pneumonia

Many aerobic gram-negative bacteria cause pneumonia.[285] The most important are the Enterobacteriaceae (notably *Klebsiella, Enterobacter, Serratia marcescens, Escherichia coli,* and *Proteus mirabilis*), *P. aeruginosa, Acinetobacter, Haemophilus influenzae,* and *L. pneumophila.* Together with *S. aureus* these organisms are by far the most frequent cause of hospital-acquired pneumonia and are a major cause of morbidity and mortality. They contaminate hospital equipment such as ventilators and the soaps, liquids, or jellies used to care for wounds and catheters. (*Klebsiella* and *Legionella* pneumonias have features that differentiate them from other gram-negative bacterial pneumonias and are discussed separately in the next section.)

Affected patients usually have a known predisposing factor such as chronic obstructive pulmonary disease, a major medical condition, or recent surgery. The bacterial flora of the the upper respiratory tract becomes colonized by various pathogens, and when aspiration occurs, the patients are in great danger of gram-negative bacterial pneumonia. Aspiration is believed to be the common method by which the organisms enter the lungs, but pneumonia following inhalation of bacteria or spread by the bloodstream is also occasionally seen.

The radiologic pattern of the gram-negative bacterial pneumonias* varies from small ill-defined nodules to patchy consolidation (Figure 6-21), which may some-

---

*References 18, 282, 307, 369-371, 375.

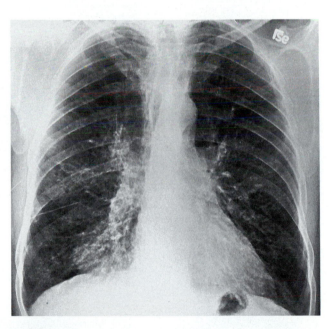

FIGURE 6-20
Anthrax pneumonia in carpet cleaner who developed pneumonia with severe fever, shaking chills, and hypotension. Bilateral basal consolidations and mediastinal lymphadenopathy are present.

FIGURE 6-21
Haemophilus influenzae pneumonia causing bilateral basal patchy consolidations predominantly in right lower lobe.

times be confluent and resemble lobar pneumonia or even pulmonary edema.[166] Usually the consolidations are multifocal, with the lower lobes nearly always affected, usually bilaterally. About half the time the upper and middle lobes are also involved.[375] Cavitation is common (Figures 6-5 and 6-22),[241] but radiographic lucencies in areas of consolidation, although often caused by abscess formation, are sometimes due to spared normal acini surrounded by pneumonia.[307] Renner and co-workers[307]

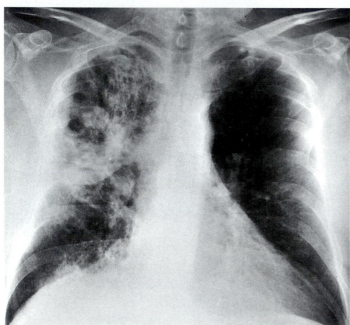

FIGURE 6-22
Acinetobacter pneumonia showing bilateral upper lobe consolidation with abscess formation.

also pointed out that the microabscesses seen at pathologic examination are not identified on plain chest radiographs; only after they coalesce to form cavities of 2 cm or more and communicate with an airway do they become visible.

Parapneumonic pleural effusions are common in most gram-negative pneumonias, with empyema an important and fairly frequent complication.[370,371]

KLEBSIELLA PNEUMONIA. Pneumonia caused by *Klebsiella pneumoniae* (Friedlander's pneumonia), like the other gram-negative pneumonias, usually affects people with chronic debilitating illnesses or alcoholism. The symptoms include high fever and toxemia and clinically resemble those of severe pneumococcal pneumonia. On radiologic examination[104,161] the consolidations are also similar to those seen with *S. pneumoniae* pneumonia: the disease is often confined to one lobe, with homogeneous nonsegmental consolidation that spreads rapidly to become a lobar pneumonia.[119] Multilobar and bilateral consolidations may occur.[161] The advancing edge of the pneumonia is sharp and distinct. In one series there was a striking predilection for the upper lobes,[161] a finding not supported by Frommhold's series,[119] and lobar expansion was a noteworthy feature in the early series,[104,161] but our impression is that both these features are unusual in the modern antibiotic era.

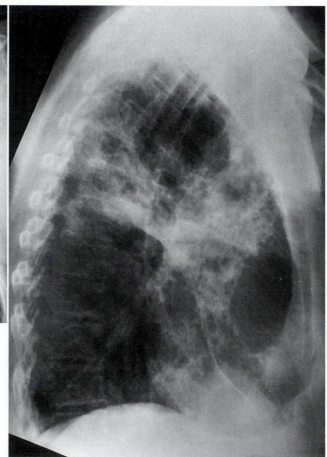

A

B

FIGURE 6-23
Klebsiella pneumonia of right upper lobe showing numerous cavities. **A,** Posteroanterior view. **B,** Lateral view.

Cavitation, which may occur early and progress quickly, is seen in 30% to 50% of cases (Figure 6-23). This feature distinguishes *Klebsiella* pneumonia from pneumococcal pneumonia, in which cavitation is rare. The cavities are frequently multiple (Figure 6-23) and may attain great size. Solitary large chronic abscesses are occasionally encountered.[303] Massive necrosis, so-called pulmonary gangrene, is a rare phenomenon. Pleural effusion and empyema are relatively uncommon.[161,285]

LEGIONELLA PNEUMOPHILA PNEUMONIA. Legionnaires' disease, which results in severe pneumonia with a high mortality, is due to *L. pneumophila,* an aerobic gram-negative bacillus found in aquatic environments such as reservoirs, cooling towers, water distribution systems, and humidifiers.[266] Infection comes from these sources rather than from person-to-person contact. The disease may be sporadic or occur in localized epidemics centered on an infected water source, such as the 1976 outbreak at an American Legion convention, in which 29 of 182 affected delegates died[113] and from which the name "Legionnaires' disease" is derived. The infection is characterized by malaise, myalgia, headache, abdominal and chest pain, nausea, vomiting, diarrhea, high fever, rigors, dyspnea, and cough; the cough is usually productive and associated with hemoptysis. Bacteremic dissemination causes a variety of extrapulmonary manifestations, including endocarditis, sinusitis, brain abscess, and pancreatitis. Predisposing chronic diseases are common and may be either pulmonary, such as chronic bronchitis

and emphysema, or systemic, such as malignant disease or renal failure. Corticosteroid therapy is a recognized risk factor, but surprisingly patients with neutropenia or AIDS do not appear to have an undue predilection for Legionnaires' disease.[266] The organism is difficult to culture from sputum and blood, and selective culture media are required. The diagnosis is usually established serologically by an indirect fluorescent antibody test. The main disadvantage is that the mean time for seroconversion is about 2 weeks.[99] Hyponatremia is common[197] and occurs more frequently in *L. pneumophila* pneumonia than in other pneumonias.[409]

The chest radiographic appearances have been reviewed in detail by Fairbank and associates.[99] The initial finding is peripherally situated patchy consolidation (Figure 6-24), which spreads rapidly, often involving more than one lobe and becoming bilateral in half the cases (Figure 6-25). There may be a slight predilection for

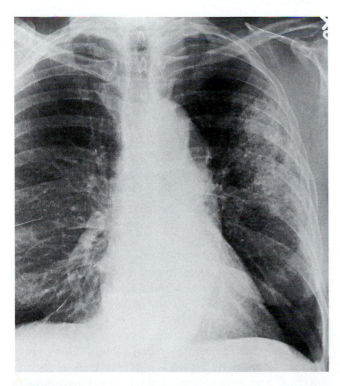

FIGURE 6-24
Legionella pneumophila pneumonia showing rounded peripheral area of consolidation in left upper lobe.

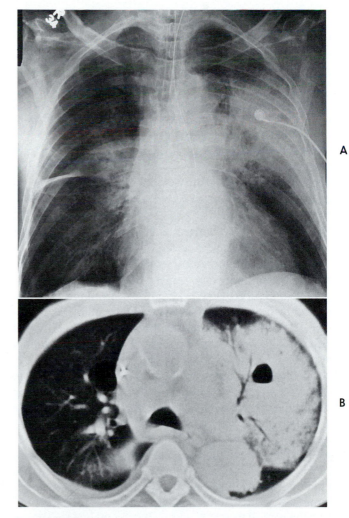

A

B

FIGURE 6-25
Legionella pneumophila pneumonia showing multilobar confluent consolidation. Cavitation, which can be seen in, **A,** plain film, is better demonstrated in, **B,** computed tomographic scan.

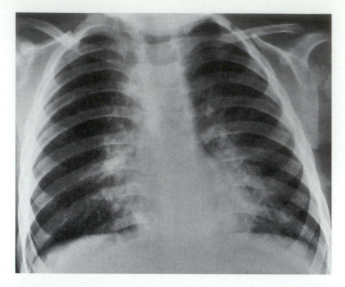

FIGURE 6-26
Pertussis pneumonia showing peribronchial consolidation adjacent to heart, giving rise to so-called shaggy heart sign.

the lower lobes, but this is not seen in all series.[246] The consolidations may assume a spherical configuration or may coalesce to resemble lobar pneumonia.[86,97] Cavitation, although reported, is unusual (Figure 6-25)[203]; it appears to be most common in immunocompromised patients.[246,255] Pleural effusions, which are usually small but occasionally massive, are documented in up to two thirds of cases,[203,246] and frank empyema formation may occur.[300] Unusual radiographic features include hilar adenopathy and spontaneous pneumothorax.[99] The radiographic resolution is slow, particularly in immunocompromised patients, and lags behind the clinical improvement. The changes usually persist for at least a month after the acute illness.

L. micdadei pneumonia is considered separately in the section on immunocompromised patients on p. 246.

PERTUSSIS (WHOOPING COUGH). Whooping cough is caused by the aerobic gram-negative coccobacillus *Bordetella (Haemophilus) pertussis*. Pneumonia caused by this organism is less common now that immunization is available.

On chest radiographs[23,37,101] the striking feature is extensive streaky peribronchial consolidation in one or more lobes. A recently reported large series, comprising 238 patients ill enough to require admission to the hospital, provides a good indication of the chest radiographic findings in the modern era.[37] Sixty-three patients (26%) had abnormal findings on chest radiography. Pulmonary consolidation, which was predominantly peribronchial in distribution, was present in 50 patients, pulmonary collapse in 9, and visible lymphadenopathy in 22. The pulmonary changes showed a tendency to involve the right lung, particularly the lower and middle lobes. The peribronchial consolidation may be maximal close to

the mediastinum, giving rise to an appearance that has been dubbed the shaggy heart sign (Figure 6-26).[23]

BRUCELLOSIS. Brucellosis, an infection transmitted by inhaling infected material from domestic animals, particularly cows, pigs, and goats, or by ingesting infected animal products, such as milk, only occasionally causes pneumonia. The responsible organism is a gram-negative coccobacillus. The symptoms include those of systemic infection: fever, malaise, and headache. Symptoms of pneumonia are seen in less than half of those with abnormalities on the chest radiograph. The chest x-ray findings are focal areas of consolidation, hilar adenopathy, nodular shadows, or miliary nodulation.[147] Spherical calcifications surrounded by thin lamellar calcifications may be seen in the spleen as a late manifestation.[7,147]

MELIOIDOSIS. Melioidosis[98] is due to the aerobic gram-negative bacillus *Pseudomonas pseudomallei*, an organism that resides in dust and soil. Pneumonia is rare except in the flooded fields and marshes of Southeast Asia.[85] Multiple organ involvement is common, with the lungs the most frequently affected organ.[85] The pneumonia may be acute or subacute. The acute form, which can be rapidly fatal, is characterized by positive blood cultures, fulminating septicemia, high fever, and acute prostration. The subacute form consists of cough, which is usually productive, occasional hemoptysis, low-grade fever, weight loss, and pleuritic chest pain. In some patients few symptoms occur and melioidosis is diagnosed only because pulmonary disease is found on chest radiography.

On chest radiographs[85,98,178,362] the acute pneumonia shows small, round, ill-defined areas of consolidation that are often unilateral and may coalesce to form segmental or lobar opacities (Figure 6-27), with a striking affinity for the upper lobes. Cavitation is frequent; the cavities may be thin walled. Pleural effusion, empyema, and pneumothorax are seen in a small proportion of patients,[85] and hilar adenopathy is reported.

In the subacute form the plain chest radiograph shows a variety of patterns, including round, segmental, or lobar consolidation, which often cavitates[85,362] and may be accompanied by empyema. In the chronic subclinical forms the chest radiograph closely resembles postprimary tuberculosis with patchy upper lobe consolidation and cavitation.

PLAGUE. Plague is due to *Yersinia (Pasteurella) pestis*, a gram-negative coccobacillus still found in some areas of Asia, Africa, South America, and the southwestern United States.[4,304] Pneumonia may be primary, resulting from inhalation of infected droplets, or may spread hematogenously from infected swollen axillary or femoral lymph nodes, sometimes known as buboes. The resulting pneumonia is severe, with high fever. In fatal cases numerous petechiae and ecchymoses develop, the appearance of which gave rise to the name "Black Death" in the fearful epidemic that swept Europe in the fourteenth century.

Radiographic examination[4,400] shows rapidly progres-

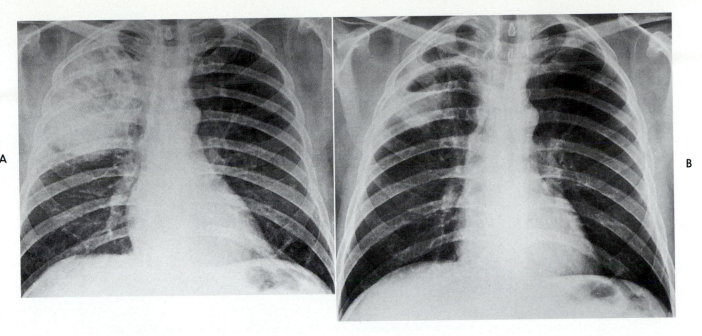

FIGURE 6-27
Melioidosis pneumonia. **A,** Large area of consolidation in right upper lobe. **B,** Six weeks later, pneumonia has partially resolved, leaving thin-walled abscess.

sive dense patchy consolidations that may be nodular, segmental, or lobar in shape. Eventually multiple lobes are involved and mediastinal adenopathy and pleural effusions may be present. In some cases of bubonic plague, mediastinal and hilar adenopathy is the only radiographic finding.

P. multocida is a gram-negative rod or coccobacillus that infects cats and dogs. Respiratory infection resulting in acute bronchitis, bronchopneumonia, lung abscess, or empyema may follow inhalation of organisms or a bite. The radiographic changes were reviewed by Winer-Muram and Rubin.[400] They include lobar, multilobar, or widespread patchy consolidation, usually sparing the upper lobes. Pleural effusions have been noted in up to 20% of patients.

TULAREMIA. Tularemia, named after Tulare County in California, is due to *Francisella tularensis,* an aerobic gram-negative coccobacillus. The disease is endemic in many parts of the world, including Europe, Asia, and North America. Human infection is acquired in a variety of ways: through the skin in individuals who handle infected animals (rabbits, squirrels, skunks, dogs, game birds, and many others) or their skins; by bites from infected insect vectors, notably ticks and fleas; by bites from the infected animals themselves; or by inhalation of organisms from infected carcasses, of dust, or following laboratory accidents. Pneumonia is a common finding in patients with tularemia.

The radiographic signs of tularemia pneumonia are lobar, segmental, rounded, oval, or patchy pulmonary consolidations, which may be unilateral or bilateral in distribution (Figure 6-28).[12,84,251,275,320] The most common pattern is unilateral patchy consolidation, but widespread bronchopneumonia, lobar consolidation, lung abscess, and apical opacities resembling tuberculosis are all encountered.[400] Cavitation may occur but is unusual, and a pattern resembling pulmonary edema may also be encountered. Miliary nodulation was seen in one case in a large series.[320] The pulmonary changes may be accompanied by cardiomegaly caused by pericarditis with pericardial effusion. Hilar adenopathy is common as are pleural effusions, both of which may be unilateral or bilateral. Empyema and bronchopleural fistula may supervene. On rare occasions the consolidations heal with fibrosis and calcification and thus resemble tuberculosis and histoplasmosis.

Anaerobic lung infection

Most anaerobic lung infections result from aspiration of infected oral contents, and overt periodontal disease is seen in the majority of patients.[26,144] Predisposing factors such as a recent episode of altered consciousness, dysphagia, or alcoholism are frequent.[26,144] Underlying bronchial carcinoma was found in 9% of patients in one large series.[26]

The infection is usually indolent or subacute,[209] although an acute febrile illness, closely resembling pneumococcal pneumonia but without shaking chills, may be seen.[25,26] Often the sputum is putrid, a feature not encountered in pneumonia caused by aerobic bacteria. In about half the cases anaerobic organisms alone are responsible (the common ones are *Bacteroides, Fusobac-*

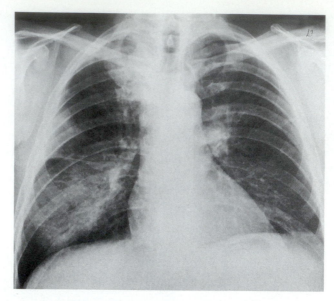

FIGURE 6-28
Tularemia pneumonia showing multiple areas of consolidation in right lung. Two weeks before this film was taken, the patient had run over a rabbit while mowing lawn.

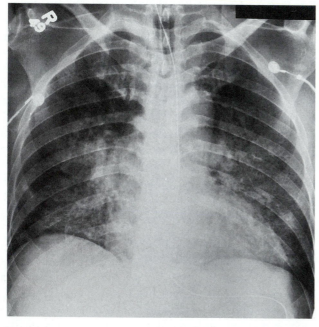

FIGURE 6-29
Anaerobic aspiration pneumonia showing bilateral middle and lower zone consolidation.

terium, Peptococcus and *Peptostreptococcus,* microaerophilic *Streptococcus,* and *Propionibacterium*), and in the other half of cases mixed anaerobic and aerobic bacteria are found on culture. A pitfall here is that the anaerobic bacteria may not be appreciated unless especially cultured, and it may therefore be assumed that aerobic organisms alone are responsible for the pneumonia.

The radiographic appearances[26,209] can be conveniently divided into pulmonary parenchymal infection, pneumonia with cavitation, and discrete lung abscess, each of which may be associated with empyema.

Anaerobic pneumonia has a strong predilection for the lower lobes (Figures 6-1 and 6-29), with the right lung more commonly affected than the left. These sites are entirely compatible with the belief that the pneumonia follows aspiration from the upper respiratory tract. There is usually one predominant focus of disease, but multilobe involvement is also common.

Cavitation within an area of pulmonary consolidation is seen in 30% to 40% of cases and may develop while the patient is in the hospital on appropriate antibiotic therapy. One third of patients have a discrete lung abscess (Figures 6-30 and 6-31). Discrete lung abscesses occur chiefly in the posterior portions of the lungs, usually in the posterior segments of the upper lobes or in the superior segments of the lower lobes. In patients with cavitation or lung abscess the disease takes longer to resolve, sometimes 6 weeks or more. Hilar and mediastinal adenopathy may accompany lung abscess,[315] and such cases may therefore closely resemble carcinoma of the lung (Figure 6-32).

One third to one half of patients have empyema.[26,209] Over half the patients in one series of anaerobic bacterial empyema had no apparent parenchymal disease.[209] If pleural effusion is seen in association with anaerobic lung infection, it is virtually certain to be an empyema.[209] The infected fluid can be mobile but is frequently loculated. Very large empyemas may be seen, and bronchopleural fistula is a recognized complication.

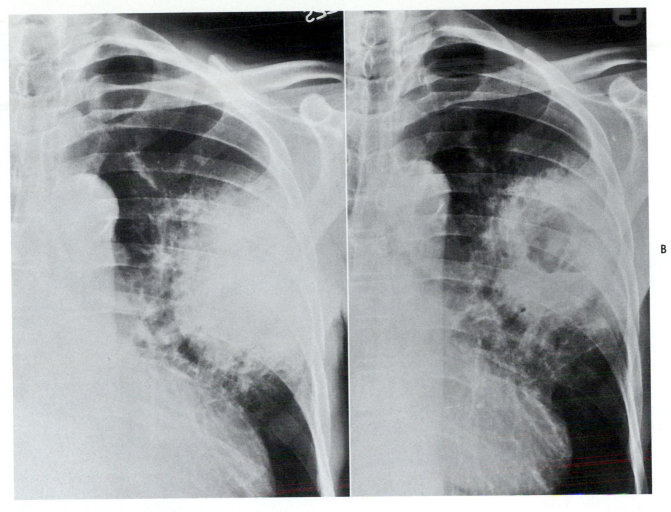

FIGURE 6-30
Anaerobic lung abscess in alcoholic patient with bad teeth. **A**, Early in course of disease, showing rounded area of pneumonia. **B**, Two days later, showing discrete lung abscess.

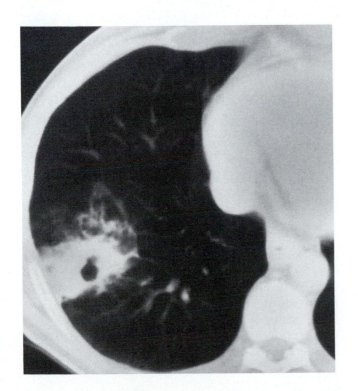

FIGURE 6-31
Computed tomographic scan of anaerobic pneumonia with cavitation.

Syphilis

Pulmonary infection caused by *Treponema pallidum* is rare. Diffuse bronchopneumonia, diffuse pulmonary fibrosis, and solitary[62] or multiple pulmonary nodules may all be seen.

Leptospirosis

Leptospirosis, caused by the spirochete *Leptospira*, is common in the tropics where it is the cause of Weil's disease, a syndrome comprising fever, jaundice, hemorrhage, nephritis, and meningitis. Leptospirosis follows contact with contaminated water or tissues of infected animals.

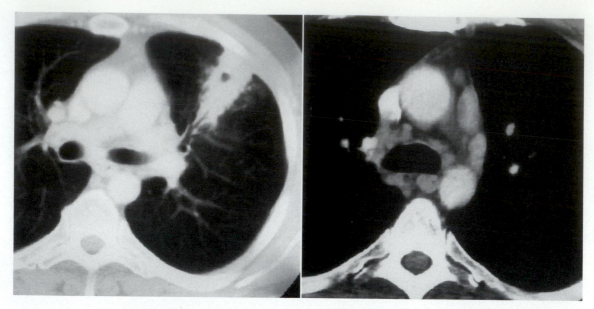

FIGURE 6-32
Anaerobic lung abscess with mediastinal adenopathy mimicking lung cancer.

Pneumonia occurs in one fifth to two thirds of patients with leptospirosis.[174] The pulmonary consolidations are due to hemorrhagic pneumonitis. Chest radiographs[174,214] show bilateral, multiple areas of pulmonary consolidation that may take the form of multiple well-defined small nodules or multifocal nonlobar consolidations with a marked tendency toward peripheral predominance. These patchy areas of consolidation in severe cases may be extensive and confluent. Patchy discoid atelectasis and small pleural effusions are common. Interlobular septal thickening (Kerley lines) is seen in a small proportion of patients.[174] Hilar and mediastinal adenopathy does not appear to be a feature.

Rickettsial infections

The most common rickettsial pneumonia is Q fever, caused by *C. burnetti.* Q fever occurs worldwide and is acquired from infected dust, from cattle or sheep products, or occasionally from the bite of infected ticks or mites. The disease occurs sporadically and in epidemics. The symptoms are sudden in onset and include a flulike illness with fever, dry cough, myalgias, arthralgias, and headache. Pneumonia develops in less than half those infected. The usual radiographic appearance of Q fever pneumonia (Figure 6-33)[137,250,284] is unifocal or multifocal, subsegmental, segmental, or lobar consolidation, with a predilection for the lower lobes. Accompanying patchy atelectasis, often discoid in shape, is common. Spherical (round) pneumonia is also common, particularly in epidemic cases.[180,229] Very occasionally these round pneumonias are confused with lung cancer.[180] Cavitation is rare.[338] Pleural effusions are seen in some patients, particularly in sporadic infection. The disease is self-limiting, but resolution of pulmonary consolidation

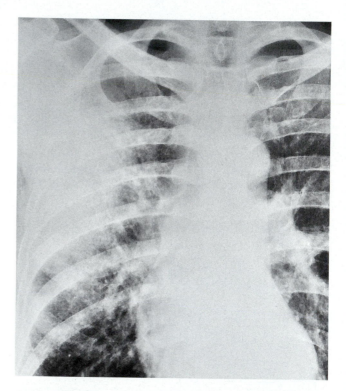

FIGURE 6-33
Q fever. There is large focal consolidation in right upper lobe.

may take up to 3 months, although the average time is 30 days.[250]

Rocky Mountain spotted fever, caused by *Rickettsia rickettsiae,* is encountered mostly in the southeastern United States, where it is transmitted through tick bites. It is an acute, often fulminant, disease in which small vessel inflammation is the basic pathologic process. The vascu-

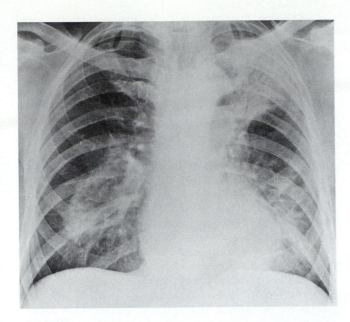

FIGURE 6-34
Psittacosis pneumonia showing multifocal bilateral consolidations.

litis is clinically most evident in the skin and central nervous system. In the lungs the resulting pulmonary vasculitis leads to a variety of patterns, varying from unifocal or multifocal consolidations, resembling bacterial pneumonia, to widespread pulmonary infection, resembling pulmonary edema, combined in some cases with pleural effusions.[215,239] The pulmonary edema pattern is probably caused by pulmonary capillary endothelial damage combined with the effect of increased hydrostatic forces owing to left heart failure.[88] The pathologic result is interstitial and alveolar edema and hemorrhage, together with a mononuclear and lymphocytic interstitial infiltrate.[239] Bacterial superinfection appears to be rare.[88] The clinical diagnosis depends on recognizing a multiorgan vasculitis, notably of the skin and meninges, in an acutely febrile patient during the tick season in endemic areas. The mortality is high in patients with widespread pulmonary consolidation.

Chlamydia infections

C. psittaci infection, so-called ornithosis or psittacosis, is usually acquired from infected birds. Infection with the psittacosis agent may result in disease of wide clinical spectrum, ranging from completely asymptomatic infections recognized only by serologic means to overwhelming illness involving multiple organ systems.[339] Usually the patient complains of fever, malaise, headache, and a nonproductive cough, and the clinical picture may be indistinguishable from other acute bacterial pneumonias with pleuritic chest pain, productive cough, hemoptysis, shortness of breath, and shaking chills. The chest radiograph reveals patchy pulmonary consolidation (Figure 6-34), which can be extensive. Another described pattern is patchy reticular shadowing with lower zone predomi-

nance that appears more severe than would be expected from the clinical features. Pleural effusions are rare.

Chlamydia trachomatis is a recently recognized cause of pneumonia in neonates and infants, where it may cause widespread streaky consolidations and air trapping similar to that seen with acute bronchiolitis of viral origin.[297] In a few reported cases in adults the chest radiographs showed focal streaky consolidation without evidence of air trapping. Pleural effusion, although reported, is not a striking feature.[92,361]

Septic emboli

The most common sources of septic pulmonary emboli are infected venous catheters, including pacemaker wires; tricuspid valve endocarditis (a major source in intravenous drug abusers)[188]; septic thrombophlebitis (again a significant problem in drug addicts); and indwelling prosthetic devices. Immunocompromised patients are a particularly vulnerable subgroup of the population.

The diagnosis is usually established by positive blood cultures and the presence of an infected source for the emboli. It is worth noting that positive radiographic findings, particularly abnormalities seen on computed tomography (CT), may be visible before blood cultures become positive[206] and the diagnosis may be first suggested at chest CT.[162]

The usual radiographic and CT scanning appearances[162,206] consist of multiple pulmonary opacities. As always, CT shows more lesions and enables the radiologist to characterize these lesions with greater accuracy than is possible from plain chest radiographs. The opacities may occur in any portion of the lungs but are usually maximal in the lower zones. The lesions are usually either round (nodular) in shape or show the shape of a pulmonary infarct, namely a wedge-shaped density based on the pleura and pointing to the hilum. Sometimes, however, the opacities are completely nonspecific in shape. They may be any size and frequently cavitate (Figure 6-35), a feature more easily recognized at CT. For example, in the series by Kuhlman, Fishman, and Teigen,[206] 50% of the visible nodules showed cavitation. Air bronchograms are frequently seen, particularly at CT, in all types of opacity, including the nodular lesions. A relatively common CT finding of both bland and infected infarcts, which may be helpful in differential diagnosis, is the "feeding vessel sign," a distinct vessel leading to the apex of a peripheral area of consolidation.[162,206,306] This sign is not specific for embolic sequelae, although it is seen more frequently with septic emboli and bland infarction than in other conditions. The combination of multiple peripheral nodules or wedge-shaped consolidations, some of which are cavitated, and a distinct feeding vessel in the appropriate clinical setting is highly suggestive of the diagnosis of septic emboli.[162,206] Accompanying pleural effusion and empyema are a common feature.[162,206]

Identification of intraluminal filling defects in the

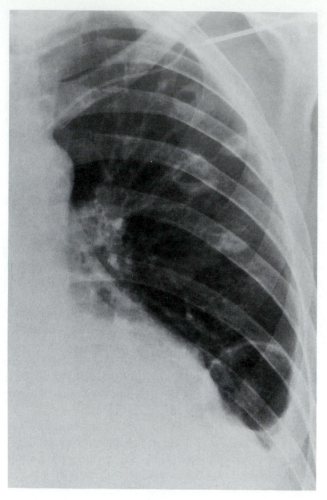

FIGURE 6-35
Septic emboli caused by staphylococcal septicemia in patient on renal dialysis with infected dialysis shunt site. Note multiple round pulmonary cavities with thin walls.

pulmonary arteries is generally not possible because peripheral, as distinct from central, emboli are rarely recognizable even with contrast-enhanced CT scans.

BACTERIAL PARAPNEUMONIC PLEURAL EFFUSIONS AND EMPYEMA

No precise definition distinguishes an uncomplicated parapneumonic pleural effusion from an empyema. By one definition, positive pleural fluid cultures are needed.[224] By another,[391] the pleural fluid must have a specific gravity greater than 1.018 and a white blood cell count greater than 500 cells/mm^3 or a protein level greater than 2.5 g/dl. Vianna[378] defined an empyema as pleural fluid with either positive cultures for the same microorganism from at least two consecutive samples or a white blood cell count greater than 15,000 cells/mm^3 and a protein level above 3 g/dl.

According to the American Thoracic Society[6] the evolution of an empyema can be divided into three stages that gradually merge. These divisions have been amplified by Light[224,225]:

First is the *exudative stage* characterized by the rapid outpouring of sterile pleural fluid into the pleural space in response to inflammation of the pleura. The associated pneumonic process is usually contiguous with the visceral pleura and results in increased permeability of the capillaries in the visceral pleura. The pleural fluid in this stage is characterized by a low white blood count, a low lactic dehydrogenase (LDH) level, a normal glucose level and a normal pH.[226] If appropriate antibiotic therapy is instituted at this stage, the pleural effusion progresses no further, and the insertion of chest tubes is not necessary. If appropriate antibiotic therapy is not instituted, bacteria invade the pleural fluid from the contiguous pneumonic process, and the second, *fibropurulent,* stage evolves. This stage is characterized by the accumulation of large amounts of pleural fluid with many polymorphonuclear leukocytes, bacteria, and cellular debris. Fibrin is deposited in a continuous sheet covering both the visceral and parietal pleura in the involved area and the tendency is to loculation. These loculations prevent extension of the empyema, but make drainage of the pleural space with chest tubes increasingly difficult. As this stage progresses, the pleural fluid pH and glucose level become progressively lower and the LDH level progressively higher. The last stage is the *organization stage,* in which fibroblasts grow into the exudate from both the visceral and parietal pleural surfaces and produce an inelastic membrane called the pleural peel [Figure 6-36]. This pleural peel encases the lung and renders it virtually functionless. At this stage the exudate is thick, and if the patient has remained untreated, the fluid may drain spontaneously through the chest wall (empyema necessitatis) or into the lung, to produce a bronchopleural fistula.

Most empyemas are associated with a recognizable pneumonia, surgery, trauma, or infradiaphragmatic infection.[2,153] The bacteria usually responsible for nontuberculous empyemas or "parapneumonic" effusions are anaerobic bacteria, *S. aureus, S. pneumoniae,* other streptococcal species, and various gram-negative bacteria.[47]

The clinical picture of patients with aerobic bacterial pneumonia and pleural effusion is similar to that of patients with pneumonia alone. The incidence of pleuritic chest pain and the degree of leukocytosis are comparable, whether or not there is an accompanying pleural effusion.[227] Patients with anaerobic bacterial infections of the pleural space usually present with a subacute illness.[26] The majority have a history of alcoholism, an episode of unconsciousness, or another reason for aspiration.

The diagnosis of parapneumonic effusion and empyema depends on recognizing the presence of fluid in the pleural cavity and performing thoracentesis to analyze the fluid. Because empyemas are rich in protein, the pleural fluid tends to loculate and therefore ultrasound or CT may be necessary to appreciate the full size of the pleural fluid collection. With free fluid, lateral decubitus views suffice to quantitate the fluid. Diagnostic thoracentesis is recommended in patients with pneumonia and pleural effusion if a layer of 1 cm or more of pleural fluid can be demonstrated on the lateral decubitus view.[226,323] Lesser quantities of fluid clear with antibiotic treatment, and therefore thoracentesis is not required.[226]

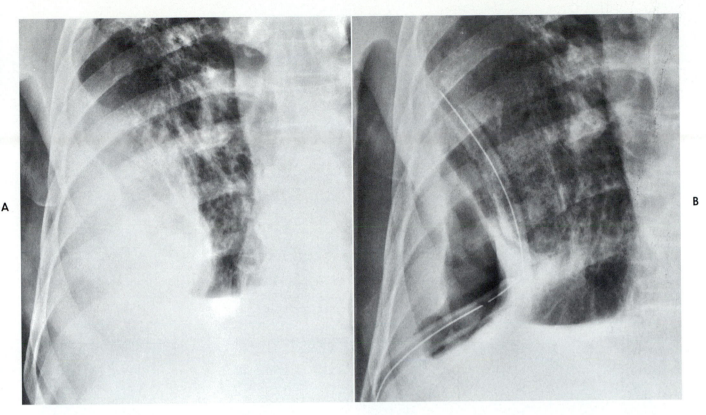

FIGURE 6-36
Pleural peel. **A,** Tuberculous empyema before tube drainage. **B,** Following tube drainage, air has entered empyema space, allowing recognition of greatly thickened parietal and visceral pleura.

The appearance on plain chest radiographs (Figures 6-37 to 6-39)[153] varies with the evolution of the parapneumonic fluid collection. Uncomplicated, sterile effusions appear identical to pleural fluid collections that may accompany noninfectious consolidations. Previous scarring of the pleural cavity may lead to loculation, but otherwise the fluid is mobile. Fibropurulent fluid collections have a strong tendency to loculate. Loculated fluid does not fall to the most dependent portion of the pleural cavity, so images taken in various positions show fixed collections of fluid density.

The distinction between pulmonary consolidation or abscess and infected loculated pleural fluid on conventional films can occasionally be difficult but has important therapeutic consequences. Empyema requires early drainage with obliteration of the space,[386] whereas adequate antibiotic therapy obviates the need for drainage in most cases of lung abscess. The radiographic features to be analyzed are shape and the appearance of any air within the opacity.[118] The shape is often the most definitive feature. Loculated collections of pleural fluid, with the exception of interlobar fluid, are based on the parietal pleura and cause an oval, lens-shaped, or rounded expansion of the pleura (Figure 6-37). When profiled the inner margin of the empyema is sharply defined and shows a curved, smooth interface with the

adjacent lung, but often one or more interfaces with the lung are not tangential to the beam and the empyema therefore has an imperceptible border. Round pneumonias do not show the very smooth, well-defined interface with the adjacent lung that is seen with empyemas. Also, although they may contact the pleura, round pneumonias are rarely as broadly based on the pleura.

Interlobar loculated pleural fluid has a unique radiographic appearance. The opacity is centered on a fissure and is lens shaped with a more pronounced bulge inferiorly than superiorly, reflecting the gravitational effect of the fluid suspended within the fissure. In the lateral projection, interlobar fluid in the major fissure appears as a well-defined lens shape, whereas in frontal projection the opacity is circular and fades off in all directions. It is therefore in the frontal view that confusion with pneumonia is most likely to occur.

If an air-fluid level is present, the comparative length in frontal and lateral projections may help distinguish lung abscess and empyema (Figure 6-38). Since empyema spaces are usually lenticular in shape, the air-fluid level is often substantially longer in one view than in the other. Intrapulmonary abscesses are usually spherical, and a spherical cavity has the same length of air-fluid level regardless of projection. Also, in empyema the air-fluid level may reach the chest wall, whereas a lung abscess is

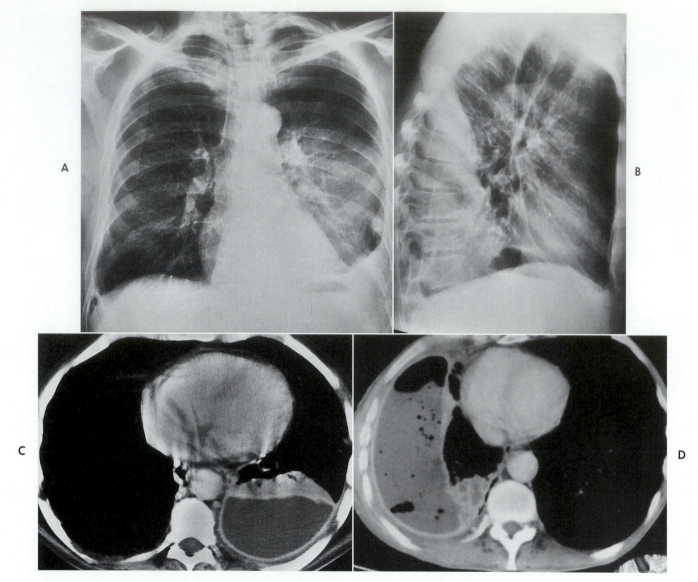

FIGURE 6-37
Typical appearances of empyema on plain film and computed tomographic (CT) scans. **A,** Frontal view. **B,** Lateral view showing lens-shaped pleural expansion. **C,** CT scan showing the pleural fluid collection displacing and compressing adjacent left lower lobe. **D,** CT scan in another patient showing lens-shaped fluid collection containing bubbles of air. Uniform thickness enhancing wall is well shown. Note also edema in adjacent extrapleural fat. (Pneumonia with abscess formation is seen in adjacent right lower lobe.)

often surrounded by lung parenchyma and the air-fluid level is therefore less likely to reach the chest wall. Proto and Merhar[290] observed that large pleural fluid collections could displace the hilar structures from the lesion, whereas lung abscesses, which destroy rather than compress lung, do not displace these structures in the same fashion. This sign, however, can be misleading in individual cases.[397]

CT can be valuable for demonstrating empyemas and for distinguishing an empyema from a peripherally positioned lung abscess. In one series of 70 patients it proved possible to correctly characterize the lesion as an empyema or lung abscess in all cases.[354] The features of empyema and lung abscess at CT are described in the following paragraphs.[14,217,341,354,397] They are illustrated in Figures 6-37 to 6-43.

1. Shape. Empyemas, unless very large, are basically lenticular in shape. The angle formed at the interface with the chest wall is obtuse or tapering. Large collections, however, may be more spherical and may then show acute angles. Lung abscesses, on the other hand, tend to be spherical and show acute angles at their margins with the chest wall. Also, fluid collections in the pleural space may change their shape as the patient changes position,

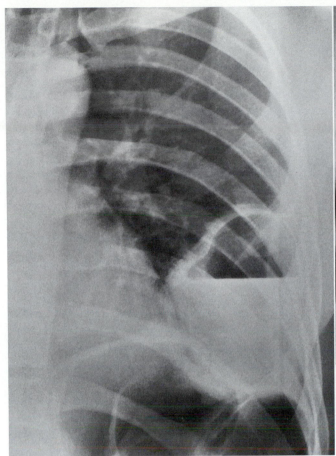

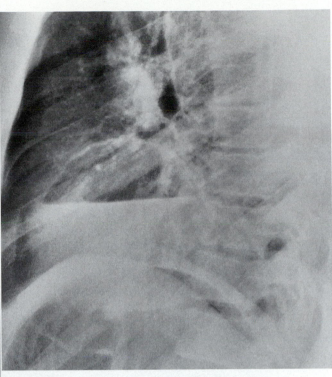

FIGURE 6-38
Air-fluid level in empyema. **A,** On frontal view, air-fluid level reaches chest wall. **B,** Lateral view. Comparison of length of air-fluid level in two projections shows disparity in length, suggesting that cavity is actually lens shaped rather than spherical.

whereas lung abscesses are fairly rigid and retain approximately the same shape in upright, supine, prone, or decubitus views.

2. Wall characteristics. The wall of an empyema is formed by thickened visceral and parietal pleura. This thickened pleura is uniform in thickness and soft tissue density, with a smooth inner and outer edge enclosing the empyema fluid; this combination of findings has been called the split pleura sign.[354] The increased thickness of the parietal pleura is particularly easy to appreciate. Normally the combined thickness of visceral and parietal pleura, together with the adjacent innermost intercostal muscle, is less than 1 to 2 mm. In empyemas the parietal pleura alone is 2 to 5 mm in some 80% of cases.[385] The thickened pleura enhances following the administration of intravenous contrast medium in almost all cases.[385]

The wall of a lung abscess usually has an irregular inner and outer margin. It also tends to be thicker than the wall of an empyema, may contain multiple dots of air, and may on occasion even show distorted air bronchograms.

3. Appearance of the adjacent tissues. The lung adjacent to an empyema may be clear but is often compressed. This compression may lead to distortion of the adjacent vessels, and if the collection is very large, hilar vessels and bronchi may be displaced away from the empyema. Since lung abscesses destroy rather than displace, the adjacent vessels and bronchi tend to remain in their normal position or are pulled toward the parenchymal destruction. Consolidation adjacent to the fluid collection is of little help in differential diagnosis, since pneumonia is the primary cause of most empyemas and lung abscesses usually form within areas of pneumonia.

The extrapleural fat adjacent to an empyema is often increased in width, and the widened fat line may show increased attenuation believed to be due to inflammatory changes in the fat.[385] Similarly, the muscles of the chest wall may be swollen because of edema.[153]

Malignant neoplasms may arise in the walls of chronic, long-standing empyema cavities; this association appears to be highest in tuberculous empyemas but is also encountered in nontuberculous infection.[253] The range of neoplasms is wide and includes non-Hodgkin's lymphoma, squamous cell carcinoma, mesothelioma, and rarely sarcoma.[253] The diagnosis of neoplasm in a chronic empyema can be difficult even with CT[253] because neoplastic tissue and chronic pleural inflammatory disease both have the same density and because nodularity is seen with chronic infection as well as neoplasm. Magnetic resonance imaging (MRI) has the potential to show a

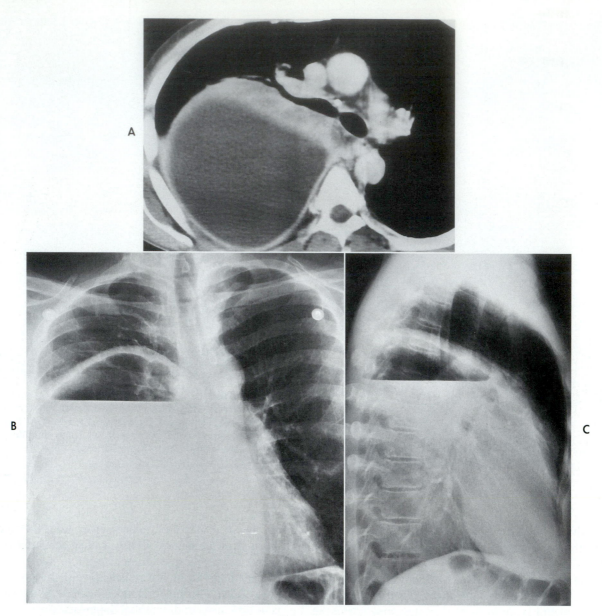

FIGURE 6-39
A, Computed tomographic (CT) scan of pleural empyema showing homogeneous oval fluid collection based on chest wall with very smooth outline and no evidence of bubbles of gas in the wall of the fluid collection. Note also forward displacement of ipsilateral central bronchi. **B**, Posteroanterior radiograph. **C**, Lateral radiograph for comparison with CT scan.

difference in signal intensity between mature fibrous tissue and neoplastic tissue,[253] although the diagnostic usefulness of this difference remains to be seen.

In summary, the CT features associated with empyema include lenticular shape, uniformly enhancing smooth wall less than 5 mm thick, compression of the adjacent lung, obtuse angles at the interface with the chest wall, and separation of pleural layers. The features associated with lung abscess include round shape; thick, nonuniform, irregular wall; acute angles at the interface of the chest wall; and absence of evidence of lung compression. Both empyemas and lung abscesses may contain one or more pockets of air and show air-fluid levels, but most empyemas do not show dots of air in their walls, whereas the wall of a lung abscess often contains bubbles of air.

PULMONARY TUBERCULOSIS

Tuberculosis was the leading cause of death in the United States at the turn of the century. Improved public health measures and specific antituberculous chemotherapy dramatically reduced the prevalence of tuberculosis, and a near eradication of the disease seemed likely. In 1985 some 22,000 new cases were reported in the United States, representing the lowest incidence since national

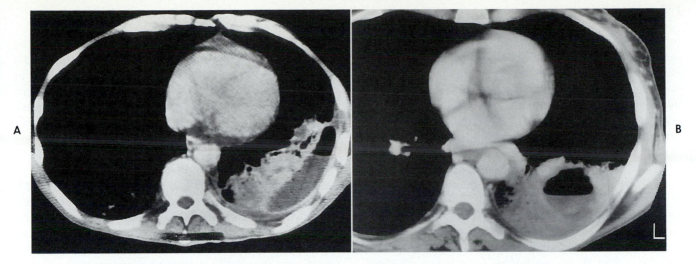

FIGURE 6-40
Comparison of lung abscess and empyema. **A,** Empyema showing lens shape, short air-fluid level, and smooth enhancing wall. There is pneumonia in underlying lung. **B,** Lung abscess showing spherical shape, with irregular poorly enhancing wall imperceptibly fading into adjacent pulmonary consolidation.

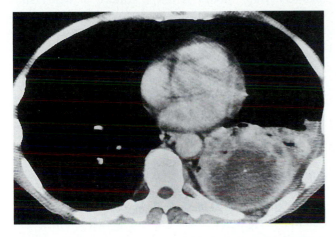

FIGURE 6-41
Lung abscess that resembles empyema at computed tomography. The wall of the abscess is relatively thick and irregular and contains bubbles of gas. The fluid collection is spherical.

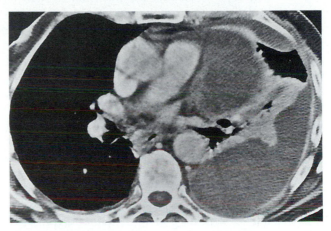

FIGURE 6-42
Multilocular pleural empyema. Each empyema space shows typical computed tomographic features of pleural empyema.

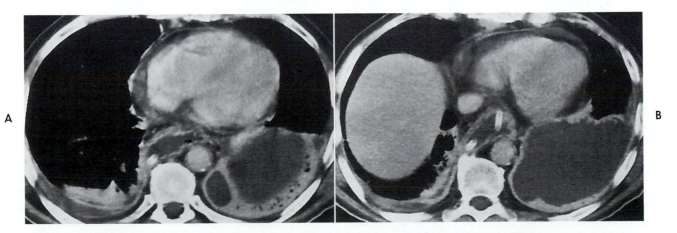

FIGURE 6-43
Potential pitfall in diagnosis of pleural empyema. The pleural empyema in this patient lies largely in a subpulmonary location. **A,** Therefore in this section, lung is draped over fluid collection and air bronchograms in compressed lung are seen between the empyema and the chest wall. **B,** Lower section shows more typical features of pleural empyema.

reporting began in 1953.[56] Since 1985, however, the incidence of tuberculosis has begun to increase again, albeit slowly. The increase has been widely attributed to the HIV epidemic. HIV-infected individuals, particularly intravenous drug abusers, are at considerable risk for reactivation of tuberculosis.[286] Nevertheless, the highest case rate for tuberculosis occurs in persons over 65 years of age, a group by and large not involved in the HIV epidemic. Tuberculosis in the elderly usually represents reactivation of previously acquired disease as a result of waning immunocompetence with advancing age.[51] These individuals acquired the disease in a time when it was far more prevalent than it is today. Tuberculosis remains a considerable health problem in Third World countries, and the United States and Europe have seen a considerable influx of immigrants and refugees from the Third World in the past two decades. Approximately one fourth of new cases of tuberculosis in the United States involve patients born outside the country.[51] Tuberculosis is now more obviously an urban disease, involving deprived population groups especially; the incidence is high in prison populations and among the indigent and the homeless.[356] Since most of the tuberculosis sanitoria are gone, treatment of tuberculosis has devolved to the general physician. Classic pulmonary tuberculosis is readily diagnosed, but increasingly tuberculosis is encountered in the elderly, who may have other serious medical problems, making the diagnosis more challenging. Furthermore, tuberculosis in adults is increasingly a primary infection and by no means classic "adult" tuberculosis. A key factor in the diagnosis of tuberculosis is simply awareness that this disease still lurks. Almost all cases are caused by infection with the human strain of *M. tuberculosis* and the remainder by the atypical mycobacteria, notably *M. kansasii* and *M. avium-intracellulare.*

The inflammatory response to tuberculous infection differs from the usual inflammatory response to infecting microorganisms in that it is modified substantially by a hypersensitivity reaction to components of the tubercle bacillus. The extent to which the hypersensitivity reaction is advantageous or deleterious in resisting and controlling infection is uncertain.

The initial response to primary tuberculous infection[288] is a polymorphonuclear leukocyte infiltration akin to the usual inflammatory reaction to bacterial infection. The response, however, devolves to a greater extent on macrophages and lymphocytes, resulting in a more indolent inflammatory reaction. The macrophages become compacted and modified to form epithelioid cells, and multinucleated giant cells and lymphocytes infiltrate the periphery of the tubercles. Delayed hypersensitivity develops some 4 to 10 weeks after the initial infection and is evidenced by a positive tuberculin reaction. The hallmark of hypersensitivity is the development of caseous necrosis in the pulmonary focus or in the involved lymph nodes. The periphery of the tubercle shows fibrocyte proliferation with the laying down of a capsule of collagen. Inflammatory involvement of the regional lymph nodes in the hilum and mediastinum is a dominant feature of primary tuberculosis, particularly in younger individuals. In primary tuberculous infections the pulmonary focus and the adenopathy may resolve without a trace or may leave a focus of caseous necrosis, scarring, or calcification.

Various terms are applied to the form of tuberculosis that develops and progresses under the influence of established hypersensitivity. These terms include postprimary, secondary, or reactivation tuberculosis. The term "reactivation tuberculosis," although not ideal because the disease sometimes evolves from primary tuberculosis without a latent interval, does serve to emphasize that most cases represent reactivation of endogenous infection rather than reinfection with *M. tuberculosis.*[355] Reactivation tuberculosis develops under the immediate influence of hypersensitivity, which accelerates the changes described previously. In particular, caseous necrosis occurs at an early stage in the process. Involvement of the regional lymph nodes is not a feature of reactivation tuberculosis; whether this is by virtue of the hypersensitivity reaction or acquired immunity is uncertain. Factors that predispose to reactivation of tuberculosis include aging, malnutrition, uremia, diabetes mellitus, alcoholism, silicosis, cancer, familial and acquired immune deficiency diseases, and drug-induced immunosuppression.[216,286]

The gross morphologic features of reactivation tuberculosis[288] can be subdivided into the following:

1. The foci of acute tuberculous infiltration in the pulmonary parenchyma.

2. Cavity formation. Airspaces in a tuberculous process may represent excavated foci of caseous necrosis or, alternatively, pneumatoceles or bullae that follow fibrous contraction or endobronchial disease.

3. Fibrosis and distortion of lung architecture. The extent of the fibrosis and damage to the lung depend on such factors as the amount of caseous necrosis and the severity of associated endobronchial and pleural disease. Fibrous tissue contracts as it matures, and even quiescent lesions may show increased contraction and distortion over an extended period of observation.

4. Calcification. Dystrophic calcification may occur in foci of caseous necrosis. Such calcification takes considerable time to become radiographically visible and is therefore often associated with pulmonary fibrosis or tuberculoma formation.

5. Tuberculoma formation, namely a focus of tuberculosis in which the processes of activity and containment are finely balanced. The result is a fairly discrete nodule or mass in which repeated extensions of infection have created a core of caseous necrosis surrounded by a mantle of epithelioid cells and collagen with peripheral round cell infiltration.

Both primary and reactivation tuberculosis may extend to extrathoracic sites such as the gastrointestinal tract, larynx, kidneys, bones, joints, and central nervous system. In these cases it is generally thought that the primary portal of entry is the lungs, even though in many instances there is no radiographic evidence of pulmonary tuberculosis. Tuberculosis of the larynx and tuberculosis of the gastrointestinal tract have a high association with visible active pulmonary tuberculosis.[16]

Radiographic appearances of pulmonary and pleural tuberculosis

Tuberculosis may involve the lungs in disease patterns that reflect a number of factors: the host's immune status, the existence of hypersensitivity from previous infection, the method of spread of disease, and an incompletely understood tendency of the disease to affect certain portions of the lungs. The radiographic appearances can be considered under the following broad headings:

1. Primary tuberculosis
2. Reactivation tuberculosis
   a. Focal pulmonary tuberculosis
   b. Tuberculous lobar pneumonia and bronchopneumonia
   c. Endobronchial tuberculosis
   d. Tuberculoma formation
   e. Miliary tuberculosis
   f. Tuberculous pleurisy

These very broad patterns of disease may overlap or undergo transformation from one pattern to another.

Primary tuberculosis

Formerly the initial infection with *M. tuberculosis* usually occurred in childhood, but primary tuberculosis has been increasingly encountered in an adult population. In a recent series[404] over half the cases of primary tuberculosis occurred in individuals 18 years of age or older and one fourth of adult cases were deemed to represent the primary form of the disease. The division between primary tuberculosis and postprimary or reactivation tuberculosis is by no means clear cut; some 10% of cases of primary tuberculosis may evolve without any interval into a chronic progressive form of the disease indistinguishable from reactivation tuberculosis.[128]

Classically the tubercle bacillus causes a nonspecific focal pneumonitis (Figure 6-44). In approximately half of cases the primary pulmonary foci are never identified or documented.[218] Indeed the chest radiograph may remain entirely normal despite definite conversion of tuberculin sensitivity or the presence of positive sputum cultures. The predominant radiographic feature of primary tuberculosis is the presence of adenopathy in the appropriate lymph drainage pathways (Figures 6-44 and 6-45). Radiographic evidence of lymphadenopathy was found in 92% of 191 children with primary tuberculosis in one series.[218] Foci of tuberculous pneumonitis when detected radiographically are almost invariably associated with lymphadenopathy. The resultant hilar adenopathy is usually unilateral, and any mediastinal adenopathy is contiguous to the affected hilum. In some patients hilar adenopathy is bilateral or mediastinal adenopathy occurs alone. The adenopathy may be strikingly severe and extensive, particularly in individuals of African or Asian origin (Figure 6-46), and may closely resemble lymphoma, metastatic disease, or sarcoidosis. In middle-aged and elderly patients lymph node enlargement is far less common and usually less apparent than it is in children.[40] Even in children lymphadenopathy is most striking in the very young.

The pulmonary foci of primary tuberculosis are randomly distributed and range from small ill-defined parenchymal shadows to segmental or lobar consolidation. Curiously there appears to be a predilection for involvement of the right lung.[218] Slight expansion of consolidated lobes may be noted. In the absence of cavitation, consolidation of segments or lobes produces a radiographic picture indistinguishable from that of the bacterial pneumonias. The time course is, however, different; tuberculous pneumonia is much more indolent, often taking weeks or months to clear. Primary tuberculosis may be masslike and in an adult may be confused with such conditions as Wegener's granulomatosis or pulmonary neoplasia (Figure 6-47). A single pulmonary focus occurs in most instances, but multiple foci may be encountered. The incidence of cavitation varies, having been found in 10%[64] to 30%[404] of cases (Figure 6-48). The pulmonary focus frequently resolves without trace, or alternatively it may evolve into a small nodule or scar that may then calcify. Such calcifications may be observed following primary tuberculosis in up to 20% of patients. Hilar or mediastinal lymph node calcification is observed in some 35% of cases (Figure 6-49).[389] Single or multiple tuberculomas may develop in primary tuberculosis, but they are seen much less frequently than in reactivation tuberculosis.

Pleural effusions occur in primary tuberculosis. In these cases, which have been studied in major hospitals, pleural effusions have been observed in approximately one fourth. On the other hand, Leung and associates,[218] studying an unselected series ranging from completely asymptomatic patients to one with a tuberculosis empyema, found pleural effusions in only 6%. The effusions are generally unilateral and are usually associated with some identifiable pulmonary parenchymal abnormality.

Segmental or lobar airway narrowing is frequent and may be caused by endobronchial tuberculosis or by extrinsic pressure from enlarged lymph nodes (Figure 6-50). The result is usually segmental or lobar atelectasis, but air trapping occurs occasionally (Figure 6-51).

CT is capable of considerable precision in the investigation of primary tuberculosis, although in most cases it is unnecessary. CT may identify foci of disease in the lung undetected on plain films and thereby assist the bronchoscopist in questionable cases.[205] Occult cavitation may be detected, particularly when obscured by a pleural effu-

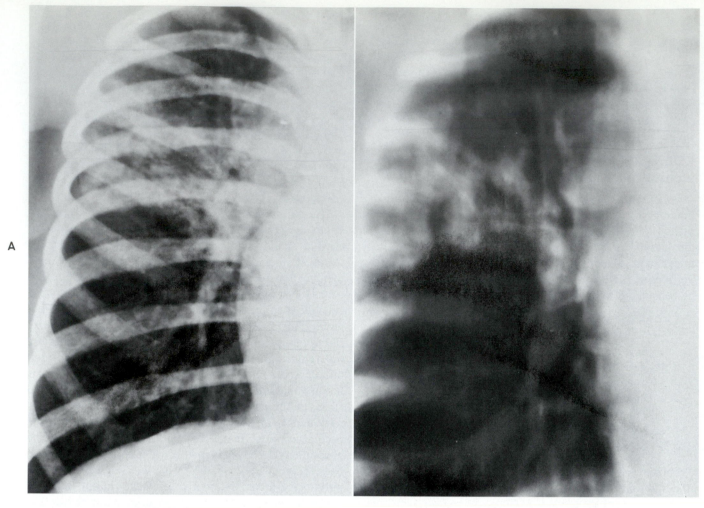

FIGURE 6-44
Ten-year-old child with primary tuberculous focus in right upper lobe. **A,** Plain film. **B,** Tomogram demonstrating hilar and mediastinal adenopathy to better advantage. Note slight constriction of right upper lobe bronchus.

FIGURE 6-45
Primary tuberculosis in 5-year-old child with right hilar adenopathy but no pulmonary consolidation. **A,** Posteroanterior view. **B,** Lateral view.

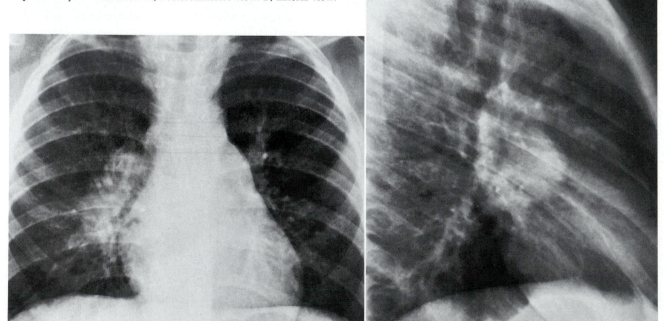

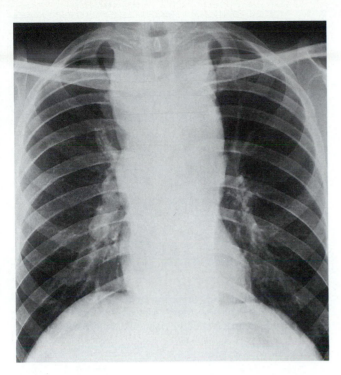

FIGURE 6-46
Massive mediastinal adenopathy and slight right hilar adenopathy in a young black man with primary tuberculosis.

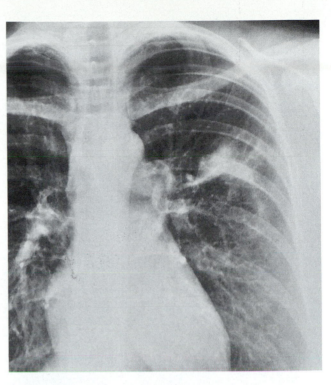

FIGURE 6-47
Primary tuberculosis resembling neoplasm in young adult. There is an area of rounded consolidation in the left upper zone together with left hilar adenopathy.

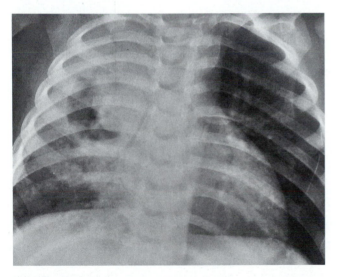

FIGURE 6-48
Fifteen-month-old Hispanic child with cavitary primary tuberculosis.

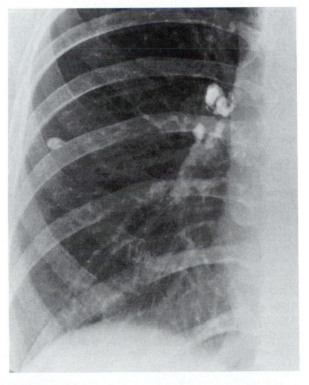

FIGURE 6-49
Calcified tuberculous focus with calcification in corresponding hilar lymph nodes.

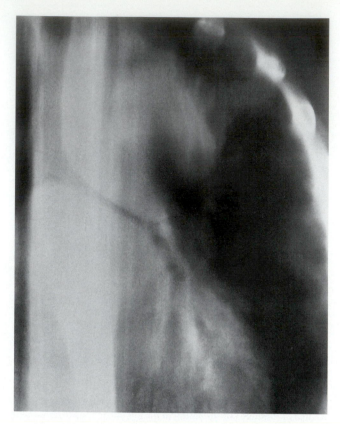

FIGURE 6-50
Primary tuberculosis in left upper lobe with elongation and narrowing of left mainstem bronchus.

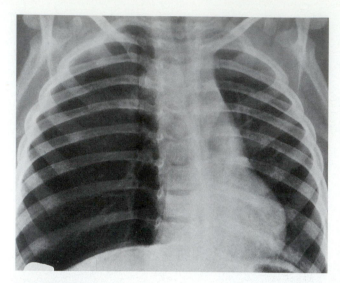

FIGURE 6-51
Radiograph of child with bronchoscopically proven primary endobronchial tuberculosis. Right paratracheal adenopathy and marked hyperexpansion of entire right lung are present.

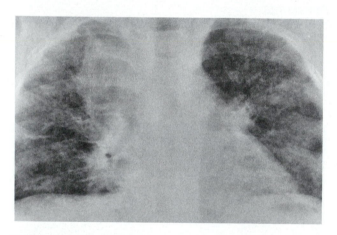

FIGURE 6-52
Three-year-old child with miliary tuberculosis complicating primary tuberculosis of right upper lobe.

sion. Bronchial stenoses, bronchial occlusions, and polypoid endobronchial tuberculous lesions, which may be responsible for atelectasis, can all be identified with CT.[61,212,213] The presence of hilar or mediastinal lymphadenopathy is readily confirmed or detected.[171,213] The lymph nodes in tuberculous lymphadenitis, particularly when over 2 cm in diameter, show a low-density center with rim enhancement of the periphery.[171] Focal adenopathy of this type in a child or young adult is highly suggestive of tuberculosis (Figure 6-52). Miliary tuberculosis may be detected by CT, particularly high-resolution CT, at a stage when the chest radiograph is normal.[155,244,270]

Pulmonary tuberculosis associated with AIDS has many of the clinical and radiographic features of primary tuberculosis, even when there is strong evidence that the disease represents reactivation of previously acquired infection.[286] The hypersensitivity reaction appears to be in abeyance, and cavitation does not usually occur. The consolidations may be noted in any part of the lungs, and hilar and mediastinal adenopathy is usual. Extrathoracic dissemination, miliary tuberculosis, and endobronchial spread are definite risks in patients with AIDS, and there is a much higher than normal incidence of sputum cultures positive for *M. tuberculosis.* Concomitant infections, for example, with *Pneumocystis carinii,* are common and may result in diagnostic confusion.

Reactivation tuberculosis

FOCAL PULMONARY TUBERCULOSIS. In the earlier phases reactivation tuberculosis gives rise to patchy subsegmental consolidations with ill-defined margins (Figure 6-53) and a tendency to coalesce so that there may be small satellite foci in the adjacent lung. There is a predilection for the posterior aspects of the upper lobes and the superior segments of the lower lobes (Figure 6-54), although no portion of the lungs is immune. For example, predominant or exclusive involvement of the anterior segments of the upper lobes has been described in a small percentage of patients (Figure 6-55).[352] Bilateral and multilobar involvement is fairly frequent.

The consolidations are usually peripheral in location, and therefore air bronchograms are not present. Some focal pleural thickening may be present in the early stages even in the absence of pleural effusions (Figure 6-56).

Cavitation is a distinct feature of reactivation tuberculosis and is a finding of considerable diagnostic significance, since it indicates a high likelihood of activity (Figure 6-57). Even quite small pulmonary foci may cavitate, and multiple cavities of varying size may be present. Fluid levels may be seen (Figure 6-57) and may aid in the recognition of cavities, the walls of which may be indistinct or obscured by overlying densities.[235] Frequently, however, fluid levels are not present. Apical bullae if present may be misinterpreted as cavitation, a mistake that can often be avoided if it is borne in mind that cavities are centered within areas of consolidation and do not merely overlap them. Additional views such as apical lordotic views, conventional tomography, or computed tomography may be employed if there is doubt about the presence of cavitation (Figure 6-58). Patients with cavitary disease represent an actual or potential threat to those who come into contact with them, and therefore immediate infective precautions may be appropriate on the basis of the radiographic findings alone.

Even in the absence of specific therapy, lesions often become contained by the granulomatous and fibrous response of the adjacent lung. In the preantibiotic era the

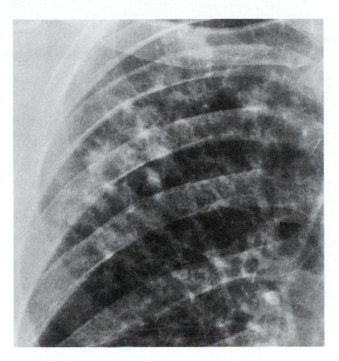

FIGURE 6-53
Early reactivation tuberculosis showing patchy small shadows with ill-defined margins.

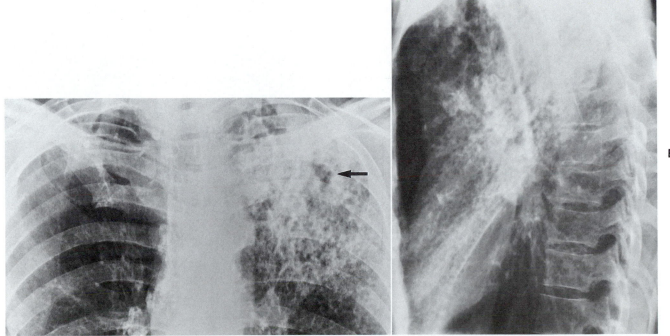

FIGURE 6-54
Reactivation tuberculosis involving left upper lobe with at least one area of cavitation *(arrow).* **A,** Frontal view. **B,** Lateral radiograph indicates predominant involvement of apical and posterior segments of left upper lobe.

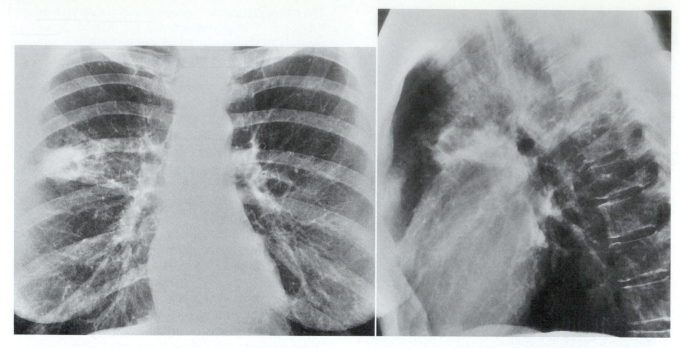

FIGURE 6-55
Reactivation tuberculosis confined to anterior segment of right upper lobe.

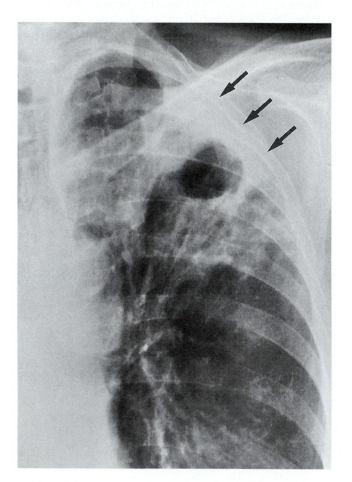

FIGURE 6-56
Cavitary reactivation tuberculosis showing localized pleural thickening *(arrows)*.

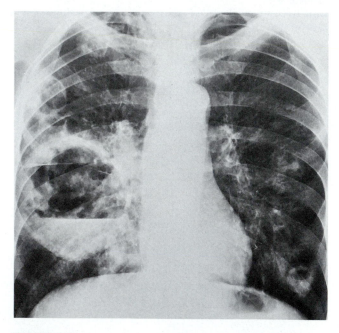

FIGURE 6-57
Reactivation tuberculosis with large right lower lobe cavitary lesion containing an air-fluid level. Other, smaller cavitary lesions are seen in other lobes.

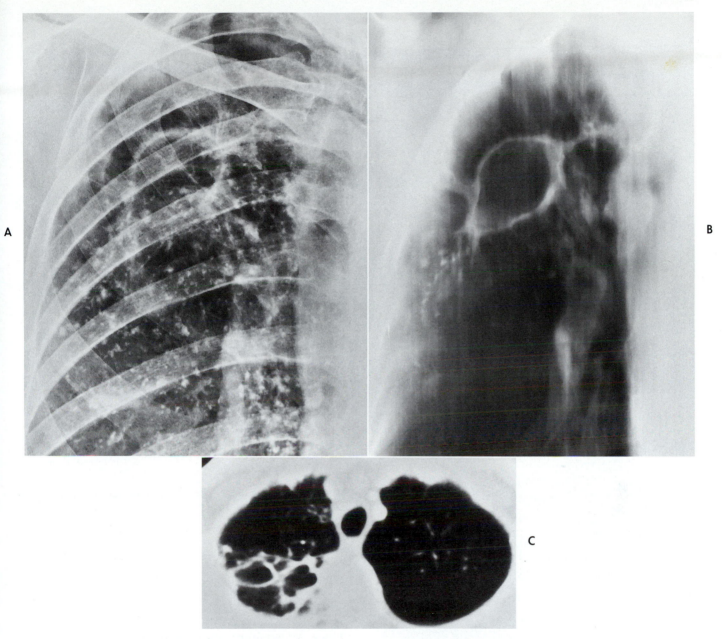

FIGURE 6-58
Fibrocalcific reactivation tuberculosis with cavitation. **A,** Plain film. **B,** Conventional tomogram in same patient clearly showing cavity. **C,** Computed tomographic examination in different patient showing cavitation in reactivation tuberculosis of posterior segment of right upper lobe.

response was prolonged and often measured in years. Specific antituberculous therapy has radically shortened the time required for healing, and the healing process is usually more complete. On radiographic examination, containment is suggested by increasing definition of the tuberculous infiltrates and the development of fibrosis in the surrounding lung. Gradual fibrous contraction of the affected segment or lobe is shown by fissural displacement or distortion of the vascular structures in the hilum. Bronchiectasis develops in the affected lung and is often much more severe than can be appreciated from plain

films (Figure 6-59). Calcification is often seen in areas of caseous necrosis coincident with the increasing fibrosis. Fluid levels in cavities, when present, disappear. The cavities themselves either disappear or become chronic, often with a relatively smooth inner wall.

TUBERCULOUS LOBAR PNEUMONIA AND BRON-CHOPNEUMONIA. An entire lobe can become consolidated (Figure 6-60), and cavitation often occurs within the affected lobe. Heavy seeding of the bronchial tree is likely, particularly in the presence of cavitation, and smaller foci of disease may be found in other parts of the

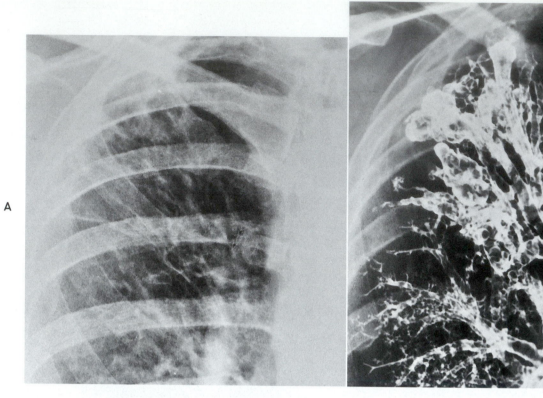

FIGURE 6-59
Fibrous contraction of right upper lobe. **A,** Plain film showing possible small peripheral cavities. **B,** Bronchogram in same patient revealing full extent and severity of underlying bronchial changes.

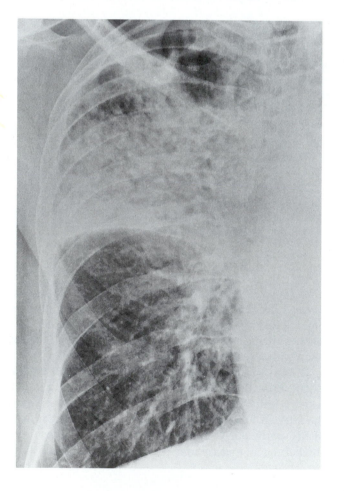

FIGURE 6-60
Tuberculous pneumonia showing lobar consolidation of right upper lobe.

lungs. Although overshadowed by the lobar pneumonia, these foci may be extremely important in indicating the true nature of the process. Sequential films show that tuberculous lobar pneumonia is more chronic and indolent than the usual cavitary pneumonias.

Widespread bronchopneumonia presumably results from a breakdown in host defenses with spread of disease via the airways. It is usually patchy and bilateral (Figure 6-61) and may involve portions of lung less commonly affected by tuberculosis, such as the middle lobe or the anterior segments of the upper lobes. Fibrocalcific changes may be seen elsewhere in the lungs if the bronchopneumonia stems from breakdown of preexisting chronic fibrocaseous tuberculosis.

In immunocompromised hosts tuberculous bronchopneumonia may become extensive and may be rapidly fatal. Cavitation may not be present in the early phases even when the patient has extensive patchy confluent perihilar consolidation.

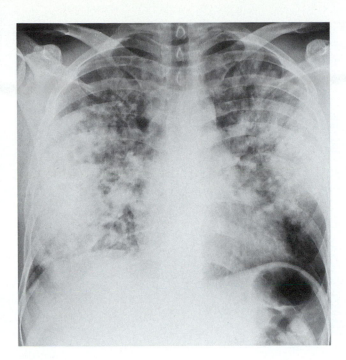

FIGURE 6-61
Tuberculous bronchopneumonia without evidence of cavitation or any identifiable originating focus.

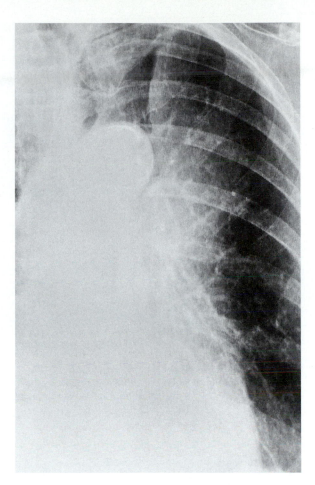

FIGURE 6-62
Endobronchial tuberculosis producing complete collapse of left upper lobe.

ENDOBRONCHIAL TUBERCULOSIS. On occasion a tuberculous focus arises in or extends into a major bronchus. Tuberculous granulations and granulomatous cicatrization may then cause a bronchial stricture, which in turn may cause obstructive emphysema or atelectasis. The associated pulmonary parenchymal lesions may be obscured by the atelectasis, and the underlying cause of the atelectasis may be difficult or impossible to ascertain from the chest radiographs (Figure 6-62).

Broncholiths represent an interesting late complication of pulmonary tuberculosis and histoplasmosis (Figure 6-63).[380] A calcified lymph node may erode into an adjacent airway and be associated with hemoptysis or pneumonia. The peripheral lung may show evidence of atelectasis resulting from bronchial obstruction or areas of consolidation related to aspiration of blood or postobstructive pneumonia. On occasion, air trapping occurs if the broncholith causes ball valve obstruction. A broncholith in one of the segmental bronchi is easy to overlook because calcifications at hilar level are assumed to be in lymph nodes outside the bronchial lumen. Broncholiths in the lobar or main bronchi may be more clearly centered within the airway, a finding that is readily confirmed by using tomography, particularly CT.[68,342] With conventional CT it can be difficult to know whether a calcified node is endobronchial in position. If there are secondary signs of endobronchial obstruction such as atelectasis or bronchiectasis and calcifications are seen in the vicinity, a series of contiguous high-resolution CT scans is advised. The node may be only partially within the lumen, but nevertheless it may be possible to forewarn the bronchoscopist even if a definite diagnosis

cannot be established. Bronchoscopic removal of broncholiths may be attended by severe hemoptysis caused by coincident erosion of the broncholith into the accompanying branch of the pulmonary artery. Hence establishing the diagnosis noninvasively has practical significance. Broncholithiasis may also be diagnosed retrospectively if a previously documented calcification disappears. On rare occasion a patient reports recurrent lithoptysis and serial radiographs show a large central calcified node disappearing as material is discharged into the bronchus and expectorated.

TUBERCULOMA FORMATION. Tuberculomas are discrete tumorlike foci of tuberculosis in which there is a fine balance between activity and repair. The margins of a tuberculoma are usually well circumscribed, although some irregularity or focal loss of definition may occur because of adjacent fibrous changes (Figure 6-64). Tuberculomas may be multiple and on occasion become large, up to 5 cm in diameter. Some growth may be perceptible over an extended period of observation. Calcification develops in the central caseous core with time and it is often detectable radiographically. It may be amorphous, and if the core is large in relation to the cellular mantle, a nodule of uniform increased density will result, whereas

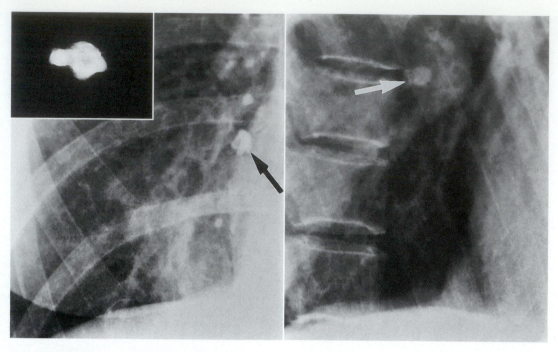

FIGURE 6-63
Peripheral broncholith in right lower lobe *(arrows)* with wedge of peripheral consolidation. Insert *(top left)* shows broncholith removed at bronchoscopy.

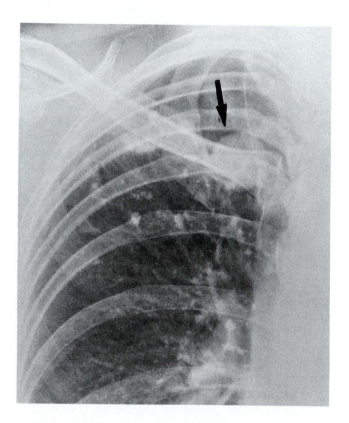

FIGURE 6-64
Tuberculoma. Note well-defined pulmonary nodule *(arrow)*, as well as associated fibrocalcific scarring in adjacent lung.

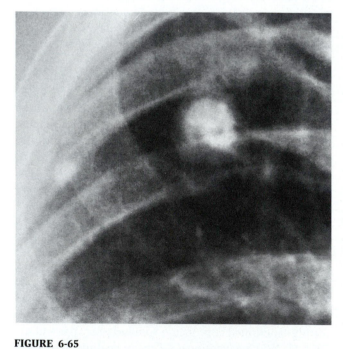

FIGURE 6-65
Two apical tuberculomas. Smaller lateral tuberculoma is uniformly dense. Contrast its density with that of adjacent ribs. Larger tuberculoma has low-density mantle around large calcified core.

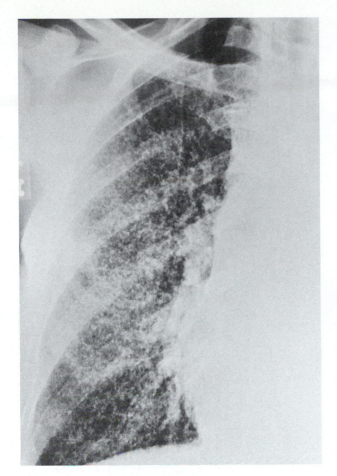

FIGURE 6-66
Miliary tuberculosis showing widespread uniformly distributed fine nodulation of lungs.

with a more confined central core of calcification a line of demarcation may be apparent (Figure 6-65). Calcifications that are more laminar, flecklike, or punctate also occur and are easier to appreciate because variable density is noted within the nodule. Tuberculomas show little tendency to break down, and cavitation is rare. Cavitation strongly suggests reactivation.

MILIARY TUBERCULOSIS. Miliary tuberculosis, which results from hematogenous dissemination of the disease, is an infrequent but feared complication of both primary and reactivation tuberculosis. The lungs are beset by myriads of 2 to 3 mm granulomas likened to millet seeds in size and appearance. The radiographic result is widespread fine nodules, which are uniformly distributed and equal in size (Figure 6-66). Because there is a threshold below which the nodules are invisible, miliary tuberculosis can be present in patients with a normal chest radiograph. Then, when the nodules reach a critical threshold in size or number, they suddenly become visible. Similarly, on or near the threshold the nodules may appear and disappear on serial radiographs. Miliary tuberculosis does not leave residual calcifications. Miliary nodulation of the lung has numerous causes other than tuberculosis (see p. 112), but tuberculosis is the preemi-

nent consideration because prompt diagnosis and treatment are vital.

Miliary tuberculosis is a rare cause of ARDS, and in such cases the diagnosis can be extraordinarily difficult because the miliary nodules are superimposed on a more diffuse, less structured background of pulmonary density.[81] Equally problematic are the rare cases in which miliary tuberculosis complicates preexisting interstitial lung disease. In the case of miliary tuberculosis complicating silicosis shown in Figure 6-67, the diagnosis was not established until autopsy. Even with successful therapy the miliary nodulation may take weeks or months to clear.

TUBERCULOUS PLEURITIS. Any tuberculous focus may involve the adjacent pleura, and some degree of focal pleural thickening and scarring is relatively common. Im and associates[172] studied apical tuberculosis with HRCT and made the interesting observation that the apical pleural thickening commonly seen with fibrocaseous tuberculosis is composed largely of extrapleural fat. Presumably the fat is a packing material that fills space as the underlying lung undergoes fibrous contraction. Pleural effusions are not uncommon in patients with widespread tuberculosis. Tuberculous pleuritis, which may occur in the absence of a visible pulmonary focus, must be considered in the differential diagnosis of any large unilateral pleural effusion for which no adequate cause can be established radiographically, clinically, or by pleural fluid analysis. CT may demonstrate a pulmonary focus that is not visible on the plain chest radiograph.[164] On occasion, pleural biopsy is necessary to establish the diagnosis of tuberculous pleuritis.

The response of tuberculous pleurisy to appropriate treatment is varied. All traces of pleural reaction may clear, but it is common to see residual pleural scarring with obliteration of the costophrenic sulcus and distortion of the diaphragm. Residual thickening may be severe, and particularly in these cases the lung can become restricted by the encompassing fibrous tissue and calcification.

Tuberculous pleurisy may become localized and form a tuberculous empyema. The empyema may break through the parietal pleura to form a subcutaneous abscess, the so-called empyema necessitans. The empyema cavity may also be connected to the bronchial tree by a fistulous track (Figures 6-68 and 6-69). Drainage of such lesions may result in a chronic bronchopleural fistula that can be extremely resistant to treatment. CT is useful in delineating foci of activity in pleural tuberculosis evidenced by fluid collections within the rind of pleural thickening. Even bronchopleural fistulae may be delineated by these axial images.[164] Tuberculosis was at one time a common cause of spontaneous pneumothorax, although today this complication is rare.

Assessment of activity on chest radiographs

Chest radiography clearly plays a vital role in the detection and control of pulmonary tuberculosis. Serial

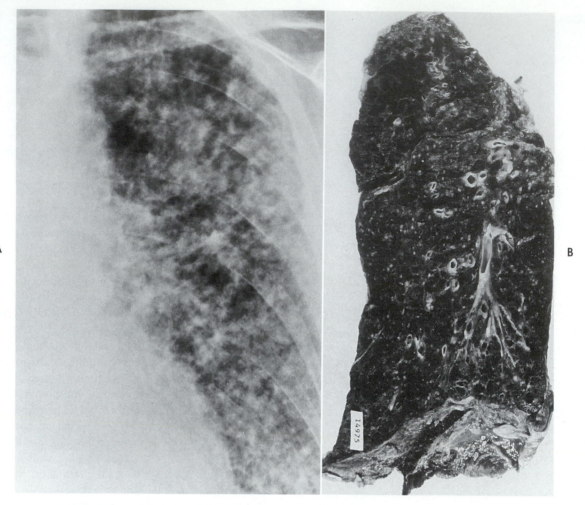

FIGURE 6-67
Silicosis in 85-year-old man. **A,** Plain chest radiograph. **B,** Autopsy specimen showing miliary tuberculosis *(white dots)* set on background of extensive nodulation.

radiography is important in gauging the activity of lesions and their response to treatment. It is hazardous to estimate activity on the basis of a single radiographic examination; even though fibrous infiltration and calcification may be prominent features, active foci may be present. Tuberculous foci that appear inactive over an extended period of observation may contain viable organisms with the potential to break down under adverse circumstances. Miliary nodulation definitely indicates activity, and cavitation is a strong indication of active disease. In practice the physician is often obliged to base certain judgments on the findings in a single radiographic examination. For example, isolation and aggressive investigation may be urged for one patient, whereas another may be allowed to proceed to routine surgery when seemingly "inactive" fibrocalcific apical scarring is present. Nevertheless, the physician cannot afford to be too cavalier about the latter type of case, and some additional study such as comparison with any previous films or a follow-up examination is advisable.

Hemoptysis in pulmonary tuberculosis

Hemoptysis is an important feature of active pulmonary tuberculosis. It may also be seen in patients in whom a complication has developed. For instance, bronchial carcinoma may have developed in an area damaged by tuberculous disease,[310] or the tuberculous lesion may have become reactivated because of an alteration in the cancer patient's immune system.[190] A mycetoma may have developed in a tuberculous cavity (see p. 206), or the bleeding may be from bronchiectasis that resulted from the tuberculous infection. The bronchial arteries supplying the bronchiectatic lung can be enormous (Figure 6-70). Finally, and very rarely, a mycotic aneurysm, the so-called Rasmussen aneurysm, may have developed (see p. 405).[301]

Effects of pulmonary collapse therapy

Some of the most remarkable radiographs result from various forms of collapse therapy dating from the preantibiotic era. The thoracoplasty involved resecting a varied

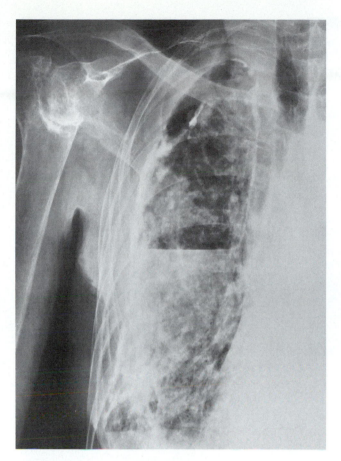

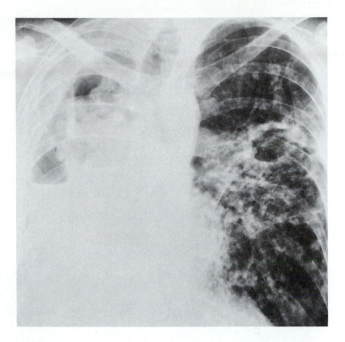

FIGURE 6-69
Middle-aged alcoholic patient with widespread reactivation tuberculosis. Right lung is almost destroyed, and a bronchopleural fistula has resulted in hydropneumothorax.

FIGURE 6-68
Elderly man with long-standing tuberculosis. There is extensive partially calcified pleural thickening, bronchopleural fistula resulting in hydropneumothorax, and tuberculous arthritis of shoulder.

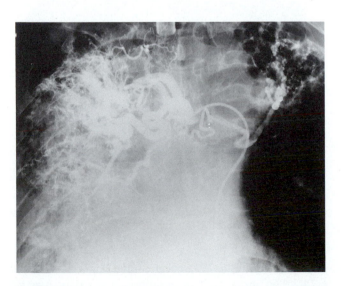

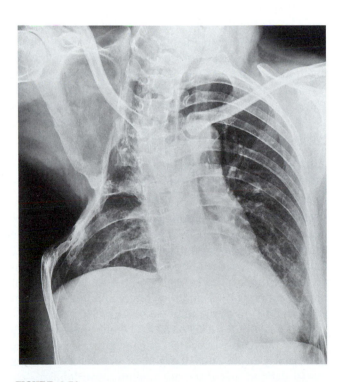

FIGURE 6-70
Selective bronchial arteriogram in patient with chronic fibrocavitary tuberculosis and hemoptysis. The bronchial artery has dimensions comparable with normal femoral artery.

FIGURE 6-71
Right thoracoplasty involving upper eight ribs with partial collapse of underlying lung. There was no evidence of active disease for many years.

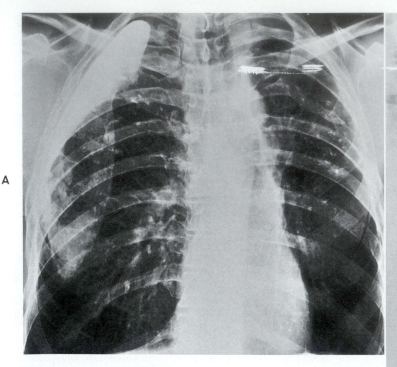

FIGURE 6-72
A, Collapse therapy by mineral oil injection (oleothorax). B, Collapse therapy using Lucite balls.

number of ribs to collapse the chest wall onto the underlying lung (Figure 6-71). In many instances only a small portion of the lung at the base remains aerated and the majority of the lung is obliterated. There is of course at least some residual fibrocalcific thickening underlying the thoracoplasty. Various other materials or objects were inserted extrapleurally to compress the underlying lung. These included paraffin, mineral oil, and Lucite balls (Figure 6-72). Collapse therapy with pneumothoraces produced pleural thickening.

Computed tomographic findings in pulmonary tuberculosis

There is little need for CT in the investigation of straightforward cases of tuberculosis when the plain film findings are consistent with the diagnosis and tubercle bacilli have been identified in the sputum. The CT findings in the various forms of tuberculosis have been established in a series of papers on the subject.* Some of the indications for CT and the possible findings are given in the following paragraphs.

DETECTION OF CAVITATION. The presence of cavities strongly suggests that the disease process is active, particularly if the outer margins of the cavitary process are ill defined and there are satellite centrilobular "ro-

---
*References 22, 61, 169-172, 205, 212, 213, 244, 256, 270.

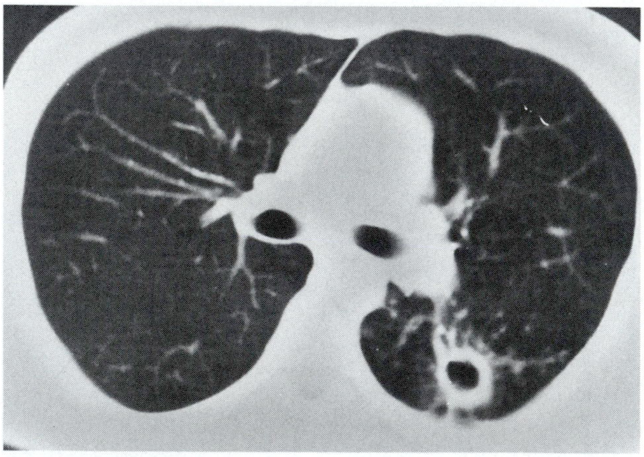

FIGURE 6-73
Convict, 33 years old, with cavitary tuberculosis involving superior segment of left lower lobe.

settes" of infiltrates in adjacent lung (Figures 6-73 and 6-74). The inner wall of a tuberculous cavity may be smooth or irregular, and the cavities usually contain only a small amount (if any) of fluid. In the series of Im and

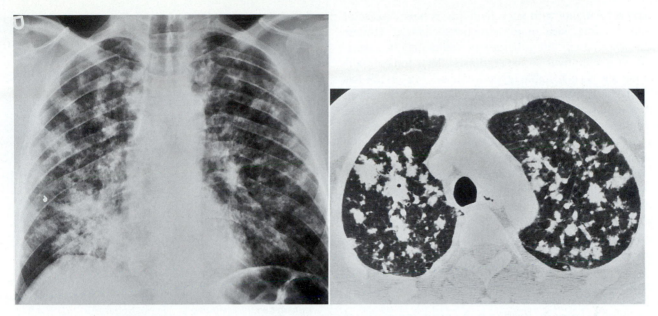

FIGURE 6-74
Tuberculous bronchopneumonia in 42-year-old man. Note centrilobular rosettes of infiltration on computed tomographic scan.

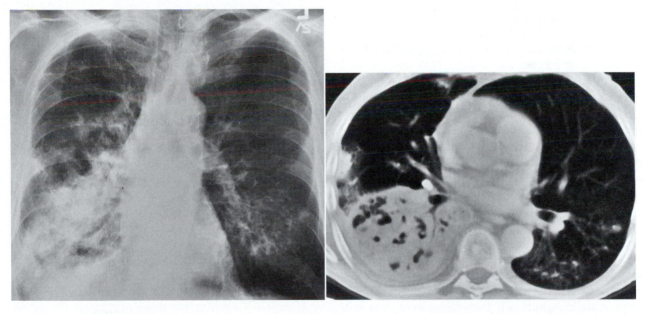

FIGURE 6-75
Tuberculosis in a 63-year-old diabetic patient previously treated for cancer of larynx, showing cavitary lower lobe tuberculosis.

associates[169] involving patients with early tuberculosis, cavities were detected in 58% of the initial CT studies, whereas the corresponding figure for the radiographs was only 22%. The CT detection of a cavitary process underlying and obscured by a large pleural effusion may be an important pointer to the diagnosis of tuberculous pleurisy. Ikezoe and co-workers[168] found an increased incidence of cavitation (and also unusual localization of disease) in diabetic and immunocompromised patients (Figure 6-75).

INVESTIGATION OF HEMOPTYSIS. Although hemoptysis is a classic symptom of tuberculosis, more profuse hemoptysis or recurrent hemoptysis may require additional imaging studies such as angiography or CT.

Generally patients with such hemoptysis have disease of some standing with major structural changes. Fungus balls within a chronic tuberculous cavity may be associated with semiinvasive aspergillosis. Such fungus balls are not always detectable on plain films.[314] Reference has already been made to the use of CT in the detection of broncholithiasis. Bronchiectasis in association with tuberculosis is readily detected by CT.[343] There does not appear to be any record of a Rasmussen aneurysm being detected by CT.

INVESTIGATION OF PRIMARY TUBERCULOSIS. CT detects infiltrates not seen on radiographs and can help to explain the presence of hilar or mediastinal adenopathy, particularly in adult patients. The nodes themselves may show the characteristic features of central low density and rim enhancement.

DETECTION OF MILIARY TUBERCULOSIS. CT is more sensitive than radiography in the detection of miliary tubercles.[155,244,270]

INVESTIGATION OF INTRATHORACIC TUBERCULOUS COMPLICATIONS. Complications include empyema, extension of infection through the chest wall (empyema necessitans), bronchopleural fistula formation, fibrosing mediastinitis, endobronchial tuberculosis leading to strictures and occlusions, pericarditis and constrictive pericarditis, and esophagomediastinal fistulas resulting from nodal erosion into the esophagus.[170]

INVESTIGATION OF PATIENTS FOLLOWING PREVIOUS THORACOPLASTY. This is done when reactivation is suspected but radiographic findings are confusing.[256]

ASSESSMENT OF "ACTIVITY." A word of caution is necessary: seemingly inactive thin-walled cavities with associated fibrous infiltrates and calcification may be associated with the presence of tubercle bacilli in the sputum. Nevertheless, there are CT features highly suggestive of activity. Thick-walled cavities with patchy satellite densities in the surrounding lung should be regarded as active. These densities represent a form of focal bronchogenic spread and are grouped around the bronchovascular bundle in a centrilobular position.[169] The result is a little rosette of infiltration. Interstitial infiltration may thicken the interlobular septa, indicating more clearly the centrilobular location of the alveolar rosettes. Extending centrally from these areas of interstitial disease may be branching linear densities, thought to represent disease involving the subsegmental bronchi. Such changes may be seen in nonfibrotic undistorted lung and indicate new disease. However, CT may identify such changes in association with fibrous contraction, calcification, and chronic cavities, and this should suggest the possibility of reactivation of previously dormant disease.

ATYPICAL MYCOBACTERIAL INFECTION

A number of mycobacteria other than *M. tuberculosis* have been identified as causes of pulmonary infection. Mycobacteria are common in the natural environment, and numerous species exist. Some of these mycobacteria have been identified as causes of pulmonary infection.

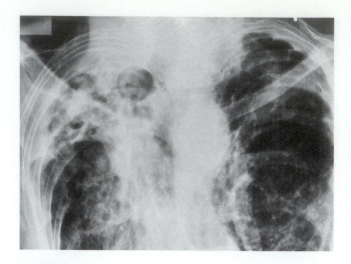

FIGURE 6-76
Elderly man with long-standing obstructive pulmonary disease. Indolent fibrocavitary disease in both lungs caused by *Mycobacterium avium-intracellulare.*

These include *M. kansasii, M. avium-intracellulare, M. fortuitum, M. xenopi,* and *M. simiae.*[73,79,267] It appears that *M. avium-intracellulare* and *M. kansasii* are the most common pathogens in nonimmunocompromised hosts. *M. avium-intracellulare* has proved to be an important pathogen in HIV-infected individuals, and the subject of *M. avium-intracellulare* infection in AIDS is dealt with in Chapter 7. The incidence of atypical mycobacterial disease in the non-HIV-infected population is approximately 2 cases per 100,000 population, an incidence one-fifth that of tuberculosis at the present time. The incidence has probably remained fairly stable because infection occurs from the natural environment and not by person-to-person transmission. The mechanisms by which these seemingly common organisms cause progressive and potentially fatal disease in isolated individuals are ill understood. The organisms have a predilection for individuals with preexisting chronic obstructive pulmonary disease or with debilitating illnesses or various forms of immunocompromise. An interesting association has been observed with achalasia of the cardia and *M. fortuitum* infection.[10] Presumably these organisms flourish in the dilated obstructed esophagus and heavily seed the lungs during episodes of aspiration. One of the problems in the study of the clinical and radiographic manifestations of atypical mycobacterial infections has been that these organisms may occur as incidental contaminants.

The classic radiologic features of atypical mycobacterial infections of the lung are those of a chronic indolent fibrocavitary process, usually involving one or both apical regions of the lungs in a middle-aged or older individual with underlying chronic obstructive pulmonary disease.[403] In many instances the radiographic features are indistinguishable from those of reactivation tuberculosis (Figure 6-76). The response to antituberculous therapy may be poor, and a seemingly inexorable progression of

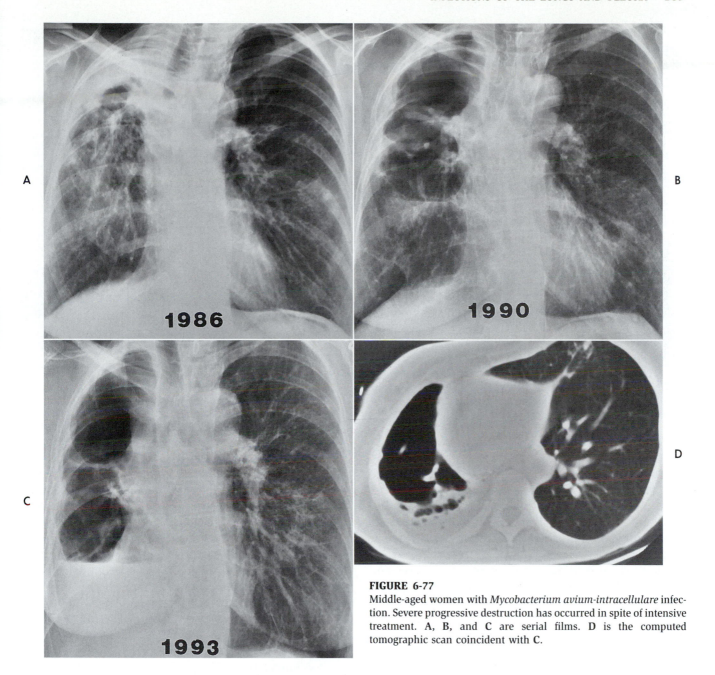

FIGURE 6-77
Middle-aged women with *Mycobacterium avium-intracellulare* infection. Severe progressive destruction has occurred in spite of intensive treatment. **A**, **B**, and **C** are serial films. **D** is the computed tomographic scan coincident with **C**.

the disease over a period of years is common (Figure 6-77). This applies especially to infections with *M. avium-intracellulare*. Localized pleural reactions occur, but pleural effusions are uncommon. Adenopathy and miliary spread of disease are unusual. The lesions have the same predilection for the posterior aspects of the upper lobes or the superior segments of the lower lobe as reactivation tuberculosis.

Cavitation is a distinct feature of atypical mycobacterial infection and occurs in up to 96% of patients.[65] Some emphasis has been placed on a tendency for the cavity or cavities to be thin walled (Figure 6-78), but this was found in only one third of Christensen and associates' cases.[65]

In their series Albelda and associates[1] placed greater

reliance on the tissue diagnosis of the atypical mycobacterioses and thus were able to identify a separate group of patients who did not match the classic radiologic description. They found a subgroup in whom patchy nodular shadows were observed in a peribronchial distribution. Upper lobe prevalence was not present. In half of the group, cavities were noted in the nodules, and this feature combined with the distribution of the lesions gave a superficial resemblance to bronchiectasis. The radiographic findings in individual cases were fairly nonspecific and unlikely to suggest more than chronic diffuse lower airway disease. Ordinarily such cases are not subjected to the aggressive investigation seemingly required for their identification. In practice it is the group with the classic features of indolent, inexorably progres-

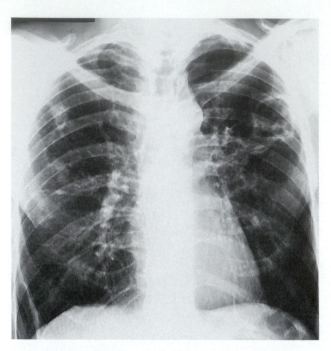

FIGURE 6-78
Atypical mycobacterial infection in alcoholic patient showing thin-walled cavities bilaterally, particularly in left upper lobe.

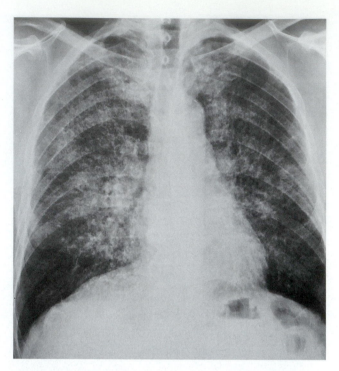

FIGURE 6-79
Nocardial infection complicating pulmonary alveolar proteinosis. Pulmonary shadowing is largely, if not totally, due to alveolar proteinosis. Complicating nocardial infection cannot be diagnosed radiologically.

sive, apical fibrocavitary disease resistant to antituberculous therapy that are likely to be aggressively investigated. Hence the radiographic descriptions may have concentrated on this group of patients to the exclusion of those with more diffuse and less obvious radiographic manifestations.

The work of Albelda and co-workers[1] has been furthered by Prince and associates,[289] who investigated a series of 21 patients with established *M. avium-intracellulare* infection but none of the traditional predisposing conditions. Four of the patients eventually died of progressive *M. avium-intracellulare* infection. The most common radiographic abnormality (70% of cases) was multiple discrete pulmonary nodules. Cavitation was found at some stage of the disease in 40% of cases. Other findings included interstitial shadowing and consolidations. Progression of disease and response to treatment were slow. These authors concluded that pulmonary infection with *M. avium-intracellulare* can occur in otherwise healthy individuals, especially elderly women. The diagnosis is made difficult by the indolent nature of the disease.

NOCARDIOSIS

Most cases of pulmonary nocardiosis are due to *Nocardia asteroides,* although other *Nocardia* species, notably *N. brasiliensis,* are occasionally implicated. *Nocardia* is a filamentous, gram-positive, weakly acid-fast bacillus that grows very slowly on aerobic cultures.

It is related to *Actinomyces israelii,* to the Mycobacteria,[381] and to the genus *Rhodococcus* (formerly known as *Corynebacterium*) and may be confused with any of these organisms.[365] Infections by the *Nocardia* species occur worldwide. The organism grows slowly and is difficult to culture, and there is no effective serologic test. Nocardiosis is seen particularly in patients on immunosuppressive therapy, in those who have received organ transplants,[202] and in individuals with chronic illness, especially AIDS, other underlying immunologic deficiency, or alveolar proteinosis (Figure 6-79).[57,278,296,319,381] In several reviews,[34,76,103] however, a substantial proportion, almost half in one large series,[396] had no recognizable underlying condition. The incidence of nocardiosis appears to be increasing, probably in part because of the increasing prevalence of immunosuppressive therapy, but the proportion of patients with nocardiosis who are immunocompromised is also expected to rise. Dissemination from the lungs to other organs, notably the brain, may occur.

In the lung, *Nocardia* typically causes single or multiple chronic abscesses similar to the lesions caused by pyogenic bacteria. Fibrosis is a late development, and pleural involvement, usually either fibrous thickening or empyema, is frequent.

The chest radiographic findings are variable.* Pulmo-

---

*References 19, 103, 116, 145, 261, 264, 333, 396.

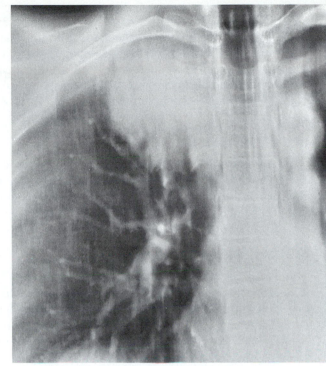

A

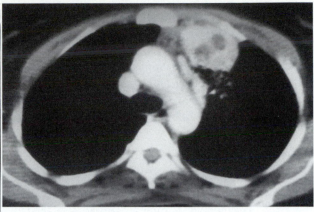

B

FIGURE 6-80
A, *Nocardia brasiliensis* pneumonia in right upper lobe. B, Computed tomographic scan of *N. asteroides* pneumonia in another patient showing central cavitation and enlarged lymph nodes in aortopulmonary window.

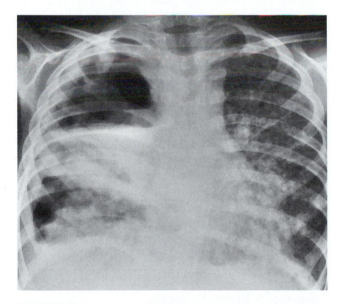

FIGURE 6-81
Nocardia asteroides pneumonia in child. These multifocal consolidations and large right lung abscess developed within 1 week.

nary consolidation is the most common. The consolidations are usually large and frequently cavitate (Figures 6-80 and 6-81). They may be unifocal or multifocal and may be patchy, segmental, or occasionally lobar. Expansion of a lobe is recorded.[145] Some patients have single or multiple round pneumonias (Figure 6-82), which can be irregular and may cavitate, giving rise to a thick-walled abscess. In such cases the distinction from bronchial

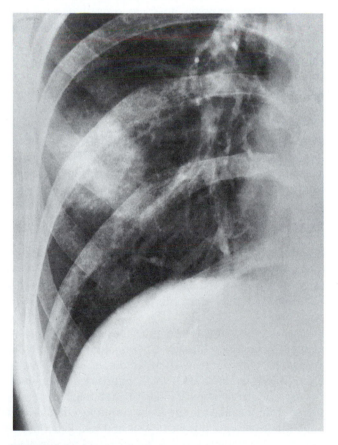

FIGURE 6-82
Round pneumonia caused by *Nocardia asteroides*. Note resemblance of this area of pneumonia to bronchial carcinoma.

carcinoma may be difficult.[48] Similarly the rare endobronchial mass caused by nocardiosis may exactly mimic a tumor radiologically and bronchoscopically.[159] Occasionally, diffuse consolidations or widespread reticulonodular shadows are encountered. Pleural effusion, which may be empyema, and hilar and mediastinal adenopathy are reported features of the disease. Rarely *Nocardia* forms a fungus ball similar to an aspergilloma.[261]

ACTINOMYCOSIS

Actinomycosis is due to *A. israelii,* an anaerobic gram-positive filamentous bacterium that was at one time erroneously classified as a fungus. Unlike the related nocardiosis, actinomycosis is not an opportunistic infection.[381] The disease occurs when local conditions favor growth, namely when organisms that reside as commensals in the mouth and oropharynx gain access to devitalized or infected tissues. Once *A. israelii* is able to proliferate within the tissues, it causes a chronic inflammatory reaction characterized by abscesses that typically contain tiny sulfur granules in thick pus.[49] The disease most commonly affects the cervicofacial region and abdomen.[381] The lungs, which are involved in less than one fourth of cases,[49] are infected either because of aspiration of oral debris containing the organism or because of direct spread from abdominal or cervicofacial disease.[49] The organism produces proteolytic enzymes that allow the infection to cross fascial planes. Therefore the pneumonia readily spreads to the pleura, producing empyema, and may spread extrapleurally to give rise to abscesses and sinus tracks in the chest wall, bones of the thorax, pericardium,[29] and mediastinum.[258] Hematogenous dissemination is rare.

The chest radiograph* and CT[3,208] usually reveal an area of persistent consolidation (Figure 6-83) or a mass (Figure 6-84), either of which may cavitate. The similarity to bronchogenic carcinoma frequently leads to diagnostic confusion.[257] As with nocardiosis, actinomycosis may cause an endobronchial mass that may be confused with bronchial carcinoma at bronchoscopy.[8] Focal fibrosis and contraction may be striking. Widespread small nodular shadowing has been reported.[29,108] The infection readily transgresses the pleura and therefore crosses fissures and extends into the chest wall. Chest wall invasion may be less common now that effective antibiotic therapy is available.[112]

Pleural involvement is manifest as pleural effusion, pleural thickening, or empyema formation but is seldom associated with large accumulations of fluid. Pleural thickening was found at CT in all eight cases reported by Kwong and co-workers[208]; the pleural thickening was smooth and localized to the pleura abutting the diseased lung. Rib involvement leads to lysis and visible periostitis (Figure 6-85), which may be demonstrated to advantage

*References 17, 29, 109, 112, 330, 349.

by CT (Figures 6-86 and 6-87). Similarly, if the spine is involved, there may be a lytic lesion in the spine adjacent to the pulmonary or pleural shadowing.[408] Both mediastinal and cardiac invasion has been reported,[258] but this is rare. CT can demonstrate chest wall,[388] pleural,[208] mediastinal, and spinal invasion to advantage.[258] It also demonstrates intrathoracic lymphadenopathy up to 2.5 cm in diameter in a high proportion of patients.[208]

BOTYROMYCOSIS

Botyromycosis is a rare chronic infectious disease caused by a variety of bacteria. It resembles actinomycosis both clinically and pathologically, in that gray-yellow granules similar to the sulfur granules of actinomycosis are a feature of the infection.[114]

FUNGAL DISEASE

Fungi are defined as mushrooms, molds, and yeasts.[149] A mold is a microscopic, multibranched tubular structure that grows at its expanding margin by the elongation of hyphal tips and by producing new branches, known as hyphae. The yeast shape is another morphologic form taken by some fungi. Yeasts are single, ovoid to spherical cells with rigid walls, in which multiplication occurs by the development of buds, with the cytoplasm and at least one nucleus moving into the bud. The distinction between certain bacteria and fungi is not clear, and some pathogenic organisms such as *Nocardia* and *Actinomyces,* often thought of as fungi, are considered to be bacteria. Pneumonias caused by *Candida, Aspergillus* and *Mucor* are predominantly seen in immunocompromised patients and are discussed on pp. 248 to 253. The following section discusses the agents responsible for most fungal pulmonary diseases, namely histoplasmosis, cryptococcosis, coccidioidomycosis, North American blastomycosis, and aspergillosis, and then briefly describes sporotrichosis and geotrichosis. It is a popular myth that fungal disease of the lung shows the same radiographic features as tuberculosis. Although this is largely true of histoplasmosis, it is a serious misstatement for cryptococcosis, coccidioidomycosis, and blastomycosis. Although these fungal diseases may resemble tuberculosis in some of their manifestations, they show a variety of patterns and may closely resemble bronchial carcinoma.

Pulmonary histoplasmosis

Histoplasmosis is caused by the fungus *Histoplasma capsulatum,* which grows as a septate mycelium in the soil in many temperate zones of the world. Birds such as chickens, starlings, and pigeons may contain the fungus in their excreta and feathers. The mixture of droppings and soil produces an enriched growth medium for the fungus. Bats are a particularly potent source of infection, but unlike birds, bats are infected and pass the yeast form in their excreta. Many reported cases occur after cleaning chicken houses or exploring bat-infested caves. Infection with the organism is particularly prevalent in the central

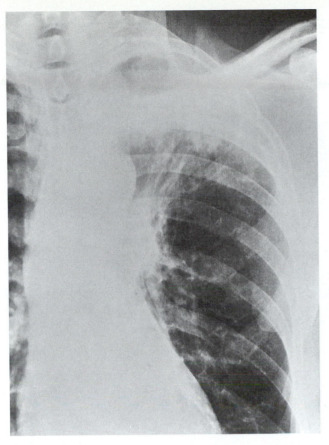

FIGURE 6-83
Pneumonia caused by actinomycosis showing extensive consolidation in apical portion of left upper lobe. Patient complained of shoulder pain, suggesting chest wall invasion.

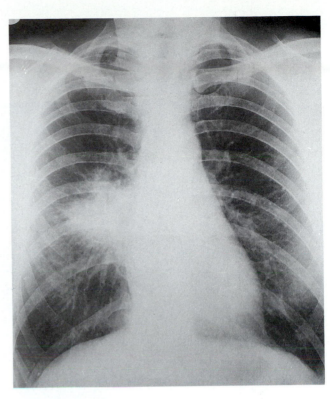

FIGURE 6-84
Round pneumonia caused by actinomycosis resembling bronchial carcinoma. (Courtesy Dr. Michael C. Pearson, London.)

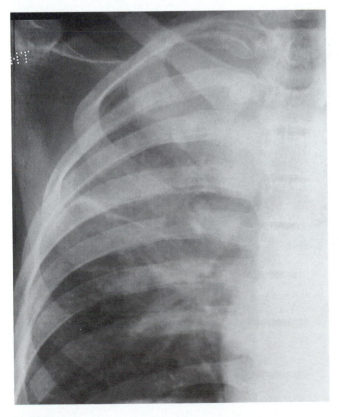

FIGURE 6-85
Actinomycosis pneumonia invading chest wall and causing periostitis of upper six ribs. (Courtesy Dr. Michael C. Pearson, London.)

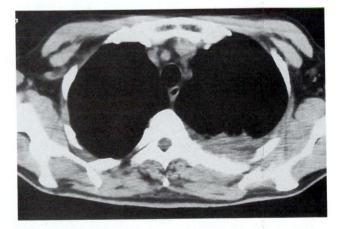

FIGURE 6-86
Actinomycosis invading chest wall. Computed tomographic scan demonstrates periostitis and soft tissue mass.

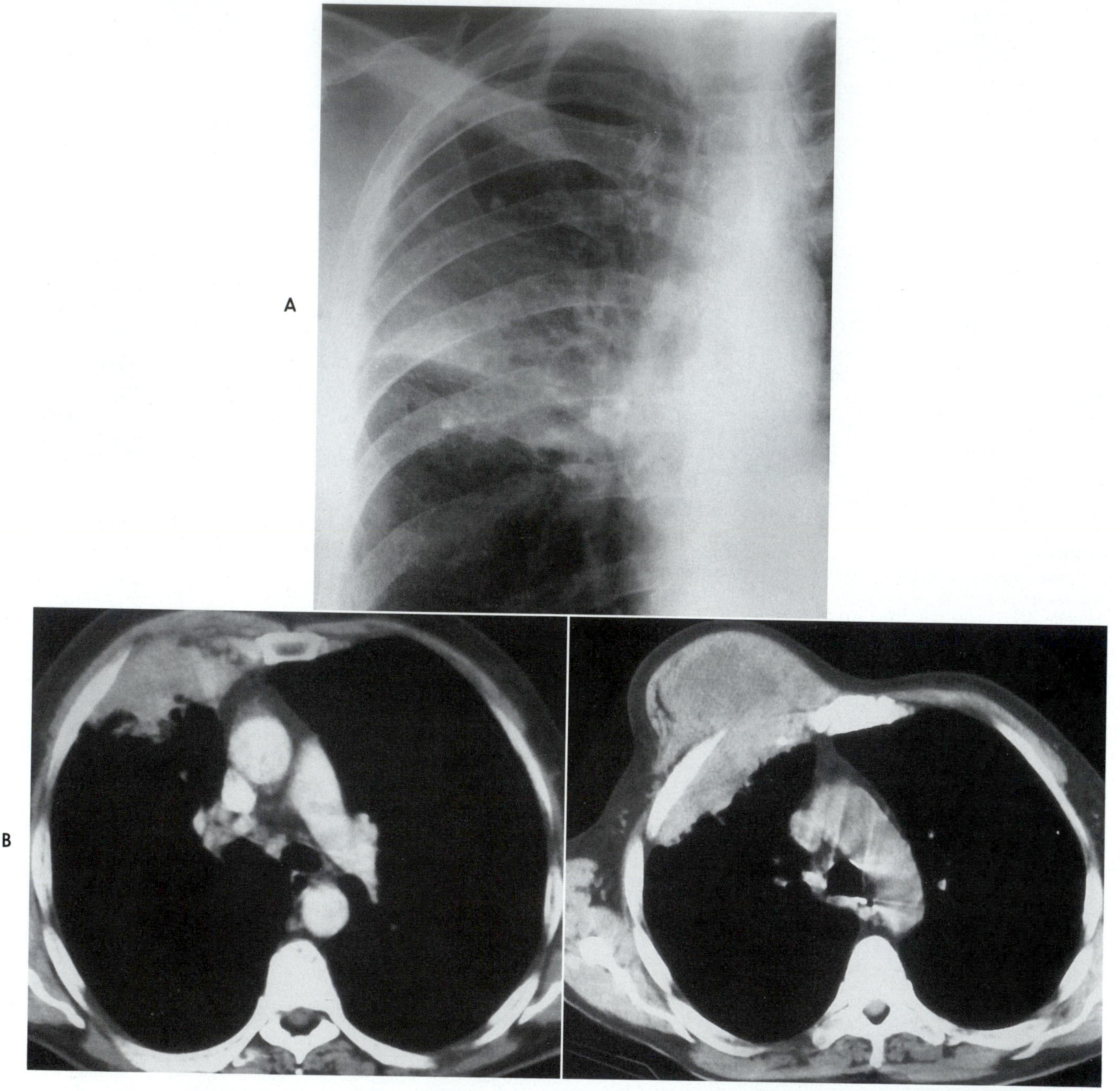

FIGURE 6-87
Actinomycosis pneumonia invading anterior chest wall. **A,** Chest radiograph showing pneumonia in right upper lobe. There is questionable destruction of anterior end of second rib. **B,** Computed tomographic (CT) scan showing consolidation and probable chest wall invasion. **C,** CT scan 2 months later showing obvious chest wall invasion with large subcutaneous mass.

and eastern United States, especially in the Mississippi, Ohio, and St. Lawrence river valleys, Texas, Virginia, Delaware, and Maryland.

Human infection results from inhalation of airborne spores that germinate and convert to the yeast form. Other routes of infection are possible but apparently infrequent. A classification of pulmonary histoplasmosis is given in the box below. Dissemination occurs via the blood and lymphatics, and organisms are removed from the blood by the cells of the reticuloendothelial system in the liver, spleen, and bone marrow. In immunocompetent individuals the fungus multiplies intracellularly until cell-mediated immunity has developed. The macrophages can then kill the fungus and produce intense inflammation. Caseous necrosis occurs, followed by calcification. In infants, as well as in patients with reduced T cell–mediated immunity (such as those who are taking steroids or immunosuppressive drugs or who have AIDS), cellular immunity is overwhelmed or fails to develop and progressive dissemination occurs.[185] Acute infection in the normal host, although common, is usually asymptomatic. Goodwin, Loyd, and Des Prez[133] suggest that most cases of symptomatic histoplasmosis occur in patients with either a structural defect in the lungs, such as emphysema, or some immunologic defect, which may or may not be definable.

The definitive diagnosis of histoplasmosis depends on growing the organism from infected sites or demonstrating it histologically in biopsy material. Culturing *H. capsulatum* is difficult, but more important, it takes time. Therefore in acutely ill patients the diagnosis has to be made histologically. In disseminated disease the bone marrow is the best source; in one relatively recent series the bone marrow examination yielded the organism in 15 of 19 cases.[80]

Several tests for histoplasmosis depend on the immune response. All have the disadvantage of sometimes being negative in disseminated disease, and all may be positive in the absence of active disease, presumably because of previous exposure. Skin testing is now recommended only for epidemiologic studies, not for diagnosing active disease.[185] The complement fixation test, immunodiffusion test, radioimmunoassay, and enzyme immunoassay give more quantitative results. The first two are insensitive but specific, whereas the latter two are very sensitive but nonspecific.[185] Radioimmunoassay of antigen (rather than antibody) in urine and serum may prove useful, particularly for diagnosing disseminated histoplasmosis in immunocompromised patients,[393] but so far these tests are still experimental.

ASYMPTOMATIC INFECTION. The widespread development of skin hypersensitivity to histoplasmin is taken as evidence that millions of people in endemic areas become infected with the fungus. More than 80% of individuals from highly endemic areas demonstrate skin test reactivity by age 20.[94] There is usually no definable clinical illness, but many adults in endemic areas show some radiographic evidence of infection, usually calcified foci of healed disease.[240]

The chest film findings (Figure 6-88) of asymptomatic infection include the following*:

1. One or more patches of pneumonia that often cluster together, may be in any lobe, and may or may not be associated with symptoms. The consolidations, particularly the larger ones, often leave a calcified remnant, although they may disappear totally.[277] In young children

*References 71, 133, 277, 309, 335, 394.

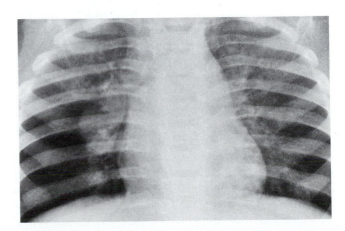

FIGURE 6-88
Asymptomatic histoplasmosis showing right hilar lymph node enlargement.

CLASSIFICATION OF PULMONARY HISTOPLASMOSIS

Histoplasmosis in normal hosts
    Asymptomatic pulmonary infection
    Symptomatic pulmonary infection
        Massive airway inoculation — acute inhalational histoplasmosis
        Single or multiple foci of pneumonia
Histoplasmoma(s)
Opportunistic infections
    Disseminated histoplasmosis (immune defect)
    Chronic cavitary histoplasmosis (structural defect)
Extrapulmonary histoplasmosis
    Mediastinal changes — adenopathy, pericarditis, esophageal involvement, fibrosing mediastinitis
    Limited systemic dissemination — granulomas in the liver and spleen
    Isolated involvement of the central nervous system, retina, bone, or skin
    Widespread systemic disease — central nervous system, liver, spleen, gastrointestinal tract, retina, skin (immune defect)

Modified from Goodwin RA, Des Prez RM: *Medicine* 60:231, 1981.

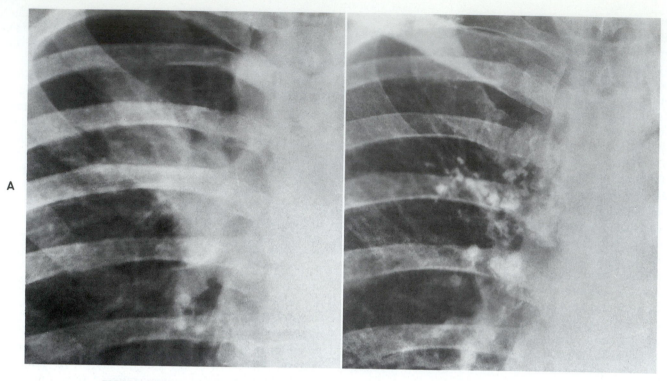

FIGURE 6-89
Symptomatic histoplasmosis in normal host. **A,** Focal area of pulmonary consolidation plus right hilar lymphadenopathy. **B,** Many years later, coarse calcification in region of previous pneumonia and in affected hilar and mediastinal lymph nodes.

the calcification takes just months to occur, but in adults it occurs more slowly.[277]

2. Regional lymph node enlargement and/or calcification, both of which can be striking. The calcifications are in areas of necrosis, and since the necrosis is focal and scattered, the result is tiny nodular calcifications sometimes called mulberry calcification.

3. One or more histoplasmomas.

These phenomena may occur singly or in combination.[394] It is generally held that cavitation is not a feature of the asymptomatic form of the disease,[309] but this assumption has been questioned[31,60] and cases of cavitation in asymptomatic patients have been reported.[71]

SYMPTOMATIC INFECTION IN THE NORMAL HOST.
The major factors determining whether symptomatic infection will occur are the quantity of the airborne inoculum and to a lesser extent the host hypersensitivity before exposure. Thus individuals from endemic areas are likely to have either a mild illness or no illness at all. Symptomatic histoplasmosis usually resolves without therapy. The chest radiograph is often normal in such patients. When abnormalities are seen, they usually consist of one or more small patchy consolidations, with or without hilar adenopathy (Figure 6-89).[185] The symptoms range from brief mild malaise to severe protracted illness. The illness resembles influenza, and the chief features are fever, headache, and muscle pains. There may also be substernal discomfort, loss of appetite, and

nonproductive cough. The liver and spleen may be enlarged, and erythema nodosum, pericarditis, and erythema multiforme may be encountered.

Exceptionally heavy exposure can occur in epidemics, often from a single source. The clinical manifestations are then more severe with higher fever. Respiratory failure and death occur on rare occasions.[185] The radiographs may show multiple small nodules or irregular shadows (Figure 6-90) (less than 1 cm in diameter), which may disappear or may leave small calcifications (Figure 6-91), or widespread fine nodular shadows 2 to 3 mm in size (miliary nodulation).[13,133,262,335,387]

DISSEMINATED HISTOPLASMOSIS. Disseminated histoplasmosis is rare. Approximately one third of cases develop during the first year of life,[309] and the rest occur in adults, especially in the sixth and seventh decades. The male predominance is approximately 4 to 1.[135]

Dissemination usually indicates a failure of immune response, either because of known processes that interfere with T cell function, such as Hodgkin's disease, AIDS, or immunosuppressive therapy, or, as conjectured by Goodwin,[132,135] as "a consequence of transient defects in the immunological apparatus such as are known to complicate certain viral infections." Dissemination may involve all organs, but it has a predilection for the reticuloendothelial system. Oropharyngeal ulcers are a particular feature of low-grade chronic disease in adults.[192]

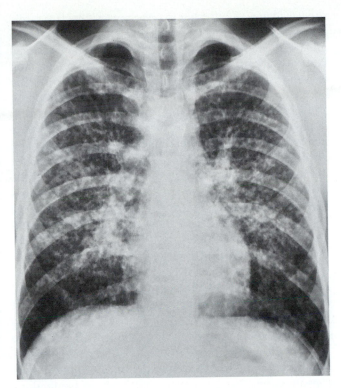

FIGURE 6-90
Acute inhalational histoplasmosis in normal host. Young man who developed fever and cough after tearing down old barn, showing widespread, ill-defined nodular shadows and bilateral hilar adenopathy.

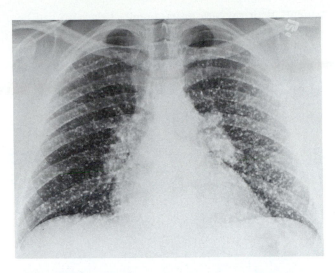

FIGURE 6-91
Innumerable small calcifications in lungs caused by previous acute inhalational histoplasmosis. There is residual hilar adenopathy.

The chest film may be normal but usually shows widespread pulmonary shadowing. The pattern varies. Widespread miliary nodules identical to miliary tuberculosis (Figure 6-92), interstitial shadowing, nodular shadowing, and patchy consolidations with or without cavities are all reported.[71,110,135,192,277] In babies the chest film may remain normal despite overwhelming disease.[309]

CHRONIC PULMONARY HISTOPLASMOSIS. Chronic pulmonary histoplasmosis is now regarded as an opportunistic infection complicating emphysema of the lungs.[134] It is believed that persistent infection occurs only in abnormal pulmonary airspaces. Such infection may then spread via the bronchi to produce chronic patchy pneumonitis. The colonization of large bullous spaces may produce infected cavities that at first are thin walled but later develop thick fibrous walls. The cavities may enlarge slowly and destroy lung, exacerbating the symptoms of underlying chronic obstructive lung disease. The majority eventually heal without treatment. In the few cases that become progressive the course is relentlessly downhill. In one large study of 50 patients with relapse following treatment, 15 died.[280]

The symptoms of chronic pulmonary histoplasmosis are similar to those of pulmonary tuberculosis, with mild to moderate malaise, fever, weight loss, and productive cough. Hemoptysis occurs in more than one third of

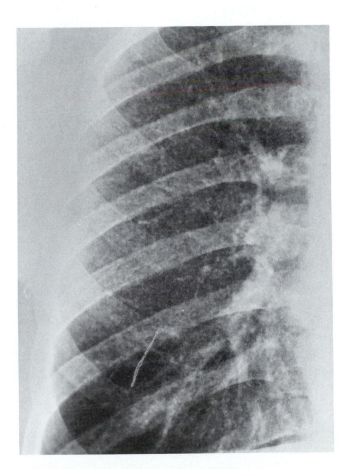

FIGURE 6-92
Disseminated miliary histoplasmosis in immunocompromised patient. Note similarity to miliary tuberculosis.

patients with cavitary disease, and chest pain can be a distinct feature.[132]

The radiographic appearances closely resemble postprimary tuberculosis. The multiple, small, patchy consolidations show a striking predilection for the upper lobes (Figures 6-93 and 6-94). Although the lower lobes may show evidence of infection in severe cases, they are rarely if ever involved in isolation. The consolidations may be unilateral but are frequently bilateral. It is now realized that cavitation, previously thought to be a common feature,[31,231] occurs in the minority (Figure 6-95). The original papers dealt with only the most severe examples, and it is now appreciated that a milder self-limiting form of the disease constitutes about 80% of the cases.[134] The infected cavities involve the upper lobes particularly and are frequently bilateral.[31,231] The cavities may resolve, but frequently they persist or progress, particularly those with a thick wall.[134] As with tuberculosis, the upper lobes contract because of scarring and destruction by the infection. Pleural effusion may occur but is rare, and lymphadenopathy is unusual.[71,335]

HISTOPLASMOMA. On histologic examination the histoplasmoma is a small necrotic focus of infection surrounded by a massive fibrous capsule.[136] On radiologic examination the typical histoplasmoma is a well-defined spherical nodule (Figure 6-96). It may be of soft tissue density or contain discrete calcifications. Calcification in the necrotic center is an early feature and may be seen 3 months after the lesion is first identified. As the fibrous capsule grows, calcification is laid down in laminations that may cause a general increase in density or may on occasion appear as concentric rings on radiologic examination. Histoplasmomas may be single or multiple (Figure 6-97). The detection of increased density caused by the presence of calcification (Figure 6-98) is the basis of the CT diagnosis of benignity in the assessment of pulmonary nodules (see p. 99).

Usually the edge of the histoplasmoma is smooth or slightly lobular. There are, however, many cases on record in which the edge is irregular, sometimes mark-

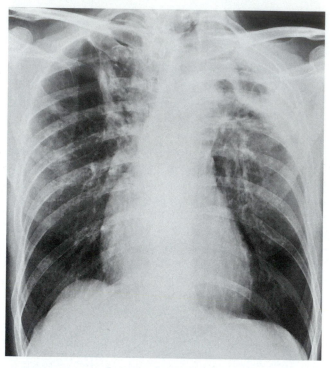

FIGURE 6-93
Chronic histoplasmosis showing upper lobe consolidation, contraction, and cavitation. Note similarity to postprimary tuberculosis.

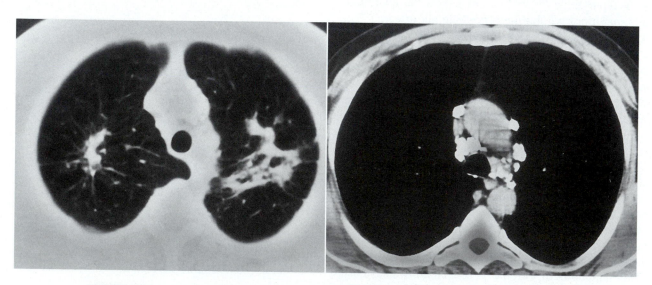

FIGURE 6-94
Middle-aged man from Shenandoah valley of Virginia with bilateral apical fibrocavitary histoplasmosis and extensive eggshell calcification of mediastinal lymph nodes.

edly so. Indeed, the edge may be so shaggy that on rare occasion it is indistinguishable from the corona radiata seen with bronchial carcinoma. Occasionally histoplasmomas, both single and multiple,[276] enlarge over the years.

The enlarging histoplasmoma, even if it is cavitary or multiple, does not appear to pose a problem of dissemi-

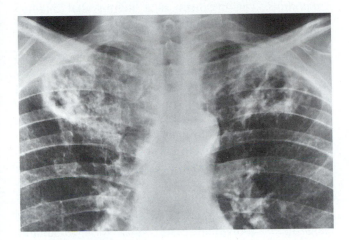

FIGURE 6-95
Chronic cavitary histoplasmosis. Note striking upper zone predominance of shadow. Multiple large cavities are present in this case.

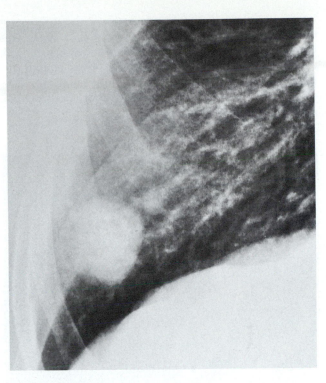

FIGURE 6-96
Histoplasmoma showing well-defined spherical nodule. The central portion of the nodule shows calcification.

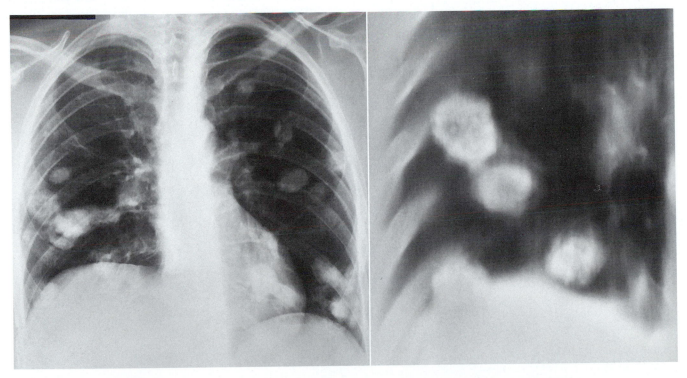

FIGURE 6-97
Multiple calcified histoplasmomas. **A,** Plain film. **B,** Conventional tomogram showing concentric organization of calcification.

nation of disease.[277,335] In one series[136] the increase in diameter averaged approximately 2 mm a year. This increase in size has at times led to confusion with carcinoma of the lung, particularly when the characteristic calcifications were not present. In general, however, the growth is far slower than that observed with malignant lesions.

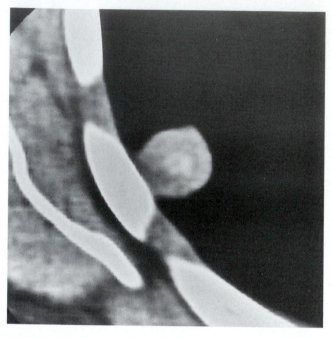

FIGURE 6-98
Computed tomographic scan of histoplasmoma showing central ringlike calcification.

MEDIASTINAL ADENOPATHY AND FIBROSIS. The subject of mediastinal adenopathy and fibrosis caused by histoplasmosis is discussed in Chapter 16.

Cryptococcosis

Cryptococcosis, also known as torulosis *(Torula histolytica)* or European blastomycosis, is an infection caused by inhaling spores that contain *Cryptococcus neoformans*. The organism is a nonmycelial budding yeast found in the soil and in bird droppings, particularly from pigeons.

The lung, the portal of entry, is a common site of disease. From here the disease may spread to many organs. Meningitis and meningoencephalitis are the most serious consequences (Figure 6-99).[222] The disease may occur at any age but is most common in adults. The prevalence is difficult to determine because there is no good skin test or serum antibody assay for cryptococcosis, and the question of saprophytic colonization as opposed to invasive disease cannot be assessed from either culture of sputum or the currently available serologic tests.[52,152] An antigen latex agglutination test can be used for diagnosis of individual cases, since it is reasonably specific; its sensitivity, however, is poor.[52]

Many patients with cryptococcal pneumonia have no symptoms, and the pulmonary lesions seen radiographically heal spontaneously. Approximately one half to two thirds of the cases of symptomatic infection are associated with immunodeficiency from conditions such as AIDS,[201] lymphoma, leukemia, diabetes mellitus, and particularly drugs; in these patients extrapulmonary dissemination is common.[194]

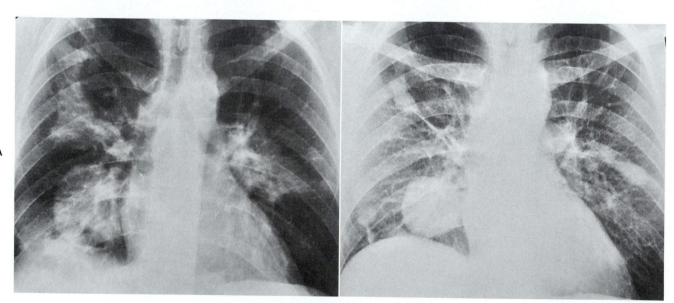

FIGURE 6-99
Cryptococcal meningitis in a 27-year-old man without known immunocompromise or pulmonary symptoms. **A,** At presentation. **B,** Eight months later.

Fever, chest pain, cough, and mucoid sputum production are the usual symptoms.[194] Cryptococcal pneumonia may be the initial manifestation of AIDS.[201] Cryptococcal meningitis develops with a greater frequency in immunocompromised patients than those without a predisposing condition.[21] Meningeal spread is extremely common in immunocompromised individuals[194]; it was seen in 18 of 27 subjects in one series of AIDS patients.[201] In another series most of those with meningeal involvement had no clinical features that specifically indicated meningeal infection.[252]

A large variety of appearances may be seen on chest radiographs. The descriptions and classifications vary considerably, as does the incidence of the various findings.* This may be due to the relative frequency and severity of immunodeficiency in the patient populations being described. As expected, patients who are immunocompromised have more extensive disease.[196] In general three patterns are encountered:

1. One or more spherical nodules or masses
2. One or more areas of patchy consolidation
3. Multiple small nodules or irregular shadows

---

*References 45, 102, 138, 177, 194, 196, 252, 402.

Hilar and mediastinal adenopathy may accompany any of these patterns, as may pleural effusions.

NODULES AND MASSES. The size of these mass lesions varies from barely visible to huge.[279] They are usually single (Figure 6-100) but may be multiple, and they vary in location with no predilection for any one lobe or zone. Some are composed largely of fungus with little associated inflammatory response,[102,138] a form of disease that produces a well-defined mass and in the few cases reported is not associated with lymphadenopathy, cavitation, or pleural effusion. The remainder are predominantly due to fibrous tissue with central caseation and abundant organisms.[353] These lesions are usually poorly defined and may show cavitation and associated lymphadenopathy, with both phenomena more common in immunocompromised patients.[196]

From the preceding description it is clear that the distinction from bronchial carcinoma is often difficult,[247] usually requiring biopsy. Sputum cultures and bronchial washings that grow *C. neoformans* do not exclude the diagnosis of carcinoma. *Cryptococcus* colonizes the respiratory tract in many chronic disorders and therefore is often found in patients with bronchial carcinoma. In one series of 28 patients with radiographic parenchymal lung lesions and *C. neoformans* in the respiratory tract, 25% had lung cancer.[90]

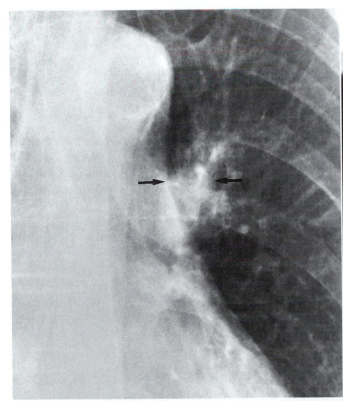

A

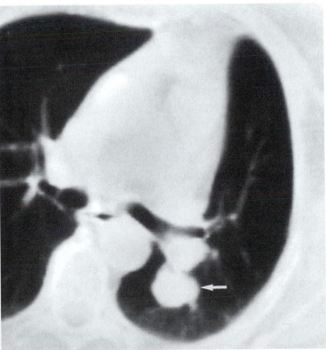

B

FIGURE 6-100
Cryptococcus nodule. **A,** Plain film (arrows point to lesion). **B,** Computed tomographic scan showing uniform soft tissue density of nodule. Nodule is indistinguishable from carcinoma.

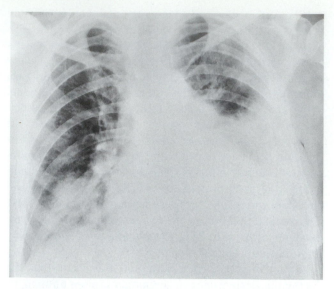

FIGURE 6-101
Cryptococcal pneumonia showing extensive bilateral middle and lower zone consolidation.

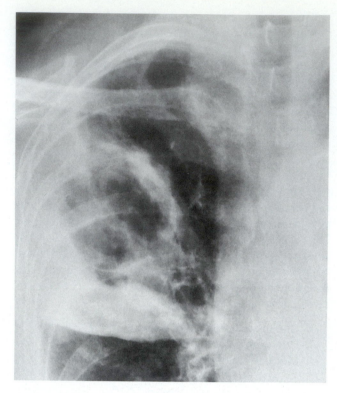

FIGURE 6-102
Cryptococcal pneumonia showing extensive cavitation in right upper lobe.

PATCHY CONSOLIDATION. As with the masses, the size, location, and multiplicity of consolidation vary greatly; even lobar consolidation has been reported.[232] Some series have shown a predilection for the lower zones (Figure 6-101)[230] and some a predominance of upper lobe presentations.[138] Air bronchograms may be present. Cavitation (Figure 6-102) and associated lymphadenopathy occur but are relatively unusual. Unlike with the consolidative lesions in histoplasmosis and tuberculosis, subsequent loss of volume and calcification do not appear to be prominent features.[353]

WIDESPREAD SMALL NODULAR OR IRREGULAR SHADOWS. This pattern is the least common and is indistinguishable from a host of other interstitial diseases. When nodular it resembles miliary tuberculosis and other fungal infections.

PLEURAL EFFUSIONS. Pleural effusions are relatively rare in pulmonary cryptococcosis.[102] When seen they typically occur in the immunocompromised host.[69] A 1980 review showed that the 30 cases reported in the English language literature were divided almost equally between localized and disseminated disease.[406]

Coccidioidomycosis

Coccidioidomycosis is caused by the fungus *Coccidioides immitis,* which is found in the soil. The disease occurs mainly in semiarid regions in the southwestern United States and northern Mexico, where it is endemic. Pulmonary infection is acquired by inhalation of the fungus, which occurs only in the endemic areas; transmission by person-to-person contact is extremely rare.[353] As with histoplasmosis, the incidence of infection, as shown by coccidioidin skin test conversion, exceeds that of clinical symptoms,[33] but the incidence of symptoms is

higher than in histoplasmosis. The infection usually occurs in adults and is mild and self-limiting, although occasionally it is severe and prolonged. Dissemination is rare but has serious consequences.

The standard diagnostic tests are precipitin and complement fixation tests. The most definitive diagnosis is made by identifying or culturing the organism in body fluids or tissues, but the success varies greatly. Organisms are almost always found in purulent drainage from skin and soft tissues, sometimes in sputum and lung or bronchial aspirates and rarely in pleural fluid, although granulomas and organisms can usually be demonstrated by biopsy of the pleura.[219]

The disease is classified in various ways. This presentation uses the same groupings for the pulmonary manifestations as those used by Drutz and Cantazaro[89] in their major review articles.

PRIMARY COCCIDIOIDOMYCOSIS. Symptoms are encountered in only 40% of patients with pulmonary coccidioidomycosis.[33,332] Usually the illness is nonspecific and resembles a mild virus infection; sometimes a severe pneumonia is seen, and very occasionally the disease become disseminated. The usual symptoms are fatigue, nonproductive cough, and pleuritic chest pain, accompanied not infrequently by dyspnea, arthralgia, headache, and sore throat. A maculopapular rash and erythema nodosum are common skin manifestations. ''Valley fever'' is a relatively specific complex consist-

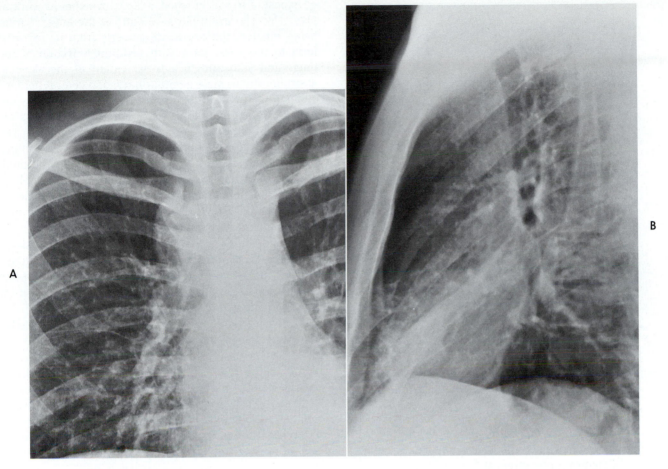

FIGURE 6-103
Primary coccidioidomycosis in patient who had visited California, showing consolidation in right middle lobe and substantial right paratracheal adenopathy. **A,** Posteroanterior view. **B,** Lateral view.

ing of erythema nodosum, erythema multiforme, and arthritis.

Radiographic examination[179,243,322] of asymptomatic patients may show fibrous scars, small, often calcified pulmonary nodules, or calcified nodal granulomas. Alternatively, the chest film may be normal.

Symptomatic patients show unifocal or multifocal segmental consolidation that may take a month or two to resolve. Hilar and mediastinal adenopathy and pleural effusion are each seen in approximately one fourth of patients,[42,140,233] usually ipsilaterally in combination with a pulmonary shadow (Figure 6-103). Such adenopathy may be pronounced[179] and if isolated should be distinguished from sarcoidosis or lymphoma.[140] Paratracheal adenopathy may rarely be associated with granulomatous masses in the trachea or major bronchi, particularly in children.[38,259]

PERSISTENT PULMONARY COCCIDIOIDOMYCOSIS.
Most patients with primary coccidioidomycosis recover within 3 weeks. Those whose symptoms or radiographic abnormalities remain after 6 to 8 weeks are considered to have persistent coccidioidomycosis. The most common

complaint is hemoptysis.[89] Patients with persistent and extensive pneumonia are often very sick. Fatal cases are usually, but not always, in immunocompromised patients.

Systemic dissemination is rare except in immunocompromised patients, occurring in less than 1% of cases, but is much more common in nonwhites than in whites.[332] Dissemination occurs most frequently to skin, followed by soft tissue, synovium, bone, lymph nodes, meninges, and urinary tract.[219] In general, dissemination is accompanied by anergy to coccidioidin and by high complement fixation titers.

The radiographic findings of persistent pulmonary coccidioidomycosis are coccidioidal nodules (coccidioidoma), persistent coccidioidal pneumonia, and miliary coccidioidomycosis. Coccidioidal nodules are areas of round pneumonia. On plain chest radiographs they are usually subpleural[312] and in an upper lobe (Figure 6-104). Cavitation is a major characteristic.[165] The wall may be thick but is often thin, in some cases strikingly so. On the whole the cavities are small, averaging 1.5 cm in diameter,[243] but they may reach 6 cm.[42] Rapid change in

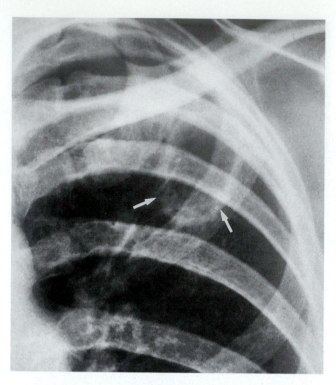

FIGURE 6-104
Thin-walled cavity *(arrow)* resulting from coccidioidal pneumonia.

size is a characteristic feature of the cavities,[179] and pneumothorax or pyopneumothorax may be a complication.[89,93] Calcification is unusual.[312,325,332]

Patients with chronic progressive coccidioidal pneumonia have prolonged symptoms and show upper lobe fibrocavitary disease with loss of volume similar to that seen with tuberculosis or histoplasmosis.[328] Miliary spread, a frequently fatal complication, may be an early manifestation of the disease or may complicate chronic pulmonary or extrapulmonary disease. Miliary nodulation has an appearance similar to that seen with miliary tuberculosis. Associated mediastinal lymph node enlargement is common.[332]

North American blastomycosis

Most cases of *Blastomyces dermatitidis* infection occur in the central and southeastern United States, but documented examples have been reported from Africa,[327] the Middle East, Canada, and Central and South America.[59] The source of the fungus is believed to be the soil.[199,327] Person-to-person transmission of the disease has not been demonstrated.[329] Blastomycosis may occur sporadically or as outbreaks from a common source. Sporadic cases show a predilection for middle-aged men, especially those exposed by occupation to the soil (for example, farmers, construction workers, and workers in the timber industry). Single-source outbreaks often follow exposure in wooded areas, particularly along rivers, and affect both sexes and all ages equally. The common thread appears to

be exposure to soil in wooded areas, whether at work or play.[55,199] The usual portal of entry is the lung.[331] After being inhaled, the organism converts from its mycelial form to the yeast form with resulting infection of the lungs and skin and to a lesser extent of the skeletal, gastrointestinal, male genitourinary, and central nervous systems.[32,327] The pulmonary infection is often asymptomatic. When symptoms occur, the manifestations are variable, in some cases resembling acute pneumonia. The symptoms may be similar to influenza with fever, chills, headache, myalgia, arthralgia, and cough. In the more chronic cases the disease may clinically and radiologically resemble carcinoma of the lung. Subcutaneous abscesses that grow to become ulcerations are the most common clinical manifestations of the disease,[327] and these ulcerations are an important clinical clue to the diagnosis. The outcome is also variable; most patients recover and remain well, but progressive pulmonary disease and dissemination may occur. A small minority of affected patients are immunocompromised.[302]

Since no general screening test is available, knowledge regarding the prevalence of disease is inadequate. The diagnosis is established by a rising antibody titer or culture of the organism. Skin tests are no longer used, and complement fixation tests are negative in 50% or more of patients.[334] However, a new enzyme immunoassay test is under development.[198] The definitive diagnosis requires the recognition of the organism on microscopic examination of smears from infected sites or, more definitively, by culture.

Pulmonary involvement is an almost constant finding at autopsy, but only 60% of patients with systemic blastomycosis demonstrate significant abnormalities on plain chest radiograph.[9] Several series and reviews have documented the radiographic findings.* A major feature of acute infection is ill-defined consolidation in the lung indistinguishable from acute pneumonia. Screening examinations in single-source outbreaks may reveal consolidations in asymptomatic individuals. The consolidation may be unifocal or multifocal. Single-lobe involvement is somewhat more frequent than multilobar pneumonia. The consolidations range from subsegmental to lobar, occurring more frequently in the upper than the lower lobes (Figures 6-105 and 6-106). In a minority of cases the consolidations are widespread bilaterally, and occasionally an interstitial pattern is present. Cavitation appears to be more a manifestation of chronic disease than acute disease, and the incidence has varied from 8%[50] to 37%[340] in two large series. A pattern closely resembling fibrocavitary tuberculosis or histoplasmosis is seen in some cases of chronic blastomycosis (Figure 6-107).[156,295,334] In a number of cases, multiple intermediate-sized nodules develop. Intermediate-sized nodules are 2 cm in diameter or less and presumably evolve from

---

*References 9, 43, 50, 156, 211, 283, 295, 334, 340, 400, 401.

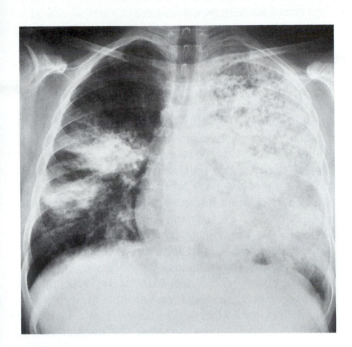

FIGURE 6-105
Blastomycosis pneumonia in 12-year-old girl, showing bilateral consolidations, predominantly in left upper lobe.

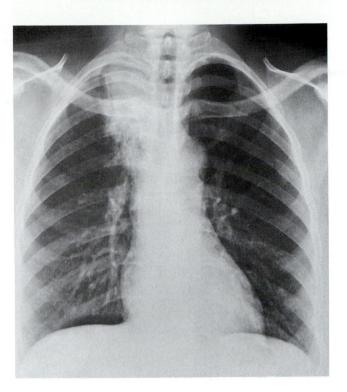

FIGURE 6-106
Blastomycosis pneumonia in middle-aged woman showing right upper lobe consolidation and loss of volume, initially thought to be postobstructive pneumonia beyond a carcinoma.

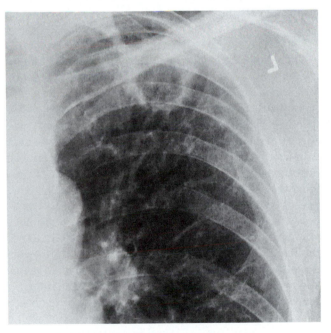

FIGURE 6-107
Blastomycosis showing fibrocavitary disease in left upper lobe.

multifocal areas of consolidation. Pleural changes are not infrequent and usually take the form of pleural thickening adjacent to the pulmonary process, but occasionally a small ipsilateral pleural effusion is present. Direct invasion of the chest wall with the development of an extrapleural mass and rib destruction is very occasionally encountered.[156] Lytic lesions in the bones caused by hematogenous spread are more frequent than direct spread,[156] a pattern identical to that seen with metastatic malignant neoplasm.

Some patients present with a spherical pneumonia, usually 3 to 8 cm in diameter. The result is a masslike lesion with ill-defined outer margins often contiguous with the hilum. The lesion is readily mistaken for a bronchial carcinoma. The presence of air bronchograms within the lesion may provide a clue that the disease is not a bronchial carcinoma, although sinister alternative diagnoses such as alveolar cell carcinoma and lymphoma remain. Halvorsen and co-workers[151] were unable to detect air bronchograms on the radiographs in any of the seven masslike lesions in their series. However, Winer-Muram and associates[399] found air bronchograms by CT in 12 of 14 such lesions. Calcification is relatively infrequent in blastomycosis and is unlikely to help in excluding a malignancy. Hilar and mediastinal adenopathy, usually mild, occurs in a minority of cases. When adenopathy is associated with a mass lesion, there is a distinct risk that the findings may be attributed to a

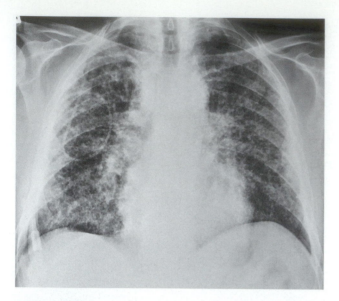

FIGURE 6-108
Blastomycosis showing widespread miliary nodulation in the lungs.

malignant process. Likewise, chest wall invasion inevitably causes confusion even in younger patients.

A variable but small proportion of cases are reported as causing miliary nodulation in the lungs (Figure 6-108), which can be indistinguishable from miliary tuberculosis. This pattern appears to be more common in immunocompromised patients.[357]

Pulmonary aspergillosis

The genus *Aspergillus* is a ubiquitous dimorphic fungus present in soil and water and is abundant in decaying and moldy vegetation. There are over 300 species of *Aspergillus,* but *Aspergillus fumigatus* is by far the most common pathogen in humans.[184] It can cause a wide spectrum of pulmonary disease, ranging from simple colonization to life-threatening invasive aspergillosis, depending on the immunologic status of the host, individual susceptibility, or preexisting lung disease. It has been suggested that pulmonary aspergillosis be considered a spectrum instead of the conventional divisions of (1) mycetoma, (2) invasive aspergillosis, and (3) allergic bronchopulmonary aspergillosis, particularly because these three entities may overlap in an individual patient and with other *Aspergillus*-related phenomena such as mucoid impaction, eosinophilic pneumonia, bronchocentric granulomatosis, extrinsic allergic alveolitis, or asthma.[141] Also, limited invasion may occur with mycetoma in patients with mild immunosuppression or underlying lung disease.[123] The subject of colonization and mycetoma is discussed here, that of invasive aspergillosis is considered on p. 245, and allergic pulmonary aspergillosis is described on p. 528.

Saprophytic colonization is seen in patients with chronic obstructive pulmonary disease who are debilitated and receiving prolonged courses of multiple antibi-

otics or corticosteroids.[184] *Aspergillus* has been found in 7% of sputum cultures in patients with a wide variety of chest diseases and in 24% of sputum cultures of asthmatic patients. Some patients show evidence of an immunologic response, such as increased total immunoglobulin E, positive precipitins, and immediate or late skin reactivity to *Aspergillus* antigen.[184]

The term "aspergilloma" (mycetoma, fungus ball) is used to describe a ball of coalescent mycelial hyphae that typically colonize preexisting chronic cavities, mainly in the lung, although mycetomas may also form in chronic pleural cavities.[74,91,249] The pulmonary cavities are usually due to old healed pulmonary tuberculosis, although cavities from a variety of other causes, including fungal infection, *P. carinii* infection, sarcoidosis, ankylosing spondylitis (Figure 6-109), interstitial pulmonary fibrosis, bronchiectasis, pulmonary sequestrations, pulmonary infarcts, lung abscesses, and pulmonary neoplasms (Figure 6-110) may also be colonized by the fungus.*

Pathologic study[58] of an intracavitary aspergilloma shows a compact, spherical conglomerate of hyphae that may be attached to the wall of the cavity but usually is not. On microscopic examination the fungus ball is composed of concentric or convoluted layers of radially arranged and intertwined hyphae. Those in the center are often nonviable. Although hyphae can be found along the surface and within the fibrous wall of the cavity, invasion into the adjacent lung parenchyma does not occur unless host defense mechanisms are compromised, in which case the condition can take a locally destructive form known variously as chronic necrotizing pulmonary aspergillosis (CPNA)[41] or "semiinvasive" aspergillosis.[123] The underlying abnormality may be locally diseased lung, such as chronic obstructive pulmonary disease, prior irradiation, or pneumoconiosis. Mild systemic immunocompromise such as connective tissue disorders, poor nutrition, diabetes mellitus, or low-dose corticosteroid therapy may also be present.

Patients with mycetoma are usually over 40 years of age and are more likely to be male than female.[242,314] The mycetoma may be asymptomatic and first discovered incidentally on a chest radiograph, but hemoptysis is seen in 50% to 80% of patients.[100,117,183,191] The mechanism of bleeding is unknown; it has been attributed to friction between the fungus ball and the hypervascular cavity wall, to endotoxins liberated from the fungus, and to type III reaction in the cavity wall.[184] Occasionally the hemoptysis is so massive as to be life threatening.[183,298] Other symptoms include productive cough, chest pain, fever, dyspnea, weight loss, and fatigue, caused mainly by the underlying condition rather than by the mycetoma itself.[298]

The diagnosis is largely established on radiographic grounds. Skin tests and sputum cultures for *Aspergillus* may be positive, but neither test is specific.[242] Positive

---

*References 91, 100, 106, 117, 176, 191, 298, 314, 336, 372, 376.

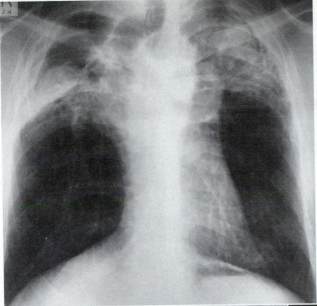

A

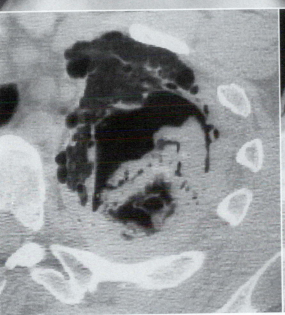

B

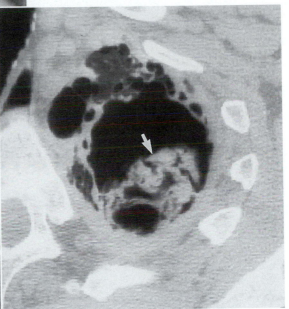

C

FIGURE 6-109
A, Bilateral mycetomas *(arrows)* within cavities secondary to upper lobe fibrosis caused by ankylosing spondylitis. **B** and **C,** Adjacent high-resolution computed tomographic scans through a mycetoma in the left upper lobe showing typical folded spongelike appearance.

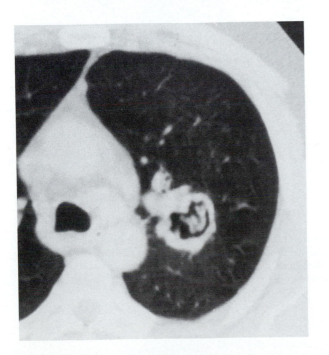

FIGURE 6-110
Mycetoma in cavitating neoplasm. "Collapsed membrane" of mycetoma is seen within cavitating squamous cell carcinoma.

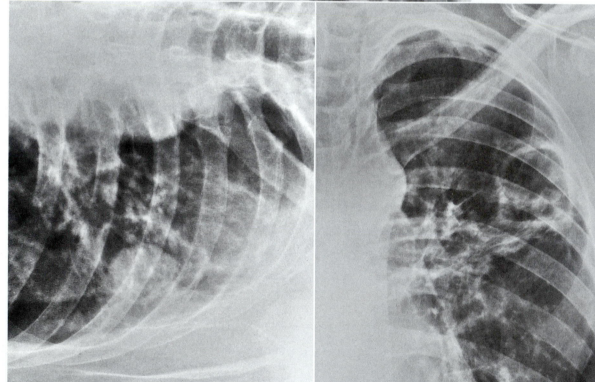

FIGURE 6-111
Mycetoma showing intracavitary ball of fungus. Note crescent of air above mycetoma, adjacent pleural thickening, and movement of fungus ball. In this case the underlying fibrocavitary disease was due to atypical mycobacterial infection. **A,** Frontal view. **B,** Lateral decubitus view. **C,** Frontal view 1 year earlier shows preexisting cavity with an air-fluid level but no recognizable mycetoma.

precipitating antibodies to *Aspergillus* antigens can be demonstrated in the serum in over 90% of patients,[117] but again the test is not specific for mycetoma, since it is also positive in many of the forms of pulmonary aspergillosis, including temporary colonization by fungal hyphae. Also, precipitin tests are species specific; therefore the occasional negative serum precipitin test result is seen when the responsible *Aspergillus* is not *A. fumigatus*.

The essential finding on plain film is the mycetoma itself,[117,175,412] a rounded mass of soft tissue density lying within a preexisting cavity (Figure 6-110). Because most of the preexisting cavities are due to old tuberculosis or histoplasmosis, mycetomas are found most often in the upper lobes or in the superior segment of the lower lobes. Usually the mass fills only a portion of the cavity, so that air is seen between the fungus ball and the wall. The air takes the shape of a meniscus and is usually referred to as the air meniscus sign or the air crescent sign (Figure 6-111). In some cases the mycetoma more or less fills the cavity and the mycetoma is no longer able to roll around.

Because the cavity wall is lined by fungus, it may appear thick (Figures 6-112 and 6-113),[228] a sign that is seen most often in long-standing mycetoma with obvious intracavitary mass, but also with early colonization before the fungus ball itself is obvious. Pleural thickening of up to 2 cm adjacent to the cavity is a frequent sign of *Aspergillus* superinfection.[223] An air-fluid level may be present within the cavity.[117,223,228]

All the plain film findings are better seen with tomography,[117] and CT scanning demonstrates the features even better. CT shows a spongelike mass that contains irregular airspaces (Figures 6-109 and 6-112).[314] The air crescent sign and the wall of the preexisting cavity are well seen, and the mobility of the fungus ball can be readily demonstrated with extra views in the prone and lateral decubitus positions, if necessary. The spongelike appearance is so characteristic that in patients with positive serum precipitins the diagnosis is secure even when the mycetoma fills the cavity and neither the air crescent sign nor evidence of mobility can be demonstrated. The diagnosis of mycetoma formation can be made with CT by noting fungal strands either lining the cavity or within the lumen (resembling a crumpled membrane) before they have formed a ball of sufficient size to be recognized on plain chest radiograph (Figures 6-112 and 6-113).

In the semiinvasive form[41,123] the fungus may produce extensive local consolidation and destruction of the lung parenchyma (Figure 6-114). There need not be a previous cavity; the appearance may simply be an area of chronic pulmonary consolidation that undergoes progressive cavitation and subsequent mycetoma formation. Once the mycetoma has formed, the appearance resembles the noninvasive form except that the cavity continues to grow slowly.[41]

There is also a stable, noncavitary, nodular or masslike form of pulmonary aspergillosis in which there is no evidence of a preexisting cavity and the lesion resembles a pulmonary neoplasm on both plain film and CT examination. None of the three reported patients in one series with this form of aspergillosis were immunocompromised[344]; the authors suggested that the lesions represented a locally invasive form of infection, but the relationship of these masses to semiinvasive or chronic necrotizing pulmonary aspergillosis is unclear.

Unusual fungi

Sporotrichosis is usually a lymphocutaneous infection acquired by direct implantation of the fungus *Sporothrix schenckii*. The highest incidence of the common lymphocutaneous form is in agricultural workers, nursery workers, and persons in similar occupations.[316] No skin tests are available, and the serologic tests are highly specialized. The best method of diagnosis is culture of the fungus from sputum specimens, bronchial brushings or washings, or pleural biopsies. Pulmonary involvement may be secondary to skin infection, but in most cases pulmonary disease is caused by inhalation of spores and occupational exposure does not play as great a role.[39,254,316] Systemic dissemination may occur. The usual symptoms of pulmonary disease are productive cough and low-grade fever. The chest radiographic findings (Figure 6-115) are variable, mostly nonspecific areas of consolidation that may give rise to thin-walled cavities and fibronodular densities in the upper lobes closely resembling pulmonary tuberculosis,[39,67] even to the extent that fungus balls may grow in sporotrichosis cavities.[316]

Geotrichosis is due to *Geotrichum candidum*, a fungus that normally inhabits the pharynx and gastrointestinal tract. It may cause bronchitis, asthma, or pneumonia. In parenchymal infection the radiograph may show upper lobe consolidation and thin-walled cavities.

MYCOPLASMA PNEUMONIA

M. pneumoniae (Eaton agent), the smallest of the free lung microorganisms, is the most common nonbacterial cause of pneumonia.[236] It usually affects previously healthy individuals between the ages of 5 and 40 years.[236] It sometimes occurs in localized outbreaks in families, schools, or military groups; the disease is spread by inhalation of droplets and has a 10- to 20-day incubation period. The symptoms resemble a viral infection, with malaise, fever, chills, headache, sore throat, nonproductive cough, and a variety of nonrespiratory manifestations.[236,260] The physical findings on examination of the chest are often less than might be expected from the chest radiograph. The diagnosis is usually established retrospectively by an elevated or rising cold agglutinin titer. The disease, which responds to tetracycline or erythromycin, usually runs a self-limiting course.[236] However, fatal cases have been recorded,[200] as has the development of interstitial fibrosis[193,364] and bronchiolitis obliterans.[75]

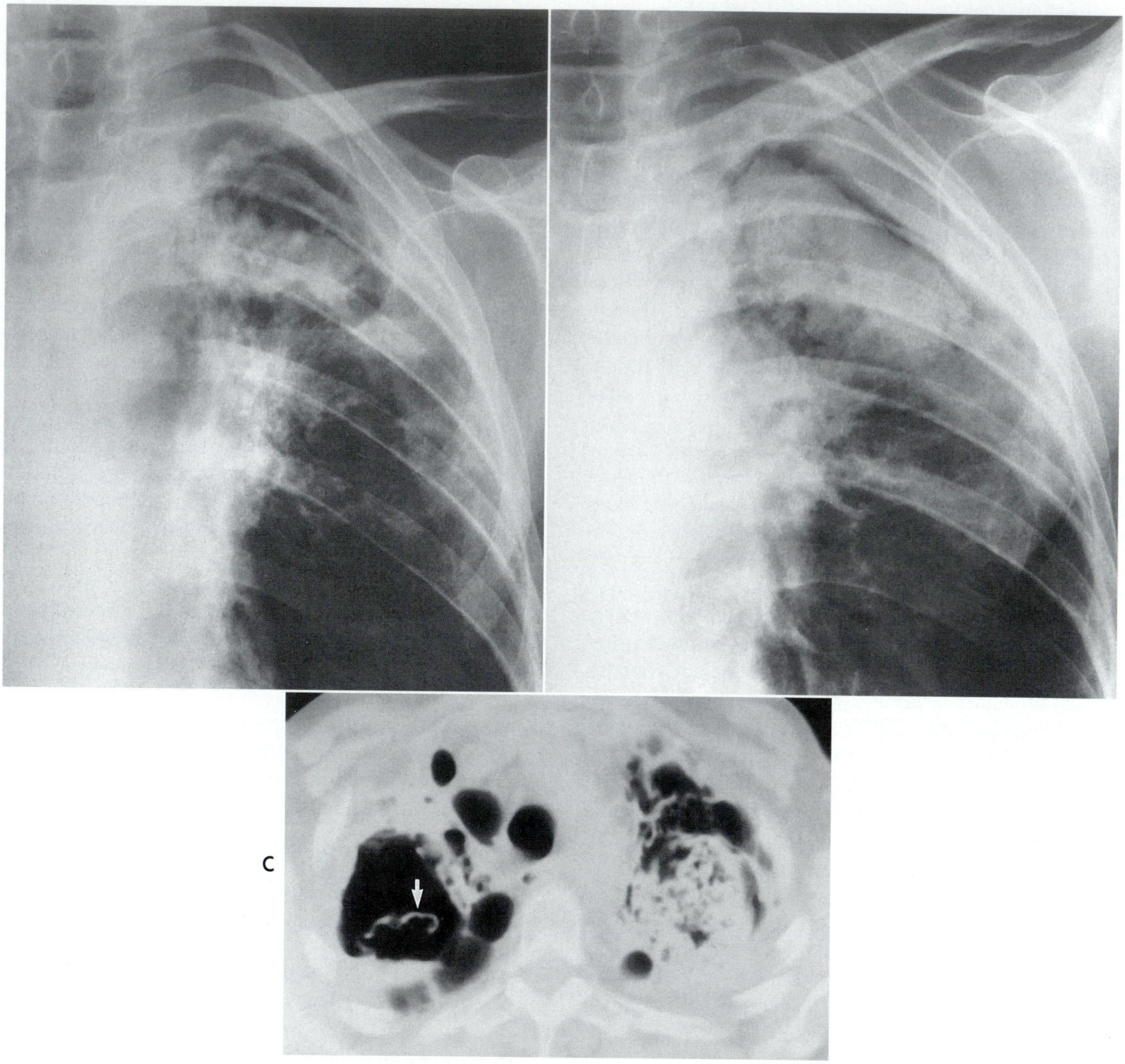

FIGURE 6-112
Growing mycetomas. **A,** Initial film showing irregular mass within a cavity. **B,** One year later, mass is larger and better defined. Air crescent sign is well demonstrated, as is thickened pleura forming lateral wall of cavity. Bubblelike and linear lucencies within the mycetoma are visible on plain film but are better seen with computed tomography. **C,** Early mycetoma showing "collapsed membrane" appearance in cavity in right upper lobe. Small amount of fluid is present in cavity. Obvious mycetoma in left upper lobe.

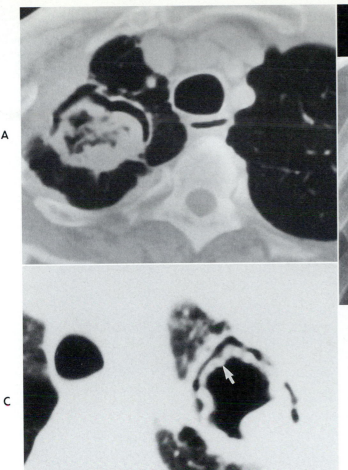

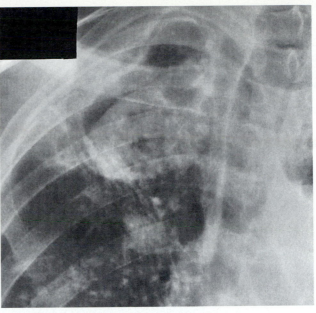

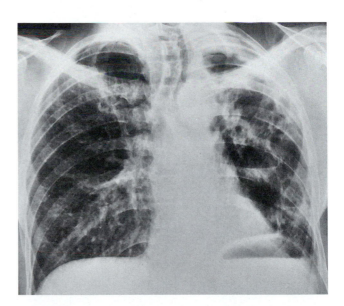

FIGURE 6-113
A, Computed tomographic (CT) scan of mycetoma showing intracavitary mass with multiple linear lucencies. Note air crescent sign and lateral wall formed by pleural thickening. **B,** Plain film on same day for comparison. **C,** CT scan in another patient shows membrane lining preexisting cavity slightly detached from cavity wall.

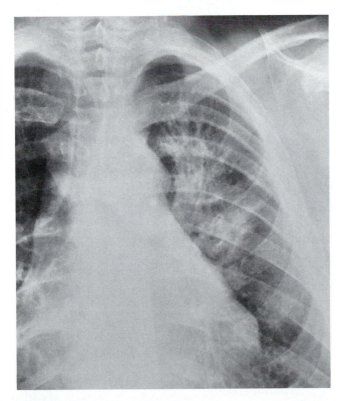

FIGURE 6-114
Semiinvasive aspergillosis showing focal ill-defined consolidation in otherwise normal-appearing lung. Patient had no known immunocompromise.

FIGURE 6-115
Sporotrichosis *(Sporothrix schenkii)* showing multiple thin-walled cavities containing air-fluid levels and adjacent pleural thickening. Note close resemblance to pulmonary tuberculosis.

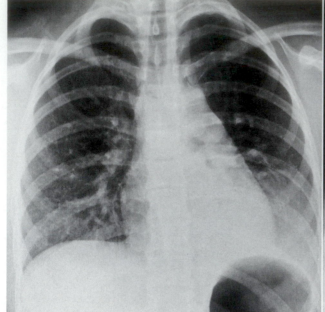

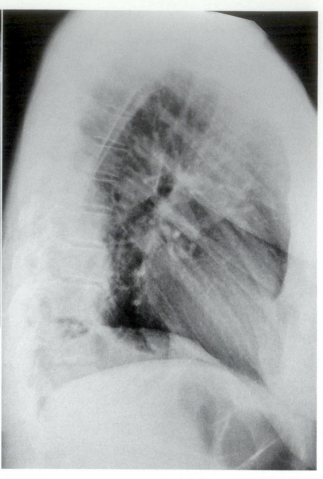

FIGURE 6-116

Mycoplasma pneumonia. **A,** Homogeneous nonsegmental "lobar-type" consolidation of left lower lobe. **B,** Bilateral lower lobe consolidations. On the right, consolidations are confluent and resemble lobar pneumonia. On the left they are patchy and interstitial in appearance. (Courtesy Dr. Michael C. Pearson, London.)

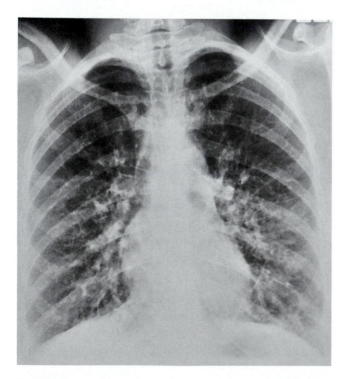

FIGURE 6-117

Mycoplasma pneumonia showing widespread linear shadowing of interstitial type.

The chest radiographic findings are variable.* The most common pattern is patchy consolidation that may coalesce to resemble lobar pneumonia.[66] Usually the pneumonia is unilateral, often involving only one lobe (Figure 6-116). Occasionally the consolidation spreads to involve other lobes.[107,139] There appears to be a predilection for the lower lobes (Figure 6-116, *B*),[146] although solitary upper lobe involvement is well recognized.[107,127,139] An alternative pattern is bilateral nodular or reticular shadowing resembling an interstitial process (Figure 6-117). In most series this pattern has been relatively uncommon, but in one large series it was seen in the majority of patients[358] and in another it was seen in one third of patients.[146] In the series by Putman and co-workers[292] an interstitial pattern was often associated with a more indolent and longer course, without high fever or cough.

Cavitation does not appear to occur. Pleural effusion is variously reported as rare or occurring in up to 20% of cases,[105] probably reflecting the use or nonuse of lateral decubitus films. Large effusions, which may be hemorrhagic, are occasionally seen.[292] Both adenopathy (Figure 6-118) and pleural effusion are more common in children.[54,83,143,358,360] Pneumatoceles have been reported

---

*References 54, 107, 111, 146, 157, 236, 292, 358.

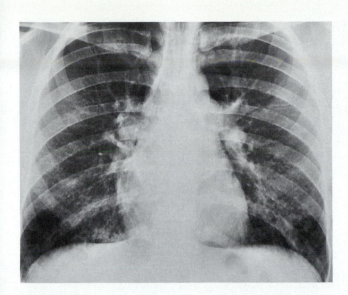

FIGURE 6-118
Mycoplasma pneumonia showing bilateral hilar lymph node enlargement as well as pulmonary changes.

but are rare.[126] The chest radiograph may take several weeks to return to normal in those few patients with interstitial fibrosis[193,364] or bronchiolitis obliterans.[75] In the series reported by Finnegan, Fowler, and White[107] only 40% had cleared by 4 weeks but almost all were clear by 8 weeks.

VIRAL PNEUMONIA

Viruses are the major cause of respiratory tract infection in the community, particularly in children. Droplet transmission from human to human is the usual mode of spread. Pneumonia is relatively uncommon. In immunocompetent infants and young children the viruses that most commonly cause pneumonia are respiratory syncytial virus, parainfluenza virus, adenovirus, and influenza virus, whereas in older children and adults influenza virus and adenovirus are the most common. Viral pneumonia in immunocompromised patients is discussed on p. 253.

The pathologic course of viral pneumonia begins with destruction and sloughing of the respiratory ciliated, goblet, and mucous cells.[72,353] The bronchial and bronchiolar walls together with the interstitial septa of the lungs become thickened owing to edema and inflammatory cells, primarily lymphocytes. This so-called interstitial pneumonitis is often patchy, affecting predominantly the peribronchial portions of the lobules. With more severe inflammation the alveoli fill with inflammatory exudate, which may be hemorrhagic, and hyaline membranes may form. Resolution is the rule, but permanent mucosal damage and chronic interstitial fibrosis may occur. Viral pneumonia is one cause of bronchiolitis obliterans.

The radiologic findings in viral pneumonia[72,181,273,318]

do not allow the diagnosis of a specific virus infection. The basic sign is widespread small, patchy shadows that may coalesce to a variable degree (Figures 6-119 and 6-120). Multilobar involvement is usual. Sometimes the pulmonary shadows are composed of multiple, poorly defined, 2 to 3 mm nodules (Figure 6-120). Bronchial wall thickening and peribronchial shadows are a striking and common feature. Such shadowing frequently radiates outward from the hila. Cavitation is not a feature. Air trapping is usually present, and therefore flattening of the diaphragm and increased retrosternal space are often apparent. Hilar adenopathy is variable; it is common in measles, pneumonia, and infectious mononucleosis but rare with other viral pneumonias. Pleural effusions are not a prominent feature, although small ones do not negate the diagnosis.

Influenza viruses

Infections with influenza virus occur in epidemics and pandemics or sporadically. Influenza A and B are the subtypes most commonly responsible for the severe outbreaks associated with pneumonia. The symptoms include fever, dry cough, myalgias, and headaches. Rhinitis, pharyngitis, bronchitis, and bronchiolitis may develop. When pneumonia occurs, it may be due to bacterial superinfection, most commonly by *S. aureus*, *Pneumococcus*, or *H. influenzae*. The virus itself may cause pneumonia, and when it does, the infection is often severe. Pneumonia is both more common and more serious in the very young, in those over 65 years of age, in late pregnancy, and in those with underlying disease, particularly cardiopulmonary disorders.

In one large series of more than 100 patients with influenzal pneumonia[120] the radiologic findings were multifocal, 1 to 2 cm, patchy consolidations that rapidly became confluent, with the majority showing bilateral consolidation and basilar predominance (Figure 6-120). Lobar and segmental consolidations were unusual, and the appearance resembled pulmonary edema in some cases. Pleural effusions, although encountered and sometimes large, were not a feature, and cavitation was notably rare. Complicating bacterial pneumonia can be difficult to distinguish from pneumonia caused by the influenza virus itself.

Parainfluenza virus

Parainfluenza virus pneumonia occurs predominantly in winter outbreaks, mainly affecting children. Usually parainfluenza infection causes upper respiratory symptoms, notably croup, and bronchiolitis; pneumonia is uncommon, particularly in adults. Pneumonia may be due to bacterial superinfection. The radiologic appearance is a patchy peribronchial consolidation mainly in the lower lobes, and pleural effusions may be seen.[392]

Respiratory syncytial virus

Respiratory syncytial virus (RSV) is a major cause of bronchiolitis and bronchopneumonia in infants and

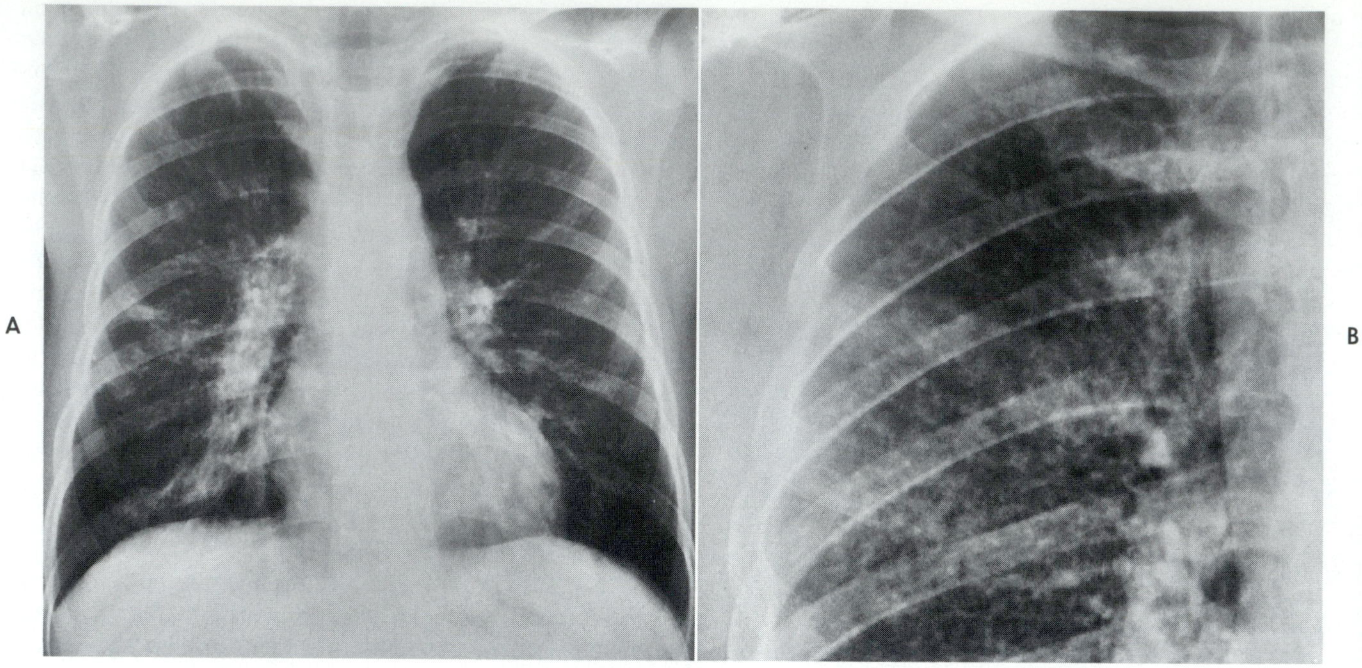

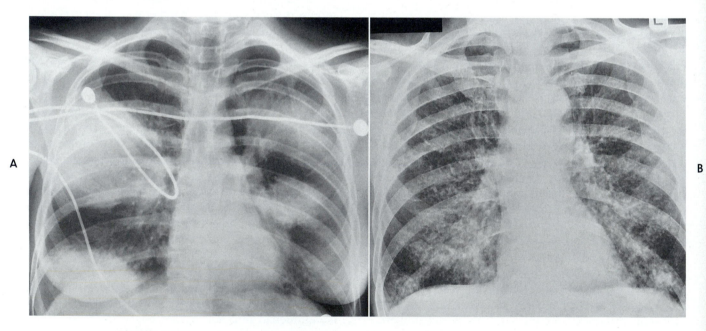

FIGURE 6-119
Viral pneumonia. **A,** In a child, showing scattered small ill-defined consolidations in both middle and lower zones. **B,** In an adult showing widespread small nodular shadows.

FIGURE 6-120
Two examples of influenzal pneumonia. **A,** Multiple focal pulmonary consolidations. **B,** Multiple small ill-defined nodular shadows scattered throughout lungs, maximal at bases.

young children. It is a recognized cause of croup. The virus can also cause pneumonia in adults. RSV pneumonia in adults can cause prolonged fever and require protracted stay in the hospital, but it rarely causes serious complications or death[379] unless the patient is immunocompromised.[95] The plain chest radiograph shows streaky peribronchial infiltrates associated with overinflation of the lungs.[308,346] Hilar adenopathy was common in some series[96,268] but rare in others.[273,308] Lobar collapse is a frequent finding,[294] and lobar consolidation is occasionally seen.[308]

Coxsackievirus, rhinovirus, and ECHO viruses

Coxsackievirus, rhinovirus, and ECHO (enteric cytopathic human orphan) viruses are all related. They usually cause a flulike illness and upper respiratory tract symptoms. Very occasionally they cause pneumonia. The ECHO viruses usually affect infants; the other two may affect children and adults.[125] The radiologic appearance[126] is nonspecific with reticulonodular shadowing radiating from the hila predominantly into the lower zones. These shadows may become confluent. Hilar adenopathy may be present.

Rubeola (measles) virus

Rubeola (measles) virus may cause pneumonia in addition to its other systemic and skin manifestations, particularly in children, but also occasionally in adults.[142,293] The pneumonia frequently contains multinucleated epithelial giant cells with inclusion bodies, a feature believed to be specific to measles and given the name "giant cell pneumonia." The pneumonia usually develops before or coincident with the measles skin rash. Chest radiographs of patients with pneumonia[101] show a widespread reticular pattern in the lungs, often accompanied by hilar adenopathy. Lobar atelectasis of varying degree is common. Usually the viral pneumonia clears with the resolution of the disease, but the radiographic changes may persist for many months.

Superinfection with *S. aureus, Pneumococcus, H. influenzae,* and *S. pyogenes* may occur, in which case the pneumonia resembles bacterial pneumonia, with more focal confluent areas and sometimes cavitation.

When children who have been immunized with inactivated measles virus are exposed to the measles virus, atypical measles may develop. The radiographic appearance of pneumonia in atypical measles[237,238,407] differs from that seen in the usual form by showing more nodular (spherical) and segmental consolidations. The nodular consolidations may persist and be confused with pulmonary masses such as metastatic neoplasm or sequestration. Hilar adenopathy and pleural effusion frequently accompany the pneumonia in atypical measles.

Infectious mononucleosis

Infectious mononucleosis caused by the Epstein-Barr virus is a common infection in the community but is a rare cause of pneumonia. The great majority of patients with infectious mononucleosis show no abnormalities on plain chest radiographs. The most frequent intrathoracic manifestation is mediastinal or hilar adenopathy, a phenomenon best seen with CT or MRI,[122,129] although these techniques are seldom indicated. Pulmonary shadows are rare. When present they are usually streaky or interstitial in appearance.[5,210]

Adenoviruses

The adenoviruses are a relatively frequent cause of mild infection of the respiratory tract. Pneumonia is uncommon and confined largely to infants, young children, and military recruits.[411] Adenovirus pneumonia in adults can be more severe than in younger patients, particularly in immunocompromised hosts.[411] The chest radiograph[130,274,345] shows patchy or confluent widespread consolidations, although consolidations confined to one lobe are also encountered. The presence of consolidation correlates poorly with the clinical severity of the pneumonia. Bronchial wall thickening and peribronchial shadowing are striking findings. Air trapping is common in young children, and lobar collapse is frequent. Small pleural effusions are seen in approximately one third of patients. The infection can be highly damaging, leaving bronchiectasis[274] or bronchiolitis obliterans, and the Swyer-James/McLeod syndrome may result.[234]

Herpes simplex viruses

Herpes simplex viruses are divided into two basic types, one that causes mucocutaneous vesicles and another that causes genital tract infection and is spread via sexual intercourse or acquired during birth.

Pneumonia is extremely uncommon except in immunocompromised patients and neonates.[163] Herpes simplex pneumonia is a particular problem for patients with AIDS (see p. 238).

Varicella-zoster virus

Chickenpox and herpes zoster (shingles) are both caused by the varicella-zoster virus. Pneumonia caused by the virus is rare in children; pneumonia in a child with chickenpox probably results from bacterial superinfection. More than 90% of cases of varicella-zoster pneumonia occur in adults, in patients with lymphoma, and in those who are immunocompromised for a variety of reasons. Symptoms of pneumonia develop 1 to 6 days after the onset of the skin rash.[373] The plain chest film[326,373] differs slightly from that seen with other viral infections: the pneumonia causes multiple 5 to 10 mm ill-defined nodules (Figure 6-121) that may be confluent and may come and go in different areas of the lungs. Hilar adenopathy and small pleural effusions occur during the acute phase of the disease but are unusual. The small, round consolidations usually resolve within a week after the disappearance of the skin lesions, but they can persist for months. In a few patients the lesions calcify and remain indefinitely as numerous, well-defined, randomly scattered, 2 to 3 mm, dense calcifications in otherwise normal lungs (Figure 4-106). The appearance resembles the calcifications seen following disseminated histoplasmosis.

PROTOZOAL INFECTIONS

Amebiasis is due to *Entamoeba histolytica,* a protozoan found worldwide. In most cases the condition is asymptomatic. Symptomatic infections are usually confined to the gastrointestinal tract and liver. Pleural effusion and lower lobe consolidation may be present contiguous to an amebic abscess in the liver or subphrenic space, just as they may accompany any other suppurative process in these sites. An amebic liver abscess may extend through the diaphragm into the pleura, giving rise to an empyema, and may even extend into the lung, causing pneumonia and lung abscess.[167] The most common symptoms are fever and cough, which may be productive of chocolate-colored pus. Hemoptysis and chest or abdominal pain are also frequent.[359] Fistulas may form, connecting the liver abscess to the airways, the pericardium, and very rarely the skin.

The radiographic findings are empyema and adjacent consolidation or lung abscess, which may be combined with signs of an elevated hemidiaphragm (Figure 6-122).[167,390,398] Signs of liver or subphrenic abscess are visible on CT or ultrasound examination.

Hematogenous spread of amebic liver abscess to the lungs is rare. When it occurs, it causes transient areas of pneumonia or lung abscess.

HELMINTHIC INFECTIONS
Roundworm, hookworm, and Strongyloides infections

Ascaris lumbricoides (roundworm), *Ancylostoma duodenale, Necator americanus* (hookworm), and *Strongyloides stercoralis* are all round worms that, as part of their life cycle, pass through the lungs.[24] *Ascaris* eggs are ingested in food contaminated by infected feces and hatched in the small intestine to penetrate the bowel wall and enter the lymphatics and blood stream. *Ancylostoma* and *Strongyloides* eggs hatch in human feces deposited in soil and penetrate the skin of the hands or feet. In some cases *Strongyloides* eggs reenter the same host via the intestinal mucosa or perianal skin. Regardless of the route by which these organisms enter the bloodstream, they are carried to the lung where they burrow through the alveolar walls to enter the airways and ascend in the tracheobronchial tree. Eventually they are swallowed into the intestine, where they grow to their adult form. *Strongyloides* may also grow to adult form within the lung itself. The clinical features are related largely to the skin and gastrointestinal tract. Pulmonary symptoms are uncommon with all three organisms and include an unproductive cough, substernal chest pain, and occasionally hemoptysis and dyspnea. *Strongyloides,* if it grows to adult form in the lung, may give rise to a syndrome resembling asthma. It may also be responsible for overwhelming infection in immunocompromised patients.[291,337]

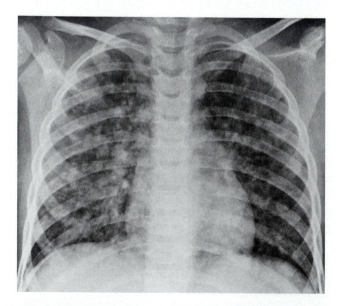

FIGURE 6-121
Chickenpox pneumonia showing widespread ill-defined 5 to 10 mm nodular shadows.

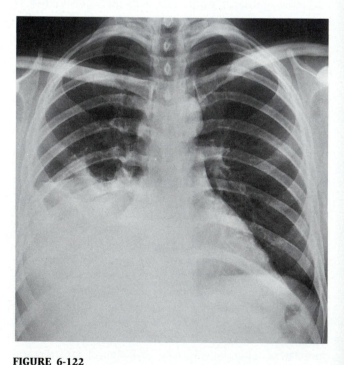

FIGURE 6-122
Intrathoracic changes secondary to amebic lung abscess. There is a large right pleural effusion with collapse and consolidation of the right lower lobe.

In most instances no pulmonary complications occur with any of these worms, but in a few patients an allergic reaction takes place in the lung parenchyma, which manifests itself radiographically as dense transient migratory pulmonary consolidations without recognizable segmental distribution.[35] Blood and sputum eosinophilia are often present, and the entity is therefore included as one of the causes of acute pulmonary infiltrates with eosinophilia (Löffler's syndrome).[124] Miliary nodulation, similar to miliary tuberculosis, may be seen.[204] Cavitation and hilar and mediastinal lymphadenopathy do not occur. Pleural effusions are also not a feature.

Other round worms that may cause a localized granulomatous reaction in the lung are the dog and cat worms, *Toxocara canis* and *Toxocara cati* (visceral larva migrans).[400] Symptoms include cough, wheezing, dyspnea, and a number of extrapulmonary manifestations. Infection, which is rarely diagnosed in humans, is caused by ingesting ova from contaminated hands, soil, or fomites. Young children are at greatest risk. Infection is often asymptomatic, but in approximately 50% of patients with pulmonary symptoms, chest radiographs show transient local or widespread patchy areas of consolidation, which are associated with peripheral blood eosinophilia (Figure 6-123).

Filariasis

The most common filarial worm to cause pulmonary manifestations is *Wuchereria bancrofti*. The major disease caused by this organism is the disfiguring condition of elephantiasis resulting from filarial obstruction of cutaneous lymphatics. *W. bancrofti* is also believed to be the cause of tropical eosinophilia, a syndrome consisting of cough, wheezing, and severe blood eosinophilia.[265] The chest radiograph[160,374] may be normal but usually shows widespread fine nodular or reticulonodular shadowing. The appearance may closely resemble miliary tuberculosis. Localized consolidation is occasionally seen. The pulmonary shadowing, which corresponds to eosinophilic and histiocytic infiltration,[374] is believed to be due to an immunologic response to microfilariae rather than to direct infection. Although pleural thickening may be demonstrated, pleural effusion does not appear to be a feature.[374] Generalized lymphadenopathy may occur, but radiographically visible mediastinal or hilar adenopathy is uncommon.[265] The radiologic changes usually resolve with treatment, but sometimes resolution takes months and interstitial fibrosis may supervene.[374] Although *W. bancrofti* is believed to be the major inciting organism in tropical eosinophilia, other filariae such as *Brugia malayi*, are thought to be responsible for a small proportion of cases.

Very rarely the filarial worm *Dirofilaria immitis* (dog heartworm) causes pulmonary infection in humans. It usually infects dogs but can be transferred to humans by mosquito bites. In the United States the condition is almost confined to the eastern and southern states.[311,313] The larvae travel to the walls of the right-sided cardiac chambers and may dislodge and embolize into the pulmonary vascular bed, where they cause a granulomatous reaction plus infarct that manifests itself as asymptomatic solitary or multiple 1 to 2 cm subpleural pulmonary nodules on chest radiograph.[63,220,313] The patients may have cough and hemoptysis.[313] Mostly the nodules occur in adults and are single, but in about 10% of patients multiple pulmonary nodules are present.[313] The early lesion may be wedge shaped. Visible calcification on plain chest radiography is not recorded. Experience with CT is limited,[63,400] but eccentric calcification within the nodule has been demonstrated.[400] Blood eosinophilia is present in 20% of patients, but since the blood eosinophil count is usually normal and there are no reliable skin or serologic tests, the granulomas are usually excised in the belief that they may be bronchial carcinoma.[311,313]

Schistosomiasis

Pulmonary disease caused by schistosomiasis is rare. Of the flukes responsible for schistosomiasis (*Schistosoma mansoni, S. japonicum,* and *S. haematobium*), *S. mansoni* and *S. haematobium* are the most likely to cause pulmonary disease. The intermediate hosts are various species of freshwater snails, which are infected by larvae hatched from eggs that reach the water in feces or urine. Cercariae, the infective larvae, leave the snails and penetrate the skin or mucous membranes of humans as they swim or paddle in the water. The cercariae migrate to the mesenteric veins or, in the case of *S. haematobium*, to the venous plexuses of the bladder, prostate, or uterus. The adult flukes mate and deposit eggs in the veins, and the eggs are carried to various sites where they induce inflammation, ulceration, and fibrosis. Deposition of eggs

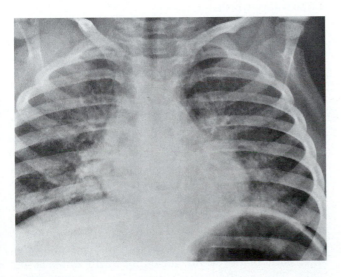

FIGURE 6-123
Toxocara canis infection with widespread pulmonary consolidation.

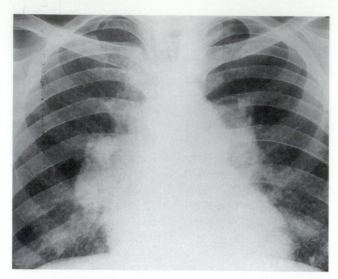

FIGURE 6-124
Schistosomiasis with widespread, basally predominant, reticulonodular shadows in both lungs. Cardiac enlargement and large central pulmonary arteries are due to associated pulmonary arterial hypertension. (Courtesy Dr. Michael C. Pearson, London.)

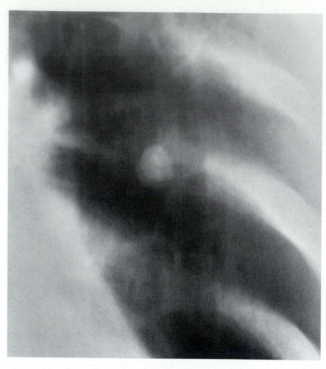

FIGURE 6-125
Schistosomiasis causing solitary pulmonary granuloma.

in the small vessels of the lungs is rare, but when it occurs, the resulting granulomatous inflammation causes luminal obliteration[182] and may result in increased pulmonary vascular resistance.[121] In these cases the major radiographic features are those of pulmonary arterial hypertension, but on occasion a widespread fine reticular nodular shadowing representing ova with surrounding inflammatory changes or fibrosis can be seen (Figure 6-124).[82,182]

Patchy consolidations caused by Löffler's syndrome may be seen early in the course of the infection as the flukes migrate through the lungs. Very rarely a solitary nodule is identified (Figure 6-125).[281]

Paragonimiasis

Paragonimiasis is usually due to infection with the lung fluke *Paragonimus westermani*. The disease, which is endemic in Southeast Asia, Indonesia, West Africa, and South America, is acquired by eating crustaceans and water snails that act as the intermediate host. The immature flukes penetrate the bowel wall, travel through the peritoneal cavity, and migrate through the diaphragm and pleura to enter the lung parenchyma. Infection, as documented by positive serologic tests, may be asymptomatic and show no radiographic abnormalities. Symptoms include hemoptysis, pleuritic chest pain, and chronic cough, which may produce sputum containing the ova of the infecting organism.

The pulmonary changes result from chronic inflammation in areas surrounding the worm. On radiographic study (Figure 6-126),[186,269,367] these areas are seen as multiple round, poorly defined areas of consolidation in any lung zone but most often in the midzones. The

consolidations may be fleeting and associated with blood eosinophilia.[15] Linear shadows 2 to 4 mm thick and 3 to 7 cm long may be seen extending inward from the pleura on both plain films and CT scans.[173] These are believed to be worm tracks. Indeed, one case of an air-filled linear track has been reported.[348] The more chronic lesions become better defined, often appear nodular, and sometimes excavate, leaving complex cystic airspaces that may contain solid material. Im and associates[173] have postulated that the intracavitary material may represent the intracavitary worm.

Because the flukes penetrate the diaphragm and pleura, pleural effusions and hydropneumothorax are common and frequently bilateral.[173,186] The disease may also spread to distant sites such as the brain.[347]

Echinococcus infections

Hydatid disease is caused by the tapeworms *Echinococcus granulosus* and *E. multilocularis (alveolaris)*. The life cycle involves primary and intermediate mammalian hosts. Dogs are the usual primary host, and the intermediate host is usually a sheep or a cow but is sometimes a human. The disease is endemic in sheep-raising areas of Australia, South America, and the Mediterranean basin, particularly North Africa and Greece. Cases are, however, occasionally encountered from infections acquired in other parts of the world, including North America and Wales. The so-called sylvatic form[77] has deer and moose as intermediate hosts and is endemic in the frozen north.

The adult worm lives in the small intestine of the

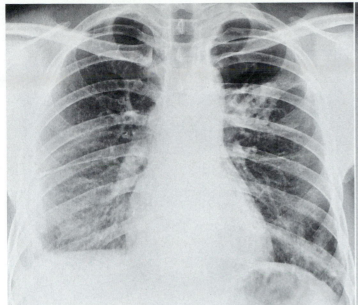

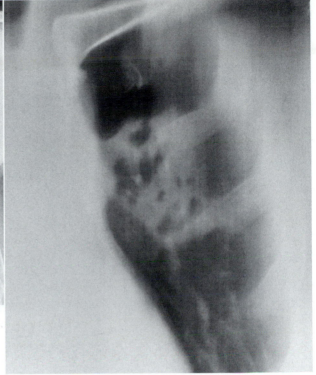

FIGURE 6-126
Paragonimiasis. A, Ill-defined consolidation. B, Tomogram shows complex central cavitation in consolidation.

primary host. Ova are passed in feces and ingested by the intermediate host. Larvae develop in the duodenum of the new host, where they enter the bloodstream and travel to the liver and lungs and occasionally even the systemic circulation. Pleural or pulmonary involvement may also be due to direct extension through the diaphragm from hydatid disease in the liver. The life cycle is completed when another primary host eats the remains of an infected intermediate host.

Disease in humans is due to the cysts that form around the parasite. The structure of these cysts is important in understanding the radiographic findings. As hydatid cysts grow, they compress the adjacent lung into a fibrotic capsule known as the pericyst. The cyst itself has a thin smooth wall composed of two adherent layers, the laminated ectocyst and the delicate lining endocyst from which hang the daughter cysts. The pulmonary cysts may grow rapidly, and approximately two thirds rupture. Most rupture into the surrounding lung and bronchial tree, causing secondary infection. Occasionally a cyst ruptures into the pleural cavity. Rupture may result in an acute allergic reaction, sometimes accompanied by life-threatening hypotension. Cysts that have not ruptured usually do not give rise to symptoms, and the diagnosis is then based on a routine chest film.

The most reliable serologic test uses partially purified hydatid antigen or antigen 5. Complement fixation, hemagglutination, latex agglutination, and bentonite flocculation tests are also available. The Casoni skin test is not recommended because of its low sensitivity and

specificity.[187] Eosinophilia (more than 5% eosinophils) occurred in 40% of patients in a series reported from Lebanon.[20]

The cardinal radiographic features[20,36,44,245,321] are one or more spherical or oval well-defined smooth masses of homogeneous density in otherwise normal lung, usually in the middle or lower zone (Figure 6-127). Multiple cysts are seen in about one third of patients and are bilateral in 20%[36]; sometimes more than 10 cysts are seen. There is a predilection for the lower lobes, the posterior segments, and the right lung.[20,36] CT scanning[324] reveals fluid contents within the cyst, with a density close to that of water; the daughter cysts when present appear as curved septations. At CT the cyst walls range in thickness from 2 mm to 1 cm, with the wall representing the combined pericyst, ectocyst, and endocyst. The cysts may be very large; cysts of 10 cm and even 20 cm have been reported. The rate of growth may be fairly rapid, with doubling times of less than 6 months. A striking feature is that the cyst is relatively pliant and molds to adjacent structures, resulting in indentation, lobulation, or flattening. Surrounding inflammation may cause the edge of the lesion to be ill defined. Calcification, which is a common feature of hydatid cysts in the liver, is extremely rare in cysts arising in the lungs. Few reports of MRI in intrathoracic hydatid disease have been published.[382,384] The complex cyst contents are well displayed, and the cyst membrane, whether collapsed or not, is clearly seen as a low-intensity curvilinear structure on both short and long TR spin-echo images.

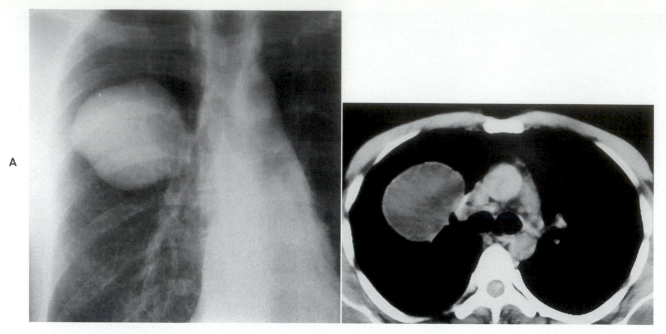

FIGURE 6-127
Hydatid cyst of lung. **A,** Plain film. **B,** Computed tomographic scan. Magnetic resonance images in this patient are shown in Figure 1-9.

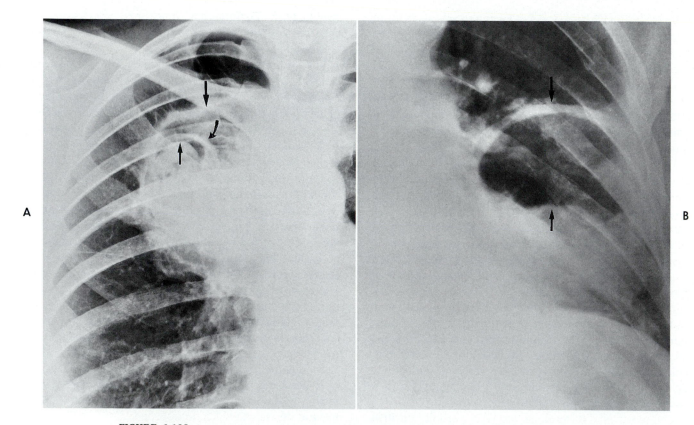

FIGURE 6-128
Ruptured hydatid cyst. **A,** Pericyst *(downward-pointing arrow),* ectocyst *(curved arrow),* and daughter cyst *(upward-pointing arrow).* There are air crescents between ectocyst and pericyst and also between daughter cyst and ectocyst. **B,** Another patient, showing pericyst *(downward-pointing arrow)* and ectocyst *(upward-pointing arrow)* with air between them.

If the pericyst ruptures (Figure 6-128), air dissecting between the fibrotic lung forming the pericyst and the ectocyst of the parasite leads to a visible crescent of air between the two, known as a meniscus or crescent sign. If the cyst itself ruptures, an air-fluid level results and daughter cysts may even be seen floating in the residual fluid. On rare occasion air is seen on both sides of the true cyst wall; a crescent is seen surrounding the cyst, and air-fluid levels are also present. Sometimes the cyst wall is seen crumpled up and floating in fluid, which lies within the noncollapsed pericyst. This pathognomonic appearance is imaginatively described as the water lily sign or the camalote sign. All these signs are particularly well demonstrated by CT and MRI (Figure 6-127).[324,382,384] With secondary infection the membranes may disintegrate and the walls thicken, so that the picture is indistinguishable from bacterial lung abscess on plain films.

Hydatid cysts may also be present in the pleura, in which case they may be secondary to seeding of the pleura following rupture. In some cases the pleura is the primary site of disease. Mediastinal cysts are relatively rare. They form smooth round or oval masses in the mediastinum that may compress adjacent mediastinal structures, such as the major airways or vascular structures, or may erode the bone of the thoracic cage.[299,383] Hydatid cysts may also on rare occasion arise in the pericardium or wall of the thoracic aorta.[158,383] On CT these mediastinal cysts, like all hydatid cysts, have a well-defined wall and fluid contents.

REFERENCES

1. Albelda SM, Kern JA, Marinelli DL, et al: Expanding spectrum of pulmonary disease caused by nontuberculous mycobacteria, *Radiology* 157:289-296, 1985.
2. Alfageme I, Munoz F, Pena N, et al: Empyema of the thorax in adults: etiology, microbiologic findings, and management, *Chest* 103:839-843, 1993.
3. Allen HA, Scatarige HA, Kim MH: Actinomycosis: CT findings in six patients, *AJR* 149:1255-1258, 1987.
4. Alsofrom DJ, Mettler FA, Mann JM: Radiographic manifestations of plague in New Mexico, 1975-1980: a review of 42 proved cases, *Radiology* 139:561-565, 1981.
5. Andiman WA, McCarthy P, Markowitz RI, et al: Clinical, virologic, and serologic evidence of Epstein-Barr virus infection in association with childhood pneumonia, *J Pediatr* 99:880-886, 1981.
6. Andrews NC, Parker EF, Shaw RR, et al: Management of nontuberculous empyema. American Thoracic Society: A statement of the subcommittee on surgery, *Am Rev Respir Dis* 85:935-936, 1962.
7. Arcomano JP, Pizzolato NF, Singer R, et al: A unique type of calcification in chronic brucellosis, *AJR* 128:135-137, 1977.
8. Ariel I, Brewer R, Kamal NS, et al: Endobronchial actinomycosis simulating bronchogenic carcinoma: diagnosis by bronchial biopsy, *Chest* 99:493-495, 1991.
9. Armstrong JD: Common fungal diseases of the lungs: blastomycosis, *Radiol Clin North Am* 11:169-173, 1973.
10. Aronchick JM, Miller WT, Epstein DM, et al: Association of achalasia and pulmonary *Mycobacterium fortuitum* infection, *Radiology* 160:85-86, 1986.
11. Asmar BI, Thirumoorthi MC, Dajani AS: Pneumococcal pneumonia with pneumatocele formation, *Am J Dis Child* 132:1091-1093, 1978.
12. Avery FW, Barnett TB: Pulmonary tularemia: a report of five cases and consideration of pathogenesis and terminology, *Am Rev Respir Dis* 95:584-591, 1967.
13. Babbit DP, Waisbren BA: Epidemic pulmonary histoplasmosis, *AJR* 83:236-250, 1960.
14. Baber EC, Hedlund LW, Oddson TA, et al: Differentiating empyemas and peripheral pulmonary abscesses: the value of computed tomography, *Radiology* 135:755-758, 1980.
15. Bahk YW: Pulmonary paragonimiasis as a cause of Loeffler's syndrome, *Radiology* 78:598-601, 1962.
16. Bailey CM, Windle-Taylor PC: Tuberculous laryngitis: a series of 37 patients, *Laryngoscope* 91:93-100, 1981.
17. Balikian JP, Chen TH, Costello P, et al: Pulmonary actinomycosis: a report of three cases, *Radiology* 128:613-616, 1978.
18. Balikian JP, Herman PG, Godleski JS: *Serratia* pneumonia, *Radiology* 137:309-311, 1980.
19. Balikian JP, Herman PG, Kopit S: Pulmonary nocardiosis, *Radiology* 126:569-573, 1978.
20. Balikian JP, Mudarris FF: Hydatid disease of the lungs: a roentgenologic study of 50 cases, *AJR* 122:692-707, 1974.
21. Balmes JR, Hawkins JG: Pulmonary cryptococcosis, *Semin Respir Med* 9:180-186, 1987.
22. Barnett SM: CT findings in tuberculous mediastinitis, *J Comput Assist Tomogr* 10:165-166, 1986.
23. Barnhard HJ, Kniker WT: Roentgenologic findings in pertussis with particular emphasis on the "shaggy heart" sign, *AJR* 84:445-450, 1960.
24. Barratt-Connor E: Parasitic pulmonary disease, *Am Rev Respir Dis* 126:558-563, 1982.
25. Bartlett JG: Anaerobic bacterial pneumonitis, *Am Rev Respir Dis* 119:19-24, 1979.
26. Bartlett JG, Finegold SM: Anaerobic infections of the lung and pleural space, *Am Rev Respir Dis* 110:56-77, 1974.
27. Bartlett JG, O'Keefe P, Tally FP, et al: Bacteriology of hospital acquired pneumonia, *Arch Intern Med* 146:868-871, 1986.
28. Basiliere JL, Bistrong HW, Spence WF: Streptococcal pneumonia: recent outbreaks in military recruit populations, *Am J Med* 44:580-589, 1968.
29. Bates M, Cruickshank G: Thoracic actinomycosis, *Thorax* 12:99-123, 1957.
30. Baum GL, Schwarz J: North American blastomycosis, *Am J Med Sci* 238:661, 1959.
31. Baum GL, Schwarz J: Chronic pulmonary histoplasmosis, *Am J Med* 33:873-879, 1962.
32. Baum GL: Cavitation in histoplasmosis: some further comments (letter), *Chest* 67:625-626, 1975.
33. Bayer AS: Fungal pneumonias; pulmonary coccidioidal syndromes: Part 1, *Chest* 79:575-583, 1981. Part 2, *Chest* 79:686-691, 1981.
34. Beaman BL, Burnside J, Edwards B, et al: Nocardial infections in the United States, 1972-1974, *J Infect Dis* 134:286-289, 1976.
35. Bean WJ: Recognition of ascariasis by routine chest or abdomen roentgenograms, *AJR* 94:379-384, 1965.
36. Beggs I: The radiology of hydatid disease: a review, *AJR* 145:639-648, 1985.
37. Bellamy EA, Johnston IDA, Wilson AG: The chest radiograph in whooping cough, *Clin Radiol* 38:39-43, 1987.
38. Beller TA, Mitchell DM, Sobonya RE, et al: Large airway obstruction secondary to endobronchial coccidioidomycosis, *Am Rev Respir Dis* 120:939-942, 1979.
39. Bennett JE: *Sporothrix schenckii*. In Mandell GL, Douglas RG, Bennett JE, eds: *Principles and practice of infectious diseases*, ed 2, New York, 1985, John Wiley & Sons.
40. Berger HW, Granada MG: Lower lung field tuberculosis, *Chest* 65:522-526, 1974.

41. Binder RE, Faling LJ, Pugatch RD, et al: Chronic necrotizing pulmonary aspergillosis: a discrete clinical entity, *Medicine* 61:109-124, 1982.

42. Birsner JW: The roentgen aspects of five hundred cases of pulmonary coccidioidomycosis, *AJR* 72:556-573, 1954.

43. Blastomycosis Cooperative Study of the Veterans Administration: Blastomycosis: a review of 198 collected cases in Veterans Administration hospitals, *Am Rev Respir Dis* 89:659-672, 1964.

44. Bonakdarpour A: Echinococcus disease: report of 112 cases from Iran and a review of 611 cases from the United States, *AJR* 99:660-667, 1967.

45. Bonmati J, Rogers JV, Hopkins WA: Pulmonary cryptococcosis, *Radiology* 66:188-194, 1956.

46. Bowton DL, Bass DA: Community-acquired pneumonia: the clinical dilemma, *J Thorac Imag* 6(3):1-5, 1991.

47. Brook I, Frazier EH: Aerobic and anaerobic microbiology of empyema: a retrospective review in two military hospitals, *Chest* 103:1502-1507, 1993.

48. Brown A, Geyer S, Arbitman M, et al: Pulmonary nocardiosis presenting as a bronchogenic tumor, *South Med J* 73:660-663, 1980.

49. Brown JR: Human actinomycosis: a study of 181 subjects, *Hum Pathol* 4:319-330, 1973.

50. Brown LR, Swensen SJ, van Scoy RE, et al: Roentgenologic features of pulmonary blastomycosis, *Mayo Clin Proc* 66:29-38, 1991.

51. Buckner CB, Leithiser RE, Walker CW, et al: The changing epidemiology of tuberculosis and other mycobacteria infections in the United States: implications for the radiologist, *AJR* 156:255-264, 1991.

52. Buechner HA, Seabury JH, Campbell CC, et al: The current status of serologic, immunologic and skin tests in the diagnosis of pulmonary mycoses, *Chest* 63:259-270, 1973.

53. Caldwell A, Glauser FL, Smith WR, et al: The effects of dehydration on the radiologic and pathologic appearance of experimental canine segmental pneumonia, *Am Rev Respir Dis* 112:651-656, 1975.

54. Cameron DC, Borthwick RN, Philp T: The radiographic patterns of acute *Mycoplasma* pneumonitis, *Clin Radiol* 28:173-180, 1977.

55. Campbell GD, Chapman SW: Blastomycosis, *Semin Respir Med* 9:164-169, 1987.

56. CDC tuberculosis — United States 1985, *MMWR* 35:669-703, 1986.

57. Chandler FW, Watts JC: Mycotic, actinomycotic, and algal infections. In Kissane JM, ed: *Anderson's pathology*, ed 8, St Louis, 1985, Mosby, pp 371-400.

58. Chandler FW, Watts JC: Fungal infections. In Dail DH, Hammar SP, eds: *Pulmonary pathology*, New York, 1988, Springer-Verlag.

59. Chick EW: Epidemiologic aspects of the pulmonary mycoses, *Semin Respir Med* 9:123-129, 1987.

60. Chick EW, Bauman DS: Acute cavitary histoplasmosis — fact or fiction (editorial), *Chest* 65:479-480, 1974.

61. Choe KO, Jeong HJ, Sohn HY: Tuberculous bronchial stenosis: CT findings in 28 cases, *AJR* 155:971-976, 1990.

62. Cholankeril JV, Greenberg AL, Matari HM, et al: Solitary pulmonary nodule in secondary syphilis, *Clin Imag* 16:125-128, 1992.

63. Cholankeril JV, Napolitano J, Ketyer S, et al: Computed tomography in the evaluation of *Dirofiliaria immitis* granuloma of the lung, *J Comput Tomogr* 7:305-309, 1983.

64. Choyke PL, Soskman HD, Curtis AM, et al: Adult-onset pulmonary tuberculosis, *Radiology* 148:357-362, 1983.

65. Christensen EE, Dietz GW, Ahn CH, et al: Radiographic manifestations of pulmonary *Mycobacterium kansaii* infections, *AJR* 131:985-993, 1978.

66. Cockcroft DW, Stilwell GA: Lobar pneumonia caused by *Mycoplasma pneumoniae*, *Can Med Assoc J* 124:1463-1468, 1981.

67. Comstock C, Wolson AH: Roentgenology of sporotrichosis, *AJR* 125:651-655, 1975.

68. Conces DJ, Tarver RD, Vix VA: Broncholithiasis: CT features in 15 patients, *AJR* 157:249-253, 1991.

69. Conces DJ, Vix VA, Tarver RD: Pleural cryptococcosis, *J Thorac Imag* 5(2):84-86, 1990.

70. Condon VR: Pneumonia in children, *J Thorac Imag* 6(3):31-44, 1991.

71. Connell JV, Muhm JR: Radiographic manifestations of pulmonary histoplasmosis: a 10 year review, *Radiology* 121:281-285, 1976.

72. Conte P, Heitzman ER, Markarian B: Viral pneumonia: roentgen pathological correlations, *Radiology* 95:267-272, 1970.

73. Contreras MA, Cheung OT, Sanders DE, et al: Pulmonary infection with nontuberculous mycobacteria, *Am Rev Respir Dis* 137:149-152, 1988.

74. Costello P, Rose RM: CT findings in pleural aspergillosis, *J Comput Assist Tomogr* 9:760-762, 1985.

75. Coultas DB, Samet JM, Butler C: Bronchiolitis obliterans due to *Mycoplasma pneumoniae*, *West J Med* 144:471-474, 1986.

76. Curry WA: Human nocardiosis: a clinical review with selected case reports, *Arch Intern Med* 140:818-826, 1980.

77. Cuthbert R: Sylvatic pulmonary hydatid disease: a radiological survey, *J Can Assoc Radiol* 26:132-138, 1974.

78. Danner PK, McFarland DR, Felson B: Massive pulmonary gangrene, *AJR* 103:548-554, 1968.

79. Davidson PT: The diagnosis and management of disease caused by *M. avium* complex, *M. kansasii* and other mycobacteria, *Clin Chest Med* 10:431-443, 1989.

80. Davies SF, McKenna RW, Sarosi GA: Trephine biopsy of the bone marrow in disseminated histoplasmosis, *Am J Med* 67:617-622, 1979.

81. Dee P, Teja K, Korzeniowski O, et al: Miliary tuberculosis resulting in adult respiratory distress syndrome: a surviving case, *AJR* 134:569-572, 1980.

82. de Leon EP, Pardo de Tavero MP: Pulmonary schistosomiasis in the Philippines, *Dis Chest* 53:154-161, 1968.

83. Demos TC, Studlo JD, Puczynski M: Mycoplasma pneumonia: presentation as a mediastinal mass, *AJR* 143:981-982, 1984.

84. Dennis JM, Bondreau RP: Pleuropulmonary tularemia: its roentgen manifestations, *Radiology* 68:25-30, 1957.

85. Dhiensiri T, Puapairoj S, Susaengrat W: Pulmonary melioidosis: clinical-radiologic correlation in 183 cases in north-eastern Thailand, *Radiology* 166:711-715, 1988.

86. Dietrich PA, Johnson RD, Fairbank JT, et al: The chest radiograph in Legionnaire's disease, *Radiology* 127:577-582, 1978.

87. di Sant' Agnese PA, Davis PB: Cystic fibrosis in adults: 75 cases and a review of 232 cases in the literature, *Am J Med* 66:121-132, 1979.

88. Donohue JF: Lower respiratory tract involvement in Rocky Mountain spotted fever, *Arch Intern Med* 140:223-226, 1980.

89. Drutz DJ, Catanzaro A: Coccidioidomycosis: state of the art. Parts 1 and 2, *Am Rev Respir Dis* 117:559-585;727-771, 1978.

90. Duperval R, Hermans PE, Brewer NS, et al: Cryptococcosis, with emphasis on the significance of isolation of *Cryptococcus neoformans* from the respiratory tract, *Chest* 72:13-19, 1977.

91. Eastridge CE, Young JM, Cole F, et al: Pulmonary aspergillosis, *Ann Thorac Surg* 13:397-403, 1972.

92. Edelman RR, Hann LE, Simon M: *Chlamydia trachomatosis* pneumonia in adults: radiographic appearance, *Radiology* 152:279-282, 1984.

93. Edelstein G, Levitt RG: Cavitary coccidioidomycosis presenting as spontaneous pneumothorax, *AJR* 141:533-534, 1983.

94. Edwards LB, Acquaviva FA, Livesay VT, et al: An atlas of sensitivity to tuberculin, PPD-B and histoplasmin in the United States, *Am Rev Respir Dis* 99(suppl 4):1-32, 1969.

95. Englund JA, Sullivan CJ, Jordan C, et al: Respiratory syncytial

virus infection in immunocompromised adults, *Ann Intern Med* 109:203-208, 1988.

96. Eriksson J, Nordshus T, Carlsen K-H, et al: Radiological findings in children with respiratory syncytial virus infection: relationship to clinical and bacteriological findings, *Pediatr Radiol* 16:120-122, 1986.

97. Evans AF, Oakley RH, Whitehouse GH: Analysis of the chest radiograph in Legionnaire's disease, *Clin Radiol* 32:361-365, 1981.

98. Everett ED, Nelson RA: Pulmonary meliodosis: observations in thirty-nine cases, *Am Rev Respir Dis* 112:331-340, 1975.

99. Fairbank JT, Patel MM, Dietrich PA: Legionnaire's disease, *J Thorac Imag* 6(3):6-13, 1991.

100. Faulkner SL, Vernon R, Brown PP, et al: Hemoptysis and pulmonary aspergilloma: operative versus non-operative treatment, *Ann Thorac Surg* 25:389-392, 1978.

101. Fawcitt J, Parry HE: Lung changes in pertussis and measles in childhood: a review of 1894 cases with a follow up study of the pulmonary complications, *Br J Radiol* 30:76-82, 1957.

102. Feigin DS: Pulmonary cryptococcosis: radiologic-pathologic correlates of its three forms, *AJR* 141:1263-1272, 1983.

103. Feigin DS: Nocardiosis of the lung: chest radiographic findings in 21 cases, *Radiology* 159:9-14, 1986.

104. Felson LB, Rosenberg LS, Hamburger M: Roentgen findings in acute Friedlander's pneumonia, *Radiology* 53:559-565, 1949.

105. Fine NL, Smith LR, Sheedy PF: Frequency of pleural effusions in mycoplasma and viral pneumonias, *N Engl J Med* 283:790-793, 1970.

106. Finegold SM, Will D, Murray JF: Aspergillosis, *Am J Med* 27:463-482, 1959.

107. Finnegan OC, Fowler SJ, White RJ: Radiographic appearances of *Mycoplasma* pneumonia, *Thorax* 36:469-472, 1981.

108. Fisher MS: "Miliary" actinomycosis, *J Can Assoc Radiol* 31:149-150, 1980.

109. Flynn MW, Felson B: The roentgen manifestations of thoracic actinomycosis, *AJR* 110:707-716, 1970.

110. Forrest JV: Common fungal diseases of the lungs. II. Histoplasmosis, *Radiol Clin North Am* 11:163-168, 1973.

111. Foy HM, Loop J, Clarke ER, et al: Radiographic study of *Mycoplasma pneumoniae* pneumonia, *Am Rev Respir Dis* 108:469-474, 1973.

112. Frank P, Strickland B: Pulmonary actinomycosis, *Br J Radiol* 47:373-378, 1974.

113. Fraser DW, Tsai TR, Orenstein W, et al: Legionnaires' disease: description of an epidemic of pneumonia, *N Engl J Med* 297:1189-1197, 1977.

114. Fraser RG, Pare JAP, Pare PD, et al: *Diagnosis of diseases of the chest*, ed 3, Philadelphia, 1989, WB Saunders.

115. Fraser RG, Wortzman G: Acute pneumococcal lobar pneumonia: the significance of nonsegmental distribution, *J Can Assoc Radiol* 3:37-46, 1959.

116. Frazier AR, Rosenow EC, Roberts GD: Nocardiosis: a review of 25 cases occurring during 24 months, *Mayo Clin Proc* 50:657-663, 1975.

117. Freundlich IM, Israel HL: Pulmonary aspergillosis, *Clin Radiol* 24:248-253, 1973.

118. Friedman PJ, Hellekant CAG: Radiologic recognition of bronchopleural fistula, *Radiology* 124:289-295, 1977.

119. Frommhold W, Lagemann K, Wolf KJ: Die akute Klebsiellenpneumonie (in German — summary in English), *Fortschr Geb Roentgenstr* 121:25-34, 1974.

120. Galloway RW, Miller RS: Lung changes in the recent influenza epidemic, *Br J Radiol* 32:28-31, 1959.

121. Garcia-Palmieri MR, Marcial-Rojas RA: The protean manifestations of schistosomiasis mansoni: a clinicopathologic correlation, *Ann Intern Med* 57:763-775, 1962.

122. Garten AJ, Mendelson DS, Halton KP: CT manifestations of infectious mononucleosis, *Clin Imag* 16:114-116, 1992.

123. Gefter WB, Weingrad TR, Epstein DM, et al: "Semi-invasive" pulmonary aspergillosis: a new look at the spectrum of *Aspergillus* infections of the lung, *Radiology* 140:313-321, 1981.

124. Gelpi AP, Mustafa A: *Ascaris* pneumonia, *Am J Med* 44:377-389, 1968.

125. George RB, Mogabgab WJ: Atypical pneumonia in young men with rhinovirus infections, *Ann Intern Med* 71:1073-1078, 1969.

126. George RB, Weill H, Rasch JR, et al: Roentgenographic appearances of viral and mycoplasmal pneumonias, *Am Rev Respir Dis* 96:1144-1150, 1967.

127. George RB, Ziskind MM, Rasch JR, et al: Mycoplasma and adenovirus pneumonias: comparison with other atypical pneumonias in a military population, *Ann Intern Med* 65:931-942, 1966.

128. Geppert EF, Leff A: The pathogenesis of pulmonary and miliary tuberculosis, *Arch Intern Med* 139:1381-1383, 1979.

129. Goddard P, Kinsella D, Duncan AW, et al: Magnetic resonance imaging of the chest in infectious mononucleosis, *Br J Radiol* 63:138-140, 1990.

130. Gold R, Wilt JC, Adhikari PK, et al: Adenoviral pneumonia and its complications in infants and childhood, *J Can Assoc Radiol* 20:218-224, 1969.

131. Gonzalez CL, Calia FM: Bacteriologic flora of aspiration-induced pulmonary infections, *Arch Intern Med* 135:711-714, 1975.

132. Goodwin RA, Des Prez RM: Histoplasmosis: state of the art, *Am Rev Respir Dis* 117:929-956, 1977.

133. Goodwin RA, Loyd JE, Des Prez RM: Histoplasmosis in normal hosts, *Medicine* 60:231-266, 1981.

134. Goodwin RA, Owens FT, Snell JD, et al: Chronic pulmonary histoplasmosis, *Medicine* 55:413-452, 1976.

135. Goodwin RA, Shapiro JL, Thurmann GH, et al: Disseminated histoplasmosis: clinical and pathological correlations, *Medicine* 59:1-33, 1980.

136. Goodwin RA, Snell JD: The enlarging histoplasmoma, *Am Rev Respir Dis* 100:1-12, 1969.

137. Gordon JD, McKeen AD, Maric TJ, et al: The radiographic features of epidemic and sporadic Q fever pneumonia, *J Can Assoc Radiol* 35:293-296, 1984.

138. Gordonson J, Birnbaum W, Jacobson G, et al: Pulmonary cryptococcosis, *Radiology* 112:557-561, 1974.

139. Grayston JT, Alexander ER, Kenny GE, et al: *Mycoplasma pneumoniae* infections: clinical and epidemiologic studies, *JAMA* 191:369-374, 1965.

140. Greendyke WH, Resnick DL, Harvey WC: Roentgen manifestations of coccidioidomycosis, *AJR* 109:491-499, 1970.

141. Greene R: Pulmonary aspergillosis: three distinct entities or a spectrum of disease, *Radiology* 140:527-530, 1981.

142. Gremillion DH, Crawford GE: Measles pneumonia in young adults, *Am J Med* 71:539-542, 1981.

143. Grix A, Giammona ST: Pneumonitis with pleural effusion in children due to *Mycoplasma* pneumonia, *Am Rev Respir Dis* 109:665-671, 1974.

144. Groskin SA, Panicek DM, Ewing DK: Bacterial lung abscess: a review of the radiographic and clinical features of 50 cases, *J Thorac Imag* 6(3):62-67, 1991.

145. Grossman CB, Bragg DG, Armstrong D: Roentgen manifestations of pulmonary nocardiosis, *Radiology* 96:325-330, 1970.

146. Gückel C, Benz-Bohm G, Widemann B: Mycoplasmal pneumonias in childhood: roentgen features, differential diagnosis and review of literature, *Pediatr Radiol* 19:499-503, 1989.

147. Gurney JW, Unger JM, Dobry CA, et al: Agricultural disorders of the lung, *Radiographics* 11:625-634, 1991.

148. Gutman E, Pongdee O, Park YS: Massive pulmonary gangrene, *Radiology* 107:293-294, 1973.

149. Halde C: Basic mycology for the clinician, *Semin Respir Med* 9:117-122, 1987.

150. Hall FM, Simon M: Occult pneumonia associated with dehydration: myth or reality, *AJR* 148:853-854, 1987.

151. Halvorsen RA, Duncan JD, Merten DF, et al: Pulmonary blastomycosis: radiologic manifestations, *Radiology* 150:1-5, 1984.

152. Hammerman KJ, Powell KE, Christianson CS, et al: Pulmonary cryptococcosis: clinical forms and treatment, *Am Rev Respir Dis* 108:1116-1123, 1973.

153. Hanna JW, Reed JC, Choplin RH: Pleural infections: clinicoradiologic review, *J Thorac Imag* 6(3):68-79, 1991.

154. Harrison BDW: Community-acquired pneumonia in adults in British hospitals in 1982-1983: a survey of aetiology, mortality, prognosis factors and outcome, *Q J Med* 62(239):195-220, 1987.

155. Hauser H, Gurret JP: Miliary tuberculosis associated with adrenal enlargement: CT appearance, *J Comput Assist Tomogr* 10:254-256, 1986.

156. Hawley C, Felson B: Roentgenographic aspects of intrathoracic blastomycosis, *AJR* 75:751-757, 1956.

157. Hebert DH: The roentgen features of Eaton agent pneumonia, *AJR* 98:300-304, 1966.

158. Hendaoui L, Siala M, Fourati A, et al: Case report: hydatid cyst of the aorta, *Clin Radiol* 43:423-425, 1991.

159. Henkle JQ, Nair SV: Endobronchial pulmonary nocardosis, *JAMA* 256:1331-1332, 1986.

160. Herlinger H: Pulmonary changes in tropical eosinophilia, *Br J Radiol* 36:889-901, 1963.

161. Holmes RB: Friedlander's pneumonia, *AJR* 75:728-747, 1956.

162. Huang RM, Naidich DP, Lubat E, et al: Septic pulmonary emboli: CT-radiographic correlation, *AJR* 153:41-45, 1989.

163. Hubbel C, Dominguez R, Kohl S: Neonatal herpes simplex pneumonitis, *Rev Infect Dis* 10:431-438, 1988.

164. Hulnick DH, Naidich DP, McCauley DI: Pleural tuberculosis evaluated by computed tomography, *Radiology* 149:759-765, 1983.

165. Hyde L: Coccidioidal pulmonary cavitation, *Chest* 54(suppl 1):273-277, 1968.

166. Iannini PB, Claffey T, Quintiliani R: Bacteremic *Pseudomonas* pneumonia, *JAMA* 230:558-561, 1974.

167. Ibarra-Perez C: Thoracic complications of amoebic abscess of the liver: report of 501 cases, *Chest* 79:672-677, 1981.

168. Ikezoe J, Takeuchi N, Johkoh T, et al: CT appearance of pulmonary tuberculosis in diabetic and immunocompromised patients: comparison with patients who had no underlying disease, *AJR* 159:1175-1179, 1992.

169. Im J-G, Itoh H, Shim Y-S: Pulmonary tuberculosis: CT findings — early active disease and sequential change with antituberculous therapy, *Radiology* 186:653-660, 1985.

170. Im J-G, Kim JH, Han MC, et al: Computed tomography of esophagomediastinal fistula in tuberculous mediastinal lymphadenitis, *J Comput Assist Tomogr* 14:89-92, 1990.

171. Im J-G, Song KS, Kang HS, et al: Mediastinal tuberculous lymphadenitis: CT manifestations, *Radiology* 164:115-119, 1987.

172. Im J-G, Webb WR, Han MC, et al: Apical opacity associated with pulmonary tuberculosis: high-resolution CT findings, *Radiology* 178:727-731, 1991.

173. Im JG, Whang HY, Kim WS, et al: Pleuropulmonary paragonimiasis: radiologic findings in 71 patients, *AJR* 159:39-43, 1992.

174. Im JG, Yeon KM, Ham MC, et al: Leptospirosis of the lung: radiographic findings in 58 patients, *AJR* 152:955-959, 1989.

175. Irwin A: Radiology of aspergillosis, *Clin Radiol* 18:432-438, 1966.

176. Israel HL, Ostrow A: Sarcoidosis and aspergilloma, *Am J Med* 47:243-250, 1960.

177. Jacobs LG: Pulmonary torulosis, *Radiology* 71:398-403, 1958.

178. James AE, Dixon GD, Johnson HF: Melioidosis: a correlation of the radiologic and pathologic findings, *Radiology* 89:230-235, 1967.

179. Jamison HW: A roentgen study of chronic pulmonary coccidioidomycosis, *AJR* 55:396-412, 1946.

180. Janigan DT, Marrie TJ: An inflammatory pseudotumor of the lung in Q fever pneumonia, *N Engl J Med* 308:86-88, 1983.

181. Janower ML, Weiss EB: Mycoplasmal, viral, and rickettsial pneumonias, *Semin Roentgenol* 15:25-34, 1980.

182. Jawahiry KI, Karpas L: Pulmonary schistosomiasis: a detailed clinicopathologic study, *Am Rev Respir Dis* 88:517-527, 1963.

183. Jewkes J, Kay PH, Paneth M, et al: Pulmonary aspergilloma: analysis of prognosis in relation to hemoptysis and survey of treatment, *Thorax* 38:572-578, 1983.

184. Johnson JS: Pulmonary aspergillosis, *Semin Respir Med* 9:187-199, 1987.

185. Johnson PC, Sarosi GA: Histoplasmosis, *Semin Respir Med* 9:145-151, 1987.

186. Johnson RJ, Johnson JR: Paragonimiasis in Indochinese refugees: roentgenographic findings with clinical correlations, *Am Rev Respir Dis* 128:534-538, 1983.

187. Jones TC: Cestodes (tapeworms). In Mandell GL, Douglas RG, Bennett JE, eds: *Principles and practice of infectious diseases,* New York, 1985, John Wiley & Sons.

188. Julander I: Staphylococcal septicaemia and endocarditis in 80 drug addicts, *Scand J Infect Dis* Suppl 41:49-54, 1983.

189. Kantor HG: Many radiologic facies of pneumococcal pneumonia, *AJR* 137:1213-1220, 1981.

190. Kaplan MH, Armstrong D, Rosen P: Tuberculosis complicating neoplastic diseases: a review of 201 cases, *Cancer* 33:850-858, 1974.

191. Karas A, Hankins JR, Attar S, et al: Pulmonary aspergillosis: an analysis of 41 patients, *Ann Thorac Surg* 22:1-7, 1976.

192. Kauffman CA, Israel KS, Smith JW, et al: Histoplasmosis in immunosuppressed patients, *Am J Med* 64:923-932, 1978.

193. Kaufman JM, Cuvelier CA, Van der Straeten M: *Mycoplasma* pneumonia with fulminant evolution into diffuse interstitial fibrosis, *Thorax* 35:140-144, 1980.

194. Kerkering TM, Duma RJ, Shadomy S: The evolution of pulmonary cryptococcosis: clinical implications from a study of 41 patients with and without compromising host factors, *Ann Intern Med* 94:611-616, 1981.

195. Khan FA, Rehman M, Marcus P, et al: Pulmonary gangrene occurring as a complication of pulmonary tuberculosis, *Chest* 77:76-80, 1980.

196. Khoury MB, Godwin JD, Ravin CE, et al: Thoracic cryptococcosis: immunologic competence and radiologic appearance, *AJR* 142:893-896, 1984.

197. Kirby BD, Snyder KM, Meyer RD, et al: Legionnaires' disease: report of sixty-five nosocomially acquired cases and review of the literature, *Medicine* 59:188-205, 1980.

198. Klein BS, Kuritsky JN, Chappell WA, et al: Comparison of enzyme immunoassay, immunodiffusion, and complement fixation tests in detecting antibody in human serum to the A antigen of *Blastomyces dermatitidis, Am Rev Respir Dis* 133:144-148, 1986.

199. Klein BS, Vergeront JM, DiSalvo AF, et al: Two outbreaks of blastomycosis along rivers in Wisconsin: isolation of *Blastomyces dermatitidis* from riverbank soil and evidence of transmission along waterways, *Am Rev Respir Dis* 136:1333-1338, 1987.

200. Koletsky RJ, Weinstein AJ: Fulminant *Mycoplasma pneumoniae* infection, *Am Rev Respir Dis* 122:491-496, 1980.

201. Kovacs JA, Kovacs AA, Polis M, et al: Cryptococcosis in acquired immunodeficiency syndrome, *Ann Intern Med* 103:533-538, 1985.

202. Krick JA, Stinson EB, Remington JS: *Nocardia* infection in heart transplant patients, *Ann Intern Med* 82:18-26, 1975.

203. Kroboth FJ, Yu VL, Reddy SC, et al: Clinicoradiographic correlation with the extent of Legionnaire's disease, *AJR* 141:263-268, 1983.

204. Krysl J, Muller NL, Miller RR, et al: Patient with miliary nodules and diarrhea, *Can Assoc Radiol J* 42:363-366, 1991.

205. Kuhlman JE, Deutsch JH, Fishman EK, et al: CT features of thoracic mycobacterial disease, *Radiographics* 10:413-431, 1990.

206. Kuhlman JE, Fishman EK, Teigen C: Pulmonary septic emboli: diagnosis with CT, *Radiology* 174:211-213, 1990.

207. Kulczycki LL, Murphy TM, Bellanti JA: *Pseudomonas* colonization in cystic fibrosis: a study of 160 patients, *JAMA* 240:30-34, 1978.

208. Kwong JS, Müller NL, Godwin JD, et al: Thoracic actinomycosis: CT findings in eight patients, *Radiology* 183:189-192, 1992.

209. Landay MJ, Christensen EE, Bynum LJ, et al: Anaerobic pleural and pulmonary infections, *AJR* 134:233-240, 1980.

210. Landen P, Palayew MJ: Infectious mononucleosis: a review of chest roentgenographic manifestations, *J Can Assoc Radiol* 25:303-306, 1974.

211. Laskey W, Sarosi GA: The radiological appearance of pulmonary blastomycosis, *Radiology* 126:351-357, 1978.

212. Lee KS, Kim YH, Kim WS, et al: Endobronchial tuberculosis: CT features, *J Comput Assist Tomogr* 15:424-428, 1991.

213. Lee KS, Song KS, Lim TH, et al: Adult-onset pulmonary tuberculosis: findings on chest radiographs and CT scans, *AJR* 160:753-758, 1993.

214. Lee REJ, Terry SI, Walker TM, et al: The chest radiograph in leptospirosis in Jamaica, *Br J Radiol* 54:939-943, 1981.

215. Lees RF, Harrison RB, Williamson BRJ, et al: Radiographic findings in Rocky Mountain spotted fever, *Radiology* 129:17-20, 1978.

216. Leff A, Geppert EF: Public health and preventive aspects of pulmonary tuberculosis: infectiousness, epidemiology, risk factors classification and preventive therapy, *Arch Intern Med* 139:1405-1410, 1979.

217. Leung AN, Muller NL, Miller RR: CT in differential diagnosis of diffuse pleural disease, *AJR* 154:487-492, 1990.

218. Leung AN, Muller N, Pineda PR, et al: Primary tuberculosis in childhood: radiographic manifestations, *Radiology* 182:87-91, 1992.

219. Levine BE: Coccidioidomycosis, *Semin Respir Med* 9:152-158, 1987.

220. Levinson ED, Ziter FMH Jr, Westcott JL: Pulmonary lesions due to *Dirofilaria immitis* (dog heartworm), *Radiology* 131:305-307, 1979.

221. Levy M, Dromer F, Brion N, et al: Community-acquired pneumonia: importance of initial noninvasive bacteriologic and radiographic investigations, *Chest* 92:43-48, 1988.

222. Lewis JL, Rabinowich S: The wide spectrum of cryptococcal infections, *Am J Med* 53:315-322, 1972.

223. Libshitz HI, Atkinson EW, Israel HI: Pleural thickening as a manifestation of *Aspergillus* superinfection, *AJR* 120:883-886, 1974.

224. Light RW: *Pleural disease*, Philadelphia, 1983, Lea & Febiger.

225. Light RW: Parapneumonic effusions and empyema, *Clin Chest Med* 6:55-62, 1985.

226. Light RW: Management of parapneumonic effusions, *Arch Intern Med* 141:1339-1341, 1981.

227. Light RW, Girard WM, Jenkinson SG, et al: Parapneumonic effusions, *Am J Med* 69:507-511, 1980.

228. Lipinski JK, Weisbrod GL, Saunders DE: Unusual manifestations of pulmonary aspergillosis, *J Can Assoc Radiol* 29:216-220, 1978.

229. Lipton JH, Fong TC, Gill MJ, et al: Q fever inflammatory pseudotumor of the lung, *Chest* 92:756-757, 1987.

230. Littman ML, Zimmerman LE: *Cryptococcosis, torulosis or European blastomycosis*, New York, 1956, Grune & Stratton.

231. Loewen DF, Procknow JJ, Loosli CG: Chronic active pulmonary histoplasmosis, *Am J Med* 28:252-280, 1960.

232. Long RF, Berens SV, Shambhag GR: An unusual manifestation of pulmonary cryptococcosis, *Br J Radiol* 45:757-759, 1972.

233. Lonky SA, Catanzaro A, Moser KM, et al: Acute coccidioidal pleural effusion, *Am Rev Respir Dis* 114:681-688, 1976.

234. MacPherson RI, Cumming GR, Chernick V: Unilateral hyperlucent lung: a complication of viral pneumonia, *J Can Assoc Radiol* 20:225-231, 1969.

235. Makanjuola D: Fluid levels in pulmonary tuberculosis cavities in a rural population of Nigeria, *AJR* 141:519-520, 1983.

236. Mansel JK, Rosenow EC, Martin JW: *Mycoplasma pneumoniae* pneumonia, *Chest* 95:639-646, 1989.

237. Margolin FR, Gandy TK: Pneumonia of atypical measles, *Radiology* 131:653-655, 1979.

238. Martin DB, Weiner LB, Nieburg PI, et al: Atypical measles in adolescents and young adults, *Ann Intern Med* 90:877-881, 1979.

239. Martin W, Choplin R, Shertzer ME: The chest radiograph in Rocky Mountain spotted fever, *AJR* 139:889-893, 1982.

240. Mashburn TD, Dawson DF, Young JM: Pulmonary calcifications and histoplasmosis, *Am Rev Respir Dis* 84:208-216, 1961.

241. Mays BB, Thomas GD, Leonard JS, et al: Gram-negative bacillary necrotizing pneumonia: a bacteriologic and histopathologic correlation, *J Infect Dis* 120:687-697, 1969.

242. McCarthy DS, Pepys J: Pulmonary aspergilloma — clinical immunology, *Clin Allergy* 3:57-70, 1973.

243. McGahan JP, Graves DS, Palmer PES, et al: Classic and contemporary imaging of coccidioidomycosis, *AJR* 136:393-404, 1981.

244. McGuinness G, Naidich DP, Jagirder J, et al: High resolution CT findings in miliary lung disease, *J Comput Assist Tomogr* 16:384-390, 1992.

245. McPhail JL, Arora TS: Intrathoracic hydatid disease, *Dis Chest* 52:772-781, 1967.

246. Meenhorst PL, Mulder JD: The chest in *Legionella* pneumonia (Legionnaires' disease), *Eur J Radiol* 3:180-186, 1983.

247. Meighan JW: Pulmonary cryptococcosis mimicking carcinoma of the lung, *Radiology* 103:61-62, 1972.

248. Melbye H, Dale K: Interobserver variability in the radiographic diagnosis of adult outpatient pneumonia, *Acta Radiol* 33:79-81, 1992.

249. Meredith HC, Cogan BM, McLaulin B: Pleural aspergillosis, *AJR* 130:164-166, 1978.

250. Millar JK: The chest film findings in Q fever — a series of 35 cases, *Clin Radiol* 29:371-375, 1978.

251. Miller RP, Bates JH: Pleuropulmonary tularemia: a review of 29 patients, *Am Rev Respir Dis* 99:31-34, 1969.

252. Miller WT, Edelman JM, Miller WT: Cryptococcal pulmonary infection in patients with AIDS: radiographic appearance, *Radiology* 175:725-728, 1990.

253. Minami M, Kawauchi N, Yoshikawa K, et al: Malignancy associated with chronic empyema: radiologic assessment, *Radiology* 178:417-423, 1991.

254. Mohr JA, Patterson CD, Eaton BG, et al: Primary pulmonary sporotrichosis, *Am Rev Respir Dis* 106:260-264, 1972.

255. Moore EH, Webb WR, Gamsu G, et al: Legionnaires' disease in the renal transplant patient: clinical presentation and radiographic progression, *Radiology* 153:589-593, 1984.

256. Moore NR, Phillips MS, Sheerson JM, et al: Appearances on computed tomography following thoracoplasty for pulmonary tuberculosis, *Br J Radiol* 61:573-578, 1988.

257. Moore WR, Scannell JG: Pulmonary actinomycosis simulating cancer of the lung, *J Thorac Cardiovasc Surg* 55:193-195, 1968.

258. Morgan DE, Nath H, Sanders C, et al: Mediastinal actinomycosis, *AJR* 155:735-737, 1990.

259. Moskowitz PS, Sae JY, Gooding CA: Tracheal coccidiodomycosis causing upper airway obstruction in children, *AJR* 139:596-600, 1982.

260. Murray HW, Masur H, Senterlit LB, et al: The protean manifestations of *Mycoplasma pneumoniae* infection in adults, *Am J Med* 58:229-242, 1975.

261. Murray JF, Finegold SM, Froman S, et al: The changing spectrum of nocardiosis, *Am Rev Respir Dis* 83:315-330, 1961.

262. Murray JF, Lurie HI, Kaye J, et al: Benign pulmonary histoplasmosis (cave disease) in South Africa, *S Afr Med J* 31:245-253, 1957.

263. Naraqui S, McDonnell G: Hematogenous staphylococcal pneumonia secondary to soft tissue infection, *Chest* 79:173-175, 1981.

264. Neu HC, Silva M, Hazen E, et al: Necrotizing nocardial pneumonitis, *Ann Intern Med* 66:274-284, 1967.

265. Neva FN, Ottesen EA: Current concepts in parasitology: tropical (filarial) eosinophilia, *N Engl J Med* 298:1129-1131, 1978.

266. Nguyen MLT, Yu VL: *Legionella* infection, *Clin Chest Med* 12:257-268, 1991.

267. O'Brien RJ: The epidemiology of nontuberculous mycobacterial disease, *Clin Chest Med* 10:407-418, 1989.

268. Odita JC, Nwankwo M, Aghahowa JE: Hilar enlargement in respiratory syncytial virus pneumonia, *Eur J Radiol* 9:155, 1989.

269. Ogakwu M, Nwokolo C: Radiological findings in pulmonary paragonimiasis as seen in Nigeria: a review based on one hundred cases, *Br J Radiol* 46:669-705, 1973.

270. Optican RJ, Ost A, Ravin CE: High-resolution computed tomography in the diagnosis of miliary tuberculosis, *Chest* 102:941-943, 1992.

271. O'Reilly GV, Dee PM, Otteni GV: Gangrene of the lung: successful medical management of three patients, *Radiology* 126:575-579, 1978.

272. Ort S, Ryan JL, Barden G, et al: Pneumococcal pneumonia in hospitalized patients, *JAMA* 249:214-218, 1983.

273. Osborne D: Radiologic appearance of viral disease of the lower respiratory tract in infants and children, *AJR* 130:29-33, 1978.

274. Osborne D, White P: Radiology of epidemic adenovirus 21 infection of the lower respiratory tract in infants and young children, *AJR* 133:397-400, 1979.

275. Overholt EL, Tiggert WE: Roentgenographic manifestations of pulmonary tularemia, *Radiology* 74:758-765, 1960.

276. Palayew MJ, Frank H: Benign progressive multinodular pulmonary histoplasmosis, *Radiology* 111:311-314, 1974.

277. Palayew MJ, Frank H, Sedlezky I: Our experience with histoplasmosis: an analysis of seventy cases with follow up study, *J Can Assoc Radiol* 17:142-150, 1966.

278. Palmer DL, Harvey RL, Wheeler JK: Diagnostic and therapeutic considerations in *Nocardia asteroides* infections, *Medicine* 53:391-401, 1974.

279. Pantongrag-Brown L: Case of the season: pulmonary cryptococcoma, *Semin Roentgenol* 26:101-102, 1991.

280. Parker JD, Sarosi GA, Doto IL, et al: Treatment of chronic pulmonary histoplasmosis: a national communicable disease center cooperative mycoses study, *N Engl J Med* 283:225-229, 1970.

281. Paul R: Pulmonary "coin" lesion of unusual pathology, *Radiology* 75:118-120, 1960.

282. Pearlberg J, Haggar AM, Saravolatz L, et al: *Hemophilus influenzal* pneumonia in the adult, *Radiology* 151:23-26, 1984.

283. Pfister AK, Goodwin AW, Squire EW, et al: Pulmonary blastomycosis: roentgenographic clues to the diagnosis, *South Med J* 59:1441-1447, 1966.

284. Pickworth FE, El-Soussi M, Wells IP, et al: The radiological appearances of Q fever pneumonia, *Clin Radiol* 44:150-153, 1991.

285. Pierce AK, Sandford JP: Aerobic gram-negative bacillary pneumonias: state of the art, *Am Rev Respir Dis* 110:647-658, 1974.

286. Pitchenik AE, Rubinson HA: The radiographic appearance of tuberculosis in patients with the acquired immune deficiency syndrome (AIDS) and pre-AIDS, *Am Rev Respir Dis* 131:393-396, 1985.

287. Pope TL, Armstrong P, Thomas R, et al: Pittsburgh pneumonia agent: chest film manifestations, *AJR* 138:237-241, 1983.

288. Pratt PC: Pathology of tuberculosis, *Semin Roentgenol* 14:196-203, 1979.

289. Prince DS, Peterson DD, Steiner RM, et al: Infection with *Mycobacterium avium* complex in patients without predisposing conditions, *N Engl J Med* 321:863-868, 1989.

290. Proto AV, Merhar GL: Central bronchial displacement with large posterior pleural collections: findings on the lateral chest radiograph and CT scans, *J Can Assoc Radiol* 35:128-132, 1984.

291. Purtilo DT, Meyers WM, Connor DH: Fatal strongyloidiosis in immunosuppressed patients, *Am J Med* 56:488-493, 1974.

292. Putman CE, Curtis A McB, Simeone JF, et al: *Mycoplasma* pneumonia: clinical and roentgenographic patterns, *AJR* 124:417-422, 1975.

293. Quinn JL: Measles pneumonia in an adult, *AJR* 91:560-563, 1964.

294. Quinn SF, Erickson S, Oshman D, et al: Lobar collapse with respiratory syncytial virus pneumonitis, *Pediatr Radiol* 15:229-230, 1985.

295. Rabinowitz JG, Busch J, Buttram WR: Pulmonary manifestations of blastomycosis, *Radiology* 120:25-32, 1976.

296. Raby N, Forbes G, Williams R: *Nocardia* infection in patients with liver transplants or chronic liver disease: radiologic findings, *Radiology* 174:713-716, 1990.

297. Radkowski MA, Kranzler JK, Beem MO, et al: *Chlamydia* pneumonia in infants: radiography in 125 cases, *AJR* 137:703-706, 1981.

298. Rafferty P, Biggs BA, Crompton GK, et al: What happens to aspergilloma? Analysis of 23 cases, *Thorax* 38:579-583, 1983.

299. Rakower J, Milwidsky H: Primary mediastinal echinococcus, *Am J Med* 29:73-83, 1960.

300. Randolph KA, Beckman JF: Legionnaire's disease presenting with empyema, *Chest* 75:404-406, 1979.

301. Rasmussen FO: Om haemoptyse, navnlig den lethale, i anatomisk og klinisk henseende, *Hospitalstidende* 11:49-52, 1868.

302. Recht LD, Davies SF, Eckman MR, et al: Blastomycosis in immuno-compromised patients, *Am Rev Respir Dis* 125:359-362, 1982.

303. Reed WP: Indolent pulmonary abscess associated with *Klebsiella* and *Enterobacter, Am Rev Respir Dis* 107:1055-1059, 1973.

304. Reed WP, Palmer DL, Williams RC, et al: Bubonic plague in the southwestern United States: a review of recent experience, *Medicine* 49:465-468, 1970.

305. Reich JM: Pulmonary gangrene and the air crescent sign, *Thorax* 48:70-74, 1993.

306. Ren H, Kuhlman JE, Hruban RH, et al: CT of inflation-fixed lungs: wedge-shaped density and vascular sign in the diagnosis of infarction, *J Comput Assist Tomogr* 14:82-86, 1990.

307. Renner RR, Coccaro AP, Heitzman ER, et al: *Pseudomonas* pneumonia: a prototype of hospital-based infection, *Radiology* 105:555-562, 1972.

308. Rice RP, Loda F: A roentgenographic analysis of respiratory syncytial virus pneumonia in infants, *Radiology* 87:1021-1027, 1966.

309. Riggs W, Nelson P: The roentgenographic findings in infantile and childhood histoplasmosis, *AJR* 97:181-185, 1966.

310. Ripstein CB, Spain DM, Bluth I: Scar cancer of the lung, *J Thorac Cardiovasc Surg* 56:362-370, 1968.

311. Risher WH, Crocker EF Jr, Beckman EN, et al: Pulmonary dirofilariasis, *J Thorac Cardiovasc Surg* 97:303-308, 1989.

312. Rivkin LM, Winn DF, Salyes JM: The surgical treatment of pulmonary coccidioidomycosis, *J Thorac Cardiovasc Surg* 42:402-412, 1961.

313. Ro JY, Tsakalakis PJ, White VA, et al: Pulmonary dirofilariasis: the great imitator of primary or metastatic lung tumor, *Hum Pathol* 20:69-76, 1989.

314. Roberts CM, Citron KM, Strickland B: Intrathoracic aspergilloma: role of CT in diagnosis and treatment, *Radiology* 165:123-128, 1987.

315. Rohlfing BM, White EA, Webb WR, et al: Hilar and mediastinal adenopathy caused by bacterial abscess of the lung, *Radiology* 128:289-293, 1978.

316. Rohwedder JJ: Pulmonary sporotrichosis, *Semin Respir Med* 9:176-179, 1987.

317. Rose RW, Ward BH: Spherical pneumonias in children simulating pulmonary and mediastinal masses, *Radiology* 106:179-182, 1973.

318. Ruben FL, Nguyen MLT: Viral pneumonitis, *Clin Chest Med* 12:223-235, 1991.

319. Rubin E, Weisbrod GL, Sanders DE: Pulmonary alveolar proteinosis: relationship to silicosis and pulmonary infection, *Radiology* 135:35-41, 1980.

320. Rubin SA: Radiographic spectrum of pleuropulmonary tularemia, *AJR* 131:277-281, 1978.

321. Sadrieh M, Dutz W, Navabpoor MS: Review of 150 cases of hydatid cyst of the lung, *Dis Chest* 52:662-666, 1967.

322. Sagel SS: Common fungal diseases of the lungs, *Radiol Clin North Am* 11:153-161, 1973.

323. Sahn SA, Light RW: The sun should never set on a parapneumonic effusion, *Chest* 95:945-947, 1989.

324. Saksouk FA, Fahl MH, Rizk GK: Computed tomography of pulmonary hydatid disease, *J Comput Assist Tomogr* 10:226-232, 1986.

325. Sargent EN, Balchum E, Freed AL, et al: Multiple pulmonary calcifications due to coccidioidomycosis, *AJR* 109:500-504, 1970.

326. Sargent EN, Carson MJ, Reilly ED: Roentgenographic manifestations of varicella pneumonia with postmortem correlation, *AJR* 98:305-317, 1966.

327. Sarosi GA, Davies SF: Blastomycosis: state of the art, *Am Rev Respir Dis* 120:911-938, 1979.

328. Sarosi GA, Parker JD, Doto IL, et al: Chronic pulmonary coccidioidomycosis, *N Engl J Med* 283:325-329, 1970.

329. Scheld WM: North American blastomycosis, *Va Med* 110:240-248, 1983.

330. Schwarz J, Baum GL: Actinomycosis, *Semin Roentgenol* 5:58-63, 1970.

331. Schwarz J, Baum GL: Blastomycosis, *Am J Clin Pathol* 21:999-1029, 1951.

332. Schwarz J, Baum GL: Coccidioidomycosis, *Semin Roentgenol* 5:29-39, 1970.

333. Schwarz J, Baum GL: Nocardiosis, *Semin Roentgenol* 5:64-68, 1970.

334. Schwarz J, Baum GL: North American blastomycosis, *Semin Roentgenol* 5:40-48, 1970.

335. Schwarz J, Baum GL: Pulmonary histoplasmosis, *Semin Roentgenol* 5:13-28, 1970.

336. Schwarz J, Baum GL, Straub M: Cavitary histoplasmosis complicated by fungus ball, *Am J Med* 31:692-700, 1961.

337. Scowden EB, Schaffner W, Stone WJ: Overwhelming strongyloidiasis: an unappreciated opportunistic infection, *Medicine* 57:527-544, 1978.

338. Seggev JS, Levin S, Schey G: Unusual radiological manifestations of Q fever, *Eur J Respir Dis* 69:120-122, 1986.

339. Shaffner W, Drutz DJ, Duncan GW, et al: The clinical spectrum of endemic psittacosis, *Arch Intern Med* 119:433-443, 1967.

340. Sheflin JR, Campbell JA, Thompson GP: Pulmonary blastomycosis: findings on chest radiographs in 63 patients, *AJR* 154:1177-1180, 1990.

341. Shin MS, Ho KJ: Computed tomographic characteristics of pleural empyema, *J Comput Tomogr* 7:179-182, 1983.

342. Shin MS, Ho KJ: Broncholithiasis: its detection by computed tomography in patients with recurrent hemoptysis of unknown etiology, *J Comput Tomogr* 7:189-193, 1983.

343. Shin MS, Ho KJ: Computed tomography of bronchiectasis in association with tuberculosis, *Clin Imag* 13:36-43, 1989.

344. Sider L, Davis T: Pulmonary aspergillosis: unusual radiographic appearance, *Radiology* 162:657-659, 1987.

345. Simila S, Ylikorkala O, Wasz-Hockert O: Type 7 adenovirus pneumonia, *J Pediatr* 79:605-611, 1971.

346. Simpson W, Hacking PM, Court SDM, et al: The radiological findings in respiratory syncytial virus infection in children, *Pediatr Radiol* 2:155-160, 1974.

347. Singcharoen T, Rawd-Aree P, Baddely H: Computed tomographic findings in disseminated paragonimiasis, *Br J Radiol* 61:83-86, 1988.

348. Singcharoen T, Silprasert W: CT findings in pulmonary paragonimiasis, *J Comput Assist Tomogr* 11:1101-1102, 1987.

349. Slade PR, Slesser BV, Southgate J: Thoracic actinomycosis, *Thorax* 28:73-85, 1973.

350. Slevin ML, Knowles GK, Phillips MJ, et al: The air crescent sign of invasive aspergillosis in acute leukemia, *Thorax* 37:554-555, 1982.

351. Smith CB, Overall JC: Clinical and epidemiologic clues to the diagnosis of respiratory infections, *Radiol Clin North Am* 11:261-278, 1973.

352. Spencer D, Yagan R, Blinkhorn R, et al: Anterior segment upper lobe tuberculosis in the adult: occurrence in primary and reactivation disease, *Chest* 97:384-388, 1990.

353. Spencer H: *Pathology of the lung*, ed 4, Oxford, Eng, 1985, Pergamon Press.

354. Stark DD, Federle MP, Goodman PC, et al: Differentiating lung abscess and empyema: radiography and computed tomography, *AJR* 141:163-167, 1983.

355. Stead WW: Pathogenesis of the sporadic case of tuberculosis, *N Engl J Med* 277:1008-1012, 1967.

356. Stead WW: Special problems in tuberculosis: tuberculosis in the elderly and in residents of nursing homes, correctional facilities, long-term health care facilities, mental hospitals, shelters for the homeless and jails, *Clin Chest Med* 10(3):397-405, 1989.

357. Stelling CB, Woodring JH, Rehm SR, et al: Miliary pulmonary blastomycosis, *Radiology* 150:7-13, 1984.

358. Stenstrom R, Jansson E, von Essen R: *Mycoplasma* pneumonias, *Acta Radiol [Diagn] (Stockh)* 12:833-841, 1972.

359. Stephen SJ, Uragoda CG: Pleuro-pulmonary amebiasis: a review of 40 cases, *Br J Dis Chest* 64:96-106, 1970.

360. Stevens D, Swift PG, Johnston PG, et al: *Mycoplasma pneumoniae* infection in children, *Arch Dis Child* 53:38-42, 1978.

361. Strutman HR, Rettig PJ, Reyes S: *Chlamydia trachomatis* as a cause of pneumonitis and pleural effusion, *J Pediatr* 104:588-591, 1984.

362. Sweet RS, Wilson ES, Chandler BF: Melioidosis manifested by cavitary lung disease, *AJR* 103:543-547, 1968.

363. Swischuk LE, Hayden CK Jr: Viral vs. bacterial pulmonary infections in children (is roentgenographic differentiation possible?), *Pediatr Radiol* 16:278-284, 1986.

364. Tablan OC, Reyes MP: Chronic interstitial pulmonary fibrosis following *Mycoplasma pneumoniae* pneumonia, *Am J Med* 79:268-270, 1985.

365. Takasugi JE, Godwin JD: Lung abscess caused by *Rhodococcus equi*, *J Thorac Imag* 6(2):72-74, 1991.

366. Taryle DA, Potts DE, Sahn SA: The incidence and clinical correlates of parapneumonic effusions in pneumococcal pneumonia, *Chest* 74:170-173, 1978.

367. Taylor CR, Swett HA: Pulmonary paragonimiasis in Laotian refugees, *Radiology* 143:411-412, 1982.

368. Tew J, Calenoff L, Berlin BS: Bacterial or nonbacterial pneumonia: accuracy of radiographic diagnosis, *Radiology* 124:607-612, 1977.

369. Tillotson JR, Lerner AM: Characteristics of pneumonias caused by *Bacillus proteus*, *Ann Intern Med* 68:287-294, 1968.

370. Tillotson JR, Lerner AM: Characteristics of nonbacteremic *Pseudomonas* pneumonia, *Ann Intern Med* 68:295-307, 1968.

371. Tillotson JR, Lerner AM: Characteristics of pneumonias caused by *Escherichia coli*, *N Engl J Med* 277:115-122, 1967.

372. Torrents C, Alvarez-Castello A, de Vera PV: Postpneumocystis aspergilloma in AIDS: CT features, *J Comput Assist Tomogr* 15:304-307, 1991.

373. Triebwasser JH, Harris RE, Bryant RE, et al: Varicella pneumonia in adults: report of seven cases and a review of the literature, *Medicine* 46:409-423, 1967.

374. Udwadia FE: Tropical eosinophilia, *Prog Respir Res* 7:35-155, 1975.

375. Unger JD, Rose HD, Unger GF: Gram-negative pneumonia, *Radiology* 107:283-291, 1973.

376. Uppal MS, Kohman LJ, Katzenstein ALA: Mycetoma within an intralobar sequestration: evidence supporting acquired origin for this pulmonary anomaly, *Chest* 103:1627-1628, 1993.

377. Vessal K, Yeganehdoust J, Dutz W, et al: Radiological changes in inhalational anthrax: a report of radiological and pathological correlation in two cases, *Clin Radiol* 25:471-474, 1975.

378. Vianna NJ: Nontuberculous bacterial empyema in patients with and without underlying diseases, *JAMA* 215:69-75, 1971.

379. Vikerfors T, Grandien M, Olcen P: Respiratory syncytial virus infection in adults, *Am Rev Respir Dis* 136:561-564, 1987.

380. Vix VA: Radiographic manifestations of broncholithiasis, *Radiology* 128:295-299, 1978.

381. von Lichtenberg F: Infectious diseases. In Robbins SL, Cotran RS, Kumar V, eds: *Pathologic basis of disease*, ed 3, Philadelphia, 1984, WB Saunders, pp 349-350.

382. von Sinner WN: New diagnostic signs in hydatid disease: radiography, ultrasound, CT and MRI correlated to pathology, *Eur J Radiol* 12:150-159, 1991.

383. von Sinner WN, Linjawi T, Al Watban J: Mediastinal hydatid disease: report of three cases, *J Can Assoc Radiol* 41:79-82, 1990.

384. von Sinner WN, Rifai A, te Strake L, et al: Magnetic resonance imaging of thoracic hydatid disease: correlation with clinical findings, radiography, ultrasonography, CT and pathology, *Acta Radiol* 31:59-62, 1990.

385. Waite RJ, Carbonneau RJ, Balikian JP, et al: Parietal pleural changes in empyema: appearance at CT, *Radiology* 175:145-150, 1990.

386. Wallenhaupt SL: Surgical management of thoracic empyema, *J Thorac Imag* 6(3):80-88, 1991.

387. Ward JI, Weeks M, Allen D, et al: Acute histoplasmosis: clinical, epidemiologic and serologic findings of an outbreak associated with exposure to a fallen tree, *Am J Med* 66:587-595, 1979.

388. Webb WR, Sagel SS: Actinomycosis involving the chest wall: CT findings, *AJR* 139:1007-1009, 1982.

389. Weber AL, Bird KT, Janower ML: Primary tuberculosis in childhood with particular emphasis on changes affecting the tracheobronchial tree, *AJR* 103:123-132, 1968.

390. Webster BH: Pleuropulmonary amebiasis: a review with an analysis of ten cases, *Am Rev Respir Dis* 81:683-688, 1960.

391. Weese WC, Shindler ER, Smith IM, et al: Empyema of the thorax, then and now, *Arch Intern Med* 131:516-520, 1973.

392. Wenzl RP, Mccormick DP, Beam WC: Parainfluenza pneumonia in adults, *JAMA* 221:294-295, 1972.

393. Wheat LJ, Kohler RB, Tewari RP: Diagnosis of disseminated histoplasmosis by detection of *Histoplasma capsulatum* antigen in serum and urine specimens, *N Engl J Med* 314:83-88, 1986.

394. Whitehouse WM, Davey WN, Engelke OK, et al: Roentgen findings in histoplasmin-positive school children, *J Mich State Med Soc* 58:1266-1269, 1959.

395. Wiita RM, Cartwright RR, Davis JG: Staphylococcal pneumonia in adults: a review of 102 cases, *AJR* 86:1083-1091, 1961.

396. Williams DM, Krick JA, Remington JS: Pulmonary infection in the compromised host: state of the art, *Am Rev Respir Dis* 114:359-394, 1976.

397. Williford ME, Godwin JD: Computed tomography of lung abscess and empyema, *Radiol Clin North Am* 21:575-583, 1983.

398. Wilson ES: Pleuropulmonary amebiasis, *AJR* 111:518-524, 1971.

399. Winer-Muram HT, Beals DH, Cole FH: Blastomycosis of the lung: CT features, *Radiology* 182:829-832, 1992.

400. Winer-Muram HT, Rubin SA: Pet-associated lung diseases, *J Thorac Imag* 6(3):14-30, 1991.

401. Witorsh P, Utz JP: North American blastomycosis: a study of 40 patients, *Medicine* 47:169-200, 1968.

402. Wolfe JN, Jacobson G: Roentgen manifestations of torulosis (cryptococcosis), *AJR* 79:216-227, 1958.

403. Woodring JH, Vandiviere HM: Pulmonary disease caused by nontuberculous mycobacteria, *J Thorac Imag* 5-2:64, 1990.

404. Woodring JH, Vandiviere JH, Fried AM, et al: Update: the radiographic features of pulmonary tuberculosis, *AJR* 146:497-506, 1986.

405. Wunderink RG, Woldenberg LS, Zeiss J, et al: The radiologic diagnosis of autopsy-proven ventilator-associated pneumonia, *Chest* 101:458-463, 1992.

406. Young EJ, Hirsch DD, Fainstein V, et al: Pleural effusions due to *Cryptococcus neoformans*: a review of the literature and report of two cases with cryptococcal antigen determinations, *Am Rev Respir Dis* 121:743-747, 1980.

407. Young LW, Smith DI, Glasgow LA: Pneumonia of atypical measles: residual nodular lesions, *AJR* 110:439-448, 1970.

408. Young WB: Actinomycosis with involvement of the vertebral column: case report and review of the literature, *Clin Radiol* 11:175-182, 1960.

409. Yu VL, Krobath FJ, Shonnard J, et al: Legionnaires' disease: new clinical perspective from a prospective pneumonia study, *Am J Med* 73:357-361, 1982.

410. Zagoria RJ, Choplin RH, Karstaedt N, et al: Pulmonary gangrene as a complication of mucormycosis, *AJR* 144:1195-1196, 1985.

411. Zahradnik JM: Adenovirus pneumonia, *Semin Respir Infect* 2:104-111, 1987.

412. Zimmerman RA, Miller WT: Pulmonary aspergillosis, *AJR* 109:505-515, 1970.

413. Ziskind MM, Schwarz MI, George RB: Incomplete consolidation in pneumococcal lobar pneumonia complicating pulmonary emphysema, *Ann Intern Med* 72:835-839, 1970.

7 AIDS and Other Forms of Immunocompromise

PAUL DEE

OPPORTUNISTIC PULMONARY INFECTIONS IN AIDS

The acquired immunodeficiency syndrome (AIDS) broke onto the medical scene in 1981.[101,102,189] Since that time there has been an appalling increase in the number of individuals harboring the human immunodeficiency virus (HIV) and in the number of patients dying of AIDS. In sub-Saharan Africa the possibility that AIDS will depopulate certain regions is seriously discussed, and HIV is now making inroads in the Indian subcontinent and Southeast Asia. The majority of AIDS patients have one or more forms of pulmonary disease during the course of their decline. Over the past decade numerous pathologic and microbiologic studies have better defined the incidence, clinical features, and outcome of these various conditions. Based in part on this experience, the increasing tendency has been to treat patients without recourse to invasive studies. However, the rapid increase in the number of AIDS patients is overwhelming the health care system in some geographic areas, necessitating more empiric therapy. Lamentably, only for a limited number of conditions, such as the bacterial pneumonias, *Pneumocystis carinii* pneumonia (PCP), and *Mycobacterium tuberculosis* infection, does specific and tolerably effective therapy exist.

Empiric treatment may be eminently reasonable in the absence of a firm microbiologic or pathologic diagnosis, but clearly the decision to treat must be based on more than a physical examination. The chest radiograph plays a key role in the diagnostic equation. In many instances the chest radiograph strongly suggests a specific diagnosis. The physician must recognize, however, that a specific diagnosis is often impossible even in the face of dramatic radiographic findings. Nevertheless, the chest radiograph has an important function in simply detecting the presence of pulmonary disease and assessing its

---

PULMONARY DISEASES ASSOCIATED WITH HIV INFECTION

INFECTIONS

Bacteria
Community-acquired bacterial pneumonias
  Streptococcus pneumoniae
  Haemophilus influenzae
  *Mycoplasma pneumoniae**
  Legionella species*
  Rhodococcus equi
Nosocomial (hospital-acquired) bacterial pneumonias
  Staphylococcus aureus
  Group B streptococci
  Aerobic gram-negative organisms
Mycobacterium tuberculosis and atypical mycobacteria

Protozoa
Pneumocystis carinii

Viruses
Cytomegalovirus
Herpes simplex virus
Epstein-Barr virus
Varicella-zoster virus*
Respiratory syncytial virus*

Higher bacteria
*Nocardia asteroides**

Fungi
Candidiasis
Cryptococcosis
Histoplasmosis
Coccidioidomycosis
Aspergillosis
Blastomycosis

Parasites
Toxoplasmosis
Cryptosporidiosis
Strongyloidiasis

MALIGNANCIES

Kaposi's sarcoma
Non-Hodgkin's lymphoma
Hodgkin's lymphoma and other malignancies*

LYMPHOPROLIFERATIVE AND ALLIED DISORDERS

Lymphocytic interstitial pneumonitis
Nonspecific interstitial pneumonitis
Lymphocytic bronchiolitis and alveolitis
Pulmonary lymphoid hyperplasia

---

*Association proposed but not definitely proved.

extent, severity, and response to treatment (see box above).

Bacterial infections

Infections with bacteria may be divided into three groups: community-acquired infections, nosocomial (hospital-acquired) infections, and tuberculous infections. Tuberculous infections are dealt with separately because of their special clinical and radiographic features,

epidemiology, and treatment. Community-acquired bacterial pneumonias in HIV-infected individuals tend to occur at less severe degrees of immunocompromise than conditions such as Kaposi's sarcoma, B cell lymphoma, or PCP.[315] Indeed, when pneumonia is diagnosed, the patient may not be known to be infected with HIV, although the presence of *Candida* infection of the oropharynx or hairy cell leukoplakia may be a strong indication of possible infection. Nosocomial infections are most commonly associated with established AIDS and are probably common in the terminal phases of the disease.[184]

The organisms most commonly causing community-acquired pneumonia in HIV-infected individuals are the encapsulated organisms *Streptococcus pneumoniae, Haemophilus influenzae,* and *Moraxella* species.[243,315] These are the same organisms that cause pneumonia in the population at large, but with four times the prevalence. Other species that have been linked to HIV infection include the *Legionella* organisms,[206] *Mycoplasma* species, and *Rhodococcus equi.*[70] The pneumonias have an abrupt onset with fever, cough, dyspnea, and possibly pleuritic chest pain.[243,291] The radiographic findings correspond to those found in the non-HIV-infected population with single or multiple segmental or lobar areas of infiltration or consolidation. HIV-infected individuals are more likely to have multilobar involvement and bacteremia. These, however, are features detected in series analysis and have less immediate diagnostic value in an individual case. Pleural effusions occur and on occasion may progress to empyema. Lymphadenopathy is not a feature. The radiographic diagnosis in uncomplicated cases is usually straightforward. However, PCP may coexist with bacterial pneumonia or alternatively the clinical and radiographic features may overlap. Magnenat and co-workers[180] and Polsky and associates[243] indicate that disseminated bacterial infections can be difficult to distinguish from PCP. In contrast, Amorosa and co-workers[10] compared 30 cases of bacterial pneumonia in AIDS with 30 cases of PCP in AIDS. Broadly speaking, lobar or segmental consolidation or rounded infiltrates with pleural effusions were found in the bacterial pneumonias, the clinical onset of bacterial pneumonia was more abrupt, and the leukocyte count was higher. However, some 20% of the patients in this series had disseminated infiltration indistinguishable from PCP. As discussed later, PCP is sometimes focal and even associated with pleural effusion. Suspicion of possible HIV infection is based largely on other extrapulmonary clinical findings and the clinical history. The spectrum of radiographic findings in community-acquired pneumonias is more fully covered in Chapter 6.

Mycobacterium tuberculosis infections

The number of notifications of tuberculosis in the United States fell by an average of 7% each year until 1985.[41] Since then there has been an upsurge of tuberculosis, almost entirely accounted for by AIDS patients.[238] It appears that tuberculosis in these individuals is usually a reactivation of previously acquired disease.[239] Thus tuberculosis particularly affects intravenous drug abusers in deprived inner cities and immigrants from Third World countries.[46,237,240,276,284] Evidence of previous infection is uncommon in more advantaged population groups. A positive tuberculin reaction has been found in as few as 1.4% of college entrants in the United States.[236] In sub-Saharan Africa a relatively high incidence of lethal tuberculosis may partly explain the lower incidence of PCP in AIDS patients.[2,55,148] Tuberculosis generally becomes manifest at less severe degrees of immunocompromise than other opportunistic infections in HIV-infected individuals.

The pathophysiology of tuberculous infection is directly related to the degree of immunocompromise. With lesser degrees of immunocompromise, tuberculin reactivity may be retained and tuberculosis usually is of the classic cavitary variety involving the apicoposterior segments of the upper lobes and the superior segments of the lower lobes. Adenopathy is not a feature.[46] However, as the immunocompromise worsens, a form of tuberculosis resembling primary tuberculosis develops, even though almost invariably the disease represents reactivation of previously acquired disease. Thus cavitation of pulmonary foci of disease is uncommon, adenopathy is a prominent, even dominant feature, and dissemination throughout the lungs and also systemically is common.[237,239] Tuberculin reactivity is lost in these patients. Dissemination of tuberculosis to kidneys, bone, and other sites may occur in the absence of evidence of pulmonary involvement.

Tuberculosis usually is eminently treatable, although an increasing incidence of drug-resistant strains of *Mycobacterium tuberculosis* is causing concern.[48] These strains are found particularly among intravenous drug abusers, who are notoriously noncompliant with long-term antituberculous therapy. Tuberculosis is often an early infection in HIV-positive individuals at a time at which a positive tuberculin reaction may be expected. Weak reactions are difficult to interpret in those who have been vaccinated with Bacillus Calmette-Guerin (BCG) or environmentally exposed in the past. Later, as tuberculin reactivity wanes, a firm diagnosis depends on identifying the organism in fluids and tissues.

The chest radiograph is important in the diagnosis of tuberculosis. As previously indicated, tuberculosis in tuberculin-positive individuals commonly manifests itself in the classic forms of disease outlined in Chapter 6. In other words, in these individuals the disease has a predilection for the apicoposterior segments of the upper lobes or the superior segments of the lower lobes. Cavitation is common and adenopathy exceptional. The disease tends to be contained, with less pleural or pericardial involvement and fewer instances of miliary disease and systemic dissemination. The tubercle bacillus because of its innate virulence strikes at a level of immunocompromise at which resistance to organisms such as *P. carinii* or *Myobacterium avium* complex is retained.[98] As the level of immunocompromise worsens in HIV-infected individuals, tuberculosis appears to develop even more virulent characteristics. Not only does the individual become anergic to tuberculin, but also the normal microscopic granulomatous response to the tubercle bacillus is dampened or even absent.[130,254] Extrapulmonary dissemination of tuberculosis becomes more common as the disease becomes less contained.

Imaging studies reflect these alterations in the immune response to tuberculous infection. Thus hilar and mediastinal adenopathy is relatively frequent. The actual incidence of adenopathy has varied widely in different series, presumably reflecting differing patient population groups. Incidences of 33%,[55] 48%,[292] 50%,[265] 59%,[238] and 82%[293] however, clearly indicate that adenopathy is a significant finding. Intrathoracic adenopathy has not been a feature of the diffuse lymphadenopathy syndrome found in HIV infection.[290] Therefore intrathoracic adenopathy inevitably signifies an active complication of HIV infection. Focal parenchymal infiltrates and cavitation are less common in this group of patients with more advanced HIV infection, and there is a greater tendency to disseminated involvement of the lungs or miliary infiltration.[45,174,265] The chest film may be normal in the presence of systemic dissemination of tuberculosis.[130,238,293] Pleural effusions are a feature of classic tuberculosis, but the likelihood of pleural involvement appears greater in HIV-infected individuals.[130,265] Tuberculosis may involve the pericardium, resulting in pericardial effusions detectable on chest radiographs or computed tomography (CT). Tuberculous infection may break out from mediastinal nodes to involve the esophagus, resulting in bronchoesophageal fistulas.[6,66] Endobronchial involvement is also a feature of tuberculosis in AIDS.[309]

Reactivation of tuberculosis in less severely immunocompromised HIV-infected individuals results in changes similar to those described in Chapter 6. The major problem is clinicians' awareness. As the incidence of tuberculosis declined, the condition became uncommon and is still unusual in many areas. In hospitals dealing with disadvantaged immigrants or drug-afflicted populations, however, the diagnosis may be regarded as commonplace. Routine testing of population groups with tuberculosis has consistently revealed a high incidence of HIV positivity.[42]

As previously indicated, worsening immunocompromise in HIV-infected individuals profoundly alters the clinical features of tuberculosis. However, this alteration is a continuum without defined thresholds or borders. The trend is toward a form of tuberculosis akin to the primary form found in non-HIV-infected individuals, with hilar and mediastinal adenopathy becoming an increasingly dominant feature. However, this concept may be too simplistic. The virulent spread of tuberculosis both locally and systemically in HIV-infected individuals is quite unlike anything found in classic primary tuberculosis. The cardinal features of tuberculosis in severely immunocompromised AIDS patients are the presence of pleural effusions, hilar and mediastinal adenopathy, and disseminated or miliary infiltration of the pulmonary parenchyma. Cavitation is not a significant feature. These features may be seen alone or in various combinations. Pleural effusions are rare with fungal, viral, or *P. carinii* infections but are common with the bacterial infections and the malignancies such as Kaposi's sarcoma. Hilar and mediastinal adenopathy is a feature of Kaposi's sarcoma and lymphoma as well as *M. avium* complex infections. Disseminated or miliary pulmonary infiltration may occur in nearly all the malignant, infective, and lymphoproliferative disorders encountered in AIDS patients. The extrapulmonary manifestations of tuberculosis may be crucial to the diagnosis. For example, bronchoesophageal fistulas appear to be specific to tuberculosis, and renal and meningeal tuberculosis have specific imaging characteristics. However, the diagnosis hinges on identification of the infecting organism.

Nontuberculous mycobacterial infections

Nontuberculous mycobacterial infections in AIDS patients differ radically from similar infections in non-HIV-infected individuals. The term "AIDS patient" is used advisedly. Unlike *M. tuberculosis,* the atypical mycobacteria infect patients who are severely immunocompromised — in effect, those with established AIDS.[44] A wide range of nontuberculous mycobacteria infect non-HIV-infected individuals, including *M. kansasii, M. fortuitum, M. gordonae,* and *M. avium-intracellulare* (MAI). In AIDS patients *M. avium-intracellulare* predominates. *M. avium-intracellulare* is the responsible organism in at least 95% of cases of atypical mycobacteriosis in HIV-positive individuals.[136] This predominance is probably related more to the ubiquity of these organisms in soil than to any vagary of immune response. Evidence suggests that the main portal of entry is the gastrointestinal tract.[135] *M. avium-intracellulare* more commonly causes enteritis than overt pulmonary disease, and mesenteric and retroperitoneal adenopathy is a frequent finding.[105,119,320] Any mediastinal, cervical, or axillary adenopathy could then simply represent extension of disease from the abdomen via the lymphatic pathways. The diffuse adenopathy could also result from bacteremia, which is common. Although primary involvement of the pulmonary parenchyma does occur, it may be less common than has been supposed. This is radically different from the atypical mycobacterioses in immunocompetent individuals where primary pulmonary involvement is virtually the rule and disseminated disease is exceptionally rare.[136,319]

The immunocompetent individual with atypical mycobacteriosis basically shows an indolent fibrocavitary process in the lung with no evidence of adenopathy or dissemination. Progression is slower than with *M. tuberculosis* infection, but response to antituberculous treatment is disappointing. In AIDS patients a severe fulminant form of the disease develops with pronounced adenopathy often extending widely outside the thorax. Dissemination to the bone marrow, liver, gastrointestinal tract, and other organs is common.

On radiographic examination the dominant feature in the chest is hilar and mediastinal adenopathy (Figure 7-1). CT scans of the chest commonly show adenopathy

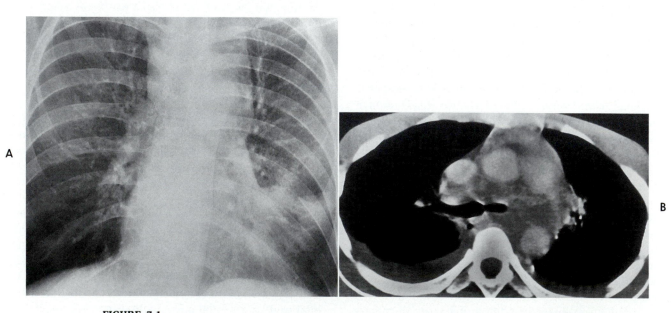

FIGURE 7-1
A, Radiograph of a young man infected with HIV. Note the lingular infiltrate and mediastinal adenopathy. B, Computed tomographic scan shows extensive mediastinal adenopathy.

extending into the abdomen, neck, and axillae. Any pulmonary parenchymal focus present in these cases may be invisible on plain radiographs or may be an entirely nonspecific focal infiltrate in a lobe or segment of a lobe.[185] On the other hand, more diffuse nodular or patchy alveolar infiltrates may occur with or without associated adenopathy.[185,296] Pleural involvement is uncommon. Cavitation in the pulmonary foci of disease is extremely uncommon.[200] Endobronchial lesions have been identified in a few patients, presumably incriminating the airways as a portal of entry.[194,224] Since the patient group with atypical mycobacteriosis has manifest AIDS, other pulmonary complications of AIDS frequently coexist. Adenopathy is a major diagnostic indicator of *M. avium-intracellulare* infection, but in patients without adenopathy the diagnosis may first be revealed by study of bronchial washings, open lung biopsy, bone marrow biopsy, or blood culture. *M. avium-intracellulare* infection in AIDS is extremely resistant to treatment, and the mortality is high.[121,135] Nevertheless, the newer macrolide antibiotic clarithromycin and the rifamycin rifabutin have shown efficacy against *M. avium-intracellulare*. Rifabutin has also shown benefit in the prophylaxis of *M. avium-intracellulare* infection. The view of disseminated MAI infection in terminally ill AIDS patients is changing. Earlier in the AIDS epidemic it was commonly believed that disseminated *M. avium-intracellulare* infection was an incidental finding in a patient dying of other causes, but current opinion is that disseminated *M. avium-intracellulare* infection actually causes morbidity and mortality in AIDS patients.[44,119,135,142]

Pneumocystis carinii pneumonia

The taxonomy of PCP is uncertain. *P. carinii* is either a unicellular protozoan or a primitive fungus.[16,74] Pneumonia caused by this organism is the most common serious complication of HIV infection.[201] Approximately 75% of patients with AIDS have at least one episode of PCP unless chemoprophylaxis is used.[187] PCP before the AIDS epidemic was confined to marasmic infants or patients undergoing chemotherapy and was uncommon even in this subset of patients. The incidence in HIV-infected individuals is so high that chemoprophylaxis against *P. carinii* is widely used in developed countries. Although morbidity and mortality from *P. carinii* infection may be reduced substantially, one outcome of such prophylaxis is that atypical presentations are more common, complicating the diagnosis. For example, fibrotic and granulomatous reactions in the lung may be encountered, whereas in the untreated host inflammatory cells are sparse in the proteinaceous alveolar exudates and reaction is limited to mononuclear infiltration of the interstitium.[25,155] In patients treated with nebulized pentamidine, extrapulmonary spread to lymph nodes, pleura, sinuses, skin, brain, and meninges may be encountered.[8,53,106,303,316]

The development of an immunofluorescence test for antibodies to *P. carinii* has clarified the epidemiology. It appears that antibodies are virtually absent in infants under 1 year, whereas they are present in a substantial majority of individuals older than 4 years.[95,196,234] Thus infestation appears to be relatively common and PCP may be the result of reactivation of latent infection. *P. carinii* organisms have been identified in the otherwise normal lungs of nonimmunocompromised individuals.[62,114,246] PCP in HIV-infected individuals occurs generally when the CD4 lymphocytic count falls below 200 cells/mm^3.[190] This relatively severe degree of immunocompromise is generally more severe than that seen in patients with reactivation of tuberculosis and with community-acquired pneumonia.

The chest radiograph plays a key role in both making the initial diagnosis and monitoring response to treatment. The chest radiograph is abnormal in more than 90% of patients with PCP.[100] The most common radiographic presentation is a diffuse opacity of the lung parenchyma, which is often finely reticular in the very early stages but progresses to more confluent airspace filling (Figures 7-2 and 7-3). The pathologic course of PCP suggests that the apparent ''interstitial'' pattern of infiltration is illusory, since PCP is preeminently an alveolar process.[310] Ordinarily the consolidation is symmetric without zonal predominance, although some perihilar accentuation may be seen (Figure 7-4). However, focal or asymmetric patterns of infiltration may occur (Figure 7-5). In some cases this is due to coincident chronic obstructive pulmonary disease (Figure 7-6). However, patients receiving aerosolized pentamidine show an increased tendency to develop focal parenchymal opacity, particularly in the upper lung zones.[1,43,73,266] It has been suggested that uneven distribution of aerosolized particles within the lung is responsible for the upper zone predominance of pneumonia in such patients.[218] *P. carinii* may, however, have a predilection to involve the apices even in patients not receiving pentamidine prophylaxis.[17] PCP may progress to a picture resembling adult respiratory distress syndrome, with extensive whiteout of major portions of lung. This is less common now that high-dose intravenous steroids are widely administered to patients whose P$_{AO_2}$ falls below 70 mm Hg.

Pneumatoceles in the lungs, particularly in the apices, have been noted with increasing frequency (Figures 7-7 and 7-8).[84,111,164,267] The term ''pneumatocele'' is used here nonspecifically to imply a macroscopic well-defined airspace in the lung parenchyma distinct from a cavity occurring within an inflammatory or neoplastic mass. As Panicek[227] has pointed out, the terminology applied to these ''air cysts'' is confused and theories about their causation vary widely. Some may simply be classic pneumatoceles resulting from a check valve mechanism, usually caused by an inflammatory response. These may be reversible. Others may represent an irreversible breakdown and coalescence of groups of alveoli, again as a result of inflammation. On the other hand, it has been suggested that the airspaces are a form of accelerated or

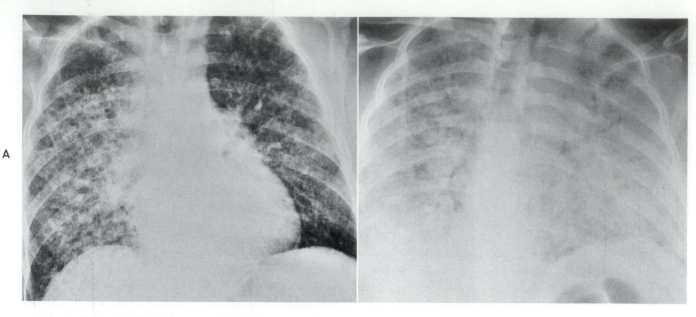

A   B

FIGURE 7-2
Pneumocystis carinii pneumonia in a hemophilic patient with AIDS shows progression to involve all parts of both lungs. **A** and **B**, Two views obtained 5 days apart.

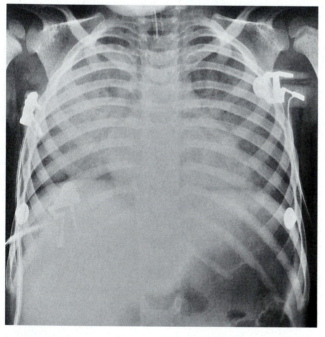

FIGURE 7-3
Two-year-old child with *Pneumocystis carinii* pneumonia showing confluent airspace shadowing.

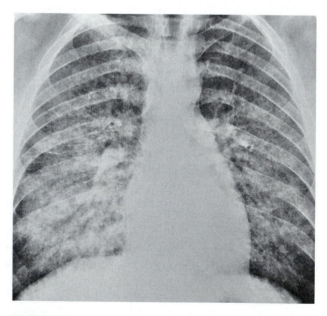

FIGURE 7-4
Twenty-five-year-old man infected with HIV and *Pneumocystis carinii* pneumonia. Note perihilar accentuation of airspace shadowing.

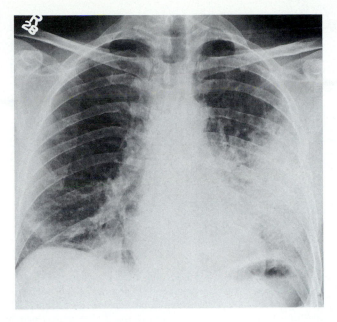

FIGURE 7-5
Pneumocystis carinii pneumonia in a young man with AIDS. Pneumonia is atypical in that it is more asymmetric and focal than usual.

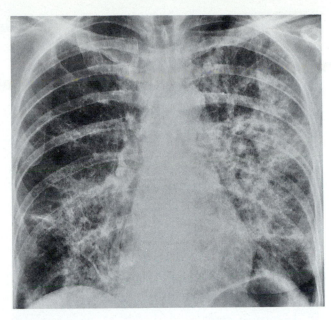

FIGURE 7-6
Pneumocystis carinii pneumonia in middle-aged woman with AIDS and a long history of smoking. Note the irregular coarse distribution of the infiltrates.

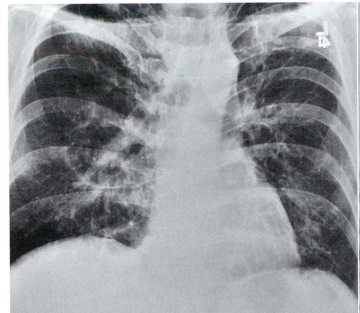

A

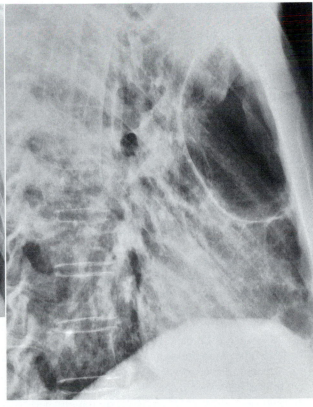

B

FIGURE 7-7
A, Posteroanterior and, **B,** lateral radiographs of an HIV-infected man with pneumatoceles. Patient had been receiving prophylactic treatment with aerosolized pentamidine.

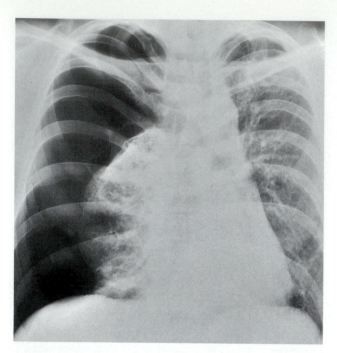

FIGURE 7-8
Pneumothorax resulting from rupture of a pneumatocele in a patient with AIDS-related *Pneumocystis carinii* pneumonia.

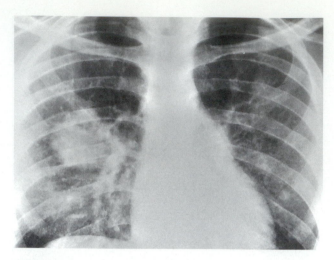

FIGURE 7-9
Radiograph of an intravenous drug abuser infected with HIV. Transbronchial biopsy of the rounded infiltrate in the right lung yielded only *Pneumocystis carinii.* Good response to co-trimoxazole (Bactrim) therapy was seen. (Courtesy Drs. P. Needelman and B. Suster, New York.)

premature aging of lung with the development of bullous emphysema.[164] In this case the unbridled activity of proteases causing alveolar damage is postulated to be the mechanism.[75] Pneumothorax is a common complication of pneumatoceles in such patients.[18,99] Evidence indicates that aerosolized pentamidine is the provoking factor, possibly by causing a more indolent fibrotic or granulomatous response to *P. carinii* infection.[217,268,277] It is also postulated that the more drawn-out response to *P. carinii* infection is related to the organism's tendency to extend to extrapulmonary sites. Within the chest, extension has been seen to the pleura in isolated cases in association with pneumothoraces or effusions[72,134,146,186] and to the lymphatic system with hilar or mediastinal adenopathy.[3,64] In several of these patients CT demonstrated calcification in hilar, mediastinal, and abdominal lymph nodes, as well as calcifications in liver, spleen, kidneys, and the adrenal glands.[107,177,248] The calcification is amorphous, cloudlike, and quite unlike the granular calcifications seen in granulomatous disease. Occasionally the calcification is sufficiently dense to be visualized on plain radiographs. Pleural effusions and adenopathy are, however, rare in association with PCP and when seen inevitably cause diagnostic confusion.

The granulomatous response to *P. carinii* may result in a pulmonary nodule or nodules (Figure 7-9).[15,25,26,118] Cavitation is described in PCP but appears to be uncommon (Figure 7-10).[25,155,205,275,288] The patient with suspected PCP and a normal chest radiograph presents a diagnostic problem. A normal chest radiograph does not exclude PCP.[92,255,301] Gallium scanning is a more sensi-

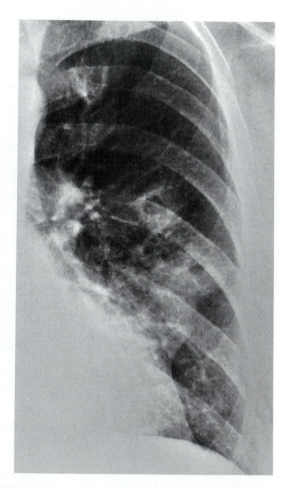

FIGURE 7-10
Example of cavitary *Pneumocystis carinii* pneumonia in a 47-year-old man with AIDS. (Courtesy Drs. P. Needelman and B. Suster, New York.)

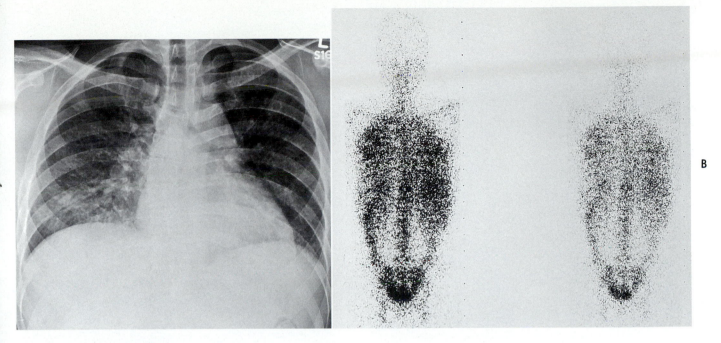

FIGURE 7-11
Pneumocystis carinii pneumonia in a man with AIDS. **A,** Chest radiograph showed early diffuse pulmonary infiltration. **B,** Gallium scan shows markedly increased uptake in lungs.

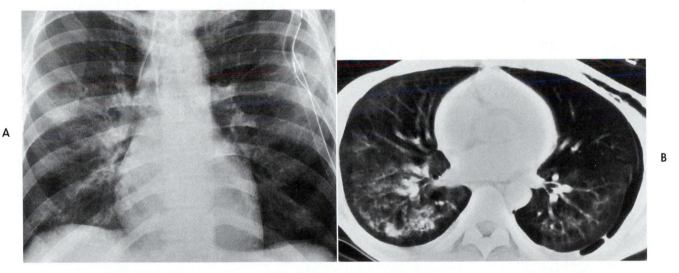

FIGURE 7-12
A, Chest radiograph of a young HIV-infected man with a left pneumothorax. Doubt existed as to the presence of pulmonary infiltrates. **B,** Computed tomographic scan clearly shows a diffuse alveolar filling process later shown to represent *Pneumocystis carinii* pneumonia.

tive method of detecting such pneumonias (Figure 7-11). Gallium-67 scintigraphy is a highly sensitive method of determining the presence of diffuse opportunistic infections of the lungs, with a 95% to 100% sensitivity in patients with PCP.[56,321] A normal ^{67}Ga scan has a predictive value greater than 90% in ruling out PCP. On the other hand, ^{67}Ga scanning has a low specificity, since other opportunistic infections can equally well result in positive scans. With other potential causes of a positive scan, such as lymphoma and lymphocytic interstitial pneumonia, the chest radiograph is unlikely to be normal. Fine-section CT scanning may also indicate the presence of diffuse alveolar opacity in these circumstances but is impractical for widespread use (Figure 7-12).[22,211]

In summary, if an HIV-infected patient has had an insidious onset of fever, cough, and dyspnea with hypoxia

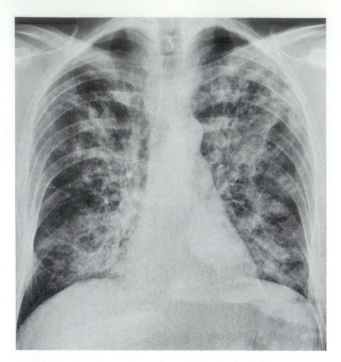

FIGURE 7-13
Pneumocystis carinii pneumonia in a homosexual man with AIDS.
Cytomegalovirus infection is also present.

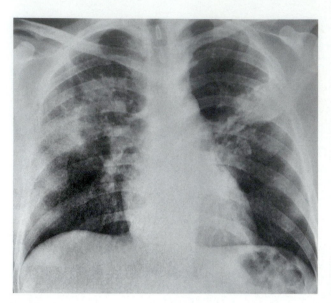

FIGURE 7-14
Nocardia pneumonia in a young homosexual man with AIDS. Note
the ill-defined consolidation in the right lung and a more masslike
consolidation in left lung. Some hilar adenopathy appears to be
present.

and has a chest radiograph showing diffuse pulmonary
infiltration, that patient probably has PCP, particularly if
the CD4 lymphocytic count is less 200 cells/mm³ and the
serum lactic dehydrogenase level is elevated.[326] The
diagnosis of PCP is more likely if the carbon monoxide
diffusing capacity is lowered and the patient shows
arterial oxygen desaturation as a result of exercise (Figure
7-12).

Viral infections of the lungs

Whether viral infection is the specific cause of clinically
evident pneumonia in an HIV-infected individual is
difficult to establish. The body's ability to contain latent
viral infections, notably the herpes simplex group, depends on cell-mediated immunity.[213] It is well recognized
that severe viral pneumonias may complicate other
non-HIV immunosuppressive disorders. By analogy
therefore the viral pneumonias should occur in association with HIV-induced immunosuppression. With an
obvious associated clinical finding such as the widely
disseminated skin eruption of varicella-zoster infection,
the cause of an associated pneumonia is scarcely in
doubt. As it happens, varicella pneumonia is relatively
uncommon in AIDS.[54] The problem arises when a virus
such as the Epstein-Barr virus, herpes simplex virus, or
cytomegalovirus (CMV) is isolated from an HIV-infected
patient with pneumonia (Figure 7-13). That these viruses
can cause pneumonia is known; the question is whether
they invariably result in pneumonia.[143,188,304,307]

The prevailing consensus is that viruses, especially

CMV, are an infrequent cause of pneumonia in HIV-
infected persons. It has been proposed that the following
criteria be met before CMV is accepted as the cause of a
pneumonia: (1) CMV recovered by culture, (2) CMV
inclusion bodies identified in lavage or biopsy samples,
and (3) progressive pneumonia responding to an antiviral
agent known to be effective against CMV.[213] With the use
of these criteria, extremely small numbers of cases have
been identified. The Epstein-Barr virus has been postulated as a cause of the lymphoproliferative disorders of
the lung in AIDS (see later discussion). Viral pneumonias
result in diffuse parenchymal infiltration often indistinguishable from noncardiogenic edema. The shadowing
may be coarser, giving a more reticular or even a slightly
reticulonodular character. Pleural effusions and adenopathy are not seen. Coarser focal airspace filling is not a
feature.

Infections by higher bacteria and the fungi

NOCARDIA ASTEROIDES. *N. asteroides* is a recognized
pulmonary pathogen in otherwise healthy persons (see p.
190).[118] However, it is most common in immunosuppressed patients, whether or not infected with
HIV.[83,169,259] The organism may disseminate to cause
central nervous system abscesses.[160] In the chest the
changes vary. The series of Feigin[83] and Kramer and
Uttamchandani[160] each included 21 patients and have
comparable findings even though Feigin's series did not
involve AIDS patients. Lobar or multilobar consolidations
often involving large portions of lungs appear to be the

most common manifestation. Solitary or multiple, irregular, ill-defined, masslike densities randomly distributed in the lungs are also frequent (Figure 7-14). Cavitation may occur in one third[83] to two thirds[160] of cases. Unilateral or bilateral pleural effusions may occur in one third[160] to one half[83] of cases. Unilateral effusions are associated with the maximally involved lung.[83] Diffuse nodular or reticulonodular infiltrates are described in a minority of cases. Hilar and mediastinal adenopathy may occur in up to one third of patients.[83] Rapid evolution of the pulmonary changes appears to be the norm as befits a bacterial pneumonia. The mortality is high in AIDS patients; nearly half the patients in the report by Kramer and Uttamchandani[160] died despite appropriate treatment.

CANDIDA ORGANISMS. *Candida* organisms, usually *C. albicans*, are a frequent finding on mucous membranes in AIDS patients. Since the organism is part of the normal flora of the skin and mucous membranes, candidiasis is assumed to be endogenous. The mere recovery of the organism is not sufficient to incriminate it as an infective agent in patients with pneumonia. Actual tissue invasion should be demonstrated histologically. Pulmonary candidiasis, when it occurs, is a late manifestation of HIV infection and therefore is commonly associated with other AIDS-related malignancies and infections. The radiographic features are thus inextricably merged with other complications of AIDS. The radiographic features of isolated *Candida* pneumonia are described on p. 251.

CRYPTOCOCCUS NEOFORMANS. The exogenously acquired fungi *Histoplasma capsulatum, Cryptococcus neoformans, Coccidioides immitis, Blastomyces dermatitidis,* and *Aspergillus* species may all cause pneumonia as well as disseminated systemic infections. Cryptococcosis is the most common fungal pulmonary infection in AIDS patients. As in non–AIDS patients, cryptococcal meningitis is more frequent than cryptococcal pneumonia, although the two conditions commonly coexist.[52,327] Cryptococcal pneumonia in HIV-infected individuals shows somewhat different features from those described in nonimmunocompromised patients in that nodular masses are uncommon and lymphadenopathy is a frequent finding.[49,203,308] It appears that the tissue response in HIV infection is altered so that the infection is less contained. Cavitation and pleural effusions tend to occur in AIDS patients.[152] The parenchymal shadowing may be focal or diffuse. When diffuse it may be reticular or reticulonodular. Miliary cryptococcosis has been described in an AIDS patient.[69] The focal infiltrates are nonspecific, ill-defined areas of shadowing, indicating an airspace filling process. There is a clear parallel with the changes of pulmonary cryptococcosis in patients rendered immunocompromised by disease processes other than AIDS.[154] The chest radiographic findings are variable and nonspecific. The associated meningitis, however, is a strong clinical clue to the diagnosis.

HISTOPLASMOSIS. Given that previous infection with histoplasmosis is common in wide areas of the United States, it is perhaps surprising that histoplasmosis is not a more common opportunistic infection in AIDS patients. Histoplasmosis is almost invariably disseminated throughout the body when it occurs in AIDS patients.[29,139,183,311,312] Involvement may include bone marrow, liver, spleen, adrenal glands, lungs, and brain and meninges. Disseminated histoplasmosis in AIDS patients is most frequently encountered in endemic areas. Patients from nonendemic areas invariably have previously traveled in endemic areas, indicating that the disease represents reactivation of latent infection. The onset is usually subacute, with fever and weight loss. Respiratory symptoms, cough, and dyspnea may be noted in up to half the patients.[312] In a small percentage of cases, perhaps 5% to 10%, the onset is acute with a clinical picture resembling gram-negative septicemia.[311] In as many as 40% of cases there is no radiographic evidence of pulmonary involvement.[311] The chest radiographs when abnormal usually indicate widely disseminated disease in contrast to the focal pneumonitis and adenopathy seen in nonimmunocompromised individuals.[57] The pulmonary opacities range from miliary nodulation through a coarser reticulonodular pattern to more extensive airspace shadowing.[38,311] Pleural effusions are rare. Adenopathy is also strikingly uncommon, a feature of some note, considering how significant a finding it is in uncomplicated histoplasmosis: Wheat and co-workers[311] described intrathoracic adenopathy in only 3% to 5% of their cases and in cases from the literature.

COCCIDIOIDOMYCOSIS. Coccidioidomycosis is the second most common endemic systemic fungal infection in the United States, having approximately one fifth of the incidence of histoplasmosis. In nonimmunocompromised individuals systemic dissemination is rare and the disease is a focal granulomatous disease of the lung and related lymph nodes. On the other hand, in AIDS patients pulmonary involvement is almost invariably diffuse, ranging from miliary nodulation to diffuse nodular or reticulonodular shadowing.[32,85,88] Nevertheless, Fish and co-workers[85] found that only 30% of patients with coccidioidomycosis had chest radiographic abnormalities. Hilar and mediastinal adenopathy may occur but is uncommon. More isolated nodular masses, sometimes with cavitation, may be seen. Pleural effusions are not a feature.

ASPERGILLOSIS. Pulmonary aspergillosis appears to be a relatively rare complication of AIDS.[65,82,210,213] The *Aspergillus* species of fungi, most commonly *A. fumigatus,* may cause pneumonia in AIDS patients. This usually occurs in the terminal stages of AIDS when almost inevitably other opportunistic infections or AIDS-related malignancies are present. A major factor contributing to the development of aspergillosis is the neutropenia caused by many of the long-term treatments used in HIV infection, such as AZT, ganciclovir, and chemotherapy for malignancies. *Aspergillus* pneumonia has been better defined in other immunocompromised states, particularly the hematologic malignancies (see pp. 248 and 249).

BLASTOMYCOSIS. Blastomycosis is a rare cause of pulmonary disease in immunocompromised patients, including HIV-infected individuals.[251] Blastomycosis is a late complication of AIDS and occurs almost invariably in association with CD4 lymphocyte counts of less than 200 cells/mm^3.[228] Thus other pulmonary manifestations of AIDS frequently predate or coexist with pulmonary blastomycosis. The condition may be confined to the lungs or be associated with disseminated disease, particularly involving the central nervous system. Pulmonary blastomycosis has been encountered in relatively few AIDS patients, and the pulmonary manifestations have been better defined in patients from the population at large.[113,278,289] The radiographic findings are variable and range from focal lobar consolidation to multiple pulmonary nodules to diffuse miliary or reticulonodular opacities. When the disease is disseminated to extrapulmonary sites, the pulmonary involvement not unexpectedly tends to be diffuse. The focal lobar consolidations may cavitate, and interestingly, pleural involvement with effusions has been described. Hilar and mediastinal adenopathy occurs. Blastomycosis has a predilection to involve the skin, a feature not seen with other opportunistic infections. Biopsy of a skin lesion may provide the diagnosis.

Protozoal infections

Infestation with *Toxoplasma gondii*, *Cryptosporidium*, and *Strongyloides stercoralis* is encountered in HIV-infected individuals. These parasites ordinarily involve extrapulmonary sites, most commonly the brain and meninges or the gastrointestinal tract. Indeed, toxoplasmosis is the most common cause of focal central nervous system lesions in AIDS patients. However, pulmonary involvement that can be ascribed to these parasites is rare. In the limited number of cases described in the literature, the pulmonary infiltration has tended to be diffuse and variably described as alveolar, nodular, or interstitial.[31,159,221,244,271] The diagnosis inevitably relies on lavage or biopsy that reveals one of these parasites in lung tissue. Even then a response to specific chemotherapy is required for confirmation of the diagnosis.

MALIGNANCIES IN AIDS
Kaposi's sarcoma

Before the AIDS epidemic, Kaposi's sarcoma was a rare condition classically involving the skin of the lower extremities in elderly men of Jewish and Mediterranean ancestry. Kaposi's sarcoma, however, is the most common malignancy in AIDS patients, and cutaneous Kaposi's sarcoma is frequently the initial manifestation of the disease.[150] The behavior of Kaposi's sarcoma in HIV-infected individuals is radically different from the classic form of the disease described by Moricz Kaposi.[151] Kaposi's sarcoma associated with HIV is usually widely distributed on the skin and may also be widely disseminated internally, frequently with pulmonary involvement.

The nature of Kaposi's sarcoma is disputed. It may not be a true neoplasm but rather a proliferative reaction to abnormal growth factors.[76] Even before the AIDS epidemic it had been recognized that Kaposi's sarcoma occurred with increased frequency in patients who had conditions associated with altered immune status such as lymphoma, leukemia, and the plasma cell dyscrasias.[264,302] In addition, immunosuppressive therapy for nonmalignant conditions such as autoimmune disease or organ transplantation can result in the development of Kaposi's sarcoma.[77,110,272] The level of immune deficiency appears to play a role. Patients whose AIDS is first manifest as isolated Kaposi's sarcoma are generally less immunosuppressed than those whose first manifestation is opportunistic infections.[162,232] Furthermore, regression of Kaposi's sarcoma may occur either with improving immune status following cessation of immunosuppressive therapy[250] or with worsening immune status in untreated AIDS.[67,144] A hitherto unexplained finding is that Kaposi's sarcoma is much more common in homosexuals than in intravenous drug abusers, suggesting the possibility of a cofactor operating in the homosexual population.[67] This idea has been strengthened by an increased incidence of Kaposi's sarcoma in HIV-negative homosexual men. Unexplained is an apparent decline in the percentage of AIDS cases in all risk groups in whom Kaposi's sarcoma is the basis of the initial diagnosis of AIDS or in whom Kaposi's sarcoma develops at some stage in the disease process.[263] During the 1980s the percentages declined from between 50% and 60% of all patients to between 10% and 20%.[67,263]

Disseminated Kaposi's sarcoma may involve any organ system, including the lung, but the gastrointestinal tract and lymph nodes are the most frequently affected. The true incidence of pulmonary Kaposi's sarcoma is hard to assess. In patients with known disseminated Kaposi's sarcoma the lungs have been found to be involved in 20% to 40% of cases diagnosed during life,[91,220] but the incidence at autopsy may be as high as 50%.[168,193] The presence of cutaneous Kaposi's sarcoma is an important pointer to the possibility of pulmonary involvement. It appears that pulmonary Kaposi's sarcoma is rare in the absence of cutaneous involvement.[168,216] Another clinical pointer is the occurrence of hemoptysis. Involvement of the tracheobronchial tree in Kaposi's sarcoma is relatively frequent, and the lesions are highly vascular. In some cases parenchymal involvement occurs in the absence of endobronchial disease.

The chest radiographic patterns in pulmonary Kaposi's sarcoma are nonspecific, and only broad general pointers can be discerned. A complicating factor is that Kaposi's sarcoma often coexists with opportunistic infections.[220] The chest radiograph may be normal even in the presence of diffuse parenchymal disease shown by biopsy or at autopsy.[61,202] Presumably the threshold for detection would be lower with CT, but it is doubtful that the use of CT would be of practical value. Pulmonary Kaposi's sarcoma may be associated with focal or more commonly with diffuse disease.[61,214,282] Focal segmental or lobar

A 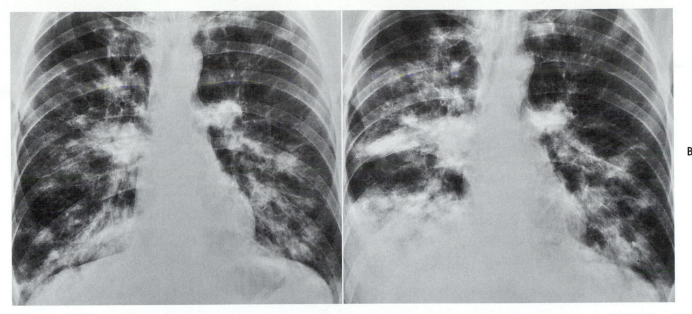 B

FIGURE 7-15
A, Kaposi's sarcoma in a young homosexual man with AIDS. Note the rounded infiltrates with a perihilar and basal distribution set upon a background of some interstitial infiltration. B, Approximately 5 weeks later there has been progression of disease, including the development of a right pleural effusion, but essential character of disease process is little changed.

infiltrates usually represent parenchymal Kaposi's sarcoma, but endobronchial Kaposi's sarcoma may result in atelectasis or postobstructive pneumonia.[214]

Radiographic evidence of diffuse disease may be broadly separated into a pattern of diffuse linear interstitial shadowing and a pattern of diffuse nodular shadowing. In both instances there is a tendency to perihilar predominance, reflecting a bronchocentric distribution of the lesions.[282] There is considerable overlap and coalescence of the changes (Figure 7-15). The diffuse linear pattern reflects an angiomatous type of infiltration of the pulmonary parenchyma, not too dissimilar from lymphangitis carcinomatosa.[61,282] The nodular pattern reflects widespread, often coalescing, parenchymal foci of Kaposi's sarcoma. The pulmonary infiltrates of Kaposi's sarcoma are not subject to significant day-to-day fluctuations in severity as may be the case with pulmonary edema or the pulmonary opportunistic infections.

Clinicians and radiologists are continually faced with patients showing radiographic evidence of diffuse pulmonary infiltration. There are two important pointers to the diagnosis of Kaposi's sarcoma involving the lungs. First, pleural involvement by Kaposi's sarcoma is common and patients may therefore have pleural effusions.[61,91,96,220] Effusions are most often bilateral and may be large. Tuberculosis is the only opportunistic infection that consistently involves the pleura, resulting in large effusions. Second, evidence of hilar and mediastinal adenopathy may be present. Hilar and mediastinal adenopathy has been detected in 25% to 60% of cases in some

series.[61,91,96,282,323] Again, adenopathy is a rare manifestation of opportunistic infections other than mycobacterial infections. On the other hand, the mycobacterial infections are not usually associated with the types of diffuse pulmonary infiltration seen in Kaposi's sarcoma.

Thus an AIDS patient with cutaneous Kaposi's sarcoma as well as pleural effusions or hilar and mediastinal adenopathy or diffuse pulmonary infiltration, or a combination of these, may have intrathoracic Kaposi's sarcoma. Involvement of other organ systems such as the gastrointestinal tract increases the likelihood of Kaposi's sarcoma, as does exclusion of mycobacterial disease by biopsy or culture. Naidich and associates[214] suggest that CT scanning, while not definitive, may be sufficiently characteristic to strongly suggest the diagnosis of pulmonary Kaposi's sarcoma. These authors point to the peribronchial and perivascular distribution of the lesions, which are distinctly nodular in character in some 40% of cases (Figures 7-16 and 7-17). Although effusions, usually bilateral, were found in some 60% of cases in this series, adenopathy was found in only a minority, contrasting with the relatively high incidence in other series. An interesting finding is relatively high CT attenuation of Kaposi's nodes on dynamic scans following a bolus infection of intravenous contrast medium.[128] The high attenuation is thought to reflect the pronounced hypervascularity of foci of Kaposi's sarcoma and was found in 80% of cases in this series. Gallium scanning provides a means of distinguishing between Kaposi's sarcoma and lymphomatous involvement of the lungs. The manifesta-

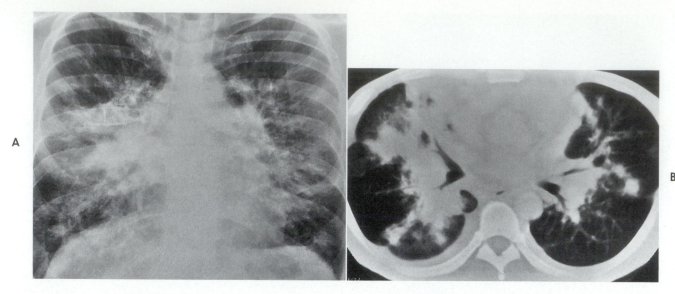

FIGURE 7-16
A, Kaposi's sarcoma in a young homosexual man with a diffuse perihilar infiltrative process. **B**, Computed tomographic scan showing dense fairly circumscribed perihilar infiltrates with central air bronchograms.

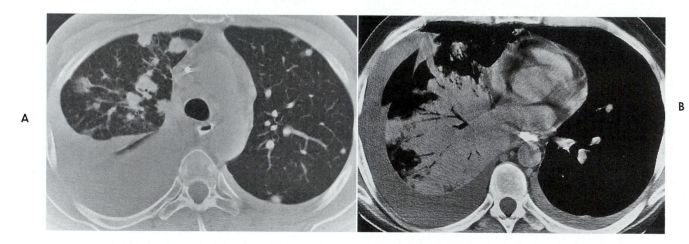

FIGURE 7-17
A, Kaposi's sarcoma in a young homosexual man. Computed tomographic (CT) scan with lung settings showing bilateral pleural effusions and discrete foci of sarcomatous infiltration. **B**, CT scan of the same patient at a lower level, showing massive perihilar infiltration in the right lung with a large associated pleural effusion. Note the air bronchograms. (Courtesy Drs. P. Needelman and B. Suster, New York.)

tions of lymphoma in the chest, especially lymph node involvement, can exactly mimic Kaposi's sarcoma. On the other hand, lymphoma shows avid uptake of gallium, whereas Kaposi's sarcoma shows no uptake or only a low grade of uptake.[165,323] A further refinement is the use of thallium-201 chloride scanning either alone or in sequence with gallium-67 citrate scanning.[166] A variety of neoplasms are thallium avid, including lymphoma, hepatocellular carcinoma, thyroid carcinoma, and bronchogenic carcinoma.[131,299] Kaposi's sarcoma is also thallium avid, whereas infective and inflammatory processes

are not.[166] Thus, with such a two-pronged approach, it is theoretically possible to separate inflammatory processes, Kaposi's sarcoma, and lymphoma. Whether this approach is practicable and cost effective remains to be seen.

Non-Hodgkin's lymphoma

Pulmonary lymphoma is the second most common intrathoracic malignancy linked to HIV infection.[150,242] In the majority of instances the lymphoma is of the B cell non-Hodgkin's type.[4,140,149,170,176] Indeed, the occurrence of non-Hodgkin's lymphoma in an individual infected

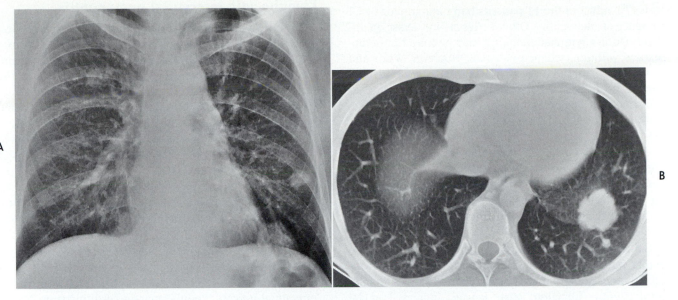

FIGURE 7-18
A, Thirty-three-year-old homosexual man with AIDS dementia and central nervous system toxoplasmosis. Chest radiograph shows pulmonary nodules. B, Computed tomographic scan shows a lobulated lower lobe mass. Biopsy showed immunoblastic lymphoma. (Courtesy Drs. P. Needelman and B. Suster, New York.)

with HIV is accepted as a diagnostic criterion for AIDS.[39] In San Francisco in 1987, non-Hodgkin's lymphoma was the criterion for the diagnosis of AIDS in 5% of cases.[149] Hodgkin's lymphoma, however, is not considered an AIDS-defining diagnosis, even though the manifestations of Hodgkin's lymphoma in HIV-infected individuals are demonstrably more atypical in location and more aggressive than in individuals without HIV infection.[30,140,141,324] Isolated cases of T cell lymphomas or leukemias have been reported, but pulmonary involvement occurs in only a minority.[117,149]

Lymphoma in AIDS is usually widely disseminated, and virtually all cases show extranodal disease. The most frequently involved extrathoracic sites are the central nervous system, bone marrow, liver, spleen, and gastrointestinal tract.[140,324] Lymphoma, non-Hodgkin's or Hodgkin's in type, in AIDS patients is usually of a high-grade aggressive form.[30,324] The clinical course generally is relatively short with a median survival of only some 10 months.[176] This reflects not only the innate aggressiveness of the malignancy but also the fact that any treatment further compromises the patient's already precarious immune system. Lymphoma is often a late feature of AIDS occurring in a severely immunocompromised host. Most patients die as a result of opportunistic infections rather than as a direct result of lymphoma.[156,176]

Although lymphoma in HIV-infected individuals is usually widely disseminated, antemortem evidence of pulmonary involvement is found in less than one third of cases. However, the incidence of pulmonary lymphoma is higher in autopsy series.[175,286] The actual incidence of

pulmonary involvement in clinical studies has varied from zero to 30%.* Primary pulmonary involvement is uncommon.[241,279]

The literature on the imaging features of AIDS-related lymphoma is sparse. Nevertheless, it appears that the chest radiographic and CT appearances in AIDS-related lymphoma do not differ radically from those in nonimmunocompromised patients.[122] The cardinal findings are pleural effusions, lymphadenopathy, and pulmonary opacities or masses occurring together or in isolation (Figure 7-18). Sider and associates[280] found pleural effusions (usually bilateral) to be the most common intrathoracic manifestation of AIDS-related lymphoma; effusions were present in 8 of the 11 patients studied. In one case a unilateral pleural effusion was the sole manifestation of intrathoracic disease.[279,280] The next most common finding in these authors' series was pulmonary parenchymal disease, either diffuse or focal. Focal nodular masses may be single[241] or multiple, resembling metastases.[280] Diffuse interstitial or alveolar shadowing, with or without the presence of pleural effusions, may be present. In Sider and associates' series[280] the radiographic and CT findings could readily have been confused with opportunistic infection or Kaposi's sarcoma. However, meticulous use of aspiration biopsy or open lung biopsy plus extensive microbiologic study in this series allowed proper analysis of the imaging features of AIDS-related lymphoma.

Intrathoracic adenopathy is said to be a distinct feature of AIDS-related lymphoma, but in Sider and associates'

---

*References 23, 140, 149, 176, 280, 324.

series[280] only 3 of the 11 patients had radiographic or CT evidence of adenopathy. Other series are imprecise on this point. Diffuse lymphadenopathy may be found in homosexuals without evidence of AIDS. However, Stern and co-workers[290] found no evidence of intrathoracic adenopathy in the diffuse lymphadenopathy syndrome, a finding confirmed by Suster and co-workers.[293] Suster and co-workers encountered 22 cases of intrathoracic adenopathy out of 106 cases of AIDS. In 21 of the 22 cases the adenopathy was deemed to be caused by opportunistic infections, most commonly *M. tuberculosis* or *C. neoformans.* There are likely to be important clinical pointers to the diagnosis of AIDS-related lymphoma, particularly because extrathoracic lymphomatous involvement is extremely common.

Gallium-67 scanning was used before the AIDS epidemic for staging lymphoreticular malignancies.[19] Another potent cause of intrathoracic adenopathy, *M. avium-intracellulare* infection, also causes increased nodal uptake of gallium-67.[158] Thus it appears that gallium-67 scanning would not be capable of distinguishing definitively between lymphoma and an opportunistic infection. As previously mentioned, Kaposi's sarcoma does not show any avidity for gallium-67 citrate, which distinguishes this entity from lymphoma.

LYMPHOPROLIFERATIVE DISORDERS OF THE LUNG IN AIDS

Individuals infected with HIV, particularly children, may manifest lymphocytic and monocytic infiltration of the airways and the pulmonary parenchyma apparently unrelated to any of the infective processes normally associated with AIDS. It is conceivable that HIV itself is the causative agent, in which case the lymphoproliferative reaction may be an immunologic response to the presence of the virus.[257] At least in HIV-infected adults such a reaction tends to occur at an earlier stage than the complicating opportunistic infections or malignancies, implying that the lymphoreticular system retains residual, although disordered, capability of mounting an immunologic response. Some investigators have incriminated the Epstein-Barr virus, possibly in association with HIV, as a cause of the lymphoproliferative disorders in children.[12,81] The evidence for both HIV and Epstein-Barr virus as a direct causal agent in the lymphoproliferative disorders remains circumstantial, however.

For the purposes of description the lymphoproliferative disorders have been divided into the following types:

1. Lymphocytic interstitial pneumonitis
2. Nonspecific interstitial pneumonitis
3. Lymphocytic alveolitis
4. Lymphocytic bronchiolitis
5. Pulmonary lymphoid hyperplasia

These conditions overlap, and the neat subdivisions are somewhat artificial.

Lymphocytic interstitial pneumonitis

Lymphocytic interstitial pneumonitis (LIP) was first described by Carrington and Liebow in 1962, well before the AIDS epidemic.[36] In the ensuing two decades before the advent of AIDS some 400 cases were described in the literature and the clinical and pathologic features were clearly defined (see p. 333). HIV infection was associated with a striking increase in the incidence of LIP, particularly in children. The occurrence of LIP in an HIV-infected individual under 13 years of age is accepted as a diagnostic criterion for AIDS.[40]

In LIP there is infiltration of the peribronchial interstitial tissues of the lung by mature polyclonal lymphocytes, plasma cells, and immunoblasts. The pleura, blood vessels, and endobronchial tissues are spared. Interstitial fibrosis may develop, but in HIV-associated cases progression of the disease usually precludes the development of much fibrosis. Although LIP is essentially a diffuse interstitial process, nodular masses resulting from coalescence of areas of alveolar airspace obliteration frequently develop, and these masses may be large. Alveolar airspace obliteration may develop as a result of atelectasis produced by peribronchial infiltration, or alternatively the interstitial infiltrates may simply encroach on the airspace.

The radiographic findings when present may be subdivided into three basic types, according to the schema of Oldham and associates[222]:

1. Diffuse fine reticular infiltrates. These are usually most prominent at the lung bases. This is a common feature of interstitial infiltration of the lung and may in part simply reflect the greater width of the lung base (Figure 7-19).

2. Diffuse reticulonodular infiltrates. The nodular component may be variable in severity, but scattered nodules up to 2 cm in diameter may be seen on the background reticulation. Again there is usually basal predominance.

3. Diffuse reticulonodular infiltrates with larger patchy areas of alveolar infiltration, usually basally positioned (Figure 7-20).

Other series have not subjected the radiographic findings to such subdivisions but have clearly indicated the occurrence of basally predominant reticulonodular infiltration.[172,208] Pleural effusions are not a feature of LIP, which reflects the sparing of the pleura in this condition. Hilar and mediastinal adenopathy is not usually found in LIP, and such a finding should immediately raise the possibility of an alternate diagnosis such as *M. avium-intracellulare* infection or malignancy. In a small number of patients bronchiectasis has developed in association with LIP.[9] Although LIP in HIV infection tends to occur at an earlier stage in the individual's immunologic decline, there is overlap with other conditions such as PCP. Nevertheless, LIP tends to wane as the patient deteriorates and more sinister complications develop.

Clinical symptoms include cough, hypoxia with club-

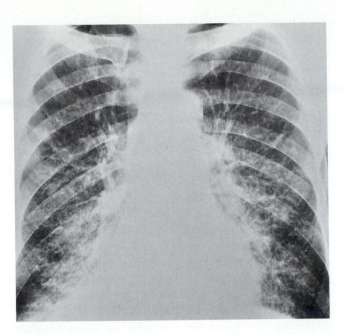

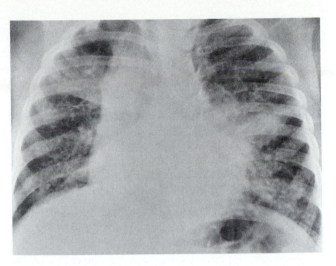

FIGURE 7-20
Radiograph of HIV-infected 3-year-old child with lymphocytic interstitial pneumonitis.

FIGURE 7-19
Radiograph of a 55-year-old Haitian man infected with HIV. Open lung biopsy showed that the pulmonary infiltrates represented lymphocytic interstitial pneumonitis. (Courtesy Drs. P. Needelman and B. Suster, New York.)

bing, dyspnea on exertion, and wheezing. Children may have peripheral adenopathy and salivary gland enlargement. There are, however, no specific hematologic markers or distinct pulmonary function abnormalities. The diagnosis is relatively easy because LIP is relatively common in HIV-infected children, particularly in the second and third years of life. Gallium scanning may be helpful, particularly if the patient also has increased uptake in the salivary glands indicating a parallel lymphoproliferative reaction.[89,270] Such increased salivary gland activity would not be associated with PCP or diffuse lymphoma, other potent causes of increased lung uptake. The chest radiographs can provide only circumstantial evidence, which must be correlated with the clinical features.

Nonspecific interstitial pneumonitis

In some patients a form of interstitial pneumonitis leading to interstitial fibrosis develops. This condition has been termed nonspecific interstitial pneumonitis (NSIP), and there are, for example, resemblances to the changes caused by drug-induced diffuse alveolar damage. In the HIV-infected individual no causal agent has been identified, although there has been speculation that HIV itself may be responsible.[314]

Histologic study shows a usually mild mononuclear infiltration of the lung with edema and fibrin deposition. Thickening of the alveolar walls, hyaline membrane formation, and hyperplasia of the alveolar lining cells

may be seen. Diffuse interstitial fibrosis may ensue. Patients may have cough, fever, and dyspnea on exertion. The chest radiographs may be normal, but a small majority of patients have diffuse reticular or reticulonodular infiltrates.[281] Gallium scans are usually normal or only weakly positive, reflecting perhaps the relatively mild mononuclear cell infiltration.[219]

NSIP is difficult to distinguish from LIP clinically and radiologically. Even the histologic features show overlap, and the distinction may be arbitrary. Exclusion of infective or malignant causes of pulmonary disease may at least allow the diagnosis of interstitial pneumonia, but a decline in the use of lung biopsies may not allow finer subdivision.

Lymphocytic alveolitis, lymphocytic bronchiolitis, and pulmonary lymphoid hyperplasia

Hyperplasia of normal lymphoid foci in the bronchial tree, the bronchial-associated lymphoid tissue (BALT), may be seen in HIV-infected individuals. Lymph nodes are normally found as far peripherally as the fourth-order bronchi, and submucosal lymphoid collections are found down to bronchoalveolar levels, particularly near points of airway bifurcation.[157] Scattered lymphocytes are normally seen in relation to the pulmonary acinus. Hyperplasia of BALT may result in mild obstructive lung disease associated with generalized lymphadenopathy. The hyperplastic BALT may just reach the threshold of radiographic visibility as a fine nodular or miliary infiltration.[78,109,325] Lymphocytic bronchiolitis and alveolitis may be identified by transbronchial biopsy or bronchoalveolar lavage. This infiltration could perhaps represent peripheral extension of lymphoid hyperplasia but also could incline toward LIP. Patients with lymphocytic bronchiolitis and alveolitis may be asymptomatic, and these individuals are likely to have normal chest radiographs as are a proportion of symptomatic patients. Increasing lymphocytic infiltration correlates with the likelihood of symptoms and the occurrence of radiographic evidence of disease. Diffuse interstitial opacities, often basally predominant, are the radiographic evidence of lymphocytic alveolitis. Both pathologic and radiologic findings merge with those of LIP.

PULMONARY INFECTION IN IMMUNOCOMPROMISED PATIENTS

The ability of an individual to combat infections may be impaired by a variety of mechanisms (Table 7-1). In summary, these mechanisms are the following:

1. Granulocytopenia. Granulocytes are an essential line of defense against microorganisms, and any deficiency of their numbers weakens the host's defenses. Granulocytopenia may be a feature of the actual disease process or a consequence of drug or radiation therapy. The incidence of pulmonary infections shows a steep rise as granulocyte counts fall below 1000 cells/mm^3.

2. Reduced cell-mediated immunity. T lymphocyte–dependent immune responses are an important line of defense, particularly against obligate intracellular parasites and nonpathogenic commensal organisms in the respiratory tract.

3. Reduced humoral immunity. Impairment of B lymphocyte function reduces the antibody response to infective agents, diminishing host resistance. A reduction in circulating antibodies may also be a serious feature of hypoglobulinemic states. Similarly, thymic aplasia, asplenia, or splenectomy can result in humoral immunodeficiency, leading to marked susceptibility to infection with organisms such as *S. pneumoniae.*

4. Incompetence of cellular elements. In chronic granulomatous disease an enzymatic defect in the granulocytes renders them incapable of combating certain microorganisms (see later discussion). It has been suggested that silica particles in some way damage pulmonary macrophages and thereby reduce the lungs' ability to mount an adequate response to microorganisms such as *M. tuberculosis* or the fungi.[5,123]

5. Nonspecific reduction in host resistance. Advanced age, alcoholism, diabetes mellitus, starvation or malnutrition, cancer, or other debilitating diseases may reduce an individual's ability to combat infection.

A commonly encountered clinical problem is the immunocompromised patient with fever and pulmonary shadows. Before the differential diagnosis is discussed in more detail, a number of generalized statements may be made in connection with pulmonary disease in the immunocompromised host[261]:

1. Seventy-five percent of pulmonary complications in these patients are due to infection (in patients with severe neutropenia or in those with focal pulmonary lesions the figure is 90%). In the remaining 25% the complications relate to pulmonary drug reactions, pulmonary manifestations of the underlying disease, or unrelated diseases such as cardiac edema or pulmonary emboli. In up to 30% of cases more than one pulmonary complication is present.

2. Diffuse pulmonary shadowing is associated with an overall mortality approaching 50%. Establishing the exact nature of the complication improves the outcome by no more than 10% to 20%. Even at autopsy the exact diagnosis is never established in 15% to 20% of cases.

3. The chest radiograph almost never provides an exact diagnosis; the most that can be expected is a list of differential diagnoses to be correlated with the clinical and laboratory findings.

The boxes on p. 248 outline conditions to be seriously considered when the radiographs indicate segmental or lobar disease, nodular or masslike consolidations, and diffuse lung disease (alveolar or interstitial or both). The large number of possibilities listed in all the boxes graphically illustrates the diagnostic problems involved but in no way diminishes the vital role of the chest radiograph.

Bacterial pneumonias

Bacteria are the most frequent cause of pneumonia in immunocompromised patients. In general terms the pneumonias caused by organisms such as *S. pneumoniae, Staphylococcus aureus,* and *Pseudomonas aeruginosa* do not differ from those in the general population. Patients with neutropenia may show a slight lag in the appearance of pulmonary consolidation, and in the group as a whole, pleural effusions and empyema are uncommon. On occasion, bacterial pneumonias become widely disseminated in the lungs of immunocompromised patients, an occurrence that is unusual in otherwise healthy individuals (Figure 7-21).

Patients receiving steroids and patients with renal transplants are particularly susceptible to *Legionella*-like organisms. These organisms include *L. pneumophila* and *L. micdadei* (Pittsburgh agent). *L. pneumophila* pneumonia shows a spreading pattern of focal consolidation involving wide areas of lung, sometimes with cavitation and pleural effusion. *L. micdadei* pneumonia is particularly prevalent in renal transplant recipients. It has a fairly characteristic radiographic pattern,[245] consisting of fairly well-circumscribed nodular densities that show a distinct tendency to central cavitation (Figure 7-22). The number of these densities is variable, and the distribution may be widespread and random.

Tuberculosis is always feared in non-AIDS immunocompromised patients but is actually rare. This presumably reflects the decline of tuberculosis in the general population. The cases encountered represent reactivation of quiescent lesions, and in these patients there is often a history of previous tuberculosis or a positive tuberculin skin test. The AIDS epidemic has resulted in a recrudescence of tuberculosis in HIV-infected individuals. In a

Table 7-1   Impairment of human immunity to infection

Impaired cell	Nature of immunocompromise	Causes of immunocompromise	Common infecting organisms
Granulocyte	Altered inflammatory response	Acute and chronic myelocytic leukemia Steroids Chemotherapeutic agents Irradiation Chronic granulomatous disease	**Bacteria** 　*Escherichia coli* 　*Staphylococcus aureus* 　*Serratia marcescens* 　*Pseudomonas aeruginosa* 　*Klebsiella pneumoniae* 　*Enterobacter* species 　*Proteus* species 　*Legionella pneumophila* 　*Nocardia asteroides* **Fungi** 　*Aspergillus* species 　*Mucor* species
T lymphocyte	Reduced cell-mediated immunity	Lymphoma Acquired immune deficiency syndrome Steroids Chemotherapeutic agents Irradiation Renal insufficiency Solid organ transplants	**Bacteria** 　*Legionella micdadei* 　*Salmonella* species 　*N. asteroides* 　*Mycobacterium tuberculosis* **Viruses** 　Cytomegalovirus 　Varicella-zoster virus 　Herpes simplex virus 　Respiratory syncytial virus **Fungi** 　*Aspergillus* species 　*Cryptococcus neoformans* 　*Histoplasma capsulatum* 　*Coccidioides immitis* **Parasites** 　*Pneumocystic carinii* 　*Toxoplasma gondii* 　Helminths 　*Strongyloides stercoralis*
B lymphocyte	Reduced antibody formation	Lymphoma Acute and chronic lymphocytic leukemia Multiple myeloma Hypogammaglobulinemia Steroids Chemotherapeutic agents	**Bacteria** 　*E. coli* 　*P. aeruginosa* 　*K. pneumoniae* 　*Streptococcus pneumoniae* 　*Haemophilus influenzae* **Viruses** 　Cytomegalovirus 　Respiratory syncytial virus **Parasites** 　*P. carinii*
Macrophage	Impaired granulomatous response	Silica	**Bacteria** 　*M. tuberculosis* **Fungi** 　*Blastomyces dermatitidis* 　*H. capsulatum*

study of patients with AIDS and complicating tuberculosis, Pitchenik and Robinson[239] found that the radiographic features most often resembled primary tuberculosis despite strong indications that most cases represented reactivation (see p. 231). Tuberculosis resulting from immunosuppressive therapy is clinically and radiographically indistinguishable from reactivation tuberculosis. On rare occasion tuberculosis disseminates in a fulminant fashion, resulting in diffuse pulmonary consolidation (Figure 7-23).

Nocardia asteroides infection is fairly common in immunocompromised hosts, particularly in patients re-

LOBAR OR SEGMENTAL DISEASE (SINGLE OR MULTIPLE FOCI WITH OR WITHOUT CAVITATION AND WITH OR WITHOUT PLEURAL EFFUSIONS)

GRAM-NEGATIVE BACILLI

Klebsiella pneumoniae
Serratia marcescens
Escherichia coli
Proteus mirabilis
Pseudomonas aeruginosa
Haemophilus influenzae
Legionella pneumophila
Legionella micdadei

GRAM-POSITIVE BACILLI

Streptococcus pneumoniae
Staphylococcus aureus

NONINFECTIVE CAUSES

Pulmonary infarction
Lymphoproliferative diseases

DIFFUSE LUNG DISEASE

Pneumocystis carinii
Viruses
    Cytomegalovirus
    Varicella-zoster virus
    Herpes simplex virus
Fungi
    Aspergillus species
    Candida species
    Histoplasma capsulatum
Toxoplasma gondii
Strongyloides stercoralis
Mycobacterium tuberculosis
Noninfective causes
    Nonspecific interstitial pneumonitis
    Drug reactions
    Pulmonary hemorrhage
    Irradiation
    Cardiac or noncardiac edema
    Lymphangitic spread of tumor
    Leukemic infiltration

NODULAR FOCI OF DISEASE WITH OR WITHOUT CAVITATION

Nocardia asteroides
Legionella micdadei
Fungi
    Aspergillus species
    Coccidioides immitis
    Cryptococcus neoformans
    Mucor species
Noninfective causes
    Pulmonary infarction
    Lymphoproliferative disease

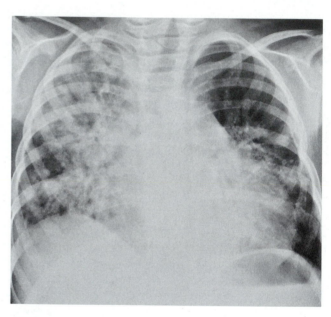

FIGURE 7-21
Disseminated *Escherichia coli* pneumonia in a child with leukemia.

ceiving corticosteroids and immunosuppressive agents. The clinical presentation is subacute, and the radiographic features are slow in development. The radiographic features are discussed on pp. 238 and 239.

Fungal infections

A. fumigatus, a rare cause of primary pneumonia in the general population, has a major role in the immunocompromised group, particularly in patients with lymphoma or leukemia.[124] The pulmonary aspergilloses are a spectrum of disease ranging from bronchopulmonary aspergillosis in the hyperimmune host (see p. 528) to pulmonary mycetoma formation in lung cavities of patients with normal immune status (see p. 206) to invasive pulmonary aspergillosis in immunocompromised hosts.[104] Overlap between these entities occurs, and "semiinvasive" pulmonary aspergillosis has been reported in chronic cavitary disease processes in patients with mild immunocompromise and underlying lung damage.[94] The following discussion is confined to the acute invasive form of pulmonary aspergillosis, which pathologically is characterized by mycotic vascular invasion, thrombosis, and infarction leading to necrosis and cavitation. The lungs may be seeded via the airways (particularly in the more localized forms of disease) or via the bloodstream.

The diagnosis of invasive aspergillosis is not easy,

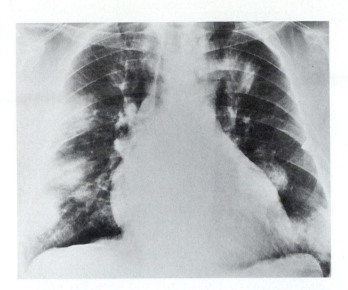

FIGURE 7-22
Renal transplant patient with multiple rounded areas of *Legionella micdadei* pneumonia.

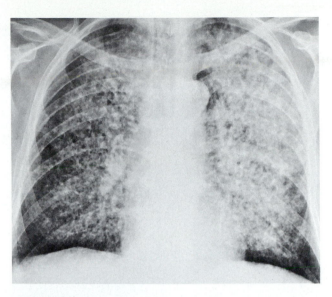

FIGURE 7-23
Leukemic patient with biopsy-proven disseminated tuberculosis. Chest radiograph 1 month earlier was normal in appearance.

particularly in the early phases before cavitation supervenes. In perhaps one third of cases the chest radiographs taken soon after the onset of symptoms are normal.[322] There are basically two initial radiographic patterns: single or multiple areas of consolidation and disseminated miliary or nodular pulmonary shadows. The areas of consolidation are usually rounded, although sometimes they are segmental in shape. The rounded consolidation pattern is by far the most frequent finding in invasive aspergillosis.[171] The regions of rounded consolidation are randomly distributed in the lung, and the margins are indistinct (Figure 7-24). The rounded consolidations appear to represent foci of infarction resulting from *Aspergillus* vascular invasion.[138,223] The result is central coagulative necrosis with a rim of hemorrhagic infarction and inflammatory reaction. CT is particularly suited to demonstrating the rounded nature of the consolidation and the indistinct invasive margin (Figure 7-25).[163] CT may also demonstrate early lesions not visualized on chest radiographs. On isolated occasion an air bronchogram may be seen within the area of consolidation.

Magnetic resonance imaging has been used to investigate invasive pulmonary aspergillosis and appears to be helpful in early diagnosis.[127] The majority of rounded consolidations had a targetlike appearance with MRI, a hypointense center, and an isointense or hyperintense rim on T1-weighted images. Areas of central hemorrhage often resulted in foci of hyperintensity within the low-density central core. Gadolinium enhancement of the rim appeared invariable. Herold and associates[127] also identified a small number of patients with hyperintense segmental disease that generally did not enhance with gadolinium.

Cavitation is not usually seen on the initial radiographs. There is evidence that cavitation occurs with recovery from neutropenia when leukocytes mobilize in the area of infiltration.[93] Thus cavitation is paradoxically a favorable sign indicating a significant defensive response. The earliest sign of cavitation is the air crescent sign in which a lucent crescent of air develops toward the margin of the rounded pneumonia.[60] The air crescent is usually seen toward the upper margin of the pneumonia. The lucency enlarges and extends to form a true cavity, often with mural nodulation (Figure 7-24).[108] An interesting precursor of the air crescent sign, which may be seen on CT, is the development of a band of decreased attenuation around the margin of rounded pneumonia.[163] This CT halo is thought to represent a zone of tissue demarcation in which the air crescent will develop.

The single or multiple areas of rounded pneumonia enlarge slowly over a period ranging from 7 to 28 days and may eventually become segmental or lobar consolidations. Hilar adenopathy is not a feature, and pleural effusions are generally seen only if hemorrhagic infarction results in bleeding into the pleural space. Invasion of the chest wall or mediastinal structures is described but is exceedingly rare.[7,178]

Disseminated pulmonary invasive aspergillosis may arise de novo or complicate the more localized form. The pulmonary shadows in these patients range from a miliary to a more coarsely nodular pattern.[27,171] Hematogenous dissemination from a distant focus, as might be expected, involves the lungs fairly evenly (Figure 7-26), whereas a heavy airway inoculum may give a more central, unevenly distributed pattern of bronchopneumonia (Figure 7-27).

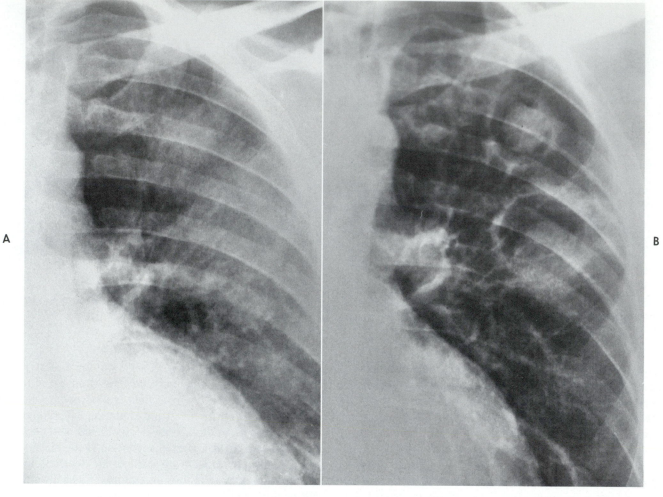

FIGURE 7-24
Aspergillus pneumonia in a leukemic patient. **A,** Nondescript area of consolidation in the lung.
B, Twelve days later two rounded cavities, each with central slough surrounded by rim of air, have
developed while the remainder of the pneumonia has cleared.

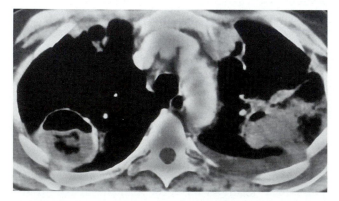

FIGURE 7-25
Leukemic patient with *Aspergillus* pneumonia. Computed tomographic scan shows a well-circumscribed thin-walled cavity containing slough in right lung. Rounded area of pneumonia in the left lung
is less well defined with very early cavitation.

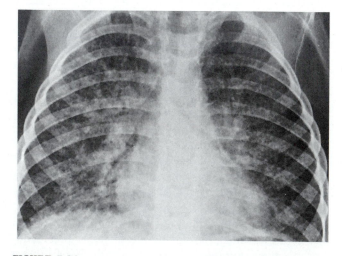

FIGURE 7-26
Disseminated aspergillosis in a child with chronic granulomatous
disease.

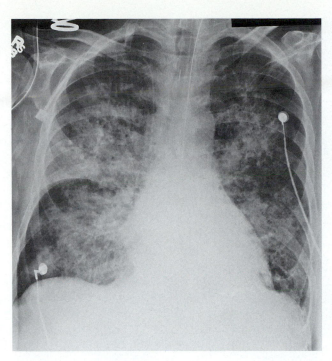

FIGURE 7-27
Disseminated *Aspergillus* pneumonia in a patient with chronic lymphatic leukemia.

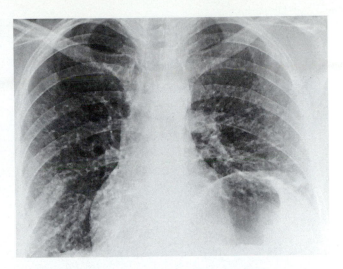

FIGURE 7-28
Biopsy-proven disseminated pulmonary candidiasis in a young man with immunoblastic leukemia.

Candida albicans species may cause pneumonia either alone or in combination with other fungi, particularly *Aspergillus* species. A significant proportion of patients with *C. albicans* pneumonia have leukemia or lymphoma, often in the later stages of treatment.[33] The majority have widespread systemic dissemination of the organism.[63] *Candida* pneumonia without systemic involvement is said to be rare.[260]

The diagnosis of *C. albicans* pneumonia is difficult, partly because pneumonia caused by other opportunistic organisms may also be present and partly because the presence of superficial colonization by *Candida* species may be discounted. Typically the patient with disseminated candidiasis has severe and prolonged neutropenia, persistent fever in spite of antibiotic therapy, hepatomegaly, obvious colonies of *C. albicans* on the mucous membranes, and pulmonary shadowing on chest radiographs. Buff and co-workers[33] have analyzed the radiographic appearances in 20 histologically proven cases of "pure" pulmonary candidiasis. The great majority were identified at autopsy, and the radiographs, obtained within 48 hours of death, presumably reflected advanced disease. Nearly half the patients had radiographic changes suggesting diffuse bilateral nonsegmental patchy disease of an alveolar or mixed alveolar-interstitial character. The remaining patients had unilateral or bilateral lobar or segmental areas of pulmonary consolidation. These authors observed that cavitation, adenopathy, masslike infiltrates, or miliary infiltrates were not observed. In contrast Pagani and Libshitz[226] described a

pattern of miliary-nodular infiltration in pulmonary candidiasis more akin to the findings shown in Figure 7-28. Possibly this pattern represents an earlier manifestation of pulmonary candidiasis. All the patients in the series of Buff and associates[33] died of disseminated candidiasis, whereas the patient illustrated in Figure 7-28 responded satisfactorily to treatment. Dubois, Myerowitz, and Allen[71] failed to find any specific radiographic patterns in pulmonary candidiasis, partly because of the high frequency of other pulmonary infections, edema, and hemorrhage. These authors stressed the need for early institution of antifungal therapy based primarily on clinical grounds.

The phycomycetes *(Rhizopus, Mucor, Mortierella, Absidia,* and *Basidiobolus)* may rarely cause pneumonia in immunocompromised patients. The commonly accepted designation for infection with these species of fungi is mucormycosis. Mucormycosis has a 100% mortality in the absence of treatment and a very high mortality even with aggressive therapy. Approximately 75% of patients with mucormycosis have leukemia or lymphoma, and diabetes mellitus figures prominently among the remainder.[212] The most striking pathologic feature of mucormycosis is fungal vascular invasion resulting in infarction.[197] An inexorable centrifugal pattern of spread is common. This is characteristically seen with infection of the paranasal sinuses, which commonly extends to involve the brain and meninges. The diagnosis of pulmonary mucormycosis is difficult. A single focus of disease in the lung is common, and this may be manifest either as a pulmonary nodule or mass or as lobar consolidation (Figure 7-29).[87,252] Cavitation is frequently seen and is probably related to vascular invasion by the phycomycetes with consequent infarction. The cavity may contain a fungus ball or a slough.[253] Foci of consolidation may be multiple and may spread centrifugally with an

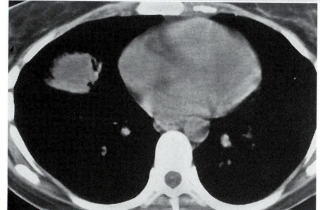

FIGURE 7-29
Mucormycosis. Isolated pulmonary consolidation is seen in the middle lobe in a patient with lymphoma. **A,** Posteroanterior (PA) radiograph. **B,** Computed tomographic scan. **C,** PA radiograph weeks later, showing progression of consolidation.

FIGURE 7-30
Mucormycosis. Widespread areas of consolidation in the lung inexplicably conforming to radiation portals for treatment of lymphoma over a year previously. *Mucor* species identified in multiple transbronchial biopsies.

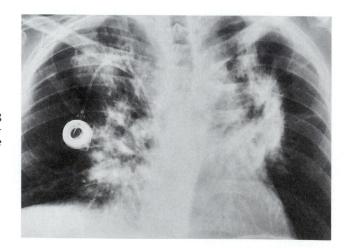

ill-defined edge until the lobar boundaries are reached (Figure 7-30). Pleural effusions are recorded, but direct spread across fissural boundaries has not been reported.

C. neoformans pneumonia occurs in immunocompromised patients (Figure 7-31), although the majority have no demonstrable cellular or humoral immunocompromise. In immunocompromised hosts the pneumonia is often overshadowed by cryptococcal meningitis. Cryptococcal pulmonary infection is discussed in detail on p. 239.

Widespread dissemination of blastomycosis, coccidioidomycosis, and histoplasmosis does occur in immunocompromised patients and has serious consequences, but given the frequency of these diseases in certain geographic areas it is surprising that these fungi are so rarely implicated as opportunistic infective agents. Specific diagnostic features are lacking, and the clinical thrust is likely to be toward excluding infection with the more common opportunistic fungi.

Viral infections

The virus that most commonly causes pneumonia in immunocompromised patients is cytomegalovirus. Infection is typically related to a defect in cell-mediated immunity and therefore occurs in patients with lymphoma or transplants. Cytomegalovirus pneumonia may coexist with or even predispose to other pneumonias, especially PCP. The radiographic appearances are of diffuse interstitial shadows with basal predominance extending from the bases to give a diffuse, patchy, often slightly nodular pattern. The overlap with PCP is considerable both radiologically and pathologically.

The other viruses capable of causing severe pneumonia, especially in patients with lymphoma, are the varicella-zoster virus and the herpes simplex virus. Varicella-zoster pneumonia is fulminant, with the development of extensive patchy areas of parenchymal consolidation that may become widely confluent (Figure 7-32). The diagnosis is much easier if the patient has coincident disseminated herpes zoster or varicella.

Parasitic infections

The protozoan *P. carinii* was first identified in 1909 by Chagas. This organism may be widespread in the animal kingdom as a commensal, and it was only in the 1960s and 1970s that it became widely recognized and sought as a pathogen in immunocompromised individuals. The advent of AIDS in the 1980s has brought PCP into public prominence, since it is the cause of up to 75% of pulmonary complications in AIDS patients and has been a major cause of death in these individuals.

Histologic studies show that PCP is predominantly an alveolar filling process with only a minor interstitial inflammatory component.[62] *P. carinii* rarely penetrates the alveolar wall, and systemic dissemination has been seen only in AIDS patients. PCP is often associated with pneumonia caused by other opportunistic organisms such as cytomegalovirus or fungi. This association may in part explain more focal patterns described in PCP.[191] Nevertheless, the most usual form of PCP is a diffuse synchronous alveolar filling process, which results in death from respiratory insufficiency rather than any systemic toxic effect. Typical or classic imaging findings in PCP are described. For consideration of the variant appearances the reader is referred to the section on AIDS (see pp. 233 to 238).

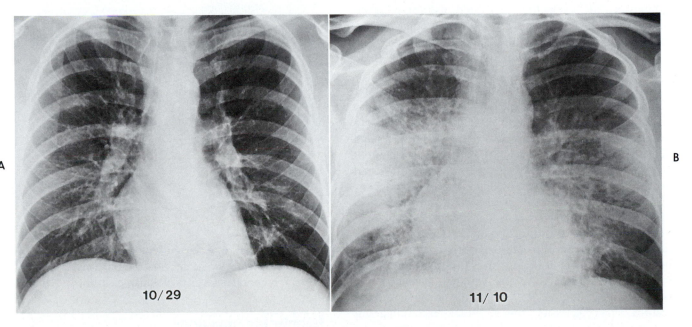

A   10/29   11/10   B

FIGURE 7-31
Cryptococcal pneumonia in a young man with lymphoma.

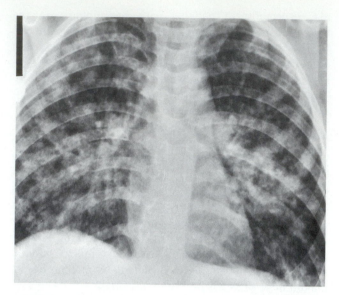

FIGURE 7-32
Varicella pneumonia in a young man with acute myelocytic leukemia.

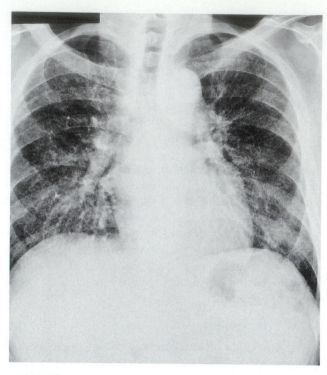

FIGURE 7-33
Pneumocystis carinii pneumonia in a leukemic patient, showing early diffuse infiltration slightly "interstitial" in character.

Patients with PCP commonly have entirely normal chest radiographs in the early phases of the disease.[92,301] In such instances the infiltrates have not reached the threshold of radiographic visibility, even though gallium-67 scans may provide unequivocal evidence of diffuse lung disease. Indeed gallium-67 scanning is a highly sensitive method of determining the presence of diffuse opportunistic infections in the lungs; it has a 95% to 100% sensitivity in patients with PCP.[56,321] A normal gallium-67 scan has a predictive value of over 90% in ruling out PCP.[321] On the other hand, gallium-67 scanning has a low specificity, since other opportunistic infections can equally well result in positive scans.

Even though PCP is predominantly an alveolar filling process, the earliest radiographic changes can appear "interstitial" (Figure 7-33). Thus a diffuse fine nodular pattern is common and there may be a slight reticular component. Progression of disease, however, leads to increasing confluence and density of the shadows, and an alveolar filling pattern becomes increasingly apparent (Figure 7-34). Typically the shadows are diffuse and symmetric with a tendency to spare the lung periphery and apices. With severe involvement, however, this perihilar predominance may be lost and the shadows may involve all parts of the lung. Certain portions of lung may be spared either because of preexisting disease such as bullous emphysema or because they lie within the field of previous irradiation.[86] Normal vascular structures become obscured, and air bronchograms may be a striking feature. This progression from a normal chest radiograph to severe diffuse airspace shadows usually occurs over a 3- to 5-day period. With successful treatment, chest radiographs that were initially normal may remain so.

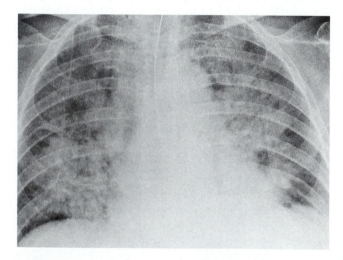

FIGURE 7-34
Autopsy-proven *Pneumocystis carinii* pneumonia in a patient with lymphoma.

Otherwise, the time for pulmonary shadowing to disappear is proportional to their initial severity, with a case of moderate severity usually clearing in 10 to 14 days.

Helminthic infections

Strongyloides stercoralis is a common intestinal parasite in many parts of the world. Infection confined to the intestinal tract may be asymptomatic or cause non-specific complaints such as diarrhea, weight loss, or abdominal pain. Immunocompromise may be associated with a massive proliferation of the organism in the gastrointestinal tract. The filariform larvae penetrate the colonic wall or the perianal skin and migrate to the lungs. An overwhelming burden of larvae may result in systemic dissemination, for example, to the central nervous system. The chest radiograph may be normal, or widespread acinar shadowing may develop.[247] Eosinophilia, a feature of helminthic infections, is often present. The organisms may be detected in the sputum, small bowel aspirates, or the stool. There may be an accompanying gram-negative bacteremia, and this together with the patient's intestinal symptoms may provide a clue to the diagnosis.

DIFFERENTIAL DIAGNOSIS OF PULMONARY SHADOWING IN IMMUNOCOMPROMISED PATIENTS

Fever and pulmonary shadows are a commonly encountered problem in immunocompromised patients. Elucidation of such cases requires consideration of the nature of the immunocompromise (Table 7-1), the results of previous tuberculin testing, whether the infection was acquired in or out of hospital, whether there is any known potential source of infection, and the results of blood or sputum cultures and serologic tests. Janzen and co-workers[145] compared the diagnostic accuracy of CT and chest radiography in immunocompromised non–AIDS patients with acute pulmonary complications. They found that CT and chest radiography have comparable sensitivity in detecting complications in this patient group. CT, however, was distinctly better in the differential diagnosis of complications. In most cases a multipronged approach is necessary to determine the likely diagnosis or decide the basis for rational therapy.

In addition to the infections discussed in the preceding pages, pulmonary shadows in immunocompromised patients may be caused by one or more of the following conditions.

Neoplastic involvement of the lung

Patients with neoplasm, particularly those with leukemia or lymphoma, may be immunocompromised because of the treatment they are receiving or because of the primary disease. In these patients the differential diagnosis of opportunistic pneumonia includes neoplastic involvement of the lung. Leukemic infiltrates, which may produce shadowing indistinguishable from opportunistic pneumonia, are discussed on p. 336. The radiographic differentiation between pneumonia and lymphomatous involvement of the lung can be difficult or impossible, particularly when the pulmonary shadowing is masslike or nodular in appearance. Pleural effusions may occur in both leukemia and lymphoma and do not necessarily indicate a complicating infection.

Pulmonary complications related to therapy

Among the pulmonary complications related to therapy are adverse drug reactions, transfusion reactions, graft versus host reactions, and radiation pneumonitis. The radiographic features of adverse drug reactions and radiation pneumonitis are discussed in Chapter 11. Adverse drug reactions are sufficiently common, particularly with the cytotoxic agents, to make these a real diagnostic possibility as a cause of focal or diffuse pulmonary infiltrates.

Transfusion reactions are usually acute, and the temporal relationship to the transfusion of blood or its fractions is clear. The reaction may simply be one of volume overload with pulmonary edema. More capricious are the agglutinin reactions resulting from an excess of antibodies in the donor serum directed against the recipient's cells, particularly granulocytes. The result is the abrupt onset of fever, chills, tachypnea, and tachycardia coincident with the development of varying patterns of pulmonary edema (Figure 7-35). The edema pattern may persist for 24 to 48 hours, and a response to corticosteroid therapy may occur.

Graft versus host disease occurs in some 25% to 50% of patients following bone marrow transplantation. Transplanted immunocompetent lymphocytes react to the patient's tissues, and in effect the transplanted cells are rejecting the host.[161] Pulmonary manifestations of graft versus host disease develop some 3 to 12 months following transplantation. Symptoms include cough, bronchospasm, and an obstructive pulmonary function pattern. Pathologic study shows a lymphocytic bronchitis and in severe cases bronchiolitis obliterans. The radiographs may, however, remain normal or show only some hyperinflation. Shadowing, usually a patchy perihilar infiltration, may develop in some cases (Figure 7-36). In severe cases a diffuse interstitial pattern is seen in the lungs.[225] The subject of the pulmonary complications of bone marrow transplantation is dealt with more fully on pp. 257 to 259.

Pulmonary hemorrhage

Leukemia may be associated with a profound bleeding tendency, and pulmonary hemorrhage may be one manifestation of this tendency. The clinical features may clearly indicate the bleeding tendency, and the abrupt appearance of patchy acinar densities with hemoptysis and a fall in the hematocrit may allow the diagnosis to be made.

The incidence of pulmonary hemorrhage in leukemia is difficult to ascertain, particularly because the coagulopathy may preclude biopsy. Pulmonary hemorrhage varying from microscopic to massive hemorrhage is seen in some three fourths of leukemic patients at autopsy.[181] Pulmonary hemorrhage may be associated not only with a bleeding tendency, but also with infection or diffuse alveolar damage.[181,285] Tenholder and Hooper[295] suggest that the incidence of pulmonary hemorrhage as a sole

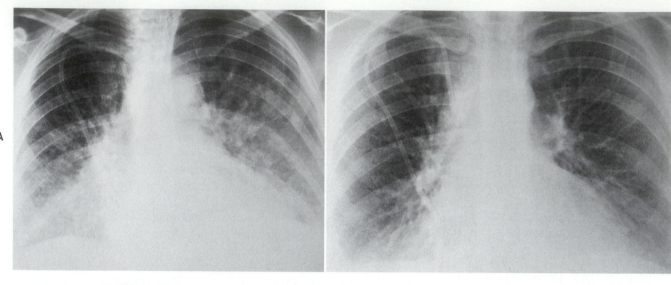

FIGURE 7-35
Agglutinin reaction in a 40-year-old woman who had had a bone marrow transplant. **A,** Chest radiograph at the height of the transfusion reaction. **B,** Chest radiograph 12 hours later following steroid therapy.

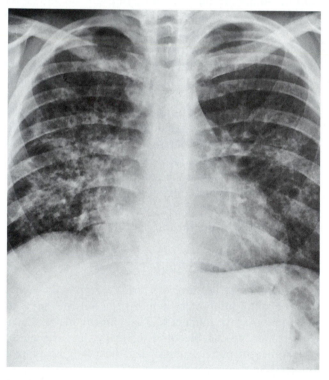

FIGURE 7-36
Graft versus host disease in a leukemic patient 4 months after bone marrow transplantation.

cause of pulmonary shadowing in leukemic patients may be as high as 40%. This seems a high figure, but it does serve to emphasize that pulmonary hemorrhage is probably underdiagnosed.

Nonspecific interstitial pneumonitis

In many cases exhaustive investigation fails to establish the cause of pulmonary densities in an immunocompromised patient. Recourse may then be made to lung biopsy, either open biopsy or by the transbronchial route. In HIV-infected individuals, particularly children, the biopsy may reveal lymphocytic interstitial pneumonitis (see pp. 244 and 245).[222] In a significant number of patients the only result is a diagnosis of nonspecific diffuse alveolar damage and interstitial pneumonitis. Cases in which biopsy is performed tend to be the problematic ones, but in this select group nonspecific interstitial pneumonitis may be found in some 30% to 45%.[153,167,262]

Nonspecific interstitial pneumonitis has been common in AIDS patients with clinically evident pneumonitis. In an exhaustive study Simmons and co-workers[281] found that although 50% of their AIDS patients had PCP, 34% had nonspecific interstitial pneumonitis. Nonspecific interstitial pneumonitis was found to be clinically and radiologically indistinguishable from PCP. Nonspecific interstitial pneumonitis is therefore a highly significant clinical "entity." It seems likely, however, that this "entity" will ultimately prove to have more than one distinct cause.

CHRONIC GRANULOMATOUS DISEASE

In chronic granulomatous disease a hereditary leukocyte defect results in recurrent infections with catalase-positive low-grade pyogenic organisms. Host defense against these organisms is provided by the macrophages with a resultant granulomatous response. The leukocyte defect, which is inherited in the majority of cases as an

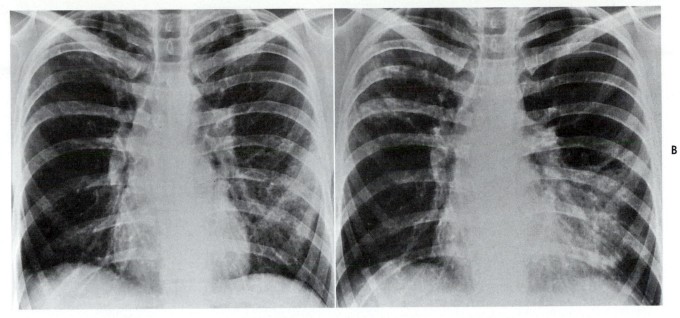

FIGURE 7-37
Chronic granulomatous disease over a 5-year-period of observation in a young man. **A,** Some patchy infiltrates in right lung and lingular pneumonia. **B,** Five years later there are patchy pulmonary infiltrates and scarring, notably in the apices and the left base.

X-linked recessive trait, appears to be an inability to produce the hydrogen peroxide necessary for the destruction of certain organisms, such as coagulase-positive staphylococci, *Escherichia coli,* and *Serratia marcescens.*[147] The defective leukocytes are capable of phagocytosing but not killing these organisms, which may indeed be protected from circulating antibiotics by their intracellular position.[132]

Clinical findings include recurrent skin infections, osteomyelitis, lymphadenopathy, hepatosplenomegaly, persistent rhinitis, and recurrent pneumonia.

The pneumonias are randomly distributed and recurrent. Response to antibiotic therapy is slow and often incomplete, with residual chronic scarring in the lungs (Figure 7-37). Hilar adenopathy is often a prominent feature.[318] Chronic granulomatous disease, however, has ordinarily been diagnosed clinically and by specialized leukocyte studies. The role of chest radiography is primarily to diagnose and follow the recurrent pneumonias.

PULMONARY COMPLICATIONS OF BONE MARROW TRANSPLANTATION

An estimated 2200 allogenic bone marrow transplants were performed in the United States in 1990, a figure that has undoubtedly been exceeded each year since then.[79] Patients are in a much more precarious position following bone marrow transplantation than recipients of solid organ transplants. Pulmonary infections occur in at least half of all bone marrow transplant recipients and are the most significant cause of death.[161] The box above outlines

---

COMPLICATIONS OF BONE MARROW TRANSPLANTATION

Acute graft versus host disease
Chronic graft versus host disease
Noninfectious complications
  Interstitial pneumonitis
  Pulmonary edema
  Pulmonary hemorrhage
  Acute tracheobronchitis
  Pulmonary venoocclusive disease
Infectious complications
  Viral, especially cytomegalovirus
  Bacterial
  Fungal, especially *Aspergillus* species
  Pneumocystis carinii

---

the potential complications of bone marrow transplantation.

Graft versus host disease results from the transplantation of immunocompetent donor lymphocytes, which then in effect attack the recipient's tissues. The common target organs are the skin, liver, and gastrointestinal tract, although other organs, including the lungs, are affected. Acute graft versus host disease occurs 20 to 100 days following the transplant procedure, and the effects are predominantly extrapulmonary with exfoliative dermatitis, diarrhea, and liver dysfunction. Chronic graft versus host disease becomes manifest at least 100 days following the transplant but may be a problem for several months after this. Chronic graft versus host disease occurs in

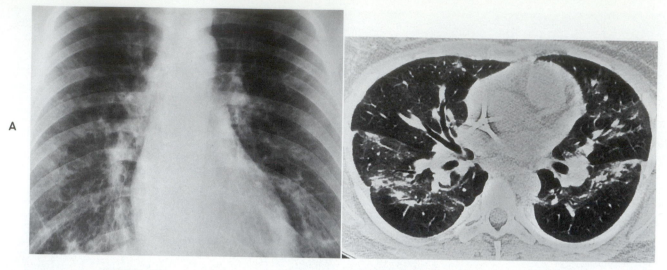

FIGURE 7-38
Graft versus host disease in a bone marrow transplant recipient. **A,** Chest radiograph showing basally preponderant peribronchial infiltration. **B,** Computed tomographic scan more clearly demonstrating peribronchial distribution of disease and also some bronchiectasis.

approximately one third of patients surviving the first 100 days,[179] and its clinical effects are akin to the autoimmune diseases. Thus scleroderma, primary biliary cirrhosis, and the sicca syndrome may be encountered. Chronic graft versus host disease results in a lymphocytic infiltration of the airways and bronchiolitis obliterans.[24,47] It is possible for chronic graphic versus host disease to have radiographic findings.[225] These consist of diffuse patchy perihilar infiltrations reflecting the airway distribution of disease (Figure 7-36). In severe cases a diffuse interstitial pattern is seen in the lungs. CT more clearly demonstrates the bronchocentric distribution of the lesions (Figure 7-38).[103] Nevertheless the chest radiograph may be normal or simply show evidence of hyperinflation. This is particularly the case in patients with bronchiolitis obliterans (Figure 7-39).[147]

Noninfectious complications are frequent. Pulmonary edema may result from drug-induced cardiac and renal damage plus the large fluid loads needed for drug administration and parenteral nutrition. Pulmonary venoocclusive disease has been described in bone marrow transplant recipients[112] and may result in cardiomegaly and signs of cardiac failure. The radiologic features of pulmonary venoocclusive disease are dealt with on p. 401. Pulmonary hemorrhage occurs, but diagnosis is difficult, particularly because hemoptysis is rare.[161] The cause of the hemorrhage is obscure, although the patients may be thrombocytopenic. However, pulmonary hemorrhage occurs most frequently in the absence of any evidence of a coagulopathy.[258] Pulmonary hemorrhage usually develops within 20 days of the transplant and is a fulminant condition with a mortality of approximately 75%. The radiographic changes are or become diffuse; a pattern of confluent alveolar density is the most common manifestation, but approximately one third of patients

show a pattern of reticular interstitial density (Figure 7-40).[317] Interstitial pneumonitis is a frequent complication of marrow transplantation. A diagnosis of interstitial pneumonitis necessitates the exclusion of infective causes as far as is reasonably possible. Patients initially have hypoxia, dyspnea, and a nonproductive cough. Radiographs show diffuse nondescript pulmonary shadowing, often with basal predominance. CT may show a mixed pattern of interstitial and airspace infiltration. The bronchovascular structures tend to remain at least partially visible, in contradistinction to the loss of their outlines in bacterial pneumonias. The pneumonitis may be drug or radiation induced, as may the frequently encountered tracheobronchitis. These patients receive radiation to the whole lung, and the chemotherapeutic doses are formidable, some 10 times greater than for other malignancies.

Infective complications are to be expected in view of the profound and prolonged immunosuppression before the graft "takes." Routine antibiotic coverage has reduced the incidence of pneumonia caused by bacteria and PCP. On the other hand, viral pneumonias, especially with cytomegalovirus, figure prominently. Although the pathogenic significance of cytomegalovirus in other immunocompromised patients is questionable, it appears to be a significant pathogen following bone marrow transplantation.[198] Of the fungi it is the *Aspergillus* species that predominate,[195,235] probably because of the marked impairment of phagocyte function and cell-mediated immunity caused by the total body irradiation and chemotherapy. The pulmonary shadowing is generally nonspecific and should not be interpreted without knowledge of the clinical situation. The alveolar densities of pulmonary hemorrhage, edema, and bacterial pneumonia may be indistinguishable. *Aspergillus* pneumonia may also cause single or multiple ill-defined areas of alveolar shadowing.

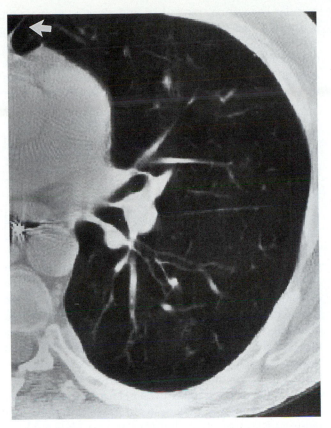

FIGURE 7-39
Bronchiolitis obliterans in a bone marrow transplant recipient. Lungs are slightly hyperinflated (arrow shows increased retrosternal space), and there is mild bronchiectasis. Chest radiograph was normal.

On occasion, highly suggestive signs such as the air crescent sign in invasive aspergillosis may be identified on plain films or by CT (see pp. 248 and 249). Pleural effusions may result from bacterial infection or fluid overload. Interstitial shadowing may result from pulmonary hemorrhage, graft versus host disease, cytomegalovirus pneumonia, and interstitial pneumonitis. CT is more precise in characterizing pulmonary disease. *Aspergillus* pneumonia is manifest as single or multiple rounded but slightly ill-defined areas of alveolar density, usually distinct from the pleural surface. The air crescent sign, when present, is virtually diagnostic. Cavitation or air bronchograms may be seen with *Aspergillus* or other fungal infections.[207] The bronchocentric distribution of the lesions of chronic graft versus host disease and bronchiolitis obliterans may be more readily appreciated. Bacterial pneumonias show diffuse airspace shadowing, usually without any tendency to be rounded or ovoid. Hilar adenopathy indicating a recurrent malignancy may be seen. Although the findings are so often nonspecific, the chest radiograph is valuable in detecting disease in the lungs or the pleura and in determining the rate of progress of response to treatment.

RADIOLOGY OF HEART TRANSPLANTATION

Approximately 2500 heart transplants are performed annually worldwide with an actuarial 5-year survival rate on the order of 70% to 80%.[80,120] By far the most common indications for transplantation are congestive cardiomyopathy and coronary artery disease. Heart-lung transplants are performed mainly for primary pulmonary hypertension, Eisenmenger's syndrome, and complex congenital heart disease. The number of such transplants performed has plateaued at about 200 cases per annum.[80]

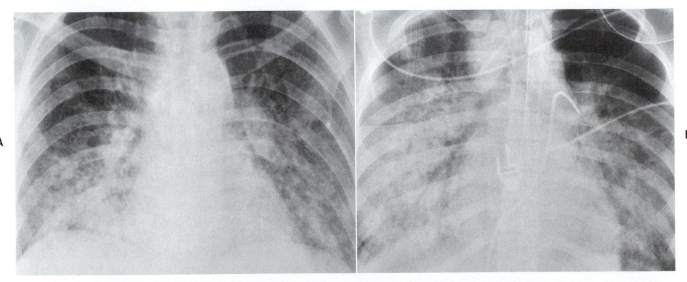

FIGURE 7-40
Pulmonary hemorrhage in a bone marrow transplant recipient. **A,** Initial radiograph showing bibasilar infiltrates. **B,** Twenty-four hours later, infiltrates have become more extensive. Blood was aspirated via the endotracheal tube. Pulmonary wedge pressures were unremarkable. Patient died.

The majority of heart and heart-lung transplant patients encounter problems common to all patients undergoing open heart surgery. A detailed analysis of the radiographic findings after thoracic surgery is beyond the scope of this text; a brief summary is given here as a prelude to a discussion of the pulmonary problems encountered with heart and heart-lung transplantation. Pleural effusions and basal atelectasis are almost inevitable, particularly at the left lung base.[37,297] Pleural effusions may be a response to the handling of the pleura during surgery. Atelectasis may be related to the local compressive effect of the effusions, although postoperative chest pain may play a part. The left lower lobe is particularly prone to atelectasis, possibly because of the compressive effect of the heart, the decreased effectiveness of endotracheal suction in this region, and the comparative frequency of a transient postoperative paresis of the left hemidiaphragm following cardioplegia.[20,313] In the immediate postoperative period the mediastinum should be observed for undue widening, which may indicate postoperative mediastinal hemorrhage.[37] Air in pleural and mediastinal spaces is routinely observed but is rarely significant unless a large pneumothorax develops. Evidence of persisting anterior mediastinal gas collections or a pericardial effusion may be seen in association with anterior mediastinitis.

The transplanted heart, particularly the right-sided chambers, may not function fully in the immediate postoperative period. This may be related to transient ischemic damage to the transplant. Inotropic support usually tides the patient over this period. Nevertheless, pulmonary edema frequently occurs in the immediate postoperative period. The edema may have other or additional causes, including renal insufficiency, excessive fluid administration, or the adult respiratory distress syndrome. However, on occasion acute right-sided failure with decline in the cardiac output ensues because of preexisting pulmonary hypertension. This acute right-sided failure cannot be detected radiographically.

Inevitably, immunosuppressed patients are at risk for infective complications, either locally in the mediastinum and pleura as a direct result of the surgery or in the lungs. The prophylactic use of antimicrobial agents substantially reduces these complications.[11] Just as important is the finer tuning of immunosuppressive regimens allowed by the more liberal use of endomyocardial biopsy to detect early rejection. The infective complications following heart transplantation have no particular features to distinguish them from infections in the other states of immunocompromise. The use of cyclosporine and prophylactic antimicrobial agents has elevated the importance of viruses, especially CMV and herpes simplex virus, as a cause of infection.[14]

Acute and chronic rejection is indicated by clinical, hemodynamic, and radiographic evidence of biventricular dysfunction. Radiographic changes include an increase in the transverse cardiac diameter with signs of pulmonary vascular congestion, interstitial and alveolar edema, and pericardial and pleural effusions. Hyperacute rejection may occur in the immediate perioperative period but is uncommon. Acute rejection commonly occurs 2 weeks to 3 months following transplantation. Chronic rejection may occur at any time in the next months or years. Other remote complications include accelerated atherosclerosis in the graft,[90,305] postpericardiectomy syndrome (Dressler's syndrome), lymphoproliferative disorders, and lymphoid malignancies.[68,116,133,232] Posttransplant lymphoproliferative disease is discussed on pp. 261 to 264.

RADIOLOGY OF LUNG TRANSPLANTATION

The first lung transplant was performed in 1963, and this attempt, like many others in the following two decades, was unsuccessful.[115] Two main problems became apparent.[58] First, it was difficult to maintain adequate immunosuppression and yet avoid infective complications. The lung, after all, is the only organ transplant exposed directly to the environment. Second, interruption of the bronchial circulation made a satisfactory bronchial anastomosis difficult to achieve. The use of steroid immunosuppression aggravated the latter problem. The introduction of cyclosporine was a major advance that ushered in the present era of successful lung transplantation. Not only was the immunosuppression more satisfactory, but the use of steroids could be radically reduced, improving tissue healing. The second decisive step was the introduction of the technique of wrapping the bronchial anastomosis in omentum brought up into the chest through an anterior diaphragmatic tunnel.[59,269] The increased vascularity in the region of the anastomosis greatly enhanced healing. More recently a technique of constructing a bronchial anastomosis after telescoping the donor bronchus into the recipient's bronchus has been applied with success.[28,34] The need for a laparotomy is obviated, and the risk of diaphragmatic herniation is removed. The tracheal anastomosis necessary for a heart-lung transplant is, however, not as susceptible to breakdown, possibly because of preservation of coronary artery to bronchial artery collateral pathways.

Double-lung transplants are now performed much less commonly than single-lung transplants. Probably the major indications for double-lung transplantation are cystic fibrosis and primary pulmonary hypertension. Single-lung transplantation in cystic fibrosis runs the significant risk of infective contamination of the transplanted lung from the native lung. Although some success has been reported with single-lung transplantation for primary pulmonary hypertension,[230] many transplant centers have encountered difficulties and the trend is back to double-lung transplantation or heart-lung transplantation. Single lung transplantation is now performed for a range of conditions that cause respiratory insufficiency, including chronic obstructive pulmonary disease, antitrypsin deficiency, emphysema, lymphangioleiomyoma-

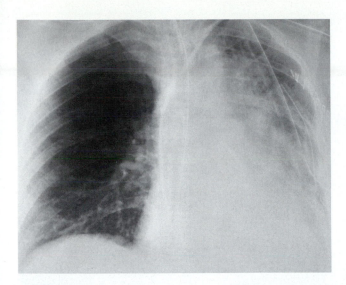

FIGURE 7-41
Radiograph of a patient obtained within 48 hours of left lung transplantation. Edema pattern in the transplanted lung represented an implantation response and gradually cleared.

tosis, and pulmonary fibrosis.[182,192,298] Initial fears that transplanting a normal-sized lung into a chest also containing a markedly hyperexpanded native lung do not appear to have been realized. The right or left lung may be used for single-lung transplantation, although there is a slight technical bias to the left lung, since the left bronchus is longer and easier to anastomose and a greater cuff of the left atrium is left, facilitating the separate use of the heart for transplantation.

Early complications

Complications of lung transplantation may be divided into those occurring in the first month after the transplant and those occurring after this time. The complications in the first month are an acute response to implantation, acute rejection, bronchial dehiscence, infective complications, and atelectasis. The transplantation response appears to be invariable in its occurrence but variable in its severity.[51,125] Alveolar and interstitial edema develops in the transplant within the first 72 hours and subsequently clears slowly (Figure 7-41). The cause of the edema is uncertain, but possibilities include the inevitable ischemia involved in the transplantation procedure, decreased lymph clearance resulting from severance of the central lymphatic pathways, and the effects of lung denervation. The most likely cause is ischemia-reperfusion injury with increased microvascular permeability in the first 24 to 48 hours after the transplantation. The result is a pattern of lung edema of variable severity but sometimes severe enough to cause complete whiteout of the lung. Strategies used to minimize this problem include limiting the ischemic time of the transplanted lung and avoiding any tendency to hypervolemia by limiting the volume of fluid administered in the first 48 to 72 hours. Acute rejection is common in the first month

and may be difficult to distinguish from the implantation response or from infection or pulmonary edema resulting from fluid overload.[126] The patient is usually febrile and hypoxic and commonly shows diffuse pulmonary shadowing. Millet and associates[204] showed that in perhaps 25% of cases the chest radiograph remains normal during episodes of acute rejection. Bergin and co-workers[21] suggest that the development of interstitial edema together with new or increasing pleural effusions in the absence of any increase in heart size or redistribution of pulmonary blood flow usually indicates acute rejection. These authors did not encounter normal chest radiographs in patients with definite biopsy evidence of rejection. The critical distinction between acute rejection and infection is established by transbronchial biopsy.[229,273,294] Additional evidence for rejection is the rapid clinical and radiographic response to bolus injections of high doses of methylprednisolone (Figure 7-42). Infection, particularly CMV or herpes simplex virus pneumonia, is a feared complication. Viral pneumonias cause diffuse pulmonary shadowing, a pattern that is clearly difficult to distinguish from acute rejection. Transbronchial biopsies are necessary for the definitive diagnosis of such infections.

Bronchial dehiscence may result in mediastinal emphysema visible on plain radiographs. CT will diagnose bronchial dehiscence with some certainty by demonstrating extrabronchial air collections in the vicinity of the anastomosis.[125,126] The omentum around the anastomosis is readily identified by CT density measurements and should not be confused with fluid collections or inflammatory masses.[97] In patients who have undergone a telescoped anastomosis the site of anastomosis may be identified on thin-section CT as a bandlike focal constriction of the bronchial lumen. Atelectasis is a frequent complication and is probably related to mucus plugging caused by impaired mucociliary clearance following the bronchial transection. Mucus plugging is readily treated by suction, particularly if the patient is intubated.

Late complications

Complications after the first month include opportunistic infections, rejection, bronchiolitis obliterans, stenosis of the bronchial and pulmonary vascular anastomoses (Figures 7-43 and 7-44), and more remotely lymphoma and lymphoproliferative disorders. As previously mentioned the lung transplant is in direct communication with the environment and the patient and the transplant are thereby exposed to exogenous organisms. However, the infection may be of endogenous origin, representing reactivation of latent infection either in the patient or in the transplanted lung. Reactivation of tuberculosis in a transplanted lung has been described,[35] and CMV and herpes simplex virus may be transmitted in the transplant. The range of opportunistic infections encountered is broadly similar to those seen in other immunocompromised hosts. The impaired mucociliary clearance from the

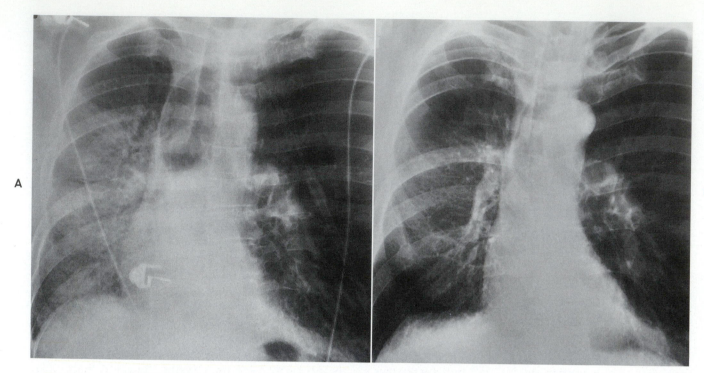

FIGURE 7-42
Episode of acute rejection in a transplanted right lung. **A,** Radiograph showing an edema pattern representing acute rejection in transplanted lung. **B,** Radiograph taken 72 hours after bolus steroid therapy showing complete resolution of the signs of rejection.

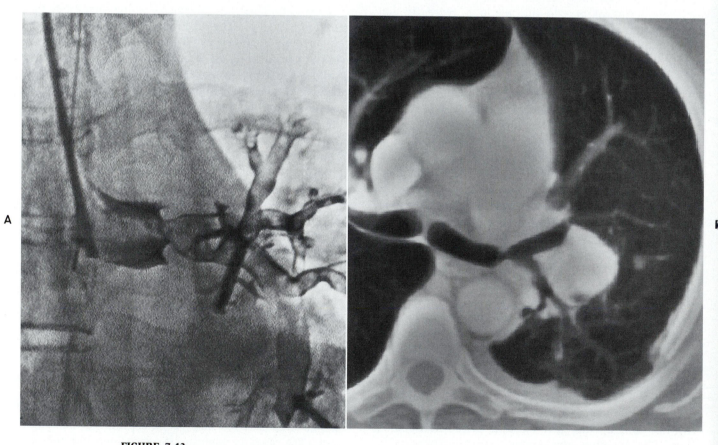

FIGURE 7-43
A, Bronchogram. **B,** Computed tomographic scan showing stenosis of the bronchial anastomosis following left lung transplantation.

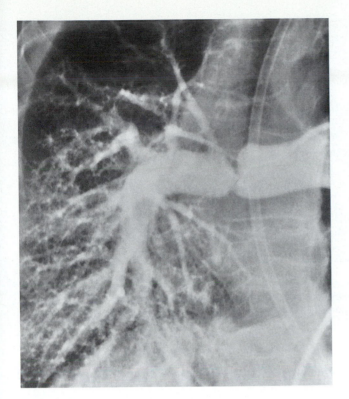

FIGURE 7-44
Pulmonary arteriogram showing a stricture of the vascular anastomosis following right lung transplantation.

transplanted lung is undoubtedly an additional factor predisposing to infection.[129]

REJECTION. Acute rejection episodes may continue to occur, albeit much less commonly than in the immediate postoperative period. Chronic rejection, as the name implies, is a much more indolent process, and in addition chronic rejection changes are usually more focal. Localized foci of pleural and parenchymal scarring with vascular sclerosis are randomly distributed in the transplant. Millet and co-workers[204] found, however, that only 25% of their patients with chronic rejection showed any radiographic evidence of disease. Even then, the focal pulmonary shadows are entirely nonspecific, and rejection can be distinguished with any certainty from pneumonitis only by biopsy.

BRONCHIOLITIS OBLITERANS. Bronchiolitis obliterans is a well-recognized complication of lung transplantation. Probably bronchiolitis obliterans is an expression of chronic rejection. Inexplicably, bronchiolitis obliterans is a much more common complication of heart-lung transplantation than single- or double-lung transplantation.[209,256] The patients have cough and dyspnea, and the pulmonary function tests show a mixture of restrictive or obstructive features. The chest radiograph is likely to be normal in the early stages. Reticular or reticulonodular densities develop, and there may be hyperinflation. The distribution of the densities may be obviously bronchocentric, and evidence of lower lobe bronchiectasis

may be seen.[283] Fine-section CT can be helpful in demonstrating bronchial wall thickening and peripheral bronchiectasis.[169]

BRONCHIAL STENOSES. Bronchial stenoses occur but are fortunately uncommon. The stenosis is readily demonstrated by CT, but bronchoscopy is a more practical method of surveying the anastomotic site. Bronchoscopy also allows laser treatment of granulations and stent placement. Stenosis at the vascular anastomotic site in the pulmonary artery may occur but usually can be corrected by balloon dilatation.

LYMPHOPROLIFERATIVE DISEASE IN ORGAN TRANSPLANT RECIPIENTS

In 2%[231] to 4%[13] of organ transplant recipients, lymphoproliferative disorders ranging from a form of benign lymphoid hyperplasia to frank lymphoma develop.[249] These lymphoproliferative disorders are the result of the immunosuppression and are believed to be induced by the Epstein-Barr virus.[173,215] Some 90% of posttransplant lymphoproliferative disorders (PTLDs) are of B cell lymphocyte origin and span a spectrum from benign polyclonal B cell hyperplasia to monoclonal non-Hodgkin's lymphoma. PTLD is a product of immunosuppression and in approximately two thirds of cases is completely reversible by reducing the level of immunosuppression and administering antiviral agents.[68,287] Nevertheless, PTLD is lethal if untreated, and early diagnosis is vital. The more aggressive forms of PTLD are believed to develop stepwise from benign lymphoid hyperplasia as the B cells proliferate unbridled by the immune system. Kidney transplant patients are less likely to suffer a fatal outcome than recipients of other organ transplants simply because immunosuppression can be completely discontinued and rejection of the transplant accepted. The immunosuppressive regimen plays a role: the more severe the immunosuppression, the earlier PTLD manifests itself. In addition, the use of cyclosporine appears to increase the risk of the development of PTLD.[232] The majority of cases of PTLD become evident within 1 year of transplantation, and children are generally affected earlier than adults.

PTLD has a high incidence of extranodal involvement with the central nervous system, tonsils, gastrointestinal tract, and lungs the common sites of disease.[116] Although involvement may be microscopic and therefore undetectable by imaging techniques, in most cases macroscopic lesions are present. In many instances PTLD is detected during routine chest radiographic follow-up of transplant patients, and observers should be alert to this possibility. In the thorax PTLD most commonly involves the lung parenchyma and the hilar and mediastinal lymph nodes. The thymus and pericardium may be involved on occasion.[68] Pleural effusions may be seen in association with pulmonary PTLD, but isolated involvement of the pleura has not been described.

The most common radiographic abnormality is the

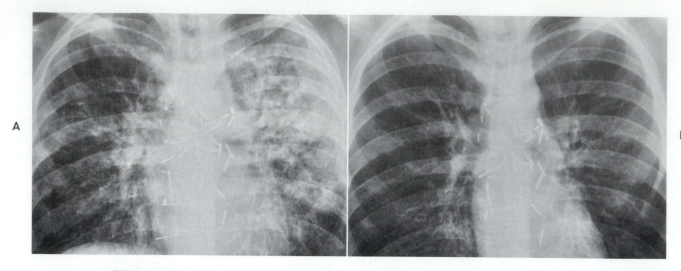

FIGURE 7-45
A, Radiograph of a heart-lung transplant recipient showing biopsy-proven lymphoproliferative disease.
B, Four months later, after adjustment of the immunosuppressive regimen, the lungs are clear.
(Courtesy Dr. C. Fuhrman, Pittsburgh.)

presence of single or multiple pulmonary nodules (Figure 7-45).[116,133,300] These nodules range in size from 1 to 5 cm and are most commonly multiple. The nodules are usually well circumscribed, and growth is relatively slow. Rounded areas of pneumonia are generally poorly circumscribed with more rapid fluctuations in size. Dodd, Ledesma-Medina, and Baron[68] found CT evidence of necrosis within the nodules to be exceptional and indicated that visible necrosis within a pulmonary nodule is more suggestive of an inflammatory process. These authors also identified a small number of cases in which PTLD caused nonspecific airspace shadowing easily confused with edema or pneumonia. Pleural involvement occurs on occasion in conjunction with pulmonary disease, resulting in pleural effusions. However, pleural effusions are commonly found in a range of benign processes, and their presence lacks specificity.[68] Chest radiographs may detect hilar adenopathy and mediastinal masses, but CT is preeminent in this regard. The association of pulmonary nodules with hilar and mediastinal adenopathy is highly suggestive of PTLD. Interestingly, Dodd and associates observed thymic enlargement in 2 of a series of 35 patients with intrathoracic PTLD. These authors suggest that thymic enlargement is an uncommon but sensitive indicator of PTLD. Pericardial effusions may occur, a finding likely to cause some confusion in the case of heart transplants. In the series of Dodd and co-workers radiographic abnormalities attributable to PTLD were found in 80% of patients, emphasizing the importance of imaging. Although some 30% of these patients had concomitant benign disease, only one had an inflammatory pulmonary nodule and none had benign hilar or mediastinal adenopathy. There are no pathognomonic signs of PTLD in the chest, and biopsy confirmation is usually required, particularly in view of the

fundamental change in therapy dictated by a diagnosis of PTLD.

The incidence of malignant neoplasms in organ transplant recipients is some 100 times that in the age-matched general population. Some 20% of these malignancies are lymphomas, and these frequently have significant intrathoracic findings. The incidence of neoplasms common in the general population, such as carcinomas of the lung, breast, prostate, colon, and cervix, is not increased. Cancers in transplant recipients tend to be uncommon ones such as squamous cell carcinomas of the lip and skin, hepatobiliary neoplasms, carcinomas of the vulva and perineum, Kaposi's sarcoma, and other sarcomas.[233] These neoplasms have no particular predilection to involve the thorax.

REFERENCES

1. Abd AG, Nierman DM, Ilowite JS, et al: Bilateral upper lobe *Pneumocystis carinii* pneumonia in a patient receiving inhaled pentamidine prophylaxis, *Chest* 94:329-331, 1988.
2. Abouya YL, Beaumel A, Lucas S, et al: *Pneumocystis carinii* pneumonia: an uncommon cause of death in African patients with acquired immunodeficiency syndrome, *Am Rev Respir Dis* 145:617-620, 1992.
3. Afessa B, Green WR, Williams WA: *Pneumocystis carinii* pneumonia complicated by lymphadenopathy and pneumothorax, *Arch Intern Med* 148:2651-2654, 1988.
4. Ahmed T, Wormser GP, Stahl RE, et al: Malignant lymphomas in a population at risk for acquired immune deficiency syndrome, *Cancer* 60:719-723, 1987.
5. Alison AC, Hart PDA: Potentiation by silica of the growth of *Mycobacterium tuberculosis* in macrophage cultures, *Br J Exp Pathol* 49:465-476, 1968.
6. Allen CM, Craze J, Grundy A: Case report: tuberculous bronchooesophageal fistulae in the acquired immunodeficiency syndrome, *Clin Radiol* 43:60-62, 1991.

7. Altman AR: Thoracic wall invasion secondary to pulmonary aspergillosis: a complication of chronic granulomatous disease of childhood, *AJR* 129:140-142, 1977.

8. Amin MB, Abrash MP, Mezger E, et al: Systemic dissemination of *Pneumocystis carinii* in a patient with the acquired immunodeficiency syndrome, *Henry Ford Hosp Med J* 38:68-71, 1990.

9. Amorosa JK, Miller RW, Laraya-Cuasay L, et al: Bronchiectasis in children with lymphocytic interstitial pneumonia and acquired immune deficiency syndrome: plain film and CT observations, *Pediatr Radiol* 22:603-607, 1992.

10. Amorosa JK, Nahass RG, Nosher JL, et al: Radiologic distinction of pyogenic pulmonary infection from *Pneumocystis carinii* pneumonia in AIDS patients, *Radiology* 175:721-724, 1990.

11. Andreone PA, Olivari MT, Elick B, et al: Reduction of infectious complications following cardiac transplantation, *J Heart Transplant* 5:13-19, 1986.

12. Andiman WA, Eastman R, Martin K, et al: Opportunistic lymphoproliferations associated with Epstein-Barr viral DNA in infants and children with AIDS, *Lancet* 2:1390-1393, 1985.

13. Armitage JM, Kormos RL, Stuart RS, et al: Post-transplant lymphoproliferative disease in thoracic organ transplant patients: ten years of cyclosporine-based immunosuppression, *J Heart Lung Transplant* 10:877-887, 1991.

14. Austin JHM, Schulman LL, Mastrobattista JD: Pulmonary infection after cardiac transplantation: clinical and radiographic correlations, *Radiology* 172:259-265, 1989.

15. Barrio JL, Suarez M, Rodriguez JL, et al: *Pneumocystis carinii* pneumonia presenting as cavitating and noncavitating pulmonary nodules in patients with the acquired immunodeficiency syndrome, *Am Rev Respir Dis* 134:1084-1086, 1986.

16. Barton EG, Campbell WG: *Pneumocystis carinii* in lungs of rats treated with cortisone acetate — ultrastructural observations related to the life cycle, *Am J Pathol* 54:209-236, 1969.

17. Baughman RP, Dohn MN, Shipley R, et al: Increased *Pneumocystis carinii* recovery from the upper lobes in *Pneumocystis* pneumonia: the effect of aerosol pentamidine prophylaxis, *Chest* 103:426-432, 1993.

18. Beers MF, Sohn M, Swartz M: Recurrent pneumothorax in AIDS patients with *Pneumocystis* pneumonia, *Chest* 98:266-270, 1990.

19. Bekerman C, Hoffer PB, Bitram JD: The role of gallium-67 in the clinical evaluation of cancer, *Semin Nucl Med* 24:296-323, 1984.

20. Benjamin JJ, Cascade PN, Wajszczuk W, et al: Lower lobe atelectasis and consolidation following cardiac surgery: the effect of topical cooling on the phrenic nerve, *Radiology* 142:11-14, 1982.

21. Bergin CJ, Castellino RA, Blank N, et al: Acute lung rejection after heart lung transplantation: correlation of findings on chest radiographs with lung biopsy results, *AJR* 155:23-27, 1990.

22. Bergin CJ, Wrath RL, Berry GJ, et al: *Pneumocystis carinii* pneumonia: CT and HRCT observations, *J Comput Assist Tomogr* 14:756-759, 1990.

23. Bermudez MA, Grant KA, Rodvien R, et al: Non-Hodgkin's lymphoma in a population with or at risk for acquired immunodeficiency syndrome: indications for intensive chemotherapy, *Am J Med* 86:71-76, 1989.

24. Beschorner WE, Saral R, Hutchins GM, et al: Lymphocytic bronchitis associated with graft-versus-host disease in recipients of bone marrow transplants, *N Engl J Med* 299:1030-1036, 1978.

25. Birley HD, Buscombe JR, Griffiths MH, et al: Granulomatous *Pneumocystis carinii* pneumonia in a patient with the acquired immunodeficiency syndrome, *Thorax* 45:769-771, 1990.

26. Bleiweiss IJ, Jagirdar JS, Klein MJ, et al: Granulomatous *Pneumocystis carinii* pneumonia in three patients with the acquired immunodeficiency syndrome, *Chest* 94:580-583, 1988.

27. Blum J, Reed JC, Pizzo SV, et al: Miliary aspergillosis associated with alcoholism, *AJR* 131:707-709, 1978.

28. Bolman RM, Shumway SJ, Estrin JA: Lung and heart-lung transplantation evolution and new applications, *Ann Surg* 214:456-470, 1991.

29. Bonner JR, Alexander J, Dismukes WE, et al: Disseminated histoplasmosis in patients with the acquired immune deficiency syndrome, *Arch Intern Med* 144:2178-2181, 1984.

30. Boring CC, Brynes RK, Chan WC, et al: Increase in high grade lymphomas in young men, *Lancet* 1:857-859, 1985.

31. Brady EM, Margolis ML, Korzeniowski OM: Pulmonary cryptosporidiosis in acquired immunodeficiency syndrome, *JAMA* 252:89-90, 1984.

32. Bronnimann DA, Adem RD, Galgiani JN, et al: Coccidioidomycosis in the acquired immunodeficiency syndrome, *Ann Intern Med* 106:372-379, 1987.

33. Buff SJ, McLelland R, Gallis HA, et al: *Candida albicans* pneumonia: radiographic appearance, *AJR* 138:645-648, 1982.

34. Calhoon JH, Grover FL, Gibbons WJ, et al: Single lung transplantation: alternative indications and technique, *J Thorac Cardiovasc Surg* 101:816-825, 1991.

35. Carlsen SE, Bergin CJ: Reactivation of tuberculosis in a donor lung after transplantation, *AJR* 154:495-497, 1990.

36. Carrington CB, Liebow AA: Lymphocytic interstitial pneumonia (abstract), *Am J Pathol* 48:36a, 1966.

37. Carter AR, Sostman HD, Curtis AM, et al: Thoracic alterations after cardiac surgery, *AJR* 140:475-481, 1983.

38. Case records of the Massachusetts General Hospital Case 43-1991, *N Engl J Med* 315:1228-1239, 1991.

39. Centers for Disease Control: Revision of case definitions of acquired immunodeficiency syndrome for national reporting — United States, *MMWR* 34:373-375, 1985.

40. Centers for Disease Control: Revision of the case definition of acquired immunodeficiency syndrome, *MMWR* 36:1-15, 1987.

41. Centers for Disease Control: Tuberculosis, final data — United States 1986, *MMWR* 36:817-820, 1987.

42. Centers for Disease Control Advisory Committee for Elimination of Tuberculosis: Tuberculosis and human immunodeficiency virus infection, *MMWR* 38:236-250, 1989.

43. Chaffey MH, Klein JS, Gamsu G, et al: Radiographic distribution of *Pneumocystis carinii* pneumonia in patients with AIDS treated with prophylactic inhaled pentamidine, *Radiology* 175:715-719, 1990.

44. Chaisson RE, Hopewell PC: Mycobacteria and AIDS mortality, *Am Rev Respir Dis* 139:1-3, 1989.

45. Chaisson RE, Schecter GF, Theuer CP, et al: Tuberculosis in patients with the acquired immunodeficiency syndrome, *Am Rev Respir Dis* 136:570-574, 1987.

46. Chaisson RE, Slutkin G: AIDS commentary: tuberculosis and human immunodeficiency virus infection, *J Infect Dis* 159:96-100, 1989.

47. Chan CK, Hyland RH, Hutcheon MA, et al: Small airways disease in recipients of allogeneic bone marrow transplants, *Medicine* 66:327-340, 1987.

48. Chawla PK, Klapper PJ, Kamholz SL: Drug resistant tuberculosis in an urban population including patients at risk for HIV infection, *Am Rev Respir Dis* 146:280-284, 1992.

49. Chechani V, Kamholz SL: Pulmonary manifestations of disseminated cryptococcosis in patients with AIDS, *Chest* 98:1060-1066, 1990.

50. Chechani V, Zaman MK, Finch PJP: Chronic cavitary *Pneumocystis carinii* pneumonia in a patient with AIDS, *Chest* 95:1347-1348, 1989.

51. Chiles C, Guthaner DF, Jamieson SW, et al: Heart lung transplantation: the post operative chest radiograph, *Radiology* 154:299-304, 1985.

52. Chuck SL, Sande MA: Infections with *Cryptococcus neoformans* in the acquired immunodeficiency syndrome, *N Engl J Med* 321:794-799, 1989.

53. Cohen OJ, Stoeckle MY: Extrapulmonary *Pneumocystis carinii* infections in the acquired immunodeficiency syndrome, *Arch Intern Med* 151:1205-1214, 1991.

54. Cohen RR, Beltrani VP, Grossman ME: Disseminated herpes zoster in patients with human immunodeficiency virus infection, *Am J Med* 84:1076-1080, 1988.

55. Colebunders RL, Ryder RW, Nzilambi N, et al: HIV infection in patients with tuberculosis in Kinshasa, Zaire, *Am Rev Respir Dis* 139:1082-1085, 1989.

56. Coleman DL, Haltner RS, Luce JM, et al: Correlation between gallium lung scans and fiberoptic bronchoscopy in patients with suspected *Pneumocystis carinii* pneumonia and the acquired immunodeficiency syndrome, *Am Rev Respir Dis* 130:1166-1169, 1984.

57. Conces DJ, Stockberger SM, Tarber RD, et al: Disseminated histoplasmosis in AIDS: findings on chest radiographs, *AJR* 160:15-19, 1993.

58. Cooper JD: The evolution of techniques and indications for lung transplantation, *Ann Surg* 212:249-256, 1990.

59. Cooper JD, Pearson FG, Patterson GA, et al: Technique of successful lung transplantation in humans, *J Thorac Cardiovasc Surg* 93:173-181, 1987.

60. Curtis A McB, Walker Smith GJ, Ravin CE: Air crescent sign of invasive aspergillosis, *Radiology* 133:17-21, 1979.

61. Davis SD, Henschke CI, Chamides BK, et al: Intrathoracic Kaposi's sarcoma in AIDS patients: radiographic-pathologic correlation, *Radiology* 163:495-500, 1987.

62. Dee P, Winn W, McKee K: *Pneumocystis carinii* infection of the lung: radiologic and pathologic correlation, *AJR* 132:741-746, 1979.

63. Degregorio MW, Lee WMF, Linker CA, et al: Fungal infections in patients with acute leukemia, *Am J Med* 73:543-548, 1982.

64. Delorenzo LJ, Huang CT, Maguise GP, et al: Roentgenographic patterns of *Pneumocystis carinii* pneumonia in 104 patients with AIDS, *Chest* 91:323-327, 1987.

65. Denning DW, Follansbee SE, Scolaro M, et al: Pulmonary aspergillosis in the acquired immunodeficiency syndrome, *N Engl J Med* 324:654-662, 1991.

66. de Silva R, Stoopack PM, Raufman JP: Esophageal fistulas associated with mycobacterial infection in patients at risk for AIDS, *Radiology* 175:449-453, 1990.

67. DesJarlais DC, Stoneburner R, Thomas P, et al: Decline in proportion of Kaposi's sarcoma among cases of AIDS in multiple risk groups in New York City, *Lancet* 2:1024-1025, 1987.

68. Dodd GD, Ledesma-Medina J, Baron RL: Post transplant lymphoproliferative disorders: intrathoracic manifestations, *Radiology* 184:65-69, 1992.

69. Douketis JD, Kesten S: Miliary pulmonary cryptococcosis in a patient with the acquired immunodeficiency syndrome, *Thorax* 48:402-403, 1993.

70. Drancourt M, Bonnet E, Gallais H, et al: *Rhodococcus equi* infection in patients with AIDS, *J Infect* 24:123-131, 1992.

71. Dubois PJ, Myerowitz RL, Allen CM: Pathoradiologic correlation of pulmonary candidiasis in immunosuppressed patients, *Cancer* 40:1026-1036, 1977.

72. Dyner TS, Lang W, Busch DF, et al: Intravascular and pleural involvement by *Pneumocystis carinii* in a patient with acquired immunodeficiency syndrome (AIDS) (letter), *Ann Intern Med* 111:94, 1989.

73. Edelstern H, McCabe RE: Atypical presentations of *Pneumocystis carinii* pneumonia in patients receiving inhaled pentamidine prophylaxis, *Chest* 98:1366-1369, 1990.

74. Edman JC, Kovacs JA, Drake JC, et al: Ribosomal RNA sequences shows *Pneumocystis carinii* to be a member of the fungi, *Nature* 33:519-522, 1988.

75. Eng RHK, Bishburg E, Smith SM: Evidence for destruction of lung tissues during *Pneumocystis carinii* infection, *Arch Intern Med* 147:746-749, 1987.

76. Ensoli B, Nakamura S, Salahuddin SZ, et al: AIDS-Kaposi's sarcoma-derived cells express cytokines with autocrine and paracrine growth effects, *Science* 243:223-226, 1989.

77. Erban SB, Sokas RK: Kaposi's sarcoma in an elderly man with Wegener's granulomatosis treated with cyclophosphamide and corticosteroids, *Arch Intern Med* 148:1201-1203, 1988.

78. Ettensohn DB, Mayer KH, Kessimian N, et al: Lymphocytic bronchiolitis associated with HIV infection, *Chest* 93:201-202, 1988.

79. Ettinger NA, Trulock EP: Pulmonary considerations of organ transplantation, Part 2, *Am Rev Respir Dis* 144:213-223, 1991.

80. Ettinger NA, Trulock EP: Pulmonary considerations of organ transplantation, Part 3, *Am Rev Respir Dis* 144:433-451, 1991.

81. Fackler JC, Nagel JE, Adler WH, et al: Epstein-Barr virus infection in a child with acquired immunodeficiency syndrome, *Am J Dis Child* 139:1000-1004, 1985.

82. Fairley CK, Kent SJ, Street A: Invasive aspergillosis in AIDS, *Aust NZ J Med* 21:747-749, 1991.

83. Feigin DS: Nocardiasis of the lung: chest radiographic findings in 21 cases, *Radiology* 159:9-14, 1986.

84. Feuerstein IM, Archer A, Peuda JM, et al: Thin-walled cavities, cysts, and pneumothorax in *Pneumocystis carinii* pneumonia: further observations with histopathologic correlation, *Radiology* 174:697-702, 1990.

85. Fish DG, Ampel NM, Galgiani JN, et al: Coocciioiomycosis during human immunodeficiency virus infection: a review of 77 patients, *Medicine* 69(6):384-391, 1990.

86. Forrest JV: Radiographic findings in *Pneumocystis carinii* pneumonia, *Radiology* 103:539-544, 1972.

87. Gale AM, Kleitsch WP: Solitary pulmonary nodule due to phycomycosis (mucormycosis), *Chest* 62:752-755, 1972.

88. Galgiani JN, Ampel NM: *Coccidioides immitis* in patients with human immunodeficiency virus infection, *J Infect Dis* 162:1165-1169, 1990.

89. Ganz WI, Serafini AN, Ganz SS, et al: Diagnostic pattern of Ga-677 uptake in lymphocytic interstitial pneumonia, *J Nucl Med* 29:887-888, 1988.

90. Gao SL, Schroeder JS, Hunt SA, et al: Retransplantation for severe accelerated coronary artery disease in heart transplant recipients, *Am J Cardiol* 62:876-881, 1988.

91. Garay SM, Belenko M, Fazzine E, et al: Pulmonary manifestations of Kaposi's sarcoma, *Chest* 91:39-43, 1987.

92. Gedroyc WMW, Reidy JF: The early chest radiographic changes of *Pneumocystis* pneumonia, *Clin Radiol* 157:331-334, 1985.

93. Gefter WB, Albeda SM, Talbot GH, et al: Invasive pulmonary aspergillosis and acute leukemia: limitations in the diagnostic utility of the air crescent sign, *Radiology* 157:605-610, 1985.

94. Gefter WB, Weingrad TR, Epstein DM, et al: "Semi-invasive" pulmonary aspergillosis: a new look at the spectrum of *Aspergillus* infections of the lung, *Radiology* 140:313-321, 1981.

95. Gerrard MP, Eden OB, Jameson B, et al: Serological study of *Pneumocystis carinii* infection in the absence of immunosuppression, *Arch Dis Child* 62:177-179, 1987.

96. Gill PS, Akil B, Colletti P, et al: Pulmonary Kaposi's sarcoma: clinical findings and results of therapy, *Am J Med* 87:57-61, 1989.

97. Glazer HS, Anderson DJ, Cooper JD, et al: Omental flap in lung transplantation, *Radiology* 185:395-400, 1992.

98. Goedert JJ, Biggar RJ, Melbye M, et al: Effect of T4 count and cofactors on the incidence of AIDS in homosexual men infected with human immunodeficiency virus, *JAMA* 257:331-334, 1987.

99. Goodman PC, Daley C, Minagi H: Spontaneous pneumothorax in AIDS patients with *Pneumocystis carinii* pneumonia, *AJR* 147:29-31, 1986.

100. Goodman PC, Gamsu G: Pulmonary radiographic findings in the acquired immunodeficiency syndrome, *Postgrad Radiol* 7:3-15, 1987.

101. Gottlieb MS, Schanker H, Fan P, et al: *Pneumocystis* pneumonia — Los Angeles, *MMWR* 30:250-252, 1981.

102. Gottlieb MS, Schroff R, Schanker HM, et al: *Pneumocystis carinii* pneumonia and mucosal candidiasis in previously healthy homosexual men: evidence of a new acquired cellular immunodeficiency, *N Engl J Med* 305:1425-1431, 1981.

103. Graham NJ, Muller NL, Miller RR, et al: Intrathoracic complications following allogeneic bone marrow transplantation: CT findings, *Radiology* 181:153-156, 1991.

104. Greene R: Pulmonary aspergillosis: three distinct entities or a spectrum of disease, *Radiology* 140:527-530, 1981.

105. Gray JR, Rabeneck L: Atypical mycobacterial infection of the gastrointestinal tract in AIDS patients, *Am J Gastroenterol* 84:1521-1524, 1984.

106. Grimes MM, LaPook JD, Bar MH, et al: Disseminated *Pneumocystis carinii* infection in a patient with acquired immunodeficiency syndrome, *Hum Pathol* 18:307-308, 1987.

107. Groskin SA, Massi AF, Randall PA: Calcified hilar and mediastinal lymph nodes in an AIDS patient with *Pneumocystis carinii* infection, *Radiology* 175:345-346, 1990.

108. Gross BH, Spitz HB, Felson B: The mural nodule in cavitary opportunistic pulmonary aspergillosis, *Radiology* 143:619-622, 1982.

109. Guillon JM, Autran B, Denis M, et al: Human immunodeficiency virus–related lymphocytic alveolitis, *Chest* 94:1264-1270, 1988.

110. Gunawardena KA, Al-Hasani MK, Haleeem A, et al: Pulmonary Kaposi's sarcoma in two recipients of renal transplants, *Thorax* 43:653-656, 1988.

111. Gurney JW, Bates FT: Pulmonary cystic disease: comparison of *Pneumocystis carinii* pneumatoceles and bullous emphysema due to intravenous drug abuse, *Radiology* 173:27-31, 1989.

112. Hackman RC, Madtes DK, Petersen FB, et al: Pulmonary veno-occlusive disease following bone marrow transplantation, *Transplantation* 47:989-922, 1989.

113. Halvorsen RA, Duncan JD, Merten DF, et al: Pulmonary blastomycosis: radiologic manifestations, *Radiology* 150:1-5, 1984.

114. Hamlin WB: *Pneumocystis carinii*, *JAMA* 204:171, 1968.

115. Hardy JD, Webb WR, Dalton ML, et al: Lung homotransplantation in man: report of an initial case, *JAMA* 186:1065-1074, 1963.

116. Harris KM, Schwartz ML, Slasky BS, et al: Post transplantation cyclosporine-induced lymphoproliferative disorders: clinical and radiographic manifestations, *Radiology* 162:697-700, 1987.

117. Harrison NK, Twelves C, Addis BJ: Peripheral T-cell lymphoma presenting with angioedema and diffuse pulmonary infiltrates, *Am Rev Respir Dis* 138:976-980, 1988.

118. Hartz JW, Geisinger KR, Scharyj M, et al: Granulomatous pneumocystosis presenting as a solitary pulmonary nodule, *Arch Pathol Lab Med* 109:466-469, 1985.

119. Hawkins CC, Gold JWM, Whimbey E, et al: *Mycobacterium avium* complex infections in patients with the acquired immunodeficiency syndrome, *Ann Intern Med* 105:184-188, 1986.

120. Heck CF, Shumway SJ, Kaye MP: The Registry of International Society for Heart Transplantation: sixth official report — 1989, *J Heart Transplant* 8:271-275, 1989.

121. Heifets LB, Iseman MD: Individualized therapy versus standard regimens in the treatment of *Mycobacterium avium* infections, *Am Rev Respir Dis* 144:1-2, 1991.

122. Heitzman ER: Pulmonary neoplastic and lymphoproliferative disease in AIDS: a review, *Radiology* 177:347-351, 1990.

123. Heppleston AG: The fibrogenic action of silica, *Br Med Bull* 25:282-287, 1969.

124. Herbert PA, Bayer AS: Fungal pneumonia. 4. Invasive pulmonary aspergillosis, *Chest* 80:220-225, 1981.

125. Herman SJ, Rappaport DC, Weisbrod GI, et al: Single-lung transplantation: imaging features, *Radiology* 170:89-93, 1989.

126. Herman SJ, Weisbrod GL, Weisbrod L, et al: Chest radiographic findings after bilateral lung transplantation, *AJR* 153:1181-1185, 1989.

127. Herold CJ, Kramer J, Sertl K, et al: Invasive pulmonary aspergillosis: Evaluation with MR imaging, *Radiology* 173:717-721, 1989.

128. Herts BR, Megibon AJ, Birnbaum BA, et al: High attenuation lymphadenopathy in AIDS patients: significance of findings at CT, *Radiology* 185:777-781, 1992.

129. Herve P, Silbert D, Cerrina J, et al: Impairment of bronchial mucociliary clearance in long-term survivors of heart-lung and double-lung transplantation, *Chest* 103:59-63, 1993.

130. Hill AR, Premkumar S, Brustein S, et al: Disseminated tuberculosis in the acquired immunodeficiency syndrome era, *Am Rev Respir Dis* 144:1164-1170, 1991.

131. Hisada K, Tonami N, Migamal T, et al: Clinical evaluation of tumor imaging with TL-201 chloride, *Radiology* 129:497-500, 1978.

132. Holmes B, Quie PG, Windhorst DB: Protection of phagocytosed bacteria from the killing action of antibiotics, *Nature (London)* 210:1131-1132, 1966.

133. Honda H, Barloon TJ, Franken EA, et al: Clinical and radiologic features of malignant neoplasms in organ transplant recipients: cyclosporine-treated vs untreated patients, *AJR* 154:271-274, 1990.

134. Horowitz ML, Schiff M, Samuels J, et al: *Pneumocystis carinii* pleural effusion: pathogenesis and pleural fluid analysis, *Am Rev Respir Dis* 148:232-234, 1993.

135. Horsburgh CR, Havlik JA, Ellis DE, et al: Survival of patients with acquired immune deficiency syndrome and disseminated *Mycobacterium avium* complex infection with and without antimycobacterial chemotherapy, *Am Rev Respir Dis* 144:557-559, 1991.

136. Horsburgh CR, Mason UG, Farhl DC, et al: Disseminated infection with *Mycobacterium avium-intracellulare*, *Medicine* 64:36-48, 1985.

137. Horsburgh C, Selik RM: The epidemiology of disseminated nontuberculous mycobacterial infection in the acquired immunodeficiency syndrome (AIDS), *Am Rev Respir Dis* 139:4-7, 1989.

138. Hruban RH, Meziane MA, Zerhouni EA, et al: Radiologic-pathologic correlation of the CT halo sign in invasive pulmonary aspergillosis, *J Comput Assist Tomogr* 11:534-536, 1987.

139. Huang CT, McGarry T, Cooper S, et al: Disseminated histoplasmosis in the acquired immunodeficiency syndrome: report of five cases from a nonendemic area, *Arch Intern Med* 147:1181-1184, 1987.

140. Ioachim HL, Cooper MC, Hellman GC: Lymphomas in men at high risk for acquired immune deficiency syndrome (AIDS), *Cancer* 56:2831-2842, 1985.

141. Ioachim HL, Dorsett B, Cronin W, et al: Acquired immunodeficiency syndrome — associated lymphomas: clinical, pathologic, immunologic, and viral characteristics of 111 cases, *Hum Pathol* 22:659-673, 1991.

142. Jacobson MA, Hopewell PC, Yajko DM: Natural history of disseminated *Mycobacterium avium* complex infection in AIDS, *J Infect Dis* 164:994-998, 1991.

143. Jacobson MA, Mills J: Cytomegalovirus infection. In White DA, Stover DE, eds: Pulmonary effects of AIDS, *Clin Chest Med* 9:443-448, 1988.

144. Janier M, Vignon MD, Cottenot F: Spontaneously healing Kaposi's sarcoma in AIDS, *N Engl J Med* 312:1638-1639, 1985.

145. Janzen DL, Padley SPG, Adler BD, et al: Acute pulmonary complications in immunocompromised non-AIDS patients: comparison of diagnostic accuracy of CT and chest radiography, *Clin Radiol* 47:159-165, 1993.

146. Jayes RL, Kamerow HN, Hasselquist SM, et al: Disseminated pneumocystosis presenting as a pleural effusion, *Chest* 103:306-308, 1993.

147. Johnston RB, Baehner RL: Chronic granulomatous disease — correlation between pathogenesis and clinical findings, *Pediatrics* 48:730-739, 1971.

148. Kamanfu G, Meika-Cabanne N, Girard P-M, et al: Pulmonary complications of human immunodeficiency virus infection in Bujumbura, Burundi, *Am Rev Respir Dis* 147:658-663, 1993.

149. Kaplan LD, Abrams DI, Feigal E, et al: AIDS-associated non-Hodgkin's lymphoma in San Francisco, *JAMA* 261:719-724, 1989.

150. Kaplan MH, Susin M, Pahwa SG, et al: Neoplastic complications of HTLV-III infection: lymphomas and solid tumors, *Am J Med* 82:389-396, 1987.

151. Kaposi M: Idiopathisches multiplex pigment sarkom der haut, *Arch Dermatol Syphilol* 4:265-273, 1872.

152. Katz AS, Niesenbaum L, Mass B: Pleural effusion as the initial manifestation of disseminated cryptococcosis in acquired immune deficiency syndrome: diagnosis by pleural biopsy, *Chest* 96:440-441, 1989.

153. Katzenstein ALA, Askin FB: Interpretation and significance of pathologic findings in transbronchial lung biopsy, *Am J Surg Pathol* 4:223-234, 1980.

154. Khoury MB, Godwin JD, Ravin CE, et al: Thoracic cryptococcosis: immunologic competence and radiologic appearance, *AJR* 141:893-896, 1984.

155. Klein JS, Warnock M, Webb WR, et al: Cavitating and noncavitating granulomas in AIDS patients with *Pneumocystis* pneumonia, *AJR* 152:753-754, 1988.

156. Knowles DM, Chamulak GA, Subar M, et al: Lymphoid neoplasia associated with the acquired immunodeficiency syndrome (AIDS): the New York University Medical Center experience with 105 patients (1981-1986), *Ann Intern Med* 108:744-753, 1988.

157. Kradin RL, Mark EJ: Benign lymphoid disorders of the lungs with a theory regarding their development, *Hum Pathol* 14:857-867, 1983.

158. Kramer EL, Sanger JH, Garay SM, et al: Gallium-67 scans of the chest in patients with acquired immunodeficiency syndrome, *J Nucl Med* 28:1107-1114, 1987.

159. Kramer MR, Gregg PA, Goldstein M, et al: Disseminated strongyloidiasis in AIDS and non-AIDS immunocompromised hosts: diagnosis by sputum and bronchoalveolar lavage, *South Med J* 83:1226-1229, 1990.

160. Kramer MR, Uttamchandani RB: The radiographic appearance of pulmonary nocardiasis associated with AIDS, *Chest* 98:382-385, 1990.

161. Krowka MJ, Rosenow EC, Hoagland HC: Pulmonary complications of bone marrow transplantation, *Chest* 87:237-246, 1985.

162. Krown SE: AIDS-associated Kaposi's sarcoma: pathogenesis, clinical course and treatment, *AIDS* 2:71-80, 1988.

163. Kuhlman JE, Fishman EK, Siegelman SS: Invasive pulmonary aspergillosis in acute leukemia: characteristic finding on CT, the CT halo sign and the role of CT in early diagnosis, *Radiology* 157:611-614, 1985.

164. Kuhlman JE, Knowles MC, Fishman Ek, et al: Premature bullous damage in AIDS: CT diagnosis, *Radiology* 173:23-26, 1989.

165. Lee VM, Fuller JD, O'Brien MJ, et al: Pulmonary Kaposi sarcoma in patients with AIDS: scintigraphic diagnosis with sequential thallium and gallium scanning, *Radiology* 180:409-412, 1991.

166. Lee VW, Rosen MP, Baum A, et al: AIDS-related Kaposi's sarcoma: finding on thallium 201 scintigraphy, *AJR* 151:1233-1235, 1988.

167. Leight GS, Michaelis LL: Open lung biopsy for the diagnosis of acute diffuse pulmonary infiltrates in the immunosuppressed patient, *Chest* 73:477-482, 1978.

168. Lemlick G, Schwam L, Lebwohl M: Kaposi's sarcoma and acquired immunodeficiency syndrome: postmortem findings in twenty-four cases, *J Am Acad Dermatol* 16:319-325, 1987.

169. Lentz D, Bergin CJ, Berry GJ, et al: Diagnosis of bronchiolitis obliterans in heart lung transplantation patients: importance of bronchial dilatation on CT, *AJR* 159:463-467, 1992.

170. Levine AM, Meyer PR, Begandy MK, et al: Development of B-cell lymphoma in homosexual men, *Ann Intern Med* 100:7-13, 1984.

171. Libshitz HI, Pagani JJ: Aspergillosis and mucormycosis: two types of opportunistic fungal pneumonia, *Radiology* 140:301-306, 1981.

172. Lin RY, Gruber PJ, Saunders R, et al: Lymphocytic interstitial pneumonitis in adult HIV infection, *NY State J Med* 88:273-276, 1988.

173. List AF, Greco FA, Vogler LB: Lymphoproliferative diseases in immunocompromised hosts: the role of Epstein-Barr virus, *J Clin Oncol* 5:1673-1689, 1987.

174. Long R, Maycher B, Scalcini M, et al: The chest roentgenogram in pulmonary tuberculosis patients seropositive for human immunodeficiency virus type 1, *Chest* 99:123-127, 1991.

175. Loureiro C, Gill PS, Meyer PR, et al: Autopsy findings in AIDS-related lymphoma, *Cancer* 62:735-739, 1988.

176. Lowenthal DA, Strauss DJ, Campbell SW, et al: AIDS-related lymphoid neoplasia: the Memorial Hospital experience, *Cancer* 61:2325-2337, 1988.

177. Lubat E, Megibow AJ, Bulthazar EJ, et al: Extrapulmonary *Pneumocystis carinii* infections in AIDS: CT findings, *Radiology* 174:157-160, 1990.

178. Luce JM, Ostenson RC: Invasive aspergillosis presenting as pericarditis and cardiac tamponade, *Chest* 76:703-705, 1979.

179. Lum LG, Storb R: Bone marrow transplantation. In Flye M et al: *Principles of organ transplantation,* Philadelphia, 1989, WB Saunders, pp 478-499.

180. Magnenat JL, Nicod LP, Auckenthaler R, et al: Mode of presentation and diagnosis of bacterial pneumonia in human immunodeficiency virus—infected patients, *Am Rev Respir Dis* 144:917-922, 1991.

181. Maile CW, Moore AV, Ulreich S, et al: Chest radiographic-pathologic correlation in adult leukemia patients, *Invest Radiol* 18:495-499, 1983.

182. Mal N, Andreassian B, Pamela F, et al: Unilateral lung transplantation in end-stage pulmonary emphysema, *Am Rev Respir Dis* 140:797-802, 1989.

183. Mandell W, Goldberg DM, Neu HC: Histoplasmosis in patients with the acquired immune deficiency syndrome, *Am J Med* 81:974-978, 1986.

184. Marchevsky A, Rosen MJ, Crystal G, et al: Pulmonary complications of the acquired immunodeficiency syndrome: a clinicopathologic study of 70 cases, *Hum Pathol* 16:659-670, 1985.

185. Marinelli DL, Albeda SM, Willimas TM, et al: Nontuberculous mycobacterial infection in AIDS: clinical, pathologic and radiographic features, *Radiology* 160:77-82, 1986.

186. Mariuz P, Raviglione MC, Gould IA, et al: Pleural *Pneumocystis carinii* infection, *Chest* 99:774-776, 1991.

187. Masur H, Clifford LH, Kovacs JA: *Pneumocystis* pneumonia from bench to clinic, *Ann Intern Med* 111:813-826, 1989.

188. Masur H, Lane HC, Palestine A, et al: Effect of DHPG on serious cystomegalovirus disease in eight immunosuppressed homosexual men, *Ann Intern Med* 104:41-44, 1986.

189. Masur H, Frederick P, Ognibene FP, et al: CD4 counts as predictors of opportunistic pneumonas in human immunodeficiency virus (HIV) infection, *Ann Intern Med* 111:223-231, 1989.

190. Masur H, Michelis MA, Green JB, et al: An outbreak of community-acquired *Pneumocystis carinii* pneumonia, *N Engl J Med* 305:1431-1438, 1981.

191. McCauley DI, Naidich DP, Leitman BS, et al: Radiographic patterns of opportunistic lung infections and Kaposi sarcoma in homosexual men, *AJR* 139:653-658, 1982.

192. McGregor CGA, Dark JH, Hilton CJ, et al: Early results of single lung transplantation in patients with end-stage fibrosis, *J Thorac Cardiovasc Surg* 98:350-354, 1989.

193. Meduri GU, Stover DE, Lee M, et al: Pulmonary Kaposi's sarcoma in the acquired immune deficiency syndrome, *Am J Med* 81:11-18, 1986.

194. Mehle ME, Adamo JP, Mehta AC, et al: Endobronchial *Mycobacterium avium-intracellulare* in a patient with AIDS, *Chest* 96:119-200, 1989.

195. Meunier F: Fungal infections in the compromised host. In Rubin R, Young L, eds: *Clinical approach to infection in the compromised host,* New York, 1988, Plenum, pp 193-220.

196. Meuwissen JHET, Tauber I, Leeuwenburg ADEM, et al: Parasitologic and serologic observations of infection with *Pneumocystis* in humans, *J Infect Dis* 136:43-49, 1977.

197. Meyer RD, Rosen P, Armstrong D: Phycomycosis complicating leukemia and lymphoma, *Ann Intern Med* 77:871-879, 1972.

198. Meyers JD, Thomas ED: Infection complicating bone marrow transplantation. In Rubin R, Young L, eds: *Clinical approach to infection in the compromised host,* New York, 1988, Plenum, pp 525-555.

199. Miamoto GY, Barlan TF, VanderEls NJ: Invasive aspergillosis in patients with AIDS, *Clin Infect Dis* 14:66-74, 1992.

200. Miller RF, Birley HDL, Fogarty P, et al: Cavitary lung disease caused by *Mycobacterium avium-intracellulare* in AIDS patients, *Respir Med* 84:409-411, 1990.

201. Miller RF, Mitchell DM: *Pneumocystis carinii* pneumonia, *Thorax* 47:305-314, 1992.

202. Miller RF, Tomlinson MC, Cattrill CP, et al: Bronchopulmonary Kaposi's sarcoma in patients with AIDS, *Thorax* 47:721-725, 1992.

203. Miller WT, Edelman JM, Miller WT: Cryptococcal pulmonary infection in patients with AIDS: radiographic appearance, *Radiology* 175:725-728, 1990.

204. Millet B, Higenbottam TW, Flower CDR, et al: The radiographic appearances of infection and acute rejection of the lung after heart lung transplantation, *Am Rev Respir Dis* 140:62-67, 1989.

205. Milligan SA, Stulbarg MS, Gamsu G, et al: *Pneumocystis carinii* pneumonia radiographically simulating tuberculosis, *Am Rev Respir Dis* 132:1124-1128, 1985.

206. Mirich D, Gray R, Hyland R: *Legionella* lung cavitation, *J Can Assoc Radiol* 41:100-102, 1990.

207. Mori M, Galvin JR, Barloon TJ: Fungal pulmonary infections after bone marrow transplantation: evaluation with radiography and CT, *Radiology* 178:721-726, 1991.

208. Morris JC, Rosen MJ, Marchevsky A, et al: Lymphocytic interstitial pneumonia in patients at risk for the acquired immune deficiency syndrome, *Chest* 91:63-67, 1987.

209. Morrish WF, Herman SJ, Weisbrod GL, et al: Bronchiolitis obliterans after lung transplantation: findings at chest radiography and high resolution CT, *Radiology* 179:487-490, 1991.

210. Morrison DL, Granton JT, Kesten S, et al: Cavitary aspergillosis as a complication of AIDS, *Can Assoc Radiol J* 44:35-38, 1993.

211. Moskovic E, Miller R, Pearson M: High resolution computed tomography of *Pneumocystis carinii* pneumonia in AIDS, *Clin Radiol* 42:239-243, 1990.

212. Murray HW: Pulmonary mucormycosis: one hundred years later, *Chest* 72:1-2, 1977.

213. Murray JF, Mills J: Pulmonary infectious complications of human immunodeficiency virus infection, *Am Res Respir Dis* 141:1356-1372, 1990.

214. Naidich DP, Tarras M, Garay SM, et al: Kaposi's sarcoma: CT-radiographic correlation, *Chest* 96:723-728, 1989.

215. Nalesnik MA, Makowkal, Starzl TE: The diagnosis and treatment of posttransplant lymphoproliferative disorders, *Curr Probl Surg* 25:367-472, 1988.

216. Nash G, Fligiel S: Kaposi's sarcoma presenting as pulmonary disease in the acquired immunodeficiency syndrome: diagnosis by lung biopsy, *Hum Pathol* 15:999-1001, 1984.

217. Newsome GS, Ward DJ, Pierce PF: Spontaneous pneumothorax in patients with acquired immunodeficiency syndrome treated with prophylactic aerosolized pentamidine, *Arch Intern Med* 180:2167-2168, 1990.

218. O'Doherty MJ, Thomas SH, Page CJ, et al: Does inhalation of pentamidine in the supine position increase deposition in the upper part of the lung? *Chest* 97:1343-1348, 1990.

219. Ognibene FP, Masur H, Rogers P, et al: Non specific interstitial pneumonitis without evidence of *Pneumocystis carinii* in asymptomatic patients infected with human immunodeficiency virus (HIV), *Ann Intern Med* 109:874-879, 1988.

220. Ognibene FP, Steis RG, Macher AM, et al: Kaposi's sarcoma causing pulmonary infiltrates and respiratory failure in the acquired immunodeficiency syndrome, *Ann Intern Med* 102:471-475, 1985.

221. Oksenhendler E, Cadronel J, Sarfati C: *Toxoplasma gondii* pneumonia in patients with the acquired immunodeficiency syndrome, *Am J Med* 88:18-21, 1990.

222. Oldham SAA, Castillo M, Jacobson FL, et al: HIV associated lymphocytic interstitial pneumonia: radiologic manifestations and pathologic correlation, *Radiology* 170:83-87, 1989.

223. Orr DP, Myerowitz RL, Dubois PJ: Patho-radiologic correlation of invasive aspergillosis in the immunocompromised host, *Cancer* 41:2028-2039, 1978.

224. Packer SJ, Cesario T, Williams JH: *Mycobacterium avium* complex infection presenting as endobronchial lesions in immunosuppressed patients, *Ann Intern Med* 109:389-393, 1988.

225. Pagani JJ, Kangarloo H, Gyepes MT, et al: Radiographic manifestations of bone marrow transplantation in children, *AJR* 132:883-890, 1979.

226. Pagani JJ, Libshitz HI: Opportunistic fungal pneumonias in cancer patients, *AJR* 137:1033-1039, 1981.

227. Panicek DM: Cystic pulmonary lesions in patients with AIDS, *Radiology* 173:12-14, 1989.

228. Pappas PG, Pottage JC, Powderly WG, et al: Blastomycosis in patients with the acquired immunodeficiency syndrome, *Ann Intern Med* 116:847-853, 1992.

229. Paradis IL, Duncan SR, Dauber JH, et al: Distinguishing between infection, rejection and the adult respiratory distress syndrome after human lung transplantation, *J Heart Lung Transplant* 11(5):232-236, 1992.

230. Pasque MK, Kaiser LR, Dresler CM: Single lung transplantation for pulmonary hypertension: technical aspects and immediate hemodynamic results, *J Thorac Cardiovasc Surg* 103:475-482, 1992.

231. Penn I: Malignancies associated with immunosuppressive or cytotoxic therapy, *Surgery* 83:492-502, 1978.

232. Penn I: Kaposi's sarcoma in organ transplant recipients, *Transplantation* 27:8-11, 1979.

233. Penn I: Cancers complicating organ transplantation, *N Engl J Med* 323:1767-1768, 1990.

234. Pifer LL, Hughes WT, Sezis S, et al: *Pneumocystis carinii* infection: evidence for high prevalence in normal and immunosuppressed children, *Pediatrics* 61:35-41, 1978.

235. Pirsch JD, Maki DG: Infectious complications in adults with bone marrow transplantation and T-cell depletion of donor marrow: increased susceptibility to fungal infections, *Ann Intern Med* 104:619-631, 1986.

236. Pitchenik AE: PPD-tuberculin and PPD-Battey dual skin testing of hospital employees and medical students, *South Med J* 71:917-922, 1978.

237. Pitchenik AE, Burr J, Suarez M, et al: Human T-cell lymphotrophic virus-III (HTLV-III) seropositivity and related disease among 71 consecutive patients in whom tuberculosis was diagnosed, *Am Rev Respir Dis* 135:875-879, 1987.

238. Pitchenik AE, Fertel D, Bloch AB: Mycobacterial disease: epidemiology, diagnosis, treatment and prevention. In White DA, Stover DE, eds: Pulmonary effects of AIDS, *Clin Chest Med* 9:425-441, 1988.

239. Pitchenik AE, Rubinson HA: The radiographic appearance of tuberculosis in patients with the acquired immuno deficiency syndrome (AIDS) and pre-AIDS, *Am Rev Respir Dis* 131:393-396, 1985.

240. Pitchenik AE, Russell BW, Cleary T, et al: The prevalence of tuberculosis and drug resistance among Haitians, *N Engl J Med* 307:162-165, 1982.

241. Poelzleitner D, Huebsch P, Mayerhofer S, et al: Primary pulmonary lymphoma in a patient with the acquired immune deficiency syndrome, *Thorax* 44:438-439, 1989.

242. Polish LB, Cohn DL, Ryder JW, et al: Pulmonary non-Hodgkins lymphoma in AIDS, *Chest* 96:1321-1326, 1989.

243. Polsky B, Gold JWM, Whimbey E, et al: Bacterial pneumonia in patients with the acquired immunodeficiency syndrome, *Ann Intern Med* 104:38-41, 1986.

244. Pomeroy C, Filice GA: Pulmonary toxoplasmosis: a review, *Clin Infect Dis* 14:863-870, 1992.

245. Pope TL, Armstrong P, Thomas R, et al: Pittsburgh pneumonia agent: chest film manifestations, *AJR* 138:237-241, 1983.

246. Price RA, Hughes WT: Histopathology of *Pneumocystis carinii* infestation and infection in malignant diseases in childhood, *Hum Pathol* 5:737-752, 1974.

247. Purtilo DT, Meyers WM, Connor DH: Fatal strongyloidiasis in immunosuppressed patients, *Am J Med* 56:488-493, 1974.

248. Radin DR, Baker EL, Klatt EC, et al: Visceral and nodal calcification in patients with AIDS-related *Pneumocystis carinii* infection, *AJR* 154:27-31, 1990.

249. Rappaport DC, Weisbrod GL, Herman SJ, et al: Cyclosporine-induced lymphoma following a unilateral lung transplant, *J Can Assoc Radiol* 40:110-111, 1989.

250. Real FX, Krown SE: Spontaneous regression of Kaposi's sarcoma in patients with AIDS, *N Engl J Med* 313:1659, 1985.

251. Recht LD, Davies SF, Eckman MR, et al: Disseminated pulmonary blastomycosis in an immunosuppressed patient, *Am Rev Respir Dis* 125:359-362, 1982.

252. Record NB, Ginder DR: Pulmonary phycomycosis without obvious predisposing factors, *JAMA* 235:1256-1257, 1976.

253. Reich J, Renzetti AD: Pulmonary phycomycosis: report of a case of bronchocutaneous fistula formation and pulmonary arterial mycothrombosis, *Am Rev Respir Dis* 102:959-964, 1970.

254. Reichman LB: HIV infection — a new face of tuberculosis, *Bull Int Union Tuberc Lung Dis* 63:19-26, 1988.

255. Reiss TF, Golden J: Abnormal lung gallium-67 uptake preceding pulmonary physiologic impairment in an asymptomatic patient with *Pneumocystis carinii* pneumonia, *Chest* 97:1261-1263, 1990.

256. Reitz BA: Heart and lung transplantation. In Baumgartner WA, Reitz BA, Achuff SC, eds: *Heart and heart lung transplant*, Philadelphia, 1990, WB Saunders, pp 319-346.

257. Resnick L, Pitchenik AE, Fisher E, et al: Detection of HTLV-III/LAV specific IgG and antigen in bronchoalveolar lavage fluid from two patients with lymphocytic interstitial pneumonitis associated with AIDS-related complex, *Am J Med* 82:553-556, 1987.

258. Robbins RA, Linder JL, Stahl MG, et al: Diffuse alveolar; hemorrhage in autologous bone marrow transplantation, *Am J Med* 87:511-518, 1989.

259. Rodriguez JL, Barrio JI, Pitchenik AE: Pulmonary nocardiasis in AIDS: diagnosis with bronchoalveolar lavage and treatment with non-sulphur containing drugs, *Chest* 90:912-914, 1986.

260. Rose HD, Sheth NK: Pulmonary candidiasis: a clinical and pathological correlation, *Arch Intern Med* 138:964-965, 1978.

261. Rosenow EC, Wilson WR, Cockerill FR: Pulmonary disease in the immunocompromised host, *Mayo Clinic Proc* 60:473-487, 1985.

262. Rossiter SJ, Miller C, Churg AM, et al: Open lung biopsy in the immunosuppressed patient: is it really beneficial? *J Thorac Cardiovasc Surg* 77:338-345, 1979.

263. Rutherford GW, Schwarcz SK, Lemp GF, et al: The epidemiology of AIDS-related Kaposi's sarcoma in San Francisco, *J Infect Dis* 159:569-572, 1989.

264. Safai B, Mike V, Beth E, et al: Association of Kaposi's sarcoma with second primary malignancies: possible idiopathogenic implications, *Cancer* 45:1472-1479, 1980.

265. Saks AM, Posner R: Tuberculosis in HIV positive patients in South Africa: a comparative radiological study with HIV negative patients, *Clin Radiol* 46:387-390, 1992.

266. Sanders TG, Northup HM, Wilf LH: Case report: bilateral upper lobe *Pneumocystis carinii* pneumonia in a patient receiving aerosolized pentamidine, *Clin Radiol* 43:356-357, 1991.

267. Sandhu JS, Goodman PC: Pulmonary cysts associated with *Pneumocystis carinii* pneumonia in patients with AIDS, *Radiology* 173:33-35, 1989.

268. Scannell KA: Pneumothoraces and *Pneumocystis carinii* pneumonia in two AIDS patients receiving aerosolized pentamidine, *Chest* 97:479-480, 1991.

269. Schafers HJ, Haydock DA, Cooper JD: The prevalence and management of bronchial anastomotic complications in lung transplantation, *J Thorac Cardiovasc Surg* 101:1044-1052, 1991.

270. Schif RG, Kabat L, Kamoni N: Gallium scanning in lymphoid interstitial pneumonitis of children with AIDS, *J Nucl Med* 28:1915-1919, 1987.

271. Schnapp LM, Glaghan SM, Campagna A: *Toxoplasma gondii* pneumonitis in patients infected with the human immunodeficiency virus, *Arch Intern Med* 152:1073-1077, 1992.

272. Schottstaedt MW, Hurd ER, Stone MD: Kaposi's sarcoma in rheumatoid arthritis, *Am J Med* 82:1021-1026, 1987.

273. Scott JP, Fradet G, Smyth RL, et al: Prospective study of transbronchial biopsies in the management of heart-lung and single-lung transplant patients, *J Heart Lung Transplant* 10:626-637, 1991.

274. Scowden EB, Schaffner W, Stone WJ: Overwhelming strongyloidiasis: an unappreciated opportunistic infection, *Medicine* 57:527-544, 1978.

275. Scully RE, Mark EJ, McNeely WF, et al: Case records of the Massachusetts General Hospital: weekly clinicopathological exercises, Case 9-1989, *N Engl J Med* 520:582-587, 1989.

276. Selwyn PA, Hartell D, Lewis VA, et al: A prospective study of the risk of tuberculosis among intravenous drug users with human immunodeficiency virus infection, *N Engl J Med* 320:545-550, 1989.

277. Shanley DJ, Luyckx BA, Haggerty MF, et al: Spontaneous pneumothorax in AIDS patients with recurrent *Pneumocystis carinii* pneumonia despite aerosolized pentamidine prophylaxis, *Chest* 99:502-504, 1991.

278. Sheflin JR, Campbell JA, Thompson GP: Pulmonary blastomycosis: findings on chest radiographs in 63 patients, *AJR* 154:1177-1180, 1990.

279. Sider L, Horton ES: Pleural effusion as a presentation of AIDS-related lymphoma, *Invest Radiol* 24:150-153, 1989.

280. Sider L, Weiss AJ, Smith MD, et al: Varied appearance of AIDS-related lymphoma in the chest, *Radiology* 171:629-632, 1989.

281. Simmons JT, Suffredini AF, Lack EE, et al: Non specific interstitial pneumonitis in patients with AIDS: radiologic features, *AJR* 149:265-268, 1987.

282. Sivit CJ, Schwartz AM, Rockoff SD: Kaposi's sarcoma of the lungs in AIDS: radiologic-pathologic analysis, *AJR* 148:25-28, 1987.

283. Skeens JL, Fuhrman CR, Yousem SA: Bronchiolitis obliterans in heart lung transplantation patients: radiologic findings in 11 patients, *AJR* 153:253-256, 1989.

284. Small PM, Schecter GF, Goodman PC: Treatment of tuberculosis in patients with advanced human immunodeficiency virus syndrome, *N Engl J Med* 324:289-294, 1991.

285. Smith LJ, Katzenstein ALA: Pathogenesis of massive pulmonary hemorrhage in acute leukemia, *Arch Intern Med* 142:2149-2152, 1982.

286. Sourour MS, Stover DE, Fels AOS: Pulmonary disease in AIDS patients with lymphoma (abstract), *Am Rev Respir Dis* 135:A168, 1987.

287. Starzl TE, Nalesnik MA, Porter KA, et al: Reversibility of lymphomas and lymphoproliferative lesions developing under cyclosporine-steroid therapy, *Lancet* 1:583-587, 1984.

288. Stein DS, Weems JJ: Cavitary *Pneumocystis carinii* pneumonia in patients receiving aerosol pentamidine prophylaxis, *South Med J* 84:273-275, 1991.

289. Stelling CB, Woodring JH, Rehm SR, et al: Miliary pulmonary blastomycosis, *Radiology* 150:7-13, 1984.

290. Stern RG, Gamsu G, Golden JA, et al: Intrathoracic adenopathy: differential feature of AIDS and diffuse lymphoadenopathy syndrome, *AJR* 142:689-692, 1984.

291. Stover DE, White DA, Romano PA, et al: Spectrum of pulmonary diseases associated with the acquired immune deficiency syndrome, *Am J Med* 78:429-437, 1985.

292. Sunderam G, McDonald RJ, Maniatis T, et al: Tuberculosis as a manifestation of the acquired immunodeficiency syndrome (AIDS), *JAMA* 256:362-366, 1986.

293. Suster B, Akerman M, Orenstein M, et al: Pulmonary manifestation of AIDS: review of 106 episodes, *Radiology* 161:87-93, 1986.

294. Tazelaar HD, Nilsson FN, Rinaldi M, et al: The sensitivity of transbronchial biopsy for the diagnosis of acute lung rejection, *J Thorac Cardiovasc Surg* 105:674-678, 1993.

295. Tenholder MF, Hooper RG: Pulmonary infiltrates in leukemia, *Chest* 78:468-473, 1980.

296. Tenholder MF, Moser RJ, Tellis CJ: Mycobacteria other than tuberculosis: pulmonary involvement in patients with acquired immunodeficiency syndrome, *Arch Intern Med* 148:953-955, 1988.

297. Thorsen MK, Goodman LR: Extracardiac complications of cardiac surgery, *Semin Roentgenol* 23:32-48, 1988.

298. Tonami N, Shuke N, Yokoyama K, et al: Thallium 201 SPECT in evaluation of suspected lung cancer, *J Nucl Med* 30:997-1004, 1989.

299. Toronto Lung Transplant Group: Experience with single lung transplantation for pulmonary fibrosis, *JAMA* 259:2258-2262, 1988.

300. Tubman DE, Frick MP, Hanto DW: Lymphoma after organ transplantation: radiologic manifestations in the central nervous system, thorax, and abdomen, *Radiology* 149:625-631, 1983.

301. Turbiner EH, Yeh HD, Rosen PP, et al: Abnormal gallium scintigraphy in *Pneumocystis carinii* pneumonia with a normal chest radiograph, *Radiology* 127:437-438, 1978.

302. Ulbright TM, Santa Cruz DJ: Kaposi's sarcoma: relationship with hematologic, lymphoid and thymic neoplasia, *Cancer* 47:963-973, 1981.

303. Unger PD, Rosenblum M, Brown SE: Disseminated *Pneumocystis carinii* infection in a patient with acquired immunodeficiency syndrome, *Hum Pathol* 19:113-116, 1988.

304. Vasudevan VP, Mascarenhas DAN, Klapper P, et al: Cytomegalovirus necrotizing bronchiolitis with HIV infection, *Chest* 97:483-484, 1990.

305. Vys CJ, Rose AG: Pathologic findings in long term cardiac transplants, *Arch Pathol Lab Med* 108:112-116, 1984.

306. Wallace JM: Pulmonary infection in human immunodeficiency disease: viral pulmonary infections, *Semin Respir Infect* 2:147-154, 1989.

307. Wallace JM, Hannah J: Cytomegalovirus pneumonitis in patients with AIDS: findings of an autopsy series, *Chest* 92:198-203, 1987.

308. Wasser L, Talavera W: Pulmonary cryptococcosis in AIDS, *Chest* 92:692-695, 1987.

309. Wasser LS, Shaw GW, Talavera W: Endobronchial tuberculosis in the acquired immunodeficiency syndrome, *Chest* 94:1240-1244, 1988.

310. Weber WR, Askin FB, Dehner LP: Lung biopsy in *Pneumocystis carinii* pneumonia: a histopathologic study of typical and atypical features, *Am J Clin Pathol* 67:11-19, 1977.

311. Wheat LJ, Connolly-Stringfield PA, Baker RL, et al: Disseminated histoplasmosis in the acquired immune deficiency syndrome: clinical findings, diagnosis and treatment, and review of the literature, *Medicine* 69:361-374, 1990.

312. Wheat LJ, Small CB. Disseminated histoplasmosis in the acquired immune deficiency syndrome, *Arch Intern Med* 144:2147-2149, 1984.

313. Wheeler EW, Rubis LJ, Jones CW, et al: Etiology and prevention of topical cardiac hypothermia-induced phrenic nerve injury and left lower lobe atelectasis during cardiac surgery, *Chest* 88:680-683, 1985.

314. White DA, Matthay RA: Noninfectious pulmonary complications of infection with the human immunodeficiency virus, *Am Rev Respir Dis* 140:1763-1787, 1989.

315. Witt DJ, Craven DE, McCabe WR: Bacterial infections in adult patients with acquired immunodeficiency syndrome (AIDS) and AIDS-related complex, *Am J Med* 82:900-906, 1987.

316. Witt K, Nielsen TN, Junge J: Dissemination of *Pneumocystis carinii* in patients with AIDS, *Scand J Infect Dis* 23:691-695, 1991.

317. Witte RJ, Gurney JW, Robbins RA, et al: Diffuse pulmonary alveolar hemorrhage after bone marrow transplantation: radiographic findings in 39 patients, *AJR* 157:461-464, 1991.

318. Wolfson J, Quie PG, Laxdol SD: Roentgenologic manifestations in children with a genetic defect of polymorphonuclear leucocyte function, *Radiology* 91:37-48, 1968.

319. Wolinsky E: Nontuberculous mycobacteria and associated diseases, *Am Rev Respir Dis* 119:107-159, 1979.

320. Wolke A, Meyers S, Adelsberg BR, et al: *Mycobacterium avium-intracellulare*–associated colitis in a patient with the acquired immunodeficiency syndrome, *J Clin Gastroenterol* 6:225-229, 1984.

321. Woolfenden JM, Carrasquilo JA, Larson SM, et al: Acquired immunodeficiency syndrome: Ga-67 citrate imaging, *Radiology* 162:383-387, 1987.

322. Young RC, Bennett JE, Vogel CL, et al: Aspergillosis — the spectrum of the disease in 98 patients, *Medicine* 49:147-173, 1970.

323. Zibrak JD, Silvestri RC, Costello P, et al: Bronchoscopic and radiologic features of Kaposi's sarcoma involving the respiratory system, *Chest* 90:476-479, 1986.

324. Ziegler JL, Beckstead JA, Volberding PA, et al: Non-Hodgkins lymphoma in 90 homosexual men: relation to generalized adenopathy and the acquired immunodeficiency syndrome, *N Engl J Med* 311:565-570, 1984.

325. Zimmerman BL, Haller JO, Price AP, et al: Children with AIDS — is pathologic diagnosis possible based on chest radiographs? *Pediatr Radiol* 17:303-307, 1987.

326. Zoman M, White DA: Serum lactate dehydrogenase levels and *Pneumocystis carinii* pneumonia, *Am Rev Respir Dis* 137:796-800, 1988.

327. Zuger A, Louie E, Holzman RS, et al: Cryptococcal disease in patients with the acquired immunodeficiency syndrome, *Ann Intern Med* 104:234-240, 1986.

8 Neoplasms of the Lungs, Airways, and Pleura

PETER ARMSTRONG

BRONCHIAL CARCINOMA
Pathology and clinical features

The most widely used histologic classifications of primary bronchial carcinoma are based on the recommendations of the 1977 Working Party for the Therapy of Lung Cancer/Lung Cancer Study Group and include the following[245,518]:

1. Epidermoid (squamous cell) carcinoma, which comprises 30% to 50% of cases. Its relative incidence appears to be falling,[22,658] however, probably because the prevalence of smoking is falling. Epidermoid carcinomas are subdivided into well, moderately, and poorly differentiated varieties.

2. Adenocarcinoma accounts for up to 35% of cases. Its relative incidence is rising,[658] and it now appears to be the predominant form of lung cancer in the United States. Bronchioloalveolar carcinoma (alveolar cell carcinoma) is sometimes classed separately and at other times included under adenocarcinoma. Bronchioloalveolar carcinoma comprised 2.8% of all cases of lung cancer in the large series of Vincent and associates[658] published in 1977, but the relative incidence appears to be rising dramatically as smoking declines and it may now comprise 10% to 20% of all lung cancers.[22] Adenocarcinomas, like epidermoid tumors, are subdivided into well, moderately, and poorly differentiated varieties.

3. Large cell anaplastic carcinoma (including the giant cell variety), which comprises 10% to 15% of cases.

4. Small (oat) cell carcinoma, which comprises 20% to 30% of cases.

The histologic distinction among these various categories is not always clear-cut: pathologists may differ in their interpretations, and different portions of the same tumor may warrant different classifications. Mixed tumors with features of both adenocarcinoma and epidermoid carcinoma may be classified separately as adenosquamous cancers.[475,604] Three rare varieties do not fit neatly into the above classification: clear cell carcinoma, carcinosarcoma, and basal cell carcinoma of the bronchus.

Primary carcinoma of the lung is usually solitary. Multiple primary tumors were said at one time to occur in less than 2% of cases,[549,608] but recent series have suggested that the incidence of synchronous multiple primary tumors is up to 10 times higher, depending on cell type, how carefully the further primary tumors are sought, and the rigidity of the criteria used to define whether or not two tumors in the lung are both regarded as primary lesions.* Difference in cell type is an accepted criterion for synchronous primary neoplasms, but tumors of the same histologic type can be accepted as synchronous provided they are of similar size and physically quite separate. Metachronous lesions are generally regarded as multiple primary lesions only if they show unique histologic features.

The presence of one lung cancer appears to predispose to the subsequent development of a second primary tumor. In the National Cancer Institute survey described on p. 303, 17% of patients with an operable lung cancer developed a second primary carcinoma of the lung. This high incidence may be related to the presence of distant bronchioloalveolar adenomas in the lungs of patients with lung carcinoma. These small, benign but possibly premalignant lesions were found in 9.3% of resection specimens in one large series.[440]

Bronchial carcinoma, particularly bronchioloalveolar carcinoma and adenocarcinoma, may develop in scarred lung or within an area of lipoid pneumonia.[175] So-called scar carcinomas develop in conditions such as old tuberculosis or old infarcts, as well as in various forms of interstitial pulmonary fibrosis (see Figure 8-6).[27,194,378,544] It may be that the presence of regenerating epithelium at the edge of a scar predisposes to malignant transformation.[436] In most so-called scar carcinomas the fibrous tissue is probably a desmoplastic response to the cancer; in other words the scar may follow, rather than precede, the development of carcinoma.[32,245,389]

Approximately 25% of patients with bronchial carcinoma are asymptomatic at the time of diagnosis.[553] Cough, wheezing, hemoptysis, and paraneoplastic syndromes (see box at right) are the cardinal symptoms when the carcinoma is still confined to the lung. Hoarseness, chest pain, brachial plexus neuropathy, Horner's syndrome, superior vena caval obstruction, dysphagia, and the problems of pericardial tamponade indicate invasion of the mediastinum or chest wall.[298]

The clinical symptoms and signs vary with cell type.[118,179] Epidermoid carcinoma is a relatively slow-growing, late-metastasizing tumor that most often arises centrally within the bronchial tree and therefore usually

---

*References 62, 88, 420, 441, 649, 706.

CLASSIFICATION OF EXTRAPULMONARY MANIFESTATIONS OF CARCINOMA OF THE LUNG

ENDOCRINE AND METABOLIC

Cushing's syndrome
Inappropriate secretion of antidiuretic hormone
Carcinoid syndrome
Hypercalcemia
Ectopic gonadotropin, gynecomastia
Insulin-like activity
Acromegaly
Cachexia of malignancy

NEUROMUSCULAR

Eaton-Lambert syndrome
Polymyositis
Peripheral neuropathy
Subacute cerebellar degeneration
Encephalomyelopathy

SKELETAL

Clubbing
Pulmonary hypertrophic osteoarthropathy
Osteomalacia

DERMATOLOGIC

Acanthosis nigricans
Scleroderma
Other dermatoses

VASCULAR

Migratory thrombophlebitis
Nonbacterial verrucous endocarditis
Arterial thrombosis

HEMATOLOGIC

Anemia
Red cell aplasia
Fibrinolytic purpura
Nonspecific leukocytosis
Polycythemia
Eosinophilia
Leukoerythroblastic reaction

Modified from Filderman AE, Shaw C, Matthay RA: *Invest Radiol* 21:80-90, 1986.

is manifest as obstructive atelectasis or pneumonia, hemoptysis, or the signs and symptoms of invasion of adjacent structures, such as the recurrent laryngeal nerve. When epidermoid tumors arise peripherally in the lung, they may grow to substantial size before symptoms develop. Hypercalcemia, usually secondary to osteolysis, is encountered with squamous cell carcinoma and may be an early manifestation. The precise mechanism of the osteolysis is not certain; parathormone production may be an important factor.

Adenocarcinoma most often arises as a peripheral pulmonary nodule and is frequently first discovered on a chest radiograph in a patient with no chest symptoms. Nevertheless, hilar and mediastinal node involvement and distant metastases, particularly in the brain and adrenal glands, are frequently present at the time of diagnosis. Dyspnea resulting from pleural effusion is a particular feature of adenocarcinoma. Adenocarcinoma is the cell type most frequently associated with preexisting chronic pulmonary disease such as asbestosis and prior lung damage. Bronchioloalveolar carcinoma, unlike other bronchial adenocarcinomas, is often an indolent tumor that metastasizes late.

Large cell anaplastic carcinoma is similar to epidermoid carcinoma in that the tumor may grow to a large size, but dissimilar in that it metastasizes early, particularly to the mediastinum and brain.[592]

Small (oat) cell carcinoma also metastasizes early and widely; metastases are usually present at initial diagnosis. Hormone production, notably adrenocorticotropic hormone, antidiuretic hormone, and melanocyte-stimulating hormone, is a feature of small (oat) cell tumors.[528]

Imaging features

The imaging appearances of lung cancer are considered in the following framework: (1) peripheral tumors (tumors arising beyond the hilum) and (2) central tumors (tumors arising at or close to the hilum).

PERIPHERAL TUMORS. Approximately 40% of bronchial carcinomas arise beyond the larger segmental bronchi,[22] and in 30% a peripheral mass is the sole radiographic finding.[80-83,356,637] The fact that peripheral tumors may grow predominantly in the direction of the hilum[372,545] may explain the variable proportions of peripheral versus central tumors reported in large surveys and the unexpectedly high number of "peripheral" masses visible at bronchoscopy. The mass can be virtually any size, but it is rare for a bronchial carcinoma to be seen on plain chest radiographs unless it is more than 1 cm in diameter.[224,338,458,610,637] Computed tomography (CT), because of its better contrast resolution, detects smaller lesions.

Shape. In general, peripheral bronchial carcinomas (except for certain bronchioloalveolar carcinomas) assume an approximately spherical or oval configuration. Bronchogenic carcinoma is therefore one of the major diagnostic considerations in adults with a solitary pulmonary nodule—a subject discussed in detail in Chapter 4.

Lobulation, a sign that indicates uneven growth rates for differing portions of the tumor, is common (Figure 8-1).[637] An equally frequent sign is a notch (umbilication), a sign that is the counterpart of lobulation because it indicates relatively slow growth of a particular portion of the tumor.[546] Occasionally a dumbbell shape is encountered or two nodules are seen next to each other (Figure 8-1). Tumors at the lung apex (Pancoast's tumors,

superior sulcus tumors) may resemble apical pleural thickening, as discussed on p. 294.

Sometimes the edge of the tumor is irregular, with one or more strands radiating into the surrounding lung (Figure 8-2). The term "corona radiata"[259] indicates the passage of multiple strands extending into the surrounding lung because of either tumor extension or a fibrotic response to the tumor. Such stranding is best seen with tomography, particularly thin section CT (Figures 8-2 and 8-3).[341] A well-developed corona radiata is a useful sign in the differential diagnosis of a solitary pulmonary nodule because it makes the diagnosis of bronchogenic carcinoma highly likely. It is not, however, entirely specific; similar very irregular margins have been encountered in a variety of lesions, including benign processes, notably chronic pneumonia and granuloma. A single linear or bandlike shadow may connect the lesion to the pleura (Figure 8-4). This so-called pleural tail sign, as discussed on p. 104, is seen with both benign and malignant pulmonary nodules.

Careful observation of the pattern of vessels in the neighboring lung parenchyma may show convergence of peripheral blood vessels leading to and entering the cancerous mass (Figure 8-3), a sign that is best appreciated with thin section CT.[341] In one small series using multiplanar reconstruction CT, all 15 bronchial cancers showed direct involvement of a draining pulmonary vein.[452]

Regardless of the irregularity of the border, the nodules or masses described thus far can be regarded as having a well-defined edge. Some peripheral cancers, 25% in one series,[637] show a very poorly defined edge similar to that seen in pneumonia (Figures 8-5 and 8-6). In such cases the spherical shape and relatively slow growth seen with carcinomas usually allow distinction from infectious processes.

Occasionally, bronchial carcinoma arising in segmental or subsegmental bronchi is seen radiographically as mucoid impaction (bronchial mucocele or bronchocele) (Figure 8-7),[17,174,693,694] in which case the resulting shadow, to a greater or lesser extent, represents dilated bronchi filled with tumor or inspissated secretions. For a mucoid impaction to be visible, the adjacent lung must be aerated by collateral air drift. Mucoid impactions result in V-shaped, Y-shaped, or branching tree densities with their stems pointing toward the hilum.

Another rare pattern is an infarct shadow extending from the primary tumor, giving two contiguous but distinct components to the opacity, the distal one being a pleural-based infarct.[402]

Air bronchograms and cavitation. Air bronchograms are usually thought of as a feature of infective consolidation or other alveolar filling processes. Kuriyama and associates,[342] however, found that with thin section CT some air-filled bronchi or bronchioles could be identified within peripherally situated small adenocarcinomas in the majority of cases. Bubblelike areas of low attenuation

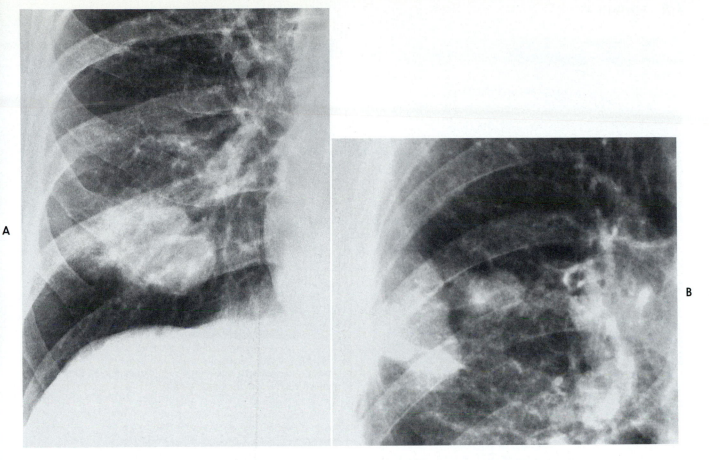

FIGURE 8-1
A, Squamous cell bronchial carcinoma occurring as solitary lobular peripheral mass. B, Two adjacent nodules caused by bronchial carcinoma. More lateral lesion shows distinct notching.

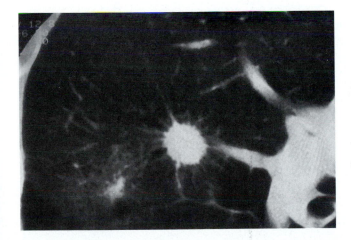

FIGURE 8-2
Bronchial carcinoma showing irregular infiltrating edge known as corona radiata.

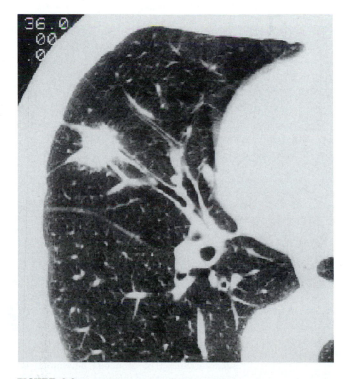

FIGURE 8-3
High-resolution computed tomographic scan of bronchial carcinoma showing distortion of adjacent vessels as well as infiltrating edges.

are seen fairly frequently within lung cancers on high-resolution CT (HRCT): they were identified in 25% of one series of 93 cases of solitary pulmonary nodule caused by lung cancer examined by HRCT.[707] These lucencies, which are seen in lung cancers of all cell types but are most frequently encountered in adenocarcinoma and

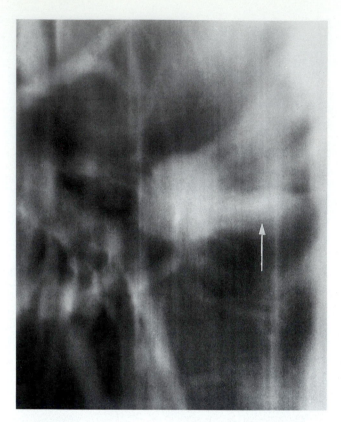

FIGURE 8-4
Bronchial adenocarcinoma showing pleural tail sign *(arrow)*.

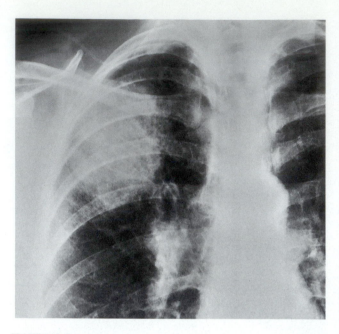

FIGURE 8-5
Poorly differentiated squamous cell carcinoma of lung with ill-defined edge resembling pneumonia.

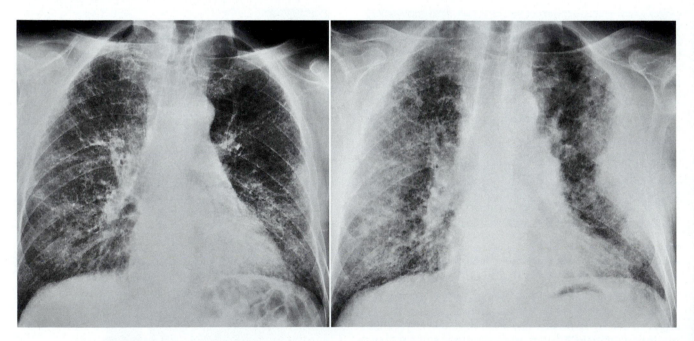

FIGURE 8-6
Adenocarcinoma of bronchus developing in patient with diffuse interstitial pulmonary fibrosis (rheumatoid lung). In this case the tumor has a very ill-defined edge resembling pneumonia. The two films were taken 6 months apart.

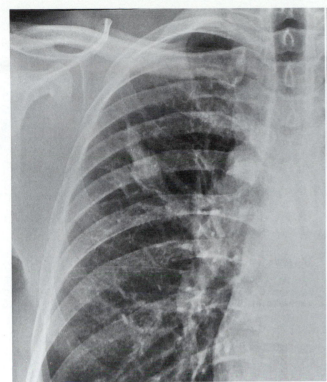

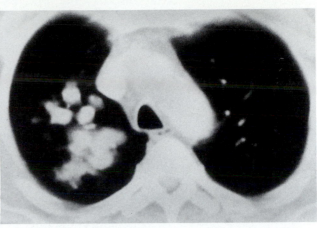

FIGURE 8-7
A, Dilated mucus-filled bronchi (mucoid impaction) in small cell bronchial carcinoma. Hilar and paratracheal nodal metastases are also present. **B,** Computed tomographic scan in another patient showing mucoid impaction beyond bronchial carcinoma.

bronchioloalveolar carcinoma, are due either to patent small bronchi or to small cystic spaces within the tumor.[707]

Approximately 16% of peripheral carcinomas show cavitation on plain chest radiography.[105,637] Squamous cell carcinoma is much more likely to cavitate than cancers of other cell types. In one series of 100 cavitary cancers, 82 were squamous cell lesions.[105] Adenocarcinomas and large cell carcinomas cavitate occasionally, whereas small cell carcinomas for practical purposes do not cavitate.[81-83,105]

Cavitation may be seen in tumors of any size and is best demonstrated by CT. The cavity is frequently eccentric, the walls are often very irregular, and tumor nodules may be visible (Figure 8-8). The wall is usually at least 8 mm thick, but on rare occasion it is notably thin, 4 mm or less (Figures 8-9 and 8-10).[695] Cavitary bronchial carcinoma may even have smooth inner and outer margins. It has been suggested that such very thin-walled cavities represent tumor cells lining bullae rather than true cavitation.[105] Fluid levels are common, and necrotic tumor fragments may be seen within the cavity. Very rarely the cavity shows an air crescent caused by air around an intracavitary tumor mass or formed debris.[176]

Calcification. Pathologists have long recognized that calcification is seen on histologic examination of bronchial carcinomas. Such calcification may be dystrophic in areas of tumor necrosis or may be intrinsic as in mucinous adenocarcinoma (Figure 8-11). The calcification is very rarely demonstrable with conven-

tional radiography except at specimen radiography.[227] It is, however, becoming increasingly apparent that CT may demonstrate calcification within cancers in vivo.[225,314,392,614,704] The incidence of visible calcification at CT was initially thought to be low, but recent studies have shown recognizable calcification within 6% to 7% of bronchogenic carcinomas (Figure 8-12).[392,704] Some of the calcifications no doubt represent preexisting granulomatous calcifications engulfed by the tumor; such granulomatous calcifications are likely to be eccentric in location, but focal central granulomatous calcifications are occasionally seen (Figure 8-13). However, amorphous or cloudlike calcification, entirely in keeping with tumor calcification, is seen in a significant minority of patients.[704] In the series reported by Mahoney and associates,[392] most calcified tumors were large with a diameter of 5 cm or more, but amorphous or cloudlike calcification can be seen in small peripheral tumors (Figure 8-11). Both small cell and non–small cell carcinomas may calcify, and there does not appear to be a predilection for cancers of any particular cell type.

Rate of growth. The volume doubling time for most bronchial carcinomas is between 1 and 18 months[205,246,473,619]; a 26% increase in diameter is equivalent to a doubling of volume. In one large series the average doubling time was 4.1 months for undifferentiated carcinomas, 4.2 months for squamous cell carcinoma, and 7.3 months for adenocarcinoma.[202] The primary tumors that grow more slowly are likely to be bronchioloalveolar carcinoma.[269]

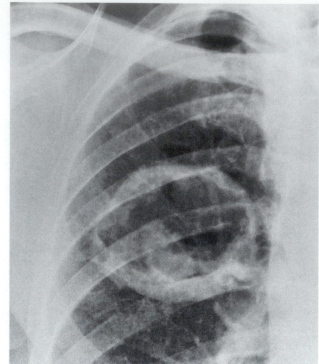

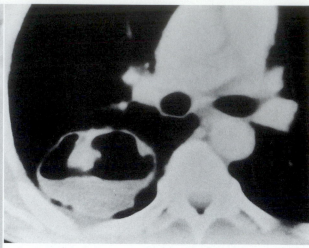

FIGURE 8-8
Squamous cell carcinoma of bronchus showing cavitation. Cavity wall is of variable thickness and shows mural nodule as well as air-fluid level. **A,** Posteroanterior radiograph. **B,** Computed tomographic scan.

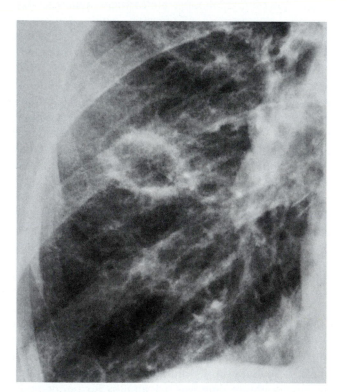

FIGURE 8-9
Squamous cell carcinoma of bronchus showing thin, uniform-thickness cavity wall.

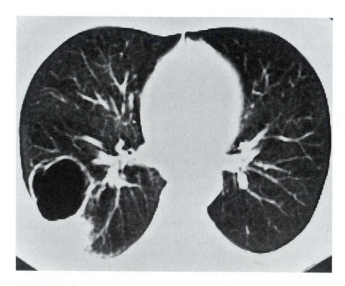

FIGURE 8-10
Bronchial adenocarcinoma showing very thin, uniform-thickness cavity wall.

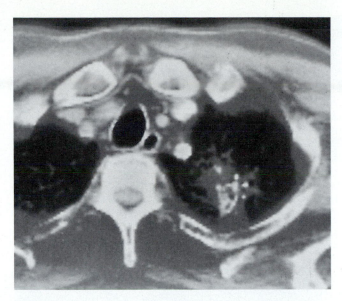

FIGURE 8-11
Adenocarcinoma of bronchus showing widespread calcification, which on histologic study was dystrophic calcification in necrotic areas of tumor, not preexisting granulomatous calcification. (Courtesy Dr. John Pitman, Williamsburg, Va.)

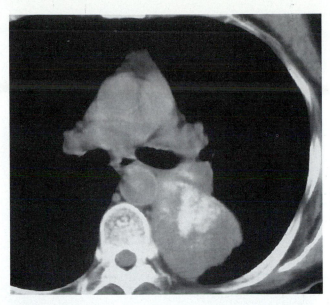

FIGURE 8-12
Extensive granular calcification in large, centrally located carcinoma. Tumor obstructed left lower lobe bronchus and caused left lower lobe collapse.

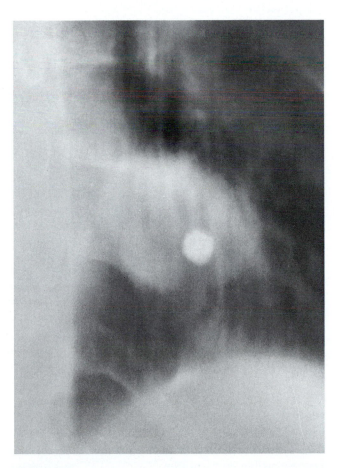

FIGURE 8-13
Calcified granuloma engulfed by bronchial carcinoma. This case is unusual in that granuloma is relatively central.

CENTRAL TUMORS. The cardinal imaging signs of a central tumor are collapse and consolidation of the lung beyond the tumor and the presence of hilar enlargement, signs that may be seen in isolation or in conjunction.

Collapse and consolidation in association with central tumors. Obstruction of a major bronchus may lead to a combination of atelectasis and retention of secretions with consequent pulmonary opacity,[77] but collateral air drift may partially or completely prevent these postobstructive changes. Obstructed portions of the lung may become secondarily infected, although this is relatively uncommon, at least in patients whose tumors are still amenable to surgical resection.[77] With time, lipid-laden alveolar macrophages accumulate within the airspaces distal to an obstruction, giving rise to an appearance known to pathologists as endogenous lipoid pneumonia ("golden pneumonia"). The interstitium thickens because of lymphocytic infiltration and collagen deposition.[77]

As might be expected, the cancer most frequently responsible for collapse and consolidation is squamous cell carcinoma, partly because it is a common cell type and partly because a larger proportion of squamous carcinomas originate centrally. In the Mayo Clinic series over half the patients with squamous cell carcinoma had collapse, consolidation, or obstructive pneumonitis.[81] The incidence of these signs with cancers of other cell types was between 15% and 37%.[82,83,356]

Collapse and consolidation, both of which can be patchy (Figure 8-14) or homogeneous, are readily recognizable radiographically. Loss of volume is usual with

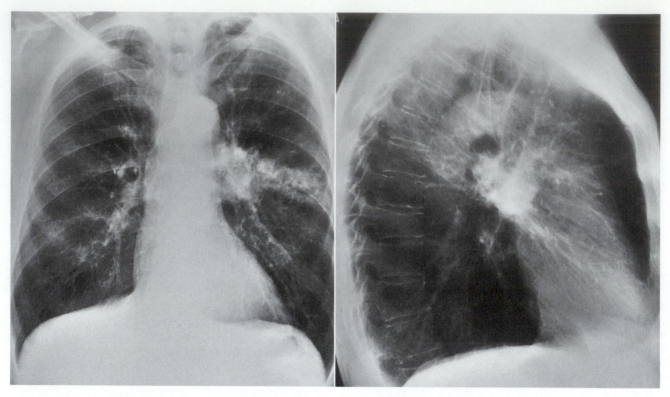

FIGURE 8-14
Collapse and consolidation beyond a hilar mass. The mass is caused by bronchial carcinoma.

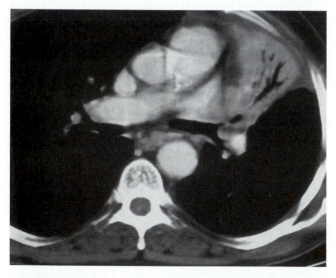

FIGURE 8-15
Air bronchogram in left upper lobe collapse beyond bronchial carcinoma in left upper lobe bronchus.

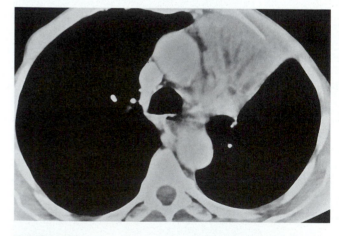

FIGURE 8-16
Dilated fluid-filled bronchi in collapsed left upper lobe beyond a central bronchial carcinoma. (Plain chest radiograph of this patient is shown in Figure 8-18.)

central tumors, but consolidation without loss of volume is not infrequent. Air bronchograms visible on plain chest radiographs are uncommon, particularly before antibiotic therapy. They are seen much more frequently at CT scanning (Figure 8-15). If the tumor regresses with

therapy, a previously invisible air bronchogram may become visible on plain film.

The most obvious retained secretion is mucus, which accumulates within and eventually distends the airways. Mucus-filled dilated bronchi, which may be visible within

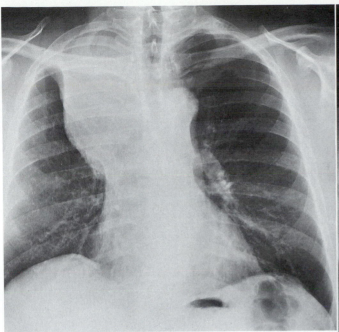

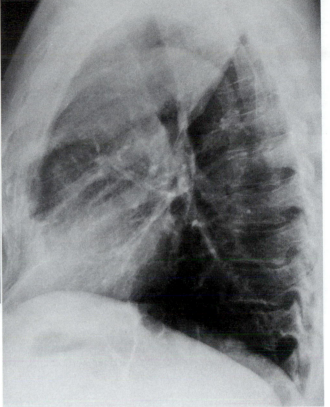

FIGURE 8-17
Golden S sign in right upper lobe collapse. Lobe has collapsed around large obstructing centrally positioned bronchial carcinoma in right upper lobe bronchus.

collapsed lobes on CT examination as branching, tubular, low-density structures (Figure 8-16), are more apparent on the postcontrast images than they are on non-contrast-enhanced images[218,591,691] and when seen should prompt a search for a central obstructing tumor.

Defining the presence or extent of the central tumor mass in the presence of postobstructive consolidation and atelectasis can be difficult, even with CT or magnetic resonance imaging (MRI). This decision can be important in making the initial diagnosis of a central tumor. Although CT or MRI may allow the tumor to be more accurately measured, the size of the lesion by itself does not change management, since both small and large tumors are surgically excised, provided they have not spread beyond the hilar nodes. On unenhanced CT scans the neoplastic and nonneoplastic tissue may be similar in density. After administration of contrast material there is differential enhancement, particularly if rapid sequential scanning is used[490,640]: the neoplastic tissue enhances to a minimal degree whereas distal atelectasis may show substantial enhancement. MRI shows a difference in signal between tumor and postobstructive pulmonary changes, particularly on T2-weighted images[306,640] or gadolinium-enhanced T1-weighted images.[328,615] Based on one small series it appears that cholesterol pneumonitis and distal bronchiectasis are seen as higher signal than tumor on T2-weighted images, whereas organizing pneu-

monia and atelectasis are isointense with tumors.[61] In two series[306,615] MRI was better than contrast-enhanced CT scanning for distinguishing tumor from postobstructive change, whereas in the series reported by Tobler and associates[640] CT proved more successful than MRI in distinguishing between the two processes.

The following features suggest that a pneumonia is secondary to an obstructing neoplasm:

1. Alteration in the shape of the collapsed or consolidated lobe because of the bulk of the underlying tumor. In a case with lobar collapse the fissure in the region of the mass may be unable to move in the usual manner, with the result that the fissure appears bulged ("Golden S" sign) (Figure 8-17). The sign indicates that the collapse is the result of an underlying mass and predicts the mass will be sufficiently central that successful bronchoscopic biopsy should be readily achievable.

2. The presence of pneumonia confined to one lobe (or more lobes if there is a common bronchus supplying these lobes) in patients over the age of 35, particularly if the lobe shows loss of volume and no air bronchograms (Figure 8-18). Occasionally the opacified lobe appears larger than normal because of buildup of secretions and infection behind the obstructing carcinoma (Figure 8-19), an appearance that has been labeled the drowned lobe. In cases of obstructive pneumonitis or atelectasis the tumor should be readily visible at bronchoscopy, an investiga-

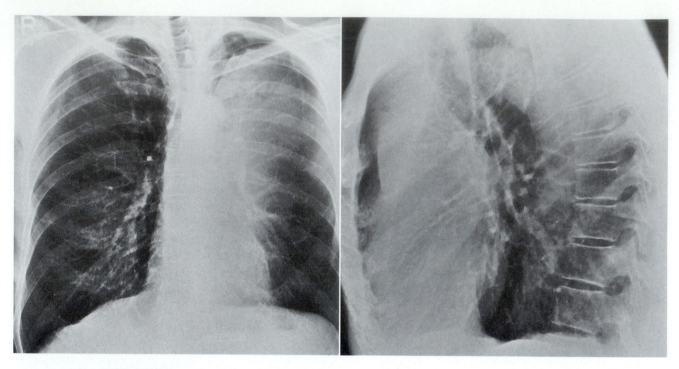

FIGURE 8-18
Left upper lobe collapse shown on posteroanterior and lateral chest radiograph beyond centrally obstructing bronchial carcinoma. (One image from the computed tomographic scan of this patient is shown in Figure 8-16.)

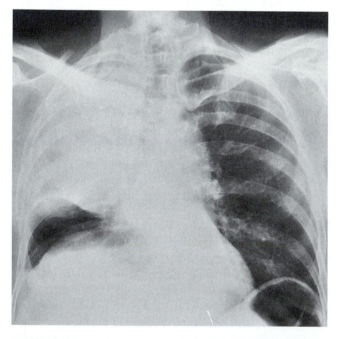

FIGURE 8-19
"Drowned lobe" beyond bronchial carcinoma in right upper lobe bronchus. Right upper lobe shows extensive consolidation and expansion.

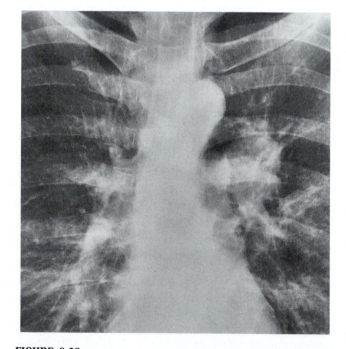

FIGURE 8-20
Small cell carcinoma of bronchus occurring as a hilar mass. As is so often the case, it is not possible to tell whether the mass is all tumor, all enlarged nodes, or mixture of the two.

tion that is usually performed without delay in patients with these radiographic findings.

3. The presence of a visible mass or irregular stenosis in a mainstem or lobar bronchus. Careful analysis of CT scans will demonstrate the presence of an obstructing tumor in virtually every case of postobstructive atelectasis caused by a lung carcinoma.[691]

4. The presence of an associated central mass (Figure 8-14). Simple pneumonia rarely causes radiographically visible hilar adenopathy, although enlarged central nodes may be seen at CT or MRI. Bacterial lung abscess can, however, be confused with bronchial carcinoma because it may result in hilar or mediastinal adenopathy.[548]

5. A localized pneumonia that persists unchanged for more than 2 weeks or one that recurs in the same lobe. Simple pneumonia often clears or spreads to other segments during this time interval. Complete resolution of pneumonia, in practice, excludes an obstructing neoplasm as cause of infection. Although consolidation may improve with appropriate antibiotic therapy, it virtually never resolves completely if it is secondary to an underlying carcinoma.

Hilar enlargement. Hilar enlargement is a common presenting feature in patients with bronchial carcinoma. In the Mayo Clinic series[80-83,356] 38% of patients had a hilar or perihilar mass and in 12% a central mass was the only radiographic abnormality (Figure 8-20). Such masses may result from the tumor itself, from enlarge-

ment of hilar nodes containing metastatic tumor, from consolidated lung, or from a combination of these phenomena. Deciding the relative contribution of tumor mass, enlarged nodes, or consolidation can be difficult. In general, the more lobular the shape, the more likely that adenopathy is present.

A mass superimposed on the hilum may lead to increased density of the hilum because of summation when the opacity of the mass is added to the density of the normal hilar shadows (Figure 8-21). This sign may be the only indication of lung cancer on a frontal chest film; when the sign is suspected, careful inspection of a lateral film is essential.

Air trapping. Expiration films to detect air trapping, although occasionally positive, have not proved useful in the diagnosis of bronchial carcinoma. Fraser and Pare[193] found only one case of carcinoma in which air trapping was evident in the 6 years that inspiratory-expiratory films were routinely obtained in their institution. Recognizable overinflation by check valve obstruction appears to be even more unusual[119]; no example was found in the 600 cases reported from the Mayo Clinic.[80-83,356]

STAGING INTRATHORACIC SPREAD OF TUMOR. Bronchial carcinoma invades locally by endobronchial and transbronchial growth,[259] spreads by way of lymphatics to hilar and mediastinal nodes, and metastasizes by means of the bloodstream to remote sites, including other thoracic structures. Only features visible at chest

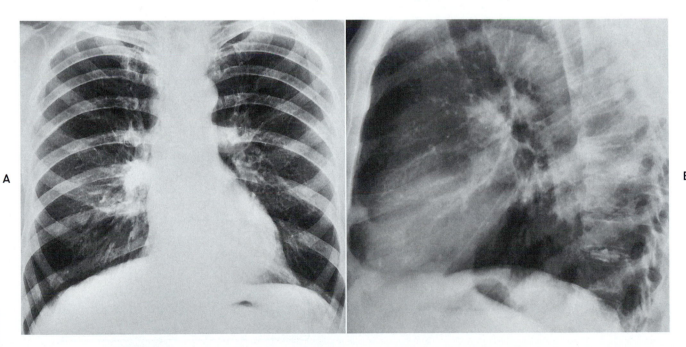

A   B

FIGURE 8-21
Dense hilum sign. Most obvious sign of carcinoma in superior segment of right lower lobe is increase in density of right hilum caused by superimposition of mass, distal pneumonia, and hilar structures.
A, Posteroanterior view. **B,** Lateral view.

TNM DEFINITIONS FOR THE INTERNATIONAL STAGING SYSTEM FOR LUNG CANCER

PRIMARY TUMOR (T)

TX Tumor proved by the presence of malignant cells in bronchopulmonary secretions but not visualized roentgenographically or bronchoscopically, or any tumor that cannot be assessed as in a retreatment staging

T0 No evidence of primary tumor

T1S Carcinoma in situ

T1* A tumor that is 3 cm or less in greatest dimension, surrounded by lung or visceral pleura, and without evidence of invasion proximal to a lobar bronchus at bronchoscopy

T2 A tumor more than 3 cm in greatest dimension, or a tumor of any size that either invades the visceral pleura or has associated atelectasis or obstructive pneumonitis extending to the hilar region. At bronchoscopy the proximal extent of demonstrable tumor must be within a lobar bronchus or at least 2 cm distal to the carina. Any associated atelectasis or obstructive pneumonitis must involve less than an entire lung

T3 A tumor of any size with direct extension into the chest wall (including superior sulcus tumors), diaphragm, or the mediastinal pleura or pericardium without involving the heart, great vessels, trachea, esophagus, or vertebral body; or a tumor in the main bronchus within 2 cm of the carina without involving the carina

T4† A tumor of any size with invasion of the mediastinum or involving the heart, great vessels, trachea, esophagus, vertebral body, or carina, or presence of malignant pleural effusion

NODAL INVOLVEMENT (N)

N0 No demonstrable metastasis to regional lymph nodes

N1 Metastasis to lymph nodes in the peribronchial or the ipsilateral hilar region, or both, including direct extension

N2 Metastasis to ipsilateral mediastinal lymph nodes and subcarinal lymph nodes

N3 Metastasis to contralateral mediastinal lymph nodes, contralateral hilar lymph nodes, ipsilateral or contralateral scalene, or supraclavicular lymph nodes

DISTANT METASTASIS (M)

M0 No (known) distant metastasis

M1 Distant metastasis present — specify sites

From Mountain CF: *Chest* 89(suppl):225S-233S, 1986.

*The uncommon superficial tumor of any size with the invasive component limited to the bronchial wall that may extend proximal to the main bronchus is classified as T1.

†Most pleural effusions associated with lung cancer are due to tumor. There are, however, some few patients in whom cytopathologic examination of pleural fluid (on more than one specimen) is negative for tumor, the fluid is nonbloody, and it is not an exudate. In such cases in which these elements and clinical judgment dictate that the effusion is not related to the tumor, the patients should be staged T1, T2, or T3, excluding effusion as a staging element.

Table 8-1 Stages for International Staging System for lung cancer

Stage	Definition*
I	T1, N0, M0
	T2, N0, M0
II	T1, N1, M0
	T2, N1, M0
IIIA	T3, N0, M0
	T3, N1, M0
	T1-3, N2, M0
IIIB	Any T, N3, M0
	T4; any N, M0
IV	Any T; any N, M1

*See box above.

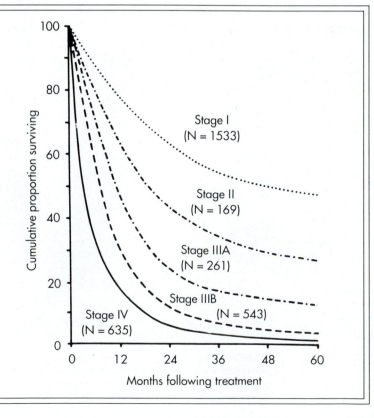

From Mountain CF: *Chest* 89(suppl):225S-233S, 1986.

imaging are discussed here. (Lymphangitis carcinomatosa is discussed separately on p. 350.)

International Staging System. The International Staging System for lung cancer,* introduced in 1986, was designed for thoracic surgeons considering patients for surgical resection, as well as for radiation therapists and oncologists trying to treat widespread disease.[455,708] The TNM system (see the upper box on the facing page) is used to describe the findings, and the stage (Table 8-1) is derived from the TNM description.

Stage I consists of T1 or T2 lesions with no hilar, mediastinal, or distant metastases. These lesions are surgically resectable, provided the patient can withstand surgery or the loss of lung tissue. Stage I tumors that are T1 have a better prognosis (greater than 75% 5-year survival)[430] than stage I tumors that are T2.

Stage II consists of the same lesions as stage I but with peribronchial or hilar involvement. These lesions are also resectable by lobectomy or pneumonectomy with the hope of cure, but the prognosis is not as good as for stage I tumors.

Stage III is divided into two substages. Stage IIIA designates patients with limited, potentially resectable, invasion of the chest wall, pericardium, or mediastinum; involvement of the proximal airways but still amenable to tracheobronchial sleeve resection; or involvement of ipsilateral mediastinal lymph nodes that may be surgically resectable. Stage IIIB identifies patients with locally extensive intrathoracic invasion beyond the limits of conventional surgical resection (invasion of the heart, great vessels, trachea, esophagus, or vertebral body and/or involvement of contralateral lymph nodes or involvement of scalene and supraclavicular nodes), but still localized in terms of planning radiation therapy.

Stage IV includes all patients with distant metastases. Patients with small cell lung cancer are usually classified as "limited" or "extensive," since they are almost invariably stage IV when initially examined. There are no universally agreed upon definitions, but limited disease typically is cancer limited to one hemithorax with hilar and mediastinal nodes encompassable within a tolerable radiotherapy portal, whereas extensive disease is any disease beyond those boundaries.[301]

The survival of patients with tumors of different stages is shown in Table 8-1, which is based on the study and treatment outcomes of 3750 patients by Mountain.[455] The dividing line between stage II and stage IIIA tumors is that with stage II lesions the entire bulk of detectable tumor can be removed by lobectomy or simple pneumonectomy, whereas with stage IIIA tumors such resection is not possible. The distinction between stages IIIA and IIIB, the dividing line between resectable and unresectable tu-

mors, is essentially the difference between (1) T2 and T3 tumors, that is, whether or not the tumor shows more than just limited, potentially resectable extension into the chest wall or mediastinum and (2) whether or not the tumor involves contralateral and supraclavicular/scalene lymph nodes.

Mediastinal lymph node involvement should preferably be designated according to the American Thoracic Society (ATS) lymph node map (see Figure 2-22). The ATS map defines lymph node groups in relation to fixed anatomic structures, such as the azygos vein, bronchi, and aortic arch, which can be easily identified at CT scanning, mediastinoscopy, and surgery. Even with the ATS map the problem of accurately distinguishing between hilar and adjacent mediastinal nodes is difficult. This distinction is of importance because one of the key differences between stage II and stage III tumors (the cutoff point for most surgeons between surgical and nonsurgical treatment) is whether mediastinal nodes are involved. The AJCC definition of hilar nodes (N1) is nodes within the lung outside the mediastinal pleura at surgery, but the visceral pleura cannot be identified at CT and surgeons may vary in their designation of nodes as hilar or mediastinal at surgery. Friedman,[195] a member of the ATS Committee on Lung Cancer, suggested that 10R nodes should be considered hilar (N1) and 10L should be considered mediastinal (N2).[195] Thus, if this recommendation is followed, a right-sided primary lung cancer with metastasis confined to 10R nodes means that the tumor is classified as stage II, whereas a corresponding situation on the left is described as stage IIIa.

Imaging in staging lung cancer. Currently the standard imaging tests used to stage the intrathoracic spread of lung cancer are the plain chest radiograph and CT scanning of the chest.[204,327,366,550,628] It must, however, be appreciated that even CT scanning (which is significantly more sensitive than plain chest radiography or conventional tomography[362,493]) disagrees with the TNM stage found at surgery in a significant proportion of patients.[344] In 40% of cases CT categorizes the extent of tumor sufficiently poorly that the overall stage is overestimated or underestimated.[363]

Several reports comparing CT and MRI for staging lung cancer have been published,* the largest of which is the multicenter prospective study of 170 patients with non–small cell bronchogenic carcinoma reported by Webb and co-workers.[674] Based on the studies reported so far, MRI has not demonstrated enough advantages to replace chest CT as a routine staging procedure, although it can, as discussed in the following sections, be useful as a problem-solving technique.[206]

A related but distinct issue is the preoperative decision

---

*Stitik, the radiologist member on the 1985 American Joint Committee on Cancer Task Force, has provided an authoritative detailed account for radiologists.[616]

*References 36, 233, 306, 405, 465, 503, 524, 615, 671.

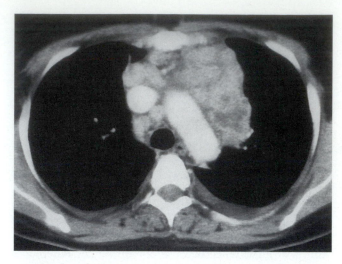

FIGURE 8-22
Computed tomographic scan of mediastinal adenopathy caused by metastases from primary large cell undifferentiated carcinoma. Enlarged nodes have enhanced to same degree as muscle following intravenous contrast enhancement.

of whether lobectomy or pneumonectomy will be required for centrally situated tumors, or whether conservative bronchoplastic surgery will be feasible. The decision depends on whether or not the tumor has crossed fissures, invaded central vessels, or spread centrally within the bronchial tree. Plain radiography, CT scanning, MRI, and bronchoscopy all provide important information, but CT scanning has not proved sufficiently accurate in predicting whether or not a pneumonectomy will be required. Therefore the surgeon still makes this decision based on bronchoscopic findings, or not infrequently on the findings at thoracotomy.[344,531] MRI, by virtue of its multiplanar imaging capability, may be helpful.[318,411]

Even with tumors amenable to surgical resection, a major problem in many patients is whether or not lung function would be adequate if a pneumonectomy is required. Pulmonary perfusion scans have a role to play here. The relative perfusion of each lung is quantitated by the number of radioactive counts in the combined anterior and posterior scans. The percentage contribution of each lung to the total counts is then multiplied by the overall forced expiratory volume in one second (FEV_1) to predict the FEV_1 of the lung that would remain after surgery.[63] Quantitative regional ventilation and perfusion can also be assessed using nuclear medicine techniques to predict postoperative loss of lung function.[561]

Intrathoracic lymph node metastases. Hilar and mediastinal nodal metastases (Figure 8-22) are often present at the time of initial diagnosis, particularly with adenocarcinoma and small cell tumors. Primary tumors greater than 3 cm in diameter have a higher incidence of nodal involvement than tumors of smaller diameter. Also, the more central the primary tumor, the more likely it is to be accompanied by nodal metastases.

The usual mode of lymph node spread is first to the ipsilateral segmental, interlobar, or lobar intrapulmonary nodes, then to the hilar nodes, and subsequently to the mediastinal nodes. Contralateral spread is not infrequent, particularly with left-sided primary lesions and most particularly with left lower lobe tumors. Also, metastases may skip a group of nodes; mediastinal nodal metastases without lobar or hilar node involvement have been reported in close to 30% of those with mediastinal metastases.[371]

Thoracic surgeons are divided over which patients, if any, with asymptomatic mediastinal nodal metastases should undergo attempts at curative surgery (symptomatic N2 disease indicates irresectable stage IIIB disease). Many surgeons exclude all patients with mediastinal nodal metastases from consideration, but others, responding to the existence of a subgroup of patients with ipsilateral mediastinal nodal involvement who seem to survive better than the overall group with stage IIIA tumors,[180] advocate surgery,[667] particularly in patients with the following conditions:

1. Metastases that are still confined within the capsule of the affected nodes rather than having spread beyond the capsule, although this point has been debated in a recent large series from Japan.[471] Pearson and associates[512] found that patients with superior mediastinal nodal metastases discovered at thoracotomy after a negative mediastinoscopy had a significantly better ultimate outcome than patients with ipsilateral nodal metastases discovered at preoperative mediastinoscopy.

2. Localized disease amenable to surgical resection, the definition of which varies among surgeons.[324,404,512,638] For some surgeons it would exclude involvement of high paratracheal or subcarinal nodes.

3. Involvement of the mediastinal nodes by squamous cell carcinoma rather than adenocarcinoma or large cell carcinoma, according to some surgeons,[324,471,559] but not all.[404]

A 5-year survival of 26% to 36% can be achieved in selected patients with stage IIIA tumors; the lower figure is for patients with, and the higher figure for those without, mediastinal nodal involvement.[454] However, when all patients with ipsilateral nodal involvement (N2 disease) are included, 5-year survival is just 3% to 6%.[588]

Currently the only useful imaging sign of hilar and mediastinal lymph node metastases is enlargement. Low-density necrotic areas within a node, a CT sign that has proved useful in diagnosing metastases from head and neck tumors in cervical lymph nodes, has not been found frequently enough to be of value in diagnosing mediastinal nodal involvement by lung cancer, and MRI has not yet permitted the recognition of tumor involvement based on signal intensity. Gallium-67 radionuclide imaging has proved to be insensitive and nonspecific in diagnosing the spread of bronchial carcinoma.[40,196,387,422,570] Recent studies have assessed positron emission tomography (PET) with fluorodeoxyglucose for staging nodal disease[237,597,662] and technetium-99m-labeled monoclonal

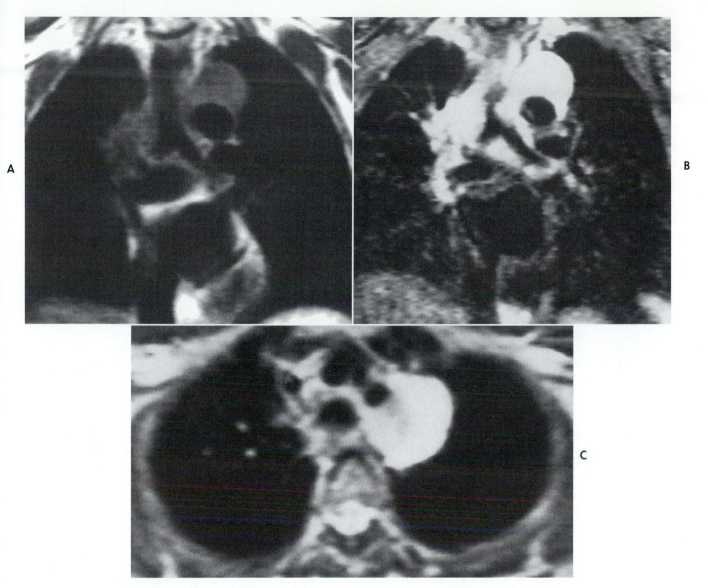

FIGURE 8-23
Magnetic resonance image of mediastinum showing extensive mediastinal adenopathy caused by involvement by small cell carcinoma of lung. **A,** T1-weighted sagittal section. **B,** T2-weighted sagittal section at same level. **C,** T2-weighted axial section above level of aortic arch. Tumor tissue can be clearly distinguished from signal void of air in bronchi and of flowing blood in major vessels. (Courtesy Dr. William C. Black, Washington, D.C.)

antibody imaging,[651] but further evaluation is required to determine the clinical value of these techniques.

Normal mediastinal lymph node size* varies according to location within the mediastinum; nodes in the subcarinal and lower paratracheal regions are up to 11 mm in short-axis diameter, with a few normal nodes reaching 15 mm, whereas nodes in the upper paratracheal regions rarely exceed 7 mm in short-axis diameter. A simple and reasonably accurate rule is that nodes smaller than 10 mm in short-axis diameter fall within the 95th percentile

and should therefore be considered normal.

MRI (Figure 8-23) appears to provide information comparable to CT regarding the presence and size of mediastinal lymph nodes. The considerable overlap of the T1 and T2 relaxation times of benign and malignant lymph nodes prevents the use of MR signal intensity for tissue characterization.[148,216,465,676] The use of MRI for staging nodal disease relies therefore on the same size criteria as CT,* and MRI is no more reliable than CT for diagnosing nodal metastases.[210,411] Advantages of MRI

---

*References 208, 215, 288, 325, 530, 572.

*References 255, 359, 405, 465, 503, 524, 615, 676.

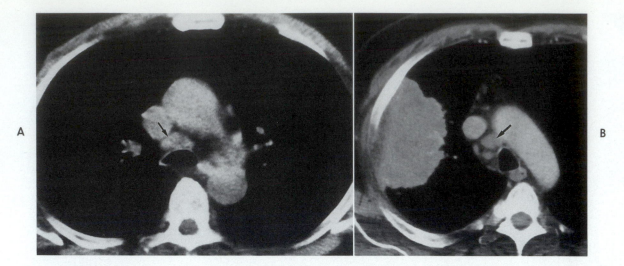

FIGURE 8-24
Benign enlargement of mediastinal nodes in patients with bronchial carcinoma. False-positive computed tomographic scan. **A,** Node *(arrow),* which measures 1.7 cm in short-axis diameter, showed only reactive hyperplasia on histologic examination. **B,** Patient with large squamous cell carcinoma of lung. Low right paratracheal node *(arrow)* measured 1.8 mm in short-axis diameter. Enlarged nodes showed only reactive hyperplasia. (Tumor had not crossed pleural space despite extensive contact with chest wall and apparent rib destruction.)

over CT are that it may be easier to distinguish lymph nodes from blood vessels owing to the different signal in areas of fast-flowing blood, a particular advantage in demonstrating hilar node involvement,[214,306,465,673] and that the coronal, or very occasionally the sagittal, imaging plane may be better for demonstrating enlargement of aortopulmonary and subcarinal nodes.[37] It should be remembered, however, that MRI has disadvantages for demonstrating mediastinal nodal enlargement: (1) respiratory or other motion may cause blurring of images, and a group of normal-sized nodes may therefore be misdiagnosed as a single large node[465,673]; (2) calcification may be overlooked,[359] and an enlarged node that would be clearly recognized as benign because of the presence of calcification may be misdiagnosed as metastatic disease; and (3) blood vessels may be misdiagnosed as lymph nodes or masses when they show signal resulting from flow.

The problem with using size as the only criterion for malignant involvement is that intrathoracic lymph node enlargement has many nonmalignant causes (Figure 8-24), including previous tuberculosis, histoplasmosis, pneumoconiosis, sarcoidosis, or reactive hyperplasia to the tumor or to associated pneumonia and atelectasis. One half to two thirds of enlarged nodes draining postobstructive pneumonia and atelectasis are free of tumor.[317,369,425] Indeed these nodes can be remarkably enlarged: in the series by McLoud and co-workers[425] 37% of nodes in the range of 2 to 4 cm were hyperplastic and did not contain metastases. Conversely, microscopic involvement by tumor can be present without causing enlargement of affected nodes. The frequency of this phenomenon varies greatly in different series.[18,132,234,317] Therefore there is no measurement above which all nodes can be assumed to be malignant and below which all can be considered benign. It is perhaps worth noting that the frequency of metastatic involvement in normal-sized nodes is significantly higher with central adenocarcinomas than with central squamous cell carcinomas.[131]

Many studies have been undertaken to establish the sensitivity and specificity of CT in diagnosing lymph node metastases.* The figures vary greatly, reflecting different size criteria and, more important, the methods used to confirm or exclude lymph node metastases. In general, CT studies on patients who have had formal, thorough lymph node sampling at thoracotomy, including sampling of normal-sized nodes, show the worst sensitivity and specificity.[369,422,425,607] The early series were not based on rigorous confirmation of data and suggested sensitivities above 85% with acceptable specificity, but nowadays, with more accurate pathologic correlation, a reasonable generalization is that in the United States (where fungal infection is endemic) sensitivity and specificity are in the 50% to low 60% range when the cutoff point for normal is a short-axis diameter of 1 cm.[425,674] Better specificity figures have been obtained in Europe[79] and Japan,[285] probably because the prevalence of coincidental histoplasmosis and other fungal disease is much lower than in the United States.

---

*References 25, 30, 131, 285, 370, 425, 492, 493, 503, 542, 607, 669, 674.

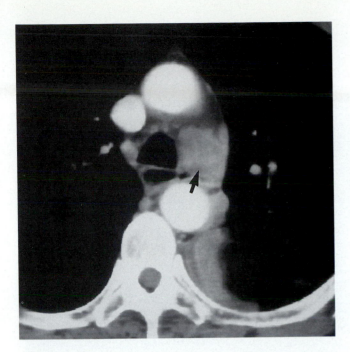

FIGURE 8-25
Enlarged nodes in patient with bronchial carcinoma: true-positive computed tomographic scan for lymph node involvement by tumor. Node *(arrow)* in aortopulmonary window has short-axis diameter in excess of 2 cm.

One method of reducing the frequency of false-positive interpretations is to ensure that nodes draining the tumor are larger than nodes elsewhere in the mediastinum. By counting only enlarged nodes (greater than 10 mm short-axis diameter) that were at least 5 mm greater in diameter than nodes in regions not draining the tumor, Buy and associates[79] were able to achieve a 95% positive predictive value for nodal metastatic disease.

In practice, CT and MRI examinations for nodal disease are used largely to decide whether to perform mediastinoscopy or mediastinotomy and, equally important, to demonstrate which nodes should undergo biopsy.[168] Nodes above 10 mm in short-axis diameter (Figure 8-25) should be subjected to some form of biopsy. Clearly there are occasions when the chances of a negative biopsy are so slim that a surgeon may decide to use the CT finding of greatly enlarged nodes as sufficient reason not to proceed with surgical resection, but these cases should be the exception to the general rule that the CT interpretation of mediastinal nodal metastases should be corroborated by biopsy before a patient is denied potentially curative surgery.[687] Routine mediastinoscopy provides access only to the paratracheal nodes, proximal tracheobronchial nodes, and superior subcarinal nodes. The other nodal sites require alternative approaches such as mediastinotomy. These other sites include nodal stations with a high propensity to early metastases, such as the aortopulmonary and anterior mediastinal nodes.

Random preoperative biopsy of normal-sized nodes, that is, nodes less than 10 mm in short-axis diameter, is unlikely to yield tumor, and most patients with normal-sized mediastinal nodes can appropriately undergo thoracotomy without prior mediastinoscopy or mediastinotomy.[132,363] That is not to say that the incidence of metastases in normal-sized lymph nodes is negligible,[18,234] but since the nodes in question are not enlarged, preoperative biopsy will necessarily be random and therefore have a low yield because of sampling error. Another argument against routine preoperative mediastinoscopy of patients with normal-sized nodes is, as discussed previously, that patients with microscopic metastases discovered only at the time of thoracotomy have an improved survival rate if the primary tumor and the affected mediastinal nodes are resected.[512]

The utility of chest CT in T1N0M0 cancers by clinical and plain chest radiographic criteria is controversial. The prevalence of mediastinal nodal involvement with such small tumors is 21% or less[123,157,251,579] and may be much less.[509] The lower the prevalence, the greater the potential for false-positive test results.[410] A cost-effectiveness analysis showed that with current surgical techniques, chest CT would be both clinically useful and cost saving, provided the CT examination was readily available and the prevalence of nodal involvement was 12.5% or greater.[52] However, Becker and associates[39] showed that routine CT scanning did not correctly alter the stage in any of their 38 patients and therefore CT did not affect management. Also, Daly and associates[131] found that the true-positive yield in 64 patients with tumors less than 2 cm in diameter was zero. Others[157,502] have found evidence for unresectable spread of disease in up to one third of patients with T1N0M0 non–small cell lung cancer based on plain chest films and therefore advocate routine preoperative CT.

Mediastinal invasion. Direct invasion of the mediastinum can often be readily detected by CT and MRI but is only occasionally diagnosable by conventional radiographic techniques. Plain film evidence relies on demonstrating phrenic nerve paralysis. Caution is needed, however, before deciding that a high hemidiaphragm is caused by phrenic nerve invasion, because lobar collapse can also lead to elevation of a hemidiaphragm and subpulmonary effusion may mimic it. Barium swallow may show esophageal displacement or invasion. Radionuclide perfusion scanning demonstrates reduced perfusion when the central pulmonary arteries have been invaded by the tumor, but the test is too insensitive and too nonspecific to be of practical value in routine staging.

The major CT and MRI sign of mediastinal invasion is visible tumor surrounding the mediastinal vessels, esophagus, or proximal mainstem bronchi (Figures 8-26 and 8-27). Mere contact with the mediastinum is not enough for the diagnosis of invasion, and apparent interdigitation with mediastinal fat can be misleading on both CT and MRI (Figure 8-28).[405] Associated pneumonia or atelecta-

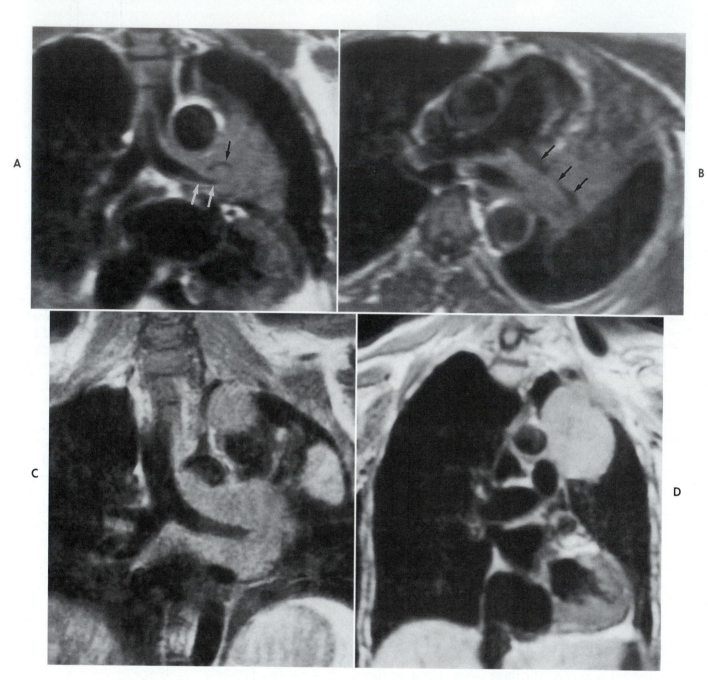

FIGURE 8-26
Magnetic resonance images of lung cancers. **A** and **B,** Invasion of tumor into mediastinum and severe narrowing of left pulmonary artery *(black arrows)* and left upper lobe bronchus *(white arrows)* is well demonstrated. T1-weighted coronal **(A)** and axial **(B)** images. **C,** Coronal T1-weighted images in another patient showing deep invasion into subcarinal and aortopulmonary window regions. **D,** Coronal T1-weighted image in different patient showing tumor growing into aortopulmonary window. (**A** and **B** courtesy Dr. William C. Black, Washington, D.C.)

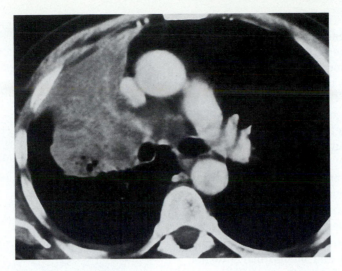

FIGURE 8-27
Mediastinal invasion by lung cancer. Tumor crosses to contact opposite mainstem bronchus.

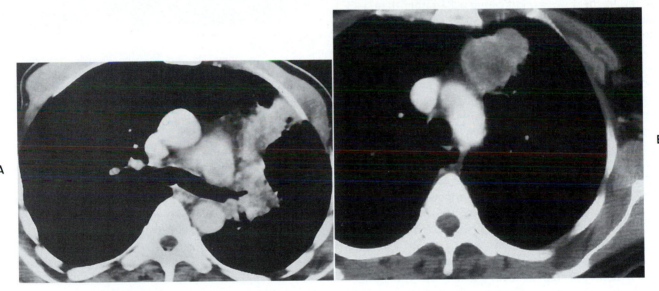

A

B

FIGURE 8-28
Mediastinal contact by bronchial carcinoma that proved to be surgically resectable. In neither case was it possible to predict preoperatively whether tumor had invaded mediastinum. **A,** Tumor had not invaded mediastinum. **B,** Mediastinal pleura was involved, but tumor proved to be resectable.

sis may make it difficult to determine whether mediastinal contact is present.

Based on a retrospective study of 80 patients with tumors categorized by CT as indeterminate for mediastinal invasion who were subsequently operated on, Glazer and co-workers[220] suggested that a tumor is likely to be technically resectable (that is, stage IIIA or less) if one or more of the following features are present: (1) less than 3 cm of contact with the mediastinum; (2) less than 90 degrees of circumferential contact with the aorta; or (3) a visible mediastinal fat plane between the mass and any vital mediastinal structures. Thirty-six of the 37 masses in their series that conformed to this description proved to be technically resectable (28 with no mediastinal invasion and 8 with mediastinal invasion). However, difficulty arises when the question is turned around to ask: what are the criteria for irresectability?[424] (This is an important question, because if the distinction could be made accurately, many patients would be spared unnecessary exploratory thoracotomy.) In the series by Glazer and associates,[220] more than 3 cm of contact with the mediastinal surface was present in almost half the tumors that proved resectable and the lack of a visible fat plane between the tumor and a major mediastinal structure did not mean that the tumor was unresectable.

The use of ultrafast "cine" CT to assess mobility of the tumor in relation to the adjacent mediastinum has been reported.[445,462] The concept is that a mobile tumor would not have invaded the adjacent mediastinum, whereas a fixed one might have.

MRI does not offer any advantages over CT for routine assessment of mediastinal invasion; the signs are basically the same, and the axial imaging plane is the standard projection for both tests.[405,465] MRI is no more accurate than CT in distinguishing between contiguity of tumor with the mediastinum and mediastinal invasion, largely because invasion of the mediastinal fat can be mimicked by adjacent inflammatory changes.[411,465,615] MRI can, however, provide unique information in certain circumstances.* It has proved superior to CT for identifying involvement of major mediastinal blood vessels[411] and the tracheal carina, indicating a T4 rather than a T3 lesion (converting the tumor from stage IIIA to an unresectable stage IIIB tumor). The superior vena cava, central pulmonary arteries and veins, and aorta are all readily identified, and encasement or invasion of the vessels is easily recognized. Here the advantage of MRI is twofold. First, an optimum imaging plane can be chosen.[306] Second, when the heart is imaged, electrocardiographic (ECG) gating can effectively stop cardiac motion. Tumor may grow along the pulmonary veins to become intrapericardial or to lie within the left atrium — features that can be well demonstrated by MRI but are difficult to show by CT. The ability to show the superior vena cava in the coronal plane without having to inject contrast medium allows easy, often exquisite, demonstration of the extent of tumor in patients with superior vena cava syndrome. Similarly, pericardial and cardiac involvement is well demonstrated on ECG-gated MRI. The normal pericardium is seen as a low-signal membrane, and its disruption can therefore be recognized. Contrast enhancement with gadolinium[328,615] does not appear to confer sufficient advantage to be recommended as a routine.

Endobronchial tumor extension remains the province of bronchoscopy, but extraluminal encasement is well seen by MRI. Tumor adjacent to the tracheal carina can be difficult to diagnose with CT, but coronal imaging at MRI shows the airway and surrounding tissues to advantage.

Chest wall invasion. A peripheral lung carcinoma may cross the pleura and invade the chest wall, but the presence of chest wall invasion alone does not preclude surgical resection, although it does adversely affect prognosis. Surgical resection, with or without adjuvant

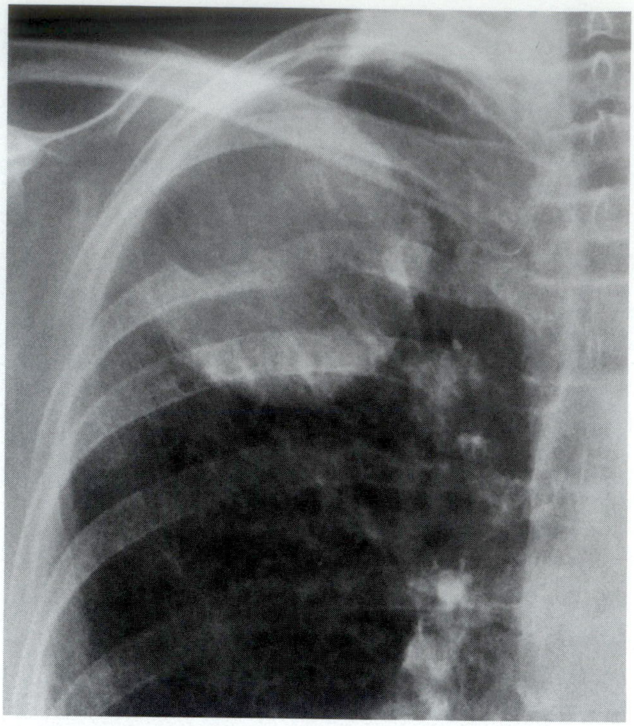

FIGURE 8-29
Bronchial carcinoma showing invasion of right fifth rib. Note irregular destruction of rib. In this case there is widening of adjacent rib interspace. Such widening is unusual in bronchial carcinoma.

radiotherapy, can achieve long-term survival in patients with chest wall involvement if the resection is complete and there are no mediastinal nodal or distant metastases.* The necessarily more extensive surgery is associated with increased morbidity and mortality, and therefore it helps the surgeon to know preoperatively whether chest wall invasion is present and the depth of any invasion.

Rib or spinal destruction is sometimes visible on plain films (Figure 8-29), but tomography or CT may be necessary to confirm this finding (Figure 8-30). Soft tissue invasion is best detected by CT or MRI.

Even CT cannot reliably show chest wall involvement adjacent to a tumor unless there is bone destruction or a large soft tissue mass.[219,510,513,578] Local chest wall pain remains the single most specific indicator of whether or not the tumor has spread to the parietal pleura or chest wall.[219] Contact with the pleura on CT examination, even if the pleura is thickened, does not necessarily indicate invasion, although the greater the degree of contact and the greater the pleural thickening, the more likely that the parietal pleura has been invaded, particularly if the extrapleural fat plane is obliterated.[537] A definite extrapleural mass that is not explicable by previous chest

---

*References 206, 346, 359, 405, 465, 674, 676.

*References 9, 416, 439, 506, 517, 537.

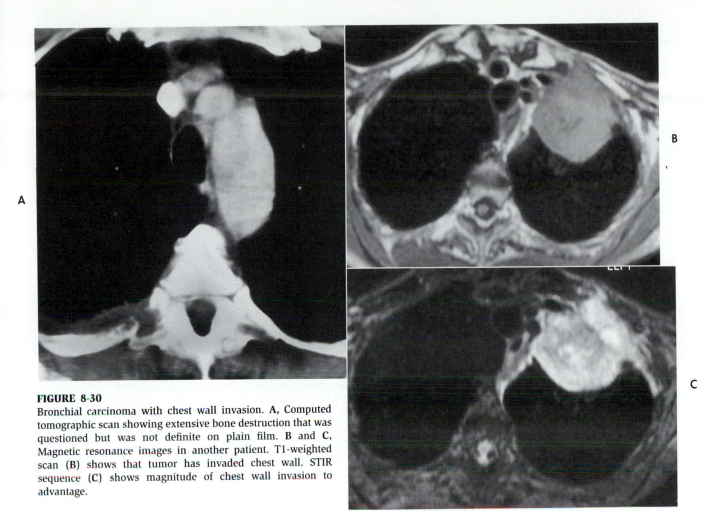

FIGURE 8-30
Bronchial carcinoma with chest wall invasion. **A,** Computed tomographic scan showing extensive bone destruction that was questioned but was not definite on plain film. **B** and **C,** Magnetic resonance images in another patient. T1-weighted scan (**B**) shows that tumor has invaded chest wall. STIR sequence (**C**) shows magnitude of chest wall invasion to advantage.

trauma is likely to be the result of invasion by tumor,[537] but even this sign may be misleading, since soft tissue swelling may be due to inflammation and fibrosis rather than neoplasm.[510] Conversely, a clear extrapleural fat plane adjacent to the mass may be helpful but again is not definitive[578] in excluding chest wall invasion.

Inducing a pneumothorax before CT has been advocated when possible chest wall invasion is assessed. The concept is that the mass will fall away from the chest wall if the tumor is confined to the lung and remain fixed to the chest wall if invasion has occurred.[668,699] Although false-positive results from benign adhesions adjacent to the primary tumor were not found in the two series reported to date,[669,699] such misinterpretations were found with tumors invading the mediastinum and are therefore likely to occur when patients are evaluated for chest wall invasion. A similar principle applies in the use of ultrafast "cine" CT to assess the relative movement of the tumor with respect to the chest wall during breathing in order to determine whether the tumor is fixed or mobile.[445,462]

MRI has similar problems to CT in diagnosing chest wall invasion. Chest wall invasion may go unrecognized when it is indeed present, and false-positive diagnoses are also a problem.[411] In some series MRI was better than CT in demonstrating chest wall[465,496] and diaphragmatic invasion. There are three basic reasons why MRI might provide more information than CT:

1. Coronal or sagittal planes may be the best imaging planes, particularly where the chest wall slopes to arch over the apex.

2. MRI provides excellent tissue contrast between a tumor and the soft tissues of the chest wall (Figure 8-31). However, care must be exercised when trying to gauge the precise edge of the tumor because surrounding edema may make the mass appear larger than it truly is. Also, it should be appreciated that on MRI, just as with CT, when the tumor mass merely contacts the chest wall, chest wall invasion must be considered indeterminate.[634]

3. The thin layer of extrapleural fat may be better shown on MRI than on CT. Tumor invasion into the chest wall must necessarily cross this fat plane, and provided the chosen sequence provides different signals for fat and tumor (T1-weighted sequences without gadolinium enhancement appear to be the best choice[496]), discontinuity of the fat line may be evident.

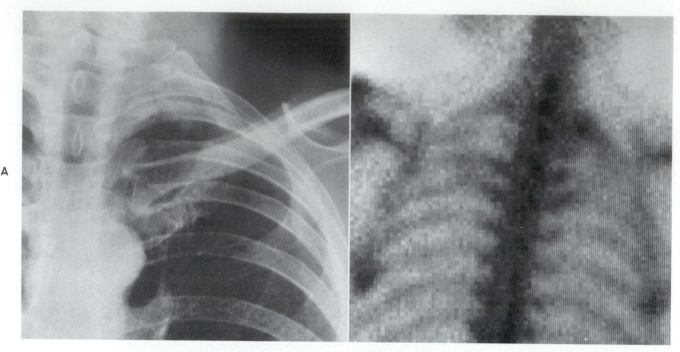

FIGURE 8-31
Pancoast's tumor. **A,** Plain film showing appearance resembling apical pleural cap. **B,** Technetium-99m
bone scan showing increased activity in invaded left first rib *(arrow)*.

Technetium-99m radionuclide bone scans are a sensitive technique with which to assess bone invasion (Figure 8-31). They are frequently positive when the plain films still show no bony abnormality.

A recent report suggests that transthoracic ultrasound can be an accurate method of identifying chest wall invasion when two of the following three findings are present: disruption of the pleura, extension into the chest wall, and fixation of the tumor during breathing.[625]

Superior sulcus (Pancoast's) tumor. Pancoast's tumor deserves special mention. The eponym nowadays refers to the symptom complex of pain in the shoulder and arm that results from an apical tumor invading the lower cords of the brachial plexus and the sympathetic chain. Pancoast's original description included ipsilateral Horner's syndrome from invasion of the sympathetic chain, and local destruction of bone by the tumor.[498] Because these tumors arise adjacent to the groove for the subclavian artery, they are also called superior sulcus tumors. They may be of any cell type.[21,302,505] They have a propensity to invade the adjacent chest wall, brachial plexus, subclavian vessels, and spine. In some centers survival has been significantly increased by combined preoperative radiation therapy and en-bloc resection of the tumor providing the tumor is technically resectable[506]; in such centers preoperative CT or MRI is essential.

On radiographic study, superior sulcus tumors appear as a mass in approximately one half to three-fourths of the cases and as an apical cap resembling pleural thickening in the remainder. Bone destruction in the adjacent ribs or spine is seen in approximately one third of cases (Figure 8-32).[21,484] These tumors are, however, often difficult to diagnose on standard plain chest radiographs because the lung apex is partly hidden by overlying ribs and clavicle. Even with lordotic apical views the diagnosis can be difficult because the tumor so often closely resembles a benign apical pleural cap (Figures 8-31 and 8-32) and the cardinal plain film sign of the lesion — bone destruction — is either absent or difficult to diagnose with confidence. Asymmetric pleural thickening, particularly if associated with appropriate symptoms, should be viewed with suspicion. A chronically enlarging unilateral apical cap strongly suggests superior sulcus carcinoma; such patients are usually symptomatic.[427]

CT scans can be helpful in diagnosing Pancoast's tumors (Figure 8-33).[243,484,675] They may demonstrate an intrapulmonary mass rather than just pleural thickening, providing extra confidence that the diagnosis is neoplasm rather than inflammatory pleural thickening. Also, CT scanning is a sensitive technique with which to diagnose the full extent of the tumor, particularly invasion of the chest wall and root of the neck.

MRI is now regarded as the optimal modality for demonstrating the extent of superior sulcus tumors,[206,253,426,632] largely because the coronal and sagittal planes are the optimal imaging planes; they demonstrate the cupula shape of the chest wall in the apical regions and also show the brachial plexus and subclavian vessels to advantage (Figures 8-34 and 8-35).[93,253] Thin

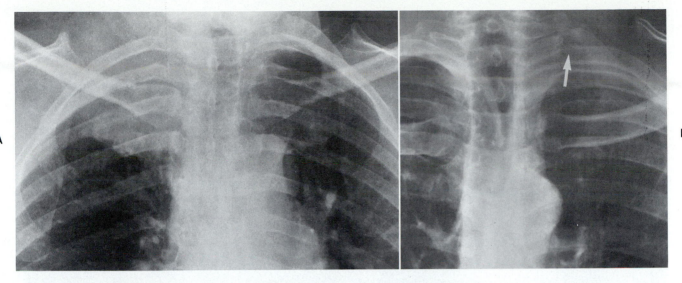

FIGURE 8-32
A, Superior sulcus carcinoma of lung destroying major portion of right first rib. The patient, a 52-year-old man, complained of chest wall pain and pain in right arm. **B,** More subtle example of superior sulcus carcinoma of lung. Apical cap is slight, and destruction of neck and head of first rib *(arrow)* is not easy to see.

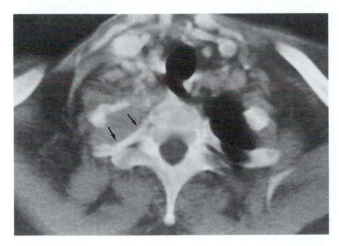

FIGURE 8-33
Computed tomographic scan of Pancoast's tumor showing tumor at lung apex invading adjacent rib *(arrows).*

sections (5 mm) are recommended,[253] and T1-weighted and STIR images in coronal and sagittal planes appear to be the optimal sequences.[253,426] Interruption of the normal extrapleural fat line over the lung apex can be readily shown, as can the contrast between tumor and normal muscle, brachial plexus, adjacent vessels, and spinal canal. Rib destruction, however, may be less well shown by MRI than by CT.[426]

Pleural involvement. Both peripheral and central bronchial carcinoma may involve the pleura by direct spread, lymphatic permeation, or tumor emboli in the pulmonary arteries.[438,601] Pleural effusions, which may be freely mobile or loculated, occur with lung carcinoma of all cell types but appear to be most frequent with adenocarcinoma.[107] Pleural effusion in association with a primary lung cancer designates the tumor as T4 except in the few patients who have clinical evidence of another cause for the effusion (such as heart failure) and in whom multiple pleural fluid cytologic examinations do not show tumor cells, in which case the effusion can be disregarded as a staging element. The presence of pleural effusion at the time of diagnosis in patients with lung cancer carries a poor prognosis, however, whether or not malignant cells are identified.[562,563] For example, Decker and co-workers[139] studied 73 patients with bronchogenic carcinoma who had cytologically negative pleural effusions and found that only 4 had surgically resectable disease. Hemorrhagic effusion on pleural aspiration is a strong indication of direct involvement by tumor.[139,438] Attempts to characterize the nature of the pleural fluid based on density measurements at CT or signal intensities at MRI have so far not proved useful.

On occasion, adenocarcinoma takes the form of a sheet of lobular pleural thickening indistinguishable from malignant mesothelioma (Figure 8-36).[696]

Staging lung cancer: a summary. Staging the intrathoracic extent of non–small cell lung cancer is a multidisciplinary process using imaging, bronchoscopy, and biopsy. Chest radiography and CT are currently the routine imaging procedures for assessing intrathoracic spread and determining resectability, with MRI and ultrasound reserved for specific indications.

The essential questions to be answered are: has the tumor spread to hilar or mediastinal lymph nodes and, if

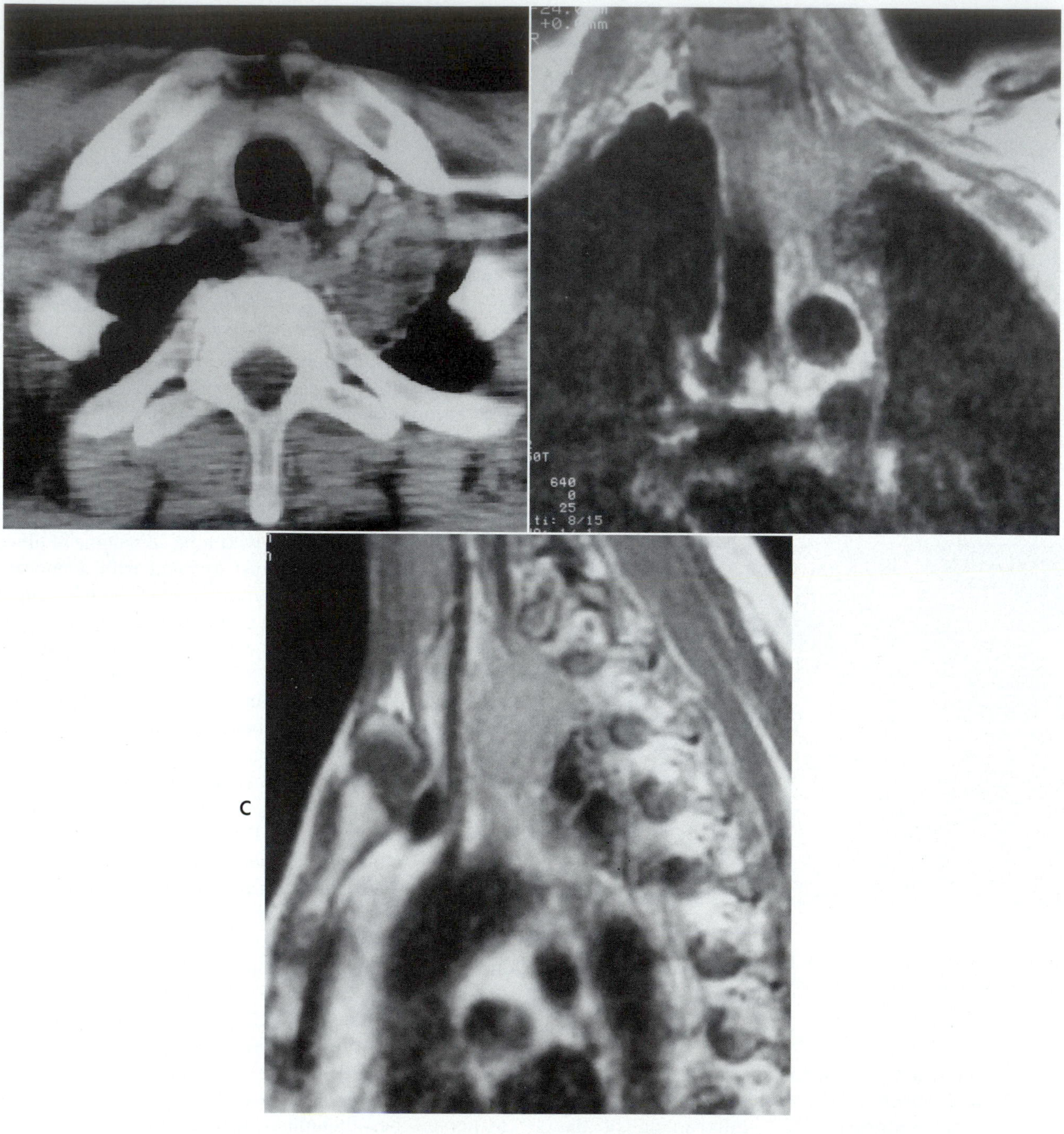

FIGURE 8-34
Comparison of, **A**, computed tomographic scan and, **B** and **C**, T1-weighted magnetic resonance (MR) images in Pancoast's tumor. This squamous cell carcinoma had invaded root of neck and encased the left subclavian and left vertebral arteries. The size and extent of extrapulmonary tumor are far easier to appreciate on the MR images.

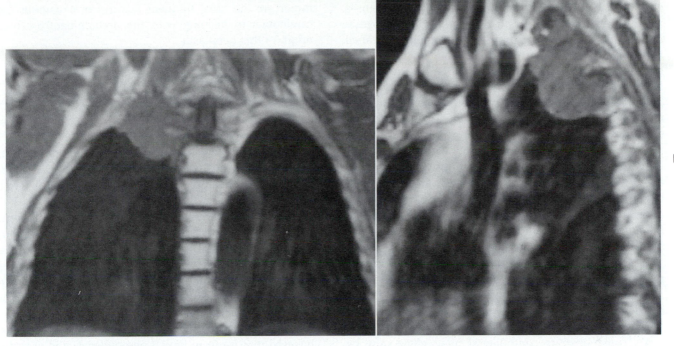

FIGURE 8-35
Magnetic resonance imaging of Pancoast's tumor (T1-weighted images). **A**, Invasion of root of neck and obliteration of extrapleural fat line of right apex are well seen on coronal view. **B**, Precise size and shape of tumor are well shown in sagittal plane.

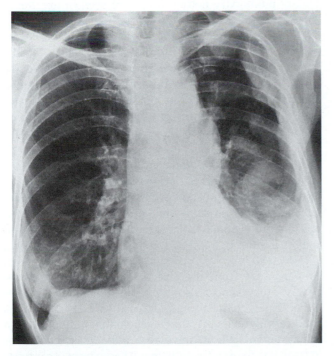

FIGURE 8-36
Extensive lobular pleural thickening and pleural effusion caused by pleural invasion by bronchial adenocarcinoma. Note resemblance to malignant mesothelioma of pleura.

so, which nodal groups are involved?, and has the tumor invaded the chest wall or mediastinum and, if so, is it still potentially surgically curable?

If chest radiography and CT show no evidence of spread beyond the lung in a patient who has no undue risks for surgery, and bronchoscopy shows that the tumor is resectable, the patient can be offered surgical resection without further preoperative invasive procedures. Patients with ipsilateral hilar node involvement are managed similarly to patients whose tumors are confined to the lung, but in the realization that the prognosis is poorer.

Spread to ipsilateral nodes, while not necessarily precluding surgical resection, has a significant adverse effect on prognosis. If surgery is undertaken, it is performed with the understanding that the figures for 5-year survival are poor, 35% at best.

The poor specificity of CT in determining nodal involvement must be appreciated. Nodal enlargement, although it may be due to metastatic carcinoma, may also be due to coincidental benign disease or to reactive hyperplasia directly connected to the presence of the tumor. Thus biopsy confirmation of neoplastic nodal involvement by mediastinoscopy, mediastinotomy, or needle aspiration is usually needed before a patient is denied surgery.

For lung cancers that have invaded the mediastinum or chest wall, the important decision is whether the tumor is nevertheless resectable for possible cure, again recognizing the poorer prognosis compared with tumors confined to the lung. CT may show definitively that the tumor is too extensive for resective surgery (that is, that it is a T4 lesion). Alternatively, CT may leave the issue in doubt, and MRI can then be used as a problem-solving modality to offer additional useful information in the following situations:

1. To demonstrate the aortopulmonary window and subcarinal region. The precise relationship of tumor to the central pulmonary artery, aorta, carina, and main bronchi is optimally displayed on coronal images or occasionally on sagittal sections. Similarly, metastases to the aortopulmonary window and subcarinal nodes may be better shown on coronal images.

2. To clarify whether the superior vena cava, central pulmonary arteries, pericardium, and heart are involved.

3. To demonstrate invasion of the brachial plexus, adjacent spine, or subclavian vessels in superior sulcus (Pancoast's) tumors.

4. To demonstrate contralateral hilar adenopathy by exploiting the better sensitivity of MRI in detecting soft tissue masses in the hilar regions.

RADIOGRAPHIC PATTERNS BASED ON CELL TYPE. The radiographic pattern of bronchial carcinoma varies with the cell type. The generalizations given here are based on a series of 600 cases of bronchial carcinoma analyzed at the Mayo Clinic[80]; clearly these observations are no substitute for histologic examination. Bronchioloalveolar carcinoma is considered separately because it shows significant differences from cancers of the other major cell types.[574]

Early, often massive lymphadenopathy and direct mediastinal invasion are well-recognized phenomena in both small cell carcinoma (Figure 8-37) and giant cell carcinoma.[191,360,511,592] Woodring and Stelling[696] have pointed out that adenocarcinoma appears to be changing its pattern and nowadays often shows hilar and mediastinal adenopathy,[371] although the nodal enlargement is not as massive as with the small cell and large cell undifferentiated tumors. A mass in, or adjacent to, the hilum is a particular characteristic of small cell carcinoma and is seen in 78% of cases (Figure 8-20).

A peripheral nodule is common in adenocarcinoma (72% of cases) and large cell tumors (63% of cases); this is approximately twice the incidence seen with squamous cell or small cell carcinomas. The largest peripheral masses are seen with squamous and large cell tumors, whereas most adenocarcinomas and small cell carcinomas are less than 4 cm in diameter. Squamous cell cancers may attain great size (Figure 8-38), and they cavitate more frequently than cancers of other cell types; cavitation was seen in 22% of squamous cell carcinomas presenting as a peripheral mass (Figure 8-39), compared with only 6% of peripheral large cell and 2% of peripheral adenocarcinomas.

Collapse and consolidation of the lung beyond the tumor are the most frequent features of squamous cell carcinoma, in keeping with the predominantly central origin of this neoplasm.

Bronchioloalveolar carcinoma

According to the World Health Organization (WHO) classification,[336] bronchioloalveolar carcinoma, also known as alveolar cell carcinoma and bronchiolar carcinoma, is a subtype of adenocarcinoma. Cigarette smoking does not appear to play a prominent etiologic role, but the prevalence of this tumor with preexisting lung scarring is striking.[165]

In most series bronchioloalveolar carcinomas account for some 2% to 5% of lung cancers, but with smoking on the decline the relative incidence of bronchioloalveolar carcinoma is rising.[22] The tumors occur equally in both sexes, and the average age at onset is 50 years. The characteristic pathologic feature is a peripheral neoplasm showing lipedic growth, the malignant cells using surrounding alveolar walls as a scaffold. These tumors are believed to arise from type II pneumocytes and probably also from bronchiolar epithelium[601] or from a common stem cell. The cells produce mucus, sometimes in such large amounts that one symptom of the consolidative form of the disease is bronchorrhea, the expectoration of large quantities of mucoid sputum.

The tumor occurs in two clinically different forms: a solitary pulmonary nodule (the form seen in just under half the patients) and unifocal or multifocal areas of pulmonary consolidation.[269] It is a matter of debate whether the multifocal form is an extension of the unifocal variety or a different and more aggressive entity.[442] The prognosis for bronchioloalveolar carcinoma when it occurs as a solitary pulmonary nodule is better than that for lung cancer of other cell types. It is more likely to be stage I and therefore surgically resectable. Also, the tumor is slower growing so that 5-year survivals are better, regardless of stage.[133] The prognoses for the larger, more ill-defined lesion, which radiographically resembles pneumonia, and for the disseminated form are both poor.[167] (The somewhat confusingly named intravascular bronchioloalveolar tumor is a separate entity and is discussed on p. 315.)

IMAGING.[50,165,269,383] Because bronchioloalveolar carcinomas arise from the alveoli and the adjacent small airways, they appear as peripheral pulmonary opacities rather than with the effects of large airway obstruction. As mentioned previously the most common finding is a solitary lobulated or spiculated pulmonary nodule or mass that is frequently indistinguishable from other types of carcinoma (Figure 8-40).[337] There is, however, a propensity to a subpleural location and the development of a pleuropulmonary tail.[269,337,586] The tail is due to desmoplastic reaction in the peripheral septa of the lung. A few such nodules have visible air bronchograms, a phenomenon that is best seen with CT,[337] particularly

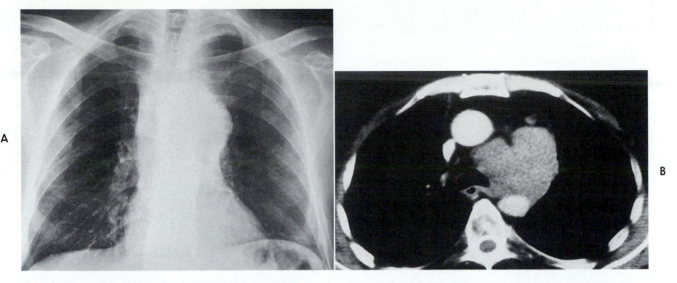

FIGURE 8-37
Small (oat) cell carcinoma showing massive mediastinal adenopathy. The primary tumor, which was centrally located in bronchial tree, is not visible radiographically. **A,** Plain film. **B,** Computed tomographic scan.

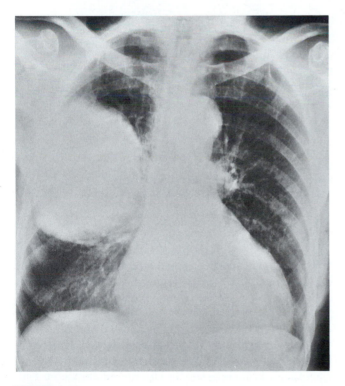

FIGURE 8-38
Squamous cell carcinoma of bronchus illustrating the huge size these tumors may have attained when first discovered.

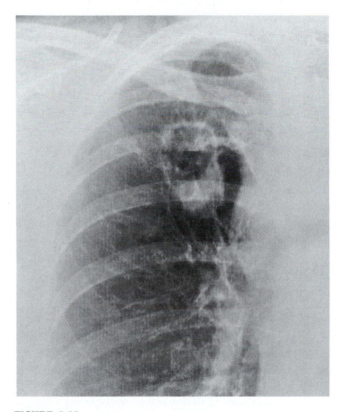

FIGURE 8-39
Squamous cell carcinoma of bronchus occurring as cavitating nodule. Part of the wall is very thin and smooth.

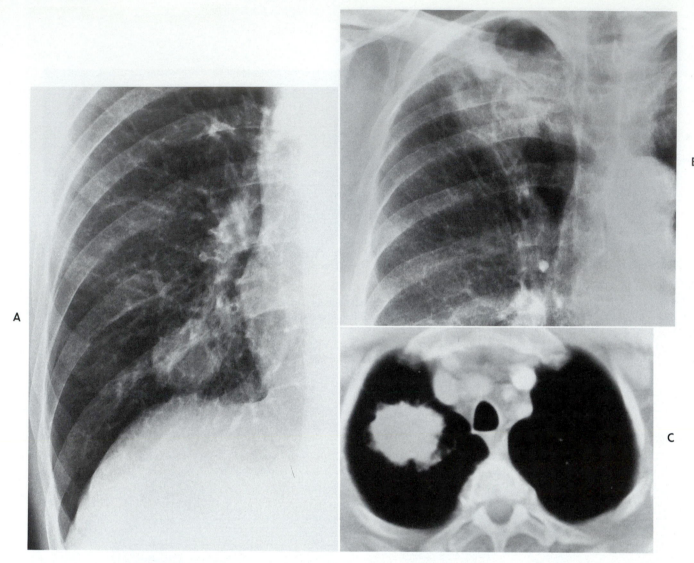

FIGURE 8-40
Two examples of bronchioloalveolar cell carcinoma occurring as a solitary pulmonary nodule or mass.
A, Plain film in 47-year-old asymptomatic man. **B,** In different patient, ill-defined tumor that resembles
pneumonia. **C,** However, on computed tomographic scan the lesion is clearly a lobular mass with
irregular edges.

HRCT.[3] Bubblelike lucencies corresponding to patent
small bronchi or air-containing cystic lucencies are a
frequent finding in bronchioloalveolar carcinoma.[3,337,707]
Bronchioloalveolar carcinomas may grow slowly, with
doubling times far greater than the 18 months usually
quoted as the upper limit for bronchial carcinoma.[269]

When bronchioloalveolar carcinoma has the radiographic appearance of ill-defined or multiple opacities, it
is easily distinguished from cancers of other cell type.
Bronchorrhea is a recognized clinical manifestation in
this form of the disease. There are a variety of appearances: an ill-defined opacity resembling a patch of
pneumonia (Figure 8-41), homogeneous consolidation of
one lobe (Figure 8-42),[167] patchy consolidation, or mul-

tiple ill-defined nodules spread widely through multiple
lobes in one or both lungs (Figure 8-43). Both atelectasis
and expansile consolidation (Figure 8-44) are reported.[279] Air bronchograms may be an obvious feature
(Figure 8-41); they are particularly well demonstrated by
CT.[3] The bronchi may show uniform narrowing, stretching, and spreading of the bronchi within the lung,[286]
whereas air bronchograms in chronic inflammation usually show normal or dilated bronchi because of the ectasia
associated with atelectasis or fibrosis. CT may show
small, rounded collections of air that correspond pathologically to small patent bronchi or cystic spaces within
the tumor; these may be seen in the consolidative form
just as they may in the nodular form.[707] Thickened septal

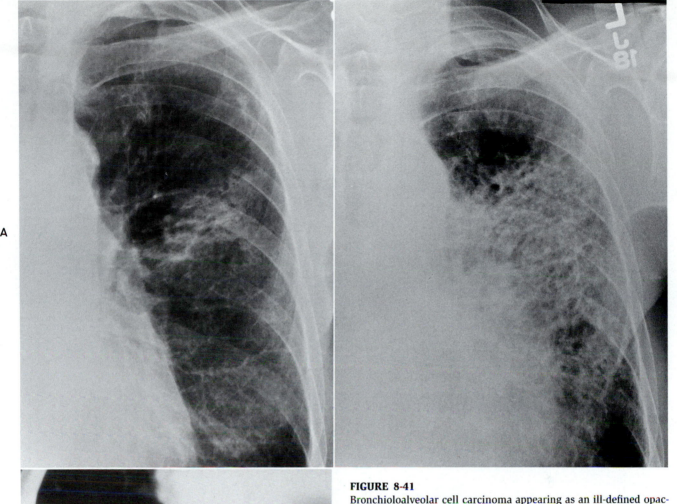

FIGURE 8-41
Bronchioloalveolar cell carcinoma appearing as an ill-defined opacity with air bronchograms. **A,** Plain film at initial examination. **B,** Plain films 7 months later. Note resemblance of each individual image to pneumonia. The time course is a major clue to the diagnosis of neoplasm. **C,** Computed tomographic scan in another patient showing the air bronchogram–bubbly pattern that is often seen with bronchioloalveolar carcinoma.

lines caused by lymphatic permeation may also be visible, as may branching tubular densities of mucoid impaction.[279] The low CT density of mucus within the tumor may be visible as low attenuation, particularly at HRCT.[3]

An interesting sign is the CT-angiogram sign, the name emphasizing the analogy with the air bronchogram sign, in which the vessels coursing through the tumor stand out clearly on contrast-enhanced images, presumably because of the contrast against the background of abundant low-density mucus within the neoplasm. This sign is present in a high proportion of patients with lobar consolidation caused by bronchioloalveolar cell carcinoma, but it is unusual in consolidation from other causes.[287,576,656,663]

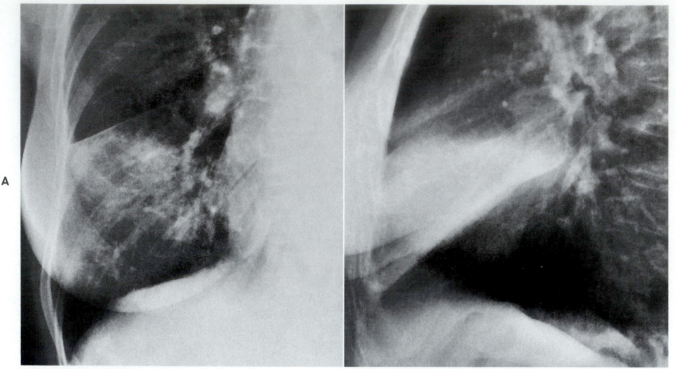

FIGURE 8-42
Bronchioloalveolar cell carcinoma occurring as lobar consolidation of middle lobe. Patient complained of coughing up copious amounts of mucoid sputum. **A**, Posteroanterior radiograph. **B**, Lateral radiograph.

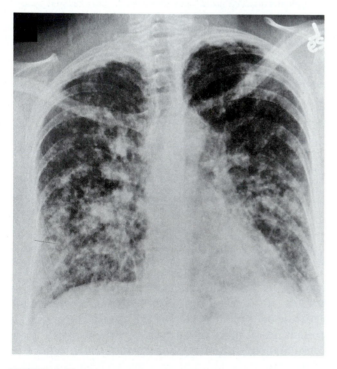

FIGURE 8-43
Bronchioloalveolar cell carcinoma presenting as widespread ill-defined patchy areas of consolidation.

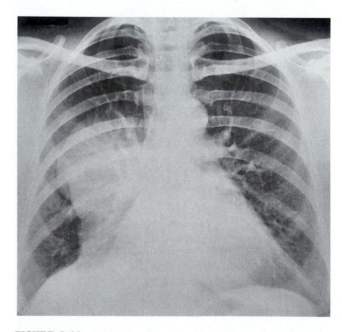

FIGURE 8-44
Bronchioloalveolar cell carcinoma presenting as expansile consolidation of right lower lobe.

Cavitation is unusual but has been recorded, as have multiple thin-walled cystic lesions within or coexistent with the consolidative form of bronchioloalveolar carcinoma.[682] In one reported case the wall of a preexisting lung cavity was thickened, presumably by tumor growing around the wall of a bronchogenic cyst.[279]

Pleural effusions are seen in up to one third of patients, and hilar and mediastinal lymphadenopathy is seen in close to one fifth.

Differentiating between the consolidative forms of bronchioloalveolar carcinoma and various nonneoplastic conditions such as pneumonia, aspiration, or pulmonary edema depends on knowing the clinical findings and appreciating the more chronic course of the disease.

CT scanning is advocated as a routine before surgery in all patients with the consolidative form of disease to make sure that the tumor is confined to one lobe, since CT frequently shows further pulmonary foci that are not appreciated on plain chest radiographs.[435]

Early diagnosis of bronchial carcinoma

The value of any cancer screening program is ultimately assessed by comparing the costs to the benefits, namely increased survival and lessened morbidity. Costs include both the monetary cost of the screening program and the overall cost of false-positive diagnoses, including unnecessary morbidity, worry, and expense. Benefit is seen only if cancer is recognized at a time when cure is possible. At present, only plain chest radiography and, to a much lesser extent, sputum cytology are of proven value in the large-scale detection of asymptomatic lung cancer. Chest radiographs for the detection and evaluation of bronchial carcinoma should be obtained with high-kilovoltage techniques, primarily because of the larger volume of lung that can be surveyed (the higher kilovoltage causes less lung to be hidden by ribs, clavicles, heart, or diaphragm). Comparison with previous normal radiographs allows greater confidence in the diagnosis of small nodules and permits recognition of smaller lesions.[72]

The basic concept of a lung cancer detection program is that more cures are achieved when small tumors, particularly peripheral ones, are found in asymptomatic individuals, since it is in this category of patients that the best surgical results are obtained.[187,268,292,495] Such presumptions are, however, fraught with difficulty because there are so many variables to consider.[280] The published surgical series refer to selected patients and are not necessarily representative of the population at large. Another problem is "lead time bias": the extra life expectancy that occurs simply from having a tumor diagnosed earlier, regardless of whether or not treatment is effective. In the series of Huhti, Saloheimo, and Sutinen,[280] for example, average survival was better in patients whose tumors were discovered by regular survey, but 5-year survival was not improved. Yet another pitfall is "length bias," the tendency for tumors with an inherently better prognosis to be found by mass screening, particularly at the first examination, thereby invalidating comparisons unless the series is carefully controlled. As Garland and co-workers[203] have pointed out, slow-growing tumors, even though large and with late-appearing symptoms, usually have a better prognosis than rapidly growing tumors, even when the latter are small and ostensibly found early.

Several large screening programs have been undertaken.* One that has attracted considerable interest is the multicenter survey conducted by the National Cancer Institute (NCI), the results of which have been conveniently summarized by Sanderson,[569] Tockman,[641] and Martini, Flehinger, and Zaman.[404] Only the briefest outline of the results is given here. From a population of approximately 10,000 high-risk patients at each of three centers (men over 45 years of age who were chronic excessive cigarette smokers), 0.73% had lung cancer diagnosed at their initial screening.[186,188,198,254] (By way of comparison, the yield for diagnosing breast carcinoma by large-scale mammography is approximately 0.7% at initial screening.) After excluding nearly 1000 individuals who were ruled ineligible because of serious medical problems, the Mayo Clinic portion of the study[189,190] randomly assigned half of those who did not have cancer at the initial screening to surveillance with chest radiography and sputum cytology every 4 months, the remaining half serving as control subjects. The rate of cancer diagnosis in the screened group was 5.5 per 1000 per year, compared with 4.3 per 1000 per year in the control group. The resectability rate was higher in the study group (46%) than in the control group (32%), but the important finding was that the lung cancer deaths were virtually identical in the two groups. The conclusion was that large-scale radiographic and cytologic screening for lung cancer is not justified. Two of the three centers, Johns Hopkins[641] and Memorial Sloane-Kettering,[431] investigated the benefit of using sputum cytology as an adjunct to plain chest radiography. Neither study showed that the addition of sputum cytology reduced lung cancer mortality.

The ultimate justification for any population screening must come from a comparison of mortality between randomly assigned screened and unscreened populations. None of the three centers participating in the comparative portion of the NCI study[161,190,430,641] showed improved overall survival as a result of screening, although whether individual subsets of patients might benefit is not clear.[161,558] The initial hope that intensive screening would detect a large proportion of early cases of squamous cell carcinoma, the cell type with the best surgical result, was not fulfilled.[188]

Two findings are of particular interest to radiologists. First, many peripherally located cancers were overlooked initially; 90% of those missed were visible in retrospect

---

*References 60, 70, 161, 166, 247, 248, 280, 472.

for months or even years. Fortunately, peripheral carcinomas often grow slowly, so despite delayed diagnosis, 70% were still within American Joint Committee stage I when finally noted.[458] Huhti, Saloheimo, and Sutinen[280] also noted that when the diagnosis was previously missed, the survival rates were better — again a reflection that the rate of tumor growth may be more important than early diagnosis. The second noteworthy finding was that some 15% to 20% of patients with cancer showed malignant cells in the sputum when the plain chest radiograph was normal. Interestingly, these patients, who all had either centrally situated squamous cell carcinoma or mixed histologic features with squamous cell carcinoma as one element, had a more favorable prognosis than those who had positive radiographic findings.[189,458]

A related issue is the difficult decision of whether failure to diagnose lung cancer on an initial chest radiograph, seen only in retrospect, constitutes malpractice or whether such "misses" are inevitable, even under the best conditions.[525,692] The magnitude of the problem is highlighted by several series.[248,254] The large review by Muhm and associates[458] showed that 45 of the 50 primary peripheral lesions had been visible but overlooked on previous films. The equivalent figure for central lesions was 12 of 16. Similarly, Heelan and co-workers[254] found that 65% of cancers in a yearly screening program had been overlooked on the previous film. Thus, if failure to diagnose a lung cancer at the first opportunity, however subtle the abnormality, were to be regarded ipso facto as malpractice, radiologists would be found guilty of malpractice even though their films and their interpretation conformed to the same standards as a group of experienced chest radiologists reporting on a large number of patients known to be at high risk for lung cancer. Clearly the dividing line between negligence and acceptable practice is difficult to define. Since there are no clear-cut criteria, these decisions, as so often in the medicolegal arena, will depend on the testimony of expert witnesses and local laws.[525] It is worth noting, however, that the legal case sometimes hinges on the technical adequacy of the radiographs and appropriate communication of the findings, as well as on the issue of film interpretation.

Austin, Romney, and Goldsmith[23] analyzed 27 patients in whom a potentially resectable lung cancer had been missed, even though it was visible in retrospect on previous films. The mean diameter of the lesions was 1.6 cm, and almost all had ill-defined edges. Most were in an upper lobe and in women. In another analysis of 17 cancers visible in retrospect, the failure to diagnose the cancers at the first opportunity was partly due to failure to see the lesion and partly due to misinterpreting the shadow as "inflammatory disease."[248] Many factors contribute to a radiologist's failure to detect a lung cancer on chest x-ray examination,[692] including the size and shape of the nodule, lesion conspicuity, viewing time,[486] and the visual search patterns used by the radiologist.[339] There may also be intentional or unintentional underreporting, driven by the desire to avoid further unnecessary, invasive, or expensive investigation.[338]

A variety of techniques to reduce errors of detection have been recommended or investigated,[655,692] including high-kilovoltage technique, the use of wide-latitude film, feedback systems,[340] and double reporting.[627]

Patients with normal chest radiographs but malignant cells in the sputum, or those strongly suspected of having lung carcinoma because of hemoptysis or a paraneoplastic syndrome, should have the upper airways examined, and bronchoscopy should be performed.[349] If the tumor is still not found, CT scanning should be undertaken, since it can demonstrate tumors too small to be identifiable on plain chest radiographs. CT can regularly demonstrate peripheral tumors smaller than 0.5 cm, whereas it is unusual to identify bronchial carcinoma on plain chest radiograph until the tumor is 1 cm or more in diameter. Even then the tumor may be difficult to see because its edge may be ill defined and more often than not it is partly obscured by overlying ribs.

BRONCHIAL CARCINOID

Bronchial carcinoids* constitute less than 5% of pulmonary tumors.[241,497] The age range is wide, stretching from teenagers[664] to old age. They show a spectrum of microscopic appearances and clinical behavior ranging from a slow-growing locally invasive tumor to a malignant metastasizing tumor with a moderately fast growth rate, but even widely metastatic carcinoids may grow very slowly.[385]

There are two well-described forms of bronchial carcinoid: typical carcinoid and atypical carcinoid. Atypical carcinoid has cellular and clinical features intermediate between those of typical carcinoid and small cell carcinoma of the lung.[111,443] All three of these tumors are believed to be of neuroendocrine origin,[459,666] being derived from the bronchial and bronchiolar amino precursor uptake decarboxylation (APUD) cells, forming a spectrum with varying degrees of malignancy.[191,443] The tumor has also been called Kulchitsky cell carcinoma (KCC).[497] KCC-1 tumors correspond to typical carcinoid, KCC-2 tumors to the more aggressive atypical carcinoids, and KCC-3 tumors to small cell carcinomas. These subtypes may be difficult to differentiate from one another in small biopsy or needle aspiration samples.[241,281] Also, individual tumors may show different patterns in different portions of a lesion. A recently described large cell neuroendocrine variant (intermediate cell neuroendocrine carcinoma) behaves intermediately between atypical carcinoid and small cell carcinoma.[245,644,666]

---

*The term "bronchial carcinoid" has now replaced "bronchial adenoma." The designation "bronchial adenoma," which covered carcinoid tumor, mucoepidermoid carcinoma,[256] and adenoid cystic carcinoma (the most frequent variety in the trachea[114]), was unsatisfactory because none of these tumors is totally benign.

Only 15% of typical carcinoids metastasize,[415] and the prognosis following surgical resection is therefore excellent.[575] Approximately half the atypical carcinoids ultimately metastasize. Spread is usually first to hilar[241] or mediastinal nodes, and blood-borne metastasis at presentation is unusual. The great majority of typical bronchial carcinomas arise centrally in the main, lobar, or segmental bronchi and may cause cough and occasionally wheezing. Repetitive bouts of pneumonia are common, and bronchiectasis and lung abscess may occur beyond the obstruction.[520] Bronchial carcinoids are vascular tumors and may present with hemoptysis.[241,281,415] Centrally located bronchial carcinoids[191] may be predominantly intraluminal, assuming a polypoid configuration, may grow along the lumen of the bronchus, or may be predominantly extraluminal, in which case they are known as "iceberg" lesions (see Figure 8-49). The surface is usually smooth; only rarely is it ulcerated to any degree. Atypical carcinoids usually arise peripherally in the lung, and both hemoptysis and pneumonitis are rare. Carcinoid syndrome is rare with bronchial carcinoids[281,478] unless liver metastases are present.[415,543]

Bronchial carcinoid tumors may secrete adrenocorticotropic hormone (ACTH) in sufficient quantities to cause Cushing's syndrome (ectopic ACTH syndrome), clinically indistinguishable from pituitary-dependent Cushing's disease.[150,182,278,657] The responsible tumors are often small, sometimes tiny, and require meticulous searching with chest CT to reveal their presence (Figure 8-45).[150,657] Some are so small that they cannot be found until they grow large enough to be visualized with imaging examinations. Small bronchial carcinoid tumors may on occasion be shown to advantage by MRI because on appropriate sequences (particularly with T2-weighted or STIR sequences) the contrast of the high signal of the tumor against the low background signal of normal lung and flowing blood in pulmonary vessels may make the lesions more conspicuous than at CT, in which the small lesions may be difficult to distinguish from the larger blood vessels.[152] It is possible to perform needle aspiration of a suspicious pulmonary nodule in a patient with Cushing's disease to analyze the sample for ACTH,[149] but analysis of bronchial lavage fluid is unhelpful.[151]

The chest radiograph is abnormal in most cases[348,478]; in approximately 10% of cases the chest radiograph is normal and the diagnosis is established only by bronchoscopy[10,213] or surgical removal of a nodule first shown by CT. The majority of bronchial carcinoids arise in the larger bronchi and cause partial or complete bronchial obstruction with consequent atelectasis (Figures 8-46 and 8-47; see Figure 8-50). Collateral air drift may keep segments aerated when the lesion is in a segmental bronchus; even whole lobes can be kept fully aerated despite complete occlusion of a lobar bronchus.[193] The consequent hypoxia of the affected lung may occasionally cause recognizable local vasoconstriction on plain film and perfusion scintigraphy.[421] The tumor itself is visible

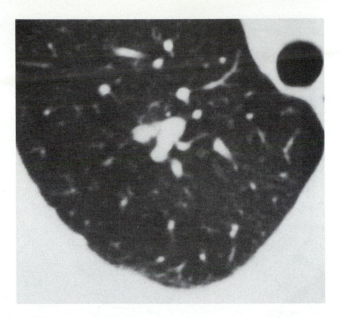

FIGURE 8-45
Bronchial carcinoid causing ectopic adrenocorticotropic hormone syndrome. Small bronchial carcinoid in this case measured only 6 to 7 mm in diameter. It caused small mucocele beyond it. Following surgical removal, the patient's Cushing's disease was cured.

on plain film as a hilar mass (Figure 8-48) in about 25% of patients with a central lesion,[10,213] but it can be demonstrated on conventional tomography (Figure 8-49) or CT (Figures 8-50 and 8-51) in many other instances. The appearance differs from carcinoma in that the bronchus may widen slightly as it approaches the mass (Figure 8-51). Bronchography shows this feature well[633] but is unnecessary because bronchoscopy provides more specific information.

Small tumors in segmental or subsegmental bronchi may result in mucous distention of the bronchi beyond the obstruction, with the surrounding lung remaining aerated by collateral air drift. The resulting bronchocele (mucoid impaction) may then be the dominant radiographic sign on plain chest radiograph or CT (Figures 8-52 to 8-54).[174,529]

Approximately 10% to 20% of bronchial carcinoids appear radiographically as a solitary pulmonary nodule (Figure 8-55). The nodules are well defined and are round, oval, lobulated, or notched, usually with a smooth edge,[478] although spiculation is reported.[111] Calcification or ossification is occasionally recognizable on plain chest radiography.[35,348] Two large series describing the chest radiographic appearances have been reported from the Mayo Clinic.[10,226] In the earlier series of 23 peripheral bronchial adenomas (bronchial carcinoid), the average diameter of the nodule was 4 cm; however, the later report on 20 similarly located tumors showed none with a diameter greater than 4 cm. Multiple lesions are a frequent pathologic finding,[601] but almost invariably they are too small to be recognized radiologically.

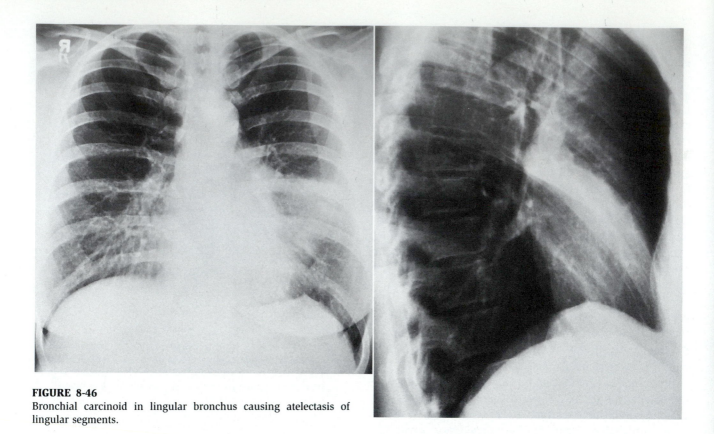

FIGURE 8-46
Bronchial carcinoid in lingular bronchus causing atelectasis of lingular segments.

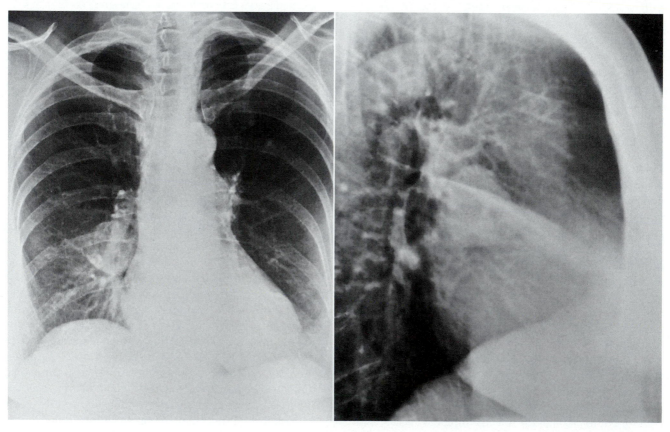

A

B

FIGURE 8-47
Bronchial carcinoid causing right middle lobe collapse. The tumor itself is visible as a hilar mass. **A,** Posteroanterior radiograph. **B,** Lateral radiograph.

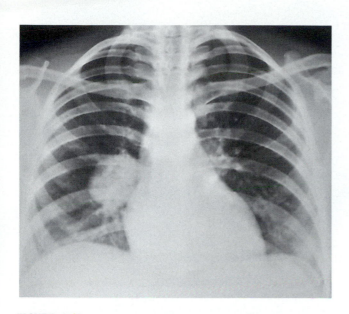

FIGURE 8-48
Bronchial carcinoid presenting as a hilar mass without distal atelectasis. (Courtesy Dr. Peter Hacking, Newcastle, U.K.)

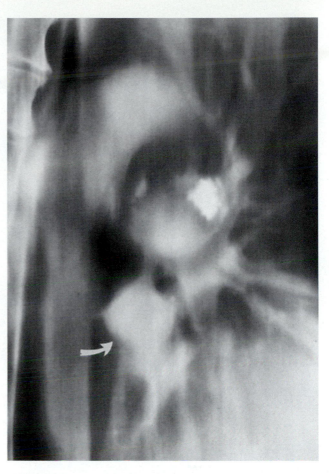

FIGURE 8-49
Bronchial carcinoid of right lower lobe bronchus with large extrabronchial *(arrow)* and small endobronchial component.

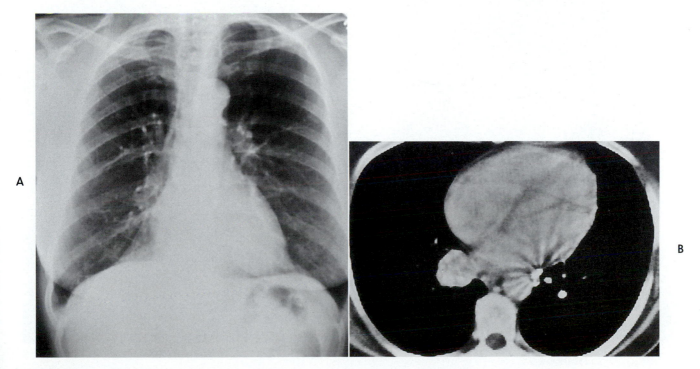

FIGURE 8-50
Bronchial carcinoid. **A,** Right lower lobe collapse. **B,** Computed tomographic scan showing tumor lying centrally. Note uniform contrast enhancement of tumor mass.

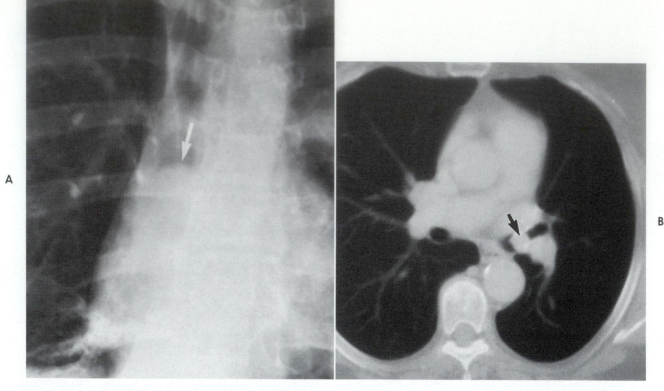

FIGURE 8-51

A, Bronchial carcinoid in intermediate stem bronchus showing widening of bronchus immediately above the tumor and the top of the intraluminal mass *(arrow).* **B,** Intraluminal bronchial carcinoid tumor *(arrow)* shown by computed tomography. (Courtesy Dr. Martin Wastie, Nottingham, U.K.)

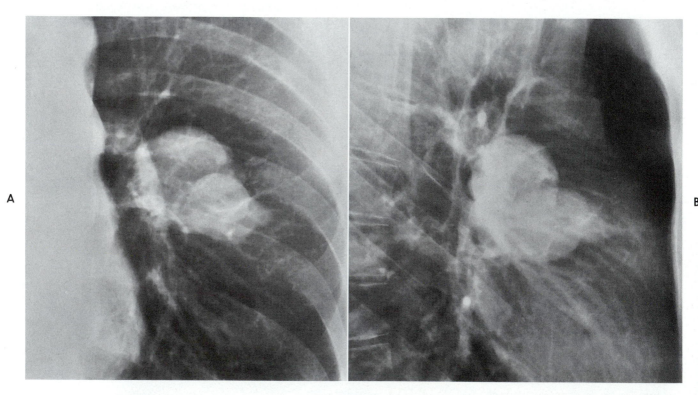

FIGURE 8-52

Bronchial carcinoid causing mucoid impaction. Mucus-filled, dilated bronchi (bronchoceles) beyond the obstruction resemble a bilobed mass, but their tubular configuration can be recognized, particularly on lateral view. **A,** Posteroanterior view. **B,** Lateral view.

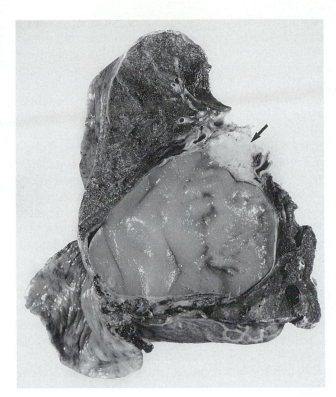

FIGURE 8-53
Operative specimen showing central bronchial carcinoid *(arrow)* and hugely dilated, mucus-filled bronchi (mucocele) mimicking large neoplastic mass beyond true tumor.

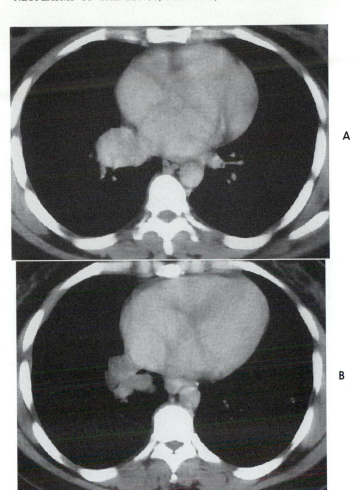

FIGURE 8-54
Bronchial carcinoid with, A, contrast-enhancing central mass and, B, lower density mucocele distal to the mass.

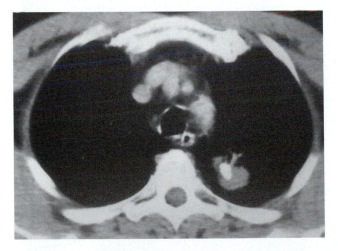

FIGURE 8-55
Dense calcification in a peripheral bronchial carcinoid shown by computed tomographic scanning (but not visible on standard plain chest radiographs).

CT scanning provides superb anatomic localization of both the intraluminal and extraluminal components of the tumors in the major bronchi,[191,469] but usually carcinoid cannot be distinguished from carcinoma unless the lesion is demonstrably ossified. The tumor may narrow, deform, or obstruct the airway. Even peripheral

carcinoids can be shown to lie adjacent to recognizable small airways.[468]

The incidence of calcification (Figure 8-55) detectable by CT appears to be considerable: 4 of 12 cases in one series[390] and 8 of 31 in another.[705] The incidence of calcification is significantly greater in centrally located tumors and in the larger tumors. A variety of patterns of calcification are seen,[705] including multiple nodular and curvilinear configurations. Sometimes the calcification takes the form of recognizable ossification[705] and is so extensive than it occupies the whole of the tumor mass.[589] Contrast enhancement, which is sometimes marked, is seen in some cases of bronchial carcinoid (Figures 8-50 and 8-54).[19,137]

Bronchial carcinoids may concentrate radionuclides. Iodine-123 *N*-isopropyl-*p*-iodoamphetamine has been shown to accumulate in sufficient quantities to demonstrate a bronchial carcinoid.[481] Carcinoids have somatostatin receptors and can therefore be imaged with radiolabeled octreotide, a somatostatin analogue. Octreotide scanning, while 96% sensitive, is also positive in a variety of other tumors, as well as inflammatory conditions.[335]

HAMARTOMA

Hamartomas are defined pathologically as tumorlike malformations composed of an abnormal mixture of the normal constituents of the organ in which they are found. Most pulmonary hamartomas contain masses of cartilage with clefts lined by bronchial epithelium, and they may also contain fat[33] or cystic collections of fluid.[447,464] Some authors prefer the term "hamartochondroma" or "chondromatous hamartoma" to distinguish these lesions from the much rarer vascular hamartomas that do not contain cartilage.[34,523] Although the precise nature of pulmonary hamartomas is debatable, they are usually classified as benign neoplasms. They grow slowly[296] and are usually solitary, although there are a few case reports of multiple pulmonary hamartomas.[46,464] Malignant transformation is either nonexistent or extremely rare,[526] but in one series a higher than expected incidence of lung carcinoma was observed in the vicinity of a hamartoma.[309] Also, malignant sarcomas arising in the wall of so-called cystic mesenchymal hamartomas have been reported in children, but cystic mesenchymal hamartomas are histologically quite different from the usual hamartoma seen in adults.[252,613,401] (It has been suggested that cystic mesenchymal hamartoma is part of the spectrum of childhood pulmonary blastoma developing in congenital cystic lung.[581])

A triad of pulmonary chondroma (often multiple), gastric epithelioid leiomyosarcoma (leiomyoblastoma), and functioning extraadrenal paraganglioma, known as Carney's triad, has been described.[92] The importance of the condition, which is seen mostly in women under 35 years of age, is that if multiple slow-growing cartilage tumors are found in the lung, the other tumors in the triad should be sought, since the other neoplasms are potentially lethal. Furthermore, patients with a smooth muscle tumor in the wall of the stomach should not automatically be assumed to have pulmonary metastases just because they have multiple pulmonary nodules. An incomplete form of the triad manifesting just the pulmonary chondromata and the gastric smooth muscle tumors is also seen.[170,412] In addition to Carney's triad, the association of pulmonary hamartomas with other developmental anomalies and benign tumors has been noted.[200]

The average age at presentation of pulmonary hamartomas is 45 to 50 years.[523] They are rarely seen in

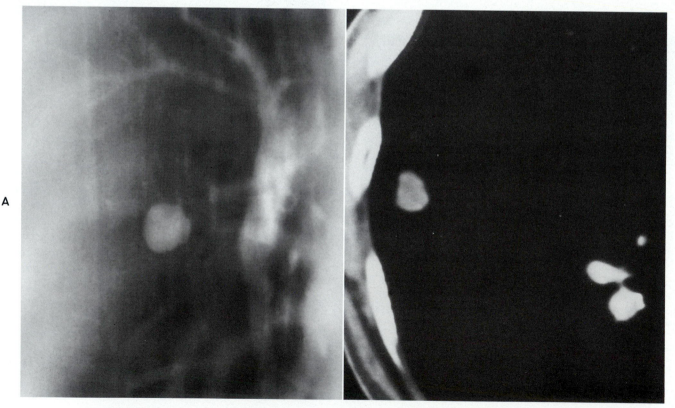

FIGURE 8-56
Hamartoma of lung presenting as a small, noncalcified, very well-defined, slightly lobulated solitary pulmonary nodule. **A,** Conventional tomogram. **B,** Computed tomographic scan.

children. Over 90% are situated peripherally, with 8% or less arising in central bronchi.[523] The peripheral lesions are asymptomatic; the endobronchial hamartomas may cause symptoms because of the consequences of bronchial obstruction or occasionally hemoptysis.

On plain chest radiographs and CT scans the peripheral lesion is seen as a spherical, lobulated, or notched pulmonary nodule with a very well-defined edge surrounded by normal lung (Figure 8-56). Pulmonary hamartomas can range up to 10 cm in diameter[134]; large lesions are unusual, however, and most are less than 4 cm.[523] The larger the lesion, the more likely that it will calcify. Definite calcification is seen on plain film in up to 15% of patients.[53,523] The calcification may show the typical popcorn configuration of cartilage calcification, in which case the diagnosis is virtually certain (Figures 8-57 and 8-58). The presence of fat density within the mass is a specific diagnostic feature (Figure 8-55). Radiologically detectable air within the tumors is exceedingly rare,[153] but central lucency caused by fat can be confused with cavitation.

The signs at CT are similar to those at plain radiography, but because of the better contrast resolution, calcium and particularly fat are easier to identify.[350,595] In a series of 47 patients with pulmonary hamartomas it was possible to identify fat (CT numbers in the range −80 HU to −120 HU) or calcium plus fat within the nodule in 28 patients by use of thin section CT; this combination appears to be specific for hamartoma, at least in nodules under 2.5 cm in diameter.[595] In 17 of the cases the hamartomas showed neither calcification nor fat, and in the remaining 2 there was diffuse calcification throughout the lesion.

Endobronchial hamartomas lead to airway obstruction. The radiologic features are identical to those seen with centrally located bronchial carcinoid.

TRACHEAL NEOPLASMS

Benign tumors of the trachea are rare. They are most frequent in children, in whom squamous papillomas are the most common. These papillomas are usually part of laryngeal papillomatosis, a condition discussed on p. 318. The next most common benign tracheal tumor of childhood is hemangioma. These tumors, which are often associated with cutaneous hemangiomas, are frequently in the subglottic region. Stridor often develops in the first year of life. On imaging examinations tracheal hemangiomas are seen as eccentrically situated nodular masses.

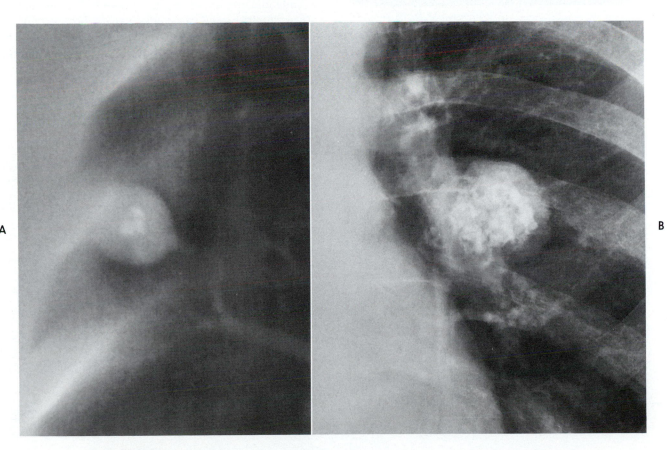

A   B

FIGURE 8-57
Hamartoma. **A,** Showing smooth edge and central cartilage calcification on conventional tomography.
B, Showing extensive popcorn calcification.

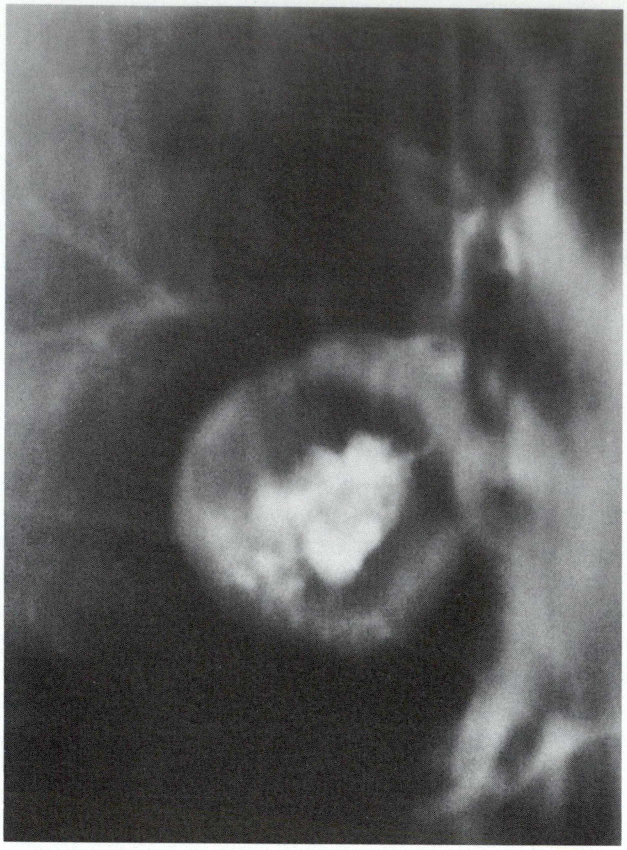

Occasionally encountered in the trachea are bronchial carcinoid and a variety of connective tissue and neural neoplasms,[8] including lipoma, fibroma, hemangioendothelioma, cartilage tumors,[137,626] granular cell myoblastoma, laryngeal papillomatosis (Figure 8-59), neurilemmoma, neurofibroma, and paraganglioma.[144,468] All these lesions produce a nonspecific focal mass in the wall of the trachea.

The most common malignant tumor of the trachea is invasion from an adjacent neoplasm, notably bronchial carcinoma. Primary malignant tumors of the trachea are rare and are virtually confined to adults. The most frequent are squamous cell carcinoma and adenoid cystic carcinoma.[144,207] Mucoepidermoid is the next most common carcinoma; it is more frequent in the major bronchi than in the trachea.[245] These three tumors make up over 90% of primary tracheal tumors. The remaining 10% consist of a wide variety of neoplasms, including sarcoma, lymphoma, adenocarcinoma, chondrosarcoma, plasmacytoma, small cell carcinoma, and metastases.[468]

Squamous cell carcinoma, like squamous cell carcinoma of the bronchus and lung, is strongly associated with smoking. By the time these tumors are diagnosed, they have often invaded the mediastinum and adjacent esophagus. Tracheoesophageal fistula may be the initial feature.

Adenoid cystic carcinomas present at an earlier age than squamous cell carcinoma, usually between 30 to 50 years. They grow slowly, tend to involve the posterior wall of the lower two thirds of the trachea, and infiltrate

FIGURE 8-58
Hamartoma. Conventional tomogram showing central cartilage calcification and surrounding fat density within lesion.

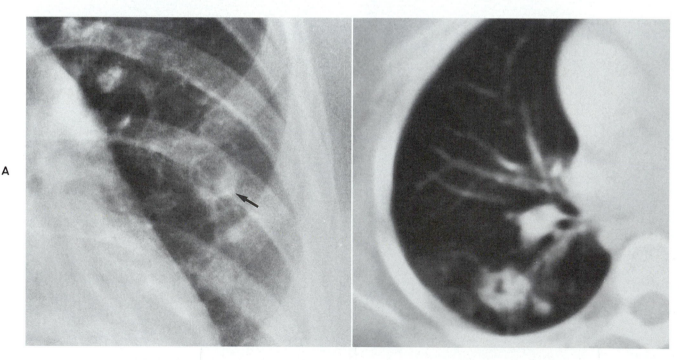

FIGURE 8-59
Laryngeal papillomatosis. **A,** In a 7-year-old child who had multiple small cavitary nodules. **B,** Computed tomographic scan in another patient with multiple cavitating nodules.

submucosally for long distances.[245,468] Therefore stridor and wheezing are common early symptoms.

All three tumors are seen on imaging studies as an intraluminal nodule (Figure 8-60) with lobular or irregular contours; low-grade mucoepidermoid carcinomas usually appear as polypoid lesions. They may grow circumferentially and are then seen as a stenosing lesion of variable length. The full extent of submucosal spread tends to be underestimated with CT[343]; the role of MRI in assessing the extent of spread has yet to be evaluated. These tumors grow through the tracheal wall to produce a paratracheal mass (Figure 8-61), a feature most frequently seen with adenoid cystic carcinoma. As with bronchial carcinoid, there may be a relatively large mediastinal mass with a much smaller intratracheal component. Although CT shows the extraluminal component of tumors of the trachea, it is poor at indicating whether or not mediastinal structures, such as the esophagus and aorta, are invaded. Obliteration of the fat planes between the tumor and these structures is sometimes caused by invasion, but at other times no invasion is found when surgery is finally performed.[603]

Like bronchial carcinoid and various benign tumors, adenoid cystic carcinomas may calcify.

RARE MALIGNANT PULMONARY NEOPLASMS

Primary pulmonary sarcomas are usually fibrosarcomas, leiomyosarcomas,[42,87,534] or sarcomas of the pulmonary artery.[143] In a large review from the Armed Forces Institute of Pathology,[236] endobronchial fibrosarcomas and leiomyosarcomas generally exhibited a relatively benign behavior compared with tumors arising within the lung parenchyma, which showed great variability in their degree of malignancy and a significant incidence of highly aggressive behavior. Chondrosarcoma, fibroleiomyosarcoma, malignant fibrous histiocytoma,[419,539,700] osteosarcoma,[514,609] rhabdomyosarcoma, myxosarcoma, and neurofibrosarcoma may also arise primarily in the lung. Most sarcomas of the lung, however, are metastases from extrathoracic primary tumors.

On imaging examinations all these sarcomas appear as a solitary pulmonary nodule or as an endobronchial mass indistinguishable from bronchial carcinoma (Figure 8-62), except that calcification is a feature of osteosarcoma and chondrosarcoma.

Hemangiopericytomas, which may be benign or malignant (the larger the lesion, the more likely it is to be malignant), occasionally arise as a primary tumor in the lung.[429] These tumors are most common in the fourth and fifth decades with no sex predominance. They are usually asymptomatic until large, but cough, hemoptysis, and chest pain are the more common symptoms. On imaging

FIGURE 8-59, cont'd
C, Patient with just one polypoid lesion *(arrow)* in trachea.

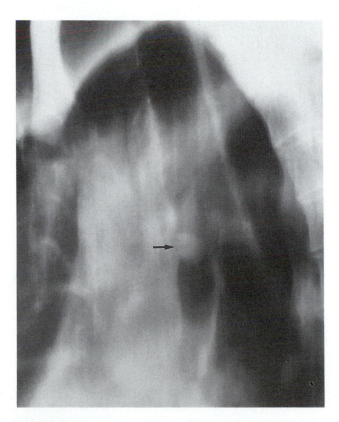

FIGURE 8-60
Small endobronchial carcinoid at bifurcation of trachea *(arrow)* shown on tomography.

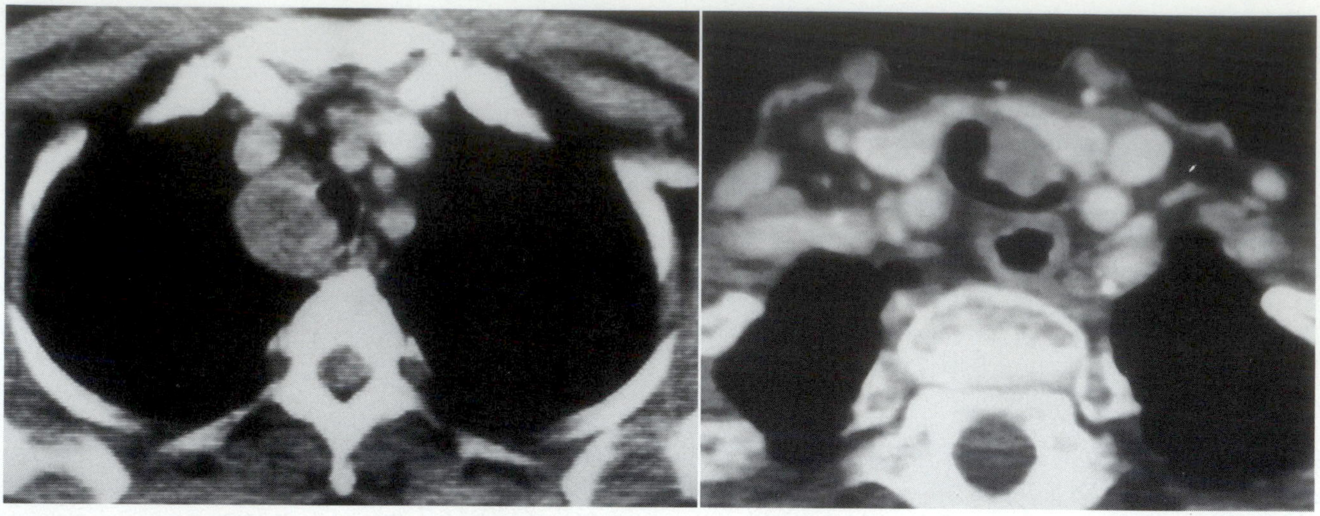

FIGURE 8-61
Tracheal carcinoma. **A,** Mucoepidermoid carcinoma showing a predominantly extraluminal mass. **B,** Squamous cell carcinoma showing a mass arising from wall and projecting into the lumen.

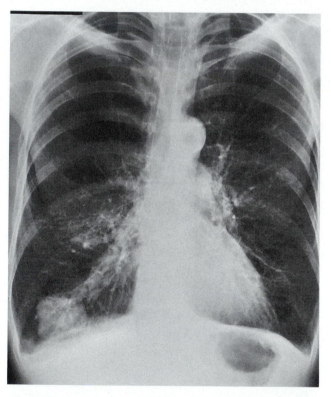

FIGURE 8-62
Primary rhabdomyosarcoma of lung. The right lower lobe mass was surgically resected on the preoperative assumption that it was a bronchial carcinoma.

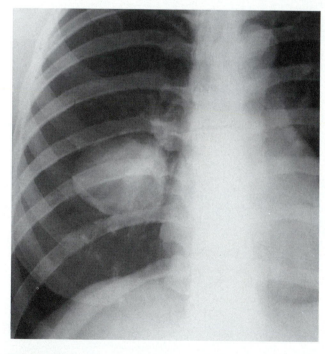

FIGURE 8-63
Hemangioendothelioma of lung presenting as an asymptomatic well-defined pulmonary mass.

examinations[240] the lesions appear as one or more well-defined pulmonary masses of any size (Figure 8-63). Speckled, eccentric calcification is seen on occasion. MRI shows a heterogeneous signal pattern corresponding to necrosis and hemorrhage with no specific features.

Neoplastic angioendotheliosis is a rare malignant neoplasm, which may be a B cell lymphoma.[453] It is characterized by proliferation of neoplastic cells in small vessels, which rarely primarily involve the lungs.[273] Chest radiography and CT show widespread, ill-defined pulmonary shadowing. Gallium scanning, which shows diffuse pulmonary activity, appears to be a sensitive technique for detecting this disease.[273]

Carcinosarcoma and pulmonary blastoma are rare tumors. Carcinosarcomas arise from two different germ cell layers and are composed of mixed malignant epithelial and connective tissue components. They are usually first found in middle-aged to elderly patients. Carcinosarcomas are often endobronchial in origin[605] and indistinguishable from other endobronchial tumors. Pulmonary blastoma is a malignant tumor that on histologic examination shows embryonic bronchial structures in a background of abundant immature sarcoma.[329,601,605] Originally blastomas were thought to arise from a multipotential mesodermal cell, but like carcinosarcomas they are now believed to arise from two germ cell layers. They are therefore now classified as a form of carcinosarcoma. Pulmonary blastoma appears at a somewhat younger age than carcinoma, with a small proportion found in children.[599] Pulmonary blastomas generally arise peripherally in the lung as a solitary well-defined mass or occasionally as multiple pulmonary masses.[244,265,507,681] Blastomas found in adults are often of moderate size but range from 2.5 to 26 cm in diameter.[73,244,316] Cavitation has been noted on plain chest radiographs,[244] and CT and ultrasound have shown a cystic structure within the mass itself.[332] Calcification has been reported on CT.[599] Pleural effusion may accompany the mass.

Senac, Wood, and Isaacs[581] reported on seven children with pulmonary blastoma, emphasizing that all the tumors were unilateral and large. Childhood blastoma may be a distinctive neoplasm.[581,397] All four patients who underwent CT examination showed similar findings: a heterogeneous mass with areas of low attenuation and whorls of high attenuation. In three cases CT showed a rounded tumor arising within an area of preexisting cystic lung. The association of pulmonary blastomas and developmental cysts of the lung has also been reported by other authors.[316]

Plasmacytoma of the lungs or major airways is an exceedingly rare tumor, even in patients with multiple myeloma. With solitary lesions the sheets of plasma cells may be difficult to distinguish histologically from a benign plasma cell granuloma, and some of the cases in the literature may have been wrongly categorized. The most common form of intrathoracic plasmacytoma is inward extension from a rib. Rarely plasmacytoma is seen radiographically as a mass arising within the trachea,[145] bronchi, or lung[11,413] or as greatly enlarged intrathoracic lymph nodes.[212,307,590] A single case with extensive ossification of a solitary pulmonary plasmacytoma has been reported,[323] although this case may have been a plasma cell granuloma, a condition in which calcification is not so rare.[307] Scattered cases of myeloma involvement of the pulmonary interstitium have also been reported.[590]

Askin's tumors are malignant small cell tumors of neuroepithelial origin seen in childhood and adolescence.[20] The great majority of these rare tumors arise in the chest wall[565]; a few are almost exclusively in the lung, but even these show pleural involvement. It would appear that all Askin's tumors are based on the pleura or clearly arise in the chest wall.[20] The intrathoracic soft tissue mass, which may show calcification, can be huge with either no visible rib destruction or only focal rib lysis. Pleural effusions and hilar adenopathy may accompany the mass.

Intravascular bronchioloalveolar tumor is a rare cause of multiple small pulmonary nodules.[130,407,554,587] There is a strong predilection for females, and the age range is 12 to 61 with a mean in the forties. The tumor is believed to be a neoplasm of blood vessels,[127] possibly related to hemangioendothelioma. The patients are often asymptomatic, and the diagnosis is established following the discovery of multiple pulmonary nodules on chest radiography or CT. The nodules are well defined or slightly ill defined in outline. Associated pleural effusion may be seen. Pathologic examination may show calcification. Metastases to hilar nodes are recorded. The course may be indolent with survival of up to 15 years.

Until the recent epidemic of acquired immunodeficiency syndrome (AIDS), Kaposi's sarcoma was regarded primarily as a skin tumor of the lower extremities. The tumor is being encountered with increased frequency in patients with AIDS and is discussed in the section on AIDS, p. 240.

RARE BENIGN PULMONARY NEOPLASMS

Amyloidoma is one of the forms of amyloidosis in which one or more nodular masses are seen in the lung parenchyma or tracheobronchial tree (Figure 8-64). The lesions occur in the elderly and are frequently asymptomatic. The nodules are round or slightly lobulated, may contain visible calcification, and may cavitate.[689] A fuller discussion of intrathoracic amyloidosis is provided in Chapter 12.

Granular cell myoblastoma is a benign tumor that is most commonly found in subcutaneous tissues but may rarely occur in the larger bronchi and even more rarely in the lung parenchyma, trachea, or mediastinum.[5,122,388] On radiologic examination it usually presents as postobstructive atelectasis or pneumonia beyond the lesion itself, occasionally as a small solitary pulmonary nodule, or as a polypoid lesion arising in a bronchus.[78,635]

Fibroma, chondroma, lipoma,[297,406] hemangioma, neurofibroma, and neurilemmoma[173] may arise in the walls of the bronchi or in the lung parenchyma. Those in the lung parenchyma are nonspecific solitary pulmonary nodules; those that arise in the larger bronchi are indistinguishable from the more common bronchial carcinoid,[573] except that it may be possible to distinguish the fat in a lipoma by CT (Figure 8-65).[108,434] Most intrathoracic lipomas arise extrapleurally from the chest wall, mediastinum, or diaphragm.[29,618] Endobronchial lipoma has been reported to contain a focus of dense calcification within the tumor, as well as fat density.[406]

Leiomyoma of the lung may be a solitary lesion,

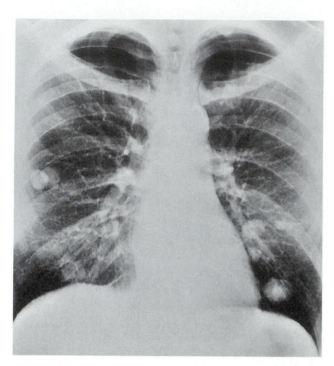

FIGURE 8-64
Multiple pulmonary nodules caused by amyloidosis. Several nodules contain a central core of calcification.

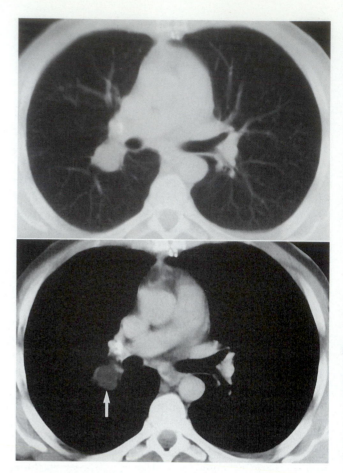

A

B

FIGURE 8-65
Endobronchial lipoma. Fat density of mass is well shown by computed tomography. **A,** At lung window settings. **B,** Narrow window settings. (Courtesy Dr. Ted A. Glass, Fredericksburg, Md.)

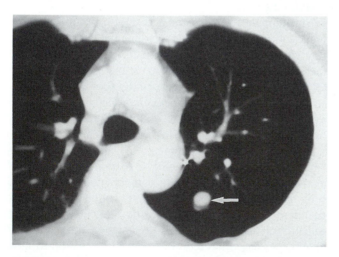

FIGURE 8-66
Benign metastasizing leiomyoma. Computed tomographic scan showing one of many pulmonary nodules *(arrow)* that developed over 15 years.

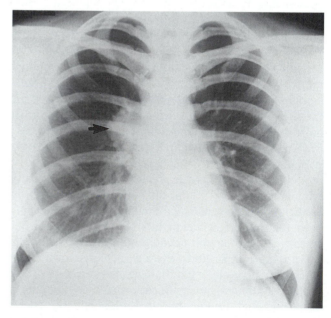

FIGURE 8-67
Intrapulmonary teratoma. This teratoma *(arrow)* was totally within lung at surgery.

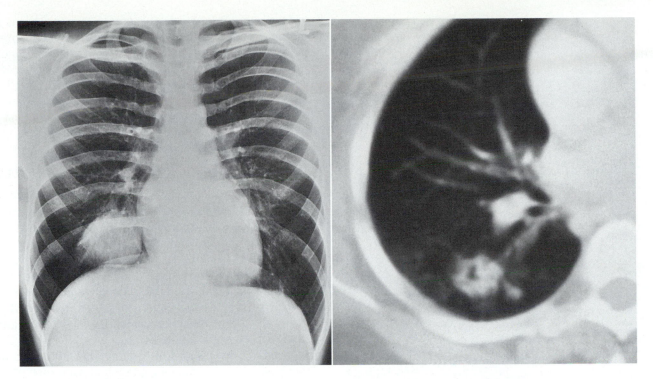

FIGURE 8-68
Plasma cell granuloma of right lower lobe bronchus. The mass shows no distinguishing features.

radiographically indistinguishable from the other benign connective tissue neoplasms. Multiple leiomyomas occur as multiple nodular lesions in the lung (Figure 8-66),[24,403,521] or very occasionally in the pleura.[75] They are given a wide variety of names, including benign metastasizing leiomyoma. Their behavior varies from that of a benign lesion to that of a low-grade sarcoma; the lesions are often hormone sensitive.[403] In women these tumors may be very slow-growing metastases from a uterine leiomyoma, and women with benign metastasizing leiomyoma often have a history of previous hysterectomy for uterine fibroids.

Chemodectomas, benign clear cell tumors, and endometriosis[264] are very occasionally encountered in the lung parenchyma. On radiologic examination all these lesions appear as nonspecific pulmonary nodules. (Pleural endometriosis is discussed on p. 692.)

Intrapulmonary teratomas are unusual. They occur equally in men and women and usually are diagnosed in the second to fourth decades. Most are benign, although malignant lesions are encountered. Chest pain, hemoptysis, and cough are the most frequent initial symptoms, and expectoration of hair (trichophysis) is the most specific. On radiographic and CT studies intrapulmonary teratomas appear as lobulated masses that may show calcification or cavitation (Figure 8-67).[451] Fat, a feature of mediastinal teratomas, has not yet been reported on imaging examinations, but the number of cases examined by CT so far is tiny.[451] The lesions are often large, and there may be bronchiectasis in the neighboring lung.

Plasma cell granuloma of the lung is the name given to what is presumed to be reactive granulomatous inflammation. Numerous other terms have been applied, notably inflammatory pseudotumor and histiocytoma. Matsubara and co-workers,[408] based on an analysis of 32 cases, believe that most or possibly all cases originate as organizing pneumonia and that these lesions are not neoplasms. The age range is wide and includes children[345] and young adults. On macroscopic study the lesions are firm, pale, sharply circumscribed masses. Histologic examination shows a localized benign proliferation of plasma cells within a background of granulation or fibrocollagenous tissue.[262] The lesion may histologically resemble plasmacytoma. Most patients are asymptomatic; the lesion is often discovered incidentally on plain chest radiographs as a solitary pulmonary nodule (Figure 8-68), which can be a large mass,[345] or as a larger ill-defined area of consolidation. Both cavitation and calcification have been described.* The occasional plasma cell granuloma arises in a central bronchus[16] and is radiologically indistinguishable from bronchial carcinoid. CT scanning shows all these features to advantage but does not allow a specific diagnosis to be made.[585]

Sclerosing hemangioma is a benign neoplasm[138,312,624] that has been confused with plasma cell granuloma in the past because of the reactive or hyperplastic changes adjacent to the neoplastic elements but is now regarded as pathologically distinct. Whether it is of endothelial or

*References 154, 262, 345, 449, 508, 577, 585, 623.

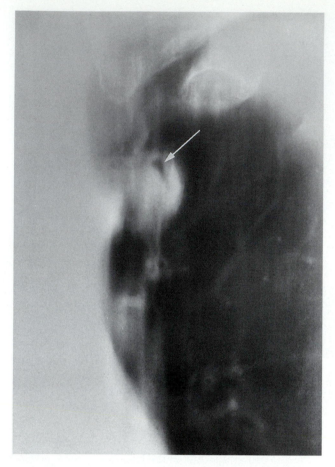

FIGURE 8-69
Plasma cell granuloma showing air meniscus sign *(arrow)*.

respiratory epithelial origin is not entirely clear, but recent opinions support an epithelial origin.[311,702] The average age at diagnosis is 42 with a range from the teenage years upwards. There is a marked female predominance. In almost all cases the reported lesion is a solitary pulmonary mass ranging in size from very small to 8 cm in diameter, with an average of 3 cm.[312] An air meniscus sign on plain film (Figure 8-69) has been reported in two patients.[26] Calcification may be seen. Only a few cases subjected to CT examination have been reported: these showed a well-defined, round pulmonary nodule of soft tissue density, with enhancement following intravenous contrast injection in one case[138] and central liquefaction in another.[624]

Squamous papillomas of the bronchi and lungs are most commonly associated with laryngeal papillomatosis, a disease that usually commences in childhood and is believed to be viral in origin.[334] Carcinomatous transformation has been reported,[113] but the incidence appears to be only about 1% of cases.[639] Papillomatosis is almost invariably confined to the larynx, but in a small minority of patients one or more papillomas are found in the trachea and bronchi, where they may cause atelectasis and bronchiectasis. Rarely they are present in the lung

and are seen on plain chest radiographs or CT scans as multiple small, widely scattered, well-defined round pulmonary nodules, frequently with cavitation (Figure 8-59).[113,217,334,489,551] The cavities, which may become several centimeters in diameter, are often thin walled. Secondary infection may lead to air-fluid levels. Atelectasis is surprisingly infrequent. Squamous cell papilloma of the trachea without laryngeal papillomatosis has been described in adults.[470]

INTRATHORACIC MALIGNANT LYMPHOMA

The lymphomas are malignant neoplasms of lymphocytes and histiocytes, together with their precursors and derivatives, set in a background of nonneoplastic, presumably normal, inflammatory cells.[547]

Hodgkin's lymphoma, a specific clinical-pathologic entity, is differentiated from the more common and more frequently fatal non-Hodgkin's lymphoma by the presence of a distinctive histologic feature, the Sternberg-Reed giant cell, a large reticulum cell with a tendency to form large, densely staining nuclei.

Hodgkin's disease is classified into four subtypes in the Rye modification of the Lukes-Butler classification[384,536]: nodular sclerosing, which comprises 40% to 75% of cases and is most common in young women, and three further categories based on the relative proportion of reactive elements to Sternberg-Reed cells (and their mononuclear counterparts); these types are the lymphocyte predominant (5% to 15% of cases), mixed cell (20% to 40% of cases), and lymphocyte depleted (5% to 15% of cases).[66,547] The lymphocyte-predominant form tends to be localized and has a less aggressive clinical course. The lymphocyte-predominant and mixed cell forms may progress to become lymphocyte depleted, the variety with the worst prognosis.

The onset of Hodgkin's disease most commonly occurs in the second or third decade with a secondary peak in the fifth or sixth decade. When initially seen the patient usually has lymph node enlargement either on physical examination or on plain chest radiographs. Intrathoracic adenopathy is common with nodular sclerosing Hodgkin's disease, and peripheral and retroperitoneal adenopathy is more common with the mixed cellularity variety.[84] The enlarged nodes are firm and nontender. The cervical nodes are the most frequently affected at initial examination. Systemic symptoms such as fever, night sweats, anorexia, fatigue, weight loss, and pruritus usually appear late. The so-called Pel-Ebstein pattern of fever, with recurrent episodes of diurnal waxing and waning, is characteristic of the disease but is only occasionally encountered. Bone pain following alcohol intake is another well-known pointer to the diagnosis. Anemia may be seen but is usually absent initially. The blood may show leukocytosis or leukopenia, and eosinophilia is occasionally seen.

Hodgkin's disease is staged using the Ann Arbor classification, which takes into account the extent of

Table 8-2 Ann Arbor staging classification for Hodgkin's disease

Stage	Definition*
I	Involvement of a single lymph node region (I) or of a single extralymphatic organ or site (I$_E$)
II	Involvement of two or more lymph node regions on the same side of the diaphragm (II) or localized involvement of an extralymphatic organ or site and of one or more lymph node regions on the same side of the diaphragm (II$_E$)
III	Involvement of lymph node regions of both sides of the diaphragm (III), which may also be accompanied by involvement of the spleen (III$_S$) or by localized involvement of an extralymphatic organ or site (III$_E$) or both (III$_{SE}$)
IV	Diffuse or disseminated involvement of one or more extralymphatic organs or tissues, with or without associated lymph node involvement

Modified from Carbone PP, Musshoff HS, Smithers EW, et al: *Cancer Res* 31:1860-1861, 1971.

*The absence or presence of fever, night sweats, or unexplained loss of 10% or more of body weight in the 6 months preceding admission are to be denoted in all cases by the suffix letters A or B, respectively.

nodal disease, the presence of extranodal disease, and clinical symptoms (Table 8-2). A modification, known as the Cotswolds classification,[380] takes into account tumor bulk and the increased use of CT for assessing the extent of disease.

In general Hodgkin's disease spreads predictably from one lymph node group to contiguous groups.[552,648] In this context the term "contiguous" does not mean physical contiguity, but a directly connected lymphatic pathway.[398] Understanding the pattern of spread is useful when considering imaging procedures for staging and when designing radiation therapy ports. The ports usually include both the areas of known disease and the adjacent node groups. Direct invasion from affected nodes into the lung or bone is another characteristic form of spread.[94] The great majority of patients are in stage I or II at diagnosis. Presentation with extranodal disease is rare in Hodgkin's disease, unlike non-Hodgkin's lymphoma in which it is a fairly common presenting feature.

The non-Hodgkin's lymphomas can be regarded as neoplasms of a lymphoreticular cell of a specific lineage: B lymphocyte, T lymphocyte, or true histiocyte.[491] These cells increase in size, and the nuclei change from a cleaved to a noncleaved appearance.[239] (AIDS-related non-Hodgkin's lymphoma is discussed in Chapter 7.)

The classification of the non-Hodgkin's lymphomas, unlike that of Hodgkin's disease, has undergone many changes.[67,86] The most widely used classification in the United States, the Working Formulation for Clinical Usage, was devised by the National Cancer Institute[474] as a compromise between histologic classifications, such as the Rappaport classification,[535] and the need to classify according to prognosis. It divides the non-Hodgkin's lymphomas on morphologic grounds into three grades that correspond to prognosis: low, intermediate, and high. The dividing lines are not clear cut: composite forms are seen in up to 10% of patients, and conversion from one grade to a more malignant grade often occurs. In general, tumors that show a follicular (nodular) architecture are clinically less aggressive than those with diffuse infiltrate, but they are often more widespread at the time of diagnosis and show a higher relapse rate on treatment, at which time they may transform to more aggressive histology. Conversely, the forms with diffuse histologic features are more likely to be localized when first diagnosed and have a lower relapse rate following treatment. The Kiel classification is used widely in Europe. The Kiel classification[211,606] is partly histologically and partly immunologically based. The division of lymphomas into high and low grade has prognostic and therefore therapeutic implications, even though the high- and low-grade classifications are based on histologic criteria. (As emphasized previously, high-grade lymphoma may be more curable than low-grade lymphoma by virtue of its lower rate of relapse following treatment.)

The interrelationship between the Working Formulation and the Rappaport classification is shown in Table 8-3.

Low-grade non-Hodgkin's lymphomas usually are first manifested as widespread adenopathy.[84] They are slowly progressive, often reaching stage III or IV by the time of clinical presentation. In one fifth to one half of patients, low-grade non-Hodgkin's lymphoma progresses to a more aggressive form, and in one fourth the disease undergoes spontaneous remission,[276] although it may recur. Intermediate- and particularly high-grade non-Hodgkin's lymphoma often shows extranodal involvement at initial presentation.

There is no generally agreed upon staging system for non-Hodgkin's lymphoma, but the Ann Arbor system is frequently applied. It has less value, however, because the course of non-Hodgkin's lymphoma depends more on histologic grade and parameters such as tumor bulk and specific organ involvement than on stage of disease.

Non-Hodgkin's lymphoma in childhood often takes a different form from that seen in adults. Most adults have low- or intermediate-grade subtypes, whereas almost all children show high-grade histologic features and many have extranodal involvement.[391,598] In the series of 80 patients with childhood non-Hodgkin's lymphoma reported by Ng and co-workers,[479] only 20% had intrathoracic lymph node enlargement as the primary site of disease.

Imaging features of the malignant lymphomas

The cardinal feature of the malignant lymphomas on chest radiographs and CT is mediastinal and hilar node enlargement, which may be accompanied by pulmonary, pleural, or chest wall involvement.

Table 8-3   Classification of non-Hodgkin's lymphomas

Working formulation	Incidence* (%)	Rappaport classification
LOW GRADE		
Small lymphocytic	3.6	Lymphocytic, well differentiated
Follicular, predominantly small cleaved cell	22.5	Nodular, poorly differentiated lymphocytic
Follicular, mixed small cleaved and large cleaved cells	7.7	Nodular, mixed lymphocytic histiocytic
INTERMEDIATE GRADE		
Follicular, predominantly large cell	3.8	Nodular, histiocytic
Diffuse, small cleaved cell	6.9	Diffuse, poorly differentiated lymphocytic
Diffuse, mixed large and small cell	6.7	Diffuse, mixed lymphocytic and histiocytic
Diffuse, large cell	19.7	Diffuse histiocytic
HIGH GRADE		
Large cell, immunoblastic	7.9	Diffuse histiocytic
Lymphoblastic	4.2	Lymphoblastic lymphoma
Small noncleaved cell	5.0	Undifferentiated, Burkitt's and non-Burkitt's lymphoma
MISCELLANEOUS		
Composite		
Mycosis fungoides		
Histiocytic		
Unclassifiable		

Modified from Robbins SL, Cotran RS, Kumar V: *Pathologic basis of disease*, ed 3, Philadelphia, 1984, WB Saunders.
*Relative incidences are from National Cancer Institute—sponsored study of classifications of non-Hodgkin lymphomas: *Cancer* 49:2112-2135, 1982. This study reviewed 1041 patients with non-Hodgkin's lymphomas.

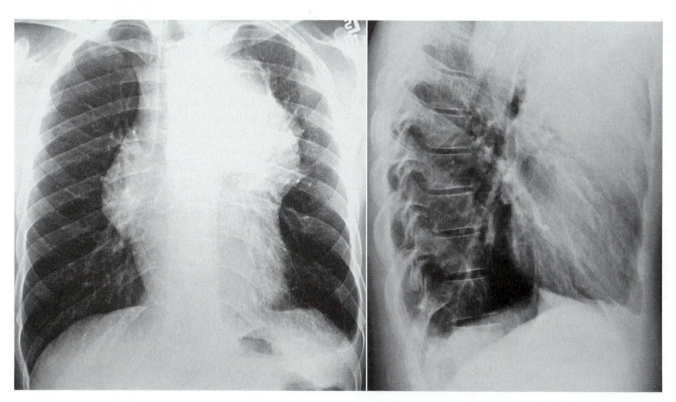

FIGURE 8-70
Anterior mediastinal node enlargement in Hodgkin's disease. Computed tomographic scan of this patient is illustrated in Figure 8-74, *A*.

INTRATHORACIC LYMPHADENOPATHY. Lymph node calcification before therapy is rare indeed, even at CT,[65,621,697] but is seen occasionally following therapy. Irregular, eggshell, and diffuse patterns of calcification may be seen.[621,698]

The appearances of intrathoracic lymphadenopathy on imaging examination are similar in Hodgkin's and non-Hodgkin's lymphoma, but the frequency and distribution of the abnormalities differ. Filly, Blank, and Castellino[181] reviewed the plain chest radiographs of patients with untreated malignant lymphomas.[181] Of the 164 patients with Hodgkin's disease, 67% had visible intrathoracic disease, and all but one of these had mediastinal or hilar adenopathy. The proportion of patients with non-Hodgkin's lymphoma showing intrathoracic abnormality on plain chest radiograph was somewhat less (43%), as was the incidence of mediastinal and hilar adenopathy (87%).

The incidence of visible mediastinal adenopathy on plain chest films in younger patients with malignant lymphomas is lower: in patients under 10 years of age, approximately 33% of those with Hodgkin's disease and only 20% to 25% of those with non-Hodgkin's lymphoma show mediastinal and hilar node enlargement.[96,235,501,479]

Any intrathoracic nodal group may be enlarged in patients with lymphoma and the possible combinations are legion, but the following generalizations regarding plain film, CT, and MRI findings may be useful[98,181,184]:

1. CT demonstrates enlarged mediastinal nodes despite normal plain chest radiographs in about 10% of those with Hodgkin's disease.[98]

2. The anterior mediastinal and paratracheal nodes are the most frequently involved groups (Figure 8-70). The tracheobronchial and subcarinal nodes are also enlarged in many cases. In most cases the lymphadenopathy is bilateral but asymmetric. Almost all patients with nodular sclerosing Hodgkin's disease have disease in the anterior mediastinum (Figure 8-70).[65] In fact, evidence of intrathoracic disease without concomitant enlargement of these nodes at CT should prompt the radiologist either to question the diagnosis of Hodgkin's disease or to raise the possibility of a second disease process.[94] Recently a form of diffuse large cell lymphoma of anterior mediastinal nodes, which tends to occur in young women and has a more favorable prognosis than the usual large cell lymphomas, has been reported.[293,568] This subtype can be difficult to distinguish from nodular sclerosing Hodgkin's disease.

3. The great majority of cases of Hodgkin's disease show enlargement of two or more nodal groups, whereas only one nodal group is involved in about half the cases of non-Hodgkin's lymphoma.

4. Hilar node enlargement is rare without accompanying mediastinal node enlargement, particularly in Hodgkin's disease.

5. The posterior mediastinum is infrequently involved. The enlarged nodes are often low in the mediastinum,

and contiguous retroperitoneal disease is likely (Figure 8-71).[235]

6. The paracardiac nodes are rarely involved but become important as sites of recurrence because they may not be included in the radiation field (Figure 8-72).[97,299] They may be visibly enlarged on plain chest radiographs, but frequently CT is needed for their demonstration (Figure 8-73).[110]

7. Compression of the pulmonary arteries,[181] superior vena cava,[568] and major bronchi[596] within the mediastinum by enlarged nodes may be seen, particularly with CT.

8. At CT scanning the enlarged nodes in any of the malignant lymphomas may be discrete or matted together, and their edges may be well defined or ill defined (Figure 8-74).[54] In general, they show only minor enhancement after intravenous administration of contrast material. Low-density areas (Figure 8-74) resulting from cystic degeneration may be seen in both Hodgkin's[274] and non-Hodgkin's lymphoma.[568] The cystic areas may per-

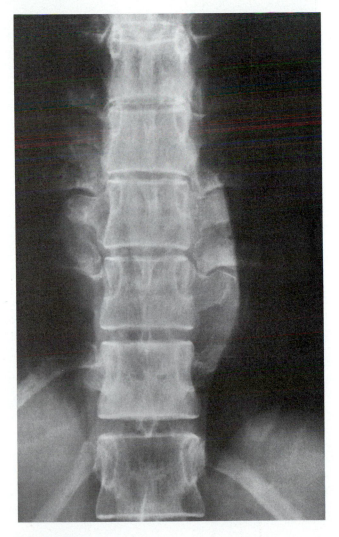

FIGURE 8-71
Posterior mediastinal nodal enlargement in Hodgkin's disease. The left paraspinal line is displaced by enlarged nodes. Note sclerosis of body of T12 resulting from lymphomatous involvement of bone.

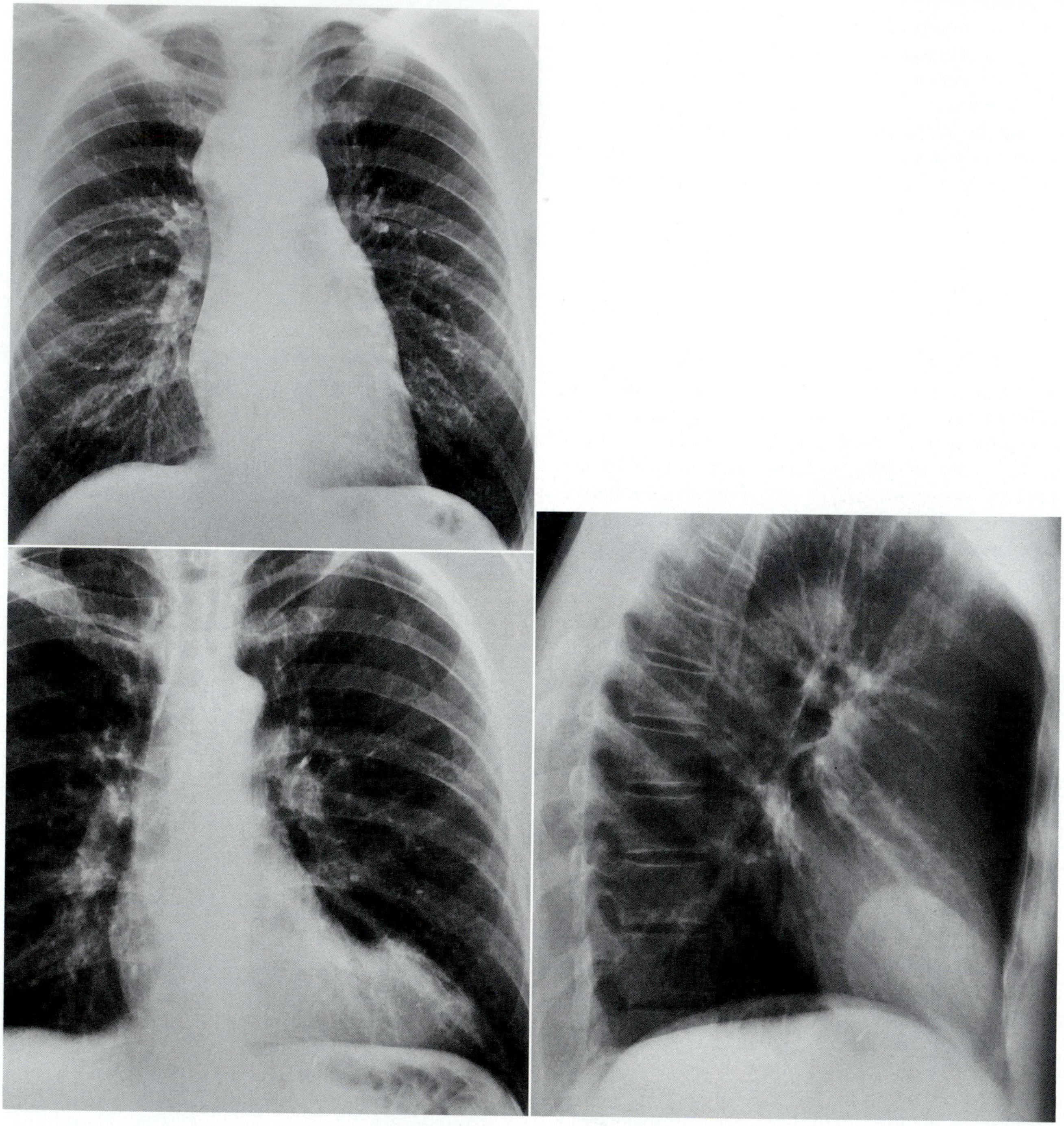

FIGURE 8-72
Pericardiac node enlargement in Hodgkin's disease. **A,** Plain film before radiation therapy. There is enlargement of paratracheal nodes bilaterally and of nodes along the left heart border. Nodes in left cardiophrenic angle are not enlarged. **B** and **C,** Four years later, at time of recurrence, posteroanterior and lateral films show massive enlargement of left cardiophrenic angle nodes but no detectable enlargement of mediastinal nodes in the original radiation field.

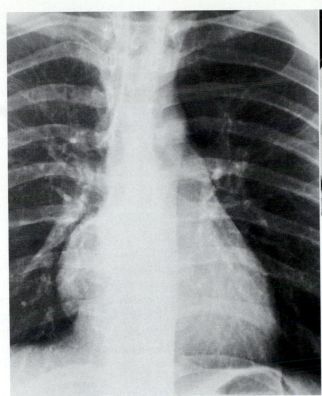

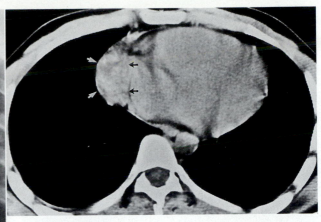

FIGURE 8-73
Paracardiac node enlargement in immunoblastic lymphoma. Distortion of right mediastinal border is difficult to distinguish from right atrial enlargement on plain film (lateral projection was unremarkable). Computed tomographic scan demonstrates enlarged lymph nodes *(arrows)* to advantage.

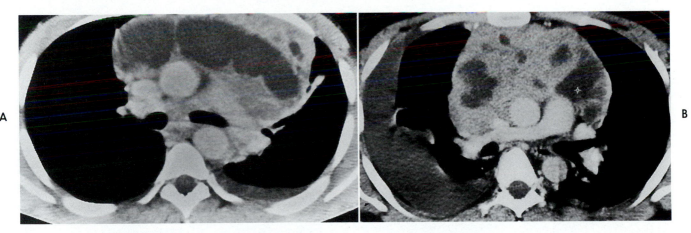

FIGURE 8-74
CT scans of enlarged lymph nodes in malignant lymphoma. **A,** Hodgkin's lymphoma. The nodes are matted together and appear as a conglomerate mass. Fluid density areas caused by necrosis are present. **B,** High-grade non-Hodgkin's lymphoma showing multiple rounded areas of low density in greatly enlarged nodes. Note large right pleural effusion.

sist following therapy, when the rest of the nodal masses shrink away.

9. MRI shows much the same anatomic features as CT, but MRI allows the demonstration of vascular and cardiac invasion or compression without the use of intravascular contrast media (Figure 8-75). The MRI signal intensity of lymphomatous masses is usually homogeneous.[476] On T1-weighted images lymphomatous tissue is slightly hyperintense compared with muscle and well below fat, whereas on T2-weighted images it is of greater signal intensity than muscle and isointense with fat. These findings appear to be independent of the grade of the tumor.[476] Negendank and co-workers[476] found that active tumor with dense fibrous tissue had unexpectedly high signal on T2-weighted images, perhaps explaining the tendency for Hodgkin's lymphoma to show higher signal on T2-weighted images than non-Hodgkin's lymphoma.

PULMONARY PARENCHYMAL INVOLVEMENT. Parenchymal involvement of the lung in malignant lymphoma at initial presentation is comparatively unusual, occurring

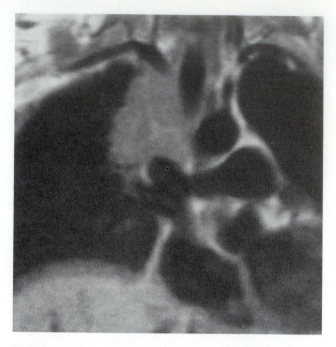

FIGURE 8-75
Hodgkin's disease (stage II) showing large lymph node masses that have compressed the right brachiocephalic vein and superior vena cava. Magnetic resonance image (T1-weighted coronal scan) shows venous compression without the need for contrast medium. (Courtesy Dr. William C. Black, Washington, D.C.)

in 10% to 15% of cases,[181] although as the disease takes hold, it becomes more common.[386] In Filly's series of plain chest radiographs in untreated cases,[181] parenchymal involvement was seen three times more frequently in Hodgkin's disease than in non-Hodgkin's lymphoma. Parenchymal involvement in Hodgkin's disease is almost invariably accompanied by visible intrathoracic adenopathy, whereas in the non-Hodgkin's lymphoma, isolated pulmonary involvement occurs with some frequency, more than 50% of the time according to Jenkins and associates.[295]

If the mediastinal and hilar nodes have been previously irradiated, recurrence confined to the lungs may be seen fairly frequently in both Hodgkin's and non-Hodgkin's lymphoma (Figures 8-76).[115]

The pulmonary opacities on plain chest radiography and CT in both Hodgkin's* and non-Hodgkin's lymphoma[28,76,181,361,593] are varied and resist easy classification. The most common pattern is one or more discrete nodules resembling primary or metastatic carcinoma, but usually rather less well defined.[76,181,361,620] Such nodules may on occasion cavitate (Figure 8-77).[181,596] Another common pattern is round or segmental, focal or patchy

---

*References 181, 183, 361, 386, 593, 596, 617, 686.

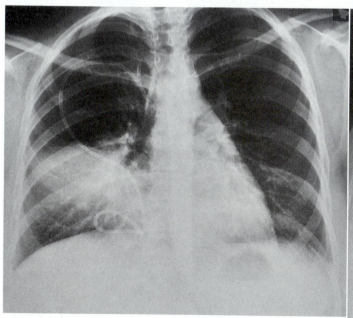
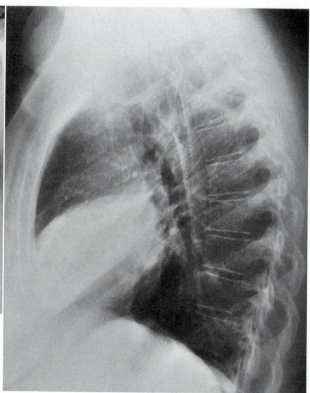

FIGURE 8-76
Hodgkin's disease of lung. The pulmonary involvement has taken the form of lobar consolidation. This young woman previously had radiation therapy to enlarged mediastinal lymph nodes. A, Posteroanterior radiograph. B, Lateral radiograph.

consolidations (Figures 8-78 and 8-79), which resemble pneumonia. Air bronchograms may be visible, particularly at CT (Figure 8-79). A pattern of peribronchial pulmonary nodules extending from the hila is sometimes seen at CT.[482] Similarly, there may be focal, streaky shadowing, which at CT can be seen to be peribronchial,[361] perhaps reflecting spread by way of the bronchopulmonary lymphatics. Widespread reticulonodular shadowing (Figure 8-80) resembling diffuse interstitial lung disease is also seen but is an uncommon pattern, particularly in Hodgkin's disease.

The pulmonary involvement is frequently perihilar or juxtamediastinal,[386] in keeping with the concept that extension into the lungs is by direct invasion from involved hilar and mediastinal nodes (Figure 8-81). However, peripheral subpleural masses or consolidations without visible connection to enlarged nodes in the mediastinum and hila (Figure 8-82) are common in both Hodgkin's disease and non-Hodgkin's lymphoma.[183,593,617] These lesions are particularly well demonstrated by CT.[361,593] Because Hodgkin's disease is believed to spread from nodal sites, it has been suggested that if the patient has Hodgkin's disease and a focal pulmonary shadow, but no evidence of hilar or mediastinal disease, the pulmonary process probably represents something other than Hodgkin's lymphoma.[65,482] A caveat here is that the patient should not previously have received radiation therapy to the hila and mediastinum.

Rapid growth of the pulmonary lesions may be seen with histiocytic lymphoma.[28,99,158] The development of large opacities or widespread disease in less than 4 weeks and even in as little as 7 days may cause great diagnostic confusion with pneumonia.

Primary (that is, isolated) pulmonary lymphoma is usually non-Hodgkin's in type. Small lymphocytic lymphoma is the most frequently encountered primary lymphoma of the lung.[315] Primary pulmonary Hodgkin's disease is rare.[701] On radiographic study[28,126,701] primary pulmonary lymphomas (Figure 8-79) usually show one or more well-defined rounded or segmental masses varying in size from small to the size of a lobe. Air bronchograms are common and are well shown by CT (Figure 8-79), on which it may be apparent that the bronchi within the lymphomatous process are stretched and narrowed,[59] similar to the appearances with bronchioloalveolar cell carcinoma. Pleural effusion is demonstrated in up to 20% of cases. A single case report of MRI in primary non-Hodgkin's lymphoma showed signal intensity similar to muscle on T1-weighted images and signal intensity higher than muscle but less than cerebrospinal fluid on T2-weighted images.[631]

In addition to lymphomatous extension from nodal disease and primary pulmonary lymphoma, non-Hodgkin's involvement of the lung can take the form of so-called mucosa-associated lymphoid tissue (MALT)[67] or the closely related bronchus-associated lymphoid tissue (BALT). In MALT and BALT, lymphomatous masses develop in multiple extranodal mucosal sites throughout the lung, giving rise to multiple pulmonary masses on imaging studies.[56]

Endobronchial disease is rare, particularly in non-Hodgkin's lymphoma,[321] but so is bronchial occlusion by neighboring lymph node enlargement. Therefore, when atelectasis is encountered, the possibility of endobronchial lymphoma should be seriously considered.

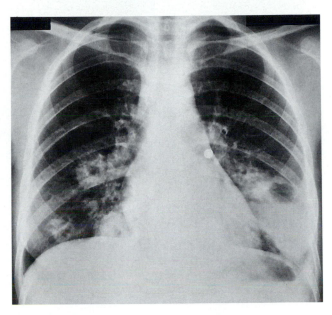

FIGURE 8-77
Hodgkin's disease showing multiple cavitating pulmonary nodules (and right paratracheal nodal enlargement).

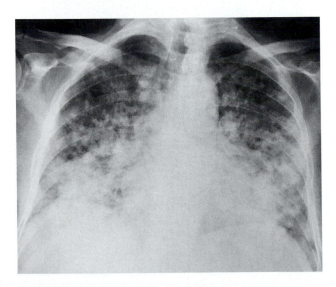

FIGURE 8-78
Histiocytic lymphoma of lung in an elderly man. The multifocal ill-defined pulmonary consolidations were originally thought to be due to pneumonia because of accompanying fever and chills, but at autopsy they were shown to be due to lymphoma.

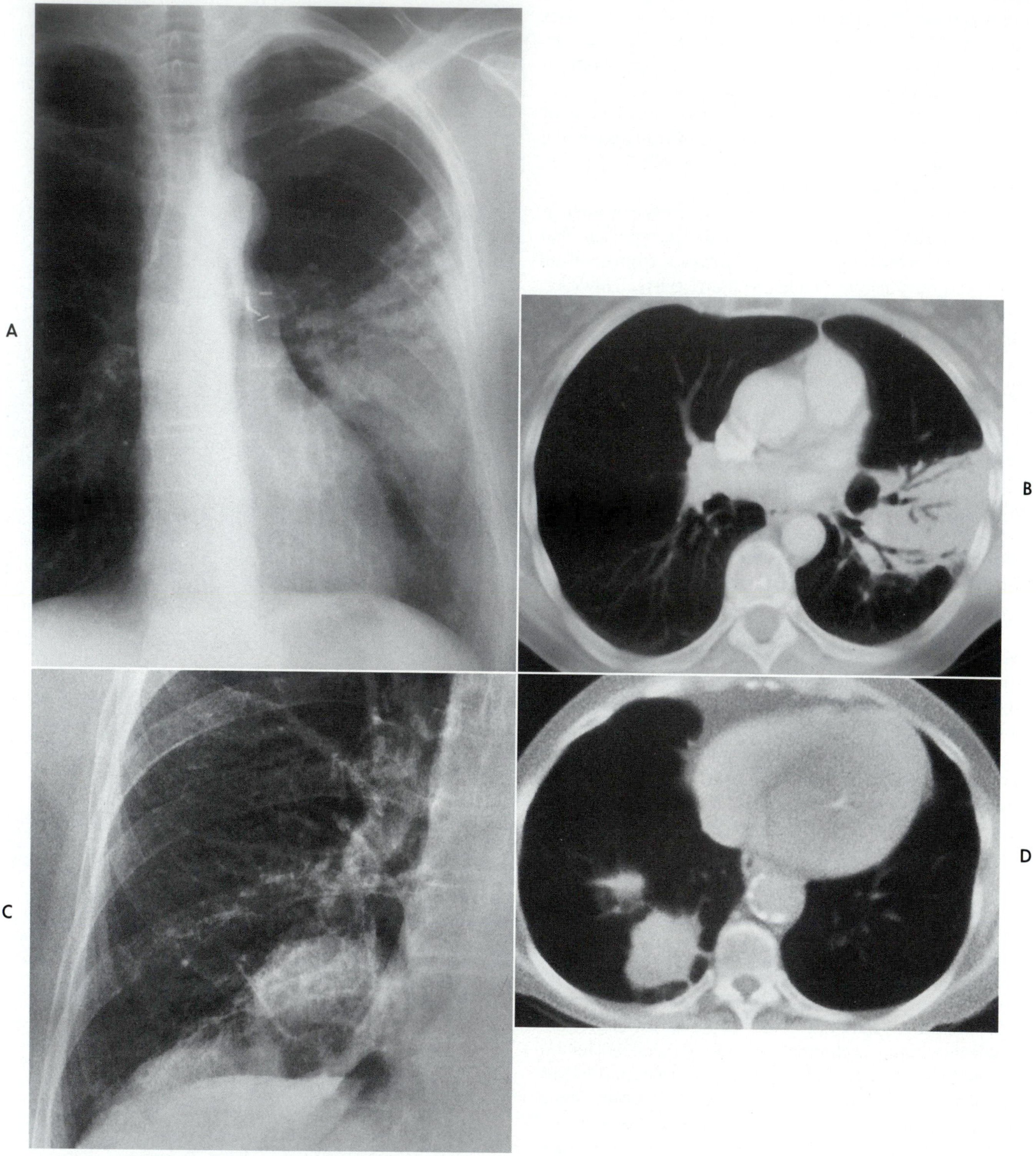

FIGURE 8-79
Primary pulmonary lymphoma taking the form of focal pulmonary consolidation. **A,** An air bronchogram can be recognized on plain film but, **B,** is much better seen on computed tomography. **C** and **D,** Large cell lymphocytic lymphoma presenting as solitary pulmonary mass.

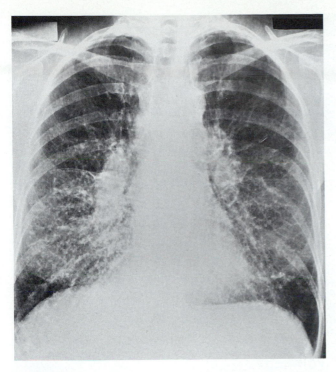

FIGURE 8-80
Histiocytic lymphoma showing widespread reticulonodular shadowing in both lungs (and enlargement of hila and right paratracheal nodes).

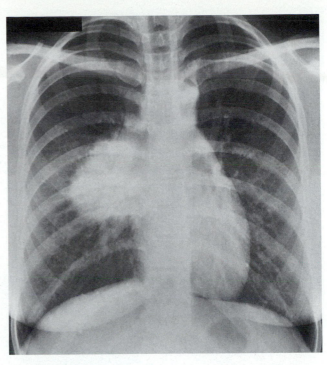

FIGURE 8-81
Pulmonary invasion in nodular sclerosing Hodgkin's disease in a 15-year-old girl.

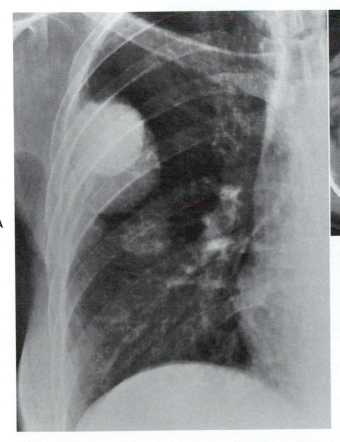

FIGURE 8-82
Subpleural lymphoma. **A**, Histiocytic lymphoma of lung showing subpleural deposits of tumor. **B**, Peripheral deposit of Hodgkin's disease *(arrow)*, which has no visible connection with mediastinal adenopathy.

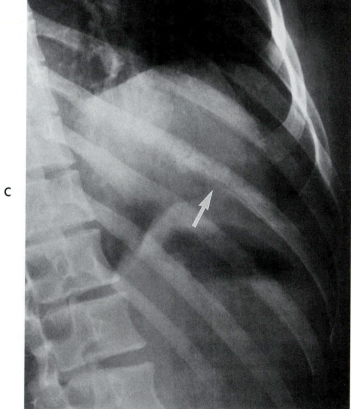

FIGURE 8-83
Solitary histiocytic lymphoma. There is a large pleural-extrapleural mass of tumor tissue. Rib view shows bone destruction and periosteal reaction of the adjacent left ninth rib *(arrow)*. **A,** Posteroanterior view. **B,** Lateral view. **C,** Oblique view of the rib.

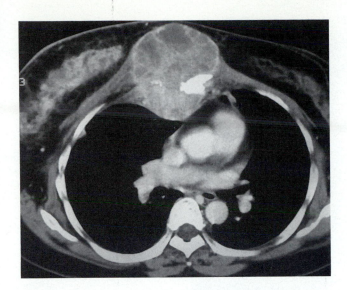

FIGURE 8-84
Massive chest wall invasion by non-Hodgkin's lymphoma.

Pleural disease

Pleural effusion is nearly always accompanied by mediastinal adenopathy visible on plain chest radiographs[181] and sometimes also by pulmonary involvement. With the more sensitive technique of CT, mediastinal adenopathy appears to be an invariable accompaniment of pleural effusion in patients with Hodgkin's disease.[98] Pleural effusions were seen in up to one fourth of patients with lymphoma on plain chest radiographs in several larger series[98,181,295,386,686] and are seen in 50% of patients with the more sensitive technique of CT.[361] Most pleural effusions are unilateral. They are usually exudates and may disappear with irradiation of the mediastinal nodes.[91,679] Such effusions are presumed to result from venous or lymphatic obstruction by enlarged mediastinal nodes rather than neoplastic involvement of the pleura[98]; pleural effusion is a frequent finding in patients with large mediastinal masses at initial presentation.[482] Chylothorax is occasionally encountered.[482] Lymphomatous pleural masses, particularly primary pleural lymphoma, are rare[160,396]; the more usual "pleural" manifestation is lymphomatous disease in the subpleural region just beneath the visceral pleura.[593]

Chest wall invasion

Chest wall invasion and rib destruction are seen on occasion, suggesting that lymphoma must either arise extrapleurally or cross the pleural cavity (Figures 8-83 and 8-84).[593] Chest wall invasion by lymphoma is well demonstrated by CT and appears to be even better shown by MRI.[48] The findings on MRI are therefore helpful when planning radiotherapy portals.[90] Chest wall tumor is more easily identified on T2-weighted than T1-weighted images but is best shown on short tau inversion recovery (STIR) sequences.[48] As with so many neoplasms that invade muscle and fat, it can be difficult to differentiate between tumor and surrounding edema, which means the true extent of tumor may be difficult to determine and the distinction between recurrence of lymphoma and postradiotherapy changes may not be possible.

Pericardial effusion

Pericardial effusions are presumptive evidence of pericardial involvement. For practical purposes pericardial effusion requires ultrasound, CT, or MRI for its recognition. In Castellino's series of 203 patients with Hodgkin's disease who had CT on initial presentation,[98] 6% had pericardial effusion, and in all these patients there was coexistent large mediastinal adenopathy extending over the cardiac margins. A nodular mass within the pericardium was seen in just one case.

Thymic lymphoma

Hodgkin's disease may rarely arise primarily in the thymus (see p. 728). Thymic enlargement, presumably representing one of the sites of neoplastic involvement, is seen on CT of 30% to 50% of patients with Hodgkin's disease.[263,685] However, since the thymus is of lymphatic origin, there is little point in determining whether an anterior mediastinal mass is of thymic or nodal origin.

Posttreatment residual masses

Successfully treated lymphomatous nodes often return to normal size and extranodal masses resolve, but bulky disease in both Hodgkin's and non-Hodgkin's lymphoma,[647] particularly nodular sclerosing or acellular forms of Hodgkin's disease, is often slow to resolve and may leave residual masses of sterilized fibrous tissue (Figure 8-85), presumably when the initial tumor mass consists chiefly of fibrous tissue.[65] The occurrence of residual mediastinal masses is considerably greater in patients with "bulky" than nonbulky disease, at least in Hodgkin's disease.[533] Determining the nature of such residual masses by imaging is difficult. CT shows soft tissue density masses, sometimes partially calcified, but cannot distinguish between tumor and fibrous tissue on density grounds alone. Gallium-67 scanning can help the observer infer residual fibrotic mass if the scan shows no uptake in a mass that previously showed substantial activity.[156,290,680] The converse conclusion, that positive uptake suggests active neoplasm, although not totally reliable (false-positive results are seen with infection and with thymic hyperplasia[156]), is generally acceptable because gallium-67 scanning is currently the best imaging test to determine active neoplasm in a residual mass.[197,423,680] At MRI, fibrotic residual mediastinal masses show low signal on T2- as well as T1-weighted images,[483] but active tumor in such masses cannot be excluded on the basis of signal intensity alone because active disease may show a similar signal pattern. Nyman and co-workers[483] have suggested that it might be possible to predict the size of the residual mass based on size of the initial mass and certain signal intensity ratios on pretreatment MRI scans, an interesting concept[670] that

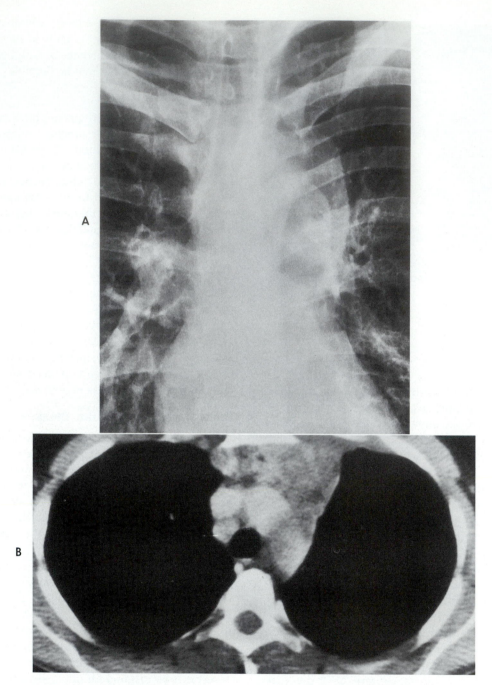

FIGURE 8-85
Residual fibrous tissue following successful radiation treatment for Hodgkin's disease. **A** and **B**, Enlarged nodes in aortopulmonary window and left paratracheal area. **C** and **D**, Residual mass of fibrous tissue in aortopulmonary window. This residual mass remained unchanged over 3 years with no further treatment.

has yet to be proved. These authors[483] found that tumors with low tumor/fat and low tumor/muscle signal intensity ratios on T2-weighted scans did not decrease in size as much as those with higher signal intensity. This finding possibly but not necessarily[670] reflects the amount of fibrous tissue in the untreated tumor.

Another posttreatment nonneoplastic radiographic abnormality that can cause confusion is cystic degeneration of the thymus.[31,322] Presumably the thymus gland undergoes cystic degeneration after radiation therapy for anterior mediastinal Hodgkin's disease. Either CT or MRI can be used to confirm the presence of cysts.

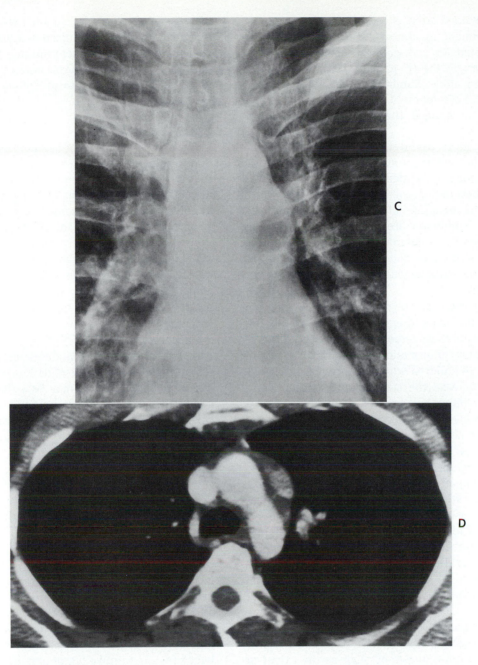

FIGURE 8-85, cont'd
For legend see opposite page.

Role of imaging in lymphoma

The plain chest radiograph can accurately demonstrate the extent of lymphomatous involvement in many patients, but chest CT is more informative.[201,319] CT shows disease not visible on plain films[566] and may show that suspected lymphomatous involvement is due to an alternative process.[275]

In general, CT scanning of the chest is more useful in the initial staging of Hodgkin's disease than it is for non-Hodgkin's lymphoma[94,556] because radiation therapy to enlarged nodes is either the only treatment for Hodgkin's lymphoma or a major component of therapy[94,437,556] and inadequate radiation therapy portals are believed to be a major cause of treatment failure. Accurate demonstration of the extent of Hodgkin's lymphoma is therefore important, whereas non-Hodgkin's lymphoma is so often disseminated at the time of initial diagnosis that demonstrating the extent of intrathoracic disease may not change management because the basic treatment for disseminated disease is chemotherapy rather than radiation therapy.

Castellino and associates[98] found that the incremental

information obtained from chest CT scans prompted a change in treatment in almost 10% of their 203 new patients with Hodgkin's disease. As expected, the impact was greatest in the 65 patients being treated with radiation therapy alone. Similarly, in the 107 new cases of Hodgkin's disease reported by Hopper and co-workers,[275] chest CT changed the stage of disease in 20 patients.

Chest CT is most useful in patients in whom the appearance of the mediastinum on plain chest radiograph is normal or equivocal. If definite lymphadenopathy is seen on plain chest radiograph but the disease is confined to the thorax, the main uses of chest CT in patients with non-Hodgkin's lymphoma are to act as a baseline to monitor treatment[95]; to demonstrate pericardial disease, which would necessitate chemotherapy; and to show paracardiac node enlargement, which would alter the radiation portals.

The role of chest CT may be rather different in children with non-Hodgkin's lymphoma. In the series by Ng and associates,[479] plain chest radiography provided the necessary management information in almost all cases; in only one of the 34 children who had chest CT did the CT scan findings increase the stage. Cohen and co-workers,[117] however, found that chest CT altered the stage in 3 of 11 children with non-Hodgkin's lymphoma.

Mediastinal sonography, using a suprasternal and parasternal approach, has been advocated as a method of following the response to treatment of lymphomatous mediastinal adenopathy.[684] Enlarged nodes become invisible in patients whose disease goes into remission. Wernecke and associates[684] claim that sonography is comparable to CT for monitoring mediastinal lymphomas and has the advantage that in some cases ultrasound can correctly predict residual disease based on the hypoechoic ultrasound texture of the affected nodes. Mediastinal sonography has not, however, become a widely used technique.[399]

So far MRI has not proved to be of greater value than CT in the routine staging of thoracic lymphoma, but it may answer highly specific questions such as the extent of pericardial, cardiac, chest wall, or spinal involvement.[48,482,636] The initial hope that MRI might be able to distinguish active or recurrent disease from posttreatment residual fibrosis based on signal characteristics has not yet been realized. It has, however, been suggested that it might be possible to predict prognostic grade in certain circumstances: Rehn and co-workers[538] found that patients with high-grade non-Hodgkin's lymphoma and a homogeneous signal pattern tended to have a better survival rate than those with an inhomogeneous pattern.

Neither radionuclide scintigraphy, with agents such as gallium-67, or PET scanning is believed to be of value for initial staging,[74,192,303,398] although ^{67}Ga has its advocates, who argue that with recent technical advances ^{67}Ga imaging is becoming sufficiently sensitive for the detection of active disease,[423] particularly when single photon emission tomography is used.[646] Gallium-67 scanning

may also be useful for predicting outcome following treatment[197,308] and, as discussed previously, can be of considerable help in determining whether or not a posttreatment residual mass contains active disease. The utility of PET scanning for predicting prognosis is under investigation.[357,487]

Mycosis fungoides

Mycosis fungoides is a T cell non-Hodgkin's lymphoma that originates in the skin and may disseminate to multiple sites, most frequently the lungs.[381,400] Such dissemination was previously thought to be a transition to another form of lymphoma, such as histiocytic lymphoma, lymphosarcoma, or Hodgkin's disease, but it is now believed that the neoplastic cells in both the cutaneous and the extracutaneous forms of the disease are distinctive to mycosis fungoides.[400] Abnormal cells known as Sézary cells are frequently found in the peripheral blood of patients with disseminated mycosis fungoides.

On chest radiographs[400,557] the lungs may show (1) one or more pulmonary nodules resembling metastases; (2) multiple areas of consolidation resembling pneumonia, a resemblance that may be striking, since in some cases the consolidations show rapid increase in size[291,557]; or (3) bilateral reticulonodular shadowing, hilar or mediastinal adenopathy, or pleural effusion.

POSTTRANSPLANT LYMPHOPROLIFERATIVE DISORDER

Posttransplant lymphoproliferative disorder (PTLD) affects approximately 2% of organ transplant recipients. The common feature of PTLD is immunosuppressive therapy, notably with cyclosporine, rather than the organ that is transplanted. It has been reported following heart, heart-lung, kidney, and liver transplantation[147] and is believed to be due to viral infection, notably by the Epstein-Barr virus.[379] The treatment is therefore antiviral therapy and, if possible, reduction in immunosuppressive therapy. Histologically the condition resembles malignant lymphoma, but unlike lymphoma it may resolve without antineoplastic treatment. The radiographic features are discussed on p. 263.

PSEUDOLYMPHOMA

Pseudolymphoma is a term coined by Saltztein[567] in 1963 to describe a localized pulmonary lesion that up until that time had been classified as a primary lymphoma, but with a better prognosis. The term denotes a tumorlike process, the precise nature of which is unknown. Pseudolymphoma shows the polyclonality of surface markers to be expected of reactive hyperplasia, whereas monoclonality is found in the neoplastic condition of small (well-differentiated) lymphocytic lymphoma.[315]

Pseudolymphoma was once considered a premalignant condition because in some cases it behaved ultimately as a malignant lymphoma.[601] It is possible, however, that the reported cases of transformation of pseudolymphoma to pulmonary lymphoma were misinterpretations, the lesions in question having been lymphoma in the first place; all the reports of malignant transformation predated or did not include immunofluorescence techniques for recognizing monoclonality or polyclonality of the lymphoid infiltration.[272] The precise relationship of pseudolymphoma and lymphoma, however, continues to be debated, and some authors still believe that pseudolymphoma is a lymphoma.[2]

The histologic appearances are inseparable from small (well-differentiated) lymphocytic lymphoma, although the cells in small lymphocytic lymphoma show a higher incidence of plasmacytoid features and a greater degree of mast cell infiltration,[315] but with modern immunofluorescence techniques it is usually possible to distinguish the two conditions. The infiltration of the lung consists mainly of mature small lymphocytes in the interstitium. This cellular infiltrate may so expand the interstitium that the adjacent alveoli are compressed, which explains the presence of air bronchograms on radiologic studies. Active germinal centers are frequently, although not invariably, present. The number of plasma cells is variable and correlates roughly with the presence and degree of the gammopathy.[333] Plasma cells may be the predominant cells, in which case confusion with solitary pulmonary plasmacytoma may arise. Some patients also have amyloid deposits.[57,622] Pseudolymphoma can also be seen in patients with dysgammaglobulinemia,[333] Sjögren's syndrome, and various collagen vascular diseases.

Holland and co-workers[272] found 54 documented cases of pseudolymphoma of the lung when reviewing the English language literature and added four cases of their own. The patients' ages ranged from 11 to 80, with a mean of 62 years. Eighty-five percent of the patients were asymptomatic; their lesions were detected incidentally on chest radiography. Those with symptoms had nonproductive cough, dyspnea, or respiratory infection.

On radiologic examination,[172,272,305] pseudolymphoma of the lung appears as solitary or multifocal, round or segmental areas of pulmonary consolidation (Figure 8-86). There is no lobar predilection, and the consolidations may be placed centrally or peripherally in the lung parenchyma. Visible air bronchograms are commonly present and may be a striking feature. A few of the lesions show cavitation, but calcification does not occur. Pseudolymphomas are rarely associated with pleural effusions despite contact with the pleura.[315]

LYMPHOCYTIC INTERSTITIAL PNEUMONITIS

Lymphocytic interstitial pneumonitis (LIP) has microscopic features similar to those of pseudolymphoma,[601] but clinically they are different.[305]

The pathogenesis of LIP is unknown. Just as with pseudolymphoma, there are doubts about whether LIP is a prelymphomatous condition or whether patients with

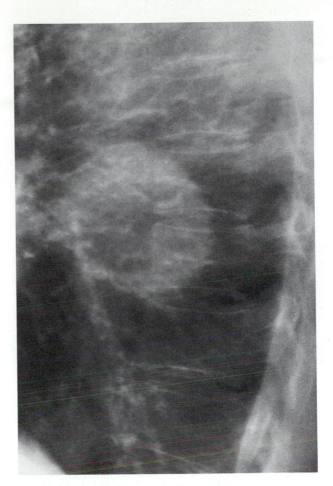

FIGURE 8-86
Pseudolymphoma. Close-up lateral view of one of three similar nodules in an asymptomatic 68-year-old man. (The lesion was behind heart in frontal view.)

LIP who develop widespread lymphoma were misclassified in the first place.[2] A variety of dysproteinemias, usually a diffuse polyclonal gammopathy but sometimes a monoclonal gammopathy or hypogammaglobulinemia, are commonly present in LIP[333,652]; dysproteinemia was found in three fourths of the Mayo Clinic series.[622] LIP may occur as an isolated entity or may be associated with AIDS, particularly in children.[124] (The association of AIDS with LIP is discussed in greater detail on p. 244.) LIP may also be associated with Sjögren's syndrome.[305,622] Other associations are much less common and include a large number of autoimmune disorders: myasthenia gravis,[448] systemic lupus erythematosus,[45] pernicious anemia,[140] autoerythrocyte sensitization syndrome,[140] chronic active hepatitis,[261] Hashimoto's thyroiditis,[305] and phenytoin therapy.[101]

On pathologic examination the lung shows diffuse interstitial thickening with occasional nodular collections of small, benign-appearing lymphocytes and plasma cells. The airways are normal, and there is no vasculitis. Interstitial fibrosis may supervene.

Patients with LIP who do not have AIDS are typically middle aged, although the range extends from childhood

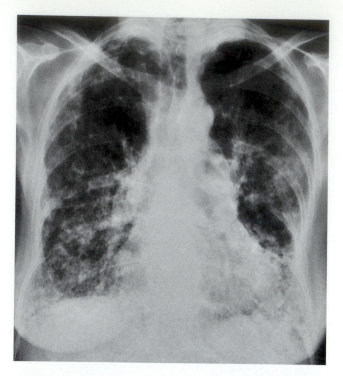

FIGURE 8-87
Lymphocytic interstitial pneumonitis showing widespread coarse reticulonodular shadowing in the lungs.

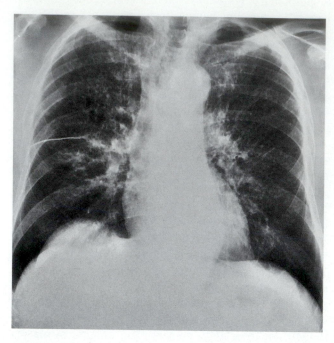

FIGURE 8-88
Waldenström's macroglobulinemia showing widespread coarse reticulonodular shadowing in the lungs.

to 77 years.[622] There is approximately a 2:1 female preponderance. The symptoms are primarily cough, chest pain, and fatigue, sometimes accompanied by low-grade fever and weight loss. The physical signs are often unimpressive and include bilateral basal crackles in the chest, occasional finger clubbing, and evidence of peripheral lymphadenopathy.[622] The onset is often insidious,[374,622] but the disease is frequently progressive and has a significant mortality.

The typical radiologic appearance of LIP* is bilateral reticulonodular opacities, the linear component of which may be quite coarse. Septal lines may also be seen (Figure 8-87). The nodular component may be fine or may show the features of acinar nodules. This latter pattern shades into multifocal, patchy consolidations that may be flame shaped and contain air bronchograms. The consolidations may be transient. Mixed alveolar and interstitial patterns are common. The shadowing, while usually maximal in the lower zone, may be more uniform in distribution or show upper zone predominance. The disease can progress into an end-stage lung with honeycomb shadowing. As with other predominantly interstitial processes, pathologic changes may be present when the chest radiograph is still normal.[242] Lymph node enlargement is not seen on plain chest radiography,[172] and if present it should suggest the development of lymphoma.[231] Pleural effusions occur in about 15% of patients.[172,374]

---

*References 172, 221, 231, 242, 258, 305, 374, 622.

WALDENSTRÖM'S MACROGLOBULINEMIA

Waldenström's macroglobulinemia is a malignant proliferation of cells with lymphoplasmacytic morphology that secrete an atypical immunoglobulin M (IgM) indistinguishable, except by immunoelectrophoresis, from the monoclonal IgM peak found in multiple myeloma. The reticuloendothelial system is diffusely infiltrated with these cells, leading to anemia, hemorrhagic phenomena, hepatosplenomegaly, and palpable lymphadenopathy. The disease therefore may clinically resemble multiple myeloma and chronic lymphocytic leukemia. Other features include osteopenia of the bones and thickening of the folds of the small bowel. The patient's symptoms commonly reflect the anemia and the high serum viscosity, which can cause headache, dizziness, drowsiness, and even coma. Bulges and constrictions of the veins of the optic fundus are a characteristic finding on physical examination.

Histologic study[690] of the lung, pleura, and intrathoracic lymph nodes shows a patchy cellular infiltrate consisting of sheets of lymphocytes and plasmacytoid forms, which may need to be differentiated from LIP. In Waldenström's macroglobulinemia the cellular infiltration of the lung is accompanied by destruction of lung architecture, whereas in LIP the lung architecture is preserved.

Lung involvement is unusual; it was seen in 4 of the 20 patients in one series.[690] When present it may be accompanied by dyspnea and cough or may be asymptomatic. The major chest radiographic finding[199,645,690] is localized or diffuse reticulonodular shadowing (Figure 8-88), which may be asymmetric; less commonly there is focal homogeneous consolidation that can be round[396] and resemble a neoplasm, even to the extent of compressing a major airway and causing atelectasis. The masslike consolidations can be single or multiple. Pleural effusion or pleural thickening is seen in about half the cases. The pleural fluid may contain the same monoclonal IgM peak found in the serum.

LYMPHOMATOID GRANULOMATOSIS

Lymphomatoid granulomatosis is a complex entity that has proved difficult to classify. It was defined by Liebow, Carrington, and Friedman[375] in 1972 as "an angiocentric, angiodestructive, lymphoreticular, proliferative and granulomatous disease involving predominantly the lungs." The infiltrate, which is intensely cellular, is composed of small lymphocytes, plasma cells, histiocytes, and atypical lymphoreticular cells.[310] Necrosis and fibrosis may be present.

In 1973 Liebow[373] grouped five entities, including lymphomatoid granulomatosis, under the heading "pulmonary angiitis and granulomatosis." These conditions* all showed necrosis of tissue accompanied by a granulomatous reaction and a vasculitis. The grouping was based on morphologic similarities, and it was thought that the five conditions might be variants of one another, although Liebow and co-workers[375] seriously considered that lymphomatoid granulomatosis might be some form of lymphoma. Subsequently lymphomatoid granulomatosis was usually considered a vasculitis with an exuberant lymphoid reaction related to, and treated similarly to, Wegener's granulomatosis. Several subsequent reviews, however, suggested that lymphomatoid granulomatosis should be regarded as pulmonary malignant lymphoma because of the similarity of the cellular elements to lymphoma, the tendency to follow lymphatic routes (a feature of lymphoma), and a high incidence of progression to true malignant lymphomas.† Vasculitis is now regarded as a feature that may be seen in lymphoma,[120] and the high rate of progression to malignant lymphoma has been repeatedly observed, occurring in up to 50% of patients.[171,221,310,375]

A large number of autoimmune or infectious diseases, as well as neoplastic diseases, are associated with lymphomatoid granulomatosis. Such associations were present in 10 of the 28 cases reported by Pisani and de Remee.[519] They suggested that lymphomatoid granulomatosis may represent a histopathologic finding that occurs transiently in several disease processes, including

lymphoma and other solid tumors. They also suggested that when true lymphoma is associated with the histopathologic findings of lymphomatoid granulomatosis, the prognosis is better than for conventional lymphoma.

Men predominate in a ratio of up to 3 to 1, and most patients are in early middle age (range 7 to 85 years).[375,466,519] Most complain of some combination of cough, often productive, fever, and dyspnea.[375,519] Massive hemoptysis from cavitating pulmonary lesions was the cause of death in three of Liebow's 40 patients.[375] Cutaneous involvement occurs in nearly half of the subjects.[519] The central nervous system is involved at least 20% of the time, and peripheral neuritis occurs with almost equal frequency.[375] The kidneys show focal nodular collections of lymphomatoid granulomatosis at autopsy, not the generalized glomerulonephritis seen with Wegener's granulomatosis; thus renal failure is not a feature of the disease. This latter feature, together with the rarity of upper airway involvement and the common presence of skin and nervous system lesions, helps to distinguish lymphomatoid granulomatosis from Wegener's granulomatosis. Surprisingly, the disease usually spares lymph nodes, spleen, and bone marrow.

On plain film and CT* the most frequent appearance, occurring in up to 80% of patients, is multiple pulmonary nodules, which are usually bilateral but may be unilateral; occasionally only a solitary pulmonary mass is seen (Figure 8-89). The nodules, which closely resemble metastases, are usually round and have ill-defined margins, although a small proportion have a well-defined edge. They may be very large; nodules up to 10 cm in diameter have been reported. Multiple, ill-defined areas of consolidation resembling pneumonia are a less common radiographic manifestation. Coalescence of the nodules or consolidations is a feature that may help in the radiographic differential diagnosis from pulmonary metastases. The lesions show a predisposition for the middle and lower lung zones, with a tendency to spare the apices. At least some of the nodules seen on plain chest radiograph are infarcts related to the angiodestructive nature of the disease.[142,289] Dee, Arora, and Innes[142] showed on histologic examination in three cases that the bulk of the lesion was an infarct, with the cellular infiltrate of lymphomatoid granulomatosis confined to the periphery and contributing little to the radiographic shadow. Cavitation was seen in approximately 10% of patients in one review of the literature,[266] but in individual series the rate of cavitation is as high as 25%.[375,678] The cavities are usually thick walled, but a thin walled cystlike cavity has been reported.[678] Cavitation appears to be associated with a poor prognosis.[375] Air bronchograms are seen in some cases (Figure 8-89), the highest reported incidence of air bronchograms being 40%.[375] Widely distributed reticulonodular shadowing has been reported

---

*The five conditions were classic Wegener's granulomatosis, limited angiitis and granulomatosis of the Wegener type, lymphomatoid granulomatosis, necrotizing "sarcoid" angiitis and granulomatosis, and bronchocentric granulomatosis.

†References 43, 112, 121, 221, 315, 333, 466.

*References 142, 155, 221, 266, 375, 519, 527, 660.

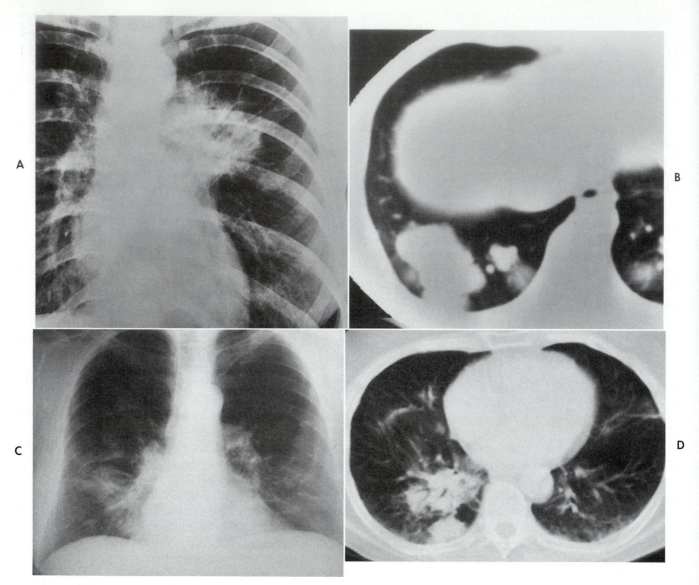

FIGURE 8-89
Various appearances of lymphomatoid granulomatosis. **A,** Large irregular, lobular mass adjacent to left hilum. **B,** Multiple lobular pulmonary masses resembling metastases on computed tomographic (CT) scanning. **C,** Multiple, ill-defined pulmonary shadows that, **D,** on CT scanning are seen to be masses with very irregular edges and air bronchograms.

in a few cases.[142,678] When examined at biopsy these lesions proved to result from cellular infiltration without infarction.[142]

The single case report of MRI of lymphomatoid granulomatosis of the lung revealed no features that permit distinction from lymphoma.[432]

Visible hilar and mediastinal adenopathy is unusual. Pleural effusion does not appear to be a major feature of the disease, although small pleural effusions are seen on plain chest radiograph in up to one third of patients. The plain chest radiograph may be normal in patients with lymphomatoid granulomatosis of the sinuses or skin.

LEUKEMIA

Several abnormalities may be seen at chest imaging in leukemic patients. These can be divided into three categories:

1. Leukemic infiltration of the lungs or pleura (Figure 8-90), defined as extravascular leukemic cells in portions of the lung parenchyma not involved by infection, infarction, or hemorrhage. Leukostasis is a separate category that may or may not be accompanied by leukemic infiltration of the lung parenchyma.

2. Intrathoracic lymph node enlargement caused by leukemia.

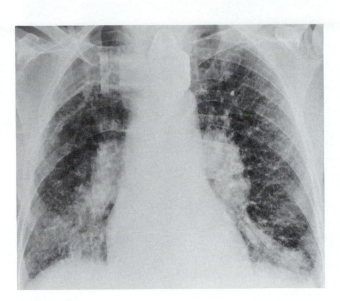

FIGURE 8-90
Leukemic infiltrates in the lungs. Note also the bilateral hilar adenopathy caused by leukemic involvement of lymph nodes.

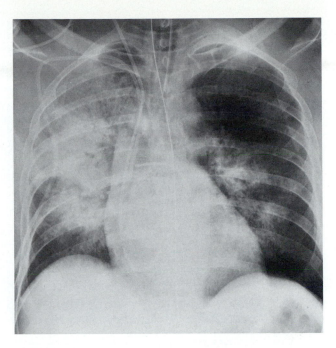

FIGURE 8-91
Acute pulmonary hemorrhage in a 39-year-old man with acute myeloid leukemia. The bilateral airspace shadowing is due to intrapulmonary bleeding.

3. Nonneoplastic complications of leukemia or its treatment, notably pulmonary infection, pulmonary hemorrhage (Figure 8-91), pulmonary edema, and drug reactions. The differential diagnosis of nonneoplastic pulmonary shadowing in leukemic patients is discussed on p. 255.

The incidence of leukemic infiltration of the lungs, mediastinal lymph nodes, and pleura varies with the course of the disease. Clearly the highest incidence is shown in autopsy series. Several large series of autopsies in patients who died of leukemia have been published.[326,393,555] In most, regardless of whether the patients were reviewed during or before the chemotherapeutic era, the incidence of leukemic infiltration of the lungs on microscopic examination was high (31% to 64%), but only rarely was this infiltration visible on plain chest radiography. In one typical series[393] 41% of the patients showed leukemic infiltrates of the lung on histologic study (ranging from 67% of patients with chronic lymphatic leukemia to 35% of patients with acute myeloid leukemia), but the leukemic infiltration was almost never visible radiologically. Ninety per cent of the patients in the study had pulmonary shadows on the chest radiographs immediately before death. In all except two the shadowing was the result of a complication of the disease, not the leukemic infiltration per se. Focal masses or consolidations are rare but are reported,[331,393] and in one case multifocal consolidation caused by leukemic infiltration showed an

air crescent sign,[582] a feature previously reported only in cases complicated by infection. Radiographically visible leukemic infiltrates are virtually confined to patients with high peripheral blast counts.[331]

In summary, provided patients with leukostasis are considered separately, leukemic infiltration of the lungs, although common pathologically, does not appear to be a cause of pulmonary symptoms and is rarely a cause of significant pulmonary opacities on chest radiographs. Indeed, the chest film frequently appears normal. When respiratory impairment is present, the leukemic infiltrates are accompanied by pulmonary infection, edema, or hemorrhage, and these are the likely cause of the patient's symptoms.[555]

Pulmonary CT, particularly HRCT, shows details of pulmonary parenchymal pathologic conditions to advantage. However, even with HRCT it is difficult to diagnose the nature of abnormal pulmonary densities in leukemic patients. In a carefully conducted correlation of HRCT and pathologic findings in postmortem lungs, Lee and associates[354] showed that the prediction of the pathologic findings from the HRCT images alone was only moderately good. Pneumonia and hemorrhage could not be distinguished from each other, and the prediction of leukemic involvement was poor. However, when diffuse shadowing was present, regardless of whether it was designated "alveolar" or "interstitial" by the radiologist, the shadowing was highly likely to represent pneumonia or hemorrhage. Focal shadows may represent a variety of

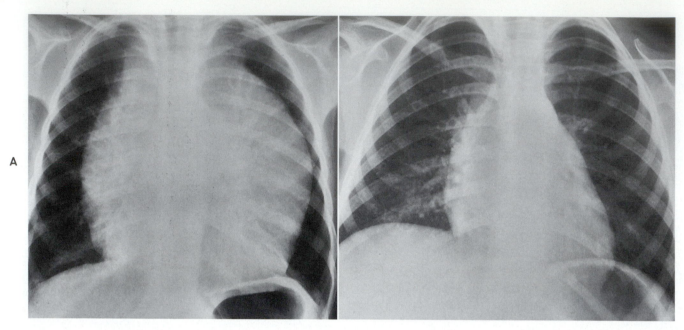

FIGURE 8-92
T cell leukemia-lymphoma in a 4-year-old girl. **A,** Massive mediastinal adenopathy. **B,** Following very
rapid response to chemotherapy. Films were taken 9 days apart.

pathologic conditions, including infarction, neoplasm, hemorrhage, and granulomatous infection.

Radiographically visible hilar and mediastinal lymph node enlargement is seen in up to 17% of adult patients at autopsy.[326,393] The distribution of nodal enlargement closely resembles that of the lymphomas. The incidence of leukemic infiltration of the nodes on pathologic examination is very high, 50% in the large series of Klatte and co-workers[326]; however, most involved nodes show little or no enlargement. T cell leukemias may show massive mediastinal adenopathy that responds rapidly to chemotherapy or radiation treatment. Huge mediastinal masses of T cell leukemia may disappear within a few days with appropriate treatment (Figure 8-92).

Pleural effusion is common in leukemia. Subpleural deposits of leukemic cells are often found at autopsy, but pulmonary infection, infarction, hemorrhage, and edema so frequently coexist with these leukemic deposits that the cause of the effusion cannot be stated with any confidence.

Pleural thickening caused by a mass of leukemic cells in patients with myeloid leukemia, so-called granulocytic sarcoma[477] or chloroma formation (because of its green appearance), may be encountered on rare occasion.[353,594] In one reported case with combined pleural and pulmonary granulocytic sarcoma, the bone marrow was normal.[267]

Leukostasis

Leukostasis is a condition seen in patients with acute myeloid leukemia who have very high white blood cell

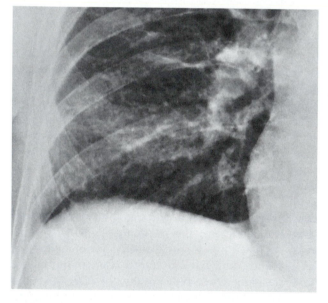

FIGURE 8-93
Leukostasis in a 43-year-old man in blast crisis, showing hazy opacity in lungs resembling pulmonary edema. The shadows cleared with leukophoresis therapy.

counts, on the order of 100,000 to 300,000 cells/mm³, together with accumulations of leukemic cells in small blood vessels, especially of the lungs, heart, brain, and testes. Central nervous system symptoms are frequent, and the patients may be dyspneic because of obliteration of small pulmonary blood vessels by the leukemic cells.[654] The chest radiograph may be normal or may show airspace shadowing (Figure 8-93). In a report on the radiographic findings in 10 patients who died with leukostasis, four had a normal-appearing chest film, four showed wide airspace disease attributed to superimposed pulmonary edema, and one showed a small area of pulmonary consolidation.[650] The radiographic shadowing in leukostasis appears to be due to pulmonary edema rather than directly to the accumulation of leukemic cells in the lungs.[467,650,654]

MESOTHELIOMA
Localized fibrous tumor of the pleura

This tumor has been given a variety of names, including pleural fibroma, fibrous mesothelioma, localized pleural mesothelioma, and benign mesothelioma. Benign mesothelioma appears to be a particularly inappropriate term, since the tumors are not mesotheliomas nor do they all behave in a benign fashion. It is probably best to regard them as a spectrum from benign to malignant.[164,564] The current term, localized fibrous tumor of the pleura, has been recommended because the lesion is thought to arise from mesenchymal cells rather than from epithelial cells.[164]

Most patients are between 45 and 65 years (range 5 to 87 years), with no significant sex difference.[71,163,164] Unlike diffuse mesothelioma the localized tumor is not asbestos related.[71] On histologic study the lesion consists of spindle-shaped cells separated by collagen.[163] It exists in benign and malignant forms; 14% to 30% are malignant.[164,564] Some workers consider that the distinction between benign and malignant forms can be made on histologic grounds,[488] but others think this distinction is not possible and consider that pedunculation is the best evidence of benignity.[71]

On macroscopic examination the tumor is seen as a mass in contact with the pleura, but a small number appear to be totally encased within lung.[488] Up to three fourths arise from visceral pleura, and the remainder from parietal pleura.[71,164] An origin from within a fissure is fairly common.[283,602] Pedunculation is present in about 50%[51]; the stalk can be up to 9 cm long.[238]

In about half the patients with localized fibrous tumors of the pleura the tumor is asymptomatic and detected incidentally at chest radiography.[71] The benign tumors behave in an indolent fashion, and some have been known to be present for 20 years before removal.[571] The most common symptoms are cough, chest pain, and dyspnea. Although hypertrophic osteoarthropathy was common in earlier series, its prevalence in series reported since 1972 has been much lower, 4% to 12%[71,164]; it appears to be more common with tumors over 7 cm in diameter. Other reported symptoms include chills and fever, weight loss, debility, and a sensation of something rolling around in the chest.[601] Symptomatic hypoglycemia is seen in up to 6% of patients.[71,164]

On plain chest radiography the usual finding is a slow-growing, rounded or oval, often lobulated, homoge-

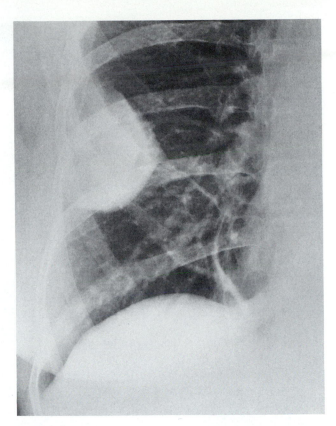

FIGURE 8-94
Localized fibrous tumor of pleura in a 61-year-old woman. At surgery this lesion was found to lie in the major fissure and was benign.

neous mass in contact with a pleural surface.[163,164,257] The lesions vary in diameter from less than 1 cm to 30 cm but are usually large, 7 cm or more when initially seen (Figures 8-94 and 8-95). They are slightly more common in the lower half of the chest.[163] When the lesions are very large, their origin from the pleura may not be obvious.[163] The wall usually shows an obtuse angle at the margin, a finding that was present in 94% of 17 cases in one series.[283] Lesions with acute angles are, however, reported.[141,163] Those tumors on pedicles may change in shape and position on images taken on different occasions and in different postures.* (Similar changes in shape, particularly with different phases of respiration, may also be seen with chest wall lipomas.[229]) If the lesion is not pedunculated, inspiration-expiration imaging may show whether the mass is in the lung or is attached to the chest wall.[163] The malignant forms may spread into soft tissue and destroy bone.[488]

On CT the lesions are usually well marginated, based on a pleural surface (Figures 8-95 and 8-96), with some 75% showing acute angles at the margins. In other words, they grow outward from a relatively narrow base or pedicle and a stalk may be visible at CT.[600] The smaller lesions show uniform soft tissue density, whereas a

---

*References 51, 163, 249, 364, 600, 683.

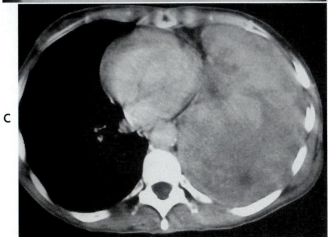

FIGURE 8-95
A and B, Huge localized fibrous tumor of pleura in an elderly woman. Despite the size of the tumor, the patient had no chest symptoms. It was histologically benign. C, Computed tomographic scan in a similar case.

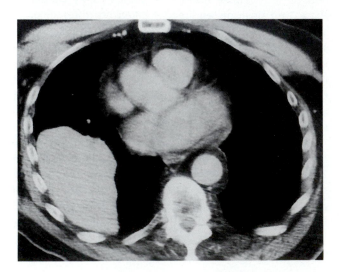

FIGURE 8-96
Computed tomographic scan of a localized benign fibrous tumor of the pleura. Note well-defined lobular mass of homogeneous soft tissue density based on pleura. (Courtesy Dr. Pablo Ros, Gainesville, Fla.)

substantial proportion of the larger lesions show low attenuation centrally owing to necrosis.[352] The soft tissue elements enhance to a much greater degree than muscle following intravenous contrast enhancement[141,352,433]; inhomogeneous contrast enhancement was a frequent feature in one small series of malignant localized fibrous tumors of the pleura.[564] Calcification is uncommon but is recorded in the benign lesions[163,352,433,516]; it appears to be more common in the localized malignant lesions.[564] Pleural effusions are occasionally present[141,163,238] and are sometimes large enough to obscure the underlying mass.[55,164,488]

Only a few reports of MRI in localized benign fibrous tumor of the pleura have been published to date.[209,351] The signal intensity on T1-weighted images is comparable to muscle. On T2-weighted images the signal intensity may be the same as or higher than muscle. The tumors enhance following intravenous administration of gadolinium.

Diffuse malignant mesothelioma

Diffuse (malignant) mesothelioma is a rare tumor. However, the incidence, approximately one to two cases per million population per year,[69,418] is expected to rise because of the increasing exposure of the population to asbestos. The etiologic role of asbestos was first suggested by Wagner, Sleggs, and Marhand[661] in a group of 33 patients with malignant mesothelioma, 32 of whom had been exposed to asbestos. Some patients were asbestos miners, but most just lived and worked in the mining community without entering the mines themselves. Asbestos exposure is now documented in about half of all patients,[14,313] but the incidence ranges in various series from under 25%[69,485] to almost 90%.[15] The contribution of asbestos in the usual urban environment is unknown. Of the various forms of asbestos, crocidolite appears to be the most carcinogenic form, followed by chrysolite and then by amosite. Because chrysolite is the most widely used form of asbestos, it is believed to account for most of the cases of diffuse mesothelioma.[270,355] Anthophyllite does not appear to induce mesothelioma.[270] The interval between first exposure to asbestos and diagnosis of the tumor is on the order of 20 to 40 years.[4] Inhalation of other substances, such as nonoccupational exposure to erionite, has been etiologically implicated,[169] and the possibility of an association with AIDS has been questioned.[41] Prior thoracic irradiation has occasionally been noted[13,69,313] and is thought to play an etiologic role.

On pathologic examination, diffuse malignant mesothelioma appears as plaques and nodules on the visceral or parietal pleura that eventually form a lobular sheet of tumor up to several centimeters thick encasing the lungs, extending through the pleural cavity, and growing into the interlobar fissures. Invasion into the adjacent chest wall, diaphragm, and mediastinal structures usually occurs relatively late[376] but may be seen early.[15] Lymphatic and hematogenous metastases are

usually late manifestations that, although present in 50% of patients at autopsy, are generally clinically silent.[14] On histologic study, malignant mesotheliomas are divided into epithelial, mesenchymal (fibrous or sarcomatous), or mixed tumors; their relative prevalence varies considerably from series to series and also varies according to the diligence with which the entire tumor is examined for mixed cell types. In Legha and Muggia's compilation of 382 cases from the literature,[355] 54% were epithelial, 21% were fibrosarcomatous, and 25% were mixed, and the proportions were very similar in the Mayo Clinic series.[1] The epithelial type consists of cuboidal cells in various arrangements, whereas the mesenchymal type shows sheets of parallel spindle-shaped cells similar to many soft tissue sarcomas. The epithelial type can be difficult to differentiate from bronchial adenocarcinoma involving the pleura. Because bronchial carcinoma also shows a higher than expected incidence in patients exposed to asbestos, these tumors can be easily confused. The complex subject of the histologic differential diagnosis of malignant mesothelioma has been reviewed by Antman and Corson.[15] Immunohistochemical techniques are often needed to distinguish between malignant mesothelioma and bronchial adenocarcinoma.[494]

The pleural fluid associated with malignant mesothelioma is an exudate that is serosanguineous in half the cases.[58] With large tumors the glucose and pH levels are low. On cytologic examination the fluid may contain malignant mesothelial cells together with varying numbers of lymphocytes and polymorphonuclear leukocytes,[355] but the cytologic distinction between benign and malignant mesothelial cells is difficult[1] and biopsy of the pleura is usually needed to establish the diagnosis.

The peak age at presentation is between 40 and 70 years, and the male-to-female ratio is 2 to 4:1.[1,69,355,418] The usual symptoms are chest pain, shortness of breath, and cough, followed by dyspnea and weight loss.[1,15,69,355] There may be intermittent low-grade fever. Clubbing of the fingers and hypertrophic pulmonary osteoarthropathy are seen but are much less common than with localized fibrous tumors of the pleura.[14]

The imaging features of diffuse malignant mesothelioma* are essentially similar on plain chest radiographs, CT, and MRI (Figures 8-97 to 8-101), but CT and MRI show the extent of the tumor with greater accuracy than plain radiography and show the accompanying pleural fluid with greater sensitivity.[347] However, because the tumor is usually so extensive at initial presentation, CT and MRI provide little advantage over conventional radiology in the initial staging of most patients.[347,560] CT and presumably MRI are useful for detecting recurrent disease following surgical treatment.[560]

The imaging findings typically consist of extensive nodular thickening of the pleura, which may conglomerate to form a circumferential lobular sheet of soft tissue

---

*References 1, 230, 260, 313, 347, 358, 365, 382, 446, 504, 677.

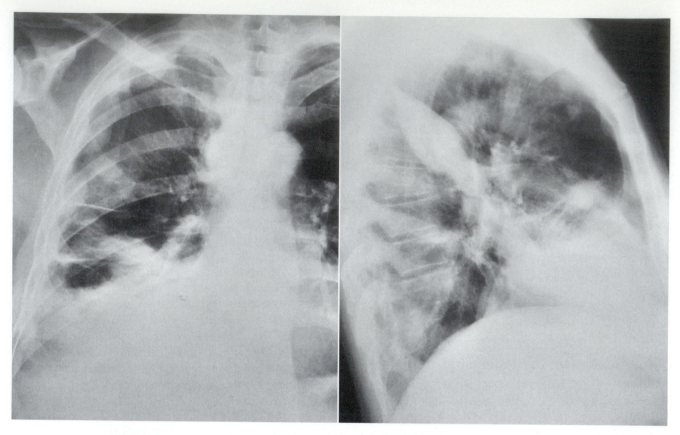

FIGURE 8-97
Malignant mesothelioma of pleura, showing lobular pleural masses. Note lobular thickening of major fissures.

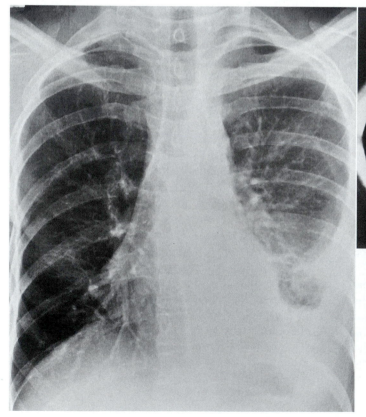

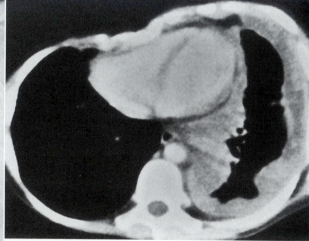

FIGURE 8-98
Malignant mesothelioma of pleura. There is lobular pleural thickening encasing the left lung and thickening of the major fissure. Patient, a 28-year-old woman, had received radiation therapy to the opposite thorax for Wilms' tumor in childhood — hence the contracted right thorax. The etiologic role of radiation therapy in this case is conjectural. A, Posteroanterior radiograph. B, Computed tomographic scan.

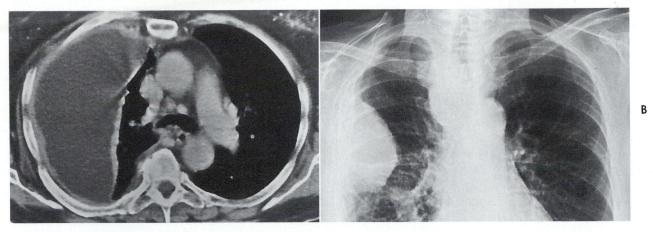

FIGURE 8-99
A, Computed tomographic appearance of malignant mesothelioma. In this 72-year-old woman there is a relatively thin rind of nodular pleural thickening and a large loculus of pleural fluid. B, Plain film of same patient for comparison.

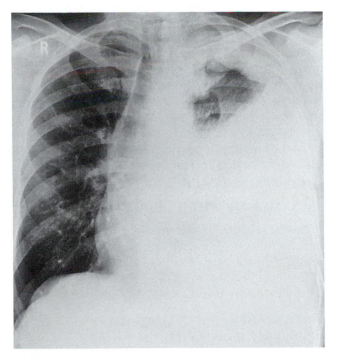

FIGURE 8-100
Malignant mesothelioma showing a very large pleural effusion that partially hides lobular neoplastic thickening of pleura.

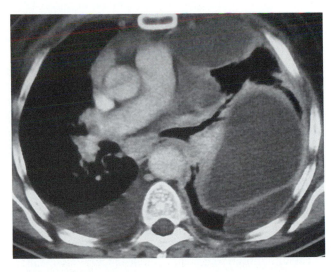

FIGURE 8-101
Malignant mesothelioma causing widespread, uniform, mild thickening of pleura and multiple fluid loculations. Note resemblance to empyema.

density encasing the lung. The tumor often runs into the fissures, accompanied by varying amounts of pleural fluid, and the adjacent lung may show evidence of invasion. The nodularity of the pleural thickening is an important diagnostic feature (Figure 8-97). The distribution of the pleural thickening may be helpful in the differential diagnosis from empyema: mediastinal pleural involvement and particularly circumferential pleural thickening are highly suggestive of malignant mesothelioma (or metastatic carcinoma).[358] Sometimes the accompanying pleural effusion is very large (Figure 8-100) and obscures the pleural masses on plain chest radiography. In such cases the chest radiographic appearances may be indistinguishable from other causes of pleural effusion. One point of distinction from other pleural effusions is that the neoplastic encasement of the lung may fix the position of the mediastinum, so that shift away from the side of the effusion is not seen as often in patients with malignant mesothelioma as it is with nonmalignant causes of large pleural effusion.[283] Indeed, the pleural shadowing is sometimes associated with ipsilateral volume loss and a fixed mediastinum,[532] and the hemithorax may even be contracted owing to encasement of the lung by the pleural tumor.[313] The tumor nodules may become evident only on plain chest radiographs if air enters the pleural space following thoracentesis. At CT scanning the soft tissue density of the tumor tissue can be readily distinguished from the adjacent pleural effusion, but the nodules may on occasion be so tiny that they are unrecognizable and the only CT feature is therefore a pleural effusion. Calcification of the tumor is extremely rare, although reported.[313,480]

Chest wall invasion, bone destruction, direct extension to the pericardium and other mediastinal structures, involvement of mediastinal lymph nodes, and invasion through the diaphragm into the upper abdomen are all best seen on CT or MRI.* They are seen in approximately 11% to 18% of patients at initial presentation, increasing to 30% or more during the course of the disease. Extension to the contralateral thoracic cavity may be seen.[230,313,365]

Asbestos-related pleural plaques may be seen in either pleural cavity, and calcified plaques may be engulfed by the tumor.[365]

The differential diagnosis includes pleural involvement by other malignant tumors, notably bronchial adenocarcinoma, breast carcinoma, malignant thymoma, and subpleural lymphoma, as well as benign conditions such as asbestos-related benign pleural effusion, tuberculous pleural thickening, empyema (Figure 8-101), and asbestos-related pleural plaques together with round atelectasis. Unless there are other features to indicate the primary tumor, the distinction between adenocarcinoma of the lung and malignant mesothelioma cannot be made

radiographically from the appearance of the pleural involvement alone, which is hardly surprising in view of the difficulty that pathologists experience when trying to distinguish between these two tumors. Although pleural involvement by breast carcinoma can also appear identical, there is usually no diagnostic difficulty because the primary tumor will have been diagnosed previously or be clinically obvious. Pleural deposits of lymphoma and thymoma usually appear as more discrete localized masses than malignant mesothelioma, and the primary thymoma or other foci of lymphoma are visible or have previously been documented. The distinction from benign pleural thickening caused by conditions such as previous tuberculosis or old hemothorax is usually made readily by noting the smoothness of the pleural shadowing in these disorders.[1] A helpful feature in distinguishing benign pleural thickening from malignant mesothelioma is that circumferential pleural thickening, that is, thickening extending over the mediastinal surfaces, is a not infrequent feature in malignant mesothelioma but is rare in benign pleural disease.[358]

The differentiation of early malignant pleural mesothelioma from noncalcified or partially calcified asbestos-related plaques can be difficult. Rabinowitz and associates[532] found that some pleural plaques associated with advanced asbestosis were large and irregular and resembled mesothelioma. They cautioned that determining the growth of the pleural plaques may be of little value, since benign plaques may enlarge on serial examinations.

LIPOMA OF THE PLEURA

Pleural and extrapleural lipomas are fairly unusual tumors. The benign lipoma is totally asymptomatic, although if it protrudes through the rib interspaces, it may produce a focal swelling and be palpable. On plain chest radiography lipomas are seen as well-marginated, oval or lens-shaped soft tissue masses based on the pleura. On CT[618] the uniform fat density, containing no more than a few linear strands of soft tissue density, makes the diagnosis straightforward.

SARCOMA OF THE PLEURA

The most common sarcomas of the pleura are metastatic. Primary pleural liposarcoma[460] and osteosarcoma[584,609] are rare tumors. The fat density within liposarcoma and the extensive calcification in osteosarcoma on CT have considerable diagnostic value.

METASTASES
Pulmonary metastases

The incidence of pulmonary metastases varies with the primary tumor and the stage of the disease. In autopsy series the most common sources of metastases to the lungs include tumors of the breast, colon, kidney, uterus, prostate, head, and neck.[125] Tumors such as choriocarcinoma, osteosarcoma, Ewing's sarcoma, testicular tumors,

---

*References 69, 230, 313, 347, 365, 382, 446, 504.

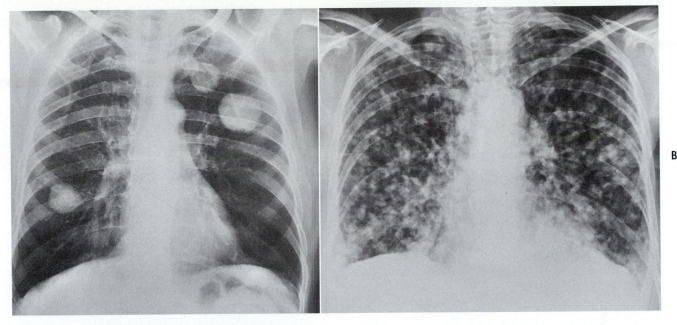

A   **B**

FIGURE 8-102
Typical hematogenous metastases. A, In a patient with colon carcinoma. B, In a patient with rhabdomyosarcoma of anterior abdominal wall.

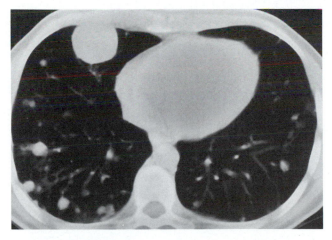

FIGURE 8-103
Computed tomographic scan showing peripheral distribution of hematogenous metastases, in this case from a germ cell tumor of testis.

melanoma, and thyroid carcinoma have a high incidence of pulmonary metastases, but because they are not as prevalent in the population, lung deposits from these tumors are encountered less frequently.[125]

The hallmark of blood-borne metastases to the lungs on imaging studies is one or more discrete pulmonary nodules, maximal in the outer portions of the lungs (Figures 8-102 and 8-103).[128,135,540] They vary in size from microscopic to many centimeters in diameter, are usually multiple, and have well- or moderately well-

defined outlines. On occasion, particularly when caused by metastatic adenocarcinoma or if the metastases have bled into the surrounding lung,[44,271] they show irregular or ill-defined edges (Figure 8-104).

Irregular, sometimes frankly nodular, thickening of the interstitial pulmonary septa is a frequent finding on specimen HRCT.[541] This finding, labeled the beaded septum sign, is regarded as highly specific for metastatic carcinoma. It corresponds to neoplastic invasion of the interlobular septa, their capillaries, and lymphatic vessels and when widespread would be called lymphangitis carcinoma.

CT makes it is possible to show pulmonary vessels leading directly to individual metastases.[444] The frequency of the sign is uncertain. It was observed in 30% to 75% of metastases in one series, depending on whether the lesion was in the upper, middle, or lower zone.[444] In a CT-pathologic correlation, however, it was found in less than 20%.[463] This variation is probably related to CT section thickness; thinner sections more accurately correlate with the macroscopic pathologic findings. The specificity of the finding is uncertain.

Cavitation is seen from time to time. It occurred in some 4% to 6% of Dodd and Boyle's large series,[146] with squamous cell carcinoma showing cavitation twice as often as adenocarcinoma, although other, similar-sized series have shown a more even distribution between the two cell types (Figure 8-105).[104] The most common sites of origin of cavitary neoplasms appear to be the uterine cervix, colon, and head and neck.[104,146] The presence of

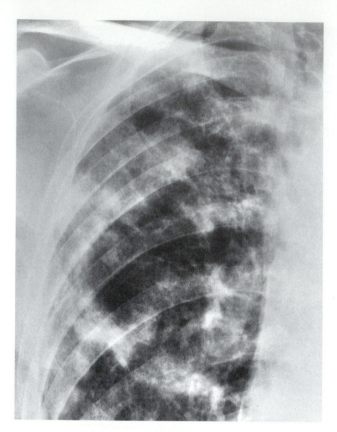

FIGURE 8-104
Metastases from adenocarcinoma of colon showing irregular outline of pulmonary nodules.

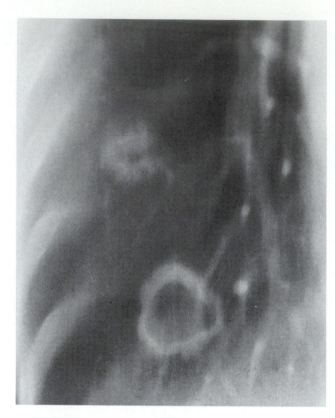

FIGURE 8-105
Cavitating metastatic carcinoma from squamous cell carcinoma of tonsil.

cavitation is unrelated to the size of the metastasis,[104,146] making it unlikely that cavitation is caused by the neoplasm outstripping its blood supply. Cavitation seems more related to cell type, dependent perhaps on processes such as liquefaction of keratin in squamous cell carcinomas, or mucoid degeneration in adenocarcinomas.[146] In general, metastases from squamous cell cancers originating in the head and neck undergo cavitation when quite small and may have strikingly thin walls,[146] although many other cell types also show thin walls.[7,222] When multiple, cavitary lesions usually coexist with solid nodules.[135]

Detectable calcification in metastases is unusual except in metastases from sarcomas, notably osteosarcoma and chondrosarcoma, in which the calcification is part of the tumor matrix just as it is in the primary tumor (Figures 8-106 and 8-107). Even in tumors such as breast, ovarian, colon, and thyroid carcinomas, where calcification can be seen in the primary tumor, calcification in pulmonary metastases has been recognized in only a few isolated cases.[394] Calcification may, however, be seen in successfully treated metastases.[116,394]

Miliary nodulation, a pattern of innumerable tiny nodules resembling miliary tuberculosis, is occasionally encountered but is decidedly rare (Figure 8-108). Miliary metastases are most likely to be due to thyroid or renal

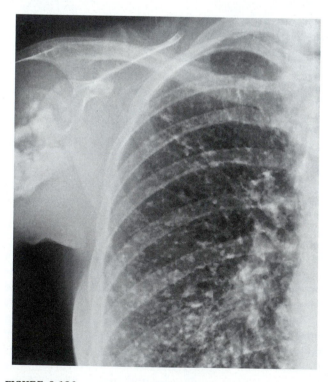

FIGURE 8-106
Calcified metastases in a case of osteosarcoma (the primary tumor is visible in upper right humerus).

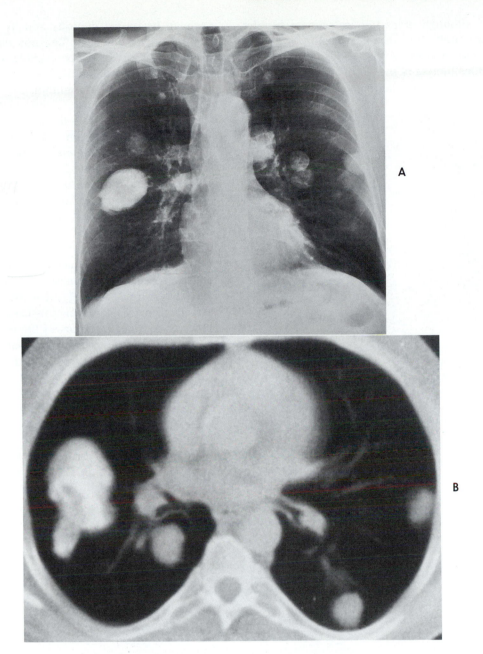

FIGURE 8-107
Calcification and ossification in metastases from osteosarcoma of leg. **A,** Posteroanterior radiograph. **B,** Computed tomographic scan.

carcinoma, bone sarcoma, trophoblastic disease,[193] or melanoma.[672]

Very occasionally, metastases are seen radiographically as myriads of tiny shadows that summate to resemble pulmonary consolidation and may then be confused with infection, edema, or drug reaction. This pattern has been seen particularly with melanoma.[106,159,672] One case has been reported in which innumerable tiny metastases resembling consolidation were confined to one lobe.[642]

In general, pulmonary metastases that respond to treatment with chemotherapy disappear and are no longer visible radiographically as nodules. Rarely, however, a residual nodule of sterilized fibrous tissue remains, and in this case there can be a major dilemma in deciding whether treatment should be continued.[368] This phenomenon has been observed particularly with choriocarcinoma[367,629] and with testicular cancer.[659]

Thin-walled air cysts, also known as pulmonary lacunae, may persist in sites of metastases that have been successfully treated. This phenomenon has been most frequently encountered with germ cell tumors of the testes (both seminoma and nonseminomatous germ cell tumors),[103,580] although other tumors such as bladder carcinomas may rarely show the phenomenon.[320] The air cysts were encountered in 7% of a series of 59 patients with teratomatous tumors of the testis.[103] They appear to be quite different from cavitating metastases in that they

seem to be healed deposits and do not contain viable tumor.[103] The diagnosis depends on noting uniformly very thin, virtually imperceptible cyst walls and no evidence of a mural nodule.

Metastases from nonseminomatous germ cell tumors may enlarge despite responding successfully to chemotherapy.[500] In such cases the masses are transforming to a mature form of teratoma. The serum tumor markers are not raised, an important point in the differential diagnosis from growing metastases.

Parenchymal metastases occur at least 10 times as often as intrathoracic nodal metastases, and nodal disease alone is unusual except in seminoma of the testis.[688] McLoud and associates[428] reviewed 1071 cases of extrathoracic malignant neoplasms. Only 2% to 3% had evidence of hilar or mediastinal lymph node metastases, and concomitant pulmonary metastases were present in almost half these cases (Figure 8-109). The authors found that the primary neoplasms consisted chiefly of tumors of the head and neck, tumors of the genitourinary system, breast cancer, and malignant melanoma.

The subject of tumor emboli is discussed on p. 393.

DETECTION OF PULMONARY METASTASES. The standard initial test for the detection of pulmonary metastases is the plain chest radiograph. High-kilovoltage technique (over 125 kV) shows more lesions than low-kilovoltage films.

CT, particularly spiral (helical) CT,[540] is currently the most sensitive technique available for the detection of pulmonary metastases. There are two principal reasons: excellent contrast resolution and few blind spots. The

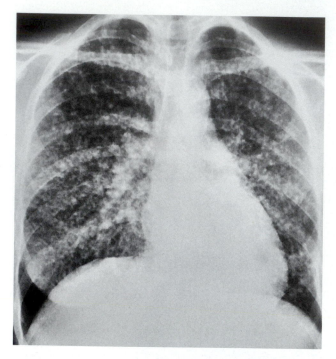

FIGURE 8-108
Miliary metastases from breast carcinoma.

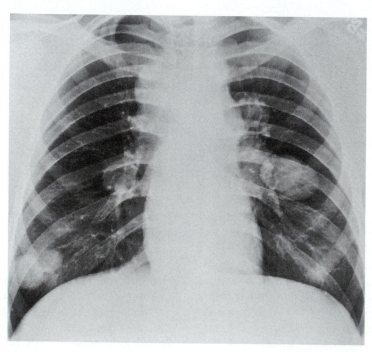

FIGURE 8-109
Concomitant pulmonary and mediastinal metastases in a 17-year-old boy with seminoma of testis.

better contrast resolution of CT compared with plain chest radiography allows smaller nodules to be demonstrated. Individual nodules as small as 3 mm in diameter may be visible on CT, whereas the lower limit for uncalcified nodules on plain film is somewhere between 7 and 9 mm. The increased sensitivity in detecting metastases carries with it a decrease in specificity, since some of the smaller nodules discovered by CT are benign granulomas, particularly in parts of the world where fungal granulomas, such as histoplasmomas, are common. Early series[102,583] suggested that a large proportion of the nodules shown only by CT would prove to be benign; however, other surveys[457,515] indicate that over 80% of nodules seen with CT that are not visible on plain chest radiographs or conventional whole lung tomograms turn out to be metastases. In countries such as the United Kingdom, where fungal granulomas are virtually nonexistent, the specificity of CT rises: in a study of 100 adult patients without known malignant disease, only two nonmetastatic nodules were encountered, both of which were calcified.[162] But even in the United Kingdom caution is needed because 6% of noncalcified nodules revealed by CT in a series of 200 patients with seminoma of the testis were nonmetastatic, presumably tuberculous granulomas,[688] and in another survey of patients with a variety of extrathoracic primary tumors the great majority of nodules detected by CT in the presence of a normal plain chest radiograph surprisingly proved to be benign.[100]

One advantage of CT is that blind areas are largely eliminated, owing to the cross-sectional technique and the lack of artifact from adjacent levels, an advantage that is particularly important because hematogenous metastases tend to occur in the outer one third of the lung and are often subpleural in location (Figure 8-103).[128] These areas, particularly the subpleural regions against the chest wall, mediastinum, and posterior costophrenic recesses, are the most difficult to assess with whole lung tomography or plain chest radiography. An additional advantage of CT is that it can demonstrate disease in the mediastinum, an anatomic region for which whole lung tomography is relatively insensitive. CT also shows the axillae, the root of the neck, and the upper abdomen on routine chest images. CT does, however, have one disadvantage: so-called contiguous sections may not be truly contiguous if the patient breathes erratically during the examination and small nodules may then be out of section on each image every time and therefore are not imaged at all. This problem is largely overcome with spiral (helical) and ultrafast scanners, because the whole chest can often be imaged during a single breath hold.[540]

CT is used only in selected cases because it is rarely necessary to demonstrate further metastases once the presence of definite pulmonary metastatic disease has been established. General indications for CT include the following:

1. Patients with a normal chest radiograph in whom the presence of pulmonary metastases would significantly alter patient management. With tumors such as osteosarcoma, choriocarcinoma, and testicular germ cell tumors,[282] all of which have a significant incidence of pulmonary metastases at presentation, but which may have no detectable metastatic spread to other sites, CT scans of the chest are often obtained to find neoplastic deposits not visible on plain chest radiography. The incidence of pulmonary metastases from seminoma is low, but since the incidence of mediastinal nodal disease can be as high as 12.5%, chest CT is recommended for initial staging as well as for follow-up for potential relapse.[688]

Locally advanced melanoma is cited as an example of a tumor with high propensity to metastasize to the lungs,[185,672] but whether routine chest CT is justified in cases with a normal chest radiograph is far from clear. In one series of 42 patients with locally advanced melanoma and either a solitary pulmonary nodule or no abnormality on chest radiographs, CT scanning showed further nodules believed to be metastases in approximately one third.[250] The authors did, however, point out that in only one of the 42 patients did the discovery of an additional nodule by CT alter the management of the patient. In a similar-sized series there was a change in management in 26% of patients following the CT scan.[330]

The incidence of pulmonary metastases in patients with head and neck carcinoma, superficial melanoma, and carcinomas of the kidney, bladder, and female genital tract is relatively low. Chiles and Ravin[109] recommended that in patients with these tumors CT should be reserved for those with advanced local disease and thoracic symptoms.

Similarly, patients with carcinoma of the gastrointestinal tract, breast, or prostate are unlikely to have pulmonary metastases in the absence of metastases to such organs as the liver and bones, and CT should therefore be reserved for patients in whom thoracic involvement is uncertain on plain chest radiograph and in whom the information would change management.[109,129]

2. Patients who are being considered for surgical resection of known pulmonary metastases. CT is clearly indicated to demonstrate all pulmonary metastases in patients for whom surgical resection of the pulmonary lesions is being considered in order to plan the surgery and to look for further occult lesions. Currently such surgery is recommended when the primary tumor has been (or can be) definitively treated and all known metastatic disease can be encompassed by the projected pulmonary resection.[456] Resection of pulmonary metastases appears most beneficial for tumors of the urinary tract, testicular and uterine neoplasms, colon and rectal carcinoma,[414,417] tumors of the head and neck, and various sarcomas,[522] notably osteogenic sarcoma.[456] How many other tumors should be added to this list is debatable.[228,450]

3. Distinguishing solitary from multiple pulmonary nodules when the diagnostic dilemma is metastasis

versus new primary bronchial carcinoma. A truly solitary pulmonary nodule may represent a primary bronchogenic carcinoma rather than a metastasis, even in a patient with a known extrathoracic primary tumor. Clearly the relative probabilities depend on the likelihood of the specific primary tumor metastasizing to the lungs and such factors as the patient's smoking habits and the interval between the original diagnosis and the appearance of the nodule. A rule of thumb suggested by Cahan and co-workers[85] states that

for patients over 35, if a patient has a squamous cancer elsewhere in the body, the solitary lung lesion is usually a separate primary (and most likely squamous cancer as well). If the patient has an adenocarcinoma elsewhere, there is an equal chance that the solitary shadow is a primary lung cancer as it is a metastasis. If there is a soft tissue or skeletal sarcoma or a melanoma elsewhere, the solitary lung lesion is most often a metastasis.

MRI currently has a limited role for detecting metastases. Even though Feuerstein and associates,[178] using a 0.5 Tesla magnet, showed that MRI was at least as sensitive as CT in detecting metastases, the general view is that CT, particularly using spiral (helical) volumetric scanning techniques, is the most cost-effective method of finding pulmonary metastases.[499] There are, however, several potential specific advantages of MRI: the absence of ionizing radiation with MRI is a clear-cut advantage over CT, particularly for young patients undergoing repeated follow-up scans. Furthermore, MRI can sometimes distinguish between small centrally located metastases and adjacent normal blood vessels, based on the signal of flowing blood in arteries and veins.

Radionuclide imaging can be useful for detecting occult intrathoracic metastases when the neoplasms concentrate on specific radionuclide,[304,630,665] such as a bone scanning agent for metastases from osteosarcoma.[64,653]

Endobronchial metastases

melanoma, ?thyroid

Metastases to the walls of a large bronchus are unusual. Bramman and Whitcomb[68] found the incidence to be only 2% in a large series of patients who had died from solid neoplasms. The most common primary sites[38] appear to be kidney, breast, colon, and rectum.[89] The clinical and radiologic features are indistinguishable from those produced by other central tumors, namely cough, wheezing, hemoptysis, atelectasis, and obstructive pneumonitis (Figure 8-110).[6,38] On plain chest radiography the lesion itself is not visible and the evidence for an endobronchial metastases is obstructive atelectasis. The endobronchial metastasis itself may be visible at CT.[284]

Lymphangitis carcinomatosa

Lymphangitis carcinomatosa is the name given to permeation of pulmonary lymphatics by neoplastic cells. The most common tumors that spread in this manner are carcinomas of the bronchus, breast, pancreas, stomach,

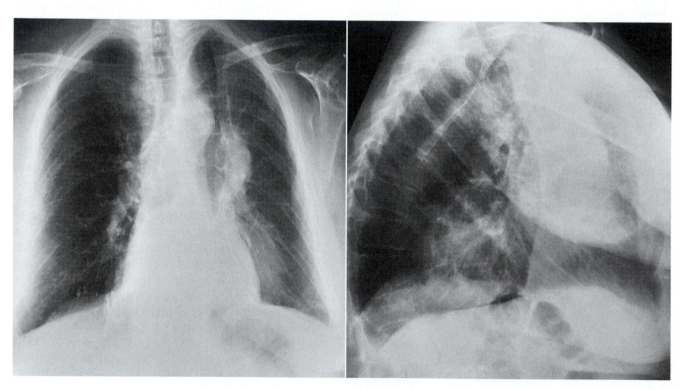

FIGURE 8-110
Endobronchial metastasis from carcinoma of kidney causing left upper lobe collapse.

colon, and prostate. The route by which tumor cells reach the intrapulmonary lymphatics is debated. Spenser,[601] when reviewing the subject, concluded that some cases are caused by blood-borne emboli that lodge in smaller pulmonary arteries and subsequently spread through the vessel walls into the lymphatic vessels. Some tumors, notably upper abdominal cancers, appear to spread by way of lymph vessels to hilar nodes and thence in retrograde fashion into the pulmonary lymphatics. Primary carcinoma of the lung can invade the pulmonary lymphatics directly and may give rise to segmental or lobar lymphangitis carcinomatosa, as well as involving one or both lungs diffusely.

Histologic study shows interstitial thickening of the interlobular septa caused by a combination of tumor cells, desmoplastic response, and dilated lymphatics. The lymphatic obstruction can lead to interstitial edema. The hilar lymph nodes may or may not show histologic evidence of tumor involvement.

The radiologic findings are fine reticulonodular shadowing and thickened septal lines (Figures 8-111 and 8-112). These signs occur because of a combination of dilated lymphatics and interstitial edema, together with shadows caused by the tumor cells themselves and any desmoplastic response that may have been induced by the tumor.[257,294,643] Another useful sign of lymphangitis carcinomatosa is subpleural edema resulting from lymphatic obstruction by tumor cells, a feature most readily visible as thickening of the fissures.[257] These changes can be unilateral (Figure 8-113), particularly in cases resulting from bronchial carcinoma. More often the pulmonary

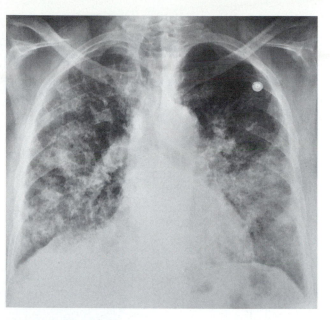

FIGURE 8-112
Lymphangitis carcinomatosa from carcinoma of breast showing randomly distributed reticulonodular shadowing with areas of confluence.

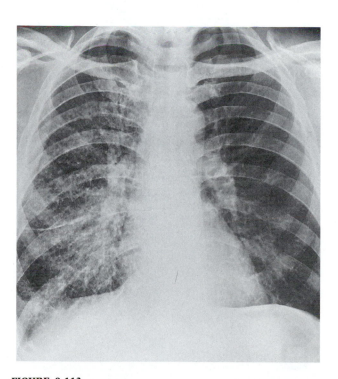

FIGURE 8-113
Unilateral lymphangitis carcinomatosa from bronchial carcinoma. Note reticulonodular shadows and subpleural thickening of minor fissure and of lung in right cardiophrenic angle. Septal lines are also present.

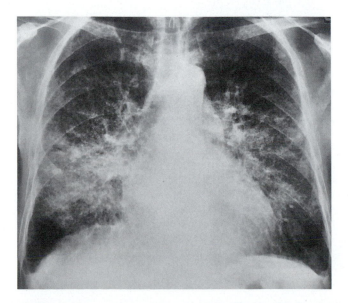

FIGURE 8-111
Lymphangitis carcinomatosa from carcinoma of prostate showing bilateral centrally predominant reticulonodular shadows.

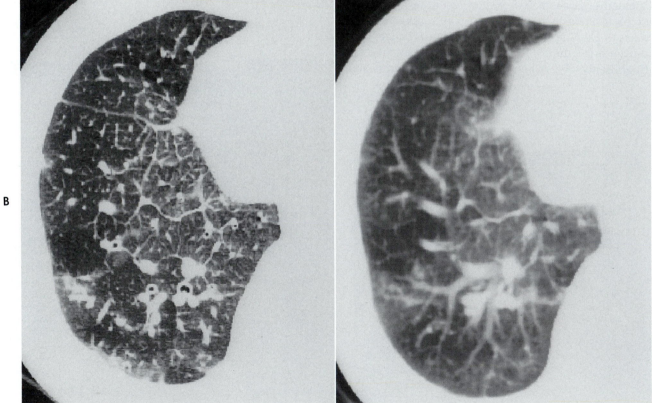

FIGURE 8-114

Lymphangitis carcinomatosa. **A,** High-resolution computed tomographic scan (1.5 mm section) showing thickened interlobular septa. Note polygonal shape of lobule and variable degree of thickening of septa. **B,** A 1.5 mm section compared with **C,** a 10 mm section of patient with lymphangitis carcinomatosa from ovarian primary tumor. Interlobular septal thickening can be diagnosed only from the thin-section image. **B** and **C** were taken on same occasion.

shadowing is bilateral and symmetric. Pleural effusion is common.

As would be expected, CT scanning is more sensitive than plain radiography in the detection of lymphangitic spread and may show changes in patients whose chest film is normal. CT, particularly HRCT scanning (Figure 8-104),[300,461,541,611] shows nonuniform, often nodular thickening of the interlobular septa and irregular thickening of the bronchovascular bundles in the central portions of the secondary pulmonary lobules (Figure 8-114).[49,461] Small, peripherally located, wedge-shaped densities are sometimes seen as well; they may represent volume averaging of the thickened septa. There is often patchy airspace shadowing, but an important differential diagnostic feature from pulmonary edema is that many of the acini subtended by thickened interlobular septa are normally aerated. Nodular shadows may be seen scattered through the parenchyma. The distribution of the changes varies greatly. The abnormalities may involve all zones of both lungs or may be centrally or peripherally predominant; sometimes they are confined to a lobe or one lung. There appears to be a correlation between the severity of the interstitial thickening observed on HRCT and pulmonary function tests.[300]

No studies have formally reported the sensitivity of HRCT for the diagnosis of lymphangitis carcinoma, but autopsy correlation shows that in patients with discrete pulmonary metastases, lymphangitis carcinomatosa is often present in areas of the lung that appear normal at HRCT.[271]

Hilar lymph node enlargement is seen in only some patients, 5 of the 12 cases in one series, supporting the supposition that lymphangitis carcinomatosa is sometimes the result of hematogenous spread of tumor to the interstitium.[294]

The major differential diagnosis of lymphangitis carcinomatosa is pulmonary edema. The nodularity of the septal thickening at thin section CT is helpful, but on plain chest radiographs, at least in patients without visible lung cancer or adenopathy, the findings may be similar to pulmonary edema, and distinguishing between the two conditions can be impossible. Clearly knowledge of the clinical or radiographic progression of disease is helpful and frequently decisive.

Malignant pleural effusion and pleural metastases

Carcinomatous metastases to the pleura can originate from almost any organ, but lung appears to be the most frequent primary site, followed by breast, pancreas, stomach, and ovary.[12,107,409,438] Carcinoma of the lung and breast, together with lymphoma, accounts for approximately 75% of malignant pleural effusions.[12] Leukemia and sarcomatous metastases are rare causes of pleural effusion[277,562] as is malignant mesothelioma. The responsible neoplasm usually involves both the visceral and parietal pleura; isolated involvement of the parietal pleura was not seen in any case in the series reported by Meyer.[438]

A malignant tumor can lead to a pleural effusion in several different ways.[376,409,563] Decreased lymphatic drainage caused by blockage of the small lymphatic stomas that drain the pleura is the probable mechanism in many cases, and obstruction to lymphatic drainage through mediastinal nodes that have been infiltrated by tumor is also believed to play a significant role. Another, probably less common mechanism is increased permeability of the pleural surfaces because of the presence of metastases so that more protein enters the pleural cavity than can be removed. Malignant tumors can also produce pleural effusions by obstructing the thoracic duct, in which case the resulting pleural effusion will be chylous.

Not all patients with pleural metastases have pleural effusions. Meyer[438] found that only 60% of autopsy patients with pleural metastases had pleural effusions and that the presence of a pleural effusion was more closely related to neoplastic invasion of the mediastinal lymph nodes than to the extent of pleural involvement by nodular metastases.

The most common symptom of pleural effusion resulting from metastases is dyspnea on exertion. Chest pain is relatively uncommon, being seen in less than one fourth of patients.[107]

Pleural effusions resulting from malignant tumor[47,107] contain high levels of protein and may show a low pH, a low glucose level, and a high lactic acid dehydrogenase level. Approximately 10% of patients with malignant pleural effusion have an elevated level of amylase in the pleural fluid, even though the primary tumor is usually not in the pancreas.[377] Bleeding may occur into the effusion, and typically the fluid contains a large number of lymphocytes. The reason for the high lymphocyte count is not entirely clear, but it is known that chronic pleural effusions in the absence of active inflammation are generally lymphocyte predominant. Unlike tuberculous effusions, which are also lymphocyte predominant, malignant effusions often contain mesothelial cells. The

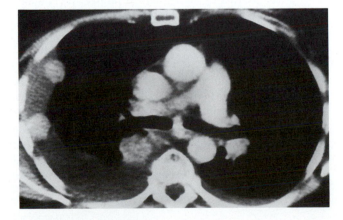

FIGURE 8-115
Pleural metastases shown as tumor nodules by computed tomography in a patient with metastatic melanoma. Tumor was widely metastatic, involving not only the pleura bilaterally but also mediastinal lymph nodes.

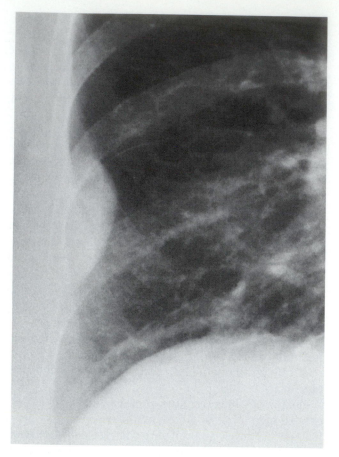

FIGURE 8-116
Pleural metastasis from carcinoma of uterus. This case is unusual in that the lesion is solitary and no pleural effusion is present.

presence of definite malignant cells on cytologic examination or pleural biopsy removes all doubt about the diagnosis. The percentage of cases in which cytologic study of the pleural fluid establishes the diagnosis ranges from 40% to 80%. The rate varies with the cell type; the yield is low with squamous tumors.[376] In general, cytologic study of the pleural fluid establishes the diagnosis more frequently than pleural biopsy, presumably because pleural biopsy samples are from the parietal pleura and parietal pleura involvement is often spotty.[376]

Usually the findings on plain chest radiograph, CT, MRI, and ultrasound are free or loculated pleural effusion that has no specific features. Tumor nodules may be recognizable in the pleura on CT (Figure 8-115), ultrasound,[223,612] or even occasionally chest radiographs (Figure 8-116). Other features of bronchogenic carcinoma or lymphoma are often present in patients whose effusion results from one of these diseases. For example, enlarged intrathoracic lymph nodes are seen in about 10% of patients with pleural effusion caused by breast cancer.[177]

REFERENCES

1. Adams VI, Unni KK, Muhm JR, et al: Diffuse malignant mesothelioma of pleura: diagnosis and survival in 92 cases, *Cancer* 58:1540-1551, 1986.

2. Addis BJ, Hyjek E, Isaacson PG: Primary pulmonary lymphoma: a re-appraisal of its histogenesis and its relationship to pseudolymphoma and lymphoid interstitial pneumonia, *Histopathology* 13:1-17, 1988.

3. Adler B, Padley S, Miller RR, et al: High-resolution CT of bronchioloalveolar carcinoma, *AJR* 159:275-277, 1992.

4. Aisner J, Wiernik PH: Malignant mesothelioma: current status and future prospects, *Chest* 74:438-444, 1978.

5. Aisner SC, Chakravarthy AK, Joslyn JN, et al: Bilateral granular cell tumors of the posterior mediastinum, *Ann Thorac Surg* 46:688-689, 1988.

6. Albertini RE, Ekberg NL: Endobronchial metastasis in breast cancer, *Thorax* 35:435-440, 1980.

7. Alexander PW, Sanders C, Nath H: Cavitary pulmonary metastases in transitional cell carcinoma of urinary bladder, *AJR* 154:493-494, 1990.

8. Allen HA, Angell F, Hankins J, et al: Leiomyoma of the trachea, *AJR* 141:683-684, 1983.

9. Allen MS, Mathisen DJ, Grillo HC, et al: Bronchogenic carcinoma with chest wall invasion, *Ann Thorac Surg* 51:948-951, 1991.

10. Altman RL, Miller WE, Carr DT, et al: Radiographic appearance of bronchial carcinoid, *Thorax* 28:433-434, 1973.

11. Amin R: Extramedullary plasmacytoma of the lung, *Cancer* 56:152-156, 1985.

12. Anderson CB, Philpott GW, Ferguson TB: The treatment of malignant pleural effusions, *Cancer* 33:916-922, 1974.

13. Anderson KA, Hurley WC, Hurley BT, Ohrt DW: Malignant pleural mesothelioma following radiotherapy in a 16-year-old boy, *Cancer* 56:273-276, 1985.

14. Antman KH: Clinical presentation and natural history of benign and malignant mesothelioma, *Semin Oncol* 8:313-320, 1981.

15. Antman KH, Corson JM: Benign and malignant pleural mesothelioma, *Clin Chest Med* 6:127-140, 1985.

16. Armstrong P, Elston C, Sanderson M: Endobronchial histiocytoma, *Br J Radiol* 48:221-222, 1975.

17. Aronberg DJ, Sagel SS, Jost GR, et al: Oat cell carcinoma manifesting as a bronchocele, *AJR* 132:23-25, 1979.

18. Aronchick JM: CT of mediastinal lymph nodes in patients with non-small cell lung carcinoma, *Radiol Clin North Am* 28:573-581, 1990.

19. Aronchick JM, Wexler JA, Christen B, et al: Computed tomography of bronchial carcinoid, *J Comput Assist Tomogr* 10:71-74, 1986.

20. Askin FB, Rosai J, Sibley RK: Malignant small cell tumor of the thoracopulmonary region in childhood: a distinctive clinicopathologic entity of uncertain histogenesis, *Cancer* 43:2438-2451, 1979.

21. Attar S, Miller SE, Satterfield J, et al: Pancoast's tumor: irradiation or surgery? *Ann Thorac Surg* 28:578-586, 1979.

22. Auerbach O, Garfinkel L: The changing pattern of lung carcinoma, *Cancer* 68:1973-1977, 1991.

23. Austin JHM, Romney BM, Goldsmith LS: Missed bronchogenic carcinoma: radiographic findings in 27 patients with a potentially resectable lesion evident in retrospect, *Radiology* 182:115-121, 1992.

24. Bachman D, Wolff M: Pulmonary metastases from benign-appearing smooth muscle tumors of the uterus, *AJR* 127:441-446, 1976.

25. Backer CL, Shields TW, Lockhart CG, et al: Selective preoperative evaluation for possible N2 disease in carcinoma of the lung, *J Thorac Cardiovasc Surg* 93:337-343, 1987.

26. Bahk YW, Shinn KS, Choi BS: The air meniscus sign in sclerosing hemangioma of the lung, *Radiology* 128:27-29, 1978.

27. Bakris GL, Mulopulos GP, Korchik P, et al: Pulmonary scar carcinoma: a clinicopathologic analysis, *Cancer* 52:493-497, 1983.

28. Balikian JP, Herman PG: Non-Hodgkin's lymphoma of the lungs, *Radiology* 132:569-576, 1979.

29. Baris YI, Kalyoncu AF, Aydiner A, et al: Intrathoracic lipomas demonstrated by computed tomography, *Respiration* 57:77-80, 1990.

30. Baron RL, Levitt RG, Sagel SS, et al: Computed tomography in the preoperative evaluation of bronchogenic carcinoma, *Radiology* 145:727-732, 1982.

31. Baron RL, Sagel SS, Baglan RJ: Thymic cysts following radiation therapy for Hodgkin's disease, *Radiology* 141:593-597, 1981.

32. Barsky SH, Huang SJ, Bhuta S: The extracellular matrix of pulmonary scar carcinoma is suggestive of a desmoplastic origin, *Am J Pathol* 124:412-419, 1986.

33. Bateson EM: Relationship between intrapulmonary and endobronchial cartilage containing tumours, so called hamartomata, *Thorax* 20:447-461, 1965.

34. Bateson EM, Abbot EK: Mixed tumours of the lung, or hamartochondromas, *Clin Radiol* 11:232-247, 1960.

35. Bateson EM, Whimster WF, Woo-Ming M: Ossified bronchial adenoma, *Br J Radiol* 43:570-573, 1970.

36. Batra P, Brown K, Collins JD, et al: Evaluation of intrathoracic extent of lung cancer by plain chest radiography, computed tomography and magnetic resonance imaging, *Am Rev Respir Dis* 137:1456-1462, 1988.

37. Batra P, Brown K, Steckel RJ, et al: MR imaging of the thorax: a comparison of axial, coronal and sagittal imaging planes, *J Comput Assist Tomogr* 12:75-81, 1988.

38. Baumgartner WA, Mark JBD: Metastatic malignancies from distant sites to the tracheobronchial tree, *J Thorac Cardiovasc Surg* 79:499-503, 1980.

39. Becker GL, Whitlock WL, Schaeffer PS, et al: The impact of thoracic computed tomography in clinically staged T1,N0,M0 chest lesions, *Arch Intern Med* 150:557-559, 1990.

40. Beckerman C, Caride VJ, Hoffer PB, et al: Noninvasive staging of lung cancer: indications and limitations of gallium-67 citrate imaging, *Radiol Clin North Am* 28:497-510, 1990.

41. Behling CA, Wolf PL, Haghigi P, et al: AIDS and malignant mesothelioma — is there a connection? *Chest* 103:1268-1269, 1993.

42. Beluffi G, Bertolotti P, Mietta A, et al: Primary leiomyosarcoma of the lung in a girl, *Pediatr Radiol* 16:240-244, 1986.

43. Bender BL, Jaffe R: Immunoglobulin production in lymphomatoid granulomatosis and relation to other "benign" lymphoproliferative disorders, *Am J Clin Pathol* 73:41-47, 1980.

44. Benditt JO, Farber HW, Wright J, et al: Pulmonary hemorrhage with diffuse alveolar infiltrates in men with high volume choriocarcinoma, *Ann Intern Med* 8:674-675, 1988.

45. Benisch B, Peison B: The association of lymphocytic interstitial pneumonia and systemic lupus erythematosus, *Mt Sinai J Med* 46:398-401, 1979.

46. Bennett LL, Lesar MSL, Tellis CJ: Multiple calcified chondrohamartomas of the lung: CT appearance, *J Comput Assist Tomogr* 9:180-182, 1985.

47. Berger HW, Maher G: Decreased glucose concentration in malignant pleural effusions, *Am Rev Respir Dis* 103:427-429, 1971.

48. Bergin CJ, Healy MV, Zincone GE, et al: MR evaluation of chest wall involvement in malignant lymphoma, *J Comput Assist Tomogr* 14:928-932, 1990.

49. Bergin CJ, Muller NL: CT of interstitial lung disease: a diagnostic approach, *AJR* 148:8-15, 1987.

50. Berkmen YM: The many faces of alveolar cell carcinoma of the lung, *Semin Roentgenol* 12:207-214, 1977.

51. Berne AS, Heitzman ER: The roentgenologic signs of pedunculated pleural tumors, *AJR* 87:892-895, 1962.

52. Black WC, Armstrong P, Daniel TM: Cost-effectiveness of chest CT in T1N0M0 lung cancer, *Radiology* 167:373-378, 1988.

53. Blair TC, McElvein: Hamartoma of the lung: a clinical study of 25 cases, *Dis Chest* 44:296-302, 1963.

54. Blank N, Castellino RA: The mediastinum in Hodgkin's and non-Hodgkin's lymphomas, *J Thorac Imag* 2(1):66-71, 1987.

55. Blount HC: Localized mesothelioma of the pleura, *Radiology* 67:822-834, 1956.

56. Bolton-Maggs PHB, Colman A, Dixon GR, et al: Mucosa associated lymphoma of the lung, *Thorax* 48:670-672, 1993.

57. Bonner H, Ennis RS, Geelhoed GW, et al: Lymphoid infiltration and amyloidosis of the lung in Sjögren's syndrome, *Arch Pathol* 95:42-44, 1973.

58. Borrow M, Couston A, Livornese L, et al: Mesothelioma following exposure to asbestos: a review of 72 cases, *Chest* 64:641-646, 1973.

59. Bosanko CMM, Korobkin M, Fantone JC, et al: Lobar primary pulmonary lymphoma: CT findings, *J Comput Assist Tomogr* 15:679-682, 1991.

60. Boucot KR, Weiss W: Is curable lung cancer detected by semiannual screening? *JAMA* 224:1361-1365, 1973.

61. Bourgouin PM, McLoud TC, Fitzgibbon JF, et al: Differentiation of bronchogenic carcinoma from postobstructive pneumonitis by magnetic resonance imaging: histopathologic correlation, *J Thorac Imag* 6(2):22-27, 1991.

62. Bower SL, Choplin RH, Muss HB: Multiple primary carcinomas of the lung, *AJR* 140:253-258, 1983.

63. Boysen PG, Harris JO, Block AJ, et al: Prospective evaluation for pneumonectomy using perfusion scanning: follow up beyond one year, *Chest* 80:163-166, 1981.

64. Brady AP, Ennis JT: The scintigraphic detection of ossific mediastinal and pulmonary metastases in osteosarcoma, *Br J Radiol* 63:978-980, 1990.

65. Bragg DG: Radiology of the lymphomas, *Curr Probl Diagn Radiol* 16:183-206, 1987.

66. Bragg DG: The clinical, pathologic and radiographic spectrum of the intrathoracic lymphomas, *Invest Radiol* 13:2-11, 1978.

67. Bragg DG, Colby TV, Ward JH: New concepts in the non-Hodgkin lymphomas: radiologic implications, *Radiology* 159:289-304, 1986.

68. Bramman SS, Whitcomb ME: Endobronchial metastasis, *Arch Intern Med* 135:543-547, 1975.

69. Brenner J, Sordillo PP, Magill GB, et al: Malignant mesothelioma of the pleura: review of 123 patients, *Cancer* 49:2431-2439, 1982.

70. Brett GZ: Earlier diagnosis and survival in lung cancer, *Br Med J* 2:260-262, 1968.

71. Briselli M, Mark EJ, Dickersin GR: Solitary fibrous tumors of the pleura: eight new cases and review of 360 cases in the literature, *Cancer* 47:2678-2689, 1981.

72. Brogdon BG, Kelsey CA, Moseley RD: Factors affecting perception of pulmonary lesions, *Radiol Clin North Am* 21:633-654, 1983.

73. Bron LP, Howarth NR, Muller AF: Pneumoblastoma in neurofibromatosis, *Chest* 103:636-638, 1993.

74. Brown ML, O'Donnell JB, Thrall JH, et al: Gallium-67 scintigraphy in untreated and treated non-Hodgkin's lymphomas, *J Nucl Med* 19:875-879, 1978.

75. Budde RB, Yankura JA: Leiomyomatosis with a solitary pleural metastasis, *Clin Imag* 13:228-230, 1989.

76. Burgener FA, Hamlin DJ: Intrathoracic histiocytic lymphoma, *AJR* 136:499-504, 1981.

77. Burke M, Fraser R: Obstructive pneumonitis: a pathologic and pathogenetic reappraisal, *Radiology* 166:699-704, 1988.

78. Butchart EG, Urquhart W, Porteous IB, et al: Granular cell myoblastoma of the bronchus, *Br J Radiol* 49:87-90, 1976.

79. Buy JN, Ghossain MA, Poirson F: Computed tomography of mediastinal lymph nodes in nonsmall cell lung cancer: a new approach based on the lymphatic pathway of tumour spread, *J Comput Assist Tomogr* 12:545-552, 1988.

80. Byrd RB, Carr DT, Miller WE, et al: Radiographic abnormalities in carcinoma of the lung as related to histological cell type, *Thorax* 24:573-575, 1969.

81. Byrd RB, Miller WE, Carr DT, et al: The roentgenographic appearance of squamous cell carcinoma of the bronchus, *Mayo Clin Proc* 43:327-332, 1968.

82. Byrd RB, Miller WE, Carr DT, et al: The roentgenographic appearance of large cell carcinoma of the bronchus, *Mayo Clin Proc* 43:333-336, 1968.

83. Byrd RB, Miller WE, Carr DT, et al: The roentgenographic appearance of small cell carcinoma of the bronchus, *Mayo Clin Proc* 43:337-341, 1968.

84. Cabanillas F, Fuller LM: The radiologic assessment of the lymphoma patient from the standpoint of the clinician, *Radiol Clin North Am* 28:683-695, 1990.

85. Cahan WG, Castro EB, Hajdu SI: The significance of a solitary lung shadow in patients with colon carcinoma, *Cancer* 33:414-421, 1974.

86. Callihan TR, Beard CW: The classification and pathology of the lymphomas and the leukemias, *Semin Roentgenol* 15:203-218, 1980.

87. Cameron EWJ: Primary sarcoma of the lung, *Thorax* 30:516-520, 1975.

88. Carey FA, Donnelly SC, Walker WS, et al: Synchronous primary lung cancers: prevalence in surgical material and clinical implications, *Thorax* 48:344-346, 1993.

89. Carlin BW, Harrell JH, Olson LK, et al: Endobronchial metastases due to colorectal carcinoma, *Chest* 96:1110-1114, 1989.

90. Carlsen SE, Bergin CJ, Hoppe RT: MR imaging to detect chest wall and pleural involvement in patients with lymphoma: effect on radiation therapy planning, *AJR* 160:1191-1195, 1993.

91. Carmel RJ, Kaplan HS: Mantle radiation and Hodgkin's disease, *Cancer* 37:2813-2825, 1976.

92. Carney JA: The triad of gastric epithelioid leiomyosarcoma, pulmonary chondroma and functioning extra-adrenal paraganglioma: a five year review, *Medicine* 62:159-169, 1983.

93. Castagno AA, Shuman WP: MR imaging in clinically suspected brachial plexus tumor, *AJR* 149:1219-1222, 1987.

94. Castellino RA: Hodgkin disease: practical concepts for the diagnostic radiologist, *Radiology* 159:305-310, 1986.

95. Castellino RA: The non-Hodgkin lymphomas: practical concepts for the diagnostic radiologist, *Radiology* 178:315-321, 1991.

96. Castellino RA, Bellani F, Gasparini M, et al: Radiographic findings in previously untreated children with non-Hodgkin's lymphoma, *Radiology* 117:657-663, 1975.

97. Castellino RA, Blank N: Adenopathy of the cardiophrenic angle (diaphragmatic) lymph nodes, *AJR* 114:509-515, 1972.

98. Castellino RA, Blank N, Hoppe RT, et al: Hodgkin disease: contributions of chest CT in initial staging evaluation, *Radiology* 160:603-605, 1986.

99. Cathcart-Rake W, Bone RC, Sobonya RE, et al: Rapid development of diffuse pulmonary infiltrates in histiocytic lymphoma, *Am Rev Respir Dis* 117:587-593, 1978.

100. Chalmers N, Best JJK: Significance of pulmonary nodules detected by CT but not by chest radiography in tumour staging, *Clin Radiol* 44:410-412, 1991.

101. Chamberlain DW, Hyland RH, Ross DJ: Diphenylhydantoin-induced lymphocytic interstitial pneumonia, *Chest* 90:458-460, 1986.

102. Chang AE, Shaner EG, Conkle DM, et al: Evaluation of computed tomography in the detection of pulmonary metastasis: a prospective study, *Cancer* 43:913-916, 1979.

103. Charig MJ, Williams MP: Pulmonary lacunae: sequelae of metastases following chemotherapy, *Clin Radiol* 42:93-96, 1990.

104. Chaudhuri MR: Cavitary pulmonary metastases, *Thorax* 25:375-381, 1970.

105. Chaudhuri MR: Primary pulmonary cavitating carcinomas, *Thorax* 28:354-366, 1973.

106. Chen JTT, Dahmash NS, Ravin CE, et al: Metastatic melanoma to the thorax: report of 130 patients, *AJR* 137:293-298, 1981.

107. Chernow B, Sahn SA: Carcinomatous involvement of the pleura, *Am J Med* 63:695-702, 1977.

108. Child SD, Staples CA, Chan N, et al: Lingular opacity with an endobronchial mass, *J Can Assoc Radiol* 42:435-437, 1991.

109. Chiles C, Ravin CE: Intrathoracic metastases from an extrathoracic malignancy; radiographic approach to patient evaluation, *Radiol Clin North Am* 23:427-438, 1985.

110. Cho CS, Blank N, Castellino RA: CT evaluation of cardiophrenic angle lymph nodes in patients with malignant lymphoma, *AJR* 143:719-721, 1984.

111. Choplin RH, Rawamoto EH, Dyer RB, et al: Atypical carcinoid of the lung: radiographic features, *AJR* 146:665-668, 1986.

112. Churg A: Pulmonary angiitis and granulomatosis revisited, *Hum Pathol* 14:868-883, 1983.

113. Clements R, Gravelle IH: Laryngeal papillomatosis, *Clin Radiol* 37:547-550, 1986.

114. Cleveland RH, Nice CM, Ziskind J: Primary adenoid cystic carcinoma (cylindroma) of the trachea, *Radiology* 122:597-600, 1977.

115. Cobby M, Whipp E, Bullimore J, et al: CT appearances of relapse of lymphoma in the lung, *Clin Radiol* 41:232-238, 1990.

116. Cockshott WP, Hendrickse JP: Pulmonary calcification at the site of trophoblastic metastases, *Br J Radiol* 42:17-20, 1969.

117. Cohen MD, Siddiqui A, Weetman R, et al: Hodgkin disease and non-Hodgkin lymphomas in children: utilization of radiological modalities, *Radiology* 158:499-505, 1986.

118. Cohen MH: Signs and symptoms of bronchogenic carcinoma, *Semin Oncol* 3:183-189, 1974.

119. Cohen S, Hossain S: Primary carcinoma of the lung: a review of 417 histologically proved cases, *Dis Chest* 49:67-74, 1966.

120. Colby TV, Carrington CB: Pulmonary lymphomas simulating lymphomatoid granulomatosis, *Am J Surg Pathol* 6:19-32, 1982.

121. Colby TV, Carrington CB: Pulmonary lymphomas: current concepts, *Hum Pathol* 14:884-887, 1983.

122. Coleman BG, Arger PH, Stephenson LW: Case report: CT features of endobronchial granular cell myoblastoma, *J Comput Assist Tomogr* 8:988-1000, 1984.

123. Conces DJ, Klink JF, Tarver RD, et al: $T_1N_0M_0$ lung cancer: evaluation with CT, *Radiology* 170:643-646, 1989.

124. Conces DJ, Tarver RD: Noninfectious and nonmalignant pulmonary disease in AIDS, *J Thorac Imag* 6(4):53-59, 1991.

125. Coppage L, Shaw C, Curtis AM: Metastatic disease to the chest in patients with extrathoracic malignancy, *J Thorac Imag* 2(4):24-37, 1987.

126. Cordier J-F, Chailleux E, Larque D, et al: Primary pulmonary lymphomas: a clinical study of 70 cases in nonimmunocompromised patients, *Chest* 103:201-208, 1993.

127. Corrin B, Manners B, Millard M, et al: Histogenesis of the so-called "intravascular bronchioloalveolar tumour," *J Pathol* 128:163-167, 1979.

128. Crow J, Slavin G, Kreel L: Pulmonary metastasis: a pathologic and radiologic study, *Cancer* 47:2595-2602, 1981.

129. Curtis AM, Ravin CE, Collier PE, et al: Detection of metastatic disease from carcinoma of the breast: limited value of full lung tomography, *AJR* 134:253-255, 1980.

130. Dail DH, Liebow AA, Gmellich JT, et al: Intravascular, bronchiolar, and alveolar tumor of the lung (IVBAT): an analysis of twenty cases of a peculiar sclerosing endothelial tumor, *Cancer* 51:452-464, 1983.

131. Daly BDT, Faling LJ, Gunars Bite PAC: Mediastinal lymph node evaluation by computed tomography in lung cancer: an analysis of 345 patients grouped by TNM staging, tumor size, and tumor location, *J Thorac Cardiovasc Surg* 94:644-672, 1987.

132. Daly BDT, Mueller JD, Faling LJ, et al: N2 lung cancer: outcome in patients with false-negative computed tomographic scans of the chest, *J Thorac Cardiovasc Surg* 105:904-911, 1993.

133. Daly RC, Trastek VF, Pairolero PC, et al: Bronchoalveolar carcinoma: factors affecting survival, *Ann Thorac Surg* 51:368-377, 1991.

134. Darke CS, Day P, Grainger RG, et al: The bronchial circulation in a case of giant hamartoma of the lung, *Br J Radiol* 45:147-150, 1972.

135. Davis SD: CT evaluation for pulmonary metastases in patients with extrathoracic malignancy, *Radiology* 180:1-12, 1991.

136. Davis SD, Zirn JR, Govoni AF: Peripheral carcinoid tumour of the lung: CT diagnosis, *AJR* 155:1185-1187, 1990.

137. Davis WK, Roberts L, Foster W, et al: Computed tomographic diagnosis of an endobronchial hamartoma, *Invest Radiol* 23:941-944, 1988.

138. Dawson WB, Muller NL, Miller RR: Pulmonary sclerosing hemangioma: unusual cause of a solitary pulmonary nodule, *J Can Assoc Radiol* 41:372-374, 1990.

139. Decker DA, Dines DE, Payne WS, et al: The significance of a cytologically negative pleural effusion in bronchogenic carcinoma, *Chest* 74:640-642, 1978.

140. De Coteau WE, Tourville D, Ambrus JL, et al: Lymphoid interstitial pneumonia and autoerythrocyte sensitization syndrome: a case with deposition of immunoglobulins on the alveolar basement membrane, *Arch Intern Med* 134:519-522, 1974.

141. Dedrick CG, McLoud TC, Shepard JP, et al: Computed tomography of localized pleural mesothelioma, *AJR* 144:275-280, 1985.

142. Dee PM, Arora NS, Innes DI: The pulmonary manifestations of lymphomatoid granulomatosis, *Radiology* 143:613-618, 1982.

143. Delany SG, Doyle TCA, Bunton RW, et al: Pulmonary artery sarcoma mimicking pulmonary embolism, *Chest* 103:1631-1633, 1993.

144. Dennie CJ, Coblentz CL: The trachea: pathologic conditions and trauma, *J Can Assoc Radiol* 44:157-167, 1993.

145. Dines DE, Lillie JC, Henderson LL, et al: Solitary plasmacytoma of the trachea, *Am Rev Respir Dis* 92:949-951, 1965.

146. Dodd GD, Boyle JS: Excavating pulmonary metastases, *AJR* 85:277-293, 1961.

147. Dodd GD, Ledesma-Medina J, Baron RL, et al: Posttransplant lymphoproliferative disorder: intrathoracic manifestations, *Radiology* 184:65-69, 1992.

148. Dooms GC, Hricak H, Moseley ME, et al: Characterization of lymphadenopathy by magnetic resonance relaxation times: preliminary results, *Radiology* 155:691-697, 1985.

149. Doppman JL, Loughlin T, Miller DL, et al: Identification of ACTH-producing intrathoracic tumors by measuring ACTH levels in aspirated specimens, *Radiology* 163:501-503, 1987.

150. Doppman JL, Nieman L, Miller DL, et al: Ectopic adrenocorticotrophic hormone syndrome: localization studies in 28 patients, *Radiology* 172:115-124, 1989.

151. Doppman JL, Pass HI, Nieman L, et al: Failure of bronchial lavage to detect elevated levels of adrenocorticotrophin (ACTH) in patients with ACTH-producing bronchial carcinoids, *J Clin Endocrinol Metab* 69:1302-1304, 1989.

152. Doppman JL, Pass HI, Nieman LK, et al: Detection of ACTH-producing bronchial carcinoid tumors: MR imaging vs CT, *AJR* 156:39-43, 1991.

153. Doppman J, Wilson G: Cystic pulmonary hamartoma, *Br J Radiol* 38:629-631, 1965.

154. Doyle AJ: Plasma cell granuloma of the lung, *Australas Radiol* 32:144-146, 1988.

155. Doyle TCA: Lymphomatoid granulomatosis — the varying lung appearances in four cases, *Australas Radiol* 27:139-142, 1983.

156. Drossman SR, Schiff RG, Kronfeld GD, et al: Lymphoma of the mediastinum and neck: evaluation with Ga-67 imaging and CT correlation, *Radiology* 174:171-175, 1990.

157. Duncan KA, Gomersall LN, Weir J: Computed tomography of the chest in T1N0M0 non-small cell bronchial carcinoma, *Br J Radiol* 66:20-22, 1993.

158. Dunnick NR, Parker BR, Castellino RA: Rapid onset of pulmonary infiltration due to histiocytic lymphoma, *Radiology* 118:281-285, 1976.

159. Dwyer AJ, Reichart CM, Woltering EA, et al: Diffuse pulmonary metastasis in melanoma: radiographic pathologic correlation, *AJR* 143:983-984, 1984.

160. Dynes MC, White EM, Fry WA, et al: Imaging manifestations of pleural tumors, *Radiographics* 12:1191-1201, 1992.

161. Eddy DM: Screening for lung cancer, *Ann Intern Med* 111:232-237, 1989.

162. Edwards SE, Kelsey-Fry I: Prevalence of nodules on computed tomography of patients without known malignant disease, *Br J Radiol* 55:715-716, 1982.

163. Ellis K, Wolff M: Mesotheliomas and secondary tumors of the pleura, *Semin Roentgenol* 12:303-311, 1977.

164. England DM, Hochholzer L, McCarthy MJ, et al: Localized benign and malignant fibrous tumors of the pleura: a clinicopathologic review of 223 cases, *Am J Surg Pathol* 13:640-658, 1989.

165. Epstein DM: Bronchioloalveolar carcinoma, *Semin Roentgenol* 25:105-111, 1990.

166. Epstein DM: The role of radiologic screening in lung cancer, *Radiol Clin North Am* 28:489-495, 1990.

167. Epstein DM, Gefter WB, Miller WT: Lobar bronchioloalveolar cell carcinoma, *AJR* 139:463-468, 1982.

168. Epstein DM, Stephenson LW, Gefter WB, et al: Value of CT in the preoperative assessment of lung cancer: a survey of thoracic surgeons, *Radiology* 161:423-427, 1986.

169. Erzen C, Eryilmaz M, Kalyoncu F, et al: CT findings in malignant pleural mesothelioma related to nonoccupational exposure to asbestos and fibrous zeolite (erionite), *J Comput Assist Tomogr* 15:256-260, 1991.

170. Evans RA, Salisbury JR, Gimson A: Indolent gastric epithelioid leiomyosarcoma in Carney's triad, *Clin Radiol* 42:437-439, 1990.

171. Fauci AS, Haynes BF, Costa J, et al: Lymphomatoid granulomatosis, prospective clinical and therapeutic experience over ten years, *N Engl J Med* 306:68-74, 1982.

172. Feigin DS, Siegelman SS, Theros EG, et al: Nonmalignant lymphoid disorders of the chest, *AJR* 129:221-228, 1977.

173. Feldhaus RJ, Anene C, Bogard R: A rare endobronchial neurilemmoma (schwannoma), *Chest* 95:461-462, 1989.

174. Felson B: Mucoid impaction (inspissated secretions) in segmental bronchial obstruction, *Radiology* 133:9-16, 1976.

175. Felson B, Ralaisomay G: Carcinoma of the lung complicating lipoid pneumonia, *AJR* 141:901-907, 1983.

176. Felson B, Wiot JF: Some less familiar roentgen manifestations of carcinoma of the lung, *Semin Roentgenol* 12:187-206, 1977.

177. Fentiman IS, Millis R, Sexton S, et al: Pleural effusion in breast cancer: a review of 105 cases, *Cancer* 47:2087-2092, 1981.

178. Feuerstein IM, Jicha DL, Pass HI, et al: Pulmonary metastases: MR imaging with surgical correlation — a prospective study, *Radiology* 182:123-129, 1992.

179. Filderman AE, Shaw C, Matthay RA: Lung cancer. I. Etiology, pathology, natural history, manifestations, and diagnostic techniques, *Invest Radiol* 21:80-90, 1986.

180. Filderman AE, Shaw C, Matthay RA: Lung cancer II. Staging and therapy, *Invest Radiol* 21:173-185, 1986.

181. Filly R, Blank N, Castellino RA: Radiographic distribution of intrathoracic disease in previously untreated patients with Hodgkin's disease and non-Hodgkin's lymphoma, *Radiology* 120:277-281, 1976.

182. Findling JW, Tyrell B: Occult ectopic secretion of corticotropin, *Arch Intern Med* 146:929-933, 1986.

183. Fisher AMH, Kendal B, Van Leuven BD: Hodgkin's disease: a radiological survey, *Clin Radiol* 13:115-127, 1962.

184. Fishman EK, Kuhlman JE, Jones RJ: CT of lymphoma: spectrum of disease, *Radiographics* 11:647-669, 1991.

185. Fishman EK, Kuhlman JE, Schuchter LM, et al: CT of malignant melanoma in the chest, abdomen, and musculoskeletal system, *Radiographics* 10:603-620, 1990.

186. Flehinger BJ, Melamed MR, Zaman MB, et al: Early lung cancer detection: results of the initial (prevalence) radiologic and cytologic screening in the Memorial Sloan-Kettering study, *Am Rev Respir Dis* 130:555-560, 1984.

187. Fontana RS: Early diagnosis of lung cancer, editorial, *Am Rev Respir Dis* 116:399-402, 1977.

188. Fontana RS, Sanderson DR, Taylor WF, et al: Early lung cancer detection: results of the initial (prevalence) radiologic cytologic screening in the Mayo Clinic study, *Am Rev Respir Dis* 130:561-565, 1984.

189. Fontana RS, Sanderson DR, Woolner LB, et al: Lung cancer screening: the Mayo program, *J Occupat Med* 28:746-750, 1986.

190. Fontana RS, Sanderson DR, Woolner LB, et al: Screening for lung cancer: a critique of the Mayo Lung Project, *Cancer* 67(4 suppl):1155-1164, 1991.

191. Forster BB, Muller NL, Miller RR, et al: Neuroendocrine carcinomas of the lung: clinical, radiologic, and pathologic correlation, *Radiology* 170:441-445, 1989.

192. Fox K, Silfen D, Alavi A: Applications of gallium-67 scintigraphy in the management of patients with malignant lymphoma, *J Nucl Med* 32:2299-2305, 1991.

193. Fraser RG, Pare JAP: *Diagnosis of diseases of the chest*, ed 2, Philadelphia, 1979, WB Saunders.

194. Freant LJ, Joseph WL, Adkins PC: Scar carcinoma of the lung: fact or fantasy? *Ann Thorac Surg* 17:531-537, 1974.

195. Friedman PJ: Lung cancer: update on staging classifications, *AJR* 150:261-264, 1988.

196. Friedman PJ, Feigin DS, Liston SE, et al: Sensitivity of chest radiography, computed tomography, and gallium scanning to metastasis of lung carcinoma, *Cancer* 54:1300-1306, 1984.

197. Front D, Ben-Haim S, Israel O, et al: Lymphoma: predictive value of Ga-67 scintigraphy after treatment, *Radiology* 182:359-363, 1992.

198. Frost JK, Ball WC, Levin ML, et al: Early lung cancer detection: results of initial (prevalence) radiologic and cytologic screening in the Johns Hopkins study, *Am Rev Respir Dis* 130:549-554, 1984.

199. Furgerson WB, Bachman LB, O'Toole WF: Waldenstrom's macroglobulinemia with diffuse pulmonary infiltration: lung biopsy and response to chlorambucil therapy, *Am Rev Respir Dis* 88:689-697, 1963.

200. Gabrail NY, Zara BY: Pulmonary hamartoma syndrome, *Chest* 97:962-965, 1990.

201. Gallagher CJ, White FE, Tucker AK, et al: The role of computed tomography in the detection of intrathoracic lymphoma, *Br J Cancer* 49:621-629, 1984.

202. Garland LH: The rate of growth and natural duration of primary bronchial cancer, *AJR* 96:604-611, 1966.

203. Garland LH, Coulson W, Wollin E: The rate of growth and apparent duration of untreated primary bronchial carcinoma, *Cancer* 16:694-707, 1963.

204. Gay SB, Black WC, Armstrong P, et al: Chest CT of unresectable lung cancer, *Radiographics* 8:735-748, 1988.

205. Geddes DM: The natural history of lung cancer: a review based on rates of tumor growth, *Br J Dis Chest* 73:1-17, 1979.

206. Gefter WB: Magnetic resonance imaging in the evaluation of lung cancer, *Semin Roentgenol* 25:73-84, 1990.

207. Gelder CM, Hetzel MR: Primary tracheal tumours: a national survey, *Thorax* 48:688-692, 1993.

208. Genereux GP, Howie JL: Normal mediastinal lymph node size and number: CT and anatomic study, *AJR* 142:1095-1100, 1984.

209. George JC: Benign fibrous mesothelioma of the pleura: MR findings, *AJR* 160:204, 1993.

210. Georgian D, Rice TW, Mehta AC, et al: Intrathoracic lymph node evaluation by CT and MRI with histopathologic correlation in non-small cell bronchogenic carcinoma, *Clin Imag* 14:35-40, 1990.

211. Gerard-Marchant R, Hamlin I, Lennert K, et al: Classification of non-Hodgkin's lymphoma, *Lancet* 2:406-408, 1974.

212. Gilroy JA, Adams AB: Extraosseus infiltration in multiple myeloma, *Radiology* 78:406-409, 1959.

213. Giustra PE, Stassa G: The multiple presentations of bronchial adenoma, *Radiology* 93:1013-1019, 1969.

214. Glazer GM, Gross BH, Aisen AM, et al: Imaging of the pulmonary hilum: a prospective comparative study in patients with lung cancer, *AJR* 145:245-248, 1985.

215. Glazer GM, Gross BH, Quint LE, et al: Normal mediastinal lymph nodes: number and size according to American Thoracic Society mapping, *AJR* 144:261-265, 1985.

216. Glazer GM, Orringer MB, Chenevert TL, et al: Mediastinal lymph nodes: relaxation time/pathologic correlation and implications of lung cancer staging with MR imaging, *Radiology* 168:429-431, 1988.

217. Glazer G, Webb WR: Laryngeal papillomatosis with pulmonary spread in a 69-year-old man, *AJR* 132:820-822, 1979.

218. Glazer HS, Anderson DJ, Sagel SS: Bronchial impaction in lobar collapse: CT demonstration and pathological correlation, *AJR* 153:485-488, 1989.

219. Glazer HS, Duncan-Meyer J, Aronberg DJ, et al: Pleural and chest wall invasion in bronchogenic carcinoma: CT evaluation, *Radiology* 157:191-194, 1985.

220. Glazer HS, Kaiser LR, Anderson DJ, et al: Indeterminate mediastinal invasion in bronchogenic carcinoma: CT evaluation, *Radiology* 173:37-42, 1989.

221. Glickstein M, Kornstein MJ, Pietra GG, et al: Nonlymphomatous lymphoid disorders of the lung, *AJR* 147:227-237, 1986.

222. Godwin JD, Webb WR, Savoca CJ, et al: Multiple thin walled cystic lesions of the lung, *AJR* 135:593-604, 1980.

223. Goerg C, Schwerk WB, Goerg K, et al: Pleural effusion: an "acoustic window" for sonography of pleural metastases, *JCU* 19:93-97, 1991.

224. Goldmeier E: Limits of visibility of bronchogenic carcinoma, *Am Rev Respir Dis* 91:232-239, 1965.

225. Goldstein MS, Rush M, Johnson P, et al: A calcified adenocarcinoma of the lung with very high CT numbers, *Radiology* 150:285-286, 1984.

226. Good CA: Asymptomatic bronchial adenoma, *Mayo Clin Proc* 28:577-586, 1953.

227. Good CA: The solitary pulmonary nodule: a problem of management, *Radiol Clin North Am* 1:429-438, 1963.

228. Gorenstein LA, Putnam JB, Natarajan G, et al: Improved survival after resection of pulmonary metastases from malignant melanoma, *Ann Thorac Surg* 52:204-210, 1991.

229. Gramiak R, Koerner HJ: A roentgen diagnostic observation in subpleural lipoma, *AJR* 98:465-467, 1966.

230. Grant DC, Seltzer SE, Antman KH, et al: Computed tomography of malignant pleural mesothelioma, *J Comput Assist Tomogr* 7:626-632, 1983.

231. Greenberg SD, Haley MD, Kenkins DE, et al: Lymphoplasmacytic pneumonia with accompanying dysproteinemia, *Arch Pathol* 96:73-80, 1973.

232. Greenfield H, Herman PC: Papillomatosis of the trachea and bronchi, *AJR* 89:45-50, 1963.

233. Grenier P, Dubray B, Carrette MF: Preoperative thoracic staging of lung cancer: CT and MRI evaluation, *Diagn Intervent Radiol* 1:23-28, 1989.

234. Gross BH, Glazer GM, Orringer MB, et al: Bronchogenic carcinoma metastatic to normal-sized lymph nodes: frequency and significance, *Radiology* 166:71-74, 1986.

235. Grossman H, Winchester PH, Bragg DG, et al: Roentgenographic changes in childhood Hodgkin's disease, *AJR* 108:354-364, 1970.

236. Guccion JG, Rosen SH: Bronchopulmonary leiomyosarcoma and fibrosarcoma: a study of 32 cases and review of the literature, *Cancer* 30:836-847, 1972.

237. Gupta NC, Frank AR, Dewan NA, et al: Solitary pulmonary nodules: detection of malignancy with PET with 2-[F-18]-fluoro-2-deoxy-D-glucose, *Radiology* 184:441-444, 1992.

238. Hahn PF, Novelline RA, Mark EJ: Arteriography in the localization of massive pleural tumors, *AJR* 139:814-817, 1982.

239. Hait WN, Farber L, Cadman E: Non-Hodgkin's lymphoma for the nononcologist, *JAMA* 253:1431-1435, 1985.

240. Halle M, Blum U, Dinkel E, et al: CT and MR features of primary pulmonary hemangiopericytomas, *J Comput Assist Tomogr* 17:51-55, 1993.

241. Hallgrimson JG, Jonsson T, Johannsson JH: Bronchopulmonary carcinoids in Iceland 1955-1984: a retrospective histopathologic study, *Scand J Thorac Cardiovasc Surg* 23:275-278, 1989.

242. Halprin GM, Ramirez RJ, Pratt PC: Lymphoid interstitial pneumonia, *Chest* 62:418-423, 1972.

243. Hamlin DJ, Burgener FA: CT including sagittal and coronal reconstruction in the evaluation of Pancoast tumors, *J Comput Tomogr* 6:35-40, 1982.

244. Han S, Wills JS, Allen O: Pulmonary blastoma: case report and literature review, *AJR* 127:1048-1049, 1976.

245. Haque AK: Pathology of carcinoma of lung: an update on current concepts, *J Thorac Imag* 7(1):9-20, 1991.

246. Hayabuchi N, Russell WJ, Murakami J: Slow-growing lung cancer in a fixed population sample: radiologic assessments, *Cancer* 52:1098-1104, 1983.

247. Hayabuchi N, Russell WJ, Murakami J, et al: Screening for lung cancer in a fixed population by biennial chest radiography, *Radiology* 148:369-373, 1983.

248. Hayabuchi N, Russell WJ, Murakami J: Problems in radiographic detection and diagnosis of lung cancer, *Acta Radiol* 30:163-167, 1989.

249. Hayward RH: Roentgenogram of the month: migrating lung tumor, *Chest* 66:77-78, 1974.

250. Heaston DK, Putman CE, Rodan BA, et al: Solitary pulmonary metastases in high risk melanoma patients: a prospective comparison of conventional and computed tomography, *AJR* 141:169-174, 1983.

251. Heavey LR, Glazer GM, Gross BH, et al: The role of CT in staging radiographic T1N0M0 lung cancer, *AJR* 146:285-290, 1986.

252. Hedlund GL, Bisset GS, Bove KE: Malignant neoplasms arising in cystic hamartomas of the lung in childhood, *Radiology* 173:77-79, 1989.

253. Heelan RT, Demas BE, Caravelli JF, et al: Superior sulcus tumors: CT and MR imaging, *Radiology* 170:637-641, 1989.

254. Heelan RT, Flehinger BJ, Melamed MR, et al: Non-small-cell lung cancer: results of New York screening program, *Radiology* 151:289-293, 1984.

255. Heelan RT, Martini N, Westcott JW, et al: Carcinomatous involvement of the hilum and mediastinum: computed tomographic and magnetic resonance evaluation, *Radiology* 156:111-115, 1985.

256. Heitmiller RF, Mathisen DJ, Ferry JA, et al: Mucoepidermoid lung tumors, *Ann Thorac Surg* 47:394-399, 1989.

257. Heitzman ER: *The lung: radiologic-pathologic correlations,* ed 2, St Louis, 1984, Mosby.

258. Heitzman ER, Markarian B, DeLise CT: Lymphoproliferative disorders of the thorax, *Semin Roentgenol* 10:73-81, 1975.

259. Heitzman ER, Markarian B, Raasch BN, et al: Pathways of tumor spread through the lung: radiologic correlations with anatomy and pathology, *Radiology* 144:3-14, 1982.

260. Heller RM, Janower ML, Weber AL: The radiological manifestations of malignant pleural mesothelioma, *AJR* 108:53-59, 1970.

261. Helman CA, Kieton GR, Benatar SR: Lymphoid interstitial pneumonia with associated chronic active hepatitis and renal tubular acidosis, *Am Rev Respir Dis* 115:161-164, 1977.

262. Herman PG, Hillman B, Pinkus G, et al: Unusual noninfectious granulomas of the lung, *Radiology* 121:287-292, 1976.

263. Heron CW, Husband JE, Williams MP, et al: Hodgkin's disease: CT of the thymus, *Radiology* 167:647-651, 1988.

264. Hertzanu Y, Heimer D, Hirsch M: Computed tomography of pulmonary endometriosis, *Comput Radiol* 11:81-84, 1987.

265. Herzog KA, Putman CE: Pulmonary blastoma, *Br J Radiol* 47:286-288, 1974.

266. Hicken P, Dobie JC, Frew E: The radiology of lymphomatoid granulomatosis in the lung, *Clin Radiol* 30:661-664, 1979.

267. Hicklin GA, Drevyanko TF: Primary granulocytic sarcoma presenting with pleural and pulmonary involvement, *Chest* 94:655-656, 1988.

268. Higgins GA, Shields TW, Keehn RJ: The solitary pulmonary nodule: ten-year follow up of Veterans Administration–Armed Forces cooperative study, *Arch Surg* 110:570-575, 1975.

269. Hill CA: Bronchioloalveolar carcinoma: a review, *Radiology* 150:15-20, 1984.

270. Hillerdal G: Malignant mesothelioma 1982: review of 4170 published cases, *Br J Dis Chest* 77:321-343, 1983.

271. Hirakata K, Nakata H, Haratake J: Appearance of pulmonary metastases on high-resolution CT scans: comparison with histopathologic findings from autopsy specimens, *AJR* 161:37-43, 1993.

272. Holland EA, Ghahremani GG, Fry WA, et al: Evolution of pulmonary pseudolymphomas: clinical and radiologic manifestations, *J Thorac Imag* 6(4):74-80, 1991.

273. Honda N, Machida K, Kamano T, et al: Gallium scintigraphy in neoplastic angioendotheliosis of the lung, *Clin Nucl Med* 16:43-46, 1991.

274. Hopper KD, Diehl LF, Cole BA, et al: Significance of necrotic mediastinal lymph nodes on CT in patients with newly diagnosed Hodgkin disease, *AJR* 155:267-270, 1990.

275. Hopper KD, Diehl LF, Lessar M, et al: Hodgkin disease: clinical utility of CT in initial staging and treatment, *Radiology* 169:17-22, 1988.

276. Horning SJ, Rosenberg SA: The natural history of initially untreated low-grade non-Hodgkin's lymphoma, *N Engl J Med* 311:1471-1475, 1984.

277. Hough DM: Multifocal osteosarcoma with extensive pleural metastatic disease, *Australas Radiol* 36:147-149, 1992.

278. Howlett TA, Drury PL, Perry L, et al: Diagnosis and management of ACTH-dependent Cushing's syndrome: comparison of the features in ectopic and pituitary ACTH production, *Clin Endocrinol* 24:699-713, 1986.

279. Huang D, Weisbrod GL, Chamberlain DW: Unusual radiologic presentations of bronchioloalveolar cell carcinoma, *J Can Assoc Radiol* 37:94-99, 1986.

280. Huhti E, Saloheimo M, Sutinen S: The value of roentgenologic screening in lung cancer, *Am Rev Respir Dis* 128:395-398, 1983.

281. Hurst R, Bates M: Carcinoid tumours of the bronchus: a 33 year experience, *Thorax* 39:617-623, 1984.

282. Husband JE, Barrett A, Peckham MJ: Evaluation of computed tomography in the management of testicular teratoma, *Br J Urol* 53:179-183, 1981.

283. Hutchinson WB, Friedenberg MJ: Intrathoracic mesothelioma, *Radiology* 80:937-945, 1963.

284. Ikezoe J, Johkoh T, Takeuchi N, et al: CT findings of endobronchial metastasis, *Acta Radiol* 32:455-460, 1991.

285. Ikezoe J, Kadowaki K, Morimoto S: Mediastinal lymph node metastases from non small cell bronchogenic carcinoma: reevaluation with CT, *J Comput Assist Tomogr* 14:340-344, 1990.

286. Im JG, Choi BI, Park JH, et al: CT findings of lobar bronchioloalveolar carcinoma — a case report, *J Comput Assist Tomogr* 10:320-322, 1986.

287. Im JG, Han MC, Yu EJ: Lobar bronchioloalveolar carcinoma: "angiogram sign" on CT scans, *Radiology* 176:749-753, 1990.

288. Ingram CE, Belli AM, Lewars MD, et al: Normal lymph node size in the mediastinum: a retrospective study in two patient groups, *Clin Radiol* 40:35-39, 1989.

289. Israel HL, Patchefsky AS, Saldana MJ: Wegener's granulomatosis, lymphomatoid granulomatosis, and benign lymphocytic angiitis and granulomatosis: recognition and treatment, *Ann Intern Med* 87:691-699, 1977.

290. Israel O, Front D, Epelbaum R: Residual mass and negative gallium scintigraphy in treated lymphoma, *J Nucl Med* 31:365-368, 1990.

291. Israel RH: Mycosis fungoides with rapidly progressive pulmonary infiltration, *Radiology* 125:10, 1977.

292. Jackman RJ, Good CA, Clagett OT, et al: Survival rates in peripheral bronchogenic carcinoma up to four centimeters in diameter presenting as solitary pulmonary nodules, *J Thorac Cardiovasc Surg* 57:1-8, 1969.

293. Jacobson JO, Aisenberg AC, Lamarre L, et al: Primary mediastinal lymphoma: an uncommon subset of adult large cell lymphoma curable with combined modality therapy, *Proc Am Soc Clin Oncol* 7:240, 1988.

294. Janower ML, Blennerhassett JB: Lymphangitic spread of metastatic cancer to the lung: a radiologic-pathologic classification, *Radiology* 101:267-273, 1971.

295. Jenkins PF, Ward MJ, Davies P, et al: Non-Hodgkin's lymphoma, chronic lymphocytic leukaemia and the lung, *Br J Dis Chest* 75:22-30, 1981.

296. Jensen KG, Schiodt T: Growth considerations of hamartoma of the lung, *Thorax* 13:233-237, 1958.

297. Jensen SM, Petersen AH: Bronchial lipoma, *Scand J Thorac Cardiovasc Surg* 4:131-134, 1970.

298. Jett JR, Cortese DA, Fontana RS: Lung cancer: current concepts and prospects, *CA* 33:74-86, 1983.

299. Jochelson MS, Balikian JP, Mauch P, et al: Peri- and paracardial involvement in lymphoma in a radiographic study of 11 cases, *AJR* 140:483-488, 1983.

300. Johkoh T, Ikezoe J, Tomiyama N, et al: CT findings in lymphangitic carcinomatosis of the lung: correlation with histologic findings and pulmonary function tests, *AJR* 158:1217-1222, 1992.

301. Johnson BE: Management of small-cell lung cancer, *Clin Chest Med* 14:173-187, 1993.

302. Johnson DH, Hainsworth JD, Greco FA: Pancoast's syndrome and small cell lung cancer, *Chest* 82:602-606, 1982.

303. Johnston GS, Go MF, Benua RS, et al: Gallium-67 citrate imaging in Hodgkin's disease: final report of cooperative group, *J Nucl Med* 18:692-698, 1977.

304. Joyce JM, Aubrey DL, MacDonald JS, et al: Lung uptake of technetium-99m HDP in giant-cell tumor metastases, *Clin Nucl Med* 14:767-768, 1989.

305. Julsrud PR, Brown LR, Li CY, et al: Pulmonary processes of mature-appearing lymphocytes: pseudolymphoma, well differentiated lymphocytic lymphoma, and lymphocytic interstitial pneumonitis, *Radiology* 127:289-296, 1978.

306. Kameda K, Adachi S, Kono M: Detection of T-factor in lung cancer using magnetic resonance imaging and computed tomography, *J Thorac Imag* 3(2):73-80, 1988.

307. Kaplan JO, Morillo G, Weinfeld A, et al: Mediastinal adenopathy in myeloma, *J Can Assoc Radiol* 31:48-49, 1980.

308. Kaplan WD, Jochelson MS, Herman TS, et al: Gallium-67 imaging: a predictor of residual tumour viability and clinical outcome in patients with diffuse large-cell lymphoma, *J Clin Oncol* 8:1966-1970, 1990.

309. Karasik A, Modam M, Jacob CO, et al: Increased risk of lung cancer in patients with chondromatous hamartoma, *J Thorac Cardiovasc Surg* 80:217-220, 1980.

310. Katzenstein AA, Carrington CB, Liebow AA: Lymphomatoid granulomatosis: a clinicopathologic study of 152 cases, *Cancer* 43:360-373, 1979.

311. Katzenstein AA, Fulling K, Weise, et al: So-called sclerosing hemangioma of the lung: evidence for mesothelial origin, *Am J Surg Pathol* 7:3-14, 1983.

312. Katzenstein AA, Gmelich JT, Carrington CB: Sclerosing hemangioma of the lung: a clinicopathologic study of 51 cases, *Am J Surg Pathol* 4:343-356, 1980.

313. Kawashima A, Libshitz HI: Malignant pleural mesothelioma: CT manifestations in 50 cases, *AJR* 155:965-969, 1990.

314. Kelly RB, Mahoney PD, Johnson JF: A calcified carcinoma of the lung and intracerebral metastasis, *CT: J Comput Tomogr* 11:389-391, 1987.

315. Kennedy JL, Nathwani BN, Burke JS, et al: Pulmonary lymphomas and other pulmonary lymphoid lesions: a clinicopathologic and immunologic study of 64 patients, *Cancer* 56:539-552, 1985.

316. Kern WH, Stiles QR: Pulmonary blastoma, *J Thorac Cardiovasc Surg* 72:801-808, 1976.

317. Kerr KM, Lamb D, Wathen CG, et al: Pathological assessment of mediastinal lymph nodes in lung cancer: implications for noninvasive mediastinal staging, *Thorax* 47:337-341, 1992.

318. Kesler KA, Conces DJ, Heimansohn DA, et al: Assessing the feasibility of bronchoplastic surgery with magnetic resonance imaging, *Ann Thorac Surg* 52:145-157, 1991.

319. Khoury MB, Godwin JD, Halvorsen R, et al: Role of chest CT in non-Hodgkin's lymphoma, *Radiology* 158:659-662, 1986.

320. Kier R, Godwin JD: Residual cavities of lung metastases following chemotherapy, *Comput Radiol* 10:293-296, 1986.

321. Kilgore TL, Chasen MH: Endobronchial non-Hodgkin's lymphoma, *Chest* 84:58-61, 1983.

322. Kim HC, Nosher J, Haas A: Cystic degeneration of thymic Hodgkin's disease following radiation therapy, *Cancer* 55:354-356, 1985.

323. Kinare SG, Parulkar GB, Panday SR, et al: Extensive ossification in a pulmonary plasmacytoma, *Thorax* 20:206-210, 1965.

324. Kirsh MM, Sloan H: Mediastinal metastases in bronchogenic carcinoma: influence of postoperative irradiation, cell type, and location, *Ann Thorac Surg* 33:459-463, 1982.

325. Kiyono K, Sone S, Sakai F, et al: The number and size of normal mediastinal lymph nodes: a postmortem study, *AJR* 150:771-776, 1985.

326. Klatte EC, Yardley J, Smith EB, et al: The pulmonary manifestations and complications of leukemia, *AJR* 89:598-609, 1963.

327. Klein JS, Webb WR: Radiologic staging of lung cancer, *J Thorac Imag* 7(1):29-47, 1991.

328. Kono M, Adachi S, Kusumoto M, et al: Clinical utility of Gd-DTPA-enhanced magnetic resonance imaging in lung cancer, *J Thorac Imag* 8(1):18-26, 1993.

329. Koss MN, Hochholzer L, O'Leary T: Pulmonary blastomas, *Cancer* 67:2368-2381, 1991.

330. Kostrubiak I, Whitley NO, Aisner J, et al: The use of computed body tomography in malignant melanoma, *JAMA* 259:2896-2897, 1988.

331. Kovalski R, Hansen-Flaschen J, Lodato R, et al: Localized leukemic pulmonary infiltrates, *Chest* 97:674-678, 1990.

332. Kovanlikaya A, Pirnar T, Olgun N: Pulmonary blastoma: a rare case of childhood malignant, *Pediatr Radiol* 22:155, 1992.

333. Kradin RL, Mark EJ: Benign lymphoid disorders of the lung with a theory regarding their development, *Hum Pathol* 14:857-867, 1983.

334. Kramer SS, Wehunt WD, Stocker JT, et al: Pulmonary manifestations of juvenile laryngotracheal papillomatosis, *AJR* 144:687-694, 1985.

335. Krenning EP, Kwekkeboom DJ, Bakker WH, et al: Somatostatin receptor scintigraphy with [^{111}In-DTPA-D-Phe^1]- and [^{123}I-Tyr^3]-octreotide: the Rotterdam experience with more than 1000 patients, *Eur J Nucl Med* 20:716-731, 1993.

336. Kreyberg L: *Histological typing of lung tumors*. Vol 1. *International histological classification of tumors*, Geneva, 1967, World Health Organization.

337. Kuhlman JE, Fishman EK, Kuhajda FP, et al: Solitary bronchioloalveolar carcinoma: CT criteria, *Radiology* 167:379-382, 1988.

338. Kundel HL: Predictive value and threshold detectability of lung tumors, *Radiology* 139:25-29, 1981.

339. Kundel HL, Nodine CF, Carmody D: Visual scanning, pattern recognition and decision-making in pulmonary nodule detection, *Invest Radiol* 13:175-181, 1978.

340. Kundel HL, Nodine CF, Krupinski EA: Computed-displayed eye position as a visual aid to pulmonary nodule interpretation, *Invest Radiol* 25:890-896, 1990.

341. Kuriyama K, Tateishi R, Doi O, et al: CT-pathologic correlation in small peripheral lung cancers, *AJR* 149:1139-1143, 1987.

342. Kuriyama K, Tateishi R, Doi O, et al: Prevalence of air bronchograms in small peripheral carcinomas of the lung on thin-section CT: comparison with benign tumors, *AJR* 156:921-924, 1991.

343. Kwong JS, Müller NL, Miller RR: Diseases of the trachea and main-stem bronchi: correlation of CT with pathologic findings, *Radiographics* 12:645-657, 1992.

344. Lahde S, Paivansalo M, Rainio P: CT for predicting the resectability of lung cancer: a prospective study, *Acta Radiol* 32:449-454, 1991.

345. Laufer L, Cohen Z, Mares AJ, et al: Pulmonary plasma-cell granuloma, *Paediatr Radiol* 20:289-290, 1990.

346. Laurent F, Drouillard J, Dorcier F: Bronchogenic carcinoma staging: CT vs MR imaging—assessment with surgery, *Eur J Cardiothorac Surg* 2:31-36, 1988.

347. Law MR, Gregor A, Husband JE, et al: Computed tomography in the assessment of malignant mesothelioma of the pleura, *Clin Radiol* 33:67-70, 1982.

348. Lawson RM, Ramanathan L, Hurley G, et al: Bronchial adenoma: review of an 18 year experience at the Brompton Hospital, *Thorax* 31:245-252, 1976.

349. Lederle FA, Nichol KL, Parenti CM. Bronchoscopy to evaluate hemoptysis in older men with nonsuspicious chest roentgenograms, *Chest* 95:1043-1047, 1989.

350. Ledor K, Fish B, Chaise L, et al: CT of pulmonary hamartomas, *J Comput Tomogr* 5:343-344, 1981.

351. Lee KS, Im JG: Benign fibrous mesothelioma of the pleura: MR findings (letter), *AJR* 160:205, 1993.

352. Lee KS, Im J-G, Choe KO, et al: CT findings in benign fibrous mesothelioma of the pleura: pathologic correlation in nine patients, *AJR* 158:983-986, 1992.

353. Lee MJ, Grogan L, Meehan S, et al: Pleural granulocytic sarcoma: CT characteristics, *Clin Radiol* 43:57-59, 1991.

354. Lee WA, Hruban RH, Kuhlman JE, et al: High resolution computed tomography of inflation-fixed lungs: pathologic-radiologic correlation of pulmonary lesions in patients with leukemia, lymphoma or other hematopoietic proliferative disorders, *Clin Imag* 16:15-24, 1992.

355. Legha SS, Muggia FM: Pleural mesothelioma: clinical features and therapeutic implications, *Ann Intern Med* 87:612-613, 1977.

356. Lehar TJ, Carr DT, Miller WE, et al: Roentgenographic appearance of bronchogenic adenocarcinoma, *Am Rev Respir Dis* 96:245-248, 1967.

357. Leskinen-Kallio S, Ruotsalainen U, Nagren K, et al: Uptake of carbon-11-methionine and fluorodeoxyglucose in non-Hodgkin's lymphoma: a PET study, *J Nucl Med* 32:1211-1218, 1991.

358. Leung AN, Muller NL, Millere RR: CT in differential diagnosis of diffuse pleural disease, *AJR* 154:487-492, 1990.

359. Levitt RG, Glazer HS, Roper CL, et al: Magnetic resonance imaging of mediastinal and hilar masses: comparison with CT, *AJR* 145:9-14, 1985.

360. Lewis E, Bernadino ME, Farha P, et al: Computed tomography and routine chest radiography: oat cell carcinoma of the lung, *J Comput Assist Tomogr* 6:739-745, 1982.

361. Lewis ER, Caskey CI, Fishman EK: Lymphoma of the lung: CT findings in 31 patients, *AJR* 156:711-714, 1991.

362. Lewis JW, Madrazo BL, Gross SC: The value of radiographic and computed tomography in the staging of lung carcinoma, *Ann Thorac Surg* 34:553-558, 1982.

363. Lewis JW, Pearlberg JL, Beaute GH, et al: Can computed tomography of the chest stage lung cancer? Yes and no, *Ann Thorac Surg* 49:591-596, 1990.

364. Lewis MI, Horak DA, Yellin A, et al: Roentgenogram of the month: the case of the moving intrathoracic mass, *Chest* 88:897-898, 1985.

365. Libshitz HI: Malignant pleural mesothelioma: the role of computed tomography, *J Comput Tomogr* 8:15-20, 1984.

366. Libshitz HI: Computed tomography in bronchogenic carcinoma, *Semin Roentgenol* 25:64-72, 1990.

367. Libshitz HI, Baber CE, Hammond CB: The pulmonary metastases of choriocarcinoma, *Obstet Gynecol* 49:412-416, 1977.

368. Libshitz HI, Jing BS, Wallace S, et al: Sterilized metastases: a diagnostic and therapeutic dilemma, *AJR* 140:15-19, 1983.

369. Libshitz HI, McKenna RJ: Mediastinal lymph node size in lung cancer, *AJR* 143:715-718, 1984.

370. Libshitz HI, McKenna RJ, Haynie TP, et al: Mediastinal evaluation in lung cancer, *Radiology* 151:295-299, 1984.

371. Libshitz HI, McKenna RJ, Mountain CF: Patterns of mediastinal metastases in bronchogenic carcinoma, *Chest* 90:229-232, 1986.

372. Liebow AA: Pathology of carcinoma of the lung as related to the roentgen shadow, *AJR* 74:383-401, 1955.

373. Liebow AA: The J. Burns Amberson lecture—pulmonary angiitis and granulomatosis, *Am Rev Respir Dis* 108:1-18, 1973.

374. Liebow AA, Carrington CB: Diffuse pulmonary lymphoreticular infiltrations associated with dysproteinemia, *Med Clin North Am* 57:809-843, 1973.

375. Liebow AA, Carrington CB, Friedman PJ: Lymphomatoid granulomatosis, *Hum Pathol* 3:457-558, 1972.

376. Light RW: *Pleural disease*, Philadelphia, 1983, Lea & Febiger.

377. Light RW, Ball WB: Glucose and amylase in pleural effusions, *JAMA* 225:257-260, 1973.

378. Limas C, Japaze H, Garcia-Bunuel R: "Scar" carcinoma of the lung, *Chest* 59:219-222, 1971.

379. List AF, Greco AF, Vogler LB: Lymphoproliferative diseases in immunocompromised hosts: the role of Epstein-Barr virus, *J Clin Oncol* 5:1673-1689, 1987.

380. Lister TA, Crowther DM, Sutcliffe SB: Report of a committee convened to discuss the evaluation and staging of patients with Hodgkin's disease: Cotswold meeting, *J Clin Oncol* 7:1630-1636, 1989.

381. Long JC, Mihm MC: Mycosis fungoides with extracutaneous dissemination: a distinct clinicopathologic entity, *Cancer* 34:1745-1755, 1974.

382. Lorigan JG, Libshitz HI: MR imaging of malignant pleural mesothelioma, *J Comput Assist Tomogr* 13:617-620, 1989.

383. Luddington LG, Verska JJ, Howard T, et al: Bronchiolar carcinoma (alveolar cell), another great imitator: a review of 41 cases, *Chest* 61:622-628, 1972.

384. Lukes RJ, Craver LF, Hall TC, et al: Report of the nomenclature committee, *Cancer Res* 26:1311, 1966.

385. Maasilta P, Tammilehto L, Mattson K, et al: Bronchial carcinoid with a twenty-four-year natural history: a case report, *Acta Oncol* 28:715, 1989.

386. MacDonald JB: Lung involvement in Hodgkin's disease, *Thorax* 32:664-667, 1977.

387. MacMahon H, Scott W, Ryan JW, et al: Efficacy of computed tomography of the thorax and upper abdomen and whole-body gallium scintigraphy for staging of lung cancer, *Cancer* 64:1404-1408, 1989.

388. Madewell JE, Feigin DS: Benign tumors of the lung, *Semin Roentgenol* 12:175-186, 1977.

389. Madri JA, Carter D: Scar cancers of the lung: origin and significance, *Hum Pathol* 15:625-631, 1984.

390. Magid D, Siegelman SS, Eggleston JC, et al: Pulmonary carcinoid tumors: CT assessment, *J Comput Assist Tomogr* 13:244-247, 1989.

391. Magrath IT: Malignant non-Hodgkin's lymphomas in children, *Hematol Oncol Clin North Am* 1:577-602, 1987.

392. Mahoney MC, Shipley RT, Corcoran HL, et al: CT demonstration of calcification in carcinoma of the lung, *AJR* 154:255-258, 1990.

393. Maile CW, Moore AV, Ulreich S, et al: Chest radiographic-pathologic correlation in adult leukemia patients, *Invest Radiol* 18:495-499, 1983.

394. Maile CW, Rodan BA, Godwin JD, et al: Calcification in pulmonary metastases, *Br J Radiol* 55:108-113, 1982.

395. Major D, Meltzer MH, Nedwich A, et al: Waldenstrom's macroglobulinemia presenting as a pulmonary mass, *Chest* 64:760-762, 1973.

396. Malatskey A, Fields S, Lisbon E: CT appearance of primary pleural lymphoma, *Comput Med Imag Graph* 13:165-167, 1989.

397. Manivel JC, Priest JR, Watterson J, et al: Pleuropulmonary blastoma: the so-called pulmonary blastoma of childhood, *Cancer* 62:1516-1526, 1988.

398. Marglin SI, Castellino RA: Selection of imaging studies for the initial staging of patients with Hodgkin's disease, *Semin Ultrasound, CT, MR* 6:380-393, 1985.

399. Marglin SI, Laing FC, Castellino RA: Current status of mediastinal sonography in the posttreatment evaluation of patients with lymphoma, *AJR* 157:469-470, 1991.

400. Marglin SI, Soulen RL, Blank N, et al: Mycosis fungoides: radiographic manifestations of extracutaneous intrathoracic involvement, *Radiology* 130:35-37, 1979.

401. Mark EJ: Mesenchymal cystic hamartoma of the lung, *N Engl J Med* 315:1255-1259, 1986.

402. Marriott AE, Weisbrod G: Bronchogenic carcinoma associated with pulmonary infarction, *Radiology* 145:593-597, 1982.

403. Martin E: Leiomyomatous lung lesions: a proposed classification, *AJR* 141:269-272, 1983.

404. Martini N, Flehinger BJ, Zaman MB: Results of resection in non-oat cell carcinoma of the lung with mediastinal lymph node metastases, *Ann Surg* 198:386-397, 1983.

405. Martini N, Heelan R, Westcott J, et al: Comparative merits of conventional computed tomographic and magnetic resonance imaging in assessing mediastinal involvement in surgically confirmed lung carcinoma, *J Thorac Cardiovasc Surg* 90:639-648, 1985.

406. Mata JM, Cáceres J, Ferrer J, et al: Endobronchial lipoma: CT diagnosis, *J Comput Assist Tomogr* 15:750-751, 1991.

407. Mata JM, Cáceres J, Prat J, et al: Intravascular bronchioalveolar tumor: radiographic findings, *Eur J Radiol* 12:95-97, 1991.

408. Matsubara O, Tan-Liu NS, Kenney RM, et al: Inflammatory pseudotumors of the lung: progression from organizing pneumonia to fibrous histiocytoma or to plasma cell granuloma in 32 cases, *Hum Pathol* 19:807-814, 1988.

409. Matthay RA, Coppage L, Shaw C, et al: Malignancies metastatic to the pleura, *Invest Radiol* 25:601-609, 1990.

410. Matthews JI, Richey HM, Helsel RA: Thoracic computed tomography in the preoperative evaluation of primary bronchogenic carcinoma, *Arch Intern Med* 147:449-453, 1987.

411. Mayr B, Lenhard M, Fink U, et al: Preoperative evaluation of bronchogenic carcinoma: value of MR in T- and N-staging, *Eur J Radiol* 14:245-251, 1992.

412. Mazas-Artasona L, Romeo M, Felices R, et al: Gastro-oesophageal leiomyoblastoma and multiple pulmonary chondromas: an incomplete variant of Carney's triad, *Br J Radiol* 61:1181-1184, 1988.

413. Mazumdar P, Abraham S, Damodaran VN, et al: Pulmonary plasmacytoma: a case report, *Am Rev Respir Dis* 100:866-869, 1969.

414. McAfee MK, Allen MS, Trastek VF, et al: Colorectal lung metastases: results of surgical excision, *Ann Thorac Surg* 53:780-786, 1992.

415. McCaughan BC, Martini N, Bains MS: Bronchial carcinoids: review of 124 cases, *J Thorac Cardiovasc Surg* 89:8-17, 1985.

416. McCaughan BC, Martini N, Bains MS, et al: Chest wall invasion of carcinoma of the lung: therapeutic and prognostic implications, *J Thorac Cardiovasc Surg* 89:836-841, 1985.

417. McCormack PM, Burt ME, Bains MS, et al: Lung resection for colorectal metastases: 10-year results, *Arch Surg* 127:1403-1406, 1992.

418. McDonald AD, Harper A, EL Attar OA, et al: Epidemiology of primary malignant mesothelial tumors in Canada, *Cancer* 26:914-919, 1970.

419. McDonnell T, Kyriakos M, Roper R, et al: Malignant fibrous histiocytoma of the lung, *Cancer* 61:137-145, 1988.

420. McElvaney G, Miller RR, Müller NR, et al: Multicentricity of adenocarcinoma of the lung, *Chest* 95:151-154, 1989.

421. McGuinnis EJ, Lull RJ: Bronchial adenoma causing unilateral absence of pulmonary perfusion, *Radiology* 120:367-368, 1976.

422. McKenna RJ, Haynie TP, Libshitz HI, et al: Critical evaluation of the gallium-67 scan for surgical patients with lung cancer, *Chest* 87:428-431, 1985.

423. McLaughlin AF, Magee MA, Greenough R, et al: Current role of gallium scanning in the management of lymphoma, *Eur J Nucl Med* 16:755-771, 1990.

424. McLoud TC: CT of bronchogenic carcinoma: indeterminate mediastinal invasion (editorial), *Radiology* 173:15-16, 1989.

425. McLoud TC, Bourgouin PM, Greenberg RW, et al: Bronchogenic carcinoma: analysis of staging in the mediastinum with CT by correlative lymph node mapping and sampling, *Radiology* 182:319-323, 1992.

426. McLoud TC, Filion RB, Edelman RR, et al: MR imaging of superior sulcus carcinoma, *J Comput Assist Tomogr* 13:233-239, 1989.

427. McLoud TC, Isler RJ, Novelline RA, et al: The apical cap, *AJR* 137:299-306, 1981.

428. McLoud TC, Kalisher L, Stark P, et al: Intrathoracic lymph node metastases from extrathoracic neoplasm, *AJR* 131:403-407, 1978.

429. Meade JB, Whitwell F, Bickford BJ, et al: Primary haemangiopericytoma of lung, *Thorax* 29:1-15, 1974.

430. Melamed MR, Flehinger BJ, Zaman MB, et al: Detection of true pathologic stage I lung cancer in a screening program and the effect on survival, *Cancer* 47:1182-1187, 1981.

431. Melamed MR, Flehinger BJ, Zaman MB, et al: Screening for early lung cancer: results of the Memorial Sloan-Kettering study in New York, *Chest* 86:44-53, 1984.

432. Mendelson DS, Apter S, Kirschner PA, et al: Magnetic resonance imaging and computed tomography findings in a patient with lymphomatoid granulomatosis, *Clin Imag* 13:130-133, 1989.

433. Mendelson DS, Meary E, Buy JN: Localised fibrous mesothelioma: CT findings, *Clin Imag* 15:105-108, 1991.

434. Mendelsohn SL, Fagelman D, Zwanger-Mendelsohn S: Endobronchial lipoma demonstrated by CT, *Radiology* 148:790-792, 1983.

435. Metzger RA, Mulhern CB, Arger PH, et al: CT differentiation of solitary from diffuse bronchioloalveolar carcinoma, *J Comput Assist Tomogr* 5:830-833, 1981.

436. Meyer EC, Liebow AA: Relationship of interstitial pneumonia, honeycombing and atypical epithelial proliferation to cancer of the lung, *Cancer* 18:322-351, 1965.

437. Meyer JA, Linggood RM, Lindfors KK, et al: Impact of thoracic computed tomography on radiation planning in Hodgkin's disease, *J Comput Assist Tomogr* 8:892-894, 1984.

438. Meyer PC: Metastatic carcinoma of the pleura, *Thorax* 21:437-443, 1966.

439. Miller JI, Mansour KA, Hatcher CR: Carcinoma of the superior pulmonary sulcus, *Ann Thorac Surg* 28:44-47, 1979.

440. Miller RR: Bronchioloalveolar cell adenomas, *Am J Surg Pathol* 14:904-912, 1990.

441. Miller RR, Nelems B, Evans KG, et al: Glandular neoplasia of the lung: a proposed analogy to colonic tumors, *Cancer* 61:1009-1014, 1988.

442. Miller WT, Husted J, Freiman D, et al: Bronchioloalveolar carcinoma: two clinical entities with one pathological diagnosis, *AJR* 130:905-912, 1978.

443. Mills SE, Walker AN, Cooper PH, et al: Atypical carcinoid tumour of the lung: clinicopathologic study in 17 cases, *Am J Surg Pathol* 6:643-654, 1982.

444. Milne ENC, Zerhouni EA: Blood supply of pulmonary metastases, *J Thorac Imag* 2(4):15-23, 1987.

445. Minami M, Kawauchi N, Matsuoka Y, et al: Cine CT with electrocardiography and respiratory gating in the evaluation of structures surrounding lung and mediastinal tumours, *Radiology* 185(P)(suppl):132, 1992.

446. Mirvis S, Dutcher JP, Haney PJ, et al: CT of malignant pleural mesothelioma, *AJR* 140:665-670, 1983.

447. Miura K, Hori T, Yoshizawa K: Cystic pulmonary hamartoma, *Ann Thorac Surg* 49:828-829, 1990.

448. Montes M, Tomasi TB, Noehren TH, et al: Lymphoid interstitial pneumonia with monoclonal gammopathy, *Am Rev Respir Dis* 98:272-280, 1968.

449. Monzon CM, Gilchrist GS, Burgert EO, et al: Plasma cell granuloma of the lung in children, *Pediatrics* 70:268-274, 1982.

450. Moores DWO: Pulmonary metastases revisited, *Ann Thorac Surg* 52:178-179, 1991.

451. Morgan DE, Sanders C, McElvein RB: Intrapulmonary teratoma: a case report and review of the literature, *J Thorac Imag* 7:70-77, 1992.

452. Mori K, Saitou Y, Tominaga K, et al: Small nodular lesions in the lung periphery: a new approach to diagnosis with CT, *Radiology* 177:843-849, 1990.

453. Mori S, Itoyama S, Mohri N, et al: Cellular characteristics of neoplastic angioendotheliosis, *Virchows Arch A* 407:167-175, 1985.

454. Mountain CF: The biological operability of stage III non-small cell lung cancer, *Ann Thorac Surg* 40:60-64, 1985.

455. Mountain CF: A new international staging system for lung cancer, *Chest* 89(suppl):225S-233S, 1986.

456. Mountain CF, McMurtrey MJ, Hermes KE: Surgery for pulmonary metastasis: a 20 year experience, *Ann Thorac Surg* 38:323-330, 1984.

457. Muhm JR, Brown LR, Crowe JK, et al: Comparison of whole lung tomography and computed tomography for detecting pulmonary nodules, *AJR* 131:981-984, 1978.

458. Muhm JR, Miller EW, Fontana RS, et al: Lung cancer detected during a screening program using four month chest radiographs, *Radiology* 148:609-615, 1983.

459. Müller NL, Miller RR: Neuroendocrine carcinomas of the lung, *Semin Roentgenol* 25:96-104, 1990.

460. Munk PL, Müller NL: Pleural liposarcoma: CT diagnosis, *J Comput Assist Tomogr* 12:709-710, 1988.

461. Munk PL, Muller NL, Miller RR, et al: Pulmonary lymphangitic carcinomatosis: CT and pathologic findings, *Radiology* 166:705-709, 1988.

462. Murata K, Takahashi M, Mori M, et al: Multiple-section dynamic CT during expiration for the evaluation of thoracic wall invasion of lung cancer, *Radiology* 185(P)(suppl):131-132, 1991.

463. Murata K, Takahashi M, Mori M, et al: Pulmonary metastatic nodules: CT-pathologic correlation, *Radiology* 182:331-335, 1992.

464. Mushtaq M, Ward SP, Hutchison JT, et al: Multiple cystic pulmonary hamartomas, *Thorax* 47:1076-1077, 1992.

465. Musset D, Grenier P, Carette MF, et al: Primary lung cancer staging: prospective comparative study of MR imaging with CT, *Radiology* 160:607-611, 1986.

466. Myers JC: Lymphomatoid granulomatosis: past, present, . . . future? (editorial), *Mayo Clin Proc* 65:274-278, 1990.

467. Myers TJ, Cole SR, Klatsky AU, et al: Respiratory failure due to pulmonary leukostasis following chemotherapy of acute non-lymphocytic leukemia, *Cancer* 51:1808-1813, 1983.

468. Naidich DP: CT/MR correlation in the evaluation of tracheobronchial neoplasia, *Radiol Clin North Am* 28:555-571, 1990.

469. Naidich DP, McCauley DI, Siegelman SS: Computed tomography of bronchial adenomas, *J Comput Assist Tomogr* 6:725-732, 1982.

470. Naka Y, Nakao K, Hamaji Y, et al: Solitary squamous cell papilloma of the trachea, *Ann Thorac Surg* 55:189-193, 1993.

471. Naruke T, Goya T, Tsuchiya R: The importance of surgery to non-small cell carcinoma of lung with mediastinal lymph node metastasis, *Ann Thorac Surg* 46:603-610, 1988.

472. Nash FA, Morgan JM, Tomkins JC: South London lung cancer study, *Br Med J* 2:715-721, 1968.

473. Nathan MH, Collins VP, Adams RA: Differentiation of benign and malignant pulmonary nodules by growth rate, *Radiology* 79:221-232, 1962.

474. National Cancer Institute—sponsored study of classifications of non-Hodgkin's lymphomas: summary and description of a working formulation for clinical usage, *Cancer* 49:2112-2135, 1982.

475. Naunheim KS, Taylor JR, Skosey C: Adenosquamous lung carcinoma: clinical characteristics, treatment, and prognosis, *Ann Thorac Surg* 44:462-466, 1987.

476. Negendank WG, Al-Katib AM, Karanes C, et al: Lymphomas: MR imaging contrast characteristics with clinico-pathologic correlations, *Radiology* 177:209-216, 1990.

477. Neiman RS, Barcos M, Berard C, et al: Granulocytic sarcoma: a clinicopathologic study of 61 biopsied cases, *Cancer* 48:1426-1437, 1981.

478. Nessi R, Ricci PB, Ricci SB, et al: Bronchial carcinoid tumors: radiologic observations in 49 cases, *J Thorac Imag* 6(2):47-53, 1991.

479. Ng YY, Healy JC, Vincent JE, et al: Non-Hodgkin's lymphoma in childhood, *Clin Radiol*, in press.

480. Nichols DM, Johnson MA: Calcification in a pleural mesothelioma, *J Can Assoc Radiol* 34:311-313, 1983.

481. Nishizawa S, Higa T, Kuroda Y, et al: Increased accumulation of N-isopropyl-(I-123) p-iodoamphetamine in bronchial carcinoid tumor, *J Nucl Med* 31:240-242, 1990.

482. North LB, Libshitz HI, Lorigan JG. Thoracic lymphoma, *Radiol Clin North Am* 28:745-762, 1990.

483. Nyman RS, Rehn SM, Glimelius BLG, et al: Residual mediastinal masses in Hodgkin's disease: prediction of size with MR imaging, *Radiology* 170:435-440, 1989.

484. O'Connell RS, McLoud TC, Wilkins EW: Superior sulcus tumor: radiographic diagnosis and workup, *AJR* 140:25-30, 1983.

485. Oels HC, Harrison EG, Carr DT, et al: Diffuse malignant mesothelioma of the pleura: a review of 37 cases, *Chest* 60:664-670, 1971.

486. Oestmann JW, Greene R, Kushner DC, et al: Lung lesions: correlation between viewing time and detection, *Radiology* 166:451-453, 1988.

487. Okada J, Yoshikawa K, Imazeki K, et al: Use of FDG-PET in the detection and management of malignant lymphoma: correlation of uptake with prognosis, *J Nucl Med* 32:686-691, 1991.

488. Okike N, Bernatz PE, Woolner LB: Localized mesothelioma of the pleura: benign and malignant variants, *J Thorac Cardiovasc Surg* 75:363-372, 1978.

489. Oleszczuk-Raszke K, Cremin BJ: Computed tomography in pulmonary papillomatosis, *Br J Radiol* 61:160-161, 1988.

490. Onitsuka H, Tsukuda M, Araki A, et al: Differentiation of central lung tumor from postobstructive lobar collapse by rapid sequence computed tomography, *J Thorac Imag* 6(2):28-31, 1991.

491. Osborne BM: Contextual diagnosis of Hodgkin's disease and non-Hodgkin's lymphoma, *Radiol Clin North Am* 28:669-682, 1990.

492. Osborne DR, Korobkin M: Detection of intrathoracic lymph node metastases from lung carcinoma (letter), *Radiology* 144:187-188, 1982.

493. Osborne DR, Korobkin M, Ravin CE, et al: Comparison of plain radiography, conventional tomography and computed tomography in detecting intrathoracic metastases from lung carcinoma, *Radiology* 142:157-161, 1982.

494. Otis CN, Carter D, Cole S, et al: Immunohistochemical evaluation of pleural mesothelioma and pulmonary adenocarcinoma: a bi-institutional study of 47 cases, *Am J Surg Pathol* 11:445-456, 1987.

495. Overholt RH, Neptune WB, Ashraf MM: Primary cancer of the lung: a 42 year experience, *Ann Thorac Surg* 20:511-519, 1975.

496. Padovani B, Mouroux J, Seksik L, et al: Chest wall invasion by bronchogenic carcinoma: evaluation with MR imaging, *Radiology* 187:33-38, 1993.

497. Paladgu RR, Benfield JR, Pak HY, et al: Bronchopulmonary Kulchitsky cell carcinomas: a new classification scheme for typical and atypical carcinoids, *Cancer* 55:1303-1311, 1985.

498. Pancoast HK: Superior sulcus tumor: tumor characterized by pain, Horner's syndrome, destruction of bone and atrophy of hand muscles, *JAMA* 99:1391-1396, 1932.

499. Panicek DM: MR imaging for pulmonary metastases? *Radiology* 182:10-11, 1992.

500. Panicek DM, Toner GC, Heelan RT, et al: Nonseminomatous germ cell tumors: enlarging masses despite chemotherapy, *Radiology* 175:499-502, 1990.

501. Parker BR, Castellino RA, Kaplan HS: Pediatric Hodgkin's disease. I. Radiographic evaluation, *Cancer* 37:2430-2435, 1976.

502. Parker LA, Mauro MA, Delany DJ: Evaluation of T1NoMo lung cancer with CT, *J Comput Assist Tomogr* 15:943-947, 1991.

503. Patterson GA, Ginsberg RJ, Poon PY, et al: A prospective evaluation of magnetic resonance imaging, computed tomography, and mediastinoscopy in the preoperative assessment of mediastinal node status in bronchogenic carcinoma, *J Thorac Cardiovasc Surg* 94:679-684, 1987.

504. Patz EF, Shaffer K, Piwnica-Worms DR, et al: Malignant pleural mesothelioma: value of CT and MR imaging in predicting resectability, *AJR* 159:961-966, 1992.

505. Paulson DL: Carcinomas in the superior pulmonary sulcus, *J Thorac Cardiovasc Surg* 70:1095-1104, 1975.

506. Paulson DL: Carcinoma in the superior pulmonary sulcus, *Ann Thorac Surg* 28:3-4, 1979.

507. Peacock MJ, Whitwell F: Pulmonary blastoma, *Thorax* 31:197-204, 1976.

508. Pearl M: Post inflammatory pseudotumor of the lung in children, *Radiology* 105:391-395, 1972.

509. Pearlberg JH, Sandler MA, Beute GH, et al: T1N0M0 bronchogenic carcinoma: assessment by CT, *Radiology* 157:187-190, 1985.

510. Pearlberg JL, Sandler MA, Beute GH: Limitations of CT in evaluation of neoplasms involving chest wall, *J Comput Assist Tomogr* 11:290-293, 1987.

511. Pearlberg JL, Sandler MA, Lewis JW: Small-cell bronchogenic carcinoma: CT evaluation, *Radiology* 150:265-268, 1988.

512. Pearson FG, DeLarue NC, Ilves R, et al: Significance of positive superior mediastinal nodes identified at mediastinoscopy in patients with resectable cancer of the lung, *J Thorac Cardiovasc Surg* 83:1-11, 1982.

513. Pennes DR, Glazer GM, Wimbish KH, et al: Chest wall invasion by lung cancer: limitations of CT evaluation, *AJR* 144:507-511, 1985.

514. Petersen M: Radionuclide detection of primary pulmonary osteogenic sarcoma: a case report and review of the literature, *J Nucl Med* 131:1110-1114, 1990.

515. Peuchot M, Libshitz HI: Pulmonary metastatic disease: radiologic-surgical correlation, *Radiology* 164:719-722, 1987.

516. Phillips CJ, Müller NL, Miller RR, et al: Large calcified pleural-based mass in the left hemithorax, *J Can Assoc Radiol* 41:232-235, 1990.

517. Piehler JM, Pairolero PC, Weiland LH, et al: Bronchogenic carcinoma with chest wall invasion: factors affecting survival following enbloc resection, *Ann Thorac Surg* 34:684-691, 1982.

518. Pietra GG: The pathology of carcinoma of the lung, *Semin Roentgenol* 25:25-33, 1990.

519. Pisani RJ, De Remee RA: Clinical implications of the histopathologic diagnosis of pulmonary lymphomatoid granulomatosis, *Mayo Clin Proc* 65:151-163, 1990.

520. Pock Steen OC: Bronchial adenoma, *Acta Radiol* 51:266-272, 1959.

521. Pocock E, Craig JR, Bullock WK: Metastatic uterine leiomyoma, *Cancer* 38:2096-2100, 1976.

522. Pogrebniak HW, Roth JA, Steinberg SM, et al: Reoperative pulmonary resection in patients with metastatic soft tissue sarcoma, *Ann Thorac Surg* 52:197-203, 1991.

523. Poirier TJ, Van Ordstrand HS: Pulmonary chondromatous hamartoma: report of seventeen cases and review of the literature, *Chest* 59:50-55, 1971.

524. Poon PY, Bronskill MJ, Henkelman RM, et al: Mediastinal lymph node metastases from bronchogenic carcinoma: detection with MR imaging and CT, *Radiology* 162:651-656, 1987.

525. Potchen EJ, Bisesi MA: When is it malpractise to miss lung cancer on chest radiographs? *Radiology* 175:29-32, 1990.

526. Poulsen JT, Jacobsen M, Francis D: Probable malignant transformation of a pulmonary hamartoma, *Thorax* 34:557-558, 1979.

527. Prénovault JMN, Weisbrod GL, Herman SJ: Lymphomatoid granulomatosis: a review of 12 cases, *J Can Assoc Radiol* 39:263-266, 1988.

528. Primack A: The production of markers by bronchogenic carcinoma: a review, *Semin Oncol* 1:235-244, 1974.

529. Pugatch RD, Gale ME: Obscure pulmonary masses: bronchial impaction revealed by CT, *AJR* 141:909-914, 1983.

530. Quint LE, Glazer GM, Orringer MB, et al: Mediastinal lymph node detection and sizing at CT and autopsy, *AJR* 147:469-472, 1986.

531. Quint LE, Glazer GM, Orringer MB: Central lung masses: prediction with CT of need for pneumonectomy versus lobectomy, *Radiology* 165:735-738, 1987.

532. Rabinowitz JG, Efremidis SC, Cohen B, et al: A comparative study of mesothelioma and asbestosis using computed tomography and conventional chest radiography, *Radiology* 144:453-460, 1982.

533. Radford JA, Cowan RA, Flanagan M, et al: The significance of residual mediastinal abnormality of the chest radiograph following treatment for Hodgkin's disease, *J Clin Oncol* 6:940-946, 1988.

534. Ramanathan T: Primary leiomyosarcoma of the lung, *Thorax* 29:482-489, 1974.

535. Rappaport H: Tumors of the hematopoietic system. In Rappaport H, ed: *Atlas of tumor pathology*, section 2, fascicle 8, Washington, DC, 1966, Armed Forces Institute of Pathology.

536. Rappaport H, Berard CW, Butler JJ: Report of the committee on histopathological criteria contributing to staging of Hodgkin's disease, *Cancer Res* 31:1864-1865, 1971.

537. Ratto GB, Piacenza G, Frola C, et al: Chest wall involvement by lung cancer: computed tomographic detection and results of operation, *Ann Thorac Surg* 51:182-188, 1991.

538. Rehn SM, Nyman RS, Glimelius BLG, et al: Non-Hodgkin lymphoma: predicting prognostic grade with MR imaging, *Radiology* 176:249-253, 1990.

539. Reifsnyder AC, Smith HJ, Mulhollan TJ, et al: Malignant fibrous histiocytoma of the lung in a patient with history of asbestos exposure, *AJR* 154:65-66, 1990.

540. Remy-Jardin M, Remy J, Giraud F, et al: Pulmonary nodules: detection with thick-section spiral CT versus conventional CT, *Radiology* 187:513-520, 1993.

541. Ren H, Hruban RH, Kuhlman JE, et al: Computed tomography of inflation-fixed lungs: the beaded septum sign of pulmonary metastases, *J Comput Assist Tomogr* 13:411-416, 1989.

542. Rendina EA, Bognolo DA, Mineo TC, et al: Computed tomography for the evaluation of intrathoracic invasion by lung cancer, *J Thorac Cardiovasc Surg* 94:57-63, 1987.

543. Ricci C, Patrassi N, Massa R: Carcinoid syndrome in bronchial adenoma, *Am J Surg* 126:671-677, 1973.

544. Richardson S, Hirsch A, Ruffie P, et al: Relationship between tuberculous scar and carcinomas of the lung, *Eur J Radiol* 17:163-164, 1987.

545. Rigler LG: A roentgen study of the evolution of carcinoma of the lung, *J Thorac Surg* 34:283-297, 1957.

546. Rigler LG: The roentgen signs of carcinoma of the lung, *AJR* 74:415-428, 1955.

547. Robbins SL, Cotran RS, Kumar V: *Pathologic basis of disease*, ed 3, Philadelphia, 1984, WB Saunders.

548. Rohlfing BM, White EA, Webb WR, et al: Hilar and mediastinal adenopathy caused by bacterial abscess of the lung, *Radiology* 128:289-293, 1978.

549. Rohwedder JJ, Weatherbee L: Multiple primary bronchogenic carcinoma with a review of the literature, *Am Rev Respir Dis* 109:435-445, 1974.

550. Romney BM, Austin JHM: Plain film evaluation of carcinoma of the lung, *Semin Roentgenol* 25:45-63, 1990.

551. Rosenbaum HD, Alavi SM, Bryant LR: Pulmonary parenchymal spread of juvenile laryngeal papillomatosis, *AJR* 90:654-660, 1968.

552. Rosenberg SA, Kaplan HS: Evidence for an orderly progression in the spread of Hodgkin's disease, *Cancer Res* 26:1225-1231, 1966.

553. Rosenow EC, Carr DT: Bronchogenic carcinoma, *CA* 29:233-245, 1979.

554. Ross GR, Violi L, Friedman AC, et al: Intravascular bronchioloalveolar tumor: CT and pathologic correlation, *J Comput Assist Tomogr* 13:240-243, 1989.

555. Ross JS, Ellman L: Leukemic infiltration of the lungs in the chemotherapeutic era, *Am J Clin Pathol* 61:235-241, 1974.

556. Rostock RA, Giangreco A, Wharam MD, et al: CT scan modification in the treatment of mediastinal Hodgkin's disease, *Cancer* 49:2267-2275, 1982.

557. Rubin DL, Blank N: Rapid pulmonary dissemination in mycosis fungoides simulating pneumonia: a case report and review of the literature, *Cancer* 56:649-651, 1985.

558. Rubin SA: Lung cancer: past, present and future, *J Thorac Imag* 7(1):1-8, 1991.

559. Rubinstein I, Baum GL, Kalter Y, et al: The influence of cell type and lymph node metastases on survival of patients with carcinoma of the lung undergoing thoracotomy, *Am Rev Respir Dis* 119:253-262, 1979.

560. Rusch VW, Godwin JD, Shuman WP: The role of computed tomography scanning in the initial assessment and follow-up of malignant pleural mesothelioma, *J Thorac Cardiovasc Surg* 96:171-177, 1988.

561. Ryo UY: Prediction of postoperative loss of lung function in patients with malignant lung mass: quantitative regional ventilation-perfusion scanning, *Radiol Clin North Am* 28:657-663, 1990.

562. Sahn SA: Malignant pleural effusions, *Clin Chest Med* 6:113-125, 1983.

563. Sahn SA: Pleural effusion in lung cancer, *Clin Chest Med* 14:189-200, 1993.

564. Saifuddin A, da Costa P, Chalmers AG, et al: Primary malignant localized fibrous tumours of the pleura: clinical, radiological and pathological features, *Clin Radiol* 45:13-17, 1992.

565. Saifuddin A, Robertson RJH, Smith SEW: The radiology of Askin tumours, *Clin Radiol* 43:19-23, 1991.

566. Salonen O, Kivisaari L, Standertskjöld-Nordenstam CG, et al: Chest radiography and computed tomography in the evaluation of mediastinal adenopathy in lymphoma, *Acta Radiol* 28:747-750, 1987.

567. Saltzstein SL: Pulmonary malignant lymphomas and pseudolymphomas: classification, therapy and prognosis, *Cancer* 16:928-955, 1963.

568. Samuels TH, Margolis M, Hamilton PA, et al: Mediastinal large-cell lymphoma, *J Can Assoc Radiol* 43:120-126, 1992.

569. Sanderson DR: Lung cancer screening: the Mayo study, *Chest* 89(suppl):324S, 1986.

570. Santiago S, Houston D, Ezer J, et al: Gallium scanning and tomography in the preoperative evaluation of lung cancer, *Cancer* 58:341-343, 1986.

571. Scharifker D, Kaneko M: Localized fibrous "mesothelioma" of pleura (submesothelial fibroma), *Cancer* 43:627-635, 1979.

572. Schnyder PA, Gamsu G: CT of the pretracheal retrocaval space, *AJR* 136:303-308, 1981.

573. Schraufnagel D, Morin JE, Wang NS: Endobronchial lipoma, *Chest* 75:97-99, 1979.

574. Schraufnagel D, Peloquin A, Pare JAP, et al: Differentiating bronchioloalveolar carcinoma from adenocarcinoma, *Am Rev Respir Dis* 125:74-79, 1982.

575. Schreurs AJM, Westermann CJJ, van den Bosch JMM, et al: A twenty-five-year follow-up of ninety-three resected typical carcinoid tumours of the lung, *J Thorac Cardiovasc Surg* 104:1470-1475, 1993.

576. Schuster MR, Scanlan KA: CT angiogram sign: establishing the differential diagnosis (letter), *Radiology* 181:903, 1991.

577. Schwartz EE, Katz SM, Mandell GA: Postinflammatory pseudotumors of the lung: fibrous histiocytoma and related lesions, *Radiology* 136:609-613, 1980.

578. Scott IR, Muller NL, Miller RR, et al: Resectable stage III lung cancer: CT, surgical and pathologic correlation, *Radiology* 166:75-79, 1988.

579. Seely JM, Mayo JR, Miller RR, et al: T_1 lung cancer: prevalence of mediastinal nodal metastases and diagnostic accuracy of CT, *Radiology* 186:129-132, 1993.

580. Sella A, Logothetis CJ, Dexeus FH, et al: Pulmonary air cyst associated with combination chemotherapy containing bleomycin (letter), *AJR* 153:191, 1989.

581. Senac MO, Wood BP, Isaacs H: Pulmonary blastoma: a rare childhood malignancy, *Radiology* 179:743-746, 1991.

582. Seynaeve P, Mathijs R, Kockx M, et al: Case report: the air crescent sign in pulmonary leukaemic infiltrate, *Clin Radiol* 45:40-41, 1992.

583. Shaner EG, Chang AE, Doppman JL, et al: Comparison of computed and conventional whole lung tomography in detecting pulmonary nodules: a prospective radiology-pathology study, *AJR* 131:51-54, 1978.

584. Shanley DJ, Mulligan ME: Osteosarcoma with isolated metastases to the pleura, *Pediatr Radiol* 21:227, 1991.

585. Shapiro MP, Gale ME, Carter BL: Variable CT appearance of plasma cell granuloma of the lung, *J Comput Assist Tomogr* 11:49-51, 1987.

586. Shapiro R, Wilson GL, Yasner R, et al: A useful roentgen sign in the diagnosis of localized bronchioloalveolar carcinoma, *AJR* 114:516-524, 1972.

587. Sherman JL, Rykwaler PJ, Tashkin DP: Intravascular bronchioalveolar tumor, *Am Rev Respir Dis* 123:468-470, 1981.

588. Shields TW: The significance of ipsilateral mediastinal lymph node metastasis (N2 disease) in non-small cell carcinoma of the lung: a commentary, *J Thorac Cardiovasc Surg* 99:48-53, 1990.

589. Shin MS, Berland LL, Myers JL, et al: CT demonstration of an ossifying bronchial carcinoid simulating broncholithiasis, *AJR* 153:51-52, 1989.

590. Shin MS, Carcelen MF, Ho KJ: Diverse roentgenographic manifestations of the rare pulmonary involvement in myeloma, *Chest* 102:946-948, 1992.

591. Shin MS, Ho KJ: CT fluid bronchogram: observation in postobstructive pulmonary consolidation, *Clin Imag* 16:109-113, 1992.

592. Shin MS, Jackson LK, Shelton RW, et al: Giant cell carcinoma of the lung: clinical and roentgenographic manifestations, *Chest* 89:366-369, 1986.

593. Shuman LS, Libshitz HI: Solid pleural manifestations of lymphoma, *AJR* 142:269-273, 1984.

594. Siegel MJ, Shackleford GD, McAlister WH: Pleural thickening: an unusual feature of childhood leukemia, *Radiology* 138:367-369, 1981.

595. Siegelman SS, Khouri NF, Scott WW, et al: Pulmonary hamartoma: CT findings, *Radiology* 160:313-317, 1986.

596. Simon G: Intrathoracic Hodgkin's disease. I. Less common intrathoracic manifestations of Hodgkin's disease, *Br J Radiol* 40:926-929, 1967.

597. Singh SK, Buonocore E, Hubner KF, et al: Quantitative F-18 FDG-PET for diagnosis and staging of chest tumors, *Radiology* 185(P)(suppl):324-325, 1992.

598. Smith SD, Rubin CM, Horvath A, et al: Non-Hodgkin's lymphoma in children, *Semin Oncol* 17:113-119, 1990.

599. Solomon A, Rubinstein ZJ, Rogoff M, et al: Pulmonary blastoma, *Pediatr Radiol* 12:148-149, 1982.

600. Soulen MC, Greco-Hunt VT, Templeton P: Migratory chest mass, *Invest Radiol* 25:209-211, 1990.

601. Spencer H: *Pathology of the lung*, ed 4, Philadelphia, 1985, WB Saunders.

602. Spizarny DL, Gross BH, Shephard JO: CT findings in localized fibrous mesothelioma of the pleural fissure, *J Comput Assist Tomogr* 10:942-944, 1986.

603. Spizarny DL, Shepard JAO, McLoud TC, et al: CT of adenoid cystic carcinoma of the trachea, *AJR* 146:1129-1132, 1986.

604. Sridhar KS, Bounassi MJ, Raub W, et al: Clinical features of adenosquamous lung carcinoma in 127 patients, *Am Rev Respir Dis* 142:19-23, 1990.

605. Stackhouse EM, Harrison EG, Ellis FH: Primary mixed malignancies of the lung: carcinosarcoma and blastoma, *J Thorac Cardiovasc Surg* 57:385-399, 1969.

606. Stansfield AG, Diebold J, Kapanci Y, et al: Updated Kiel classification for lymphomas, *Lancet* 1:292-293, 1988.

607. Staples CA, Muller NL, Miller RR, et al: Mediastinal nodes in bronchogenic carcinoma: comparison between CT and mediastinoscopy, *Radiology* 167:367-372, 1988.

608. Stark P: Multiple independent bronchogenic carcinomas, *Radiology* 145:599-601, 1982.

609. Stark P, Smith DC, Watkins GE, et al: Primary intrathoracic extraosseous osteogenic sarcoma: report of three cases, *Radiology* 174:725-726, 1990.

610. Steele SD: The solitary pulmonary nodule: report of a cooperative study of resected asymptomatic solitary pulmonary nodules in males, *J Thorac Cardiovasc Surg* 46:21-39, 1963.

611. Stein MG, Mayo J, Muller N, et al: Pulmonary lymphangitic spread of carcinoma: appearance on CT scans, *Radiology* 162:371-375, 1987.

612. Steinberg HV, Erwin BC: Metastases to the pleura: sonographic detection, *J Clin Ultrasound* 15:276-279, 1987.

613. Stephanopoulos C, Catsaras H: Myxosarcoma complicating a cystic hamartoma of the lung, *Thorax* 18:144, 1963.

614. Stewart JG, MacMahon H, Viborny CJ, et al: Dystrophic calcification in carcinoma of the lung: demonstration by CT, *AJR* 149:29-30, 1987.

615. Stiglbauer R, Schurawitzki H, Klepetko W, et al: Contrast-enhanced MRI for the staging of bronchogenic carcinoma: comparison with CT and histopathologic staging — preliminary results, *Clin Radiol* 44:293-298, 1991.

616. Stitik FP: Staging of lung cancer, *Radiol Clin North Am* 28:619-630, 1990.

617. Stollberg HO, Patt NL, MacEwen KF, et al: Hodgkin's disease of the lung, *AJR* 92:96-115, 1964.

618. Storey TF, Narla LD: Pleural lipoma in a child — CT evaluation, *Pediatr Radiol* 21:141-142, 1991.

619. Strauss MJ: The growth characteristic of lung cancer and its application to treatment design, *Semin Oncol* 1:167-174, 1974.

620. Strickland B: Intrathoracic Hodgkin's disease. II. Peripheral manifestations of Hodgkin's disease in the chest, *Br J Radiol* 40:930-938, 1967.

621. Strijk SP: Lymph node calcification in malignant lymphoma: presentation of nine cases and a review of the literature, *Acta Radiol[Diagn] (Stockh)* 26:427-431, 1985.

622. Strimlan CV, Rosenow EC, Weiland LH, et al: Lymphocytic interstitial pneumonitis: review of 13 cases, *Ann Intern Med* 88:616-621, 1978.

623. Strutynsky N, Balthazer EJ, Klein RM: Inflammatory pseudotumours of the lung, *Br J Radiol* 47:94-96, 1974.

624. Sugio K, Yokoyama H, Kaneko S, et al: Sclerosing hemangioma of the lung: radiographic and pathologic study, *Ann Thorac Surg* 53:295-300, 1992.

625. Suzuki N, Saitoh T, Kitamura S: Tumor invasion of the chest wall in lung cancer: diagnosis with US, *Radiology* 187:39-42, 1993.

626. Swain ME, Coblentz CL: Tracheal chondroma: CT appearance, *J Comput Assist Tomogr* 12:1085-1086, 1988.

627. Swennson RG, Theodore GH: Search and nonsearch protocols for radiograph consultation, *Radiology* 177:851-856, 1990.

628. Swensen SJ, Brown LR: Conventional radiography of the hilum and mediastinum in bronchogenic carcinoma, *Radiol Clin North Am* 28:521-538, 1990.

629. Swett HA, Wescott JL: Residual nonmalignant pulmonary nodules in choriocarcinoma, *Chest* 65:560-562, 1974.

630. Swift JE, Blend MJ, Bekerman C, et al: Detection of pulmonary metastases in a patient with synovial cell sarcoma using In-III labeled monoclonal antibody 19-24, *Clin Nucl Med* 15:227-230, 1990.

631. Takashima S, Fujita N, Morimoto S, et al: MR imaging of primary pulmonary lymphoma, *Australas Radiol* 34:353-355, 1990.

632. Takasugi JE, Rapoport S, Shaw C: Superior sulcus tumors: the role of imaging, *J Thorac Imag* 4(1):41-48, 1989.

633. Templeton AW, Moffat R, Nelson D: Bronchography and bronchial adenoma, *Chest* 59:59-61, 1971.

634. Templeton PA, Caskey CI, Zerhouni EA: Current uses of CT and MR in staging of lung cancer, *Radiol Clin North Am* 28:631-646, 1990.

635. Teplick JG, Teplick SK, Haskin ME: Granular cell myoblastoma of the lung. *AJR* 125:890-894, 1975.

636. Tesoro-Tess JD, Balzarini L, Ceglia E, et al: Magnetic resonance imaging in the initial staging of Hodgkin's disease and non-Hodgkin lymphoma, *Eur J Radiol* 12:81-90, 1991.

637. Theros EG: Varying manifestations of peripheral pulmonary neoplasms: a radiologic-pathologic correlative study, *AJR* 128:893-914, 1977.

638. Thomas PA, Piantadosi S, Mountain CF: Should subcarinal lymph nodes be routinely examined in patients with non-small cell lung cancer, *J Thorac Cardiovasc Surg* 95:883-887, 1988.

639. Thurlbeck WM: In *Pathology of the lung.* New York, 1988, Thieme.

640. Tobler J, Levitt RG, Glazer HS, et al: Differentiation of proximal bronchogenic carcinoma from postobstructive lobar collapse by magnetic resonance imaging: comparison with computed tomography, *Invest Radiol* 22:538-543, 1987.

641. Tockman MS: Survival and mortality from lung cancer in a screened population: the John Hopkins study, *Chest* 89(suppl):324S-325S, 1986.

642. Toye R, Jones DK, Armstrong P, Richman PI: Case report: numerous pulmonary metastases from renal cell carcinoma confined to the middle lobe, *Clin Radiol* 42:443-444, 1990.

643. Trapnell DH: The radiological appearances of lymphangitis carcinomatosa of the lung, *Thorax* 19:251-260, 1964.

644. Travis WD, Linnoila RI, Tsokos MG, et al: Neuroendocrine tumors of the lung with proposed criteria for large-cell neuroendocrine carcinoma, *Am J Surg Pathol* 15:529-553, 1991.

645. Tsuji M, Yoshii Y, Taka T, et al: Waldenstrom's macroglobulinemia: report of an autopsy case presenting with a pulmonary manifestation, *Virchows Arch A Pathol Anat* 415:169-173, 1989.

646. Tumeh SS, Rosenthal DS, Kaplan WD, et al: Lymphoma: evaluation with Ga-67 SPECT, *Radiology* 164:111-114, 1987.

647. Uematso M, Kondo M, Tsutsui T, et al: Residual masses on follow-up computed tomography in patients with mediastinal non-Hodgkin's lymphoma, *Clin Radiol* 40:244-247, 1990.

648. Urba WJ, Longo DL: Hodgkin's disease: review article, *N Engl J Med* 326:678-687, 1992.

649. van Bodegom PC, Wagenaar SS, Corrin B, et al: Second primary lung cancer: importance of long term follow-up, *Thorax* 44:788-793, 1989.

650. van Buchem MA, Wondergem JH, Kool LJS, et al: Pulmonary leukostasis: radiologic-pathologic study, *Radiology* 165:739-741, 1987.

651. Vansant JP, Johnson DH, O'Donnell DM, et al: Staging lung carcinoma with a Tc-99m labeled monoclonal antibody, *Clin Nucl Med* 17:431-438, 1992.

652. Vath RR, Alexander CB, Fulmer JD: The lymphocytic infiltrative lung disease, *Clin Chest Med* 3:619-634, 1982.

653. Velchik NG, Wegener W: Osteogenic sarcoma with pulmonary metastasis visualised by bone imaging, *Clin Nucl Med* 14:662-665, 1989.

654. Vernant JP, Brun B, Mannoni P, et al: Respiratory distress of hyperleukocytic granulocytic leukemias, *Cancer* 44:264-268, 1979.

655. Vincent JM, Armstrong P: Detection and diagnosis of the primary tumor in lung cancer, *Curr Opin Radiol* 3:341-350, 1991.

656. Vincent JM, Ng YY, Norton AJ, et al: CT "angiogram sign" in primary pulmonary lymphoma, *J Comput Assist Tomogr* 16(5):829-831, 1992.

657. Vincent JM, Trainer PJ, Reznek RH, et al: The radiological investigation of occult ectopic ACTH-dependent Cushing's syndrome, *Clin Radiol* 48:11-17, 1993.

658. Vincent RG, Pickien JW, Lane WW, et al: The changing histopathology of lung cancer: a review of 1682 cases, *Cancer* 39:1647-1653, 1977.

659. Vogelzang NJ, Stenlund R: Residual pulmonary nodules after combination chemotherapy of testicular cancer, *Radiology* 146:195-197, 1983.

660. Voyvodic F, Whyte A: Lymphomatoid granulomatosis, *Australas Radiol* 36:163-164, 1992.

661. Wagner JC, Sleggs CA, Marhand P: Diffuse pleural mesothelioma and absestos exposure in North Western Cape Province, *Br J Industr Med* 17:260-271, 1960.

662. Wahl RL, Quint LE, Orringer M, et al: Staging non-small-cell lung cancer in the mediastinum: comparison of FDG-PET, CT and hybrid "anatometabolic" fusion images with pathology, *Radiology* 185(P)(suppl):324, 1992.

663. Walkey MM: And what is your sign (letter)? *Radiology* 178:894, 1991.

664. Wang LT, Wilkins EW, Bode HH, et al: Bronchial carcinoid tumors in pediatric patients, *Chest* 103:1426-1428, 1993.

665. Wang PW, Tai DI, Chen HY: Tc-99m HIDA hepatobiliary agent in the diagnosis of pulmonary metastases from hepatocellular carcinoma, *Clin Nucl Med* 16:120-123, 1991.

666. Warren WH, Gould VE, Faber LP: Neuroendocrine neoplasms: a clinicopathologic update, *J Thorac Cardiovasc Surg* 98:321-332, 1989.

667. Watanabe Y, Shimizu J, Oda M, et al: Aggressive surgical intervention in N2 non-small cell cancer of the lung, *Ann Thorac Surg* 51:253-261, 1991.

668. Watanabe A, Shimokata K, Saka H, et al: Chest CT combined with artificial pneumothorax: value in determining origin and extent of tumor, *AJR* 156:707-710, 1991.

669. Watanabe Y, Shimizu J, Tsubota M, et al: Mediastinal spread of metastatic lymph nodes in bronchogenic carcinoma, *Chest* 97:1059-1065, 1990.

670. Webb WR: MR imaging of treated mediastinal Hodgkin disease, *Radiology* 170:315-316, 1989.

671. Webb WR: The role of magnetic resonance imaging in the assessment of patients with lung cancer: a comparison with computed tomography, *J Thorac Imag* 4(2):65-75, 1989.

672. Webb WR, Gamsu G: Thoracic metastases in malignant melanoma: a radiographic survey of 65 patients, *Chest* 71:176-181, 1977.

673. Webb WR, Gamsu G, Stark DD, et al: Magnetic resonance imaging of the normal and abnormal pulmonary hila, *Radiology* 152:89-94, 1984.

674. Webb WR, Gatsonis C, Zerhouni EA, et al: CT and MR imaging in staging non-small cell bronchogenic carcinoma: report of the Radiologic Diagnostic Oncologic Group, *Radiology* 178:705-713, 1991.

675. Webb WR, Jeffrey RB, Godwin JD: Thoracic computed tomography in superior sulcus tumors, *J Comput Assist Tomogr* 5:361-365, 1981.

676. Webb WR, Jensen BG, Sollitto R, et al: Bronchogenic carcinoma: staging with MR compared with staging with CT and surgery, *Radiology* 156:117-124, 1985.

677. Wechsler RJ, Rao VM, Steiner RM: The radiology of malignant mesothelioma, *CRC Crit Rev Diagn Imaging* 20:283-310, 1984.

678. Wechsler RJ, Steiner RM, Israel HL, et al: Chest radiograph in lymphomatoid granulomatosis: comparison with Wegener granulomatosis, *AJR* 142:79-83, 1984.

679. Weick JK, Kiely JM, Harrison EG, et al: Pleural effusion in lymphoma, *Cancer* 31:848-853, 1973.

680. Weiner M, Leventhal B, Cantor A, et al: Gallium-67 scans as an adjunct to computed tomography scans for the assessment of a residual mediastinal mass in pediatric patients with Hodgkin's disease, *Cancer* 68:2478-2480, 1991.

681. Weisbrod GL, Chamberlain DW, Tao LC: Pulmonary blastoma, report of three cases and a review of the literature, *J Can Assoc Radiol* 39:130-136, 1988.

682. Weisbrod GL, Towers MJ, Chamberlain DW, et al: Thin-walled cystic lesions in bronchioloalveolar carcinoma, *Radiology* 185:401-405, 1992.

683. Weisbrod GL, Yee AC: Computed tomographic diagnosis of pedunculated fibrous mesothelioma, *J Can Assoc Radiol* 34:147-148, 1983.

684. Wernecke K, Vassallo P, Hoffmann G, et al: Value of sonography in monitoring the therapeutic response of mediastinal lymphoma: comparison with chest radiography and CT, *AJR* 156:265-272, 1991.

685. Wernecke K, Vassalo P, Rutsch F, et al: Thymic involvement in Hodgkin's disease: CT and sonographic findings, *Radiology* 181:375-385, 1991.

686. Whitcomb ME, Schwartz MJ, Keller AR, et al: Hodgkin's disease of the lung, *Am Rev Respir Dis* 106:79-85, 1972.

687. Whittlesey D: Prospective computed tomographic scanning in the staging of bronchogenic carcinoma, *J Thorac Cardiovasc Surg* 95:876-882, 1988.

688. Williams MP, Husband JE, Heron CW: Intrathoracic manifestations of metastatic testicular seminoma: a comparison of chest radiographic and CT findings, *AJR* 149:473-475, 1987.

689. Wilson SR, Sanders DE, Delarie NC: Intrathoracic manifestations of amyloid disease, *Radiology* 102:283-289, 1976.

690. Winterbauer RH, Riggins RCK, Griesman FA, et al: Pleuropulmonary manifestations of Waldenstrom's macroglobulinemia, *Chest* 66:368-375, 1974.

691. Woodring JH: Determining the cause of pulmonary atelectasis: a comparison of plain radiography and CT, *AJR* 150:757-763, 1988.

692. Woodring JH: Pitfalls in the radiologic diagnosis of lung cancer, *AJR* 154:1165-1175, 1990.

693. Woodring JH: Unusual radiographic manifestations of lung cancer, *Radiol Clin North Am* 28:599-618, 1990.

694. Woodring JH, Bernady MO, Loh FK: Mucoid impaction of the bronchi, *Australas Radiol* 29:234-239, 1985.

695. Woodring JH, Fried AW, Chuang VP: Solitary cavities of the lung: diagnostic implications of cavity wall thickness, *AJR* 135:1269-1271, 1980.

696. Woodring JH, Stelling CB: Adenocarcinoma of the lung: a tumor with a changing pleomorphic character, *AJR* 140:657-664, 1983.

697. Wycoco D, Raval B: An unusual presentation of mediastinal Hodgkin's lymphoma on computed tomography, *J Comput Tomogr* 7:187-188, 1983.

698. Wyman S, Weber AL: Calcification in intrathoracic nodes in Hodgkin's disease, *Radiology* 93:1021-1024, 1969.

699. Yokoi K, Mori K, Miyazawa N, et al: Tumor invasion of the chest wall and mediastinum in lung cancer: evaluation with pneumothorax CT, *Radiology* 181:147-152, 1991.

700. Youssem SA, Hochholzer L: Malignant fibrous histiocytoma of the lung, *Cancer* 60:2532-2541, 1987.

701. Youssem SA, Weiss LM, Colby TV: Primary pulmonary Hodgkin's disease: a clinicopathologic study of 15 cases, *Cancer* 57:1217-1224, 1986.

702. Youssem SA, Wick MR, Singh G, et al: So-called sclerosing hemangiomas of lung: an immunohistochemical study supporting a respiratory epithelial origin, *Am J Surg Pathol* 12:582-590, 1988.

703. Zerhouni EA, Stitik FP: Controversies in computed tomography of the thorax: the pulmonary nodule — lung cancer staging, *Radiol Clin North Am* 23:407-426, 1985.

704. Zerhouni EA, Stitik FP, Siegelman SS, et al: CT of the pulmonary nodule: a cooperative study, *Radiology* 160:319-327, 1986.

705. Zwiebel BR, Austin JHM, Grimes MM: Bronchial carcinoid tumours: assessment with CT of location and intratumoral calcification in 31 patients, *Radiology* 179:483-486, 1991.

706. Zwirewich CV, Miller RR, Müller NL: Multicentric adenocarcinoma of the lung: CT-pathologic correlation, *Radiology* 176:185-190, 1990.

707. Zwirewich CV, Vedal S, Miller RR, et al: Solitary pulmonary nodule: high-resolution CT and radiologic-pathologic correlation, *Radiology* 179:469-476, 1991.

708. Zwischenberger JB, Cox CS: Staging and surgery for lung cancer, *J Thorac Imag* 7(1):57-69, 1991.

9 Pulmonary Vascular Diseases and Pulmonary Edema

DAVID M. HANSELL
A. MICHAEL PETERS

PULMONARY THROMBOEMBOLISM

Pulmonary thromboembolism is a common cause of death in hospitalized patients. Accurate incidence figures are difficult to obtain because they depend on how carefully embolism is searched for,[107] but pulmonary thromboembolism appears to be the sole or major cause of death in 10% to 15% of adults dying in the acute care wards of general hospitals.[226] It is particularly common in patients who die after severe burns or trauma.

Almost all emboli lodge within the branches of the pulmonary arteries, a few straddle the bifurcation of the main pulmonary artery (saddle emboli), and the occasional one lodges in the right side of the heart. Their effects[225,377] are due primarily to mechanical obstruction. Reflex responses by the vessels and bronchi are transient and are probably clinically unimportant.[284] Virchow demonstrated, and it has since been repeatedly confirmed, that the bronchial circulation alone can sustain the lung parenchyma without infarction occurring.[76] Animal studies have shown that bronchial arteries start to dilate within days after pulmonary arterial occlusion[200,360] and are hypertrophic within 1 month.[301] Exactly why some emboli cause pulmonary infarction whereas others do not is uncertain, but it would appear that infarction occurs only when the combined bronchial and pulmonary arterial circulation is inadequate, a

369

situation that applies particularly when emboli lodge peripherally in the pulmonary arterial tree and also when emboli occur in patients with heart failure or circulatory shock.[76,345] It has been estimated that fewer than 15% of thromboemboli cause true infarction.[225]

On pathologic study, pulmonary infarction is characterized by ischemic necrosis of alveolar walls, bronchioles, and blood vessels within an area of hemorrhage. Most infarcts occur in the lower lobes, and the majority are multiple. Usually they are cone-shaped areas of hemorrhage and edema that point toward the hilum and are based on the pleura, which is often covered by a fibrinous exudate. Following infarction, fibrous replacement converts the infarct into a contracted scar with indrawing of the pleura. In some cases hemorrhage is the dominant finding and there is no evidence of tissue necrosis; these lesions resolve without residual scar formation.

Pulmonary edema is a rare consequence of pulmonary embolism. Such patients usually have heart disease, and it seems probable that in these patients the pulmonary emboli precipitate left ventricular failure.[382] In massive pulmonary embolism the edema may be due to overperfusion of nonoccluded portions of the pulmonary circulation.[164,358]

Emboli usually resolve, and the vessel lumen is restored.[74,105,206,225] The main mechanism is presumed to be intravascular lysis and fragmentation.[290] In a few patients the emboli do not lyse[50,340] and the presence of repeated, unresolved emboli may lead to chronic pulmonary hypertension.[74,102,285]

The clinical manifestations of pulmonary embolism are protean and often nonspecific.[326] They range from no symptoms to sudden death. The symptoms and signs include dyspnea, chest pain that is often pleuritic but is sometimes anginal, cough, hemoptysis, tachypnea, hypotension, tachycardia, fever, and a pleural friction rub.[22,377] Most patients have an underlying disorder, such as congestive heart failure, recent surgery, or carcinomatosis, or are immobilized.[22,377] Because so many of the symptoms and signs of pulmonary embolism are nonspecific, the diagnosis is frequently overlooked.[281]

The standard laboratory tests are nonspecific. Arterial P_{O_2} values are often, but not always, low. Serum lactic dehydrogenase values tend to be high, and although the electrocardiogram may show right axis shift, $S_1Q_3T_3$ pattern, or a new incomplete right bundle branch block, the test is often within normal limits or shows only preexisting or nonspecific changes.[121]

Accurate diagnosis is important because anticoagulant[201,258] and thrombolytic[120] therapy carries significant risks that would not be justified in the absence of pulmonary embolism.

Imaging of pulmonary emboli

Plain chest radiography, radionuclide lung scanning, and pulmonary angiography are the major methods of establishing the diagnosis of pulmonary embolism. In most instances plain chest films and radionuclide lung scans are obtained first and pulmonary angiography is reserved for cases in which the risks of misdiagnosis outweigh the risks of the procedure.

PLAIN CHEST RADIOGRAPHY. Many plain film signs of pulmonary embolism and infarction have been described.* Before discussion of these signs it is important to state clearly that none is specific and that the sensitivity of the signs is poor.[42,129,332,334] Even in patients with life-threatening pulmonary embolism, the plain chest radiograph can appear normal.[362] In one large series of 152 patients suspected to have pulmonary emboli, the overall sensitivity of the plain chest radiograph was 0.33 and the overall specificity was 0.59.[129] Therefore the major role of the chest film is to exclude other diagnoses that might mimic pulmonary embolism, such as pneumothorax, pneumonia, or rib fractures, and to provide information that helps in interpreting the radionuclide scans. There will, however, be some cases in which the chest radiograph will suggest the diagnosis, and it is therefore important to appreciate the plain film signs, despite their low sensitivity and specificity. A useful framework for discussing the radiographic abnormalities in acute pulmonary emboli is to divide them into (1) pulmonary embolism without infarction and (2) pulmonary embolism with infarction.[54]

Acute pulmonary embolism without infarction. As discussed earlier, most emboli do not cause infarction. The few plain film signs of acute pulmonary embolism without infarction or hemorrhage are oligemia of the lung beyond the occluded vessel (Westermark's sign) (Figure 9-1), increase in the size of the main pulmonary artery or of one of the descending pulmonary trunks, and elevation of a hemidiaphragm.† The nonspecificity of these signs is self-evident; emphysema may cause similar pulmonary vascular changes, and the position of the diaphragm is influenced by numerous factors, pulmonary embolism being just one.

Linear or disk-shaped densities[103] may be seen in patients with pulmonary emboli (Figure 9-2). These shadows represent discoid atelectases, not pulmonary infarcts,[346,365] and are secondary to elevation of the diaphragm, inhibition of ventilation, and possibly depletion of surfactant.[226]

Repetitive emboli may cause pulmonary arterial hypertension, a phenomenon that can be recognized radiologically (see the section "Pulmonary Arterial Hypertension" later in this chapter).

Acute pulmonary embolism with infarction. Pulmonary infarction gives rise to radiographically detectable consolidation, which is usually multifocal in distribution and

---

*References 54, 100, 180, 188, 212, 231, 247, 298, 303, 334, 336, 342, 366, 371.
†References 55, 100, 180, 188, 247, 298, 336, 366.

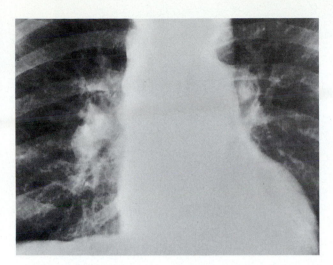

FIGURE 9-1
Westermark's sign of pulmonary embolism. The right hilum is large, and vessels beyond the hilum in the right lower lobe are small.

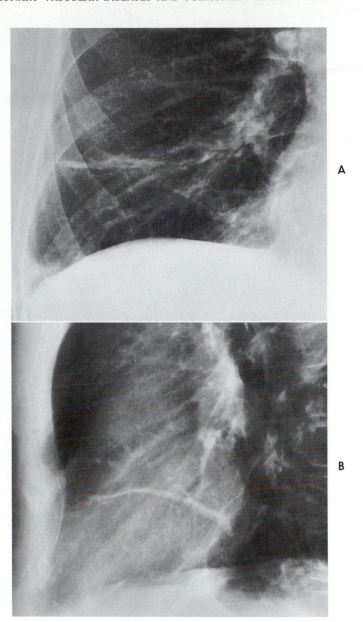

FIGURE 9-2
A, Posteroanterior and, B, lateral radiographs showing discoid atelectasis in a patient with pulmonary embolism.

predominant in the lower lung fields.[76] Such shadows usually occur 12 to 24 hours after the embolic episode, although their appearance may be delayed for several days.[353] The resulting opacity (Figure 9-3) may assume a variety of shapes depending on the location and underlying lobular architecture of the lung.[135,148] Lobar consolidation is, however, unusual[168] and a pattern resembling pulmonary edema is only occasionally encountered.

Hampton and Castleman[135] described their famous "hump" in an early paper that correlated the pathologic findings with the postmortem chest radiograph. They emphasized that "infarcts are always in contact with pleural surfaces and that the shadows are rarely, if ever, triangular in shape." They noticed that the central margin of the infarct shadow may be rounded, hence the term "hump" (Figure 9-3). In fact, a Hampton's hump is unusual[147] and is in any event a nonspecific finding. Air bronchograms are rarely seen on plain films,[12] an observation that could help in the differential diagnosis from pneumonia and other causes of consolidation. Frequently, the clinical features point to one or another diagnosis; if they do not, the radiographic appearance of the opacity cannot be relied on to offer a distinction between the various causes of consolidation.

Where the consolidation is the result of pulmonary hemorrhage without true infarction, radiographic clearing occurs quickly, often within a week, whereas infarction takes several months to resolve[96] and frequently leaves permanent linear scars.[304] By three months infarct shadows either are totally resolved or show no more than linear scarring or pleural thickening.[210] As infarcts resolve, they may "melt away like an ice cube" (Figure 9-3), whereas acute pneumonia disappears in a patchy fashion.[375] It may therefore be possible to suggest the diagnosis retrospectively, but this sign has no value at the

time when it is most needed.

Cavitation within the infarct is rare (Figures 9-4 and 9-5). It may be seen in the absence of infection,[130,293] but usually cavitary infarcts are either secondarily infected or result from septic emboli. (Septic emboli are discussed in Chapter 6). Aseptic cavitation is more likely to occur in an area of infarction greater than 4 cm in diameter and usually happens 2 weeks after the appearance of the consolidation.[373]

Pleural effusions commonly accompany pulmonary embolism.[37,96,231,332] In a carefully conducted prospective study, Bynum and Wilson[46] showed that approximately

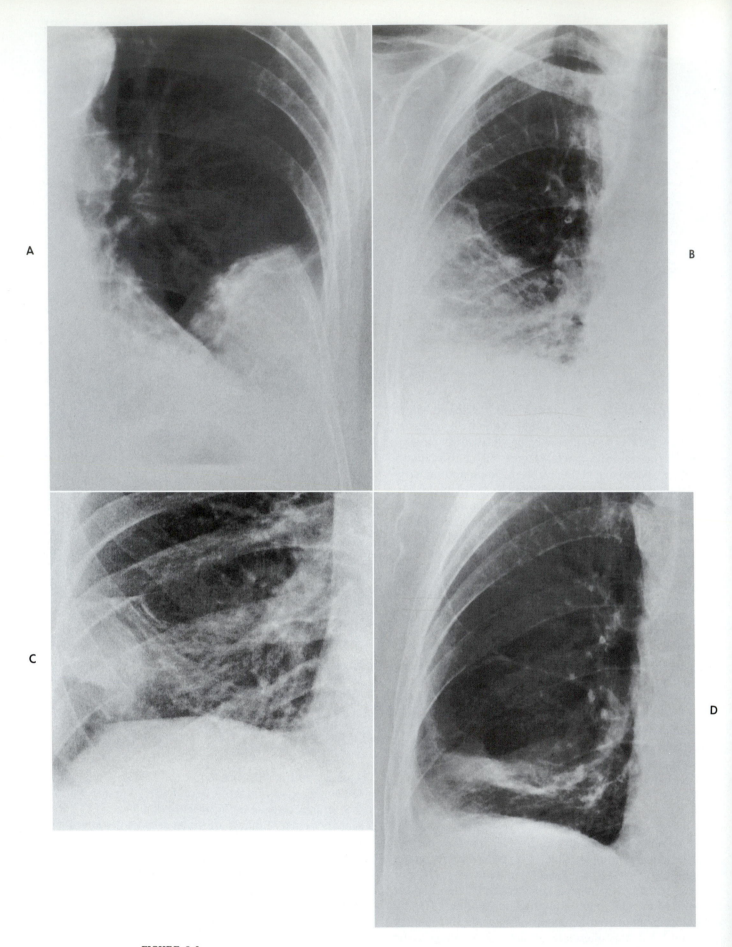

FIGURE 9-3
Pulmonary consolidation caused by pulmonary embolism. **A,** Consolidation at the left base shows a rounded, truncated, cone shape known as Hampton's hump. **B,** Consolidation in the right lung in the same patient, showing segmental configuration. Appearance of right-sided consolidation, **C,** 2½ weeks later and, **D,** 5½ weeks later showing gradual resolution "from the periphery."

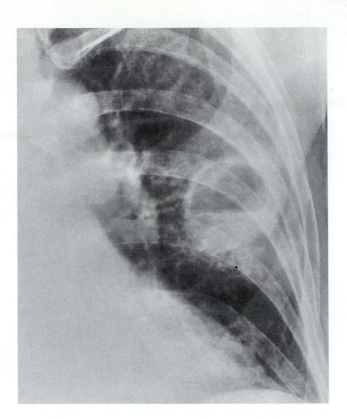

FIGURE 9-4
Cavitating pulmonary infarct.

50% of patients with pulmonary embolism also had a pleural effusion, and these were often bloody. In one third of their cases the effusion was an isolated finding, and in the remaining two thirds it was accompanied by radiographic evidence of pulmonary infarction or hemorrhage. Typically the effusions are small and unilateral and appear soon after the onset of symptoms, but occasionally the effusions are bilateral and large.[334] It is interesting to note that almost all patients who had a pleural effusion had chest pain on the same side.[46] It appears probable that pleural effusions following pulmonary embolism are caused by infarction of the lung and that, in those cases in which no infarct shadow is visible on plain chest radiograph, the infarct is there but either is hidden from view or is not identifiable on the plain radiograph.[46]

RADIONUCLIDE IMAGING. The conventional radionuclide technique for imaging the lung in suspected pulmonary thromboembolism involves simultaneous imaging of the distribution of pulmonary blood flow (perfusion imaging) and the distribution of alveolar ventilation. The combined study is called a ventilation-perfusion (V/Q) scan. The principle underlying the diagnosis of pulmonary vascular disease, usually pulmonary embolism, is that whereas pulmonary perfusion is abnormal, the pulmonary parenchyma usually remains intact and ventilation remains normal. This gives rise to the so-called mismatched perfusion defect, the hallmark of pulmonary embolism. If embolism results in pulmonary infarction, a defect of ventilation, corresponding to the perfusion defect, appears.

A
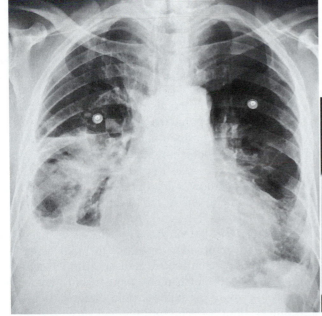

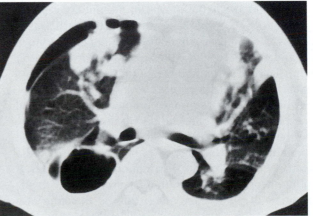
B

FIGURE 9-5
Cavitating pulmonary infarcts. **A,** Plain film. **B,** Computed tomographic scan showing a mixture of cavitating and noncavitating infarcts, which on autopsy were not infected.

Whereas V/Q lung scanning attempts to identify defects of tracer uptake in the lung, other radiolabeled tracers for imaging thromboembolism attempt to identify positive uptake of tracer by the thromboembolic material — "hot spot" in contrast to "cold spot" imaging. Such agents are generally active components of the clotting process and include radiolabeled platelets, fibrinogen, monoclonal antibodies recognizing platelets or fibrinogen, fragments of fibrin that recombine with preformed fibrin but not fibrinogen, and peptides that bind to activated fibrinogen receptors on platelets. These approaches constitute an active biotechnologic approach to imaging thrombus and are briefly discussed later.

PERFUSION LUNG SCANNING. Perfusion lung imaging can be performed by the intravenous injection of a radiotracer, which is trapped in the lung on first pass. There are two available classes of tracer: (1) microparticles of human protein labeled with technetium-99m (Tc-99m), which microembolize in the lung vascular bed, and (2) radioactive inert gases, which, because of their low aqueous solubility, rapidly enter alveolar gas following intravenous injection. The first approach with microparticles is the one generally used in the routine clinical diagnosis of pulmonary embolism. The particles may be either of macroaggregated human serum albumin (MAA), which have a size range of 10 to 100 μm, or microspheres of denatured human serum albumin, which are available with an intermediate and narrower size range (20 to 45 μm). MAA is cheaper, more widely available, and much more frequently used than microspheres, although in some clinical circumstances the latter are preferred because of their narrower size range. For instance, in patients with a right-to-left shunt there is a theoretic risk of systemic tissue ischemia as a result of vessel occlusion from the larger shunted particles. With either particle, some departments use a smaller number in patients with pulmonary hypertension because of the potential for further occlusion of an already depleted vascular bed. However, the number of capillaries (normally 300 million) far outnumbers the number of particles administered (200,000 to 500,000), even in pulmonary vascular disease, so there is a wide safety margin. The particles are biodegradable and have a biologic half-time in the lung of 6 to 8 hours. The Tc-99m elutes from the particles faster than this, and by 24 hours most of the remaining activity is visible in the gut and kidneys.

Provided the particles mix completely in the blood before microembolization, the distribution of radioactivity is proportional to the distribution of pulmonary blood flow (Figure 9-6). Not only is photon emission itself a random event, but so is the distribution of the particles. A distribution of radioactivity that is proportional to the distribution of pulmonary blood flow is therefore also dependent on the injection of a sufficiently large number of particles.[145]

The particles should be injected with the patient supine during a series of deep inspirations and without withdrawing blood into the syringe before injection. The latter promotes clumping of the particles, while deep inspiration ensures a more even distribution of blood flow. The supine position is used to promote delivery of particles to the apex, which otherwise in the erect position are poorly visualized because of the normal gravity-dependent distribution of pulmonary blood flow. Ninety-five percent of the administered Tc-99m is trapped in the lungs. Up to 5% may pass through[369]; the majority of the nontrapped radioactivity is probably unbound Tc-99m, which may give rise to faint thyroid and gastric activity. Free Tc-99m is excreted in the urine and taken up by the renal parenchyma, and if present in significant amounts (usually as a result of poor labeling of the protein) it also gives images of the kidneys. This, however, can be distinguished from anatomic right-to-left shunting of the particles by an absence of splenic and cerebral activity.

A Tc-99m lung perfusion scan, whether performed with MAA or with microspheres, gives an effective radiation dose equivalent of 1 mSv/100 MBq. The usual imaging dose is 75 MBq (about 2 mCi). Since the material is "sticky," injection through long lines should be avoided because a considerable fraction is likely to be retained in the line. Injection through a butterfly needle is acceptable, especially for children, although up to one third of the dose may be retained within the tubing.

Inert gases, such as xenon-133 (Xe-133), krypton-81m (Kr-81m), and the positron emitter, nitrogen-13 (N-13), rapidly enter alveolar gas following intravenous injection, and it is possible to obtain images depicting the distribution of pulmonary blood flow to *aerated* alveoli during a period of breath holding following injection. Although practical disadvantages exclude the routine use of Xe-133 for this purpose, Kr-81m can be given by continuous intravenous infusion[64] and perfusion images obtained in multiple projections. Although radioactive inert gases are infrequently used to assess regional perfusion, many of the original investigations that defined the gravitational distribution of pulmonary blood flow were based on intravenous Xe-133.[157]

Gravity influences the distribution of pulmonary blood flow because the pulmonary circulation is at low pressure. In the erect position, mean alveolar pressure in the apices exceeds both pulmonary arterial and venous pressures, and there is very little apical flow. In the midzones blood flow is determined by the arterioalveolar pressure gradient, and in the lower zones by the arteriovenous gradient.

VENTILATION IMAGING. Two classes of agents are available for ventilation imaging: the radioactive inert gases and the radiolabeled aerosols. Until recently the inert gases were much more popular, but now aerosols are being more frequently used, largely because of technical improvements in the delivery systems and reductions in aerosol particle size.

Worldwide, Xe-133 is the most widely used inert gas for imaging ventilation. In the United Kingdom the ultra

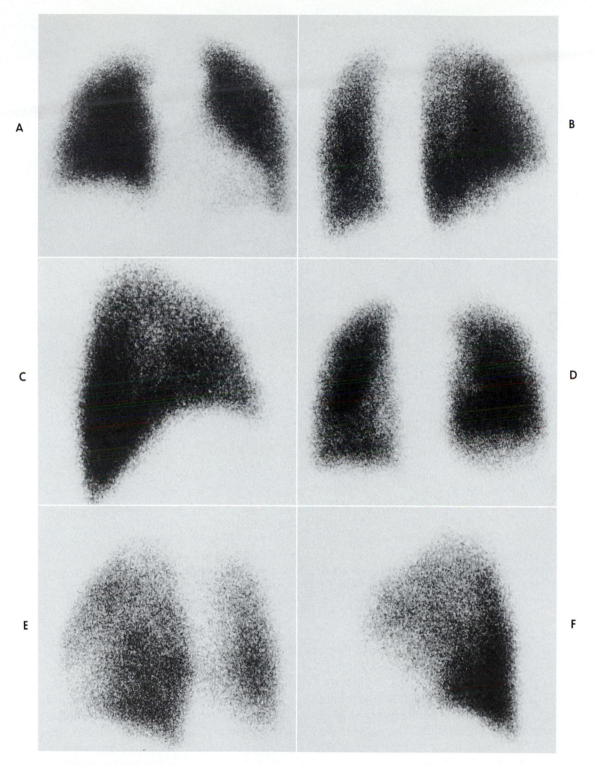

FIGURE 9-6
Normal ^{99m}Tc perfusion scans of the lungs. **A,** Anterior. **B,** Right posterior oblique. **C,** Right lateral. **D,** Posterior. **E,** Left posterior oblique. **F,** Left lateral view.

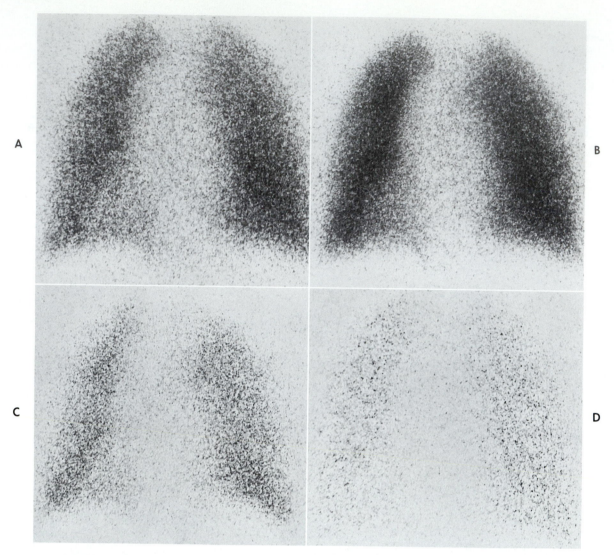

FIGURE 9-7
Normal ^{133}Xe ventilation scan. Posterior scans: **A**, ½ to 1 minute after the beginning of wash-in; **B**, 2 to 2½ minutes after the beginning of wash-in (equilibrium); **C**, 1 to 1½ minutes after the beginning of wash-out; and, **D**, 2 to 2½ minutes after the beginning of wash-out.

short-lived inert gas, Kr-81m, is more widely used,[367] but, although probably the optimal agent for ventilation imaging, it is expensive and has limited availability. A few centers use Xe-127,[237] which has a half-life of 36 days. Because of the very short half-life of Kr-81m, the technique of Kr-81m imaging is fundamentally different from that of xenon imaging.

Xe-133 has a half-life of 5.3 days and, although cheap and easily available, gives images of poor resolution because of its low photon energy of 80 KeV. Following a short period of inhalation, the so-called wash-in phase, it gives an image of the regional distribution of ventilation (Figure 9-7). With continuing inhalation the distribution of radioactivity increasingly reflects regional lung vol-

ume. Eventually the wash-in rate becomes equal to the wash-out rate, and during this equilibrium phase the image portrays regional lung volume. After the administration of Xe-133 has been terminated, the equilibrium phase is followed by the wash-out phase. Regions of air trapping within the lung then become evident as areas of increased count rate. Although this dynamic approach may give useful information, particularly regarding air trapping, it can only be conveniently performed in one projection. This is a disadvantage because, owing to its low energy, Xe-133 (80 KeV) has to be administered before Tc-99m (140 KeV), that is, at a time when the location of any perfusion abnormalities if present is unknown. Nevertheless, wash-in images acquired during limited periods of inhalation can be obtained in multiple projections — posterior and both posterior obliques.[83] Alternatively, the lungs can be imaged in these three projections during the wash-out phase, since regional hypoventilation is often associated with air trapping. Xe-127 has a higher energy (203 KeV) than Tc-99m and so can be administered following perfusion imaging in a selected projection, namely the one that best shows any perfusion defects, a significant advantage over Xe-133.

Because of its very short half-life of 13 seconds, Kr-81m (190 KeV) can effectively be used only for wash-in studies. The gas is obtained as the metastable daughter of rubidium-81(Rb-81), which is delivered in a cannister from a cyclotron unit. Rb-81 has a half life of 4.7 hours, giving a Kr-81m generator a useful life span of 1 working day. The count rate from the lung during continuous Kr-81m inhalation is proportional to regional ventilation, but inversely proportional to the arithmetic sum of ventilatory turnover (the ratio of ventilation to lung volume, $\dot{V}/V$) and the rate constant of decay, δ, of the radionuclide. If δ is large compared with $\dot{V}/V$ (that is, the radionuclide decays very rapidly), the count rate over the lung becomes proportional only to $\dot{V}/\delta$ (that is, the regional count rate represents regional ventilation). If δ is small compared with $\dot{V}/V$, as for xenon, then, at equilibrium, regional count rate is proportional to regional lung volume. The attraction of Kr-81m is that it can be continuously administered and images acquired in any projection with minimal patient cooperation. Perfusion and ventilation images can be obtained without moving the patient, either in sequence by alternating the photopeak settings on the gamma camera between Kr-81m and Tc-99m, or simultaneously by dual photon acquisition. For the sequential approach, "down-scatter" of the higher energy photons of Kr-81m into the Tc-99m window is prevented simply by switching off the Kr-81m supply. Residual gas clears rapidly, mainly by radioactive decay, and does not therefore interfere with the Tc-99m images. Kr-81m is ideal for physiologic studies of the lung because of its ability to provide moment to moment (real time) information on regional ventilation and its facility for single photon emission computerized tomography (SPECT).[361]

Aerosols are generally made from Tc-99m DTPA, although some centers have used aerosolized Tc-99m-labeled colloid or albumin microspheres. Their administration requires the cooperation of the patient, who is asked to breathe through a mouthpiece, with a nose clip in place, for several minutes. Most users give the aerosol before the administration of Tc-99m MAA, although some give it after, only to patients with abnormal perfusion scans. If they are given in close succession, some form of image subtraction may be necessary. As with Kr-81m, images can be acquired in multiple projections, facilitating comparison with the subsequent perfusion images. Aerosols also provide the opportunity of SPECT. The regional distribution of radioactivity depicts regional ventilation at the instant of inhalation. In this respect, aerosol imaging is similar to Tc-99m MAA perfusion imaging in that the distribution of perfusion is "frozen" at the time of injection, but unlike Kr-81m, which continuously and dynamically depicts the distribution of ventilation as the patient breathes the gas. The value of Kr-81m imaging is underlined by patients shown to have an unstable distribution of ventilation (that is, different from one projection to another). This may give rise to diagnostic confusion but is difficult to detect with any other ventilation agent. Unstable ventilation has been noted particularly in children[249] and may be posture dependent. It calls into question the reliability of injecting MAA in the supine position and administering the ventilation agent in the erect position.

A recent advance in aerosol technology has been the introduction of an agent called "Technegas."[43] This is an ultrafine dispersion of Tc-99m-labeled carbon particles generated by combustion of pertechnetate at 2500° C in a graphite crucible in an atmosphere of 100% argon within the Technegas "generator." This agent gives ventilation images with a quality approaching that of Kr-81m,[169] but is otherwise similar to the conventional DTPA aerosols in terms of convenience and availability. Once the generator has been purchased, ventilation imaging can be performed immediately on request. Deposition of particles in the central airways, which is a problem with conventional DTPA aerosols, particularly in patients with chronic lung disease, appears to be less with Technegas because of the smaller particle size. As with Tc-99m DTPA aerosols, subtraction of the aerosol signal from the subsequent perfusion signal (or vice versa) may be necessary.

Movement of gas in the peripheral airways, beyond the sixteenth generation of airway,[363] is by molecular diffusion, at a rate that is inversely proportional to molecular size. Aerosol particles are therefore presumably deposited mainly in distal airways rather than alveoli, although their kinetic energy may carry them into the alveolar sac. The Tc-99m DTPA complex then diffuses across the distal airway epithelium into the pulmonary circulation. This rate of diffusion is also inversely proportional to molecular size and to the permeability of the epithelium.[65] In normal, nonsmoking subjects, Tc-99m DTPA clears from the lung by this route with a half-time of about 80 minutes. In smokers it is considerably faster. By the time the perfusion scans are performed, activity is often already visible in the renal collecting systems. It is also usually visible, as swallowed activity, in the upper gastrointestinal tract as a result of particle deposition in the mouth. In patients with chronic lung disease it is also visible in the proximal airways as a result of particle deposition caused by turbulent airflow. Larger particles tend to be deposited in the proximal airways, and it is toward the elimination of this problem that the technical improvements in aerosol production and delivery have largely been aimed. Radioactivity doses of the ventilation agents are difficult to estimate and depend on the

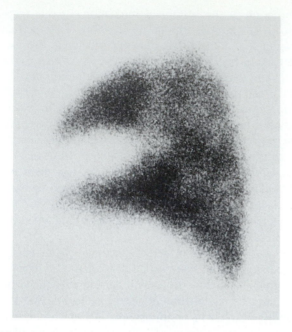

FIGURE 9-8
Perfusion defect. ^{99m}Tc scan; right lateral view. The typical segmental-shaped perfusion defect is pointing to the hilum and is based on the pleura. The defect in this case corresponds to all of the middle lobe and is due to a pulmonary embolus. The ventilation scan was normal.

efficiency of the delivery. Nevertheless, they are generally less than those from perfusion imaging, and from Kr-81m they are negligible.

Some positron-emitting radiopharmaceuticals are also available for imaging perfusion and ventilation by positron emission tomography (PET). A positron is the positively charged equivalent of an electron and is emitted from the nucleus of the atom. After emission it almost immediately encounters an electron, whereupon there is mutual annihilation of the two particles with transformation of their energy into two gamma photons, each of 511 KeV, emitted in opposite directions (180 degrees) to each other. The PET camera essentially consists of a ring of scintillation probes, each one paired with another, opposing one. As a result of coincident detection of the two 511 KeV photons, the PET camera is able to reconstruct the point within the body from which the positron originated, and thereby construct an image "slice" of the patient. The positron-labeled gases of interest in respiratory medicine are N-13 and carbon monoxide and carbon dioxide, both labeled with oxygen-15. They all have very short physical half-lives, measurable in minutes. N-13 is an inert gas with properties similar to xenon, although, because it is less soluble in both water and fat, it actually has better physical properties than xenon for imaging ventilation.

A minimum of four views is recommended for V/Q lung scanning: anterior, posterior, and both posterior obliques. Occasionally laterals and anterior obliques are

also useful. SPECT may have a role in V/Q lung scanning,[195,243] particularly when combined with Kr-81m ventilation imaging and dual photon acquisition. SPECT applied only to perfusion imaging has little value. If clinically relevant, V/Q lung imaging should be performed with little hesitation in pregnant women because of the obvious undesirability of anticoagulation in such circumstances. The radiation dose to the fetus is small, especially if Kr-81m is used for ventilation imaging. Since the clinical need is usually one of excluding pulmonary embolism, perfusion only lung imaging may be adequate, provided the patient is a nonsmoker, has a normal chest radiograph, and has no history of chronic lung disease. Reducing the injected dose to less than about 40 MBq provides an opportunity for a follow-up scan, although for statistical reasons the number of particles injected should not be reduced.[145] Tc-99m is excreted in breast milk,[232] so nursing mothers should express their milk and save it for 2 days from the time of injection to allow for radionuclide physical decay.

Interpretation. The diagnostic feature of pulmonary embolism in a V/Q lung scan is a perfusion defect in a region of normally ventilated lung — the so-called mismatched perfusion defect (Figure 9-8). The size of the defect may range from appreciably smaller than a segment (subsegmental), to about the size of a segment (segmental), or even a lobe or whole lung. A nonsegmental defect is one that does not correspond to segmental anatomy. The pathologic basis of the mismatched perfusion defect is that in uncomplicated pulmonary embolism the pulmonary architecture remains intact and ventilation therefore continues normally. However, when embolism is followed by lung infarction, a ventilation defect appears, although it is usually smaller than the perfusion defect because the lung around the periphery of the perfusion defect continues to ventilate. The diagnostic feature of a pulmonary infarct, therefore, is an incompletely matched perfusion defect (Figure 9-9) in association with an appropriate radiographic abnormality. The positive identification of a pulmonary infarct on a V/Q lung scan depends on high-quality, multiprojection ventilation imaging and is understressed in the literature, probably because of the predominant use of single projection Xe-133 imaging.

A perfusion scan showing multiple segmental defects in the presence of a normal ventilation scan and the appropriate clinical setting, such as recent surgery, signifies a high probability (greater than 90%) of recent pulmonary embolism. In a more equivocal clinical setting, unmatched perfusion defects may be the result of previous unresolved pulmonary embolism, and in these circumstances it is often necessary to repeat the scan after an interval, usually 1 to 3 weeks, after which complete or partial resolution of the perfusion defect supports recent pulmonary embolism. Pulmonary emboli resolve at variable rates, broadly dependent on the patient's age and fitness. In young fit patients the scan can be repeated

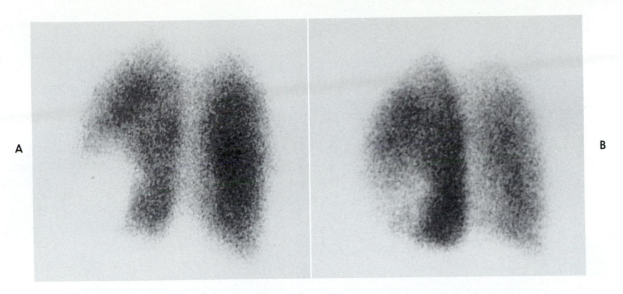

FIGURE 9-9
Pulmonary infarct. A, A perfusion defect is visible in lingular region of the left lung (left posterior oblique view). B, Kr-81m ventilation scan shows a defect at same site, but it is clearly smaller than the corresponding perfusion defect, typical of pulmonary infarction.

CAUSES OF A REVERSED VENTILATION-PERFUSION MISMATCH

Basal pleural effusion
Lobar pneumonia
Lobar collapse
Cardiomegaly
Acute partial bronchial obstruction
Chronic obstructive airway disease
Bronchiectasis

---

within about 1 week, although in older patients 2 to 3 weeks is appropriate.

Very often, patients with suspected pulmonary embolism have coincidental cardiopulmonary disease and the interpretation of the V/Q scan is then more difficult. Several matched defects may be seen on the ventilation and perfusion scans. Complete matching is seen in obstructive airways disease, either acute, as in bronchial asthma, or chronic, as in chronic obstructive airways disease. It is complete because of efficient hypoxic vasoconstriction, a defense mechanism that prevents pulmonary arterial blood from circulating through non-ventilated lung. Hypoxic vasoconstriction may nevertheless be incomplete, in which case a region of lung may be better perfused than ventilated—a so-called reversed mismatch (see box above). Reversed mismatching is a characteristic feature of several chest diseases, including pleural effusions (and fluid in the fissures, Figure 9-10), lobar pneumonia, collapsed and consolidated lung, and gross cardiomegaly, and is also seen in acute partial

bronchial obstruction, in which the chest radiograph may appear normal, and in chronic obstructive airway disease, especially in acute exacerbations.[48,72,190] In these conditions hypoxic vasoconstriction fails or is incomplete. If the patient is imaged with gas or inhales aerosol in the erect posture, pleural effusion typically gives a complete absence of ventilation at the base as a result of lung compression, as well as a variable reduction in perfusion. If the patient is imaged supine, pleural effusions may produce confusing images as a result of fluid accumulating in the posterior pleural space and attenuating both ventilation and perfusion signals as well as compressing the lung. In lobar pneumonia, perfusion is maintained, albeit at an abnormally reduced level, and, since the lobe is airless, ventilation is completely absent (Figure 9-11). Cardiomegaly has more recently been shown to be associated with a reversed mismatched defect in the left lower lobe.[2] Like pleural effusion, the mechanism is essentially regional lung compression. The effect of cardiomegaly on left lower lobe ventilation depends on posture, being greatest in the supine position, when lung compression is maximal, and least in the prone. Its effect on perfusion is minimal in all positions. Thus, on lying down, patients with cardiomegaly develop a physiologic right-to-left shunt, and this presumably contributes to the orthopnea experienced by these patients. The importance of reversed mismatching has been understated in the literature, particularly regarding lobar pneumonia, which, with high-quality ventilation imaging, can be distinguished from pulmonary infarction.

Completely matched defects are seen in destructive parenchymal lung disease, such as pulmonary granulomatous disease and pulmonary abscess. A completely

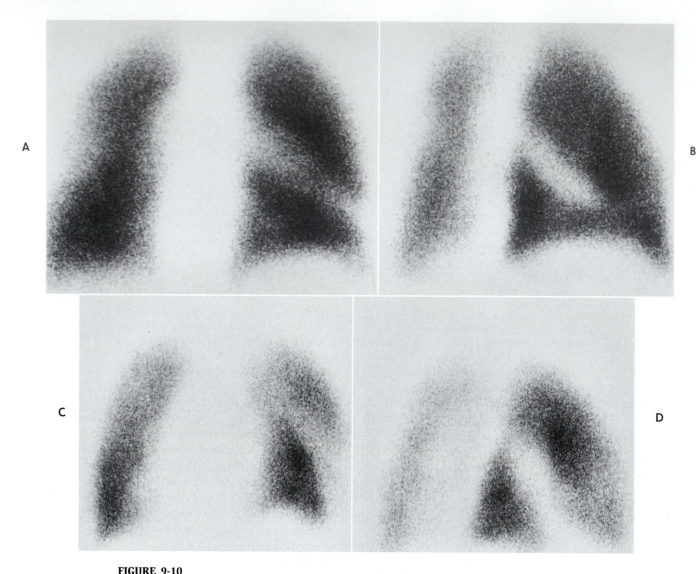

FIGURE 9-10

Two examples of the fissure sign on ^{99m}Tc perfusion scans. **A** and **B,** The only perfusion defect in this 43-year-old man, in whom there was a strong clinical suspicion of pulmonary emboli, was a linear band of low activity corresponding to position of right major fissure. A right pleural effusion was present on the chest radiograph. The pulmonary angiogram was normal. **A,** Posterior. **B,** Right posterior oblique. **C** and **D,** Similar findings in a 78-year-old woman with congestive cardiac failure. In this example, the pleural effusion produces a strikingly large perfusion defect. **C,** Posterior. **D,** Right posterior oblique.

matched defect in a patient with lobar consolidation on chest radiography should arouse suspicion of pulmonary abscess formation.[190]

Notwithstanding pulmonary angiography's limitations in the detection of small peripheral emboli,[262] it has been used as the "gold standard" in many reported comparisons with V/Q scanning. From these, several diagnostic algorithms have been proposed for the interpretation of V/Q lung scans performed for suspected pulmonary thromboembolism.* These algorithms are based on a comparison of the perfusion-ventilation images and the

chest radiograph, and they express the likelihood of embolism as low, intermediate, and high.[174,276] The probability that an abnormal scan is due to pulmonary embolism represents the positive predictive value of the test, which is highly dependent on the prevalence of the disease in the patient population studied.[214] A normal V/Q scan excludes pulmonary embolism with a probability of about 95%.[182,253] Before discussion of these algorithms, it should be emphasized that they have been based largely on ventilation imaging using Xe-133 and have generally assumed a fixed pretest clinical likelihood for pulmonary embolism.

Summarizing the literature, an abnormal V/Q scan

---

*References 29, 32, 38, 60, 158, 159, 160, 213, 253, 317.

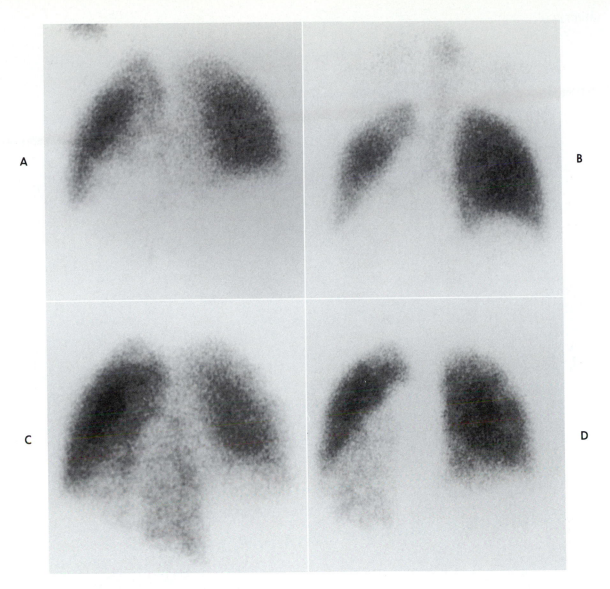

FIGURE 9-11
Lobar pneumonia. There is complete absence of ventilation of the left lower lobe, as seen on, **A,** left posterior oblique and, **B,** posterior views. Perfusion to the left lower lobe shown on, **C,** left posterior oblique and, **D,** posterior views, although markedly reduced, is present. There is therefore evidence of a physiologic right-to-left shunt.

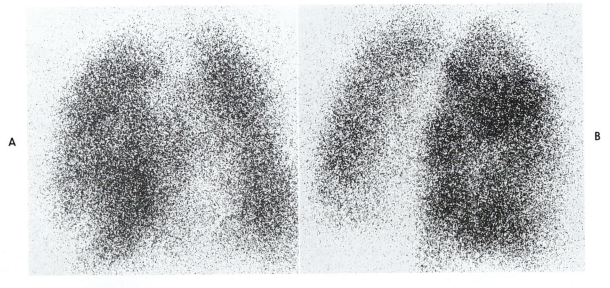

FIGURE 9-12
Low-probability scan. Scattered perfusion defects are all smaller than 25% of a segment. The images are ⁹⁹ᵐTc perfusion scans. **A,** Left posterior oblique. **B,** Right posterior oblique.

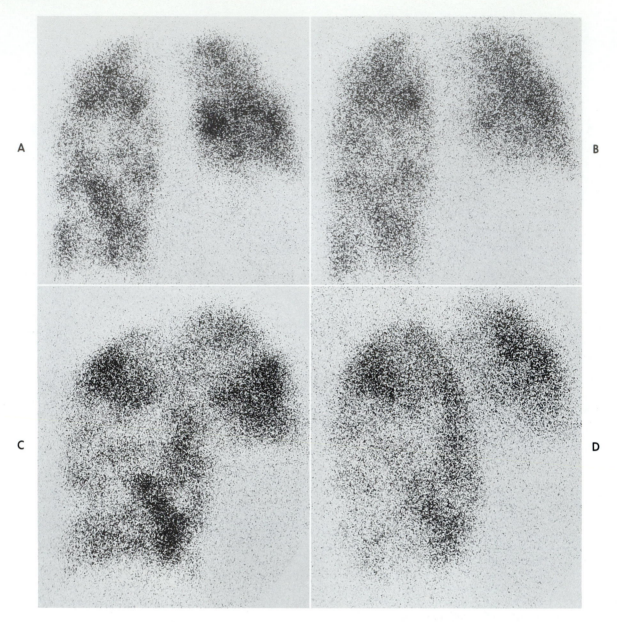

FIGURE 9-13
Low-probability scan. Multiple perfusion defects are matched by corresponding ventilation defects. The images are paired ^{99m}Tc perfusion and ^{81m}Kr ventilation scans. Four of the six standard projections are illustrated. Perfusion scans (**A, C, E, G**) are arranged in left column; corresponding ventilation scans, in right column (**B, D, F, H**).

indicating a low probability for *recent* pulmonary embolism is one in which the individual perfusion defects are (1) smaller than 25% of a segment (that is, subsegmental; Figure 9-12), regardless of the chest radiographic and ventilation scan appearances; or (2) are matched on the ventilation scan (Figure 9-13) or are accompanied by larger chest radiographic abnormalities. Prominent, non-pulmonary structures, such as an enlarged hilum, cardiac chamber, or aorta, are capable of producing matched defects, but they are readily identifiable from the chest radiograph and should not be confused with pulmonary defects.

A V/Q scan indicating a high probability of recent pulmonary embolism is one in which there are two or more perfusion defects, not matched by corresponding ventilation defects or chest radiographic abnormalities, including at least one of segmental or larger size, that were not present in any scan obtained before the clinical episode (Figure 9-14). In the appropriate clinical setting a high probability V/Q scan indicates a probability of

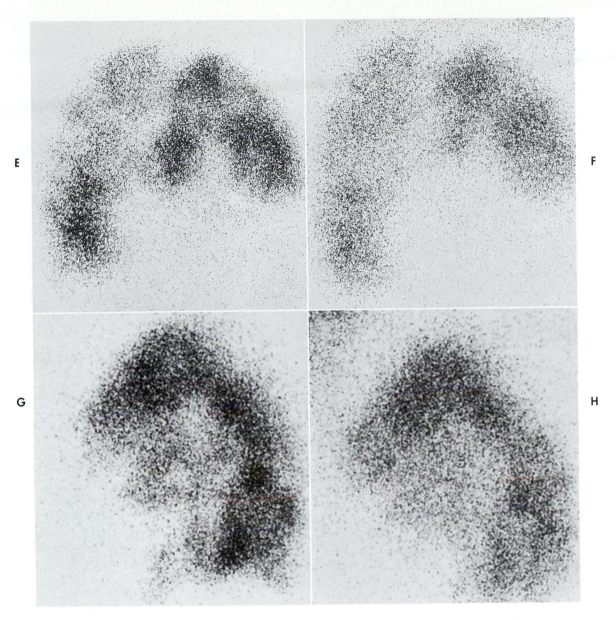

FIGURE 9-13, cont'd
For legend see opposite page.

pulmonary embolism exceeding 90%,[60,213,317,253] although the second criterion for a high probability scan, above, would have to apply; thus, without a scan predating the clinical episode, the probability would be somewhat lower. Conversely, segmental or larger defects resolving within 1 to 3 weeks carry a very high probability of recent embolism.

An intermediate-probability V/Q scan, also described in the literature as an indeterminate scan, is an abnormal scan that does not fit into the low- or high-probability categories. In essence the probability of pulmonary embolism in patients with intermediate-probability scans is likely to be similar to what it was before the scan, which consequently is unlikely to effect a change in management. In general, V/Q scans indicating an intermediate probability for recent pulmonary embolism have been classified in the literature as those (1) with perfusion defects that, although matched, correspond in size and shape to an area of consolidation on the chest radiograph (and may therefore represent infarction), or (2) with perfusion defects in areas of severe obstructive lung disease, pulmonary edema, or pleural effusion. In practice, with Kr-81m ventilation imaging or the current aerosols, the number of scans placed in the intermediate,

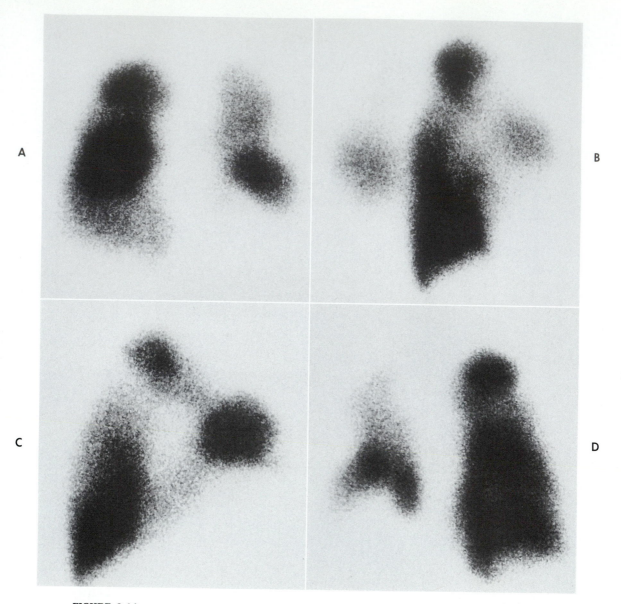

FIGURE 9-14
High-probability scan. Six views of a ^{99m}Tc perfusion scan. **A,** Anterior. **B,** Right posterior oblique. **C,** Right lateral. **D,** Posterior.

or indeterminate, category should be minimal; for example, in the second of the above criteria for intermediate probability, the perfusion abnormalities should be seen, on multiple projection ventilation imaging, to be matched by, or smaller than, the corresponding ventilation defects and so be categorized as "low probability."

Within nuclear medicine reporting practice, the probability stratification approach, with its specified criteria, is exclusive to the V/Q scan performed for suspected pulmonary embolism. This has grown out of the philosophy that the only reason for performing a V/Q lung scan is to diagnose pulmonary embolism. Several reported

comparisons with pulmonary angiography have failed to take into account the clinical and radiologic evidence of deep venous thrombosis, early follow-up of abnormal scans, and the pretest likelihood of the disease.[214,253] This last consideration was brought out by the PIOPED study in which it was shown that the incidence of abnormal pulmonary angiography was greater, in all probability categories, when the prescan clinical likelihood of pulmonary embolism was high compared with when it was it low. The original classifications were based on Xe-133 for ventilation imaging, which, although it could have been performed with multiple projections, was generally based

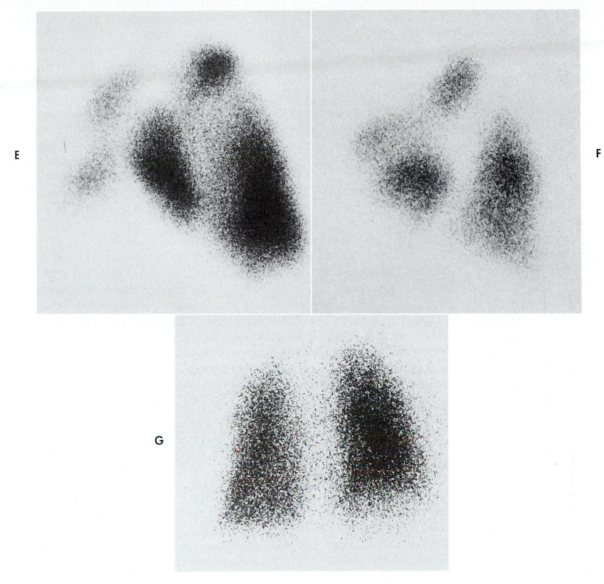

FIGURE 9-14, cont'd
E, Left posterior oblique. F, Left lateral. The ventilation scan was a normal study. G, Selected image of
posterior ^{133}Xe scan at 1 minute after beginning of the wash-in.

on posterior imaging only. With the advent of high-quality ventilation imaging the importance of which cannot be overstressed, the chest radiograph should become less important in determining the probability of pulmonary embolism from the V/Q scan, although it must be viewed at the same time as the scan and correlated with whatever abnormalities are present on the scan, whether or not the presence of suspected pulmonary embolism is being investigated.

Hull and co-workers[160] suggested a relatively high incidence of pulmonary embolism in patients with low-probability scans. They demonstrated the value of com-

bining the V/Q scan with impedance plethysmography for the simultaneous diagnosis of deep venous thrombosis. Patients with low probability V/Q scans who had no evidence of deep venous thrombosis, and were not receiving anticoagulants, had a very low incidence of recurrent thromboembolism on follow-up. In other words, even though they came from a group ("low probability") with an incidence of abnormal pulmonary angiography of about 40% in this series, their pulmonary embolic disease was apparently of minor clinical significance. This observation emphasizes the value of viewing V/Q lung scanning (combined with an objective assessment of venous thrombosis) as a means of identifying patients who require anticoagulation rather than making a diagnosis of pulmonary embolism per se.[174] The purpose of anticoagulation is, after all, not to treat embolism, but to prevent further embolization.

In the context of the patient with suspected pulmonary embolism, an important function of the chest radiograph, apart from providing anatomic landmarks, is to avoid missing pulmonary infarction. A matched defect without a corresponding radiographic abnormality has a low probability for pulmonary embolism: the appearance of a corresponding radiographic abnormality moves the V/Q scan into the intermediate category because it increases the likelihood of infarction. Partial mismatching typical of infarction with an appropriate radiographic abnormality further increases the likelihood. An important question that remains unanswered is how often an infarct can give a completely matched defect. If uncommon, the matched defect could be relegated to low probability, irrespective of the chest radiograph.

Rather than listing the criteria for categorizing a lung scan as low, intermediate, or high probability, it may be more useful to identify those features on the V/Q lung scan that cause the most difficulty in diagnosing pulmonary embolism. These are the solitary unmatched perfusion defect, symmetric segmental unmatched perfusion defects, the matched perfusion defect with a similar-sized corresponding radiographic opacity, multiple unmatched but subsegmental perfusion defects, and unmatched segmental perfusion defects not clearly seen on any projection to extend to the periphery of the lung (the so-called stripe sign). In this setting it is important to appreciate that the unmatched perfusion defect points to pulmonary vascular disease and not specifically to embolic disease. The solitary unmatched perfusion defect has been reported to be due to proven embolism only about 50% of the time.[127,279,317] In a population with a high prevalence of pulmonary embolism, it would indicate a high probability of the disease, as would symmetric segmental unmatched defects. On the other hand, if the patient is known to have a medium-sized arteritis, or is a smoker and the unmatched perfusion defect involves an entire lung with a normal contralateral lung, the diagnosis of pulmonary embolism would be considerably less certain. The matched perfusion defect with corresponding radiographic opacity is classified as indeterminate because it may or may not represent pulmonary infarction, although again the literature is not clear on how many are actually partially mismatched, as a result of infarction, and likely to be seen on Xe-133 imaging as a matched defect. Multiple unmatched subsegmental perfusion defects are unlikely to represent recent pulmonary embolism, since, after multiple emboli, at least one would be expected to produce a segmental defect. Furthermore, multiple unmatched subsegmental perfusion defects are seen in primary pulmonary hypertension, Eisenmenger's syndrome, and venoocclusive disease (see later discus-

sion). The fifth of these features, the "stripe" sign, does not carry the diagnostic weight of the defect that clearly interrupts the normal contour of the lung.[315]

Another controversial area is the confidence with which pulmonary embolism is excluded in patients with multiple matched defects. Although most experts seem to agree that the probability *is* low, Hull and co-workers[159,160] found a surprisingly high incidence of abnormal pulmonary angiograms in patients with such scans. They proposed that regional bronchoconstriction in response to pulmonary vascular occlusion may result in matched V/Q defects in pulmonary embolism. This physiologic phenomenon has been demonstrated experimentally but is not widely accepted in clinical practice as a cause of a matched defect.

There are several diseases other than pulmonary embolism in which the V/Q scan may show mismatched perfusion abnormalities. A mismatched defect indicates pulmonary vascular disease, which usually, although not always, is due to pulmonary embolism. The causes of mismatched perfusion defects are listed in the box below. Important causes include carcinoma of the bronchus, which often gives rise to the characteristic finding of a completely nonperfused lung or lobe with a normally perfused opposite lung and normal ventilation (Figure

---

CAUSES OF VENTILATION-PERFUSION MISMATCHING

Pulmonary embolism
  Acute
  Chronic
Pulmonary thrombosis
External compression of pulmonary artery
  Carcinoma of the bronchus
  Lymphoma
Primary pulmonary hypertension
Pulmonary venoocclusive disease
Vasculitis of medium-sized arteries
Ventilated bullae
Focal obliteration of pulmonary capillaries
  Fibrosing alveolitis
  Emphysema
  Tuberculosis
  Irradiation
Congenital pulmonary artery hypoplasia
Sequestered segment
Artifact (may be posture dependent)
  Unstable ventilation
  Related to pleural fluid
Upper lobe diversion (in heart disease)
Previous vascular surgery with creation of intravascular shunts.
Intraluminal obstruction (e.g., catheters, *Dirofilaria immitis*)
Pulmonary arteriovenous malformations (especially following therapeutic embolization)

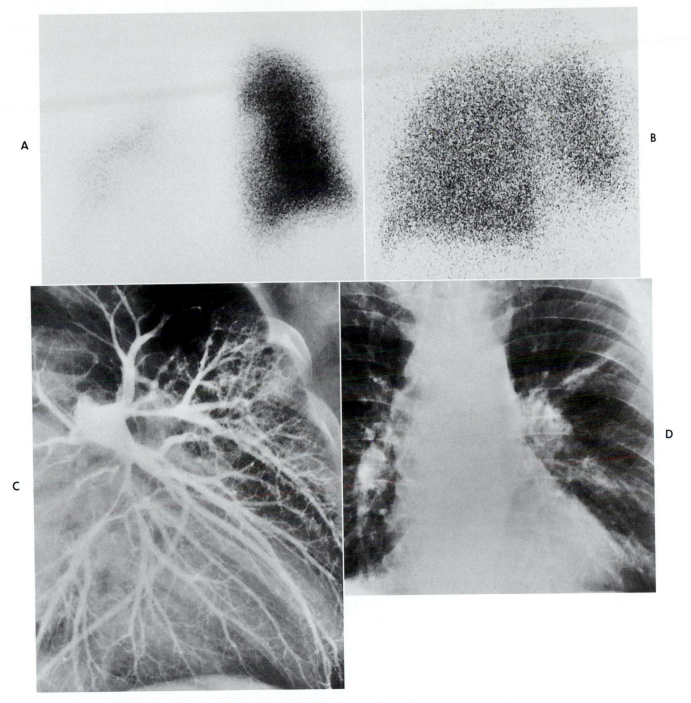

FIGURE 9-15
Mismatched perfusion defect resulting from a carcinoma of the bronchus involving the major divisions of the left pulmonary artery. **A**, ^{99m}Tc scan, posterior view. **B**, ^{133}Xe ventilation scan, left posterior oblique. **C**, Pulmonary arteriogram illustrates involvement of the central pulmonary arteries by the tumor. **D**, Posteroanterior radiograph.

9-15); bullae, which occasionally ventilate[73] but are usually evident on the chest radiograph; pulmonary vasculitis involving medium-sized arteries, which may be indistinguishable from embolism; and fibrosing alveolitis, which usually involves the lower zones symmetrically (Figure 9-16). In children, in whom pulmonary embolism is rarely diagnosed, unmatched perfusion defects are more likely to be due to sequestered lobes or segments, congenital anomalies of the pulmonary artery, and previous surgery for congenital cardiovascular anomalies.

The indeterminate scan, as distinct from the intermediate-probability scan, is a category that should perhaps

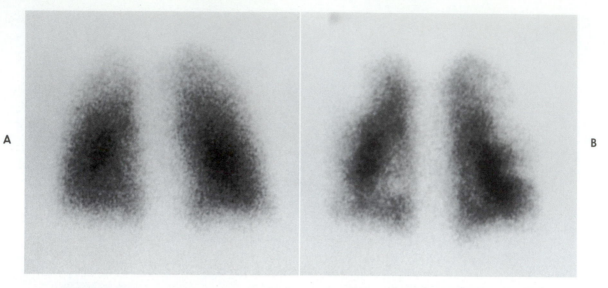

FIGURE 9-16
Fibrosing alveolitis. This disease is one of several, other than pulmonary embolic disease, that may give rise to unmatched perfusion defects. This V/Q scan (posterior view) shows extensive perfusion abnormalities (**B**) but normal ^{81m}Kr ventilation images (**A**).

be reserved for one particular finding: the presence of a perfusion defect in a region of lung in which ventilation has been abolished. Thus it is not unusual to find a perfusion defect in a lobe that has been compressed by a pleural effusion, which itself may be the result of an embolic episode (Figure 9-17). In this instance, since there is no ventilation signal, it is impossible to determine whether the perfusion defect is matched or not, and if there are no other unmatched perfusion defects elsewhere in the lung, the significance of the perfusion defect in terms of pulmonary embolism is truly indeterminate.

IMAGING THROMBOEMBOLISM WITH RADIOLABELED COMPONENTS OF THE CLOTTING SYSTEM. Positive imaging of thromboembolism was first achieved with indium-111 (In-111) labeled platelets.[124] However, it did not become a routine clinical procedure, mainly because it is labor intensive, but more fundamentally because thrombus must be active to accumulate platelets. In-111 platelets must be administered before heparinization, which reduces platelet accumulation on thrombus. A promising approach is the use of P256, a radiolabeled monoclonal antibody to platelets,[328] which has been shown to be successful for localizing DVT and pulmonary emboli in postoperative patients.[181]

Another approach under investigation is the use of agents that bind to fibrin and therefore have the theoretic advantage of being effective in relatively older thrombus and after anticoagulation. One such agent is an In-111-labeled monoclonal antibody against fibrin.[81] An agent that uses a similar principle is fragment E1, which is a fragment of fibrin that recombines with fibrin but not fibrinogen. Since this, a peptide, is a smaller molecule than an antibody, it has a theoretic advantage of faster

blood clearance and therefore an increased target-to-background ratio.[183] Even more recent is a tripeptide that is a "molecular recognition unit" of fibrinogen and binds to the fibrinogen receptor of platelets following their activation. This agent has the theoretic advantage of being selective for platelets that have already accumulated in thrombus and so should bind preformed thrombus in patients receiving anticoagulants.

PULMONARY ANGIOGRAPHY. Accurate morbidity and mortality statistics for pulmonary angiography are difficult to obtain. In the PIOPED study there were five deaths (0.5%) out of the 1111 patients who underwent pulmonary angiography.[323] In some large series there are no deaths,[60,239,264,349] and in others the rate is less than 1%, usually under 0.5%.* When all these series are combined, 15 deaths, in a total of 5320 patients, can be attributed to pulmonary angiography.[323] Pulmonary hypertension was a major predisposing factor; nine of the ten patients surveyed by Goodman[123] had proved or presumed pulmonary hypertension. Of the nonfatal complications, arrhythmias are the most common, followed by cardiac perforation. Cardiac perforation, although it may lead to pericardial tamponade, frequently resolves without incident, particularly if there is no associated myocardial intravasation. Such nonfatal complications can be expected in 1% to 5% of patients.[323] Elderly patients are more at risk of renal failure but otherwise have the same low complication rate as younger patients.[324] It should be borne in mind that patients subjected to angiography tend to be more acutely ill and are therefore less likely to recover from physical insults. When a perfusion lung

---

*References 21, 75, 106, 202, 219, 231.

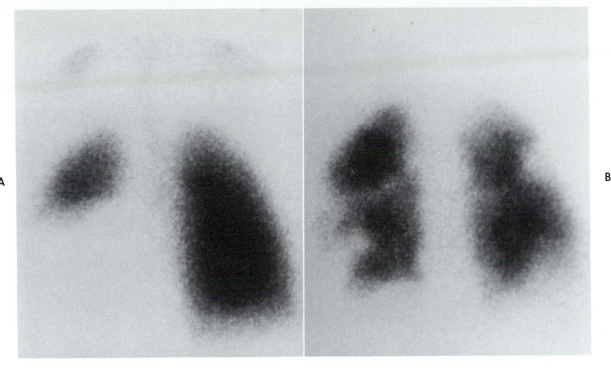

FIGURE 9-17
Pleural effusion in association with pulmonary embolism. **A,** There are multiple perfusion defects in both lungs (posterior view). **B,** Those in the right lung are clearly unmatched on the [81mKr] ventilation image (posterior view), which shows normal ventilation to the right lung but absence of ventilation in the left lower lobe owing to the effusion. Although the overall picture suggests high probability of pulmonary embolic disease, perfusion defects in the left lower lobe would put the left lung scan in the indeterminate category if there had been no unmatched defects in the right lung.

scan has been performed, the angiographic examination can be tailored to search for emboli in the areas of perfusion defect. Thus the perfusion scan helps in performing the study and may also reduce complications by justifying a more limited examination than would otherwise be necessary.[87] In critically ill patients a technique for performing pulmonary angiography on the intensive care unit has been described.[280]

Interpretation. The two major angiographic signs of acute pulmonary embolism are (Figures 9-18 and 9-19)[75,95,325,371]:

1. Intraluminal filling defects within the opacified arterial tree seen on two or more films during the angiographic study. These filling defects are caused by opacified blood flowing around the thrombus. Sometimes, the contrast medium flows past the thrombus to opacify the distal vessels. At other times only the trailing edge of a thrombus impacted in a downstream arterial branch is seen.

2. Occlusion of a pulmonary artery branch. Occlusion is a nonspecific sign and may be seen in a variety of conditions, including congenital malformations, organized thrombus from a previous embolus, in situ thrombosis, mediastinal fibrosis, occlusion from direct involvement by neoplasm, inflammatory disease (such as lung abscess or granulomatous infection), progressive massive fibrosis, or pneumoconiosis.

The other arteriographic sign of pulmonary embolism is focal reduction or delay in the opacification of the pulmonary arterial branches,[75] equivalent to the perfusion defect seen at radionuclide imaging. Clearly, reduced perfusion, regardless of how it is demonstrated, is a less specific sign than an intraluminal filling defect or an abrupt occlusion of a vessel.[35,286] It will be seen in any condition that destroys lung parenchyma, notably emphysema, bronchiectasis, or pulmonary scarring, and in any condition that leads to focal hypoxic constriction.

Pulmonary thromboemboli usually lyse following the embolic episode. In dogs, experimentally produced emboli can disappear within days,[77,229] and rapid resolution has also been recorded in humans.[291] In general, however, it appears that thromboemboli are detectable angiographically for weeks or months following the acute event. Goodman[123] recently reviewed the literature on the subject and warned that pulmonary angiography should not be withheld simply because of a few days' delay in the onset of symptoms.

Some emboli do not lyse completely. They may leave residual webs, which can be seen angiographically,[186,251] or they may form permanent occlusions. Pulmonary

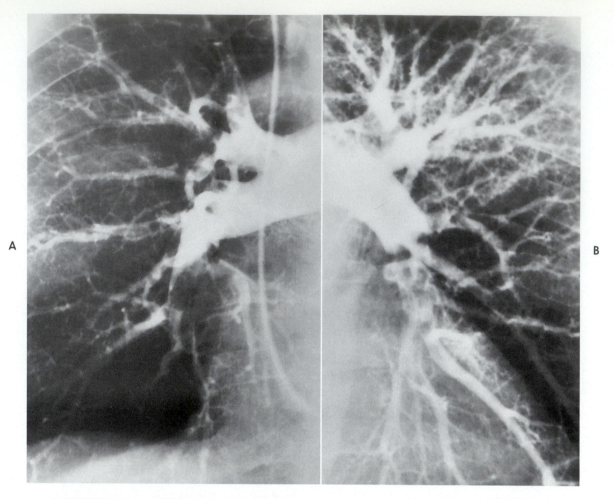

FIGURE 9-18
Pulmonary emboli. There are multiple filling defects and occlusions of branches of the pulmonary arteries on pulmonary angiography. **A**, Right and, **B**, left pulmonary arteriograms.

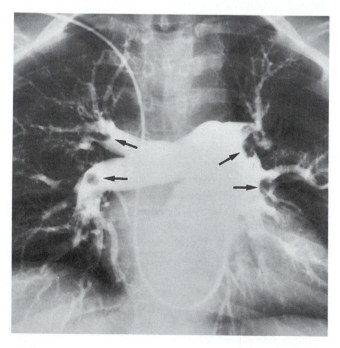

FIGURE 9-19
Pulmonary emboli. Pulmonary angiogram shows multiple filling defects. Trailing ends of the occluding thromboemboli are particularly well shown *(arrows)*.

arterial hypertension may result[379] when multiple vessels are occluded. In chronic pulmonary embolism the occlusion of vessels dominates the picture; the filling defects of recent emboli are then often more difficult to find and may not be detectable.

Indications. Which patients should have angiography? Practice varies,* but, in general, pulmonary angiography is recommended for patients with suspected pulmonary embolism in the following circumstances:

1. When the V/Q scan is abnormal but cannot be placed into either high- or low-probability categories. This is a particularly common dilemma in patients with underlying chronic obstructive lung disease.[192]

2. When the V/Q scan result is significantly at variance with the clinical probability of pulmonary embolism.

3. When thrombolytic therapy or long-term anticoagulation is contemplated, or when drug therapy would carry a high risk.

4. Before embolectomy, vena caval interruption, or filter insertion.

---

*References 60, 70, 236, 274, 281, 316.

In practice these criteria are not strictly adhered to. It has been argued that physicians should realize that the risks of pulmonary angiography performed by experienced operators, although not negligible, are often less than those of anticoagulant therapy, particularly in patients whose V/Q scan findings are nonspecific,[60] and that pulmonary angiography should therefore be performed more readily, not just as a last resort.[274] The fact that practice varies so much reflects the inherent difficulties of assigning risks and benefits in the entity of pulmonary embolism.

Pulmonary angiography is the currently accepted "gold standard" for the diagnosis of pulmonary embolism during life.[21,75,274] It is self-evident, however, that there must be both false-positive and false-negative interpretations. Nevertheless, it appears that life-threatening emboli are not missed. Novelline and associates,[239] Cheely and co-workers,[60] and the PIOPED study[253] all followed large groups of patients clinically suspected of having pulmonary embolism who had normal pulmonary angiograms. Had significant pulmonary emboli been overlooked, it seems likely that some of these patients would have had further embolic episodes in the ensuing years. In fact, none of Novelline's 167 patients did, even though they were not receiving anticoagulant therapy; in three cases small incidental emboli were found in patients dying from other causes.[239] In Cheely's series, 4 of 144 patients with negative angiograms subsequently developed emboli, but in none were they the cause of death.[60] In the PIOPED study, surveillance of 675 patients with negative angiograms revealed 4 (0.06%) patients with pulmonary embolism.[253] The problem of false-positive diagnoses is more difficult to evaluate.[325] Despite the reiteration that pulmonary angiography is relatively safe and highly sensitive, the provision of pulmonary angiography is often lacking.[70]

DIGITAL SUBTRACTION ANGIOGRAPHY. The advantages of digital subtraction angiography are increased contrast resolution and greater safety, but these advantages are currently offset by the poor spatial resolution of the imaging system and, particularly, motion artifact from misregistration of mask frames.[31,94,155] The technique is increasingly available in clinical practice and has its advocates.[234] It appears to be significantly better at diagnosing emboli in the proximal two thirds of the pulmonary arterial tree than for emboli lodged distally, and may be a good alternative to radionuclide imaging, particularly in patients with chronic obstructive lung disease.[196]

COMPUTED TOMOGRAPHY, MAGNETIC RESONANCE IMAGING, AND ECHOCARDIOGRAPHY. Large thrombi in the main pulmonary arteries and their major branches may be visible on both contrast-enhanced CT (Figures 9-20 and 9-21)[13,63,119,175,179] and electrocardiographically gated MRI.* Most reports have concentrated on the

detection of central emboli in patients with pulmonary arterial hypertension, although individual cases with peripheral emboli have been demonstrated as intraluminal filling defects on contrast-enhanced CT scans.[39] Neither technique is currently used on a routine basis, and there are no data on sensitivity and specificity. Ultrafast CT can be used to identify intraventricular thrombi that may be responsible for pulmonary emboli,[223] and spiral volumetric CT scanning seems to be an effective way of demonstrating pulmonary emboli in central to fourth division pulmonary arteries.[267] MRI appears to be the more promising of the two techniques because no contrast agent is needed and because blood clots in the pulmonary arteries generate a different signal from fast-flowing blood. Care must be taken not to misinterpret the signal generated from slow-flowing blood on MR images, a phenomenon that is particularly common in patients with pulmonary arterial hypertension. The distinction between slow-flowing blood and thrombus is best made by comparing the change in signal intensity during the cardiac cycle.[97,368] Intraluminal clot produces signal intensity that remains fixed in distribution during the cardiac cycle and demonstrates little or no increase in relative intensity from first to second echo in spin-echo sequences,[368] whereas the signal from slow-flowing blood varies with the cardiac cycle and increases in relative intensity from the first to second echo. At its current stage of development MRI does not appear to be clinically useful in the diagnosis of peripheral pulmonary emboli.[259,368] There is experimental evidence that a blood pool macromolecular contrast agent may enable MRI to detect more peripheral perfusion defects.[27] Increasingly sophisticated MRI techniques are being developed so that high-resolution, three-dimensional pulmonary angiograms showing sixth- and seventh-order vessels are now possible.[104,140,370]

Infarcts in the lung may show a pleura-based truncated cone or triangular configuration on CT scans—a shape that corresponds to the Hampton's hump described earlier in this chapter (Figure 9-22). While the cross-sectional images of CT show the wedge shape of pulmonary infarction to advantage,[308] a postmortem HRCT study of 83 fixed lungs with subpleural densities (12 contained pulmonary infarcts and 71 a variety of pathologic conditions including pneumonia, hemorrhage, and tumor) showed that there was no significant difference in the incidence of wedge-shaped opacities on CT between the lungs with infarcts and those with other disorders. A "vascular sign" (a vessel running into the apex of the wedge) was slightly more common in the infarct group.[268] In the in vivo CT study of Balakrishnan and co-workers,[13] the vascular sign was not so prevalent. Furthermore, some infarcts did not have the truncated wedge configuration but had a more rounded form without a broad base in contact with the pleura.[13,63]

The high signal intensity of T1-weighted MR images of acute hemorrhage associated with pulmonary infarc-

---

*References 110, 224, 259, 322, 333, 339.

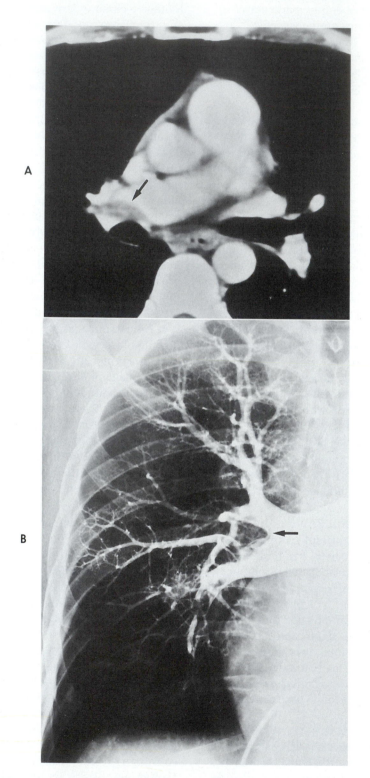

FIGURE 9-20
Pulmonary emboli. **A,** Arrow points to an intraluminal defect in the right pulmonary artery on
contrast-enhanced computed tomography scan. **B,** Corresponding pulmonary angiogram shows a large
embolus straddling the bifurcation of the right pulmonary artery *(arrow)* and multiple emboli
occluding the right lower lobe artery and its branches.

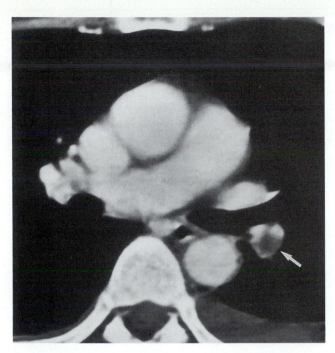

FIGURE 9-21
Contrast-enhanced computed tomography scan showing a filling defect as result of an embolus lodged in the left lower lobe artery (arrows).

tion[269] is nonspecific and may be seen in other hemorrhagic conditions, including lung contusion.

Both transthoracic and transesophageal echocardiography can be used to evaluate central pulmonary emboli and the direct hemodynamic effects of embolism on right ventricular and tricuspid valve function.[69,109,115] Transesophageal echocardiography is reported to be more reliable than transthoracic echocardiography in demonstrating pulmonary emboli in transit.[163]

TUMOR EMBOLISM

Tumor emboli sufficiently large to be hemodynamically significant are sometimes encountered[52,134,374] and can on occasion be the presenting feature of the neoplastic disease.[44,79] They occlude small pulmonary vessels and can give rise to severe dyspnea, which usually develops over a matter of days[314] but sometimes builds up over several weeks.[144] Pleuritic chest pain is relatively common, and fatigue, weight loss, cough, hemoptysis, and syncope are seen in a few patients.

On physical examination most patients show signs of right ventricular overload, but just as with pulmonary thromboembolism there may be relatively few respiratory findings. The condition differs from widespread, bloodborne metastases in that a metastasis represents tumor that has invaded the vessel wall and acquired its own blood supply, whereas tumor emboli are clumps of cells that are lodged within the lumen of the pulmonary vessels and have not yet invaded the vessel wall but are acting as obstructing emboli similar to thromboemboli. The pa-

tients are hypoxemic, have increased alveolar-arterial oxygen gradients, and have pulmonary arterial hypertension, sometimes severe.[51] Tumor emboli are a fairly frequent finding at autopsy, but the condition is rarely diagnosed ante mortem. Chan and co-workers,[52] in their extensive review of the literature on the subject, found a wide distribution of types of malignancy. The primary tumors frequently associated with tumor embolism are hepatoma, breast and renal carcinoma,[79] gastric and prostate cancers, and choriocarcinoma.[91,125] The diagnosis of pulmonary endovascular choriocarcinoma in young female patients is important because it is potentially curable with chemotherapy.[295]

The plain chest radiographs are usually normal. Pulmonary arterial hypertension is rarely recognizable. A few patients show nonspecific pulmonary shadows. Radionuclide lung scans show multiple, small, peripheral, subsegmental perfusion defects with a normal ventilation scan. Pulmonary angiography shows delayed filling of segmental arteries, reduction in number of branch vessels, and occasionally 1 to 2 mm filling defects.

The mortality of the condition is very high, and the role of intervention is not clear. Surgical resection of the primary tumor without specific treatment of the emboli has been attempted, and good results have been claimed.[79] Whether these emboli will respond to chemotherapy has not yet been investigated; the number of patients whose disease is diagnosed ante mortem is very low.

PULMONARY ARTERIAL HYPERTENSION

Pulmonary artery pressure is a function of blood flow and the resistance across the pulmonary vascular system, the resistance to flow depending predominantly on the cross-sectional area of the perfused vascular bed. The pulmonary vascular bed has a much lower resistance than the systemic circuit and can respond to increasing flow by opening up additional vascular channels. Pulmonary arterial hypertension occurs when the flow increases to such an extent that the available extra channels are saturated, or because of vasoconstriction or structural change in the small pulmonary vessels. It is defined as pulmonary artery pressures above the normal systolic value of 30 mm Hg or above the mean value of 18 mm Hg.

The radiographic features of pulmonary arterial hypertension are discussed before the various causes are described (see box on p. 394) because the same signs are seen regardless of the cause of the hypertension. The basic signs are cardiac enlargement, right ventricular enlargement, and enlargement of the central pulmonary arteries with rapid tapering of the vessels as they proceed distally (Figure 9-23). The distal vessels may be large, normal, or reduced in caliber. The important point is the disparity in the relative size of the central and distal vessels. The terms "central" and "distal" are inevitably vague because there is no precise anatomic definition of central and distal (peripheral) vessels, but the term

CLASSIFICATION OF PULMONARY HYPERTENSION

INCREASED RESISTANCE TO PULMONARY VENOUS DRAINAGE

Congenital narrowing of pulmonary veins
Mediastinal fibrosis
Pulmonary venoocclusive disease
Left atrial obstruction — mitral valve disease, cor triatriatum, left atrial myxoma
Left ventricular dysfunction
Constrictive pericarditis

INCREASED RESISTANCE DUE TO DISEASE IN THE ARTERIAL-ARTERIOLAR WALL OR LUMEN

Emboli: thrombotic and other
Primary pulmonary hypertension
Eisenmenger's syndrome
Persistence of fetal circulation
Arteriopathy in hepatic cirrhosis
Drug or chemically induced
Pulmonary vasculitis
Schistosomiasis
Congenital stenosis
Hypogenesis or aplasia
Surgical resection of lung

INCREASED PULMONARY VASCULAR RESISTANCE SECONDARY TO PLEUROPULMONARY DISEASE

Chronic obstructive pulmonary disease
Interstitial fibrosis of the lungs
Sarcoidosis
Pneumoconioses
Granulomatous infections
Pleural fibrothorax

INCREASED PULMONARY BLOOD FLOW

Left-to-right shunts (atrial septal defect, ventricular septal defect, patent ductus arteriosus)

HYPOVENTILATION

Obesity hypoventilation syndrome
Pharyngeal and tracheal obstructions
High altitude
Neuromuscular disorders of breathing
Chest wall deformity, kyphoscoliosis

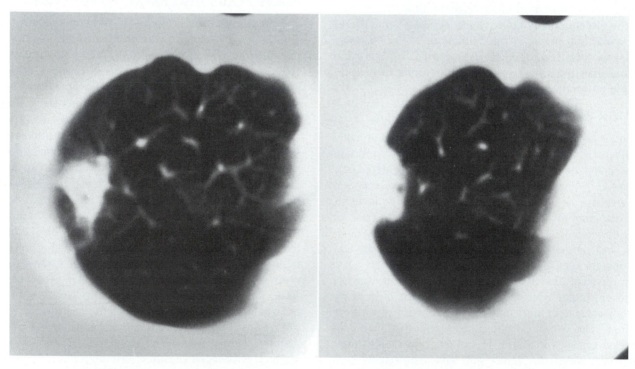

A   B

FIGURE 9-22
Computed tomography scans of a pulmonary infarct in the right upper lobe. **A** and **B,** Adjacent sections illustrating a truncated cone shape based on the pleura (same patient as in Figure 9-20).

"central arteries" refers to the main pulmonary artery and its branches approximately down to segmental level. The term "distal vessels" refers to vessels beyond the segmental level. The criteria of central vessel dilatation on plain chest radiographs are with one exception also poorly defined. On plain film the main pulmonary artery forms the border for less than half of its circumference, and this border represents a portion of the vessel that is traveling obliquely upward and backward. Thus, diagnosing dilatation based on increased prominence or convexity of the main pulmonary artery segment of the cardiac contour is at best a crude measurement. CT scanning provides a more accurate indication of size. One well-documented measurement of the size of the pulmonary arterial tree on plain films is that of the right descending pulmonary artery.[53] The upper limit of normal for transverse diameter at the midpoint of this vessel is 16 to 17 mm. Thus measurements of 17 mm or greater indicate dilatation (Figure 9-24).

The degree of dilatation of the central pulmonary arteries varies considerably, not only among the various entities that cause pulmonary arterial hypertension, but also from patient to patient with the same condition. Therefore, although the radiographic changes are reasonably specific, they are neither sensitive nor well correlated with the severity of the hypertension. Indeed, severe pulmonary arterial hypertension can be present in pa-

tients with a normal-appearing chest radiograph. Possibly because more precise measurement of the main pulmonary artery is possible with CT, Kuriyama and associates[187] found good correlation between the calculated cross-sectional area of the main pulmonary artery, adjusted for body surface area, and mean pulmonary artery pressure. Pulmonary artery distensibility, as judged by changes in pulmonary artery caliber on MRI, is significantly diminished in patients with pulmonary arterial hypertension.[33,114] Furthermore, velocity mapping with cine MRI shows inhomogeneity of flow in the main pulmonary arteries in pulmonary hypertension.[185]

Prolonged severe pulmonary arterial hypertension may lead to atheroma formation in the central pulmonary arteries or their branches (Figure 9-25). (Atheroma is not seen in the pulmonary circuit with normal pulmonary artery pressures.) The atheroma reveals itself radiographically by curvilinear calcification identical to that seen with atheromatous change in the aorta and its branches. In practice, atheromatous calcification of the pulmonary

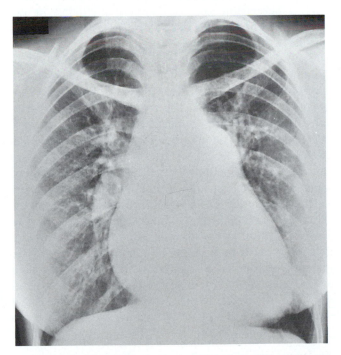

FIGURE 9-23
Pulmonary arterial hypertension illustrating cardiomegaly and enlargement of the main pulmonary artery and hilar arteries. Vessels beyond the hilum are normal or small, notably in the lower zones. The patient, a 19-year-old woman, had severe primary pulmonary hypertension.

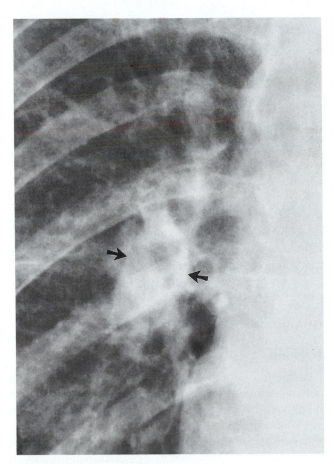

FIGURE 9-24
Pulmonary arterial hypertension caused by chronic pulmonary thromboembolism showing the method of measuring the size of the lower lobe arteries. Transverse diameter of the right lower artery in this patient *(arrows)* measures 19 mm.

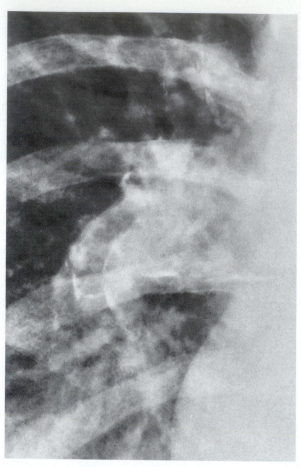

FIGURE 9-25
Atheromatous calcification in the pulmonary arteries in a patient with prolonged severe pulmonary hypertension caused by a patent ductus arteriosus with Eisenmenger's syndrome.

artery is very rare and is seen only in Eisenmenger's syndrome and in a few patients with very prolonged pulmonary hypertension. Dissection of the pulmonary artery is even rarer and may be recognized on echocardiography or, as described in a single case report, on cine MRI.[327]

Pulmonary hypertension secondary to increased resistance to pulmonary venous drainage

Restriction of flow through the pulmonary venous system or through the left atrium and mitral valve raises pulmonary venous pressure, which in turn leads to elevation of pulmonary arterial pressure. With a healthy right ventricle, increases in mean left atrial pressure up to 25 mm Hg are accompanied by a proportional increase in pulmonary artery pressure to maintain a constant mean gradient of approximately 10 mm Hg. When the mean venous pressure is chronically greater than 25 mm Hg, a disproportionate elevation of pulmonary arterial pressure is observed, indicating an increase in pulmonary arteriolar resistance. (Mitral stenosis is a good example; just

under one third of patients with stenosis sufficiently severe to chronically elevate pulmonary venous pressure above 25 mm Hg develop systolic pressures of 80 mm Hg or greater.) The mechanism for the elevation of pulmonary arterial pressure is unclear. Both vasoconstriction and structural changes play a part. Microscopic examination shows distention of the pulmonary capillaries, thickening and rupture of the basement membranes of the endothelial cells, and minor degrees of hemorrhage into the alveoli. The appearance of the arteries depends on whether the venous obstruction has been present since birth or was acquired later in life. In adult-onset pulmonary arterial hypertension there is medial hypertrophy and intimal fibrosis of the smaller pulmonary arteries and arterioles. Necrotizing arteritis may occasionally be seen.

The changes of pulmonary arterial hypertension secondary to chronic impedance of pulmonary venous drainage are visible radiologically only when the pulmonary arterial pressures are very high. Such high pressures are almost never encountered in left ventricular failure, reduced left ventricular compliance, or constrictive pericarditis. Thus, when pulmonary arterial hypertension can be diagnosed radiologically in an adult, the conditions to be considered in the category of increased impedance to pulmonary venous drainage are mitral valve disease, left atrial myxoma, cor triatriatum (which may develop in adulthood), and pulmonary venoocclusive disease. (Pulmonary venoocclusive disease has been grouped by the World Health Organization [WHO] with primary pulmonary hypertension and is therefore discussed in the section "Pulmonary Venoocclusive Disease" later in this chapter).

The radiographic changes reflect a combination of pulmonary arterial and pulmonary venous hypertension together with the features of the primary condition (Figures 9-26 and 9-27). The central pulmonary arteries are dilated, tapering to normal caliber at or beyond segmental level. The peripheral lower zone arteries may even be reduced in caliber. The upper zone vessels are enlarged because of upper zone blood diversion. In mitral stenosis the left atrium is enlarged and may show calcification either in its wall or in left atrial thrombus. Although the left atrium is almost invariably enlarged in cases of mitral valve disease with pulmonary arterial hypertension, it may not be strikingly big, and enlargement should therefore be looked for carefully on the plain chest radiograph. The chest radiograph in left atrial myxoma is identical to that of mitral stenosis except that occasionally it is possible to recognize focal calcifications within the tumor mass.

Pulmonary hypertension secondary to thromboembolism

Pulmonary hypertension may follow acute pulmonary embolism when the emboli occlude enough of the pulmonary arterial bed. The mechanisms are complex, consisting of a mixture of mechanical obstruction and

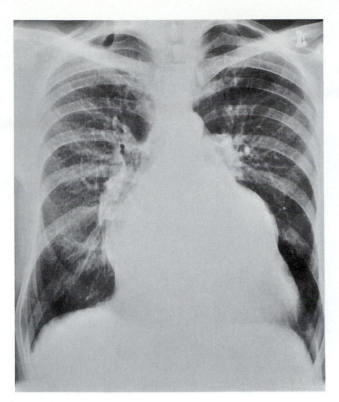

FIGURE 9-26
Pulmonary arterial hypertension secondary to mitral stenosis. Note the large hilar arteries and small arteries beyond the hila. The upper zone vessels are large because of elevation of the pulmonary venous pressure, and the left atrium is massively dilated.

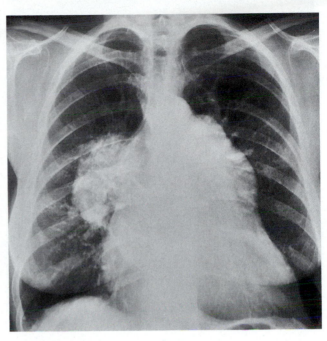

FIGURE 9-27
Pulmonary arterial hypertension caused by mitral stenosis. Dilatation of the central pulmonary arteries is particularly striking in this 59-year-old woman with systemic pressures in her pulmonary circuit. Note the enlarged left atrium.

vasoconstriction. These acute changes in pulmonary artery pressure do not produce radiographically visible pulmonary arterial hypertension, in part because a previously normal right ventricle can only produce right ventricular systolic pressures up to 45 to 55 mm Hg. Higher pressures require preexisting right ventricular hypertrophy.

Repetitive thromboemboli without intervening lysis of thrombi may lead to chronic elevation of pulmonary artery pressure. The condition is rare, being seen in less than 1% of patients following acute emboli. Sometimes there is an obvious source for recurrent pulmonary emboli, such as a ventriculoatrial shunt catheter.[252] There is, however, debate about whether pulmonary hypertension caused by chronic obstruction of the pulmonary arterial blood flow is the result of recurrent pulmonary emboli rather than thrombotic occlusion of the pulmonary microvasculature.[270] Infarction is not usually a feature, and the condition frequently is not diagnosed until the progressive occlusion of the pulmonary vascular bed has led to symptomatic pulmonary arterial hypertension.[137] It is these patients who may show the radiographic changes of pulmonary arterial hypertension. Surgical thromboendarterectomy may be undertaken in carefully selected patients with substantial success.[227,228,285] A few patients with unilateral chronic

thromboembolic occlusion have all the radiographic features reminiscent of pulmonary artery agenesis; the correct diagnosis is important because these patients may otherwise be denied the appropriate treatment, thromboendarterectomy.[230]

At pathologic study, organized thrombi are seen in both elastic and muscular arteries. The thrombi in the smaller vessels show recanalization, forming a lattice of fibrous trabeculae lined by endothelium. New blood vessels may form within the thrombi, and medial hypertrophy occurs secondarily. Plexiform lesions (see the description in the following section) are absent, although organizing thrombi may on occasion be difficult to distinguish from plexiform lesions.[89]

The plain chest radiograph shows cardiomegaly and central vessel dilatation, with patchy peripheral oligemia in the majority of patients (Figure 9-28).[4,379] Oligemic areas correspond well with the distribution of emboli, although normal vascularity may be seen in areas perfused by vessels that contain sizable emboli.[379] A few patients have normal or near-normal studies; others show only changes such as atelectasis, pleural thickening, or pleural effusion, with no radiographic signs of pulmonary hypertension.

On CT there may be well-defined areas of low attenuation of the lung parenchyma caused by hypoperfusion

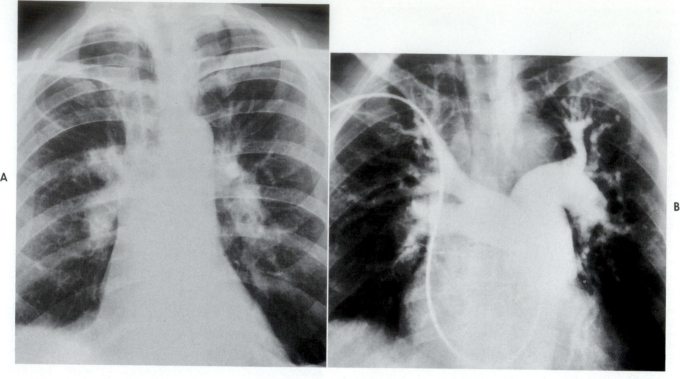

FIGURE 9-28
Pulmonary arterial hypertension caused by chronic thromboemboli. **A,** Plain film showing enlargement of the hilar arteries with patchy peripheral oligemia. **B,** Pulmonary angiogram showing central vessel dilatation with occlusion of multiple branch vessels and an increase in size of the unobstructed pulmonary arterial branches.

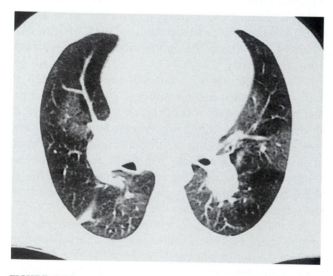

FIGURE 9-29
Computed tomographic sign of "mosaic oligemia" in a patient with chronic thromboembolic disease. There is increased transradiancy in areas of underperfused lung peripherally; note more prominent vessels in the denser (relatively overperfused) central regions of lung.

secondary to the pulmonary emboli, so-called mosaic oligemia (Figure 9-29). The intervening normal lung may appear abnormally dense, probably because of increased perfusion, and these areas may be misinterpreted as having an abnormal ground-glass pattern.[204]

An increase in lung density on CT in the central part of the lung, in contrast to the middle and peripheral regions, has been reported in patients with chronic thromboembolic pulmonary hypertension[92]; in this study, half of the segmental pulmonary arteries were dilated (ratio of the diameter of the segmental artery to the accompanying bronchus greater than 1). Furthermore, dilated bronchial arteries in the posterior mediastinum were identified in half of the patients.

Ventilation-perfusion lung scans in pulmonary hypertension secondary to chronic thromboembolic disease show multiple segmental mismatched perfusion defects indistinguishable from high-probability scans in acute pulmonary embolism.[78,98,193,379] The appearances remain unchanged on sequential imaging. It is not uncommon to find patients referred for V/Q scintigraphy for the first time with suspected acute pulmonary embolism who show mismatched perfusion defects that do not resolve on repeat scans performed a few weeks later. The true incidence of patients with high-probability lung scans who have nonresolving defects and no previous V/Q scans, and who may therefore have chronic disease, is not known.

Pulmonary angiography[4,379] reveals filling defects caused by thrombi in the lobar or segmental arteries, with occlusions of large and medium-sized vessels. If the thrombus in the main pulmonary arteries is laminated, the typical angiographic signs of filling defects may be absent.[41] The central vessels are frequently dilated, with rapid distal tapering. Web-shaped filling defects are occasionally seen. "Pouching" of partially or completely occluded pulmonary arteries is a more recently described sign of chronic thromboembolic disease.[9]

Primary pulmonary hypertension

The term "unexplained" or "primary pulmonary hypertension" refers to a group of patients who have pulmonary arterial hypertension with no clinically discernible cause, a normal pulmonary arterial wedge pressure, and no evidence of left-to-right shunt on cardiac catheterization. Patients with major emboli are excluded from the designation primary pulmonary hypertension.[89,137,355] Primary pulmonary hypertension was classified by the WHO[141] into three subtypes based on the histologic appearances of the vascular bed: (1) plexogenic arteriopathy, (2) recurrent pulmonary thromboembolism, and (3) pulmonary venoocclusive disease. In this chapter we treat recurrent pulmonary thromboembolism and pulmonary venoocclusive disease separately because they often, although by no means always, have distinguishing features on imaging tests.

Prolonged vasoconstriction is believed to be the first stage of plexogenic pulmonary arteriopathy (classic primary pulmonary hypertension); the next stage is structural change in the arterial wall. On pathologic study,[30,89,355] the initial structural manifestations are medial hypertrophy of the muscular pulmonary arteries and muscularization of the arterioles. This is followed by concentric laminar fibrosis in a so-called onion skin configuration. The walls of the muscular pulmonary arteries may show necrotizing arteritis with fibrinoid necrosis. Plexiform lesions are a striking and diagnostically important finding, consisting of a network of capillary-like channels within a dilated segment of a muscular pulmonary artery. The lesions are seen only in patients with severe pulmonary arterial hypertension. Plexiform lesions are not specific to primary pulmonary hypertension but are seen also in patients with pulmonary hypertension secondary to left-to-right shunts, both natural and postsurgical, as well as in those with pulmonary hypertension secondary to liver disease. They are not seen in pulmonary venoocclusive disease or in recurrent pulmonary thromboemboli.

A number of theories have been proposed to explain the etiology of classic primary pulmonary hypertension.[355] These include recurrent venous thromboembolism, in situ thrombosis secondary to a coagulation defect, effect of drugs, a congenital defect of the arterial walls, and an arteritis or some form of collagen vascular disease. Venous thromboemboli are considered an unlikely cause of the plexogenic form,[137,355] partly because of the absence of plexiform lesions in cases that show definite histologic features of large thromboemboli, and also because of the predominance of children and young adults, an unlikely age group to predominate if venous thromboembolism were the cause. Aminorex fumarate, an appetite suppressant, produced an identical picture to primary pulmonary hypertension in those few subjects who used the drug, as does the "bush tea" of native West Indians, in which *Crotolaria fulva* is believed to be responsible. Identical clinical and pathologic features to those encountered in primary pulmonary hypertension have been reported in patients with the toxic oil syndrome.[122] The striking female-to-male ratio of patients with primary pulmonary hypertension and the fact that the disease is often encountered shortly after puberty suggest that female sex hormones may be important in the etiology of the condition. Familial cases of primary pulmonary hypertension have also been reported, and it has been postulated that the disease may be related to an inherited tendency to increased pulmonary vascular reactivity: there is an increased prevalence of Raynaud's phenomenon in these patients.[56]

The age range is wide; most patients are adults or older children, but cases have been described in young children and infants. In a large series of 156 patients the average age was 33 (range 16 to 69) and the female-to-male ratio was 4:1.[355] The patients complain of weakness, dyspnea, and chest pain. Hemoptysis may occur. Arrhythmias are common in the later stages. Physical examination reveals all the expected signs of right ventricular pressure overload and elevated systemic venous pressure. The murmur of pulmonary regurgitation may be heard on auscultation. Cyanosis is a late finding.

The radiographic features of primary pulmonary hypertension (Figures 9-23 and 9-30) (excluding pulmonary venoocclusive disease) are dilatation of the main pulmonary artery and the other central arteries with rapid tapering to oligemic peripheral lung. The peripheral lung vessels are narrow and inconspicuous. The average width of the right descending pulmonary artery was twice the diameter of that in normal control subjects in one review of 54 patients with primary pulmonary hypertension,[176] but as with all types of pulmonary hypertension, the plain chest radiographs may show relatively little dilatation of central vessels (Figure 9-31).

V/Q scintigraphy in primary pulmonary hypertension may be normal or show multiple small unmatched perfusion defects throughout both lungs (Figure 9-32).* The appearances are, in other words, quite different from those in chronic, unresolved, pulmonary embolism. Wil-

---

*References 56, 80, 98, 193, 260, 271, 372.

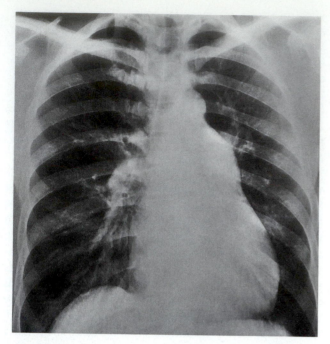

FIGURE 9-30
Primary pulmonary hypertension in a 37-year-old man. There is cardiomegaly, an enlarged main pulmonary artery, and enlarged hilar arteries. In this instance, the arteries beyond hila are normal in size.

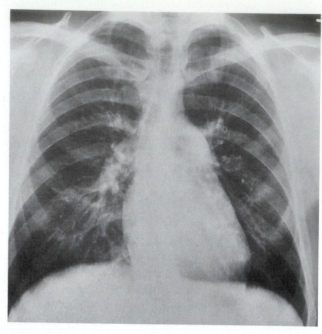

FIGURE 9-31
Primary pulmonary hypertension in a 25-year-old man. The chest is almost normal despite a pulmonary artery pressure of 93 mm Hg systolic and a mean pressure of 62 mm Hg. The heart is normal in size and shape. The only abnormal finding is enlargement of the main pulmonary artery.

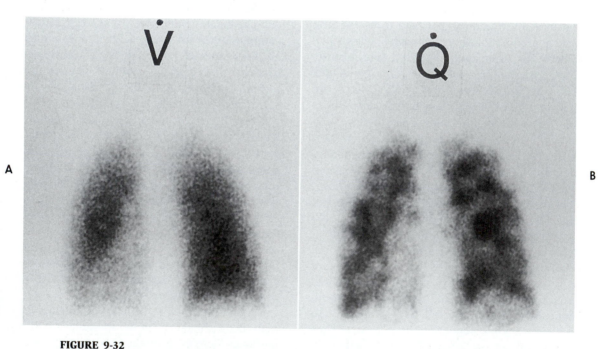

FIGURE 9-32
Primary pulmonary hypertension. This V/Q scan in a young woman with idiopathic pulmonary hypertension shows multiple widespread subsegmental perfusion defects (B) and a normal ^{81m}Kr ventilation scan (A). It is a striking example of the appearances of primary pulmonary hypertension. In some cases, the V/Q scan is normal. In contrast, pulmonary hypertension resulting from chronic pulmonary thromboembolism is usually associated with lung scan criteria of high probability of embolic disease.

son and co-workers[372] noted that patients with normal scans were predominantly young women, whereas there was an equal sex distribution in those with multiple perfusion defects. This observation is consistent with a later one by Rich and associates,[271] who correlated the perfusion scan with the histology of the lung. Their category of plexogenic hypertension was seen in women and associated with a normal scan, while their histologic category, microthrombotic, was seen in both sexes, was associated with multiple small defects, and seems to correspond to Wilson's group with a similar perfusion pattern. The concept that this latter form of primary pulmonary hypertension arises from previously unrecognized microthrombosis is an attractive one but not established. Nor is it clear whether the microthrombus arises in situ or is embolic.

Cardiac catheterization is required for the diagnosis. The pulmonary vascular resistance is extremely high. The pulmonary capillary wedge pressure, if it can be measured, is normal, and the left-sided pressures are also normal. Right-to-left shunting through a patent foramen ovale may be present. Pulmonary arteriography is used to exclude intraluminal filling defects caused by thromboemboli rather than to make the diagnosis. The pulmonary arterial tree shows dilatation of the central vessels. The peripheral vessels taper to an abnormal degree[36] and are reduced in number. Delayed clearance of contrast material from the arterial tree was seen in 22 of 25 patients in one series.[132]

Pulmonary venoocclusive disease

Pulmonary venoocclusive disease is a very rare disorder, and its cause is unknown. The entity was included by the WHO as one of the subtypes of primary pulmonary hypertension along with plexogenic pulmonary arteriopathy (classic primary pulmonary hypertension) and recurrent pulmonary thromboembolism.[141] The pulmonary veins thrombose and develop intimal fibrosis. It is often suggested that the initial pulmonary venous thromboses follow infection, presumably by an as yet unidentified virus.[337,354,356] Occlusion of the pulmonary veins leads to pulmonary venous and capillary congestion, pulmonary edema, rarely acute pulmonary hemorrhage,[66] alveolar hemosiderin deposits, and pulmonary arterial hypertension that may be very severe.[356] The muscular pulmonary arteries develop medial hypertrophy, and there is muscularization of the small pulmonary veins and arterioles.[137] Thrombi, which may be recent, organized, or recanalized, may be seen in these vessels, but plexiform lesions are absent. Patchy interstitial fibrosis and interstitial pneumonia are often present, although honeycomb lung is not a feature.[89,137] The pulmonary arteriolar wedge pressure is usually normal—and if abnormal, is only mildly elevated.[47,59,263,282,297] It is primarily for this reason that pulmonary venoocclusive disease is included in the category of primary pulmonary hypertension. The outcome is almost invariably fatal, and in most cases the only

curative treatment is lung transplantation.[82] Apart from two patients who developed venoocclusive disease following bone marrow transplantation and who responded to high-dose methylprednisolone,[133] steroid therapy seems to be ineffective. There are a few reports of individual patients showing sustained response to vasodilators[246] and specifically nifedipine.[287]

The chest radiographic appearances[263,297] are those of pulmonary arterial hypertension together with, in some cases, signs of pulmonary edema. Both alveolar edema and interstitial edema are commonly seen in this condition (Figure 9-33). In one review of the radiographic features of 26 cases, 20 patients showed pulmonary edema.[263] It has been suggested that part of the radiographic shadowing is due to an interstitial pneumonitis and this, but not the venulopathy, may respond to steroid treatment.[117] The left atrium is not enlarged, an important point of difference from mitral valve disease, left atrial myxoma, and cor triatriatum. Surprisingly, there is usually no evidence of upper zone blood diversion.

Radionuclide lung scans are either normal or show small bilateral wedge-shaped perfusion defects.[189,337] Pulmonary angiography shows dilatation of the proximal pulmonary arteries and slow circulation through the pulmonary vascular bed.[337] The venous phase does not help in making the diagnosis but does help to exclude other causes of pulmonary arterial hypertension, such as congenital stenosis of the pulmonary veins, left atrial myxoma, and cor triatriatum.[297]

Pulmonary hypertension secondary to pulmonary vasculitis

Pulmonary arterial hypertension may be caused by a large variety of extremely rare pulmonary vasculitides. Mostly these conditions affect the small vessels and these are discussed in Chapter 12. Large vessel vasculitis is recognized but is much less common.[241] Takayasu's disease is the best known example of a large vessel vasculitis causing pulmonary hypertension.

Takayasu's arteritis (Takayasu's disease, pulseless disease) is an arteritis of medium and large arteries that most commonly affects segments of the aorta and its main branches. The vessel wall becomes fibrosed and thickened, usually causing luminal stenosis rather than aneurysm. Takayasu's arteritis occurs chiefly in women, and is manifested between 10 and 20 years of age in 75% of patients.[198] The presenting features are constitutional symptoms, fever, arthralgia, and symptoms of local ischemia with absent pulses or bruits. Moderate systemic hypertension is common and is usually due to renal ischemia.[198] The course is variable, with episodic remissions or progression; death occurs in about 25% of cases.

Involvement of pulmonary arteries occurs in approximately half the patients.[178,197] The pulmonary hypertension is usually mild, and pulmonary symptoms are unusual.[197] The plain chest radiograph, in addition to showing the features of pulmonary arterial hypertension,

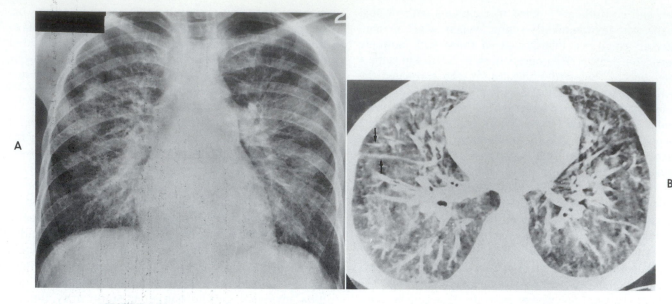

FIGURE 9-33
Pulmonary venoocclusive disease in a 16-year-old boy with a 4-month history of increasing dyspnea. The patient died 3 days later. Note alveolar and interstitial edema and signs of pulmonary arterial hypertension. Computed tomographic (CT) scan shows interlobular septal thickening *(downward-pointing arrow)* and subpleural pulmonary edema *(upward-pointing arrow)* to advantage. **A,** Posteroanterior radiograph. **B,** CT scan.

may reveal oligemic areas beyond the obstructed arteries.[380] The plain chest radiograph may also show the features of aortic arteritis, namely irregular outline to the aorta, aortic ectasia, calcification of the aortic wall, or even rib notching.[24,380] Abnormal perfusion scans, resembling the pattern in pulmonary embolism, are seen in up to 80% of patients.[178] Angiography reveals obstructions or stenoses of the lobar and segmental branches of the pulmonary arteries, and there may also be focal areas of dilatation.[197,380]

Radiolabeled granulocyte scanning in systemic vasculitis, including Wegener's and microscopic polyarteritis, is interesting in that it shows prominent abnormal increased diffuse granulocyte margination in the pulmonary vasculature.[173] This is also a prominent feature of the adult respiratory distress syndrome (see later discussion), as well as other conditions, such as graft versus host disease and inflammatory bowel disease, in which overt lung damage is absent. Its significance in terms of lung injury in systemic vasculitis is uncertain.

Pulmonary hypertension secondary to pleuropulmonary disease

Pulmonary hypertension is a common phenomenon in chronic pulmonary diseases, notably in chronic bronchitis, emphysema, and interstitial fibrotic lung disease (Figures 9-34 and 9-35). The acquired immunodeficiency syndrome is a rare but recognized cause of pulmonary hypertension.[143,154,313] The mechanism by which HIV infection causes pulmonary hypertension is unclear.[215] Fibrothorax and lung destruction resulting from infection are less frequent causes of pulmonary hypertension.

The common factor responsible for the elevated pulmonary vascular resistance in all these conditions is probably hypoxia, the most efficient known vasoconstrictor. Hypercapnia, acidemia, erythrocythemia, and increased blood volume may all contribute to the pulmonary hypertension. In disorders such as emphysema and interstitial fibrosis there is the added possibility that destruction of the lung vasculature may play a role.[208] The relationship between lung destruction and raised pulmonary vascular resistance is not simple. No direct correlation between the severity of the emphysema and the degree of right ventricular hypertrophy (the pathologist's criterion of long-standing pulmonary arterial hypertension) at autopsy has been shown.[71,153] However, recent in vivo studies using MRI have demonstrated right ventricular hypertrophy in patients considered to have mild and even trivial chronic obstructive pulmonary disease.[248,347] Pulsed Doppler echocardiography may also give indirect evidence of pulmonary arterial hypertension in patients with chronic obstructive pulmonary disease,[217] but there are problems in consistently obtaining pressure gradient readings with continuous wave Doppler.[341] Interestingly, more lung can be destroyed by panacinar emphysema than by centrilobular emphysema without raising pulmonary arterial pressure, yet centrilobular emphysema is associated with particularly severe forms of cor pulmonale (the "blue bloater").

The radiologic features consist of a combination of the signs of the responsible pleuropulmonary disease and the signs of pulmonary arterial hypertension, often with evidence of associated biventricular cardiac failure.

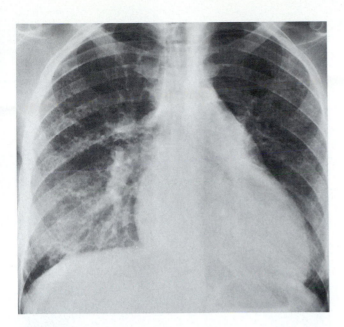

FIGURE 9-34
Pulmonary arterial hypertension secondary to interstitial fibrosis, in this instance caused by polymyositis and dermatomyositis.

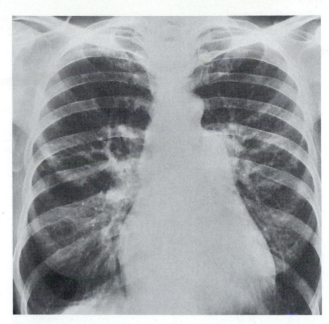

FIGURE 9-35
Pulmonary arterial hypertension secondary to chronic bronchitis and emphysema showing signs of pulmonary hypertension — cardiomegaly, central arterial dilatation, and upper zone vessel enlargement — and signs of emphysema — overinflated lungs and patchy vessel deficiency.

Pulmonary hypertension secondary to increased pulmonary blood flow

Pulmonary artery pressure can be elevated even without a rise in pulmonary vascular resistance if the pulmonary arterial blood flow is large enough. Sustained very high flows of this order are seen only with left-to-right shunts. The increased vessel size resulting from the massive blood flow dominates the radiographic picture. The elevations of pulmonary artery pressure are mild and do not contribute in a recognizable fashion to the radiographic appearances.

The term "Eisenmenger reaction" refers to raised pulmonary vascular resistance secondary to left-to-right shunting of blood, the usual causes of which are atrial septal defect (ASD), ventricular septal defect (VSD), and patent ductus arteriosus (PDA). The appearances on histologic examination are identical to those seen in primary pulmonary hypertension. The arterial changes consist of varying degrees of hypertrophy of the media of the small muscular arteries and arterioles, together with intimal cellular proliferation in the more severe cases. Plexiform lesions and necrotizing arteritis may also be seen in the advanced cases. The medial hypertrophy and any vasoconstrictive element that may be present are potentially reversible, whereas necrotizing arteritis and the plexiform lesions are regarded as irreversible.

The radiographic features of left-to-right shunt are cardiac enlargement and enlargement of all the pulmonary vessels, both central and peripheral, in all lung zones. With normal pulmonary vascular resistance the distention of the pulmonary vascular tree is approximately proportional to the increased flow. With a fully established Eisenmenger's syndrome (reversal of shunt owing to elevation of pulmonary vascular resistance) the central vessels show disproportionate enlargement with rapid tapering at segmental level and beyond. It can be difficult to recognize mild or moderate elevation of pulmonary vascular resistance because the diagnosis depends on evaluating the relative size of the vessels and there are no acceptable measurements or ratios on which to base this decision. The pattern varies according to the defect. Rees and Jefferson[265] noted that in Eisenmenger's ASD the chest radiograph shows massive enlargement of the central vessels with rapid tapering beyond hilar level (Figure 9-36), whereas with Eisenmenger's VSD the degree of dilatation of the central vessels is usually mild and sometimes even unrecognizable (Figure 9-37). Thus, with ventricular septal defect, even in cases with systemic pressures in the pulmonary circuit, the rapid tapering of vessel size is often not present. In fact, the appearances are often similar to a mild or moderate left-to-right shunt with no recognizable evidence of pulmonary arterial hypertension. It is even possible to see a normal or near-normal radiograph in Eisenmenger's VSD. Eisenmenger's PDA shows moderate dilatation of the aortic

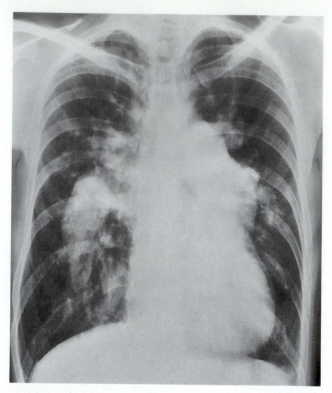

FIGURE 9-36
Pulmonary arterial hypertension in a middle-aged man caused by an atrial septal defect with Eisenmenger's syndrome, showing truly massive enlargement of the central pulmonary arteries.

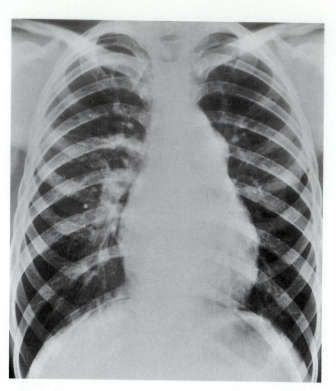

FIGURE 9-37
Pulmonary arterial hypertension in a 14-year-old boy caused by ventricular septal defect with Eisenmenger's syndrome, illustrating the relatively mild dilatation of the main pulmonary artery and hilar arteries seen with this condition even when, as in this case, the pulmonary arterial pressure is at systemic levels.

arch and the main pulmonary artery, and mild dilatation of the right and left hilar arteries. (The ductus itself may calcify.) The explanation for the different appearances of Eisenmenger's ASD, VSD, and PDA is conjectural. In the fetus the arterioles have a relatively thick muscular wall and a small lumen. In the normal individual the thickness of the muscle layer decreases and the relative size of the lumen increases after birth. In a patient with an ASD, even a sizable one, the pulmonary vascular resistance drops to normal and rises again only much later in life, whereas in a patient with a large VSD the pulmonary vascular resistance remains high from early infancy on. It seems likely that in such patients the constant pulmonary hypertension during early life prevents the involution of elastic tissue in the main pulmonary artery and its proximal branches. These arteries are therefore less distensible than in patients with ASD.[137]

Pulmonary hypertension caused by alveolar hypoventilation without underlying lung disease

Alveolar hypoventilation can lead to hypoxia, and hypoxia is the most potent known stimulus for pulmonary vasoconstriction.[99] Hypoxic pulmonary vasoconstriction normally helps match blood flow and ventilation, diverting blood flow away from poorly ventilated areas.[216] When only a small portion of the lung is

hypoxic, this response improves arterial oxygen saturation by reducing blood flow to the poorly ventilated segments without increasing pulmonary artery pressure. However, with widespread alveolar hypoxia, this normally protective response causes a large fraction of the pulmonary vasculature to constrict, increasing pulmonary artery pressure.[216]

Alveolar hypoventilation without underlying disease is seen in morbid obesity — an entity that used to be called the Pickwickian syndrome, but is now more frequently labeled the alveolar hypoventilation syndrome. (The term "Pickwickian syndrome" was coined in 1956 by Burwell and associates[45] when describing an obese middle-aged executive with fatigue and somnolence; they likened the syndrome to the fat boy in Charles Dickens' novel *The Pickwick Papers*.) The effects of morbid obesity on lung ventilation are complex, consisting of (1) obstructive sleep apnea and (2) hypoventilation (hypoxemia and hypercapnia) even while awake and breathing room air. The mechanisms of hypoventilation include a marked increase in abdominal contents that push the diaphragm up, increased chest wall compliance, weakness of inspiratory muscles, and altered hypoxic and hypercapnic responsiveness.[277,329,385] Most patients with the sleep apnea and alveolar hyperventilation syndromes are markedly obese, but there are exceptions. Conversely, many very obese patients do not suffer from either syndrome.

On radiographic study the appearances are those of pulmonary arterial hypertension with cardiomegaly and dilatation of the central pulmonary arteries in an obese subject.

PULMONARY ARTERY ANEURYSM

Pulmonary artery aneurysms are rare. They may be congenital in origin or acquired. Mycotic aneurysms are the most frequently encountered.[266] Those that develop in the walls of tuberculous cavities are known as Rasmussen's aneurysms.[8] Mycotic aneurysms may also occur in association with lung abscess or septicemia, particularly in drug addicts. Behçet's disease, described on p. 501, is a potent cause of lobar and segmental artery aneurysms,[116] and segmental pulmonary artery aneurysms are a feature of the rare Hughes-Stovin syndrome (see p. 502). Posttraumatic false aneurysm,[84,331] dissecting aneurysm of a pulmonary artery,[302] postembolic aneurysm,[139] and myxomatous emboli from a right atrial myxoma[113] are all very rare causes of pulmonary artery aneurysm.

Hemoptysis is the principal complication and is frequently fatal. The largest series were reported before the advent of antituberculous therapy. In one autopsy series,[8] rupture of the aneurysm was the immediate cause of death in 38 of the 45 tuberculosis patients examined. In only two cases were the aneurysms believed to be incidental. Even today, fatalities occur.[266]

It is rare to see the aneurysm as a discrete mass in an otherwise normal lung. Usually the aneurysm is adjacent to, or surrounded by, the infection that caused it, and it may therefore be very difficult to appreciate. On plain radiographs and conventional tomograms, Rasmussen's aneurysms may closely resemble mycetomas growing in cavities. Because both cause hemoptysis, the true diagnosis is easily overlooked. The clue may be the rapid change in size of a mass resulting from an aneurysm. CT scanning clearly showed the vascular nature of the mass in one of the cases reported by Remy and associates.[266]

ANGIODYSPLASIA IN HEPATIC CIRRHOSIS

Patients with severe, long-standing hepatic cirrhosis of any cause may develop an angiodysplasia of the lungs. These lesions, which have been likened to spider nevi, are spidery vessels randomly distributed through the lungs with a predilection for the subpleural regions.[25,240,275] They are difficult to demonstrate microscopically. The best way to demonstrate the angiodysplasia at pathologic study is with latex or gelatin casts of the vascular tree.[25,240] They are believed to be responsible for right-to-left shunting of blood with consequent hypoxia. Shunting of blood from the portal system to the pulmonary veins has been suggested as a possible mechanism in some patients.[137,240,288] Most of the reports in the litera-

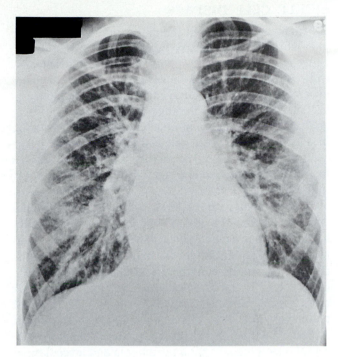

FIGURE 9-38
Angiodysplasia of the lungs in a 20-year-old man with juvenile cirrhosis who was very hypoxic. The lungs show a widespread increase in vessel size.

ture consist of small groups of patients,* but one prospective study of 170 patients with various types of liver disease showed gas transfer defects in 20%. The patients may develop severe enough hypoxemia to be cyanotic, and clubbing of the fingers and toes may be evident. Most of the patients, but not all, have spider nevi of the skin.[16]

The chest radiograph may be normal or may show increased vascular markings and small nodular shadows (Figure 9-38).[25,275] In the 170 patients referred to previously, nodular shadowing was found on the chest radiograph in 6%.[319] Radionuclide perfusion lung scanning shows extensive extrapulmonary uptake caused by the bypassing of the pulmonary arteriolar bed.[3,16] Radionuclide shunt calculations have shown that more than 50% of the pulmonary blood flow may bypass the alveoli.[376] In one reported case, substantial fluctuation in the degree of right-to-left shunting was observed and corresponded to changes in arterial oxygen tension.[61] Pulmonary angiography shows dilatation of the large and medium-sized arteries, with a myriad of abnormal spidery branches in the lung periphery and rapid filling of enlarged pulmonary veins. It is noteworthy that lung biopsy may be negative for disease, even in patients with very abnormal radiographic findings.[90] The lungs do not show interstitial fibrosis, nor is there any thickening of the alveolar walls.[25]

*References 16, 25, 90, 136, 177, 240, 283.

SICKLE CELL DISEASE

Patients with sickle cell anemia are at increased risk for pneumonia and pulmonary infarction.[142] Distinguishing between these two entities both clinically and radiologically can be difficult.[19] Because of this difficulty the more general term "acute chest syndrome" is often applied to describe fever, clinical findings of a pulmonary process, and radiologic evidence of new pulmonary consolidation in a patient with sickle cell hemoglobinopathy.[256] The acute chest syndrome is one of the most common reasons for hospitalization and is a significant cause of mortality in these patients.[18,256]

A large survey of children who required hospital admission during the period 1958 to 1968[18] showed that bacterial pneumonia, particularly pneumococcal pneumonia, was responsible for the acute event in some 40% of patients, and the authors speculated that the true incidence of bacterial pneumonia was much higher. A more recent survey revealed a similar incidence of pulmonary infections but a much lower proportion of bacterial pneumonia and relatively few cases of pneumococcal pneumonia.[256] Viral pneumonia and mycoplasmal pneumonia were about as frequent as bacterial pneumonia. The lower incidence of bacterial pneumonia in the more recent study may have reflected the use of penicillin prophylaxis and pneumococcal immunization.[256] In both of these series the precise cause of more than half the episodes could not be determined, and they were presumed to result from pulmonary infarction, atelectasis, or missed infection.

Pulmonary infarction, which is much more frequent in adults than in children,[57,80] is often associated with other evidence of sickle cell crisis such as abdominal or musculoskeletal pain.[18] Pulmonary infarction is rare in children under 12 years of age. Autopsy series, which clearly represent the severe end of the spectrum of pulmonary disease, show a high prevalence of pulmonary infarcts, even in infants and young children.[242] The autopsy findings consist of (1) pneumonia, (2) pulmonary infarction with necrosis of alveolar walls, (3) pulmonary vascular thrombosis with pulmonary hypertension, and (4) bone marrow embolization from areas of ischemic bone necrosis.[142]

On radiographic examination[311] there are confluent lobar or segmental consolidations that may be accompanied by pleural effusion (Figure 9-39). The consolidations resolve more slowly than in the general population, and recurrence is common. Distinguishing consolidation resulting from infection from that caused by infarction is often impossible. Pulmonary angiography is not recommended, and radionuclide lung scanning is of limited diagnostic value because so many of the scans fall into the intermediate-probability category. One clue to the diagnosis of infarction may be the late development of a pulmonary shadow; consolidation resulting from pneumonia is likely to be present on the initial film. If the shadowing is clearly interstitial in character and the

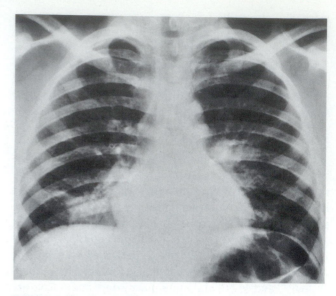

FIGURE 9-39
Sickle cell disease, with probable pulmonary infarcts, in a 17-year-old boy with left-sided chest pain. Radionuclide scan showed mismatched ventilation-perfusion defects in the lung regions that were clear on this chest radiograph.

patient has fever, viral or mycoplasmal pneumonia is the likely diagnosis. Pulmonary edema, either interstitial or alveolar, may be present and can be confused with pneumonia and infarction. The edema may be the result of treatment with analgesics such as morphine or may be the consequence of heart failure.

In a CT study of 10 patients with acute chest syndrome, 9 patients had segmental or lobar consolidations, and 9 had areas of ground-glass opacification or hypoperfusion.[28] No patient had definitive evidence of concurrent pulmonary infection, although 2 patients had elevated mycoplasma titers. Without pathologic confirmation the nature of the ground-glass densities remains a matter of speculation, but the authors suggest that they represent areas of early edema; in 3 patients who were later rescanned the ground-glass densities resolved.

In addition to the pulmonary features of the acute chest syndrome, the heart may show nonspecific enlargement and the pulmonary blood vessels are frequently enlarged. Several hemodynamic factors are at work, and the relative role of each may be difficult to unravel in an individual case. Chronic anemia of any cause gives rise to a sustained increase in cardiac output even when the patient is at rest.[350] Chronic high cardiac output can be recognized on plain chest radiographs as nonspecific cardiomegaly and increase in the size of the pulmonary blood vessels. Increased left ventricular mass has been well documented by echocardiography.[14] Myocardial damage or ischemia from sickle cell disease may also contribute to the cardiac enlargement and to cardiac dysfunction, although the evidence for this is tenuous.[191] Very rarely, pulmonary hypertension similar to that seen

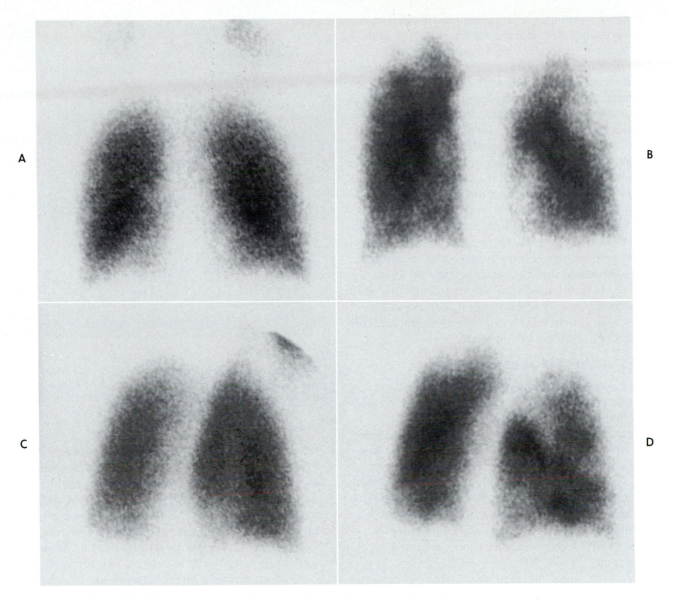

FIGURE 9-40
Sickle cell disease. **A** and **B**, Posterior ventilation-perfusion scan. **C** and **D**, Right posterior oblique ventilation-perfusion scan. Several unmatched perfusion defects, especially in the upper lobes, can be seen in the V/Q scan of this patient.

in primary pulmonary hypertension may develop secondary to obstruction of the pulmonary vascular bed.[68]

With high-quality ventilation imaging, such as with Kr-81m, the majority of patients with sickle cell disease who have an acute chest syndrome have V/Q lung scan appearances more suggestive of lobar pneumonia than infarction, that is, with lobar ventilation defects more complete than perfusion, which is only partially reduced (Figure 9-40). This is somewhat surprising in view of the frequency with which plugging of pulmonary vessels by sickled cells has been demonstrated pathologically.

PULMONARY EDEMA

Pulmonary edema is usually due to one of two mechanisms[10,166,207,318]: elevated pulmonary venous pressure or increased permeability of the alveolar-capillary membrane. In some instances a combination of factors contributes to the development of pulmonary edema; for example, patients receiving interleukin-2 therapy for advanced malignancy often have renal insufficiency, fluid overload, and increased alveolar-capillary permeability.[292] Occasionally the edema is related to decreased plasma oncotic pressure or lymphatic insufficiency. Finally there are those disorders in which the mechanism is unknown or incompletely understood; even here, increased vascular permeability is often a major factor.

This division of pulmonary edema into "cardiogenic" and "noncardiogenic," although convenient, is not always clear-cut,[318] nor is there general agreement about all the conditions to be included in these catch-all terms. Objective methods to distinguish between the different types of pulmonary edema by analysis of MRI signals of lung water have been similarly inconclusive.[352] In an experimental model the timing and distribution of lung enhancement on MRI after administration of a macromolecular paramagnetic contrast agent discriminated between pulmonary capillary leak and hydrostatic pulmonary edema.[26] Despite the imprecision, the concept of dividing pulmonary edema into conditions in which the cause is primarily hydrostatic and those in which the cause is primarily capillary damage (such as adult respiratory distress syndrome; see discussion in a later section) has considerable merit for the clinician, since the treatment is fundamentally different.

Raised pulmonary venous pressure

Because the signs of raised pulmonary venous pressure frequently precede or accompany cardiogenic pulmonary edema, they are described first.

Normally, in the upright subject, particularly on a film taken with deep inspiration, the vessels in the lower zones are larger than the equivalent vessels in the upper zones. With elevation of the pulmonary venous pressure the upper zone vessels enlarge.[306] If when the patient is erect the upper zone vessels have a diameter equal to or larger than the equivalent lower zone vessels, elevation of the pulmonary venous pressure should be strongly considered (Figure 9-41).[348]

It has been suggested that, as an absolute measurement, vessels in the first intercostal space on standard upright films should not exceed 3 mm in diameter.[170] In some patients one can measure the diameter of the vessels that accompany a bronchus. For example, the anterior segmental bronchus of one or the other upper lobe can often be identified end on as a ring shadow. The accompanying artery is normally much the same diameter as the bronchus, depending on the zone. Woodring has established that the pulmonary artery/bronchus (seen end on) ratio on the erect chest radiograph in normal individuals is 0.85 (standard deviation 0.15) in the upper zones and 1.34 (standard deviation 0.25) in the lower zones.[378] In patients with left ventricular failure the ratios reverse and become 1.5 in the upper zones and 0.87 in the lower zones; this relationship is maintained on supine radiographs of patients with left ventricular failure. However, reliably identifying an end-on pulmonary artery and its accompanying bronchus in both the upper and lower zones on a portable radiograph may be impossible.

The sign of upper zone vessel dilatation is believed to

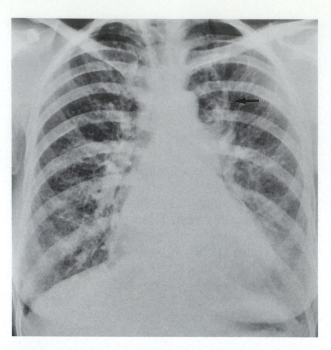

FIGURE 9-41
Raised pulmonary venous pressure in a patient with mitral stenosis. Note that the vessels in the first and second rib interspace *(arrow)* are large compared with equivalent vessels in the lower zones.

reflect increased blood flow to the upper zones.[108,273,364] The most widely accepted explanation for redistribution of pulmonary blood flow in subjects with elevated pulmonary venous pressure is that of West and associates,[364] who suggested that in the upright subject there is preferential development of pulmonary edema in the lower lobes. This basal interstitial edema, although not visible radiographically, is believed to form a perivascular cuff, which acts as a buffer between the vessels and the distending forces being transmitted through the lungs, with resultant redistribution of blood flow to the upper zones.[364] This explanation has, however, been disputed.[131,273,330]

The assessment of the signs of redistribution of blood flow requires technically good radiographs and is therefore easier when films obtained with fixed equipment are used, although acceptable interpretations can often be made from images taken with portable equipment. It is not surprising that there is considerable interobserver variation for the signs of mild raised pulmonary venous pressure.[238] It is essential that the patient be upright and that the film be exposed on inspiration. In normal supine subjects blood flow is fairly equal in the upper and lower zones, and redistribution of blood flow is therefore much more difficult to recognize on examinations with the patient supine. Also, it should be realized that a similar pattern of redistribution occurs in several other conditions, notably raised pulmonary arteriolar resistance,[131] basal lung disease, particularly emphysema,[220,221] and basal pulmonary emboli.

The radiographic sign of upper zone redistribution of blood flow has proved accurate in predicting the pulmonary venous pressure in chronic valvular heart disease[20,305] and reasonably accurate in acute and chronic ischemic heart disease,[20,23,146,211] although it should be appreciated that there are a significant proportion of patients with chronic ischemic heart disease causing left ventricular end-diastolic pressures higher than 24 mm Hg who do not show visible upper zone vessel dilatation or for that matter any of the other radiographic signs of congestive heart failure.[152] The presence of upper lobe redistribution of flow is of limited value in the differential diagnosis of pulmonary shadows, when pulmonary edema is just one of several diagnoses being considered. In one large series only 50% of the patients with pulmonary edema resulting from heart disease showed redistribution of flow.[222] We also have seen many examples of cardiogenic pulmonary edema in which the vascular redistribution could not be recognized. Frequently the vessels cannot be adequately seen because of surrounding edema; sometimes they can be readily identified, but no redistribution is present.

Cardiogenic pulmonary edema

Under normal circumstances the pulmonary interstitium and alveoli are kept relatively dry. Increased quantities of tissue fluid resulting from elevated pulmonary venous pressure lead at first to increased lymphatic drainage. Once the capacity of the pulmonary lymphatics is exceeded, pulmonary edema results. Fluid collects first in the interstitium and then spills into the airspaces.

The major causes of cardiogenic (hydrostatic) pulmonary edema are cardiac disease, overhydration, and fluid retention as a result of renal failure. Clinically the major effects are dyspnea and tachypnea. With the development of alveolar flooding, severe hypoxemia and hypocapnia or hypercapnia occur. In extreme cases blood-tinged foam is expectorated. Wheezing, the demand for an upright posture, and sweating are all prominent symptoms.

The radiologic signs of cardiogenic pulmonary edema are usually divided into interstitial and alveolar patterns, even though these phenomena are in reality a continuum. Interstitial edema may be seen without alveolar fluid, but if alveolar edema is present, the interstitium must also be edematous, whether or not it can be seen on the radiograph.

Plain chest films are highly sensitive for the diagnosis of pulmonary edema and can even demonstrate edema in patients who have not yet developed symptoms.[49,138] Conversely, it should be realized that pulmonary edema may be visible radiographically long after the hemodynamic factors have returned to normal.[255]

Cardiogenic interstitial pulmonary edema

Interstitial pulmonary edema causes a variety of radiographic signs,[126,149,254] the most readily recognized of which are septal lines, bronchial wall thickening, and subpleural pulmonary edema (Figure 9-42).

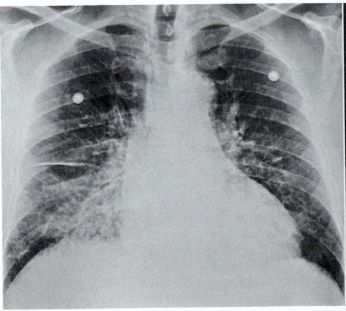
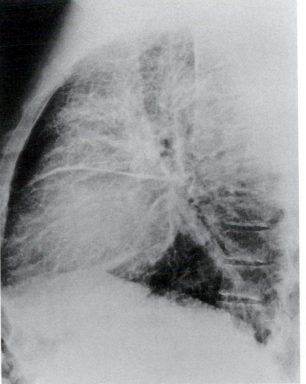

FIGURE 9-42
Cardiogenic pulmonary edema following myocardial infarction in a 52-year-old man, illustrating widespread fissural thickening and lack of clarity of the intrapulmonary vessels and septal lines. There is frank alveolar edema in the right lower zone. The fissural thickening caused by subpleural edema is particularly striking. **A,** Frontal view. **B,** Lateral view.

SEPTAL LINES. The appearance of septal lines is discussed in detail in Chapter 4. Because thickened septal lines occur in few conditions (see box on p. 111), their identification is an extremely useful indicator of pulmonary edema. If transient or rapid in development, they are virtually diagnostic of interstitial pulmonary edema. Septal lines are not, however, a particularly frequent finding even in florid pulmonary edema.[49,138] On occasion they persist after pulmonary edema has resolved.

BRONCHIAL WALL THICKENING. In normal chest radiographs the walls of the bronchi within the lung substance are invisible unless end on to the x-ray beam, when they are seen to have a very thin and well-defined ringlike wall. If edema collects in the peribronchial interstitial space, the combined shadow of the edematous bronchial wall and the thickened interstitium results in visible bronchial wall thickening.[86] Not only do the end-on bronchial walls become much thicker, those that are not end on may have visible walls. The posterior wall of the bronchus intermedius, as seen in the lateral chest radiograph, is another useful site at which to assess thickening caused by edema; it should normally measure less than 3 mm.[294]

SUBPLEURAL PULMONARY EDEMA. Fluid can accumulate in the loose connective tissue beneath the visceral pleura. The pulmonary septa communicate freely with this space, and edema can therefore flow peripherally to dissect beneath the pleura. Subpleural edema is seen radiographically as a sharply defined band of increased density that, when adjacent to a fissure, makes the fissure appear thick (Figure 9-42),[147] and when in the costophrenic angles produces a lamellar-shaped fluid collection resembling pleural effusion. It is the lamellar shape with the shadow conforming to the pleural boundary that suggests pulmonary rather than pleural fluid (Figure 9-43). A well-defined curvilinear opacity in a subpleural distribution on CT has been described in some patients with left ventricular failure. The bandlike opacity, possibly representing engorged lymphatics, is separated from the visceral pleural surface by a few millimeters and disappears after diuretic therapy.[7]

LACK OF CLARITY OF THE INTRAPULMONARY AND HILAR VESSELS (HILAR HAZE). The hilar and pulmonary blood vessels may appear indistinct because of surrounding edema. This sign, which is one of the most consistent findings with interstitial pulmonary edema,[138,254] may be difficult to evaluate. Comparison with previous radiographs to establish the normal appearance for a particular patient is frequently needed. Often the sign can only be appreciated retrospectively on follow-up films once the edema has resolved.

GENERALIZED INCREASE IN DENSITY OF THE LUNG PARENCHYMA. This is another subtle feature of pulmonary edema. The density of the lung on a plain chest radiograph is dependent on so many anatomic and technical factors that the sign is of little use in clinical

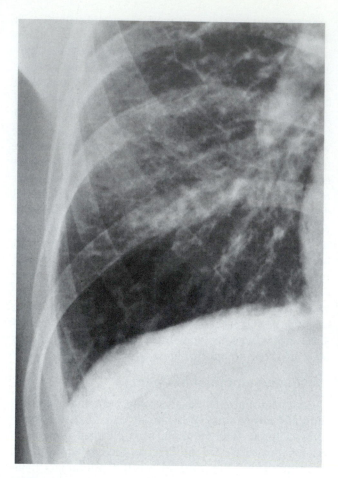

FIGURE 9-43
Subpleural pulmonary edema producing a lamellar homogeneous density parallel to the chest wall.

management, although it has been used in experimental animals.[312] Density measurement by CT and signal characteristics at MRI are more objective methods of quantitating the amount of fluid present in the lungs.[309,310,352]

Cardiogenic alveolar edema

Alveolar edema represents spill of fluid from the interstitium into the alveolar airspaces. The cardinal radiographic sign is therefore shadowing with the characteristics of airspace filling (Figure 9-44). The margins are poorly defined, although larger collections may show a well-defined boundary. The distribution is patchy and widespread, and the shadows tend to coalesce. Usually the shadowing is bilateral, occasionally unilateral, and rarely lobar. When unilateral, there is a striking and unexplained predisposition for the right lung (Figure 9-45).[235,381] Air bronchograms or air alveolograms may be evident, particularly when the edema is confluent. The acinar shadow of pulmonary edema has been emphasized. The appearance is due to the contrast between fluid-filled acini surrounded by aerated acini. The result-

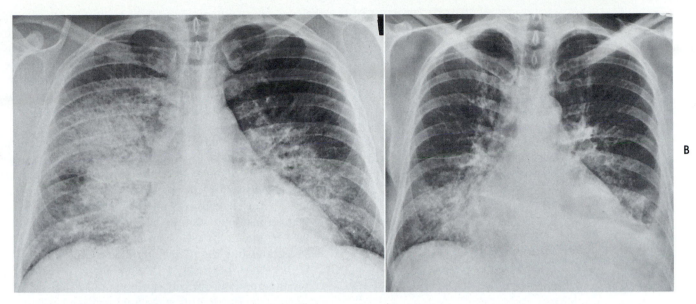

FIGURE 9-44
Cardiogenic alveolar edema. **A,** Butterfly pattern. **B,** Bibasilar edema in a different patient showing septal lines and a left pleural effusion. Note also the bronchial wall thickening and thickening of the minor fissure.

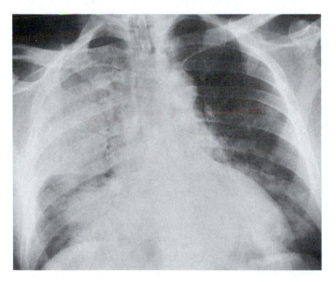

FIGURE 9-45
Unilateral pulmonary edema following overtransfusion with intravenous fluids, showing an alveolar filling process almost entirely confined to the right lung. Note the air bronchograms.

ing shadow is a 5 to 10 mm moderately ill-defined nodule. Sometimes the nodules are smaller and resemble the miliary pattern seen in miliary tuberculosis.

The terms "bat's wing"[156] and "butterfly" shadowing were coined to describe the appearance of perihilar shadowing that is predominantly in the central portions of the lobes and fades out peripherally, leaving an aerated outer "cortex" (Figure 9-44). This pattern is best seen on frontal views; the distribution is less easy to define on the lateral views.[118] The mechanism responsible for this characteristic distribution is uncertain. One suggestion is that lymphatic drainage is better in the outer portions of the lungs. Another is that the greater change in volume of the outer lung during each respiratory cycle in some way helps prevent edema.[101] Despite the emphasis given to the bat's wing pattern, it should be realized that most patients show a more diffuse and random distribution, with some lobes more severely affected than others. True, the shadowing often spares the extreme upper and lower zones, but the classic bat's wing pattern is seen in only a minority of patients.

Whatever the pattern, a striking feature of cardiogenic pulmonary edema is rapid change on films taken over short intervals; rapid clearing is particularly suggestive of the diagnosis. An extension of this phenomenon is the change in distribution of pulmonary edema when patients alter their position for a few hours, for example, by lying on one side.[383]

Adult respiratory distress syndrome

Adult respiratory distress syndrome (ARDS), often referred to as noncardiogenic pulmonary edema, is a common disorder with a very high mortality.[85] It is due to increased pulmonary vascular permeability and develops in response to lung injury. A large variety of insults may precipitate the disorder, particularly bacterial sepsis, pneumonia, aspiration of gastric contents, circulatory shock, trauma, burns, and drug overdose. A full list of causes is given in the box on p. 412.

The clinical syndrome[15,85,128] is characterized by acute, severe, progressive respiratory distress, widespread pulmonary opacity on chest radiographs, significant

---

CLINICAL DISORDERS CAUSING OR ASSOCIATED WITH THE ADULT RESPIRATORY DISTRESS SYNDROME

Septicemia — notably bacterial and viral pneumonia, gram-negative septicemia

Hemodynamic shock of any cause

Circulating toxins or vasoactive substances — notably bacterial endotoxins

Trauma, including radiation damage

Major surgery, notably following cardiopulmonary bypass

Burns

Bowel infarction

Fat embolism

Amniotic fluid embolism

Aspiration of liquids
  Gastric contents
  Near drowning
  Hydrocarbon fluids

Inhaled toxins, notably
  Smoke
  Oxygen
  Chemicals (NO_2, NH_3, war gases)
  Metal fumes (cadmium, mercury)

Metabolic disorders
  Acute pancreatitis
  Diabetic ketoacidosis
  Uremia

Hematologic disorders, notably
  Disseminated intravascular coagulation
  Leukoagglutinin reactions of drugs

Drug related, notably
  Heroin
  Salicylates
  Methadone
  Ethchlorvynol

Modified from Balk R, Bone RC: *Med Clin North Am* 67:685-700, 1983; and Matthay MA: *Clin Chest Med* 6:301-314, 1985.

hypoxemia despite high inspired oxygen concentration, and decreased compliance of the lungs. In most cases these features are present within 24 hours of the inciting events, and in 90% of patients the syndrome is evident within 72 hours.

The mechanism of damage to the pulmonary vascular endothelium is under intensive investigation, but the factors mediating ARDS have proved frustratingly difficult to unravel.[272] It appears clear that the inciting condition activates an injurious cascade.[128] The neutrophil appears to be an important agent in producing increased capillary permeability, but the inciting and inhibiting forces are unclear. Complement byproducts, alveolar macrophages, platelets, arachidonic acid metabolites, free radicals of oxygen, proteolytic enzymes, and inflammatory mediators such as prostaglandins may all play a part,[5,128] but no known pathogenetic sequence completely accounts for the acute alveolar damage that characterizes ARDS.[128]

Whatever the mechanism, the end result is damage to the alveolar capillary membrane leading to increased permeability to protein and interstitial edema. As the process continues, proteinaceous fluid spills into the alveoli. Eventually alveolar disruption and hemorrhage occur; surfactant is reduced and the alveoli tend to collapse. Unlike cardiogenic pulmonary edema, the edema is prolonged because the oncotic forces for reabsorption of fluid are not present.

On pathologic study[11] the alveoli and the perivascular and peribronchial spaces are congested and edematous. Widespread pulmonary microthrombosis is a feature of approximately 75% of patients with posttraumatic ARDS.[351] The alveoli are inhomogeneously filled with proteinaceous fluid, white cells, debris, and often hemorrhage. Greene, in his review article, divided the morphologic features into the following three stages[128]:

1. In stage 1 (first 24 hours) there is capillary congestion, endothelial cell swelling, and extensive microatelectasis. During this stage fluid leakage is minimal and limited to the interstitium. The respiratory distress is largely due to decreased pulmonary compliance.

2. In stage 2 (1 to 5 days) there is fluid leakage and fibrin deposition and hyaline membranes develop. Alveolar consolidation by hemorrhagic fluid becomes extensive, and severe hypoxemia develops.

3. In stage 3 (after 5 days) there is alveolar cell proliferation, collagen deposition, and microvascular destruction. The type II pneumonocytes become hyperplastic in an attempt to cover the denuded alveolar surfaces.

The radiographic changes may be delayed by 12 hours or more following the onset of clinical symptoms,[165,172,244] an important difference from cardiogenic pulmonary edema, where the chest radiograph is frequently abnormal before or coincident with the onset of symptoms. Some patients never develop significant pulmonary shadowing even though they become profoundly hypoxemic.[359]

The major features on plain chest radiograph (Figures 9-46 and 9-47)[88,165,172,255,261] are bilateral, widespread, patchy, ill-defined densities resembling cardiogenic pulmonary edema, usually without cardiomegaly, upper zone blood diversion, or pleural effusion. The densities progress in severity to produce confluent opacification, the distribution of which is variable, but usually all lung zones are involved both centrally and peripherally, and air bronchograms may be a prominent feature. CT scans, however, show that the distribution of the pulmonary shadowing is patchy with preservation of normal lung regions.[209] It has been reported that the increased density, partially collapsed parts of the lung are concentrated in the dependent regions.[111,112] Signs of interstitial edema, namely hilar haze and lack of clarity of lung vessels, may also be present. Occasionally the shadowing appears exclusively interstitial,[88] but septal lines are very rare.[255] Pistolesi and co-workers[255] have pointed out that the main pulmonary artery may appear bulged and that enlargement of the right side of the heart is frequently seen.

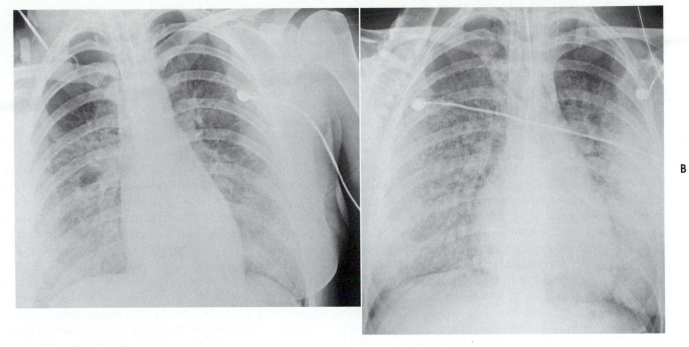

FIGURE 9-46
Adult respiratory distress syndrome in a 19-year-old woman. **A,** Early phase showing perihilar airspace shadowing. **B,** Twenty-four hours later there is widespread, fairly uniformly distributed airspace shadowing.

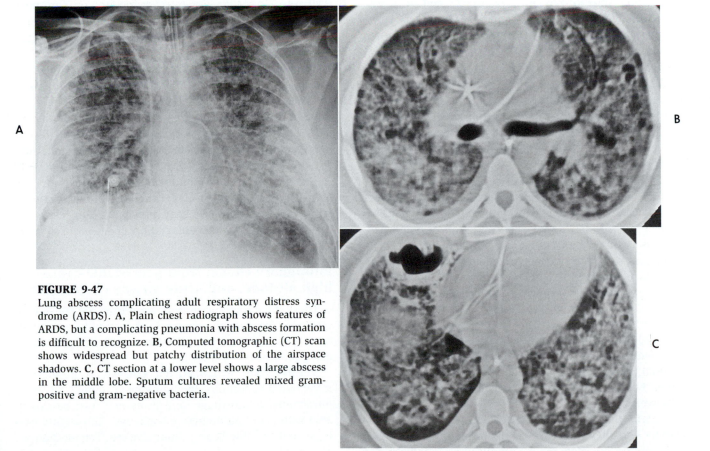

FIGURE 9-47
Lung abscess complicating adult respiratory distress syndrome (ARDS). **A,** Plain chest radiograph shows features of ARDS, but a complicating pneumonia with abscess formation is difficult to recognize. **B,** Computed tomographic (CT) scan shows widespread but patchy distribution of the airspace shadows. **C,** CT section at a lower level shows a large abscess in the middle lobe. Sputum cultures revealed mixed gram-positive and gram-negative bacteria.

Patients with abnormal radiographs are all severely hypoxic and require assisted ventilation. There is usually a good correlation between the radiographic severity of the pulmonary edema and the arterial P_{O_2}. Furthermore, the extent of lung involvement as judged by standardized reading of chest radiographs has been shown to correlate well with densitometric measurements on CT.[34] As well as showing complications not visible on portable radiographs, CT can detect microcystic lung changes that indicate a worse prognosis in patients with ARDS.[320]

The acute lung injury of ARDS is associated with diffuse pulmonary granulocyte accumulation. In experimental ARDS, increased pulmonary In-111-labeled granulocyte uptake early after injection reflects increased intravascular delay, but the later accumulation reflects migration, which is probably more closely related to the lung injury.[151,335] The injury to the blood-gas barrier in ARDS can be quantified from the clearance rate from the lung of inhaled Tc-99m DTPA aerosol.[65] Small hydrophilic solutes, such as Tc-99m DTPA (molecular weight 492 daltons), diffuse through the epithelium of the distal airways into pulmonary capillary blood and are cleared from the lung in normal nonsmoking subjects with a half-time of about 80 minutes. The clearance rate is markedly increased in ARDS but normal in cardiogenic edema.[205] The permeability of the pulmonary endothelium can be measured with a radiolabeled protein, such as In-113m-labeled transferrin, which accumulates in the pulmonary interstitium as a result of, and at a rate proportional to, the degree of endothelial "leak."[278]

DISTINGUISHING CARDIOGENIC AND NONCARDIOGENIC PULMONARY EDEMA. The distinction between cardiogenic and noncardiogenic pulmonary edema on radiographic grounds alone can be difficult, but certain features may point in one direction or another.[255] In cardiogenic edema the shadows caused by pulmonary edema are present coincident with the onset of symptoms, show a central predominance, and may be associated with peribronchial cuffing and septal lines. Air bronchograms are relatively rare, occurring one third as frequently as in ARDS. The severity of the shadows changes rapidly on serial films. The pulmonary vascular pedicle is often enlarged, and upper zone diversion of blood flow may be visible. Pleural effusions are common.

In noncardiogenic pulmonary edema the shadows may be delayed compared with the onset of symptoms and may show relatively uniform zonal distribution. ARDS is rarely associated with septal lines, and peribronchial cuffing is less common than with the cardiogenic pulmonary edema. Air bronchograms are common in ARDS. The central and peripheral pulmonary vascular pattern is normal, though the main pulmonary artery may appear large. Pleural effusions are small and are only occasionally seen.[222]

COMPLICATIONS OF ADULT RESPIRATORY DISTRESS SYNDROME. ARDS results in high mortality and, as might be expected, many complications. Septicemia is common and in many instances results from a pneumonia that complicates the ARDS. Multiple organ failure is a major cause of death. It is not clear whether organs such as the kidney, liver, and central nervous system are damaged by the same process that initiates the ARDS or whether multiple organ failure results from complications that follow the pulmonary injury, but it would appear that with modern critical care facilities death from respiratory failure is less common than death from multiple organ failure.

Diagnosing pneumonia from the chest radiograph in the presence of extensive pulmonary edema is clearly difficult (Figure 9-47).[6] Increasing consolidation in one area of the lung in a patient with clinical features to indicate pneumonia is the important radiographic finding. The distinction from edema and atelectasis is often impossible. Cavitation is fairly specific to pneumonia, but even here there is still the difficulty of distinguishing abscess formation from pneumatocele formation. CT scanning may be helpful in this regard (Figure 9-47). Pulmonary hemorrhage resulting from trauma, for example, caused by the balloon of a Swan-Ganz catheter, has to be included in the differential diagnosis.

During the acute phase many patients suffer barotrauma caused by positive-pressure ventilation with relatively noncompliant lungs. Pneumothorax and pneumomediastinum are common, and in severe cases air dissects from the mediastinum into the neck and chest wall and even into the retroperitoneum or peritoneal cavity (Figure 9-48). Interstitial emphysema is common, and pneumatoceles may develop within the lungs (Figure 9-49).

The long-term outlook for survivors of ARDS is poorly documented. Alberts, Priest, and Moser[1] in their review of the literature could find descriptions of follow-up chest radiographs in only 81 patients. In the great majority the chest radiograph returned to normal, a few showed some degree of hyperinflation, and 11% showed residual interstitial shadowing. The true rate of conversion of ARDS to interstitial fibrosis is unknown, since follow-up lung biopsy is so rarely performed. However, follow-up studies with high-resolution CT may provide insights into the nature of the residual morphologic damage in survivors of ARDS.[245]

Pulmonary edema from neurogenic causes, high altitude, and acute airway obstruction

These three forms of pulmonary edema are considered separately because the edema in these conditions shows certain differences from the other varieties of noncardiogenic pulmonary edema.

NEUROGENIC PULMONARY EDEMA. A number of intracranial conditions, including head trauma, seizures, intracranial hemorrhage, and tumors,[307] can be associated with acute pulmonary edema, even in patients who have no detectable heart or lung disease. The mechanism of the edema is debated.[67,338] Because the edema can

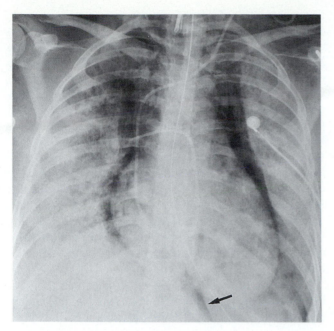

FIGURE 9-48
Pneumomediastinum in a patient with ARDS receiving positive-pressure ventilation. Air has tracked into the neck and retroperitoneum *(arrow)*.

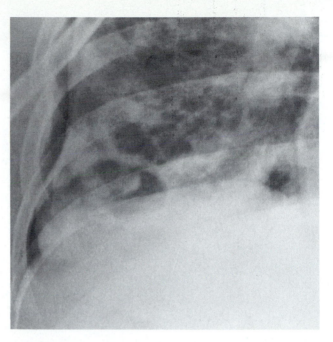

FIGURE 9-49
Pneumatoceles that developed in a patient with adult respiratory distress syndrome. (There is also a right pneumothorax and a chest drainage tube.)

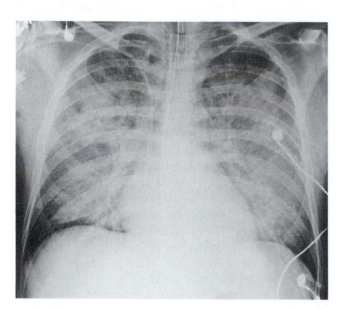

FIGURE 9-50
Pulmonary edema caused by increased intracranial pressure following a subarachnoid hemorrhage caused by a ruptured aneurysm.

occur within a minute, it has been suggested that a sudden burst of neural activity stimulates the sympathetic nervous system, increasing the pulmonary blood volume and raising the pulmonary venous pressure.[338] The edema becomes proteinaceous, suggesting that endothelial damage also plays a part, but the cause of this damage is obscure.

The radiographic picture[93] is indistinguishable from that of cardiogenic pulmonary edema except that the heart is not enlarged (Figure 9-50). Although the edema may appear quickly, it may take up to 24 hours to be radiologically apparent. Unlike the usual forms of noncardiogenic pulmonary edema, the lungs usually clear within 24 to 48 hours.[67]

HIGH-ALTITUDE PULMONARY EDEMA. High-altitude pulmonary edema (mountain sickness) is seen predominantly in children or young adults who rapidly ascend to heights of 2700 to 3500 m or greater. The entity is seen more frequently in individuals who undertake heavy physical exercise shortly after arrival at altitude, and there seems to be an individual susceptibility.[194] Symptoms of pulmonary edema develop 3 to 48 hours after achieving high altitude, and the majority of patients experience symptoms within 24 hours.[203] The most frequent early symptoms are shortness of breath, dry cough, and restlessness. The edema is extremely responsive to treatment with oxygen and a return to lower altitudes.[203]

The mechanism is debated. Lockhart and Saiag,[194] in their review, while acknowledging that the pathogenesis was elusive, divided the potential causes into the consequences of high pulmonary arterial pressure secondary to hypoxia and the effect of increased capillary permeability. Pulmonary capillary wedge pressures are near normal,[161] although transient elevations at the time of edema cannot be excluded. The protein content of the edema, which, if high would indicate increased vascular permeability, is not known, but the presence of hyaline membranes and

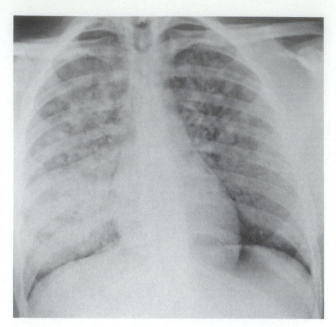

FIGURE 9-51
Pulmonary edema caused by acute severe laryngospasm following general anesthesia.

fibrinlike material in the alveoli at autopsy suggests a protein-rich edema fluid.[203,233]

The chest radiographic appearances are those of acute alveolar edema.[199] The heart remains normal in size, but the main pulmonary artery becomes prominent, decreasing in size with recovery.[203]

PULMONARY EDEMA ASSOCIATED WITH UPPER AIRWAY OBSTRUCTION. Pulmonary edema can on rare occasion be associated with acute upper airway obstruction caused by such conditions as laryngospasm (Figure 9-51),[167] croup,[344] epiglottitis,[344] sleep apnea,[58] or strangulation.[58] The mechanism is not clear. The possibilities include hypoxia, sympathomimetic overactivity, and negative intrapleural pressure. Clearly these processes may act in concert.[344] The extremely negative intrathoracic pressures in a patient struggling to overcome upper airway obstruction may lead to transudation of fluid on a mechanical basis, whereas severe hypoxemia may damage the small intrapulmonary vessels directly or may act by means of extreme vasoconstriction, elevation of pulmonary pressure, and excess sympathomimetic activity.

Reexpansion pulmonary edema

Following drainage of a pneumothorax the reexpanded lung may become acutely edematous. A similar sequence of events can follow drainage of a pleural effusion. The mechanism is obscure, some authors suggesting it is related to surfactant depletion[218,250,296,343] and others that it results from anoxic capillary damage, leading to increased capillary permeability.[296] The edema usually develops within 2 hours of reexpansion and can progress for 1 or 2 days, resolving within 5 to 7 days. Reexpansion edema generally causes little morbidity, but patients can become hypotensive and hypoxic,[150,171] and at least one death has been recorded.[289] It is generally held that complete pneumothoraces with gross lung collapse, chronicity of the pneumothorax, and high negative aspiration pressures are predisposing factors. Most pneumothoraces have been complete and present for at least 3 days,[218,343] but exceptions of shorter duration have been reported.[300] In many patients expansion has been rapid because negative aspiration pressure was used,[62,289,384] but this has by no means been universal.[40,162,337,357] The chest radiograph shows ipsilateral air space shadowing (Figure 9-52). Exceptional cases are reported with contralateral edema[150,321] and recurrent edema with recurrent pneumothorax.[299]

It is worth noting that rapid reperfusion of a lung, for example, after thrombolysis of a massive pulmonary embolus, may also cause acute pulmonary edema.[358]

Amniotic fluid embolism

Under normal circumstances no amniotic fluid enters the maternal circulation during pregnancy or labor. Amniotic fluid contains fetal cellular debris and mucin, and it is the squames from the fetal skin and the mucin from fetal meconium that appear to be responsible for the syndrome of amniotic fluid embolism.[250] On reaching the lungs these materials incite hemodynamic shock with dyspnea, frothy blood-tinged sputum, cyanosis, and central nervous system irritability. Right-sided heart catheterization characteristically shows elevated central venous pressure, elevated pulmonary arterial pressure, and elevated capillary wedge pressure, and it may be possible to identify amniotic fluid debris in blood samples taken through the right heart catheter.[233]

The condition is rare but frequently fatal (in a recent review of the literature the fatality rate was found to be 86%[233]) and is responsible for approximately 10% of maternal deaths.[233] Peterson and Taylor[250] suggested that in the majority of patients the amniotic fluid gains access through the site of placental attachment, the placenta having prematurely separated. In some cases uterine laceration is present. There is a high correlation with intrauterine death and fetal distress, suggesting that it is the amniotic fluid contents—particularly mucin—that do the harm. In patients who die of amniotic fluid embolism, labor is usually rapid with evidence of strong uterine contractions, implicating uterine hypertonicity as an important etiologic factor.[171,181] The condition is most often seen late in the course of pregnancy, and the babies are rarely premature, although the syndrome was recently found to be an important cause of illegal abortion–related deaths.[171] At autopsy the lungs are edematous with widespread atelectasis. It is not possible on gross examination to recognize that amniotic fluid embolism has occurred, but histologic examination with special

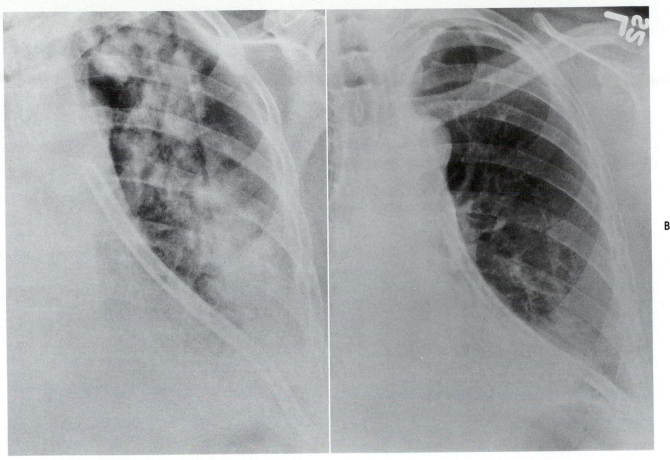

FIGURE 9-52
Reexpansion pulmonary edema. A, Plain chest radiograph showing acute pulmonary edema that developed after a large left pleural effusion was drained. B, Twenty-five hours later, the pulmonary edema has cleared.

stains reveals fetal squames or mucin in all cases.[181]

The radiologic appearances are those of pulmonary edema, which is indistinguishable from the two other conditions that need to be considered in women during labor, acute cardiogenic edema and massive gastric aspiration.

REFERENCES

1. Alberts WM, Priest GR, Moser KM: The outlook for survivors of ARDS, *Chest* 84:272-274, 1983.
2. Alexander MSM, Peters AM, Cleland J, Lavender JP: Impaired left lower lobe ventilation in patients with cardiomegaly: an isotope study of mechanisms, *Chest* 101:1189-1193, 1992.
3. Andersen BL, Gordon L, Buse MG: Intrapulmonary shunting associated with cirrhosis: incidental diagnosis by perfusion lung scan, *Clin Nucl Med* 7:108-110, 1982.
4. Anderson G, Reid L, Simon G: The radiographic appearances in primary and in thromboembolic pulmonary hypertension, *Clin Radiol* 24:113-120, 1973.
5. Andreadis NA, Petty TL: New basic and clinical science in adult respiratory distress syndrome, *Semin Respir Med* 8(suppl):1-74, 1986.
6. Andrews CP, Coalson JJ, Smith JD, et al: Diagnosis of nosocomial bacterial pneumonia in acute diffuse lung injury, *Chest* 80:254-258, 1981.
7. Arai K, Takashima T, Matsui O, et al: Transient subpleural curvilinear shadow caused by pulmonary congestion, *J Comput Assist Tomogr* 14:87-88, 1990.
8. Auerbach O: Pathology and pathogenesis of pulmonary arterial aneurysm in tuberculous cavities, *Am Rev Tuberc* 39:99-115, 1939.
9. Auger WR, Fedullo PF, Moser KM, et al: Chronic major-vessel thromboembolic pulmonary artery obstruction: appearance at angiography, *Radiology* 182:393-398, 1992.
10. Ayres SM: Mechanisms and consequences of pulmonary edema: cardiac lung, shock lung, and principles of ventilatory therapy in adult respiratory distress syndrome, *Am Heart J* 103:97-112, 1982.
11. Bachofen M, Wiebel ER: Structural alterations of lung parenchyma in the adult respiratory distress syndrome, *Clin Chest Med* 3:35-56, 1982.
12. Bachynski JE: Absence of air bronchogram sign: a reliable finding in pulmonary embolism with infarction or hemorrhage, *Radiology* 100:547-552, 1971.
13. Balakrishnan J, Meziane MA, Siegelman SS, et al: Pulmonary infarction: CT appearance with pathologic confirmation, *J Comput Assist Tomogr* 13:941-945, 1989.

14. Balfour IC, Covitz W, Davis H, et al: Cardiac size and function in children with sickle cell anemia, *Am Heart J* 108:345-350, 1984.

15. Balk R, Bone RC: The adult respiratory distress syndrome, *Med Clin North Am* 67:685-700, 1983.

16. Bank ER, Thrall JH, Dantzker DR: Radionuclide demonstration of intrapulmonary shunting in cirrhosis, *AJR* 140:967-969, 1983.

17. Baron MG: Fleischner lines and pulmonary emboli, *Circulation* 45:171-178, 1972.

18. Barrett-Connor E: Acute pulmonary disease and sickle cell anemia, *Am Rev Respir Dis* 104:159-165, 1971.

19. Barrett-Connor E: Pneumonia and pulmonary infarction in sickle cell anemia, *JAMA* 224:997-1000, 1973.

20. Baumstark A, Swensson RG, Hessel SJ, et al: Evaluating the radiographic assessment of pulmonary venous hypertension in chronic heart disease, *AJR* 141:877-884, 1984.

21. Bell WR, Simon TL: Current status of pulmonary thromboembolic disease: pathophysiology, diagnosis, prevention and treatment, *Am Heart J* 103:239-262, 1982.

22. Bell WR, Simon TL, deMetz DL: The clinical features of submassive and massive pulmonary emboli, *Am J Med* 62:355-360, 1977.

23. Bennett ED, Rees S: The significance of radiological changes in the lungs in acute myocardial infarction, *Br J Radiol* 47:879-881, 1974.

24. Berkmen YM, Lande A: Chest roentgenography as a window to the diagnosis of Takayasu's arteritis, *AJR* 125:842-846, 1975.

25. Berthelot P, Walker JG, Sherlock S, et al: Arterial changes in the lungs in cirrhosis of the liver — lung spider nevi, *N Engl J Med* 274:291-298, 1966.

26. Berthezene Y, Vexler V, Jerome H, et al: Differentiation of capillary leak and hydrostatic pulmonary edema with a macromolecular MR imaging contrast agent, *Radiology* 181:773-777, 1991.

27. Berthezene Y, Vexler V, Price DC, et al: Magnetic resonance imaging detection of an experimental pulmonary perfusion deficit using a macromolecular contrast agent, polylysine-gadolinium-DTPA40, *Invest Radiol* 27:346-351, 1992.

28. Bhalla M, Abboud MR, McLoud TC, et al: Acute chest syndrome in sickle cell disease: CT evidence of microvascular occlusion, *Radiology* 187:45-49, 1993.

29. Biello DR, Mattar AG, McKnight RC, et al: Ventilation-perfusion studies in suspected pulmonary embolism, *AJR* 133:1033-1037, 1979.

30. Bjornsson J, Edwards WD: Primary pulmonary hypertension: a histopathologic study of 80 cases, *Mayo Clin Proc* 60:16-25, 1985.

31. Blinder RA, Coleman RE: Evaluation of pulmonary embolism, *Radiol Clin North Am* 23:391-405, 1985.

32. Bogren HG, Berman DS, Vismara LA, et al: Lung ventilation-perfusion scintigraphy in pulmonary embolism: diagnostic specificity compared to pulmonary angiography, *Acta Radiol [Diagn] (Stockh)* 19:933-944, 1978.

33. Bogren HG, Klipstein RH, Mohiaddin RH, et al: Pulmonary artery distensibility and blood flow patterns: a magnetic resonance study of normal subjects and of patients with pulmonary arterial hypertension, *Am Heart J* 118:990-999, 1989.

34. Bombino M, Gattinoni L, Pesenti A, et al: The value of portable chest roentgenography in adult respiratory distress syndrome: comparison with computed tomography, *Chest* 100:762-769, 1991.

35. Bookstein JJ, Silver TM: The angiographic differential diagnosis of acute pulmonary embolism, *Radiology* 110:25-33, 1974.

36. Boxt LM, Rich S, Fried R, et al: Automated morphologic evaluation of pulmonary arteries in primary pulmonary hypertension, *Invest Radiol* 21:906-909, 1986.

37. Branch WT, McNeil BJ: Analysis of the differential diagnosis and assessment of pleuritic chest pain in young adults, *Am J Med* 75:671-679, 1983.

38. Braun SD, Newman GE, Ford K, et al: Ventilation-perfusion scanning and pulmonary angiography: correlation in clinical high-probability pulmonary embolism, *AJR* 143:977-980, 1984.

39. Brealnach E, Stanley RJ: CT diagnosis of segmental pulmonary artery embolism, *J Comput Assist Tomogr* 8:762-764, 1984.

40. Brennan NJ, FitzGerald MX: Anatomically localised re-expansion pulmonary oedema following pneumothorax drainage, *Respiration* 38:233-237, 1979.

41. Brown KT, Bach AM: Paucity of angiographic findings despite extensive organized thrombus in chronic thromboembolic pulmonary hypertension, *J Vasc Intervent Radiol* 3:99-102, 1992.

42. Buckner CB, Walker CW, Purnell GL: Pulmonary embolism: chest radiographic abnormalities, *J Thorac Imag* 4:23-27, 1989.

43. Burch WM, Sullivan PJ, McLaren CJ: Technegas — a new ventilation agent for lung scanning, *Nucl Med Commun* 7:865-871, 1986.

44. Burchard KW, Carney WI: Tumor embolism as the first manifestation of cancer, *J Surg Oncol* 27:26-30, 1984.

45. Burwell CS, Robin ED, Whaley RD: Extreme obesity associated with alveolar hypoventilation — a Pickwickian syndrome, *Am J Med* 21:811-818, 1956.

46. Bynum LJ, Wilson JE: Radiographic features of pleural effusions in pulmonary embolism, *Am Rev Respir Dis* 117:829-834, 1978.

47. Carrington CB, Liebow AA: Pulmonary venoocclusive disease, *Hum Pathol* 1:322-324, 1970.

48. Carvalho P, Lavender JP: The incidence and etiology of the ventilation perfusion reverse mismatch defect, *Clin Nucl Med* 14:571-576, 1989.

49. Chait A, Cohen HE, Meltzer LE, et al: The bedside chest radiograph in the evaluation of incipient heart failure, *Radiology* 105:563-566, 1972.

50. Chait A, Summers D, Krasnow N, et al: Observation on the fate of large pulmonary emboli, *AJR* 100:364-373, 1967.

51. Chakeres DW, Spiegel PK: Fatal pulmonary hypertension secondary to intravascular metastatic tumor emboli, *AJR* 139:997-1000, 1982.

52. Chan CK, Hutcheon MA, Hyland RH, et al: Pulmonary tumor embolism: a critical review of clinical, imaging and hemodynamic features, *J Thorac Imag* 2:4-14, 1987.

53. Chang CH: The normal roentgenographic measurement of the right descending pulmonary artery in 1,085 cases, *AJR* 87:929-935, 1962.

54. Chang CH: Radiological considerations in pulmonary embolism, *Clin Radiol* 18:301-309, 1967.

55. Chang CH, Davis WC: A roentgen sign of pulmonary infarction, *Clin Radiol* 16:141-147, 1965.

56. Chapman PJ, Bateman ED, Benatar SR: Primary pulmonary hypertension and thromboembolic pulmonary hypertension — similarities and differences, *Respir Med* 84:485-488, 1990.

57. Charache S, Scott JC, Charache P: "Acute chest syndrome" in adults with sickle cell anemia: microbiology, treatment, and prevention, *Arch Intern Med* 139:67-69, 1979.

58. Chaudhary BA, Ferguson DS, Speir WA: Pulmonary edema as a presenting feature of sleep apnea syndrome, *Chest* 82:122-124, 1982.

59. Chawla SK, Kittle CF, Faber LP, et al: Pulmonary veno-occlusive diseases, *Ann Thorac Surg* 22:249-253, 1976.

60. Cheely R, McCartney WH, Perry JR, et al: The role of noninvasive tests versus pulmonary angiography in the diagnosis of pulmonary embolism, *Am J Med* 70:17-22, 1981.

61. Chen NS, Barnett CA, Farrer PA: Reversibility of intrapulmonary arteriovenous shunts in liver cirrhosis documented by serial radionuclide perfusion lung scans, *Clin Nucl Med* 9:279-282, 1984.

62. Childress ME, Moy G, Mottram M: Unilateral pulmonary edema resulting from treatment of spontaneous pneumothorax, *Am Rev Respir Dis* 104:119-121, 1971.

63. Chintapilli K, Thorsen MK, Olson DL, et al: Computed tomography of pulmonary thromboembolism and infarction, *J Comput Assist Tomogr* 12:553-559, 1988.

64. Ciofetta G, Pratt TA, Hughes JMB: Comparison of krypton-81m and technetium-99m human serum albumin for measurement of pulmonary perfusion distribution. In Lavender JP, ed: Clinical and experimental applications of krypton-81m, Br J Radiol Special Report no. 15, BIR 1978, pp 46-51.

65. Coates G, O'Brodovich H: Measurement of pulmonary epithelial permeability with Tc-99m DTPA aerosol, *Semin Nucl Med* 16:275-284, 1986.

66. Cohn RC, Wong R, Spohn WA, Komer M: Death due to diffuse alveolar hemorrhage in a child with pulmonary veno-occlusive disease, *Chest* 100:1456-1458, 1991.

67. Colice GL, Matthay MA, Bass E, et al: Neurogenic pulmonary edema: clinical commentary, *Am Rev Respir Dis* 130:941-948, 1984.

68. Collins FS, Orringer EP: Pulmonary hypertension and cor pulmonale in the sickle hemoglobinopathies, *Am J Med* 73:814-821, 1982.

69. Come PC: Echocardiographic evaluation of pulmonary embolism and its response to therapeutic interventions, *Chest* 101:151S-162S, 1992.

70. Cooper TJ, Hayward MW, Hartog M: Survey on the use of pulmonary scintigraphy and angiography for suspected pulmonary thromboembolism in the UK, *Clin Radiol* 43:243-245, 1991.

71. Cromie JB: Correlation of anatomic pulmonary emphysema and right ventricular hypertrophy, *Am Rev Respir Dis* 84:657-662, 1961.

72. Cunningham DA, Lavender JP: Kr-81m ventilation scanning in chronic obstructive airways disease, *Br J Radiol* 54:110-116, 1981.

73. Cunningham DA, Mitchell DM: Well ventilated bullae: a potential confusion on ventilation/perfusion scanning, *Br J Radiol* 64:56-60, 1991.

74. Dalen JE, Alpert JS: Natural history of pulmonary embolism, *Prog Cardiovasc Dis* 17:259-270, 1975.

75. Dalen JE, Brooks HL, Johnson LW, et al: Pulmonary angiography in acute pulmonary embolism: indications, techniques, and results in 367 patients, *Am Heart J* 81:175-185, 1971.

76. Dalen JE, Haffajee CI, Alpert JS, et al: Pulmonary embolism, pulmonary hemorrhage and pulmonary infarction, *N Engl J Med* 296:1431-1435, 1977.

77. Dalen JE, Mathur VS, Evans H, et al: Pulmonary angiography in experimental pulmonary embolism, *Am Heart J* 72:509-520, 1966.

78. D'Alonzo GE, Bower JS, Dantzkes DR: Differentiation of patients with primary and thromboembolic hypertension, *Chest* 85:457-461, 1984.

79. Daughtry JD, Stewart BH, Golding LAR, et al: Pulmonary embolus presenting as the initial manifestation of renal cell carcinoma, *Ann Thorac Surg* 24:178-181, 1977.

80. Davies SC, Luce PJ, Win AA, et al: Acute chest syndrome in sickle-cell disease, *Lancet* 1:36-38, 1984.

81. de Fauca P, Peltier P, Planchon B, et al: Evaluation of indium-111 labeled antifibrin monoclonal antibody for the diagnosis of venous thrombotic disease, *J Nucl Med* 32:785-791, 1991.

82. de Vries TW, Weening JJ, Roorda RJ: Pulmonary veno-occlusive disease: a case report and a review of therapeutic possibilities, *Eur Respir J* 4:1029-1032, 1991.

83. Diffey BL, Gibson CJ, Scott LE: A new technique for xenon-133 ventilation imaging in the diagnosis of pulmonary embolism, *Br J Radiol* 59:1179-1184, 1986.

84. Dillon WP, Taylor AT, Mineau DE, et al: Traumatic pulmonary artery pseudoaneurysm simulating pulmonary embolism, *AJR* 139:818-819, 1982.

85. Divertie MB: The adult respiratory distress syndrome: subject review, *Mayo Clin Proc* 57:371-378, 1982.

86. Don C, Johnson R: The nature and significance of peribronchial cuffing in pulmonary edema, *Radiology* 125:577-582, 1977.

87. Dunnick NR, Newman GE, Perlmutt, et al: Pulmonary embolism, *Curr Prob Diagn Radiol* 6:197-229, 1988.

88. Dyck DR, Zylak CJ: Acute respiratory distress in adults, *Radiology* 106:407-501, 1973.

89. Edwards WD, Edwards JE: Clinical primary pulmonary hypertension: three pathologic types, *Circulation* 56:884-888, 1977.

90. El Gamal M, Stoker JB, Spiers EM, et al: Cyanosis complicating hepatic cirrhosis, *Am J Cardiol* 25:490-494, 1970.

91. Evans KT, Cockshott WP, Hendrickse P de V, et al: Pulmonary changes in malignant trophoblastic disease, *Br J Radiol* 38:161-171, 1965.

92. Falaschi F, Palla A, Formichi B, et al: CT evaluation of chronic thromboembolic pulmonary hypertension, *J Comput Assist Tomogr* 16:897-903, 1992.

93. Felman AH: Neurogenic pulmonary edema: observations in 6 patients, *AJR* 112:393-396, 1971.

94. Ferris EJ, Holder JC, Lim WN, et al: Angiography of pulmonary emboli: digital studies and balloon-occlusion cineangiography, *AJR* 142:369-373, 1984.

95. Ferris EJ, Steinzler RM, Rowke JA, et al: Pulmonary angiography in pulmonary embolic disease, *AJR* 100:355-363, 1967.

96. Figley MM, Gerdes AJ, Ricketts HJ: Radiographic aspects of pulmonary embolism, *Semin Roentgenol* 2:389-405, 1967.

97. Fisher MR, Higgins CB: Central thrombi in pulmonary arterial hypertension detected by MR imaging, *Radiology* 158:223-226, 1986.

98. Fishman AJ, Moser KM, Fedullo PF: Perfusion lung scans vs. pulmonary angiography in evaluation of suspected primary pulmonary hypertension, *Chest* 84:679-683, 1983.

99. Fishman AP: Chronic cor pulmonale: state of the art, *Am Rev Respir Dis* 114:775-794, 1976.

100. Fleischner FG: Pulmonary embolism, *Clin Radiol* 13:169-182, 1962.

101. Fleischner FG: The butterfly pattern of acute pulmonary edema, *Am J Cardiol* 20:39-46, 1967.

102. Fleischner FG: Recurrent pulmonary embolism and cor pulmonale, *N Engl J Med* 176:1213-1220, 1967.

103. Fleischner FG, Hampton AO, Castleman B: Linear shadows in the lung, *AJR* 46:610-618, 1941.

104. Foo TKF, MacFall JR, Hayes CE, et al: Pulmonary vasculature: single breath-hold MR imaging with phased-array coils, *Radiology* 183:473-477, 1992.

105. Fred HL, Axelrad MA, Lewis JM, et al: Rapid resolution of pulmonary thromboemboli in man, *JAMA* 196:1137-1140, 1966.

106. Fred HL, Burdine JA, Gonzales DA, et al: Arteriographic assessment of lung scanning in the diagnosis of pulmonary embolism, *N Engl J Med* 275:1025-1032, 1966.

107. Freiman DG, Suyemoto J, Wessler S: Frequency of pulmonary thromboembolism in man, *N Engl J Med* 272:1278-1280, 1965.

108. Friedman WF, Braunwald E: Alterations in regional blood flow in mitral valve disease studied by radioisotopic scanning, *Circulation* 34:363-376, 1966.

109. Gabrielsen F, Schmidt A, Eggeling T, et al: Massive main pulmonary artery embolism diagnosed with two-dimensional Doppler echocardiography, *Clin Cardiol* 15:545-546, 1992.

110. Gamsu G, Hirji M, Moore EH, et al: Experimental pulmonary emboli detected using magnetic resonance, *Radiology* 153:467-470, 1984.

111. Gattinoni L, Presenti A, Baglioni S, et al: Inflammatory pulmonary edema and positive end-expiratory pressure: correlations between imaging and physiologic studies, *J Thorac Imag* 3:59-64, 1988.

112. Gattinoni L, Pesenti A, Thorresin A, et al: Adult respiratory distress syndrome profiles by computed tomography, *J Thorac Imag* 1:25-30, 1986.

113. Geddes DM, Kerr IH: Pulmonary arterial aneurysms in association with a right ventricular myxoma, *Br J Radiol* 49:374-376, 1976.

114. Gefter WB, Hatabu H, Dinsmore BJ, et al: Pulmonary vascular cine MR imaging: a noninvasive approach to dynamic imaging of the pulmonary circulation, *Radiology* 176:761-770, 1990.

115. Gelernt MD, Mogtader A, Hahn RT: Transesophageal echocardiography to diagnose and demonstrate resolution of an acute massive pulmonary embolus, *Chest* 102:297-299, 1992.

116. Gibson RN, Morgan SH, Krauz T, et al: Pulmonary artery aneurysms in Behcet's disease, *Br J Radiol* 58:79-82, 1985.

117. Gilroy RJ Jr, Teague MW, Lloyd JE: Pulmonary veno-occlusive disease: fatal progression of pulmonary hypertension despite steroid-induced remission of interstitial pneumonitis, *Am Rev Respir Dis* 143:1130-1133, 1991.

118. Gleason DC, Steiner RE: The lateral roentgenogram in pulmonary edema, *AJR* 98:279-290, 1966.

119. Godwin JD, Webb WR, Gamsu G, Ovenfors CO: Computed tomography of pulmonary embolism, *AJR* 135:691-695, 1980.

120. Goldhaber SZ: Recent advances in the diagnosis and lytic therapy of pulmonary embolism, *Chest* 99:173S-179S, 1991.

121. Goldhaber SZ, Braunwald E: Pulmonary embolism. In Braunwald E, ed: *Heart disease: a textbook of cardiovascular medicine*, ed 3, Philadelphia, 1988, WB Saunders.

122. Gomez-Sanchez MA, Mestre de Juan MJ, Gomez-Pajuelo C, et al: Pulmonary hypertension due to toxic oil syndrome: a clinicopathologic study, *Chest* 95:325-331, 1982.

123. Goodman PC: Pulmonary angiography, *Clin Chest Med* 5:465-477, 1984.

124. Goodwin DA, Bushberg JT, Doherty PW, et al: In-111 labeled autologous platelets for location of vascular thrombi in humans, *J Nucl Med* 19:626-634, 1978.

125. Graham JP, Rotman HH, Weg JG: Tumor emboli presenting as pulmonary hypertension, *Chest* 69:229-230, 1976.

126. Grainger RG: Interstitial pulmonary oedema and its radiological diagnosis: a sign of pulmonary venous and capillary hypertension, *Br J Radiol* 31:201-217, 1958.

127. Gray HW: The single perfusion abnormality: quo vadis? *Nucl Med Commun* 12:377-379, 1991.

128. Greene R: Adult respiratory distress syndrome: acute alveolar damage, *Radiology* 163:57-66, 1987.

129. Greenspan RH, Ravin CE, Polansky SM, et al: Accuracy of the chest radiograph in diagnosis of pulmonary embolism, *Invest Radiol* 17:539-543, 1982.

130. Grieco MH, Ryan SF: Aseptic cavitary pulmonary infarction, *Am J Med* 45:811-816, 1968.

131. Guintini C, Mariani M, Barsotti A, et al: Factors affecting regional pulmonary blood flow in left heart valvular disease, *Am J Med* 57:421-436, 1974.

132. Gupta BD, Moodie DS, Hodgman JR: Primary pulmonary hypertension in adults: clinical features, catheterization findings and long-term follow-up, *Cleve Clin Q* 47:275-284, 1980.

133. Hackman RC, Madtes DK, Petersen FB, Clark JG: Pulmonary veno-occlusive disease following bone marrow transplantation, *Transplantation* 47:989-992, 1989.

134. Hadfield JW, Sterling JC, Wraight EP: Multiple tumour emboli simulating a massive pulmonary embolus, *Postgrad Med J* 58:792-793, 1982.

135. Hampton AO, Castleman B: Correlations of post mortem chest teleroentgenograms with autopsy findings with special reference to pulmonary embolism and infarction, *AJR* 43:305-326, 1940.

136. Hansoti RC, Shah NJ: Cirrhosis of liver simulating congenital cyanotic heart disease, *Circulation* 32:71-77, 1966.

137. Harris P, Heath D: *The human pulmonary circulation*, ed 3, Edinburgh, 1986, Churchill Livingston.

138. Harrison MO, Conte PJ, Heitzman ER: Radiological detection of clinically occult cardiac failure following myocardial infarction, *Br J Radiol* 44:265-272, 1971.

139. Hartshorne MF, Eisenberg B: CT diagnosis of a giant central pulmonary artery aneurysm arising quickly after pulmonary embolic disease (letter), *AJR* 153:190-191, 1989.

140. Hatabu H, Gefter WB, Listerud J, et al: Pulmonary MR angiography utilizing phased-array surface coils, *J Comput Assist Tomogr* 16:410-417, 1992.

141. Hatano S, Strasser T, eds: *Primary pulmonary hypertension: WHO committee report*, Geneva, 1975. World Health Organization.

142. Haupt HM, Moore W, Bauer TW, et al: The lung in sickle cell disease, *Chest* 81:332-337, 1982.

143. Hays MD, Wiles HB, Gillette PC: Congenital acquired immunodeficiency syndrome presenting as cor pulmonale in a 10 year old girl, *Am Heart J* 121:929-931, 1991.

144. He XW, Tang YH, Luo ZQ, et al: Subacute cor pulmonale due to tumor embolization to the lungs, *Angiology* 40:11-17, 1989.

145. Heck LL, Duley JW: Statistical considerations in lung imaging with Tc-99m albumin particles, *Radiology* 113:675-679, 1974.

146. Heikkila J, Hugenholtz PG, Tabakin BS: Prediction of left heart filling pressure and its sequential change in acute myocardial infarction from the terminal force of the P wave, *Br Heart J* 35:142-151, 1973.

147. Heitzman ER: *The lung: radiologic-pathologic correlations*, ed 2, St Louis, 1984, Mosby.

148. Heitzman ER, Markarian B, Dailey ET: Pulmonary thromboembolic disease: a lobular concept, *Radiology* 103:529-537, 1972.

149. Heitzman ER, Ziter FM: Acute interstitial pulmonary edema, *Radiology* 98:291-299, 1966.

150. Henderson AF, Banham SW, Moran F: Reexpansion pulmonary oedema: a potentially serious complication of delayed diagnosis of pneumothorax, *Br Med J* 291:593-594, 1985.

151. Henson PM, Larsen GL, Webster RO, et al: Pulmonary microvascular alterations and injury induced by complement fragments: synergistic effect of complement activation, neutrophil sequestration and prostaglandins, *Ann NY Acad Sci* 384:287-300, 1982.

152. Herman PG, Khan A, Kallman CE: Limited correlation of left ventricular end-diastolic pressure with radiographic assessment of pulmonary hemodynamics, *Radiology* 174:721-724, 1990.

153. Hicken P, Heath D, Brewer D: The relation between the weight of the right ventricle and the percentage of abnormal air space in the lung in emphysema, *J Pathol Bacteriol* 92:519-528, 1966.

154. Himelman RB, Dohrmann M, Goodman P, et al: Severe pulmonary hypertension and cor pulmonale in the acquired immunodeficiency syndrome, *Am J Cardiol* 64:1396-1399, 1989.

155. Hirji M, Gamsu G, Webb WR, et al: EKG-gated digital subtraction angiography in the detection of pulmonary emboli, *Radiology* 152:19-22, 1984.

156. Hodson CJ: Pulmonary oedema and bats-wing shadows, *J Fac Radiol* 1:176-186, 1950.

157. Hughes JMB, Glazier JB, Maloney JE, West JB: Effect of lung volume on the distribution of pulmonary blood flow in man, *Respir Physiol* 4:58-72, 1968.

158. Hull RD, Hirsh J, Carter CJ, et al: Pulmonary angiography, ventilation lung scanning, and venography for clinically suspected pulmonary embolism with abnormal perfusion lung scan, *Ann Intern Med* 98:891-899, 1983.

159. Hull RD, Hirsh J, Carter CJ, et al: Diagnostic value of ventilation perfusion lung scanning in patients with suspected pulmonary embolism, *Chest* 88:819-828, 1985.

160. Hull RD, Raskob GE, Coates G, et al: A new noninvasive management strategy for patients with suspected pulmonary embolism, *Arch Intern Med* 149:2549-2555, 1989.

161. Hultgren HN, Lopez CE, Lundberg E, et al: Physiologic studies of pulmonary edema at high altitude, *Circulation* 29:393-408, 1985.

162. Humphreys RL, Berne AS: Rapid re-expansion of pneumothorax: a cause of unilateral pulmonary edema, *Radiology* 96:509-512, 1970.

163. Hunter JJ, Johnson KR, Karagianes TG, Dittrich HC: Detection of massive pulmonary embolus-in-transit by transesophageal echocardiography, *Chest* 100:1210-1214, 1991.

164. Hyers TM, Fowler AA, Wicks AB: Focal pulmonary edema after massive pulmonary embolism, *Am Rev Respir Dis* 123:232-233, 1981.

165. Iannuzzi M, Petty TL: The diagnosis, pathogenesis, and treatment of adult respiratory distress syndrome, *J Thorac Imag* 1:1-10, 1986.

166. Ingram RH, Braunwald E: Pulmonary edema: cardiogenic and noncardiogenic. In Braunwald E, ed: *Heart disease: a textbook of cardiovascular medicine*, ed 3, Philadelphia, 1988, WB Saunders.

167. Jackson FN, Rowland V, Corssen G: Laryngospasm-induced pulmonary edema, *Chest* 78:819-821, 1980.

168. Jacoby CG, Mindell HJ: Lobar consolidation in pulmonary embolism, *Radiology* 118:287-290, 1976.

169. James JM, Lloyd JJ, Leahy BC, et al: Tc-99m technegas and krypton-81m ventilation scintigraphy: a comparison in known respiratory disease, *Br J Radiol* 65:1075-1082, 1992.

170. Jefferson K, Rees S: *Clinical cardiac radiology*, London, 1973, Butterworths.

171. Jenkinson SG: Pneumothorax, *Clin Chest Med* 6:153-161, 1985.

172. Joffe N: The adult respiratory distress syndrome, *AJR* 122:719-732, 1974.

173. Jonker N, Peters AM, Gaskin G, et al: A retrospective study of granulocyte kinetics in patients with systemic vasculitis, *J Nucl Med* 33:491-497, 1992.

174. Juni JE, Alavi A: Lung scanning in the diagnosis of pulmonary embolism: the emperor redressed, *Semin Nucl Med* 21:281-296, 1991.

175. Kalebo P, Wallin J: Computed tomography in massive pulmonary embolism, *Acta Radiol* 30:105-107, 1989.

176. Kanemoto N, Furuya H, Etoh T, et al: Chest roentgenograms in primary pulmonary hypertension, *Chest* 76:45-49, 1979.

177. Karlish AJ, Marshall R, Reid L, et al: Cyanosis with hepatic cirrhosis: a case with pulmonary arteriovenous shunting, *Thorax* 22:555-561, 1967.

178. Kawai C, Ishikawa K, Kato M, et al: "Pulmonary pulseless disease": pulmonary involvement in so-called Takayasu's disease, *Chest* 73:651-657, 1978.

179. Kereiakes DJ, Herfkens RJ, Brundage BH, et al: Computerized tomography in chronic thromboembolic pulmonary hypertension, *Am Heart J* 106:1432-1436, 1983.

180. Kerr IH, Simon G, Sutton GC: The value of the plain radiograph in acute massive pulmonary embolism, *Br J Radiol* 44:751-757, 1971.

181. King AD, Bell SD, Stuttle AWJ, et al: The natural history of post-operative deep venous thrombosis and pulmonary embolism illustrated in a case report using the In-111 labelled platelet-specific monoclonal antibody P256, *Chest* 101:1597-1601, 1992.

182. Kipper MS, Moser KM, Kortman KE, et al: Long-term follow up of patients with suspected pulmonary embolism and a normal lung scan, *Chest* 82:411-415, 1982.

183. Knight LC, Maurer AH, Robbins PS, et al: Detection of venous thrombosis by I-123-fragment E1, a new thrombus imaging agent, *Radiology* 156:509-514, 1985.

184. Kollath J, Riemann H: Pulmonary digital subtraction angiography, *Cardiovasc Intervent Radiol* 6:233-238, 1983.

185. Kondo C, Caputo GR, Masui T, et al: Pulmonary hypertension: pulmonary flow quantification and flow profile analysis with velocity-encoded cine MR imaging, *Radiology* 183:751-758, 1992.

186. Korn D, Gore I, Blenke A, et al: Pulmonary arterial bands and webs: an unrecognized manifestation of organised pulmonary emboli, *Am J Pathol* 40:129-151, 1962.

187. Kuriyama K, Gamsu G, Stern RG, et al: CT determined pulmonary artery diameters in predicting pulmonary hypertension, *Invest Radiol* 19:16-22, 1984.

188. Laur A: Roentgen diagnosis of pulmonary embolism and its differentiation from myocardial infarction, *AJR* 90:632-637, 1963.

189. Lavender JP, Finn JP: V/Q patterns in nonthromboembolic lung diseases. In Loken MK, ed: *Pulmonary nuclear medicine*, Norwalk, Conn, 1987, Appleton & Lange, pp 103-131.

190. Lavender JP, Irving H, Armstrong JD: Kr-81m ventilation scanning: acute respiratory disease, *AJR* 136:309-316, 1981.

191. Lindsay J, Meshel JC, Patterson RH: The cardiovascular manifestations of sickle cell disease, *Arch Intern Med* 133:643-651, 1974.

192. Lippmann M, Fein A: Pulmonary embolism in the patient with chronic obstructive pulmonary disease: a diagnostic dilemma, *Chest* 79:39-42, 1981.

193. Lisbona R, Kreisman H, Novales-Diaz J, et al: Perfusion lung scanning: differentiation of primary from thromboembolic pulmonary hypertension, *AJR* 144:27-30, 1985.

194. Lockhart A, Saiag B: Altitude and the human pulmonary circulation, *Clin Sci* 60:599-605, 1981.

195. Loken MK: *Pulmonary nuclear medicine*, Norwalk, Conn, 1987, Appleton & Lange.

196. Ludwig JW, Verhoeven LAJ, Kersbergen JJ, et al: Digital subtraction angiography of the pulmonary arteries for the diagnosis of pulmonary embolism, *Radiology* 147:639-645, 1983.

197. Lupi EH, Sanchez GT, Horwitz S, et al: Pulmonary artery involvement in Takayasu's arteritis, *Chest* 67:69-74, 1975.

198. Lupi-Herrera E, Sanchez-Torres G, Marcushamer J, et al: Takayasu's arteritis: clinical study of 107 cases, *Am Heart J* 93:94-103, 1977.

199. Maldonado D: High altitude pulmonary edema, *Radiol Clin North Am* 16:537-549, 1978.

200. Malik AB, Tracy SE: Bronchovascular adjustments after pulmonary embolism, *J Appl Physiol* 49:476-481, 1980.

201. Mant MJ, O'Brien BD, Thony KL, et al: Haemorrhagic complications of heparin therapy, *Lancet* 1:1133-1135, 1977.

202. Marsh JD, Glynn M, Torman HA: Pulmonary angiography: application in a new spectrum of patients, *Am J Med* 75:763-770, 1983.

203. Marticorena E, Tapia FA, Dyer J, et al: Pulmonary edema by ascending to high altitudes, *Dis Chest* 45:273-283, 1964.

204. Martin KW, Sagel SS, Siegel BA: Mosaic oligemia simulating pulmonary infiltrates on CT, *AJR* 147:670-673, 1986.

205. Mason GR, Effros RM, Uszler JM, Mena I: Small solute clearance from the lungs of patients with cardiogenic and non-cardiogenic edema, *Chest* 88:327-334, 1985.

206. Mathur VS, Dalen JE, Evans H, et al: Pulmonary angiography one to seven days after experimental pulmonary embolism, *Invest Radiol* 2:304-312, 1967.

207. Matthay MA: Pathophysiology of pulmonary edema, *Clin Chest Med* 6:301-314, 1985.

208. Matthay RA, Berger HJ: Cardiovascular function in cor pulmonale, *Clin Chest Med* 4:269-295, 1983.

209. Maunder RJ, Shuman WP, McHugh JW, et al: Preservation of normal lung regions in the adult respiratory distress syndrome: analysis by computed tomography, *JAMA* 255:2463-2465, 1986.

210. McGoldrick PJ, Rudd TG, Figley MM, et al: What becomes of pulmonary infarcts? *AJR* 133:1039-1045, 1979.

211. McHugh TJ, Forrester JS, Adler L, et al: Pulmonary vascular congestion in acute myocardial infarction: hemodynamic and radiologic correlations, *Ann Intern Med* 76:29-33, 1972.

212. McLeod JG, Grant IWB: A clinical, radiographic, and pathological study of pulmonary embolism, *Thorax* 9:71-83, 1954.

213. McNeil BJ: A diagnostic strategy using ventilation-perfusion studies in patients suspect for pulmonary embolism, *J Nucl Med* 17:613-616, 1976.

214. McNeil BJ: Ventilation perfusion studies and the diagnosis of pulmonary embolism: concise communication, *J Nucl Med* 21:319-323, 1980.

215. Mette SA, Palevsky HI, Pietra GG, et al: Primary pulmonary hypertension in association with human immunodeficiency virus infection: a possible viral etiology for some forms of hypertensive pulmonary arteriopathy, *Am Rev Respir Dis* 145:1196-1200, 1992.

216. Michael JR, Summer WR: Pulmonary hypertension, *Lung* 163:65-82, 1985.

217. Migueres M, Escamilla R, Coca F, et al: Pulsed Doppler echocardiography in the diagnosis of pulmonary hypertension in COPD, *Chest* 98:280-285, 1990.

218. Miller WC, Toon R, Palat H, et al: Experimental pulmonary edema following re-expansion of pneumothorax, *Am Rev Respir Dis* 108:664-666, 1973.

219. Mills SR, Jackson DC, Older RA, et al: Incidence, etiologies and avoidance of complications of pulmonary angiography in a large series, *Radiology* 136:295-299, 1980.

220. Milne ENC: Some new concepts of pulmonary blood flow and volume, *Radiol Clin North Am* 16:515-536, 1978.

221. Milne ENC, Bass H: Roentgenologic and functional analysis of combined chronic obstructive pulmonary disease and congestive cardiac failure, *Invest Radiol* 4:129-147, 1969.

222. Milne ENC, Pistolesi M, Miniati M, et al: The radiologic distinction of cardiogenic and noncardiogenic edema, *AJR* 144:879-894, 1985.

223. Minor RL, Oren RM, Stanford W, Ferguson DW: Biventricular thrombi and pulmonary emboli complicating idiopathic dilated cardiomyopathy: diagnosis with cardiac ultrafast CT, *Am Heart J* 122:1477-1481, 1991.

224. Moore EH, Gamsu G, Webb WR, et al: Pulmonary embolus: detection and follow-up using magnetic resonance, *Radiology* 153:471-472, 1984.

225. Moser KM: Pulmonary embolism: state of the art, *Am Rev Respir Dis* 115:829-852, 1977.

226. Moser KM: Venous thromboembolism: state of the art, *Am Rev Respir Dis* 141:235-249, 1990.

227. Moser KM, Auger WR, Fedullo PF, Jamieson SW: Chronic thromboembolic hypertension: clinical picture and surgical treatment, *Eur Respir J* 5:334-342, 1992.

228. Moser KM, Daily PO, Peterson KL, et al: Thromboendarterectomy for chronic, major vessel thromboembolic pulmonary hypertension in 42 patients: immediate and long-term results, *Ann Intern Med* 107:560-565, 1987.

229. Moser KM, Guisan M, Bartimmo EE: In vivo and post mortem dissolution rates of pulmonary emboli and venous thrombi in the dog, *Circulation* 48:170-178, 1973.

230. Moser KM, Olson LK, Schlusselberg M, et al: Chronic thromboembolic occlusion in the adult can mimic pulmonary artery agenesis, *Chest* 95:503-508, 1989.

231. Moses DC, Silver TM, Bookstein JJ: The complementary roles of chest radiography, lung scanning, and selective pulmonary angiography in the diagnosis of pulmonary embolism, *Circulation* 49:179-188, 1974.

232. Mountford PJ, Coakley AJ: A review of the secretion of radioactivity in human breast milk: data, quantitative analysis and recommendations, *Nucl Med Commun* 10:15-27, 1989.

233. Mulder JI: Amniotic fluid embolism: an over view and case report, *Am J Obstet Gynecol* 152:430-435, 1985.

234. Musset D, Rosso J, Petitpretz P, et al: Acute pulmonary embolism: diagnostic value of digital subtraction angiography, *Radiology* 166:455-459, 1988.

235. Nessa CB, Rigler LG: The roentgenological manifestations of pulmonary edema, *Radiology* 37:35-46, 1941.

236. Newman GE: Pulmonary angiography in pulmonary embolic disease, *J Thorac Imag* 4:28-39, 1989.

237. Nimmo MJ, Merrick MV, Millar AM: A comparison of the economics of xenon 127, xenon 133 and krypton 81m for routine ventilation imaging of the lungs, *Br J Radiol* 58:635-636, 1985.

238. Norgaard H, Gjorup T, Brems-Dalgaard E, et al: Interobserver variation in the detection of pulmonary venous hypertension in chest radiographs, *Eur J Radiol* 11:203-206, 1990.

239. Novelline RA, Baltarowich OH, Athanasoulis CE, et al: The clinical course of patients with suspected pulmonary embolism and a negative pulmonary arteriogram, *Radiology* 126:561-567, 1978.

240. Oh KS, Bender TM, Bowen A, et al: Plain radiographic, nuclear medicine and angiographic observations of hepatogenic pulmonary angiodysplasia, *Pediatr Radiol* 13:111-115, 1983.

241. Okubo S, Kunieda T, Ando M, et al: Idiopathic isolated pulmonary arteritis with chronic cor pulmonale, *Chest* 94:665-666, 1988.

242. Oppenheimer EH, Esterly JR: Pulmonary changes in sickle cell disease, *Am Rev Respir Dis* 103:858-859, 1971.

243. Osborne D, Jaszczak RJ, Greer K, et al: SPECT quantification of technetium-99m microspheres within the canine lung, *J Comput Assist Tomogr* 9:73-77, 1985.

244. Ostendorf P, Brizle H, Vogel W, et al: Pulmonary radiographic abnormalities in shock, *Radiology* 115:257-263, 1975.

245. Owens CM, Evans TW, Keogh BF, Hansell DM: Computed tomography in established adult respiratory distress syndrome, *Chest*, in press.

246. Palevsky HI, Pietra GG, Fishman AP: Pulmonary veno-occlusive disease and its response to vasodilator agents, *Am Rev Respir Dis* 142:426-429, 1990.

247. Palla A, Donnamaria V, Petruzzelli S, et al: Enlargement of the right descending pulmonary artery in pulmonary embolism, *AJR* 141:513-517, 1983.

248. Pattynama PM, Willems LN, Smit AH, et al: Early diagnosis of cor pulmonale with MR imaging of the right ventricle, *Radiology* 182:375-379, 1992.

249. Peters AM, Gordon I, Kaiser AM, et al: Spontaneous abrupt changes in the distribution of ventilation: scintigraphy, *Br J Radiol* 62:536-543, 1988.

250. Peterson EP, Taylor HB: Amniotic fluid embolism, *Obstet Gynecol* 35:787-793, 1970.

251. Peterson KL, Fred HL, Alexander JK: Pulmonary arterial webs: a new angiographic sign of previous thromboembolism, *N Engl J Med* 277:33-35, 1967.

252. Piatt JH Jr, Hoffman HJ: Cor pulmonale: a lethal complication of ventriculoatrial CSF diversion, *Childs Nerv Syst* 5:29-31, 1989.

253. The PIOPED investigators: Value of the ventilation/perfusion scan in acute pulmonary embolism: results of the prospective investigation of pulmonary embolism diagnosis (PIOPED), *JAMA* 263:2753-2759, 1990.

254. Pistolesi M, Giuntini C: Assessment of extravascular lung water, *Radiol Clin North Am* 16:551-574, 1978.

255. Pistolesi M, Miniati M, Milne ENC, et al: The chest roentgenogram in pulmonary edema, *Clin Chest Med* 6:315-344, 1985.

256. Poncz M, Kane E, Gill FM: Acute chest syndrome in sickle cell disease: etiology and clinical correlations, *J Pediatr* 107:861-866, 1985.

257. Pond GD: Pulmonary digital subtraction angiography, *Radiol Clin North Am* 23:243-260, 1985.

258. Porter J, Jick H: Drug-related deaths among medical inpatients, *JAMA* 237:879-881, 1977.

259. Posteraro RH, Sostman HD, Spritzer CE, Herfkens RJ: Cine-gradient-refocused MR imaging of central pulmonary emboli, *AJR* 152:465-468, 1989.

260. Powe JE, Palevsky HI, McCarthy KE, et al: Pulmonary arterial hypertension: value of perfusion scintigraphy, *Radiology* 164:727-730, 1987.

261. Putman CE, Minagi H, Blaisdell FW: Roentgen appearance of disseminated intravascular coagulation (DIC), *Radiology* 109:13-18, 1972.

262. Quinn MF, Lundell CJ, Klotz TA, et al: Reliability of selective pulmonary arteriography in the diagnosis of pulmonary embolism, *AJR* 149:469-471, 1987.

263. Rambihar VS, Fallen EL, Cairns JA: Pulmonary veno-occlusive disease: antemortem diagnosis from roentgenographic and hemodynamic findings, *Can Med Assoc J* 120:1519-1522, 1979.

264. Ranniger K: Pulmonary arteriography: a simple method for demonstration of clinically significant pulmonary emboli, *AJR* 106:588-592, 1962.

265. Rees RSO, Jefferson KE: The Eisenmenger syndrome, *Clin Radiol* 18:366-371, 1967.

266. Remy J, Lemaitre L, Lafitte JJ, et al: Massive hemoptysis of pulmonary artery origin: diagnosis and treatment, *AJR* 143:963-969, 1984.

267. Remy-Jardin M, Remy J, Wattinne L, Giraud F: Central pulmonary thromboembolism: diagnosis with spiral volumetric CT with the single breath-hold technique — comparison with pulmonary angiography, *Radiology* 185:381-387, 1992.

268. Ren H, Kuhlman JE, Hruban RH, et al: CT of inflation-fixed lungs: wedge-shaped density and vascular sign in the diagnosis of infarction, *J Comput Assist Tomogr* 14:82-86, 1990.

269. Revel D, Daville O, Cordier JF, et al: Magnetic resonance imaging (MRI) of hemorrhagic lesions of lung parenchyma, *Diagn Intervent Radiol* 2:35-38, 1990.

270. Rich S, Levitsky S, Brundage BH: Pulmonary hypertension from chronic pulmonary thromboembolism, *Ann Intern Med* 108:425-434, 1988.

271. Rich S, Pietra GG, Kieras K, et al: Primary pulmonary hypertension: radiographic and scintigraphic patterns of histologic subtypes, *Ann Intern Med* 105:449-502, 1986.

272. Rinaldo JE, Rogers RM: Adult respiratory distress syndrome, *N Engl J Med* 315:578-580, 1986.

273. Ritchie BC, Schauberger G, Staub NC: Inadequacy of perivascular edema hypothesis to account for distribution of pulmonary blood flow in lung edema, *Circ Res* 24:801-814, 1969.

274. Robin ED: Overdiagnosis and overtreatment of pulmonary embolism: the emperor may have no clothes, *Ann Intern Med* 87:775-781, 1977.

275. Robin ED, Horn B, Goris ML, et al: Detection, quantitation and physiology of lung spiders, *Trans Assoc Am Physicians* 88:202-216, 1975.

276. Robinson PJ: Lung scintigraphy: doubt and certainty in the diagnosis of pulmonary embolism, *Clin Radiol* 40:557-560, 1989.

277. Rochester DF, Enson Y: Current concepts in the pathogenesis of the obesity hypoventilation syndrome, *Am J Med* 57:402-420, 1974.

278. Rocker GM, Pearson D, Stephens M, Shale DJ: An assessment of a double isotope method for the detection of transferrin accumulation in the lungs of patients with widespread pulmonary infiltrates, *Clin Sci* 75:47-52, 1988.

279. Rosen JM, Biello DR, Siegel BA, et al: Kr-81m ventilation imaging: clinical utility in suspected pulmonary embolism, *Radiology* 154:787-790, 1985.

280. Rosengarten PL, Tuxen DV, Weeks AM: Whole lung pulmonary angiography in the intensive care unit with two portable chest x-rays, *Crit Care Med* 17:274-278, 1989.

281. Rosenow EC III, Osmundson PJ, Brown ML: Pulmonary embolism: subject review, *Mayo Clin Proc* 56:161-178, 1981.

282. Rosenthal A, Vawter G, Wagenvoort CA: Intrapulmonary veno-occlusive disease, *Am J Cardiol* 31:78-83, 1973.

283. Rydell R, Hoffbauer FW: Multiple arteriovenous fistulas in juvenile cirrhosis, *Am J Med* 21:450-460, 1956.

284. Sabiston DC: Pathophysiology, diagnosis, and management of pulmonary embolism, *Am J Surg* 138:384-391, 1979.

285. Sabiston DC, Wolfe WG, Oldham HN, et al: Surgical management of chronic pulmonary embolism, *Ann Surg* 185:699-712, 1977.

286. Sagel SS, Greenspan RH: Nonuniform pulmonary arterial perfusion: pulmonary embolism? *Radiology* 99:541-548, 1970.

287. Salzman GA, Rosa UW: Prolonged survival in pulmonary veno-occlusive disease treated with nifedipine, *Chest* 95:1154-1156, 1989.

288. Sano A, Kuroda Y, Moriyasu F, et al: Portopulmonary venous anastomosis in portal hypertension demonstrated by percutaneous transhepatic cine-portography, *Radiology* 144:479-484, 1982.

289. Sautter RD, Dreher WH, MacIndoe JH, et al: Fatal pulmonary edema and pneumonitis after reexpansion of chronic pneumothorax, *Chest* 60:399-401, 1971.

290. Sautter RD, Fletcher FW, Emanuel DA, et al: Complete resolution of massive pulmonary thromboembolism, *JAMA* 189:948-949, 1964.

291. Sautter RD, Fletcher FW, Ousley JL, et al: Extremely rapid resolution of a pulmonary embolus: report of a case, *Dis Chest* 52:825-827, 1967.

292. Saxon RR, Klein JS, Bar MH, et al: Pathogenesis of pulmonary edema during interleukin-2 therapy: correlation of chest radiographic and clinical findings in 54 patients, *AJR* 156:281-285, 1991.

293. Scharf J, Nahir AM, Munk J, et al: Aseptic cavitation in pulmonary infarction, *Chest* 59:456-458, 1971.

294. Schnur MJ, Winkler B, Austin JHM: Thickening of the posterior wall of the bronchus intermedius, *Radiology* 139:551-559, 1981.

295. Seckl MJ, Rustin GJ, Newlands ES, et al: Pulmonary embolism, pulmonary hypertension, and choriocarcinoma, *Lancet* 338:1313-1315, 1991.

296. Sewell RW, Fewel JG, Grover FL, et al: Experimental evaluation of reexpansion pulmonary edema, *Ann Thorac Surg* 26:126-132, 1978.

297. Shackleford GD, Sacks EJ, Mullins JD, et al: Pulmonary veno-occlusive disease: case report and review of the literature, *AJR* 128:643-648, 1977.

298. Shapiro R, Rigler LE: Pulmonary embolism without infarction, *AJR* 60:460-465, 1948.

299. Shaw TJ, Caterine JM: Recurrent re-expansion pulmonary edema, *Chest* 86:784-786, 1984.

300. Sherman S, Ravikrishnan KP: Unilateral pulmonary edema following reexpansion of pneumothorax of brief duration, *Chest* 77:714, 1980.

301. Sherrier RH, Chiles C, Newman GE: Chronic multiple pulmonary emboli: regional response of the bronchial circulation, *Invest Radiol* 24:437-441, 1989.

302. Shilkin KB, Low LP, Chen BTM: Dissecting aneurysm of the pulmonary artery, *J Pathol* 98:25-29, 1969.

303. Short DS: A radiological study of pulmonary infarction, *Q J Med* 79:233-245, 1951.

304. Simon G: Further observations on the long line shadow across a lower zone of the lung, *Br J Radiol* 43:327-332, 1970.

305. Simon G: The value of radiology in critical mitral stenosis — an amendment, *Clin Radiol* 23:145-146, 1972.

306. Simon M: The pulmonary vessels: their hemodynamic evaluation using routine radiographs, *Radiol Clin North Am* 1:363-376, 1963.

307. Simon RP, Gean-Marton AD, Sander JE: Medullary lesion inducing pulmonary edema: a magnetic resonance imaging study, *Ann Neurol* 30:727-730, 1991.

308. Sinner WN: Computed tomographic patterns of pulmonary thromboembolism and infarction, *J Comput Assist Tomogr* 2:395-399, 1978.

309. Skalina S, Kundel HL, Wolf G, et al: The effect of pulmonary edema on proton nuclear magnetic resonance relaxation times, *Invest Radiol* 19:7-9, 1984.

310. Slutsky RA, Long S, Peck WW, et al: Pulmonary density distribution in experimental noncardiac canine pulmonary edema evaluated by computed transmission tomography, *Invest Radiol* 19:168-173, 1984.

311. Smith JA: Cardiopulmonary manifestations of sickle cell disease in childhood, *Semin Roentgenol* 22:160-167, 1987.

312. Snashall PD, Keyes SJ, Morgan BM, et al: The radiographic detection of acute pulmonary oedema: a comparison of radiographic appearances, densitometry and lung water in dogs, *Br J Radiol* 54:277-288, 1981.

313. Speich R, Jenni R, Opravil M, et al: Primary pulmonary hypertension in HIV infection, *Chest* 100:1268-1271, 1991.

314. Soares FA, Landell GA, de Oliveira JA: Pulmonary tumor embolism to alveolar septal capillaries: an unusual cause of sudden cor pulmonale, *Arch Pathol Lab Med* 116:187-188, 1992.

315. Sostman HD, Gottschalk A: The stripe sign: a new sign for diagnosis of nonembolic defects in pulmonary perfusion scintigraphy, *Radiology* 142:731-741, 1982.

316. Sostman HD, Ravin CE, Sullivan DC, et al: Use of pulmonary angiography for suspected pulmonary embolism: influence of scintigraphic diagnosis, *AJR* 139:673-677, 1982.

317. Spies WG, Burstein SP, Dillchan GL, et al: Ventilation-perfusion scintigraphy in suspected pulmonary embolism: correlation with pulmonary angiography and refinement of criteria for interpretation, *Radiology* 159:383-390, 1986.

318. Sprung CL, Rackow EC, Fein IA, et al: The spectrum of pulmonary edema: differentiation of cardiogenic, intermediate and non-cardiogenic forms of pulmonary edema, *Am Rev Respir Dis* 124:718-722, 1981.

319. Stanley NN, Woodgate DJ: Mottled chest radiograph and gas transfer defect in chronic liver disease, *Thorax* 27:315-323, 1972.

320. Stark P, Jasmine J: CT of pulmonary edema, *Crit Rev Diagn Imag* 29:245-255, 1989.

321. Steckel RJ: Unilateral pulmonary edema after pneumothorax, *N Engl J Med* 289:621-622, 1973.

322. Stein MG, Crues JV, Bradley WG, et al: MR imaging of pulmonary emboli: an experimental study in dogs, *AJR* 147:1133-1137, 1986.

323. Stein PD, Athanasoulis C, Alavi A, et al: Complications and validity of pulmonary angiography in acute pulmonary embolism, *Circulation* 85:462-468, 1992.

324. Stein PD, Gottschalk A, Saltzman HA, Terrin ML: Diagnosis of acute pulmonary embolism in the elderly, *J Am Coll Cardiol* 18:1452-1457, 1991.

325. Stein PD, O'Connor JF, Dalen JE, et al: The angiographic diagnosis of acute pulmonary embolism: evaluation of criteria, *Am Heart J* 73:730-741, 1967.

326. Stein PD, Saltzman HA, Weg JG: Clinical characteristics of patients with acute pulmonary embolism, *Am J Cardiol* 68:1723-1724, 1991.

327. Stern EJ, Graham C, Gamsu G, et al: Pulmonary artery dissection: MR findings, *J Comput Assist Tomogr* 16:481-483, 1992.

328. Stuttle AWJ, Klosok J, Peters AM, Lavender JP: Sequential imaging of postoperative thrombus using the In-111 labelled platelet specific monoclonal antibody P256, *Br J Radiol* 62:963-969, 1989.

329. Sugerman JH: Pulmonary function in morbid obesity, *Gastroenterol Clin North Am* 16:225-237, 1987.

330. Surrette GD, Muir AL, Hogg JC, et al: Roentgenographic study of blood flow redistribution in dogs, *Invest Radiol* 10:109-114, 1975.

331. Symbas P, Scott HW: Traumatic aneurysm of the pulmonary artery, *J Thorac Cardiovasc Surg* 45:645-649, 1963.

332. Szucs MM, Brooks HL, Grossman W, et al: Diagnostic sensitivity of laboratory findings in acute pulmonary embolism, *Ann Intern Med* 74:161-166, 1971.

333. Szucs RA, Rehr RB, Tatum JL: Pulmonary artery thrombus detection by magnetic resonance imaging, *Chest* 95:232-234, 1989.

334. Talbot S, Worthington BS, Roebuck EJ: Radiographic signs of pulmonary embolism and infarction, *Thorax* 28:198-203, 1973.

335. Tate RM, Repine JE: Neutrophils and the adult respiratory distress syndrome, *Am Rev Respir Dis* 128:552-559, 1983.

336. Teplick JG, Haskin ME, Steinberg SB: Changes in the main pulmonary artery segment following pulmonary embolism, *AJR* 92:557-560, 1964.

337. Thadani V, Burrow C, Whitaker W, et al: Pulmonary veno-occlusive disease, *Q J Med* 173:133-159, 1975.

338. Theodore J, Robin ED: Editorial: speculations on neurogenic pulmonary edema (NPE), *Am Rev Respir Dis* 113:405-411, 1976.

339. Thickman D, Kressel HY, Axel L: Demonstration of pulmonary embolism by magnetic resonance imaging, *AJR* 142:921-922, 1984.

340. Tilkian AG, Schroeder JS, Robin ED: Chronic thromboembolic occlusion of main pulmonary artery or primary branches: case report and review of the literature, *Am J Med* 60:563-570, 1976.

341. Torbicki A, Skwarski K, Hawrylkiewicz I, et al: Attempts at measuring pulmonary arterial pressure by means of Doppler echocardiography in patients with chronic lung disease, *Eur Respir J* 2:856-860, 1989.

342. Torrance DJ: Roentgenographic signs of pulmonary artery occlusion, *Am J Med Sci* 237:651-662, 1959.

343. Trapnell DH, Thurston JGB: Unilateral pulmonary oedema after pleural aspiration, *Lancet* 1:1367-1369, 1970.

344. Travis KW, Tordres ID, Shannon DC: Pulmonary edema associated with croup and epiglottitis, *Pediatrics* 59:695-698, 1977.

345. Tsao MS, Schraufnagel D, Wang NS: Pathogenesis of pulmonary infarction, *Am J Med* 72:599-606, 1982.

346. Tudor J, Maurer BJ, Wray R, et al: Lung shadows after acute myocardial infarction, *Clin Radiol* 24:365-369, 1973.

347. Turnbull LW, Ridgway JP, Biernacki W, et al: Assessment of the right ventricle by magnetic resonance imaging in chronic obstructive lung disease, *Thorax* 45:597-601, 1990.

348. Turner AF, Lau FYK, Jacobson G: A method for the estimation of pulmonary venous and arterial pressures from the routine chest roentgenograms, *AJR* 116:97-106, 1972.

349. Urokinases Pulmonary Embolism Trial: A national cooperative study, *Circulation* 47(suppl II):38-45, 1973.

350. Varat MA, Adolph RJ, Fowler NO: Cardiovascular effects of anemia, *Am Heart J* 83:415-426, 1972.

351. Vesconi S, Rossi GP, Pesenti A, et al: Pulmonary microthrombosis in severe adult respiratory distress syndrome, *Crit Care Med* 16:111-113, 1988.

352. Vinitski S, Steiner RM, Wexler HR, Rifkin M: Assessment of lung water by magnetic resonance in three types of pulmonary edema, *Heart Vessels* 4:88-93, 1988.

353. Vix VA: The usefulness of chest radiographs obtained after a demonstrated perfusion scan defect in the diagnosis of pulmonary emboli, *Clin Nucl Med* 8:497-500, 1983.

354. Wagenvoort CA: Pulmonary veno-occlusive disease: entity or syndrome? *Chest* 69:82-86, 1976.

355. Wagenvoort CA, Wagenvoort N: Primary pulmonary hypertension: a pathologic study of the lung vessels in 156 clinically diagnosed cases, *Circulation* 42:1163-1184, 1970.

356. Wagenvoort CA, Wagenvoort N: The pathology of pulmonary veno-occlusive disease, *Virchows Arch [Pathol Anat]* 364:69-79, 1974.

357. Waqaruddin M, Bernstein A: Re-expansion pulmonary oedema, *Thorax* 30:54-60, 1975.

358. Ward BJ, Pearse DB: Reperfusion pulmonary edema after thrombolytic therapy of massive pulmonary embolism [published erratum appears in *Am Rev Respir Dis* 139(2):572, 1989], *Am Rev Respir Dis* 138:1308-1311, 1988.

359. Wegenius G, Erikson U, Borg T, et al: Value of chest radiography in adult respiratory distress syndrome, *Acta Radiol* 25:177-184, 1984.

360. Weibel ER: Early stages in the development of collateral circulation to the lung in the rat, *Circ Res* 8:353-376, 1960.

361. Weiner C, McKenna WJ, Myers MJ, et al: Lung ventilation is reduced in patients with cardiomegaly in the supine but not in the prone position, *Am Rev Respir Dis* 141:150-155, 1990.

362. Wenger NK, Stein PD, Willis PW: Massive acute pulmonary embolism: the deceivingly nonspecific manifestations, *JAMA* 220:843-844, 1972.

363. West JB. Uptake and delivery of the respiratory gases. In West JB, ed: *Physiological basis of medical practice*, Baltimore, 1985, Williams & Wilkins, pp 546-571.

364. West JB, Dollery CT, Heard BE: Increased pulmonary vascular resistance in the dependent zone of isolated dog lung caused by perivascular edema, *Circ Res* 17:191-206, 1965.

365. Westcott JL, Cole S: Plate atelectasis, *Radiology* 155:1-9, 1985.

366. Westermark N: On the roentgen diagnosis of lung embolism, *Acta Radiol* 19:357-372, 1938.

367. White PG, Hayward MWJ, Cooper T: Ventilation agents — what agents are currently used? *Nucl Med Commun* 12:349-352, 1991.

368. White RD, Winkles ML, Higgins CB: MR imaging of pulmonary arterial hypertension and pulmonary emboli, *AJR* 149:15-21, 1987.

369. Whyte MKB, Peters AM, Hughes JMB, et al: Quantification of right to left shunt at rest and on exercise in patients with pulmonary arteriovenous malformations, *Thorax* 47:790-796, 1992.

370. Wielopolski PA, Haacke EM, Adler LP: Three dimensional MR imaging of the pulmonary vasculature: preliminary experience, *Radiology* 183:465-472, 1992.

371. Wiener SN, Edelstein J, Charms B: Observations on pulmonary embolism and the pulmonary angiogram, *AJR* 98:859-873, 1966.

372. Wilson AG, Harris CN, Lavender JP, et al: Perfusion lung scanning in obliterative pulmonary hypertension, *Br Heart J* 35:917-930, 1973.

373. Wilson AG, Joseph AEA, Butland RJA: The radiology of aseptic cavitation in pulmonary infarction, *Clin Radiol* 37:327-333, 1986.

374. Winterbauer RH, Elfenbein IB, Ball WC: Incidence and clinical significance of tumor embolisation to the lungs, *Am J Med* 45:271-290, 1968.

375. Woesner ME, Sanders I, White GW: The melting sign in resolving transient pulmonary infarction, *AJR* 111:782-790, 1971.

376. Wolfe JD, Taskkin DP, Holly FE, et al: Hypoxemia of cirrhosis: detection of abnormal pulmonary vascular channels by a quantitative radionuclide method, *Am J Med* 63:746-754, 1977.

377. Wolfe WG, Sabiston DC: *Pulmonary embolism*, Philadelphia, 1980, WB Saunders.

378. Woodring JH: Pulmonary artery-bronchus ratios in patients with normal lungs pulmonary vascular plethora, and congestive heart failure, *Radiology* 179:115-122, 1991.

379. Woodruff WW, Hoeck BE, Chitwood WR, et al: Radiographic findings in pulmonary hypertension from unresolved embolism, *AJR* 144:681-686, 1985.

380. Yamato M, Lecky JW, Hiramatsu K, et al: Takayasu arteritis: radiographic and angiographic findings in 59 patients, *Radiology* 161:329-334, 1986.

381. Youngberg AS: Unilateral diffuse lung opacity, *Radiology* 123:277-281, 1977.

382. Yuceoglu YZ, Rubler S, Eshwar K, et al: Pulmonary edema associated with pulmonary embolism: a clinicopathological study, *Angiology* 22:501-510, 1971.

383. Zimmerman JE, Goodman LR, St Andre AC, et al: Radiographic detection of mobilizable lung water: the gravitational shift test, *AJR* 138:59-64, 1982.

384. Ziskind MM, Weill H, George RA: Acute pulmonary edema following the treatment of spontaneous pneumothorax with excess negative intrapleural pressure, *Am Rev Respir Dis* 92:632-636, 1965.

385. Zwillich CW, Sutton FO, Pierson DJ, et al: Decreased hypoxic ventilatory drive in the obesity-ventilation syndrome, *Am J Med* 59:343-348, 1975.

10 Inhalational Lung Diseases

PAUL DEE
PETER ARMSTRONG

PNEUMOCONIOSIS

The term "pneumoconiosis" means dusty lungs. Nowadays it is used to describe the nonneoplastic reactions of the lungs to inhaled dust particles. By definition the term pneumoconiosis excludes asthma, bronchitis, and emphysema,[123] all of which may in some instances be due to dust inhalation. Although some authors include organic as well as mineral dust,[123] many limit the term to inorganic dust, notably coal, silica, and asbestos.

The character and severity of the reaction of lung tissue are determined by three basic factors[123]: (1) the nature and properties of the inhaled dust, particularly the size of the particles and the degree to which the dust is fibrogenic; (2) the amount of dust retained in the lungs and the duration of exposure to it; and (3) individual idiosyncrasy and immunologic reactivity of the subject.[22,87] Individuals with positive circulating rheumatoid factor show a response different from that normally encountered.

The pneumoconioses are best classified according to the mineral dust responsible. This classification is not always easy because the industrial exposure may involve more than one dust known to be fibrogenic. Silica is so plentiful in the rocks of the earth's crust that some exposure to silica is inevitable in many forms of mining.

The pneumoconioses are therefore classified according to the predominant dust responsible. Thus coal worker's pneumoconiosis should not be referred to as silicosis even though silica may in some circumstances be partly responsible for the reaction of the lungs.

Radiographic classification of the pneumoconioses

The need for standard interpretations of plain chest radiographs of subjects with pneumoconiosis led to the development of the International Labor Office/University of Cincinnati (ILO/UIC) international classification. The ILO/UIC classification, which is now the standard internationally recognized descriptive system, has been modified periodically, most recently in 1980.[29,85] It is accompanied by a set of standard radiographs because the primary aim is to encourage reproducible radiographic interpretation. The system does not take clinical features into account.

The ILO/UIC classification is complex. Put simply, the opacities caused by dust inhalation are divided into two major groups: multiple small opacities up to 1 cm in diameter and opacities larger than 1 cm in diameter. The multiple small opacities are subdivided into categories 1, 2, and 3 according to the profusion of small opacities in the lungs. Films in which the number of opacities is too small to justify inclusion in category 1 are relegated to category zero.

Category 1. Small opacities definitely seen but few in number.

Category 2. Numerous small opacities with normal lung vasculature still visible.

Category 3. Very numerous opacities where the lung vasculature is partly or totally obscured.

A system with 12 categories has been introduced to try and overcome the difficulty of deciding among categories 1, 2, and 3. It uses two numbers. The first number is the category finally chosen, and the second is the alternate category considered; for example, 1/2 would indicate that category 2 was considered but that the final choice was category 1.

The opacities in categories 1, 2, and 3 are further subdivided according to whether they are round or irregular in shape. Those that are round are classified according to size as p, q, or r (p, up to about 1.5 mm in diameter; q, about 1.5 to 3 mm in diameter; r, about 3 to 10 mm in diameter). Those classified as irregular cannot be meaningfully measured, so they are designated as fine, medium, or coarse, using the letters s, t, and u, respectively. As might be expected, the interobserver variability in categorizing small opacities is great. In one study it occurred in two thirds of the cases.[8]

Opacities larger than 1 cm in diameter are categorized as A, B, or C according to the size of the opacity. (A, one or more opacities whose combined diameter is 1 to 5 cm; B, one or more opacities whose combined diameters are greater than 5 cm but whose combined area does not exceed the equivalent of the right upper zone; C, one or more opacities whose combined area is larger than the equivalent of the right upper zone [that is, greater than B].) When opacities of different categories are present on a single film, one category is usually predominant, and this is the one quoted.

Additional descriptors are given for pleural thickening and calcification, as well as for lack of definition of the diaphragm and cardiac outline.

It is important to realize that the ILO/UIC classification is a method of describing chest radiographs. Small opacities, particularly those in category 1, are seen in diseases other than the pneumoconioses and even on a proportion of routine radiographs in patients with no dust exposure.

Silicosis

Free silica (silicon dioxide) is present in many rocks in the earth's crust. It occurs in amorphous and crystalline forms, with quartz the most important crystal. The entity "silicosis" refers to lung disease caused primarily by free silica; the term should not be used for coal worker's pneumoconiosis or other pneumoconioses, even if free silica plays some part in the pathogenesis.[123]

The incidence of silicosis has fallen since its peak during World War II. Exposed individuals usually work in quarries, drill or tunnel quartz-containing rocks, cut or polish masonry, clean boilers or castings in iron and steel foundries (fettlers), or are exposed to sandblasting. The usual chronic form of the disease requires 20 years or more exposure to high dust concentrations before radiographic abnormality is visible.[189] With very high concentrations of dust, radiographic changes may be visible in 4 to 8 years.[158,189] Acute silicosis is a somewhat different entity that occurs with severe exposure, particularly in enclosed spaces (see later discussion).

Dust particles of appropriately small size are deposited on the alveolar walls and ingested by macrophages. They may enter the pulmonary lymphatics, or they may be transported to bronchioles by the mucociliary escalator. The macrophages die and produce fibrosis by releasing their contents, including the particulate silica. The precise mechanism of fibrogenesis is debatable, as is the role of autoimmunity.[123,189]

The basic lesion of silicosis is the hyalinized nodule.[97] The silica particles, nearly all of which are 1 to 2 μm in diameter, are found fixed within the silicotic nodules. These nodules are usually more prominent in the upper zones and lie close to the bronchioles, small vessels, and lymphatics. They consist of concentric layers of collagen containing silica particles surrounded by a fibrous capsule. The outer zone is made up of irregularly dispersed connective tissue that also contains crystalline silica. Silica in this peripheral zone sets up further reaction, resulting in enlargement of nodules and creation of new nodules. The fibrosis seen with silicosis is both more abundant and more collagenous than that seen with other mineral dusts, such as coal. The airways are not usually involved, provided that most of the nodules are smaller than 5 mm.[188] Silica-laden macrophages that reach the hilar and mediastinal nodes form granuloma-like lesions in the nodes.

Silicosis is often complicated by massive fibrotic lesions that are the result of the conglomeration of nodules matted together by fibrosis. These masses, which contain obliterated blood vessels and bronchi, may cavitate. Tuberculous infection coexists in some cases.

RADIOGRAPHIC APPEARANCE.[16,127] Between 10 and 20 years' exposure is usually necessary before the chest radiograph becomes abnormal.[189] Early in the course of the disease 1 to 3 mm nodules are seen, especially in the posterior portions of the upper two thirds of the lungs (Figure 10-1). A reticular pattern may also be seen, either alone or in combination with the nodules. As the process advances, the nodules increase in size and number and become more widespread, involving all zones. Usually the nodulation is symmetric. Sometimes the nodules are calcified.[51]

Progressive massive fibrosis is defined as nodules greater than 1 cm in diameter. These masses, which are identical to those seen with coal worker's pneumoconiosis, develop when the silicotic nodules coalesce. As the nodules coalesce, contraction of the upper lobes is observed and bullae are seen in the vicinity of the conglomerate masses. Emphysematous changes are also seen in the lower lobes.[189]

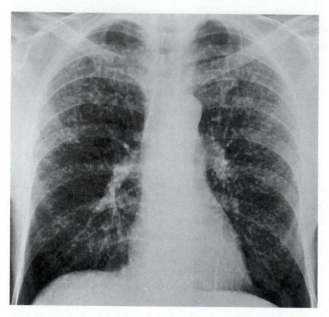

FIGURE 10-1
Silicosis. There is widespread 2 to 3 mm nodulation in lungs, with middle and upper zone predominance.

The conglomerate nodules may have sharp margins but more often are irregular in shape, with strands of density extending into the surrounding lung. They usually appear in the periphery of the lungs and either remain there or slowly migrate toward the hila,[64] leaving emphysematous lung between the fibrotic mass and the chest wall.[127] Cavitation may be visible, and the cavities may empty and fill over a period of time.[64] Pleural thickening is frequently seen in association with progressive massive fibrosis.

Hilar and mediastinal lymph node enlargement is not uncommon. Calcification, sometimes of the eggshell type, may be seen in the nodes (Figure 10-2).[88]

ACUTE SILICOPROTEINOSIS. Intense exposure to silica dust may result in lung damage after only weeks or months, so-called acute silicosis. In these cases, usually in sandblasters, there is a marked cellular and exudative alveolar reaction[169] and death may ensue within 2 to 3 years. The dominant feature is the presence of an alveolar proteinaceous exudate, hence the term "acute silicoproteinosis."[21]

On radiographic examination there is widespread alveolar shadowing that progresses rapidly over a period of months.[38] There is reasonable side-to-side symmetry, but a tendency to central and upper zone predominance is frequent (Figure 10-3). Air bronchograms may be noted,

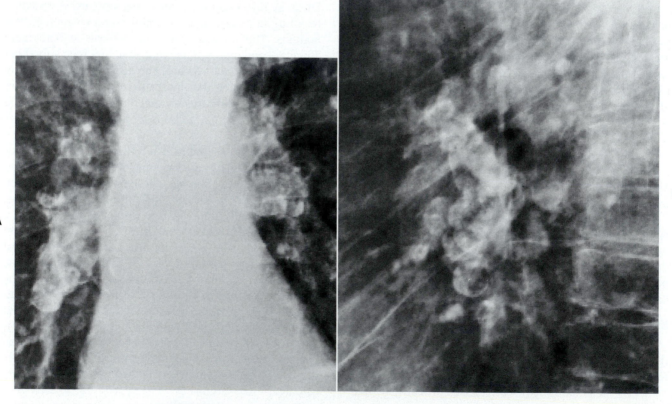

FIGURE 10-2
Eggshell calcification in silicosis. **A,** Anteroposterior view. **B,** Lateral view.

and contraction of the lungs may be minimal at first, suggesting consolidation of the lungs. Hilar and mediastinal adenopathy may be seen, but the hila are often obscured by the parenchymal shadows. Peripheral air trapping, bulla formation, lung volume loss, and distortion of mediastinal structures all indicate increasing fibrosis. Pneumothorax may occur.

Coal worker's pneumoconiosis

The factors governing the degree of lung damage caused by inhaling coal dust are not fully understood. Probably the most important factor is the amount of dust of suitable particle size that is inhaled.[82,123] What is less certain is the importance of the silica content of the dust. That coal dust alone could cause classic progressive massive fibrosis (PMF) was shown many years ago in coal trimmers who, because they worked in the hulls of ships, were exposed only to coal dust containing virtually no free silica. At postmortem examination their disease was found to be due to coal dust alone.[60] Later epidemiologic studies showed that the radiographic changes in miners are closely related to coal dust exposure[136] but poorly related to the silica content of the coal. It is generally agreed that silica plays little part in simple pneumoconiosis,[83,112] although some dispute this.[87,157] Hence the role of silica in the production of PMF remains uncertain.[112,123] Suffice it to say that there is reasonable evidence that silica plays a part in the development of PMF in some cases[115,116,126] and that PMF can develop in miners exposed to coal dust with negligible quantities of silica.[117]

PATHOLOGY.[37,112] With excessive dust load of appropriate size, clearance by the mucociliary escalator is overwhelmed and dust-laden macrophages aggregate in the respiratory bronchioles and alveoli. After a time fibroblasts lay down reticulin. The aggregation of dust and fibroblasts leads to the basic lesion of simple pneumoconiosis — the coal macule. If silica is released, collagenous fibrosis is stimulated. The coal macule develops around bronchioles, weakening the bronchiolar wall and leading to a form of centrilobular emphysema known as proximal acinar or focal emphysema,[74,148] a form of emphysema believed to be clinically unimportant.[112] The extent to which clinically important panacinar emphysema is caused by coal dust is debated.[26,103,106,123,148]

Despite the similarity of their radiographic appearances, coal worker's pneumoconiosis (CWP) and silicosis are different pathologically. The coal macule does not have a hyaline center, nor does it show the laminated collagen typical of the silicotic nodule.

The massive nodules (defined as those with a diameter greater than 1 cm) in CWP are ill-defined, amorphous, inhomogeneous collections of proteinaceous material, mineral dust, and calcium phosphates. The mass lesions may cavitate with or without infection.

The pathogenesis of PMF in coal workers is poorly understood. PMF is related to the severity of dust exposure, and it has recently been postulated that the fibrosis occurs in response to dust-laden macrophages that have ruptured from the mediastinal lymph nodes into the bronchi or pulmonary vessels.[153]

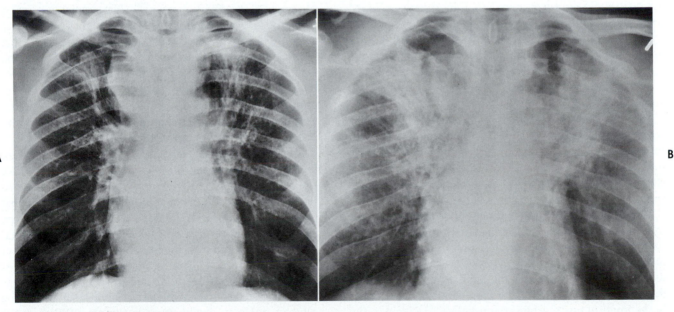

A   B

FIGURE 10-3
Acute silicoproteinosis in a young man employed for 2 years as a sandblaster. **A,** Mediastinal adenopathy and upper zone shadowing after 2 years of exposure. **B,** One year later there is dense consolidation of upper zones with air bronchograms. Death ensued shortly thereafter.

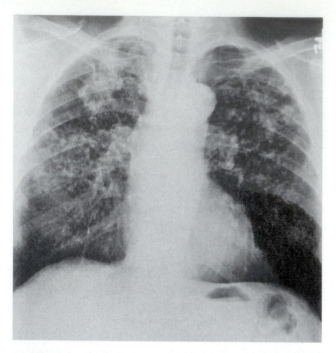

FIGURE 10-4
Coal worker's pneumoconiosis. Typical example showing widespread middle and upper zone small nodules with category A progressive massive fibrosis (PMF). PMF shadows are larger on right than on left.

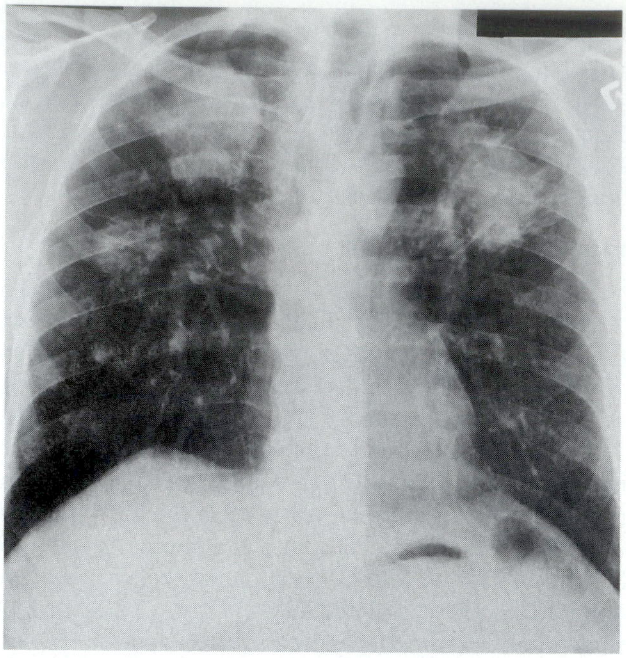

FIGURE 10-5
Category B progressive massive fibrosis in a coal miner in whom background lung nodulation is minimal.

CWP in patients with rheumatoid arthritis (Caplan's syndrome) is considered in Chapter 12.

CLINICAL FEATURES. It has been stated that simple CWP is symptom free.[112,123] It should be remembered, however, that bronchitis and emphysema, features that are so frequently encountered in miners, are excluded from the definition of pneumoconiosis. The extent to which these two processes are due to coal dust exposure or other factors such as smoking is a contentious issue. The interested reader is referred to the reviews by Parkes,[123] Morgan and Lapp,[112] and Oxman and associates.[122]

PMF category A appears not to cause symptoms or signs. PMF categories B and C may be associated with respiratory disability and deterioration in ventilatory function tests.[112] Cough and sputum are sometimes seen. Hemoptysis is rare. Jet-black sputum caused by ischemic rupture of PMF into a bronchus is occasionally reported.

RADIOLOGY. The chest radiograph reflects fairly well the extent and severity of the macules and masses found pathologically and is thus a good tool for diagnosing and following the progression of CWP.* The radiographic findings correlate well with the amount of dust to which the worker was exposed[87] and the quantity of dust found in the lungs at postmortem examination.[141] Except in the most obvious cases, those in Categories B and C, the correlation between the chest radiograph and lung func-

tion is poor,[119] probably because the radiograph substantially underdiagnoses the associated emphysema.[116,148] This latter point is important because the degree of functional disability appears to correlate far better with the severity of emphysema than it does with the presence of macules or PMF.[16,73,105,148] The etiologic role of smoking in emphysema is debated. Some studies have shown that coal miners have a degree of emphysema that is excessive even if allowance is made for age and smoking history.[30,146] This applies particularly to patients with progressive massive fibrosis. At lesser degrees of pulmonary involvement, smoking may play a more significant role in the causation of the emphysema and hence the patient's symptoms.[16,94]

The radiographic signs of CWP are similar to, and often indistinguishable from, those described for silicosis. Like silicosis, CWP is divided into simple and complicated forms based on the chest radiograph. Nodules, at first barely visible, appear in the upper two thirds of the lungs. A reticular pattern may also be seen, either in combination with the nodules or in isolation, and septal (Kerley) lines may be seen.[176] The significance of the reticular or linear shadows has been debated over the years.[7] It has been suggested that the irregular opacities (s, t, u) may be a better guide to disablement in simple CWP than the purely rounded opacities because they correlate better with the extent of emphysema.[105]

PMF is uncommon in coal workers with less than 20 years' experience in and around the mines.[185] Typically

---

*References 25, 56, 61, 64, 72, 73, 127, 136, 145.

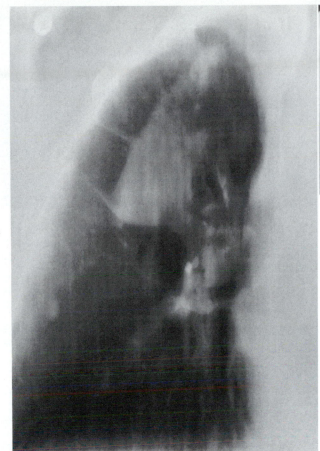

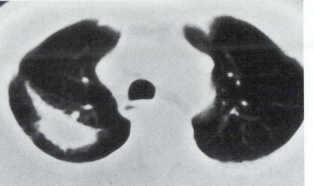

FIGURE 10-6
Progressive massive fibrosis. **A,** Tomogram shows the well-defined outer margin paralleling chest wall. **B,** Computed tomographic scan in a different patient shows characteristic shape, with outer margin parallel to chest wall and axis of density parallel to major fissure.

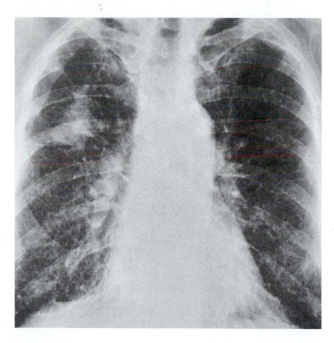

FIGURE 10-7
Unilateral progressive massive fibrosis in a West Virginia coal miner.

(Figure 10-4), PMF starts as a mass near the periphery of the lung. The shape varies. It may be round or oval with lobular or irregular edges (Figure 10-5). There is often a well-defined lateral border that parallels the lateral chest wall (Figure 10-6, *A*). In contrast the medial border is frequently ill defined. The depth of the mass may be significantly less than the side-to-side diameter; in other words, it may show a lens-shaped opacity, a feature that is best appreciated in a lateral or oblique view or at CT (Figure 10-6, *B*). Since PMF is frequently bilateral and accompanied by widespread nodulation in the remainder of the lungs (Figure 10-4), the diagnosis is rarely in doubt. There are cases, however, where the mass is completely or predominantly unilateral (Figure 10-7) and background nodulation may not exist or may be difficult to appreciate. In such cases the differential diagnosis from lung carcinoma becomes particularly important. In a patient with a long history of coal dust exposure, a lens-shaped density is virtually diagnostic of PMF if it is peripherally situated in an upper lobe close to and parallel to the major fissure and has a well-defined outer margin paralleling the chest wall.[185] Another important feature that distinguishes PMF from bronchial carcinoma is small irregular calcifications that may be seen within PMF; sometimes the mass has a calcified rim (Figure 10-8). PMF masses may cavitate (Figure 10-9).

PMF masses, as the name implies, enlarge with time. The rate of growth is, however, very slow, an observable increase in diameter taking years, not months, as is the case with carcinoma. In some cases PMF lesions migrate medially toward the hilum (Figure 10-10). The migration is slow, taking 10 or more years to reach the hilum. Severe emphysema accompanies such migration (Figure 10-11).

Computed tomography in the evaluation of silicosis and coal worker's pneumoconiosis

Computed tomography (CT), particularly high-resolution CT (HRCT), has added another dimension to the

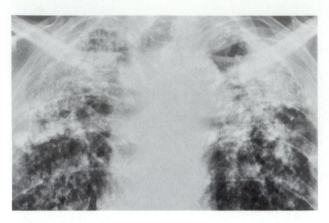

FIGURE 10-8
Extensive punctate calcification in coal worker's pneumoconiosis with progressive massive fibrosis.

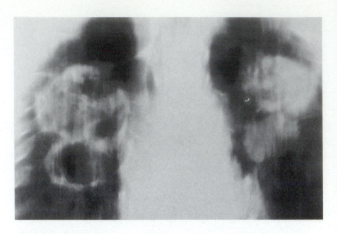

FIGURE 10-9
Cavitation in progressive massive fibrosis. Tomogram shows bilateral masses with thick-walled irregular cavitation, worse on right than on left.

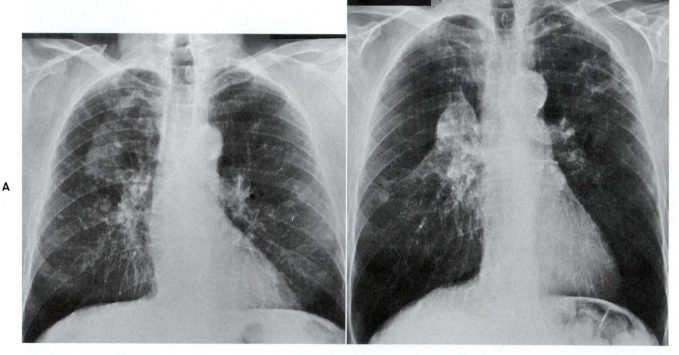

FIGURE 10-10
Coal worker's pneumoconiosis showing medial migration of progressive massive fibrosis. Film in **A** was obtained 7 years before **B**.

evaluation of diffuse interstitial lung disease. HRCT performed with optimal technique is capable of resolving structures as small as 200 μm in diameter.[114] Studies in a range of diffuse infiltrative lung diseases have clearly demonstrated that HRCT frequently detects disease in patients with normal chest radiographs,* whereas the converse does not appear to be true. On the other hand,

*References 2, 3, 69, 121, 134, 166.

HRCT may be normal in the presence of pathologically proven infiltrative lung disease.[121] This has long been recognized to occur with plain chest radiographs[47,55] but to a far greater extent than with HRCT. HRCT using thin sections and special reconstruction algorithms is demonstrably better than conventional CT in detecting and diagnosing diffuse infiltrative lung disease.[134] A common practice is to survey the chest with contiguous thick section CT scans supplemented by a series of five or six

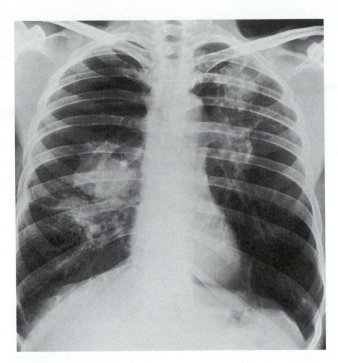

FIGURE 10-11
Coal worker's pneumoconiosis with progressive massive fibrosis (PMF). There has been substantial medial migration of the right PMF shadow. Note the punctate calcification in the left-sided masses and also accompanying severe emphysema.

appropriately spaced HRCT scans. HRCT not only allows more sensitive detection of diffuse infiltrative lung disease but also is more accurate in the diagnosis of specific pathologic entities.[121,170] The use of HRCT is more fully covered in Chapter 5.

The ILO classification of the radiographic patterns in the pneumoconioses cannot be readily transposed to HRCT. A more suitable standard is that devised by the College of American Pathologists,[140] in which nodules up to 7 mm in diameter are termed micronodules, lesions between 7 and 20 mm are classified as nodules, and lesions greater than 20 mm are regarded as progressive massive fibrosis. The CT findings in silicosis and CWP are indistinguishable. The findings on standard CT and HRCT are as follows:

1. Centrilobular micronodules (Figure 10-12, *A* and *C*). Although the interlobular septa are not visualized in early pneumoconiosis, micronodules in a centrilobular location are the earliest feature of silicosis and CWP. In silicosis the micronodules correspond to the periadventitial silicotic nodules, and in CWP they correspond to the coal macule.[3,15,133] The lesions show a distinct tendency to involve the upper lung zones and the posterior aspects of the lungs. As the disease process evolves, there is spread anteriorly and inferiorly, although the upper zone preponderance is usually maintained. The reason for the upper zone preponderance is uncertain.[66]

2. Subpleural micronodules and subpleural plaque formation (Figure 10-12, *A* and *C*). Small nodules may be visualized on the pleural margin of the lung, particularly posteriorly and laterally. Confluence of these nodules may lead to linear narrow subpleural densities or plaques. Subpleural micronodules are in no way specific for pneumoconiosis and may be found in normal persons, particularly smokers.[132] Such micronodules may also be found in sarcoidosis and lymphangitic spread of cancer.

3. Nodules. Growth of the micronodules to exceed 7 mm in diameter occurs in the evolution of silicosis and CWP. The nodules are set on a background of centrilobular and subpleural micronodulation, and there are likely to be subpleural plaques. Calcification may occur within the nodules.

4. Emphysema. Emphysema appears to be common in association with silicosis and CWP. The deterioration of pulmonary function in patients with silicosis and CWP correlates with the severity of the associated emphysema and not with the profusion of nodules.[16] The emphysema may be centrilobular, panacinar, or bullous. Bullous emphysema occurs particularly in association with progressive massive fibrosis. The subject of emphysema is covered more fully in Chapter 17.

5. Progressive massive fibrosis (Figure 10-12, *B*). Growth and coalescence of nodules result in progressive massive fibrosis. PMF usually develops in the periphery of the upper and posterior lung zones and shows a distinct tendency to central contraction toward the hilar regions with further growth of the nodules. A peripheral zone of bullous emphysema frequently develops, although there may also be fibrous bands extending to the pleural surface. PMF may be rounded in contour, but ovoid masses are more usual. The outer margin of PMF often parallels the contour of the adjacent chest wall. Large lesions (5 cm or greater in diameter) often show irregular low-attenuation regions indicative of avascular necrosis, and cavitation may occur. Lesions may also show irregular punctate calcifications. Asymmetry between the lungs may occur in early PMF, with unilateral involvement on occasion. The larger lesions exhibit reasonable side-to-side symmetry.

6. Diffuse interstitial pulmonary fibrosis. Diffuse interstitial pulmonary fibrosis leading to honeycombing may develop in silicosis and CWP. There is no way to distinguish this from fibrosis of nonoccupational origin on the basis of the CT appearance alone.

7. Lymphadenopathy and lymph node calcification. Lymphadenopathy involving the hilar and mediastinal nodes is a regular feature of silicosis and CWP. Necrosis frequently occurs in the nodes, and eggshell calcification is a characteristic finding. Erosion may occur into adjacent bronchovascular structures.[156]

Asbestos-related diseases

Asbestos is composed of a group of fibrous silicates with differing chemical and physical properties but with the notable common property of heat resistance. Chemi-

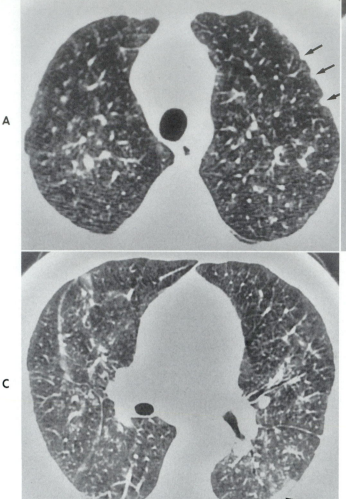

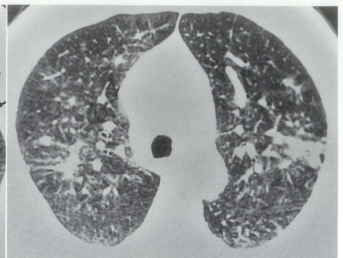

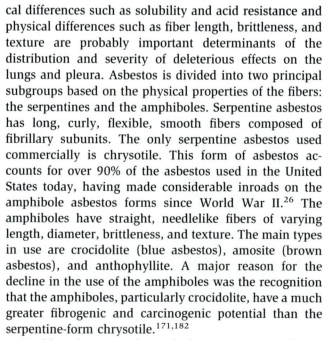

FIGURE 10-12
A, High-resolution computed tomography (HRCT) shows subpleural nodules *(arrows)* and micronodulation. **B,** HRCT shows developing conglomerate shadows of progressive massive fibrosis in the posterior and lateral aspects of the upper lobes. **C,** HRCT shows a plaque of subpleural parenchymal density *(arrow)* as well as micronodulation. (Courtesy Dr. Martin Wastie, Nottingham, U.K.)

cal differences such as solubility and acid resistance and physical differences such as fiber length, brittleness, and texture are probably important determinants of the distribution and severity of deleterious effects on the lungs and pleura. Asbestos is divided into two principal subgroups based on the physical properties of the fibers: the serpentines and the amphiboles. Serpentine asbestos has long, curly, flexible, smooth fibers composed of fibrillary subunits. The only serpentine asbestos used commercially is chrysotile. This form of asbestos accounts for over 90% of the asbestos used in the United States today, having made considerable inroads on the amphibole asbestos forms since World War II.[26] The amphiboles have straight, needlelike fibers of varying length, diameter, brittleness, and texture. The main types in use are crocidolite (blue asbestos), amosite (brown asbestos), and anthophyllite. A major reason for the decline in the use of the amphiboles was the recognition that the amphiboles, particularly crocidolite, have a much greater fibrogenic and carcinogenic potential than the serpentine-form chrysotile.[171,182]

World production and use of asbestos have expanded to an extraordinary degree over the past century. Production expanded from 50 tons per annum in the 1860s to a peak of over 5 million tons per annum in the early 1970s.[7] Asbestos production has now declined somewhat as alternative materials have become available, and at the same time there has been a distinct switch to the white asbestos chrysotile as more information about the health hazards of the various forms of asbestos has become available. Nevertheless, with the long time lags known to exist before the adverse effects of asbestos exposure become manifest, and with the vast tonnages of the material now in place or in use, asbestos is likely to remain one of the major environmental hazards well into the twenty-first century.

BENIGN ASBESTOS PLEURAL EFFUSION. The association of asbestos exposure with benign, possibly recurrent pleural effusions was firmly established only in the last 25 years.[45,46,57] The transient, often asymptomatic nature of these effusions and the lack of specific markers to indicate their cause undoubtedly accounted for the delayed recognition of this condition. Indeed the diagnosis is one of exclusion and should conform to the following criteria: (1) a history of occupational or environmental asbestos exposure; (2) no other cause for the effusion; and (3) no evidence of malignancy within 3 years of detecting of the effusion.

In the noteworthy epidemiologic study of Epler, McLoud, and Gaensler,[46] the overall incidence of benign pleural effusion was 3.1%, with a 7% incidence among individuals having a heavy occupational exposure and a

0.2% incidence in environmentally exposed individuals. Effusions may be unilateral or bilateral and tend to recur. The amount of fluid is usually small; effusions greater than 500 ml are uncommon. The fluid has the characteristics of an exudate and may be blood tinged. Symptoms include pleuritic pain, fever, and an elevated white blood cell count, but many patients have only mild symptoms or no symptoms at all.

Benign pleural effusion is the most common abnormality seen within 10 years of the onset of asbestos exposure. No direct causal relationship between benign effusions and the subsequent development of malignant pleural effusion has been postulated, but in one study of 70 cases of malignant mesothelioma,[39] 5 cases were preceded by what were regarded as successive benign pleural effu-

sions for up to 7 years. A long latent period together with a history of heavy exposure should make the physician less ready to accept a diagnosis of a benign effusion without thorough investigation and extended follow-up. In the series of Cookson and associates,[34] 12 years was the shortest latent period for the development of an effusion related to a malignant pleural mesothelioma. On the other hand, these authors do record a latent period of 22 years in one patient with a benign, asbestos-related effusion.

Benign pleural effusions are associated with the subsequent development of diffuse pleural thickening (Figures 10-13 and 10-14). McLoud and co-workers[108] found that just over 50% of their patients with benign pleural effusions subsequently developed diffuse basal pleural

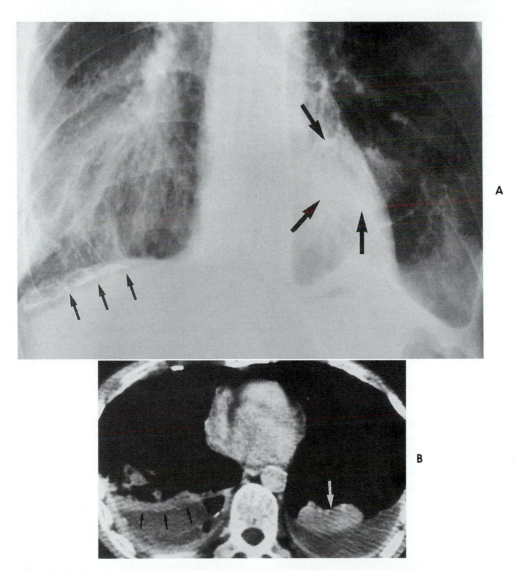

FIGURE 10-13
A, Diffuse basal pleural thickening in an asbestos-exposed individual. Note also pleural calcification *(small arrows)* and left basal rounded atelectasis *(large arrows)*. B, Computed tomographic scan shows bilateral pleural effusions with a rind of pleural thickening on right *(black arrows)*. There is also an area of rounded atelectasis on left *(white arrow)*.

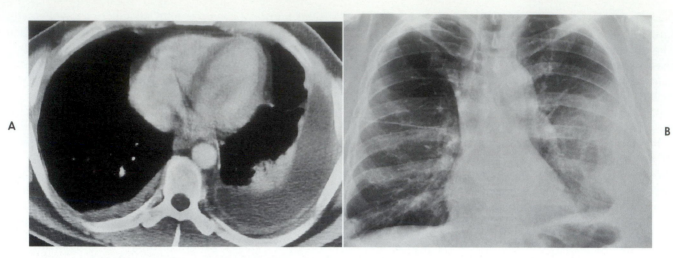

FIGURE 10-14
A, Large benign asbestos-related pleural effusion. B, One year later the patient required a decortication procedure for "trapped" lung.

thickening, an association also emphasized by Cookson and associates.[34] As will be discussed later, there is a possible association between benign pleural effusions and the subsequent development of rounded atelectasis.[86] On rare occasion the degree and extent of the subsequent pleural thickening may be such that the resulting impairment of lung function necessitates a decortication procedure.[56,58,152]

PLEURAL THICKENING AND CALCIFICATION RE-LATED TO ASBESTOS EXPOSURE. Irregular pleural thickening and calcification were first positively related to exposure to asbestos in 1955,[86] and the occurrence of noncalcified asbestos-induced plaques was first reported in 1967.[9] Considerable attention has since been paid to these changes, since they represent the most frequent radiographic manifestation of exposure to asbestos. Although the incidence of pleural plaque formation increases with dose, the elapsed time from initial exposure is a more important factor.[179] Pleural plaques are usually first identified more than 20 or 30 years after the initial asbestos exposure. Asbestos-induced pleural plaques occur on the parietal pleura, especially over the diaphragm and along the posterolateral chest wall. The apices and the costophrenic sulci tend to be spared. The plaques are composed of hyalinized fibrous tissue and frequently lie beneath the ribs. Although often isolated pleural elevations, they may enlarge, spread, and coalesce. Dystrophic calcification within plaques is common and is more frequent as the plaques age and enlarge. Electron microscopy studies have identified asbestos fibers in the plaques on the parietal pleura, indicating that transpleural migration and assimilation of inhaled asbestos fibers must occur.[90] There is evidence that the widely used, more benign form of asbestos, chrysotile, is particularly associated with this transpleural migration, while the more fibrogenic and carcinogenic amphiboles, crocidolite and

amosite, tend to get held up in the lung parenchyma.[159] This may account for the widespread finding of asbestos-related pleural disease unassociated with parenchymal fibrosis or intrathoracic malignancy. Population surveys in industrial regions and in asbestos-mining areas have revealed a surprisingly high incidence of pleural plaques even in individuals who have only a remote connection with asbestos.[5,80,161] The use of asbestos is so widespread that many individuals are exposed unwittingly and unknowingly, and therefore accurate data are difficult to obtain. Hillerdal[75] was not able to find any association with asbestos in some 20% of patients with autopsy-proven plaque formation. One should not discount the possibility of other, as yet unidentified environmental agents as a cause of pleural plaque formation. In an exhaustive study of pleural plaque formation in a rural region of Czechoslovakia, Rous and Studeny[143] were adamant that asbestos could not be implicated in their cases. Pleural plaque formation and calcification have been noted to occur after contact with other nonasbestos fibrous minerals such as erionite in Turkey[13] and sepiolite in Bulgaria.[168]

On radiographic examination, pleural plaques are irregular, smooth elevations of the pleura most easily identified in profile along the margins of the lungs or over the diaphragm (Figure 10-15). Plaques are less easily seen en face unless they are larger. Plaques seen en face are relatively flat in relation to their width, and the density of the shadow projected over the lungs is therefore less than would be expected for a parenchymal lesion of equivalent size. Furthermore, one margin of the lesion is likely to be indistinct as it smooths off into normal pleura. Plaques are multiple, and there is reasonable side-to-side symmetry. Sparing of the costophrenic sulci and the mediastinal contours is characteristic. Calcification is linear when seen in profile (Figure 10-16),

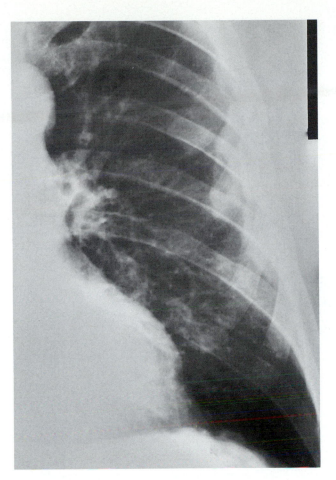

FIGURE 10-15
Typical noncalcified pleural plaques in an asbestos-exposed individual. Note the sparing of the costophrenic sulcus.

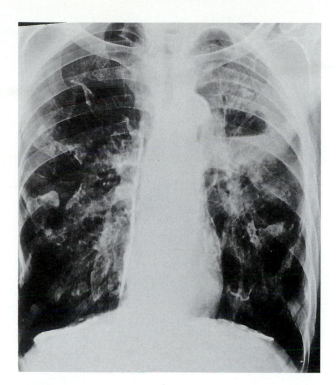

FIGURE 10-16
Linear calcification in pleural plaques over the diaphragm and in the right paravertebral region. There is also calcified plaque formation seen en face, as well as a left upper lobe bronchial carcinoma.

but when it is seen en face, the appearance is variable, the most common type being so-called holly leaf calcification (Figure 10-17). Extensive pleural calcification in association with parenchymal fibrosis may be lacelike (Figure 10-18). Enlargement and spreading of plaques result in thick irregular sheets of pleural thickening, which are often calcified (Figure 10-19). Pleural plaques do occur on the visceral pleura, especially in association with parenchymal fibrosis,[138,181] a position that can be inferred by identifying pleural thickening or calcification in an interlobar fissure (Figure 10-20).

Visualization of pleural plaques is improved by optimal radiographic technique. Oblique views can substantially increase the rate of plaque detection by throwing posterolateral plaques into profile.[12] CT further increases plaque detection rates, by virtue of both the axial nature of the images and greater sensitivity in the detection of calcification (Figure 10-21).[54,99] The differential diagnosis of pleural plaques includes extrapleural fat deposition in obesity,[150] extrapleural thickening in relation to multiple rib fractures, postinflammatory pleural thickening (especially when calcified), pleural metastases, and over-

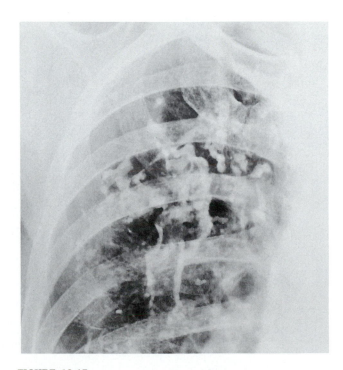

FIGURE 10-17
"Holly leaf" calcification in asbestos-related plaques seen en face.

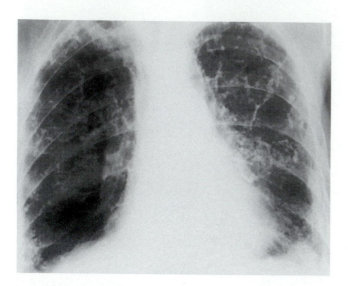

FIGURE 10-18
Lacelike asbestos-related pleural plaque formation seen en face.

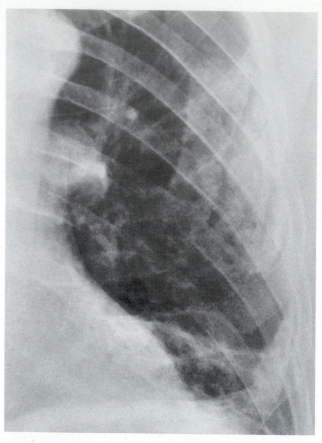

FIGURE 10-19
Extensive calcifications in sheetlike pleural plaque formation.

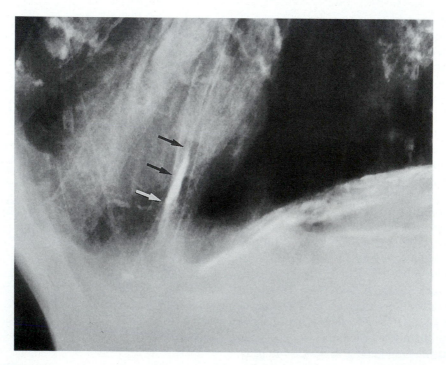

FIGURE 10-20
Calcified plaque formation in a major fissure *(arrows)*. Calcification must be in the visceral pleura.

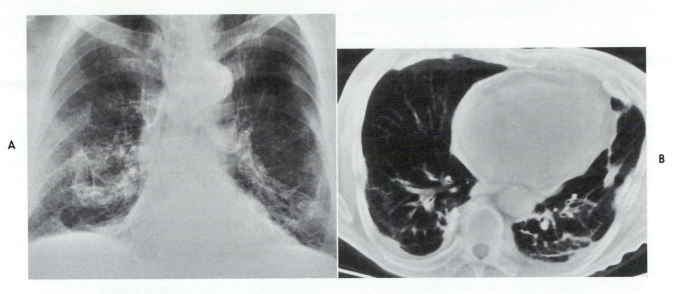

FIGURE 10-21
A, Chest radiograph and, B, computed tomographic scan showing calcified pleural plaques resulting from asbestos exposure. Some coarse linear fibrotic bands are noted in the subjacent lung parenchyma.

projected densities representing unusually prominent costal insertions of the serratus anterior muscle.[32,59]

The most important differential diagnosis is from diffuse pleural thickening related to previous benign asbestos-induced pleural effusions, because diffuse post-effusion thickening is more likely to be associated with parenchymal fibrosis and intrathoracic malignancy. Diffuse pleural thickening involves and obliterates the costophrenic sulci, whereas pleural plaques tend to spare these regions. Extensive sheetlike plaque formation may simulate diffuse posteffusion thickening. McLoud and co-workers[108] found evidence to suggest that diffuse pleural thickening could be attributed to extensive sheet-like plaque formation in approximately one fourth of the cases in which it was found. Patients with diffuse pleural thickening may have some impairment of pulmonary function, and on rare occasion the impairment may be severe enough to warrant decortication of the lung.

The pleural changes associated with asbestos exposure have attracted inordinate interest, possibly because of their epidemiologic implications, but from a purely practical clinical standpoint, isolated asbestos-related pleural changes usually have only minor significance.[155] The changes are rarely confused with more significant disease processes, and indeed in many cases the changes either are overlooked or are below the limits of radiographic visibility. Studies have shown that only 12.5% of asbestos-related pleural changes found at autopsy are identified on plain chest films even by trained observers using the strictest criteria.[79]

Three fundamental questions are related to pleural plaques and associated disease:

1. Does pleural plaque formation in environmentally exposed individuals still raise the possibility of potentially significant fibrosis even in the absence of radiographic evidence of parenchymal disease? Studies of such individuals identified through health surveys indicate that minor lung function abnormalities suggestive of inhomogeneously distributed fibrosis may occur.[28] However, it has not been suggested that these changes progress to become clinically significant. Although patients with asbestos-induced fibrosis frequently have pleural plaques and calcifications, these changes are not invariable. Indeed, in 20% to 25% of such cases pleural changes are conspicuously absent.[53] Two parallel processes, both related to asbestos exposure but of differing clinical and pathologic significance, may therefore be operating.

2. Do pleural plaques ever degenerate into malignant mesotheliomas or, alternatively, are pleural plaques an indicator of an increased risk of mesothelioma? There is no evidence of the former, although certainly evidence supports a small but statistically significant incidence of mesothelioma in individuals with occupational exposure and radiographically detectable pleural plaques.[43,52] On the other hand, pleural plaques are not invariably found in patients with mesotheliomas. An autopsy study by Scully, Mark, and McNeely[154] found pleural plaques in 27 (58%) of 47 mesothelioma cases. It appears that environmentally exposed individuals with pleural plaques and calcification are not at risk for the development of mesothelioma.

3. Is the incidence of bronchogenic carcinoma increased in patients with asbestos-related pleural plaque formation? Again analysis is distorted because two parallel processes may be under comparison. In occupationally exposed individuals, Fletcher[52] found the mortality from

bronchogenic carcinoma in individuals with plaques to be 2.4 times greater than expected, in contrast to a 1.2 times greater incidence in individuals without plaques. However, Kiviluoto, Meurman, and Hakama[96] could find no such association in environmentally exposed individuals. Data from autopsy studies relating the incidence of bronchial carcinoma to coincident pleural plaques are conflicting.[76,155,175] A prospective study with control subjects matched for age, occupational exposure, and smoking habits is lacking. Again, it appears that the environmentally exposed individual with pleural plaques and calcification is not at risk for the development of bronchogenic carcinoma.

BENIGN ASBESTOS-RELATED PARENCHYMAL MASSES. Rounded atelectasis is an unusual form of juxtapleural lung collapse that may simulate a pulmonary neoplasm. A definite association exists between this condition and asbestos exposure, and it has been widely accepted that benign, asbestos-induced effusions are an essential precursor in such cases.[110] However, Hillerdal and Hemmingsson[78] have challenged this concept, and the mechanism of origin of rounded atelectasis must remain conjectural. The condition was first described in patients who had undergone therapeutic pneumothorax for tuberculosis.[137] Other conditions such as pulmonary infarction, Dressler's syndrome, congestive cardiac failure, and nonspecific pleurisy can precede the formation of rounded atelectasis.[167] Alternative designations for rounded atelectasis include folded lung,[18] atelectatic pseudotumor,[100] and pleuroma.[162]

Hanke and Kretzschmar[68] have proposed a sequence of events to account for the development and appearance of rounded atelectasis. First, a pleural effusion causes atelectasis in the underlying lung. An infolding of the visceral pleura isolates an area of atelectasis, which floats in the effusion and is thereby elevated and tilted. The development of fibrous adhesions suspends the rounded atelectatic area in the elevated and tilted position. The pleural effusion resorbs, and the lung reexpands except for the now sequestered, rounded area of atelectasis. Kretzschmar[100] added that organization and contraction of the fibrinous pleural exudate together with fibrous contraction in the surrounding lung parenchyma produce additional distortion. Hillerdal and Hemmingsson[78] suggest that, at least in asbestos-related cases, the condition may result from contraction of diffuse visceral pleural thickening, plus retraction caused by parenchymal fibrosis. These authors point out that rounded atelectasis may arise long after the normal time during which benign asbestos-related pleural effusions occur.

The radiographic findings are characteristic (Figures 10-13 and 10-22). Rounded atelectasis may be a single, masslike lesion, although more than one lesion is frequently seen in a lung.[151] The mass lesion is juxtapleural in position and is most commonly found in one of the lower lobes posteriorly or posteromedially. The upper lobes, particularly the lingula or the middle lobe, may be involved (Figure 10-23).[27,78] Rounded atelectasis forms a rounded or oval mass 2.5 to 5 cm in diameter in contact with the pleural surface. Acute angles are usually visible at the pleural margins and indicate an intraparenchymal location. The mass is usually separated from the diaphragm by interposed lung. The pleura is thickened, particularly in the vicinity of the lesion, and the costo-

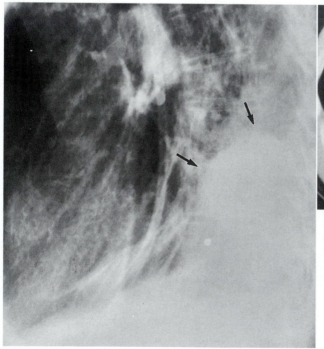

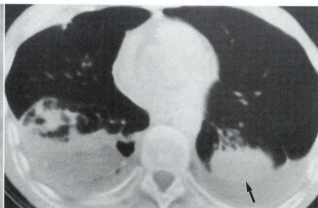

FIGURE 10-22
Rounded atelectasis. A, Lateral chest radiograph shows pleural thickening at the lung bases plus a rounded juxtapleural mass (arrows). B, Computed tomographic scan shows the juxtapleural mass (arrow) with underlying pleural thickening and fluid. Note the characteristic "parachute cord" divergence of the pulmonary vessels as they merge into the rounded atelectasis.

phrenic sulci are usually blunted or obliterated. The pathognomonic feature, however, is the characteristic pattern of distortion of the vessels and bronchi in the vicinity of the lesion. The vessels leading toward the mass are crowded, but as they reach the mass, they tend to diverge and arc around the undersurface of the mass before merging with it. This appearance has been variously described as the "vacuum cleaner effect,"[162] the "comet tail,"[151] and the helical effect. Conventional tomography is an excellent method of demonstrating this vital sign (Figure 10-24), although CT is now more usually employed in the diagnosis of rounded atelectasis.[27,104,107] The most important and highly characteristic finding on CT is a pattern of curving and divergence of the vessels and bronchi as they approach and merge with the atelectatic mass. The appearance simulates the cords of a parachute. This finding is essential for the diagnosis of rounded atelectasis. Rounded atelectasis on the diaphragmatic surface may cause problems because the axis of the "cords" is perpendicular to the plane of the CT scan. Overlying pleural thickening is an invariable feature, but the lesion can be seen to be intraparenchymal because of the acute angles it forms with the pleural surface. The margin directed toward the hilum is usually indistinct, although the other margins are well defined. An air bronchogram may be noted in the lesion. Rounded atelectasis enhances homogeneously after intravenous administration of contrast material. The main differential diagnosis is of course a peripheral bronchogenic carcinoma, and biopsy may indeed be necessary in atypical cases (Figure 10-25). Rounded atelectasis is ordinarily a static or very slowly growing process as can be readily determined by serial radiographs or a follow-up CT scan. The appearance of rounded atelectasis on magnetic resonance imaging has been described.[178] The lesion had a signal intensity similar to liver on T1-weighted images, and blood vessels and bronchi were seen to curve into the mass.

ASBESTOSIS. Asbestosis was first identified with some certainty at the turn of the century.[33] By the mid-1980s an estimated 65,000 persons in the United States had clinically diagnosable asbestosis.[180] The term "asbestosis" is generally reserved for asbestos-induced pulmonary fibrosis and associated visceral pleural fibrosis. Thus the commonly found parietal pleural changes associated with asbestos exposure are excluded, being regarded more as an indication of such exposure than as a significant disease entity. Asbestosis is related to the cumulative dust exposure, whereas the parietal pleural changes are more related to the length of time since the initial exposure.[28] The time interval between the initial exposure and the development of evidence of asbestosis is extremely vari-

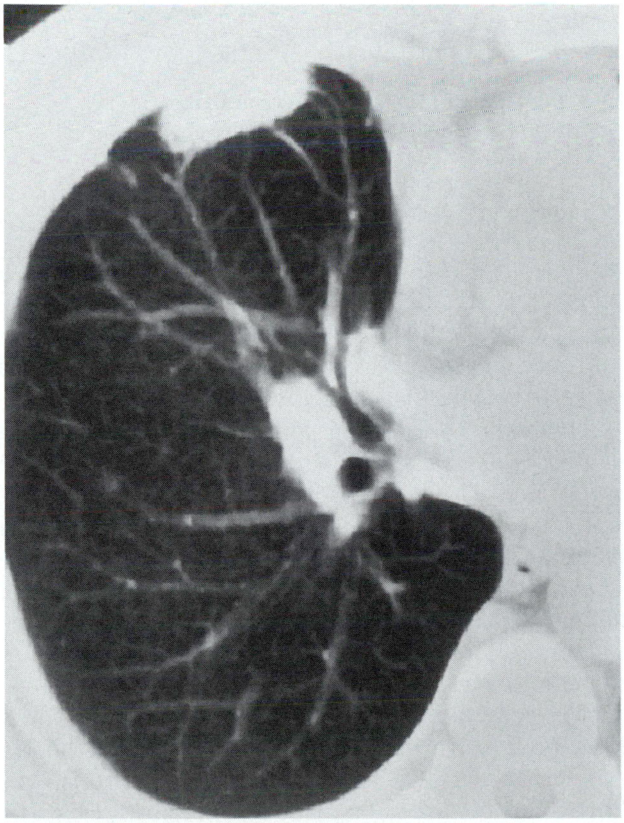

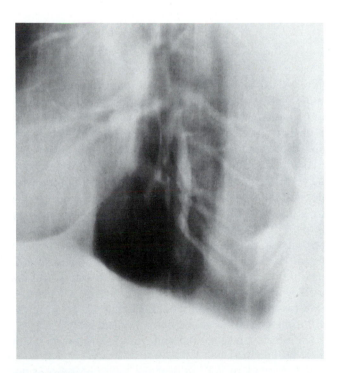

FIGURE 10-23
Rounded atelectasis in the middle lobe of a middle-aged man with a previous asbestos-related pleural effusion.

FIGURE 10-24
Tomogram demonstrates rounded atelectasis at the lung base posteriorly, showing characteristic arching of vessels as they merge into the density.

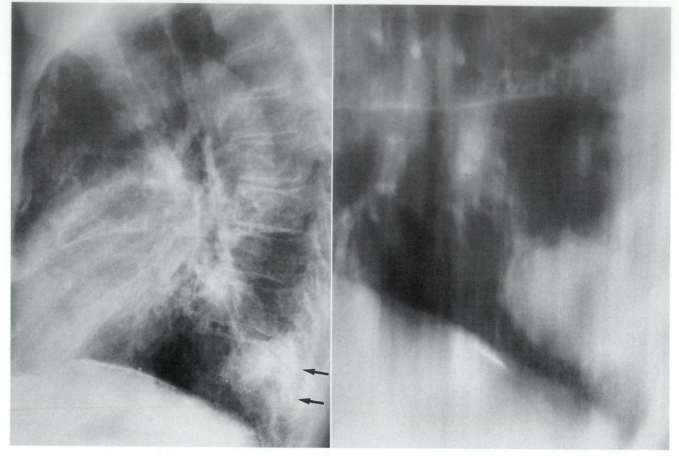

FIGURE 10-25
A, Radiograph of shipyard worker with asbestosis and a posterobasal mass *(arrows)*. Note also pleural calcification and plaque formation. B, Conventional tomogram showing a juxtapleural mass without distortion of the lung vessels. Biopsy proved bronchogenic carcinoma.

able, but 20 to 30 years is usual. Intense exposures can cause asbestosis in as short a period as 3 years, but this is exceptional. The most fibrogenic form of asbestos is crocidolite, and in descending order of fibrogenicity are amosite, anthophyllite, and chrysotile.

Asbestos causes interstitial pulmonary fibrosis, spreading centrifugally from the region of the terminal bronchioles and the alveolar ducts,[36] with histologic features that are indistinguishable from those of idiopathic pulmonary fibrosis. The changes predominate in the subpleural portions of the lungs and at the lung bases. Visceral pleural thickening occurs, particularly over the regions of maximum fibrosis. Mild to moderate fibrosis correlates broadly with increasing cumulative exposure. Established asbestos-induced pulmonary fibrosis tends to progress with time even after cessation of exposure.[65,144]

Asbestosis presents the following features on plain chest radiographs:

1. A ground-glass haze over the lower portions of the lungs may be seen.[163] The early changes at the level of the terminal bronchioles are far below the resolving power of the x-ray beam, but the resultant diffuse thickening can summate, attenuating the x-ray beam in much the same way as a layer of pleural fluid along the posterior chest wall on a supine chest radiograph. This radiographic feature is nonspecific and highly subjective.

2. Interstitial shadowing develops, particularly at the lung bases and in a subpleural location (Figures 10-26 and 10-27). The shadows are a mixture of opacities, pinpoint to 4 mm in diameter. These are interspersed with linear opacities, some of which represent septal lines. The subpleural location of the fibrosis over the diaphragm and the mediastinum tends to obscure these soft tissue contours. Laterally, the fibrotic changes may be seen to extend up the chest wall toward the axillae. The fibrotic changes may become severe, with upper lobe involvement, progressive lung volume loss, and even "honeycombing," indicative of severe end-stage fibrosis. The fibrotic changes are not specific for asbestosis; comparable changes may be seen, for example, in idiopathic pulmonary fibrosis. However, pleural changes suggestive of asbestos exposure are present in all but some 20% of

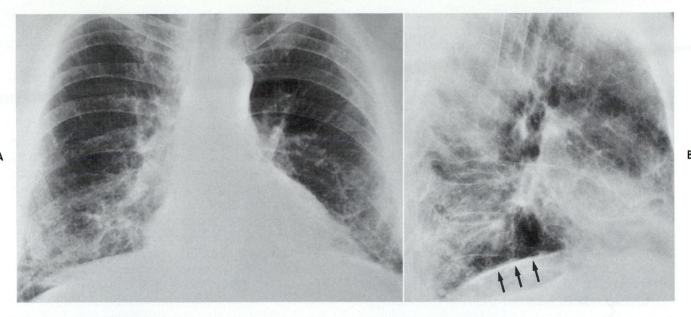

FIGURE 10-26

A, Frontal and, B, lateral radiographs of a shipyard worker with asbestosis showing basally predominant interstitial pulmonary fibrosis. There is widespread pleural calcification.

cases of asbestosis, providing an important clue to the underlying cause (Figures 10-25 and 10-26).

3. Pleural plaques, diffuse pleural thickening, and pleural calcification are to be found in 80% of patients with asbestosis. The radiographic features of these pleural changes are discussed on pp. 436 to 440. Plain radiographs cannot distinguish visceral from parietal pleural thickening and calcification except when these occur in the interlobar fissures (Figure 10-22).

4. Asbestosis may be associated with coarse bands of fibrous tissue extending into the lung from the pleural surface. These bands usually occur in the middle and lower zones of the lungs, and there is usually some associated pleural thickening. On occasion the bands radiate into the lung from a particular point on the pleural surface. The relationship of these fibrous bands to the development of rounded atelectasis is unknown. Conglomerate shadowing or benign fibrous masses akin to progressive massive fibrosis in silicosis have been reported.[63,77] However, such changes may in fact relate to concomitant exposure to silica or talc.[49] The major differential diagnosis of these lung masses is bronchogenic carcinoma, particularly in view of the close association between asbestosis and primary lung malignancies. Caplan's syndrome (multiple rheumatoid necrobiotic nodules associated with occupational exposure to dust) has also been reported.[62,174] This cause of benign pulmonary masses must be uncommon in asbestosis, even if a true association could be proved.

Computed tomography in the evaluation of asbestosis.
The chest radiograph is the mainstay in the evaluation of

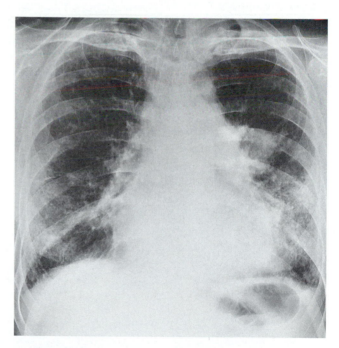

FIGURE 10-27

Asbestosis with a bronchogenic carcinoma in the left lung. Note basally predominant pulmonary fibrosis. There is slight blunting of the costophrenic sulci; otherwise, pleural changes are lacking in this case.

patients with a history of asbestos exposure. CT has some contribution to make in this field, although cost restricts its use for screening. The main indications for the use of CT in established or suspected asbestosis are (1) the identification of pulmonary fibrosis as distinct from emphysema or diffuse pleural disease; (2) the identification of pulmonary fibrosis for compensation purposes when the chest radiographs and pulmonary function tests give conflicting results; and (3) the investigation of suspected pleural or parenchymal masses and guidance for their biopsy.

Pleural plaques are readily detected with CT, particularly HRCT.[1,2,54,91,99] This particularly applies to the posterior and paravertebral regions of the chest, notoriously difficult regions in which to detect plaques by chest radiography. CT is also more sensitive in detecting calcification in plaques than are plain radiographs.[164] The extrapleural fat layers should be studied with care; the plaques indent the subjacent lung, leaving the fat layer intact. Diffuse pleural thickening resulting from previous asbestos-related pleurisy is usually located at one or both bases posteriorly and laterally with obliteration of the costophrenic sulcus. Rounded atelectasis, calcification, pleural plaques in other locations, and subpleural fibrosis are frequent accompaniments of diffuse pleural thickening.

The chest radiograph has been recognized to be insensitive in the detection of early asbestos-related pulmonary fibrosis.[47,56,95,139] Conventional CT has been shown to be more sensitive than chest radiography in the detection of early asbestosis.[91,99,177] HRCT has been found by Aberle and co-workers[2] to be considerably more sensitive than conventional CT in the detection of asbestos-related fibrosis. Staples and associates[166] have shown that HRCT is capable of detecting pulmonary fibrosis in asbestos-exposed workers with normal chest radiographs. Conventional CT and HRCT are, however, complementary methods of imaging in many patients, particularly if the mediastinum and upper abdomen are to be evaluated.

The findings in asbestosis on HRCT are as follows (Figures 10-28 to 10-31):

1. Thickening of the interlobular septa in the peripheral portions of the lung, particularly at the lung bases.[3]

2. Concomitant intralobular line densities representing fibrosis in the peribronchiolar tissues.[4]

3. Subpleural, fine nodulation representing foci of subpleural fibrosis.[4] These nodules often connect with the intralobular line densities, and this represents extension of the peribronchiolar fibrosis to the periphery. Short linear densities extending into the lung perpendicular to the pleural surface result.

4. Curvilinear line density paralleling the chest wall in a subpleural location. First described by Yoshimura and co-workers,[187] this line has since been noted by a number of authors.[3,4,54,166] However, such lines are not specific to asbestosis and occur in other diffuse interstitial lung diseases.[135] They can also occur transiently in normal lungs in the dependent position, clearing rapidly with alteration in position. Al-Jarad and associates[6] and Aberle, Gamsu, and Ray[1] did not find that the presence of curvilinear subpleural lines correlated significantly with asbestosis. When present in asbestosis the lines represent peribronchiolar fibrosis on the margin of a series of subpleural honeycomb spaces.

5. Parenchymal bands. These densities are linear structures up to 5 cm in length, coursing into the lung from the pleural surface. They appear to represent condensations of fibrous tissue along the bronchovascular bundles and interlobular septa.[3] Parenchymal bands are associated with at least moderate pulmonary fibrosis.

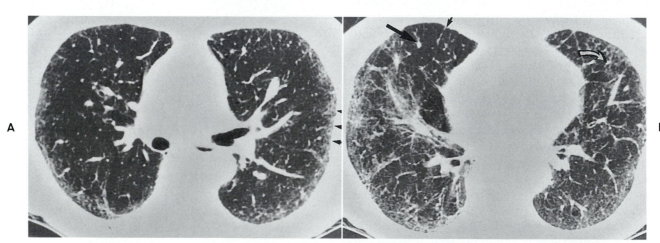

FIGURE 10-28
Asbestosis. **A,** High-resolution computed tomographic (HRCT) scan at midchest level showing circumferential subpleural fibrosis. Arrows show fine subpleural nodulation. **B,** HRCT scan on same patient at the lung base showing more extensive fibrosis but still with maximal involvement of the subpleural zone. Large arrow shows centrilobular vessel. Small arrow shows irregular thickening of the interlobular septum. White arrow shows peribronchiolar fibrosis. (Courtesy Dr. Martin Wastie, Nottingham, U.K.)

6. Honeycombing. Multiple cystlike spaces with thickened walls are a feature of more advanced disease and are not specific to asbestosis. The distribution in the posterior and basal subpleural regions of the lungs in association with pleural plaque formation and calcification, however, is highly suggestive of asbestosis.

7. Ground-glass density. Diffuse, mild alveolar wall fibrosis and edema cannot be resolved by HRCT. Never-theless, the changes may summate to give a ground-glass opacity to involved regions of the lung. This density is a fixed abnormality and is unaffected by positional changes, unlike the dependent density seen so frequently on normal CT scans. Ground-glass opacity, however, is not specific to asbestosis nor even a particularly obvious or frequent finding. Al-Jarad and co-workers[6] found ground-glass opacity to be common in fibrosing alveolitis

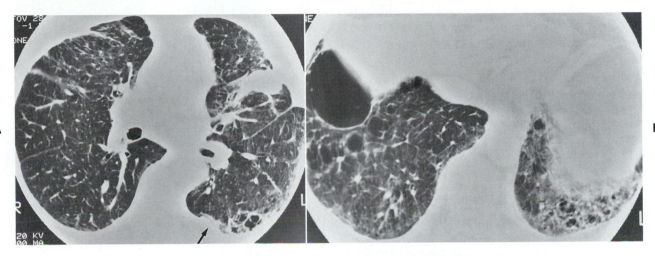

FIGURE 10-29
Asbestosis. **A,** Interstitial pulmonary fibrosis with coarse bands of fibrous tissue extending into the lung from the pleural surface. Pleural plaque is indicated *(arrow)*. **B,** Same patient. Computed tomographic scan at the lung base showing bleb formation and some diffuse parenchymal haze, particularly in left lung. (Courtesy Dr. C. Fuhrman, Pittsburgh.)

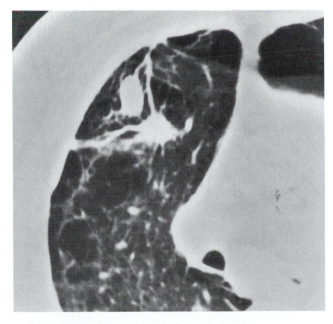

FIGURE 10-30
Pulmonary nodules in a patient with asbestosis. Excisional biopsy revealed squamous cell carcinoma. Note subpleural bleb formation and a subpleural linear density paralleling chest wall. There are also coarse linear fibrotic bands in the vicinity of nodules.

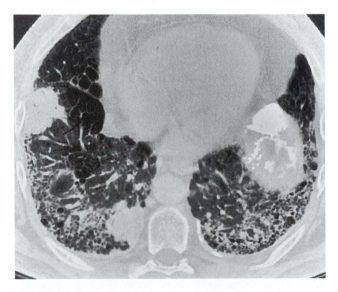

FIGURE 10-31
High-resolution computed tomography in a pipe fitter with asbesto-sis. Two synchronous primary bronchial carcinomas are seen in right lung. Note honeycombing and a large calcified pleural plaque on left diaphragm.

but relatively uncommon in a parallel study of asbestosis.

8. Benign fibrotic masses. These are masses of fibrous tissue in the lung parenchyma usually connected to the pleural surface by parenchymal bands. It is essential to rule out bronchial carcinoma by biopsy or close follow-up.

9. Mediastinal adenopathy. Sampson and Hansell[149] found mediastinal adenopathy to be a frequent finding in patients with uncomplicated asbestosis. The adenopathy was thought to represent a form of reactive hyperplasia. That adenopathy may be directly associated with asbestosis should be borne in mind when such a patient is being evaluated for an intrathoracic malignancy.

In summary, the diagnosis of asbestosis requires consideration of the occupational history or possible environmental exposure, the clinical features (breathlessness, clubbing, lung crackles), the results of pulmonary function tests, and the chest radiographic and CT appearances. The correlation between pulmonary function and radiographic abnormalities is better in asbestosis than in silicosis or CWP.[42] Nevertheless, the chest radiograph may be normal in the face of CT, clinical, or pulmonary function indications of the presence of asbestosis. Pulmonary function tests are more sensitive than chest radiography in detecting early or subclinical asbestosis,[57,125] but they lack specificity. Chest radiography remains an essential tool in grading the severity of asbestosis and is clearly of vital importance in the diagnosis of the benign and malignant complications of this condition.

Talcosis

Talc is a hydrated magnesium silicate that has widespread use as a cosmetic, an industrial lubricant, and a filling agent, for example, in the tire and pharmaceutical industries. Geologically, talc is often associated with asbestos and silica, and this has resulted in problems in determining the extent to which radiographic and pathologic changes can be attributed to talc exposure. Feigin[49] correlated the radiographic and pathologic findings in a series of individuals exposed to talc of varying degrees of purity. Mineralogic analysis of the talc gave an estimate of the extent of contamination by asbestos and silica. Feigin[49] described four categories of disease: talcoasbestosis, talcosilicosis, pure talcosis, and intravenous talcosis. Intravenous talcosis is considered on p. 474. Talcoasbestosis and talcosilicosis show the classic features of exposure to asbestos and silica discussed earlier in this chapter; the changes attributable to talc are completely overshadowed. On radiologic study pure talcosis is seen as a reticulonodular infiltration of the lungs, either diffuse or lower zone predominant. Hilar adenopathy may occur. Pleural thickening and calcification are not features of pure talcosis, contrary to previous description.

Kaolinosis

Kaolin, a hydrated aluminum silicate, causes a pneumoconiosis with features similar to CWP, including a

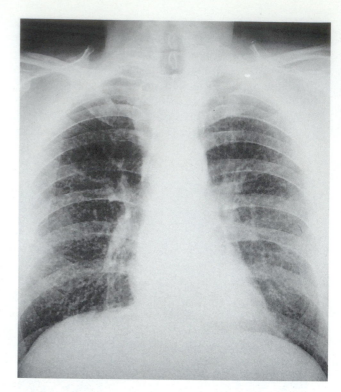

FIGURE 10-32
Uncomplicated kaolinosis in a Cornish china clay worker. (Courtesy Dr. Irving Wells, Plymouth, U.K.)

tendency to develop progressive massive fibrosis and even Caplan's syndrome.[183] The radiographic changes of kaolinosis occur in a minority of exposed workers, and progression of the lesions is slow.[92,120] The most frequent abnormality is a fine nodulation of the lungs with some basal predominance (Figure 10-32). The nodules become larger and more numerous with prolonged exposure, and a reticular element may become apparent. Enlargement and condensation of the nodules into progressive massive fibrosis occur in only a small minority of cases, some 1% in Oldham's estimate (Figure 10-33).[120]

Inert dust pneumoconioses

A number of inorganic dusts are inert and fail to excite any fibrous response when taken up into the lung parenchyma. The dust accumulates in the lung parenchyma and may become radiographically visible, often dramatically so. The most frequently encountered inert dusts are the following:

1. Iron (siderosis). Classically found in electric arc welders, oxyacetylene cutters, and silver polishers (Figure 10-34).

2. Tin (stannosis). The main occupational exposure occurs during the smelting of tin ores (Figure 10-35).

3. Barium (baritosis). This condition is encountered in miners and handlers of the ore baryta.

4. Antimony. Antimony pneumoconiosis is encountered as a result of the mining, milling, and refining of antimony ores (Figure 10-36).

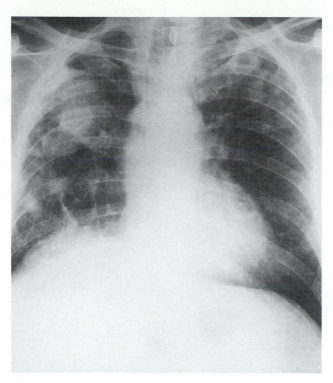

FIGURE 10-33
Kaolinosis with progressive massive fibrosis in a patient from the same region as the patient in Figure 10-31. (Courtesy Dr. Irving Wells, Plymouth, U.K.)

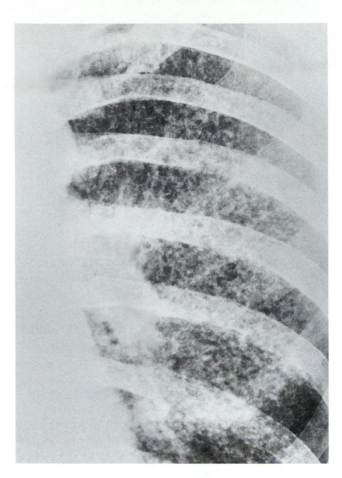

FIGURE 10-34
Siderosis in a hematite miner from Cumberland, England. (Courtesy Dr. Peter Hacking, Newcastle upon Tyne, U.K.)

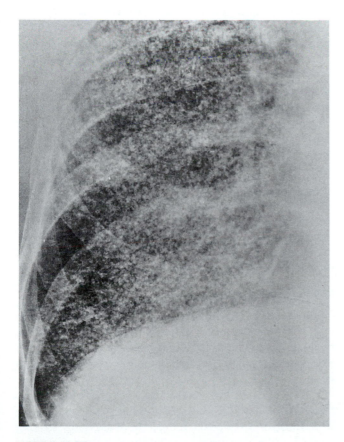

FIGURE 10-35
Stannosis in an apparently healthy middle-aged man.

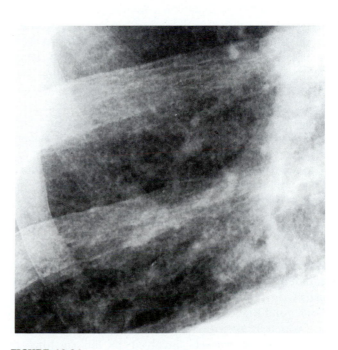

FIGURE 10-36
Detailed view of right lung base in an antimony refiner. Note the fine diffuse increase in the lung markings, representing antimony dust deposition.

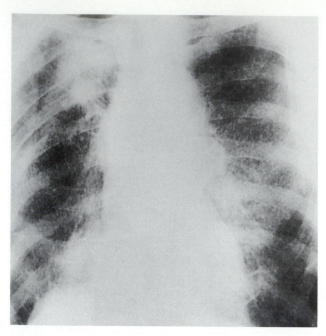

FIGURE 10-37
Siderosilicosis in a hematite miner from Cumberland, England.

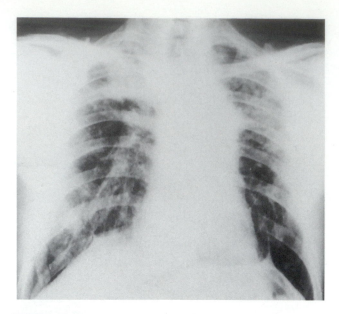

FIGURE 10-38
Aluminosis in a bauxite smelter, showing dense upper zone pulmonary fibrosis.

Pathologic examination shows some dust at the alveolar level, but the major accumulations are seen in aggregations of dust-laden macrophages in the interstitium of the lung and along the lymphatic pathways. Radiographic visibility depends on the atomic number of the dust and the severity of dust accumulation. Relatively small dust accumulations may be visible as a very fine, low-density stippling of the lung parenchyma, which may be vaguely referred to as "dirty looking lungs." Dusts of high atomic number, such as iron, may result in much more remarkable radiographic changes if the dust accumulation is considerable. The pattern tends to be reticulonodular with the nodular element predominating. The changes are most pronounced in the central portion of the lungs, reflecting perhaps the greater amount of interstitial tissue in the perihilar regions. The unusually high radiographic density of the nodules may be more evident if comparison is made with the density of the ribs.

In many industrial circumstances the workers receive a concomitant exposure to silica dust and therefore the changes of silicosis may also be present (Figure 10-37).

Aluminosis

The inhalation of aluminum and its oxides has been associated with the development of pulmonary fibrosis in aluminum workers. Only a few are affected, and these are usually involved with particular processes. For example, Shaver and Riddell[160] described a form of pneumoconiosis, which is basically the prototype of the condition aluminosis, in workers involved in the smelting of aluminum ore (bauxite) to produce corundum. The condition is therefore frequently known as Shaver's disease.

The role of aluminum and aluminum oxides in causing pulmonary disease is difficult to assess because workers are also exposed to silica and mineral oils in dusts and fumes, a complex subject well reviewed by Brooks.[19] Exposure to the fumes may be acute and intense, resulting in acute tracheobronchitis and possibly even pulmonary edema. The pulmonary edema pattern in such individuals usually evolves over subsequent weeks or months into a diffuse reticulonodular pattern, indicating diffuse lung damage with fibrosis. Shaver's patients[160] were subjected to chronic exposure to fumes over periods ranging from 3 to 15 years, and the result was a coarse interstitial pulmonary fibrosis with reduced lung volumes. The upper zones were more severely involved, and honeycombing and bleb formation were frequent findings (Figure 10-38). Pneumothorax was strikingly common. Widening of the mediastinum with distortion of the tracheobronchial structures was common and was presumably related to the fibrosis. Less intense exposures may cause an asthmalike syndrome after single or repeated exposures.

Berylliosis

Awareness of the serious toxic effects of beryllium has restricted its use and brought about improved industrial hygiene. The condition of berylliosis is therefore much less common today, although sporadic cases continue to be reported.[11,35,81,98]

The lesions of berylliosis are characterized by the presence of noncaseating granulomas indistinguishable from those of sarcoidosis. Indeed there are many striking clinical and radiographic similarities between these two conditions.[165] Granulomatous skin lesions, lymphaden-

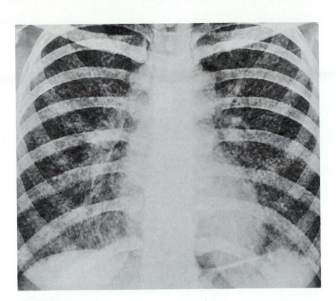

FIGURE 10-39
Chronic berylliosis. There is diffuse, finely nodular, interstitial infiltration of the lungs with hilar and mediastinal adenopathy.

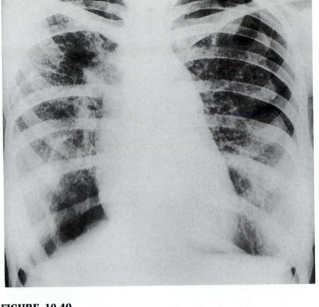

FIGURE 10-40
Radiograph of a young female metallurgist with chronic berylliosis. Note cardiomegaly with pulmonary artery dilatation, interstitial pulmonary fibrosis, and a left pneumothorax.

opathy, nephrocalcinosis and hypercalcemia, granulomatous involvement of the liver and spleen, and diffuse lung disease are seen in both diseases. However, the salivary glands, eyes, bones, and central nervous system are not involved in berylliosis. Berylliosis is encountered in two forms, the acute and the chronic.

Acute berylliosis results from a single intense exposure and manifests as an acute tracheobronchitis and pulmonary edema. In some cases the pulmonary parenchymal changes are seen radiographically as miliary nodulation of the lungs rather than the patchy alveolar filling pattern of pulmonary edema. In the majority of cases the radiographic findings resolve over a period of 2 to 4 weeks, and only in some 10% of cases is there a transition to chronic berylliosis.

In chronic pulmonary berylliosis, hilar and mediastinal adenopathy is a frequent finding. The parenchymal lesions may be miliary in type in the early stages, although this stage may go unobserved (Figure 10-39). Symmetric reticulonodular shadowing without zonal predominance is characteristic. With progression of disease the lungs lose volume and the fibrosis becomes coarser and more honeycombed. Bleb formation occurs, and pneumothorax is a potential complication (Figure 10-40). With further progression the hilar shadows become increasingly prominent, reflecting a combination of central pulmonary artery dilatation and adenopathy. CT findings are variable and nonspecific and include pulmonary nodularity, upper zone or diffuse interstitial fibrosis, emphysema with bleb formation, and hilar and mediastinal adenopathy (Figure 10-41).[70] The patient eventually dies of respiratory failure or cor pulmonale.

INHALATION OF NOXIOUS GASES, VAPORS, AND FUMES

The deleterious effects of noxious gases and fumes are mediated by several different mechanisms. These mechanisms include the following:

1. Asphyxiation. The oxygen in the ambient air is displaced by gas or vapor, and the subject suffers from acute lack of oxygen. Examples include asphyxiation by carbon dioxide, nitrogen, methane, and freon. Alternatively, the transport of oxygen may be interfered with, as for example in carbon monoxide or cyanide poisoning. There are no radiographic features.

2. Toxic absorption. Absorption of toxic materials may affect the lung directly or more distant body systems. Aluminum and beryllium are examples of substances that may damage the lungs acutely. These conditions are discussed on pp. 448 and 449.

3. Allergy. Certain (inorganic) substances, notably compounds of platinum, may excite an allergic response resulting in an occupational asthma without specific radiographic features. Many inhaled organic substances are responsible for allergic manifestations, a subject discussed further in Chapter 12.

4. Surface irritants. Many substances, when inhaled, have a direct irritant or damaging effect on the airways and lungs. The resulting inflammatory and edematous changes can be life threatening. Notable examples were seen following the use of chlorine and other gases during World War I. A single identifiable agent is usually involved in industrial accidents. The list of potentially hazardous substances is long and includes sulfur dioxide, zinc chloride, hydrogen fluoride, ammonia, osmium

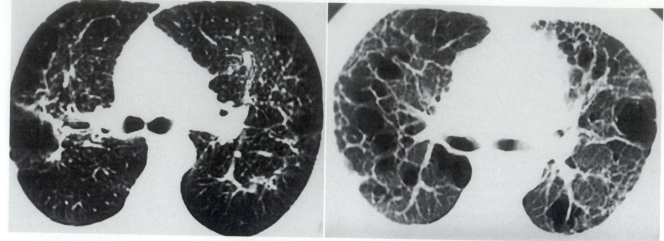

FIGURE 10-41
Chronic berylliosis. **A,** Computed tomographic (CT) scan showing central nodulation and some fibrosis with peripheral emphysema. **B,** CT scan showing coarse honeycombing and fibrosis in a more advanced case (Courtesy Dr. Haydn Adams, Penarth, U.K. From Harris KM, McConnochie K, Adams H: *Clin Radiol* 47:26-31, 1993.)

tetroxide, vanadium pentoxide, chromates, nitrogen dioxide, phosgene, and many others. The principal cause of nonindustrial inhalational injury is fire.

ACUTE INHALATIONAL INJURY

Injury to the airways and lung parenchyma may result from the inhalation of a variety of noxious substances. The result may be chemical pulmonary edema and pneumonia severe enough in some cases to cause death. Fire accidents are the most frequent cause of severe acute inhalational injury. In other cases the changes may be attributed to a single noxious agent such as beryllium (acute berylliosis; see pp. 448 and 449) or nitrogen dioxide (as in silo-filler's disease; see p. 452). The physician should not overlook the possibility that patients might have aspirated gastric contents during the course of rescue and resuscitation or have manifestations of blunt thoracic trauma.

Approximately 6000 persons die in fires in the United States every year, and a much greater number require hospital treatment. More than 50% of the deaths occur as a result of inhalational injury.[71] Victims of fire accidents may be divided into three categories: those suffering only cutaneous injury, those with cutaneous and inhalational injury, and those with inhalational injury alone. Extensive or severe cutaneous injury may result in sepsis and fluid balance problems with possible pulmonary edema or adult respiratory distress syndrome (ARDS). The greatest problems are, however, encountered with inhalational injury to the airways.

The pathophysiology of inhalational injury is complex, but three main causes of injury can be identified[50]:

1. Thermal injury to the upper airways. Except in the rare cases when inhalational injury is caused by steam or explosive gases, thermal damage below the subglottic region does not appear to occur. Nevertheless, thermal damage to the larynx may lead to serious respiratory compromise requiring tracheotomy. Lee and O'Connell[102] found radiographic evidence of subglottic edema in nearly one third of 45 patients from a major fire disaster. In part the subglottic edema may have resulted from thermal injury.

2. Carbon monoxide poisoning. Carbon monoxide poisoning is thought to be an important direct or indirect cause of death from fire. As an indirect cause it may cause loss of consciousness or disorientation, preventing the victim from escaping the fire. There are no direct radiographic manifestations of carbon monoxide poisoning. Severe hypoxic injury may also result when the products of combustion replace the ambient oxygen.

3. Noxious effects of the products of combustion. The composition of smoke may be extremely complex and may include volatolized plastics and their breakdown products, as well as simpler noxious agents such as oxides of nitrogen, cyanides, and aldehydes.[40]

The noxious products of combustion induce a laryngotracheobronchitis that may be severe enough to be hemorrhagic, ulcerative, or necrotizing. Less severe degrees of damage may show edema, bronchospasm, and inhibition of ciliary action. At alveolar level there may be damage to the alveolar macrophages, increasing the susceptibility to infection. Surfactant and the surfactant producing type III alveolocytes may be destroyed or damaged, leading to a loss of lung compliance. Finally, the vascular endothelium may be damaged, leading to an increased microvascular permeability with resultant edema.

Radiographic findings are variable in their severity and extent. Some 60%[172] to 75%[102] of patients in specialized burn units have some chest radiographic abnormality

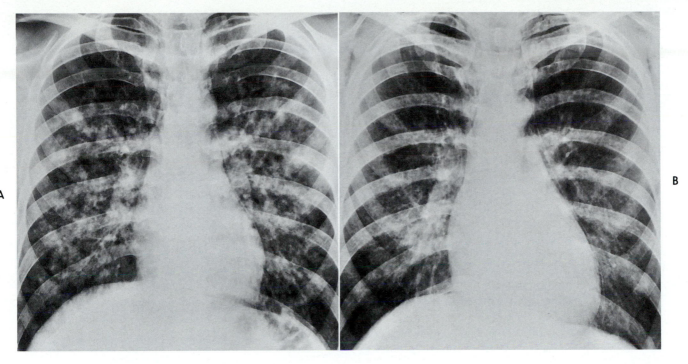

FIGURE 10-42
A, Radiograph of a young man admitted after accidentally setting his kitchen on fire while intoxicated.
B, Prompt recovery after 72 hours. (Courtesy Dr. K. Simpkins, Leeds, U.K.)

during the course of their hospitalization (Figure 10-42). The radiographic findings may be divided into those occurring immediately (within the first 24 hours) and those occurring in a delayed fashion. The significance of the presence or absence of radiographic findings in the immediate postinjury period is disputed. Earlier reports suggested that the chest radiograph is an insensitive indicator of the severity of inhalational injury.[128] Other authors have placed more reliance on the radiograph as a predictor of outcome and the likely need for ventilation support.[89,102,172,173]

The immediate radiographic findings include subglottic edema, diffuse peribronchial infiltration, frank interstitial or alveolar pulmonary edema, areas of atelectasis developing as a result of bronchial occlusions, and barotrauma resulting from intubation and positive-pressure ventilation. Lee and O'Connell[102] found subglottic edema that caused a conical narrowing of the airway in nearly one third of patients from a major fire disaster. In two thirds of patients there was evidence of diffuse peribronchial thickening, which progressed to frank edema in 7 of 45 cases. Teixidor and associates[173] found evidence of alveolar and mixed interstitial and alveolar edema in nearly one half of cases admitted for smoke inhalation to a burn unit over a 1-year period (Figure 10-42). Areas of atelectasis may develop rapidly and may be present on admission. Patients with only airway damage may never develop radiographic changes. On the other hand, severe inhalational injury involving the pulmonary parenchyma produces more widespread radiographic changes that may be present on admission or wax during the first 24 hours (Figure 10-43).[172]

Delayed pulmonary manifestations of inhalational injury include pneumonia, ARDS, barotrauma, atelectasis, and fluid overload. The radiographic appearances may become complex, and in severely or critically injured patients in intensive care units it may be difficult to sort out the various components of the radiographic picture. The various processes and factors that can contribute to the final radiographic picture include the following[89,173]:

1. Reaction to the initial insult
2. Severity and extent of secondary pneumonitis
3. Development of noncardiogenic edema (ARDS)
4. Fluid imbalances in severely burned patients or patients with secondary renal failure
5. Patchy atelectasis resulting from bronchial mucosal damage and mucus plugging
6. The patient's preexisting medical status, such as preexisting chronic obstructive pulmonary disease

Even with the aid of various clinical data such as the pulmonary wedge pressures, the nature of the tracheal aspirates, the ventilatory pressures, and the blood gas data, anything more than an educated guess may not be possible.

In general, the more rapid the radiographic improve-

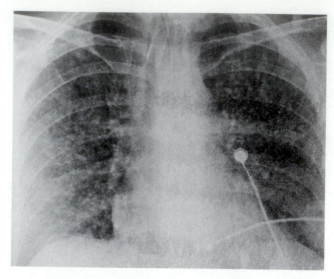

FIGURE 10-43
Radiograph of a patient who had sustained severe smoke inhalation injury 36 hours previously.

ment, the more favorable the prognosis. Bronchiolitis obliterans may still develop at a later stage despite a rapid immediate response. In such cases patients may manifest fine patchy interstitial shadowing — mainly peripheral in location and fairly symmetric in distribution (Figure 10-44). These changes wane over a period of days or weeks, leaving no visible sequelae, although the patient may continue to have respiratory defects.

SILO-FILLER'S DISEASE

Silo-filler's disease is discussed separately because of the circumstances of exposure and because it has a characteristic two-phase pattern of disease.[113,131,153] The patients are exposed to oxides of nitrogen from silage in the closed environment of a silo. The initial phase occurs immediately following the exposure. Cough and dyspnea develop, and the radiographic features vary from normal to classic pulmonary edema (Figure 10-45). Death may ensue quickly.[41,190] Most patients, however, recover steadily with steroid therapy and have no sequelae. In the absence of treatment the patient may recover only to have a recrudescence of symptoms some 2 to 3 weeks later, at which time a diffuse miliary or fine nodular pattern develops in the lungs, an appearance that corresponds to diffuse bronchiolitis obliterans. Occasionally patients are in this secondary phase when first examined, having not sought medical attention following the initial injury.[190] Some patients die during the secondary phase, and in these individuals the pulmonary infiltrates may become coarser and confluent before death. In the majority of cases, however, the pulmonary shadowing gradually clears, leaving no visible sequelae. Occasional patients show clinically evident pulmonary damage either after the edema phase or as a result of bronchiolitis obliterans.

DROWNING OR SUBMERSION INJURY

Each year an estimated 150,000 persons worldwide lose their lives as a result of drowning.[186] The number of episodes of near drowning cannot be estimated. Unless prevented by laryngeal spasm, the drowning fluid penetrates the lungs, where it may be radiographically demonstrable as pulmonary edema. Laryngeal spasm, which is particularly common in children, may prevent ingress of fluid but may be fatal because of cerebral hypoxia from inadequate ventilation. In one series of 12 children requiring mechanical ventilation, 4 did not have radiographic evidence of pulmonary edema on admission.[48] Nevertheless, 2 of these 4 children subsequently died.

The initial radiographic appearances vary from complete normality through varying degrees of pulmonary edema (Figure 10-46).[82] However, an initially normal chest radiograph may be associated with significant hypoxia, and furthermore radiographic deterioration may occur in the first 72 hours.[129] Mechanical ventilation, aspiration of gastric contents during resuscitation, neurologic damage, prolonged hypoxia, and so on may modify the radiographic picture during subsequent examinations. The aspiration of gastric contents could, for example, lead to a secondary aspiration pneumonia. Pneumothorax and pneumomediastinum occur commonly in victims of near drowning on ventilator support. Neurogenic pulmonary edema or even frank adult respiratory distress syndrome (ARDS) may supervene.[44] Although the common drowning fluids, fresh and salt water, are capable of damaging the pneumocytes and dispersing or inactivating lung surfactant, no effect is demonstrable in most cases of near drowning and the aspirated fluid may be promptly absorbed or otherwise dispersed.[124] Nevertheless, in more severe cases there may be a significant

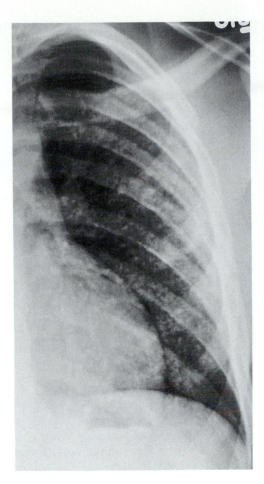

FIGURE 10-44
Bronchiolitis obliterans (biopsy proven) in a young man who had made heroic attempt to rescue a person from a burning car some 3 weeks previously.

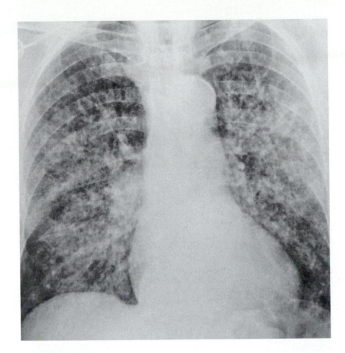

FIGURE 10-45
Radiograph of a patient overcome by fumes in a silo several hours previously.

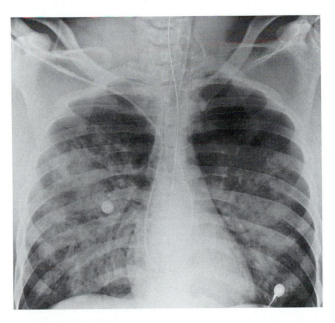

FIGURE 10-46
Radiograph of a young man following an episode of near drowning, showing pulmonary edema pattern.

decrease in lung compliance and alterations in ventilation-perfusion matching, necessitating mechanical ventilation. It is in such a case that the secondary pulmonary problems and more severe neurologic defects are most likely to be encountered.

ASPIRATION OF GASTRIC CONTENTS

Massive aspiration of gastric contents is sometimes known as Mendelson's syndrome. Mendelson,[109] in fact, described massive aspiration of gastric contents in a particular patient group, women during parturition. A number of factors make pregnant patients more liable to aspiration. During pregnancy the volume and acidity of gastric secretions increase and relative atony of the stomach with delayed emptying occurs. The gastroesophageal sphincter is relatively lax, and the administration of some form of anesthetic, often with the patient in an "unprepared" state, is common. However, massive aspiration of gastric contents may occur in other patients, almost invariably during periods of altered conscious-

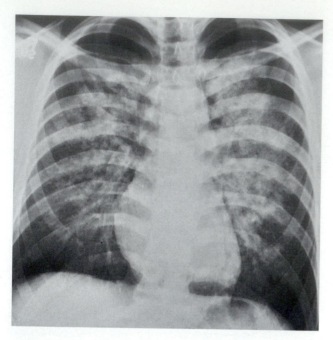

FIGURE 10-47
Radiograph of a young man who suffered massive aspiration of gastric contents while under general anesthesia.

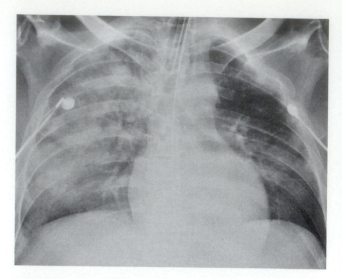

FIGURE 10-48
Predominantly unilateral shadowing following episode of massive gastric aspiration in a 43-year-old man.

ness. The clinical features are abrupt in onset and consist of cough, wheezing, cyanosis, dyspnea, and tachypnea. Initially the pathologic changes consist of a chemical tracheobronchitis and pneumonia. Secondary bacterial infection, however, is common, and the clinical course may be further complicated by pulmonary embolism and ARDS.

The classic radiographic finding is diffuse perihilar alveolar consolidation similar to cardiogenic pulmonary edema (Figure 10-47). Landay, Christensen, and Bynum[101] reviewed 60 patients who had suffered acute aspiration of gastric contents and found a remarkable variability in the radiographic findings.[101] This study showed that the severity of the pulmonary changes depended on the volume of fluid aspirated, and experimental evidence indicates that the severity of the process is also related to the pH of the aspirate.[23] Almost all patients have radiographic abnormalities following an episode of massive aspiration, and some worsening is usual in the first 36 hours. In uncomplicated cases the chest radiograph clears over the next 4 to 5 days. Secondary bacterial pneumonia with severe underlying pulmonary disease and the development of ARDS are adverse features that may lead to a fatal outcome even after an initial period of improvement. The parenchymal densities are often ill-defined acinar airspace shadows, which are frequently confluent. Small irregular shadows are, however, common. The distribution of the densities is generally perihilar or bibasilar, although there is considerable variation, possibly dependent on the patient's position during the episode of aspiration. The

pulmonary shadows may even be entirely unilateral (Figure 10-48).[188] Pleural effusions are uncommon, which is presumably a reflection of the more central location of the inflammatory process. The more severe and extensive the shadowing on the initial examination, the worse the prognosis. However, relatively minor initial changes may progress to a fatal outcome.

HYDROCARBON PNEUMONIA

Volatile hydrocarbons, when aspirated, may result in a widespread chemical pneumonia. In the past, there has been debate as to whether ingested hydrocarbons cause pneumonia in the absence of aspiration. Volatile hydrocarbons, when absorbed from the gut, are excreted via the lungs, and it has been suggested that this excretion may cause toxic damage to the lungs. However, the consensus is that ingested hydrocarbons have minimal or no effect on the lungs and that the pulmonary toxic effects are overwhelmingly caused by aspirated hydrocarbons.[42] Ingested hydrocarbons may have low pulmonary toxicity because they are poorly absorbed from the gut and also undergo some detoxification during their transit through the liver. Toxic lung damage caused by intravenously administered hydrocarbons has, however, been observed both experimentally[84] and in clinical practice.[118]

Radiographic abnormalities are commonly present on admission or develop within the first 12 hours. These radiographic abnormalities correlate poorly with clinical symptoms and signs. Many patients with radiographic abnormalities have no symptoms, or their symptoms resolve before the radiographic changes clear. Chest radiographs show scattered pulmonary densities that are almost invariably bilateral with middle and lower zone predominance (Figure 10-49). Initially the densities are

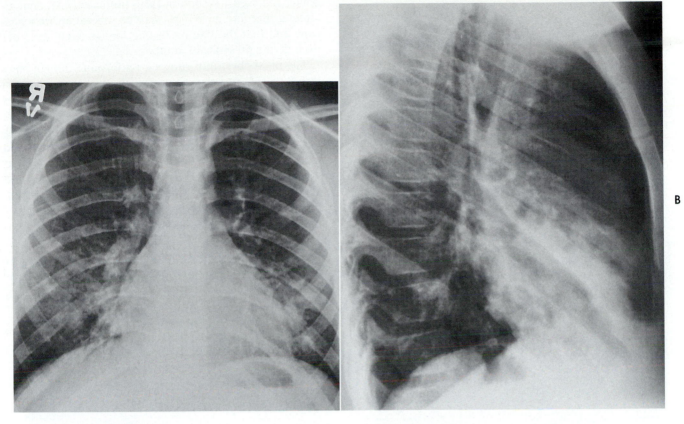

FIGURE 10-49
Kerosene pneumonia in a 12-year-old boy shows extensive patchy bibasilar infiltration. **A,** Posteroanterior view. **B,** Lateral view.

often mottled, but with time they may become confluent. The pulmonary shadowing commonly worsens somewhat over the first 72 hours following aspiration. Usually the pulmonary densities then clear over the next few days. On occasion, however, radiographic changes take weeks or months to clear, particularly in adults. Obstructive emphysema with air trapping peripherally may be seen, and pneumatoceles are occasionally observed. Segmental or subsegmental atelectasis is common.

The majority of cases of hydrocarbon pneumonia occur in children, particularly young children. The prognosis, both immediate and long term, is good. Few of these children have damage to the lungs, although there may be minor residual pulmonary function abnormalities.[67] Some adults suffer permanent damage, with chronic organizing pneumonia, fibrosis, and bronchiectasis.

INHALATION OF FOREIGN BODIES

The usual foreign materials inhaled into the airways are food and broken fragments of teeth; a nut is the single most common object. Inhalation of foreign bodies occurs most frequently in the first 3 years of life, with a peak incidence at 1 to 2 years of age. It is rare before 6 months of age. Foreign bodies usually lodge in the left or right main bronchus; neither side is involved significantly more often than the other. The next most common site is the trachea, followed by a lobar bronchus.[17,31,93]

Although in most cases aspiration of a foreign body is diagnosed within 2 to 3 days of the event, the diagnosis may not be made for weeks or sometimes even months, as was the case in approximately one third of children in two large series.[17,31] In more than 80% of cases,[17,20,93,142] a definite event of aspiration or choking is followed by cough or wheezing, which may persist, usually without respiratory distress. In time the cough may disappear. However, an interval of hours, months, or years may occur during which the child is asymptomatic following the initial event.[130]

The most common complication of foreign body aspiration is pneumonia or atelectasis, which occurs in approximately one fourth of the cases when the foreign body lodges in a bronchus but is rare when the object lodges in the trachea. Bronchiectasis may follow prolonged retention of a bronchial foreign body. Pneumothorax and pneumomediastinum are rare.

Bronchoscopy is the usual method of final diagnosis and also permits removal of the foreign body in almost all cases. Thoracotomy or other surgical intervention is rarely required. Blazer, Naveh, and Friedman[17] emphasized that 15% of their patients who had inhaled foreign

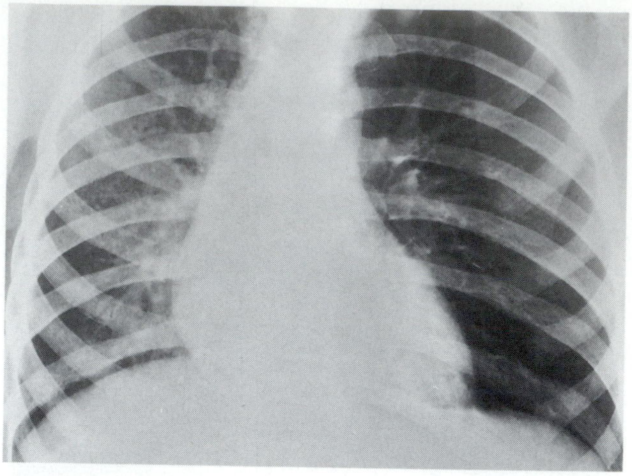

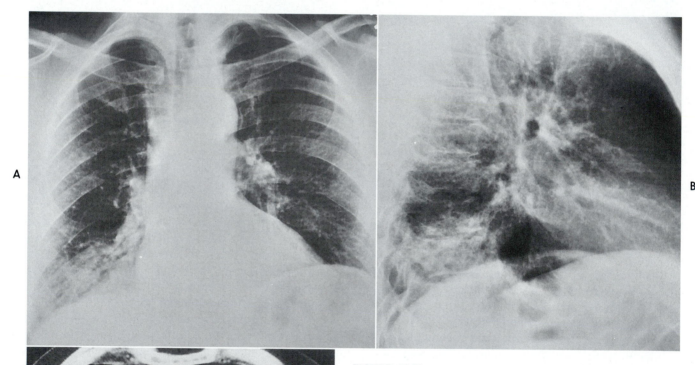

FIGURE 10-50
Inhaled foreign body lodged in left main bronchus in a young child, causing obstructive air trapping in the left lung.

bodies required a second or third bronchoscopy, demonstrating that foreign bodies may be missed at bronchoscopy and that the finding of one foreign body does not exclude the presence of another.

The plain chest film shows a radiopaque foreign body in 5% to 15% of cases. Occasionally the foreign body is seen as a shadow of soft tissue density in one of the larger airways.

The cardinal sign of inhalation soon after aspiration is obstructive overinflation or air trapping of the affected lobe or lobes (Figure 10-50).[17,20,142] Air trapping with or without contralateral shift of the mediastinum is best demonstrated on films taken during expiration. Such films can be difficult to obtain in young children, and air trapping and mediastinal shift are often easier to demonstrate with fluoroscopy.

Alternative techniques that do not require fluoroscopy include assisted expiratory films and lateral decubitus

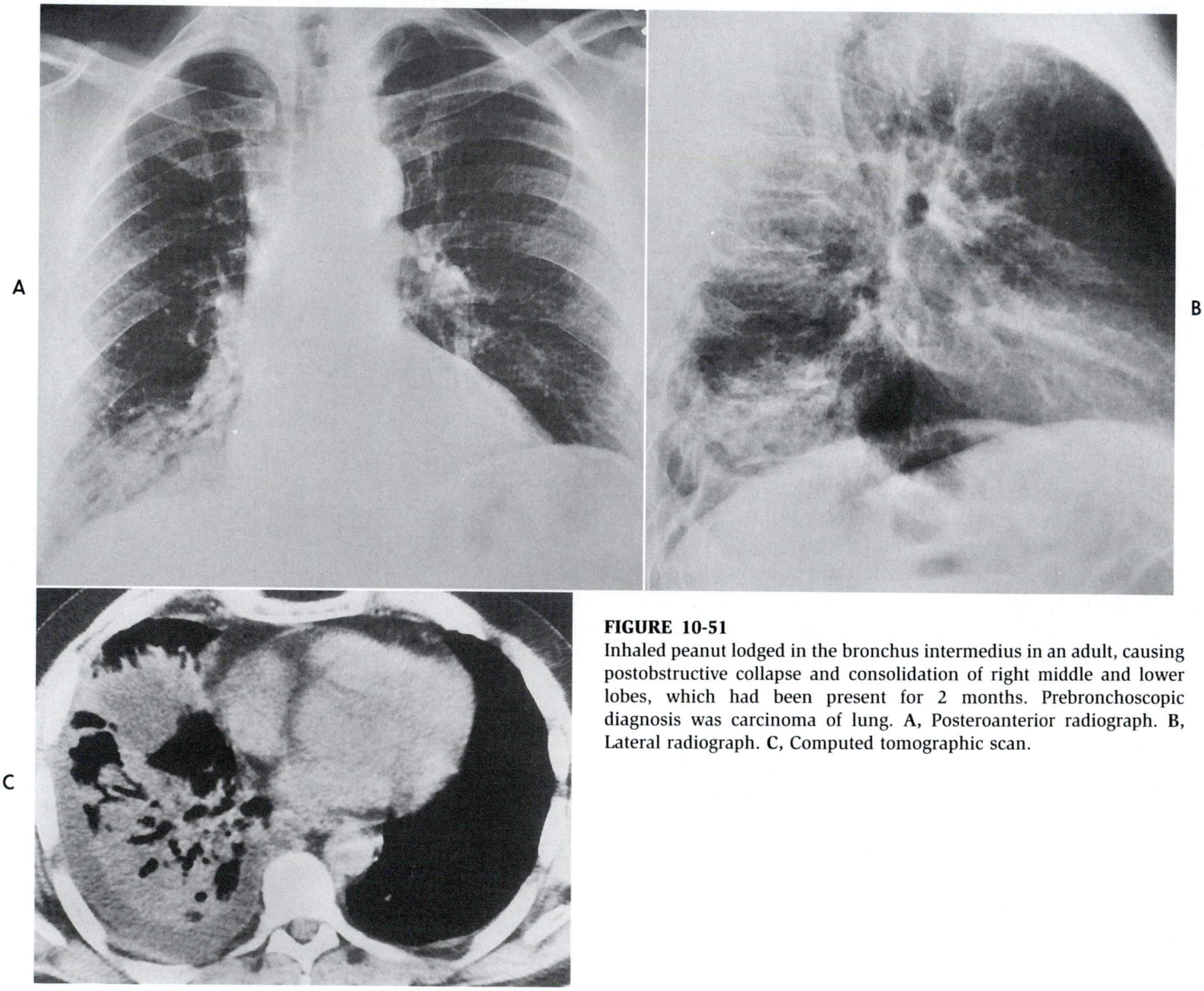

FIGURE 10-51
Inhaled peanut lodged in the bronchus intermedius in an adult, causing postobstructive collapse and consolidation of right middle and lower lobes, which had been present for 2 months. Prebronchoscopic diagnosis was carcinoma of lung. **A,** Posteroanterior radiograph. **B,** Lateral radiograph. **C,** Computed tomographic scan.

examinations.[24] An assisted expiratory film consists of a chest radiograph exposed while gentle pressure is applied to the epigastrium with a lead-gloved hand.[184] Air trapping is demonstrated by the contrast between the relatively lucent affected lobe and the more opaque normal lobes. The idea behind the use of lateral decubitus films to detect inhaled foreign bodies is that the dependent lung is normally less inflated than the uppermost lung regardless of the degree of inspiration, whereas air trapping renders the dependent lung hyperlucent. Radionuclide perfusion scanning of the lungs has been used to demonstrate reduced blood flow to areas of the lung in which the airway has been partially occluded by a foreign body.[10,111,147]

The other major feature of foreign body aspiration into the airway is atelectasis or pneumonia distal to the obstructing foreign body (Figure 10-51). These signs were seen in 20% to 45% of patients in the larger series.[17,20,93,142] A pneumothorax or a pneumomediastinum may be present, but both are surprisingly uncommon (less than 2% of patients) following aspiration of a foreign body.[17,142]

Normal inspiratory and expiratory chest radiographs can be expected in about one fourth of cases. In the series of 200 patients reported by Blazer, Naveh, and Friedman,[17] 15.6% of those with bronchial foreign bodies and 60.6% of those with tracheal foreign bodies showed no abnormalities on inspiratory and expiratory films, and even with fluoroscopy almost half the patients with tracheal foreign bodies showed no abnormality.

REFERENCES

1. Aberle DR, Gamsu G, Ray CS: High-resolution CT of benign asbestos-related diseases: clinical and radiographic correlation, *AJR* 151:883-891, 1988.
2. Aberle DR, Gamsu G, Ray CS, et al: Asbestos-related pleural and parenchymal fibrosis: detection with high-resolution CT, *Radiology* 166:729-734, 1988.
3. Akira M, Higashihara T, Yokoyama K, et al: Radiographic type p. pneumoconiosis: high resolution CT, *Radiology* 171:117-123, 1989.
4. Akira M, Yokoyama K, Yamamoto S, et al: Early asbestosis: evaluation with high-resolution CT, *Radiology* 178:409-416, 1991.
5. Albeda SM, Epstein DM, Gefter WB, et al: Pleural thickening: its significance and relationship to asbestos dust exposure, *Am Rev Respir Dis* 126:621-624, 1982.
6. Al-Jarad N, Strickland B, Pearson MC, et al: High resolution computed tomographic assessment of asbestosis and cryptogenic fibrosing alveolitis: a comparative study, *Thorax* 47:645-650, 1992.
7. Amandus HE, Lapp NL, Jacobson G, et al: Significance of irregular small opacities of coal miners in the USA, *Br J Ind Med* 33:13-17, 1976.
8. Amandus HE, Prendergrass EP, Dennis JM, et al: Pneumoconiosis: interreader variability in the classification of the type of small opacities in the chest roentgenogram, *AJR* 122:740-743, 1974.
9. Anton HC: Multiple pleural plaques, *Br J Radiol* 40:685-690, 1967.
10. Apau RL, Saenz R, Siemsen JK: Bloodless lung due to bronchial obstruction, *J Nucl Med* 13:561-562, 1972.
11. Aronchick JM, Rossman MD, Miller WT: Chronic beryllium disease: diagnosis, radiographic findings and correlation with pulmonary function tests, *Radiology* 163:677-682, 1987.
12. Baker EL, Greene R: Incremental value of oblique chest radiographs in the diagnosis of asbestos-induced lung disease, *Am J Ind Med* 3:17-22, 1982.
13. Baris I, Simonato L, Artvinli M, et al: Epidemiological and environmental evidence of the health effects of exposure to erionite fibers: a four year study in the Cappadocian region of Turkey, *Int J Cancer* 39:10-17, 1987.
14. Becklake MR: Asbestos-related diseases of the lung and other organs: their epidemiology and implications for clinical practice, *Am Rev Respir Dis* 114:187-227, 1976.
15. Begin R, Ostiguy G, Fillion R, et al: Computed tomography scan in the early detection of silicosis, *Am Rev Respir Dis* 144:697-705, 1991.
16. Bergin CJ, Muller NL, Vedal S, et al: CT in silicosis: correlation with plain films and pulmonary function tests, *AJR* 146:477-483, 1986.
17. Blazer S, Naveh Y, Friedman A: Foreign body in the airway, *Am J Dis Child* 134:68, 1980.
18. Blesovsky A: The folded lung, *Br J Dis Chest* 60:19-22, 1966.
19. Brooks SM: Lung disorders resulting from the inhalation of metals, *Clin Chest Med* 2:235-254, 1981.
20. Brown BSTJ, Ma H, Dunbar JS, et al: Foreign bodies in the tracheobronchial tree in childhood, *J Can Assoc Radiol* 14:158-171, 1963.
21. Buechner HA, Ansari A: Acute silico proteinosis: a new pathologic variant of acute silicosis in sandblasters, characterized by histologic features resembling alveolar proteinosis, *Dis Chest* 55:274-278, 1969.
22. Burrell R: Immunological aspects of coal workers pneumoconiosis, *Ann NY Acad Sci* 200:94-105, 1972.
23. Bynum LJ, Pierce AK: Pulmonary aspiration of gastric contents, *Am Rev Respir Dis* 114:1129-1136, 1976.
24. Capitanio MA, Kirkpatrick JA: The lateral decubitus film, an aid in determining air trapping in children, *Radiology* 103:460-462, 1972.
25. Caplan A: Correlation of radiological category with lung pathology in coal workers' pneumoconiosis, *Br J Ind Med* 19:171-179, 1962.
26. Caplan A, Simon G, Reid L: The radiological diagnosis of widespread emphysema and categories of simple pneumoconiosis, *Clin Radiol* 17:68-70, 1966.
27. Carvalho PM, Carr DH: Computed tomography of folded lung, *Clin Radiol* 41:86-91, 1990.
28. Casey KR, Rom WN, Moatamed F: Asbestos-related diseases, *Clin Chest Med* 2:179-202, 1981.
29. Classification of radiographs of the pneumoconioses, *Med Radiogr Photogr* 57:2-17, 1981.
30. Cockcroft AE, Wagner JC, Ryder R, et al: Post-mortem study of emphysema in coal workers and non-coal workers, *Lancet* 2:600-603, 1982.
31. Cohen SR, Herbert WI, Lewis GB, et al: Foreign bodies in the airway: five-year retrospective study with special reference to management, *Ann Otol Rhinol Laryngol* 89:437-442, 1980.
32. Collins JD, Brown RKT, Batra P: Asbestosis and the serratus anterior muscle, *J Natl Med Assoc* 75:296-300, 1983.
33. Cooke WE: Pulmonary asbestosis, *Br Med J* 2:1024-1025, 1927.
34. Cookson WO, Deklerk NH, Musk AW, et al: Benign and malignant pleural effusions in former Wittenoom crocidolite millers and miners, *Aust NZ J Med* 15:731-737, 1985.
35. Cotes E, Gibson JC, McKerrow CB, et al: A long term follow-up of workers exposed to beryllium, *Br J Ind Med* 40:13-21, 1983.
36. Craighead JE, Mossman BT: The pathogenesis of asbestos-associated diseases, *N Engl J Med* 306:1446-1455, 1982.

37. Davis JMG, Chapman J, Collings P, et al: *Autopsy study of coal miner's lungs,* Institute of Occupational Medicine Edinburgh Report, No. TM/79/9 (Eur. P27), 1979.

38. Dee PM, Suratt P, Winn W: The radiographic findings in acute silicosis, *Radiology* 126:359-363, 1978.

39. DeLajartre M, deLajartre AY: Mesothelioma on the coast of Brittany, France, *Ann NY Acad Sci* 330:323-332, 1979.

40. Demling RH: Smoke inhalation injury, *Postgrad Med* 82:63-68, 1987.

41. Douglas WW, Hepper NGG, Colby TV: Silo-fillers disease, *Mayo Clin Proc* 64:291-304, 1989.

42. Eade NR, Taussig LM, Marks MI: Hydrocarbon pneumonitis, *Pediatrics* 54:351-357, 1974.

43. Edge JR: Incidence of bronchial carcinoma in shipyard workers with pleural plaques, *Ann NY Acad Sci* 330:289-294, 1979.

44. Effmann EL, Merten DF, Kirks DR, et al: Adult respiratory distress syndrome in children, *Radiology* 157:69-74, 1985.

45. Eisenstadt HB: Asbestos pleurisy, *Dis Chest* 46:78-81, 1964.

46. Epler GR, McLoud TC, Gaensler EA: Prevalence and incidence of benign asbestos pleural effusion in a working population, *JAMA* 247:617-622, 1982.

47. Epler GR, McCloud TC, Gaensler EA, et al: Normal chest roentgenograms in chronic diffuse infiltrative lung disease, *N Engl J Med* 298:934-939, 1978.

48. Fandel I, Bancalari E: Near drowning in children: clinical aspects, *Pediatrics* 58:573-579, 1976.

49. Feigin DS: Talc: understanding its manifestations in the chest, *AJR* 146:295-301, 1986.

50. Fein A, Leff A, Hopwell PC: Pathophysiology and management of the complications resulting from fire and the inhaled products of combustion: review of the literature, *Crit Care Med* 8:84-98, 1980.

51. Felson B: *Chest roentgenology,* Philadelphia, 1973, WB Saunders.

52. Fletcher DE: A mortality study of shipyard workers with pleural plaques, *Br J Ind Med* 29:142-145, 1972.

53. Freundlich IM, Greening RR: Asbestosis and associated medical problems, *Radiology* 89:224-229, 1967.

54. Friedman AC, Fiel SB, Fisher MS, et al: Asbestos-related pleural disease and asbestosis: a comparison of CT and chest radiography, *AJR* 150:269-275, 1988.

55. Gaensler EA, Carrington CB: Open biopsy for chronic diffuse infiltrative lung disease: clinical, roentgenographic and physiological correlations in 502 patients, *Ann Thorac Surg* 30:411-426, 1980.

56. Gaensler EA, Carrington CB, Coutre RE, et al: Pathological, physiological and radiological correlations in the pneumoconioses, *Ann NY Acad Sci* 200:574-607, 1972.

57. Gaensler EA, Kaplan AI: Asbestos pleural effusion, *Ann Intern Med* 74:178-191, 1971.

58. Gefter WB, Conant EF: Issues and controversies in the plain-film diagnosis of asbestos-related disorders in the chest, *J Thorac Imag* 3:11-28, 1988.

59. Gilmartin D: The serratus anterior muscle on chest radiographs, *Radiology* 131:629-635, 1979.

60. Gough J: Pneumoconiosis of coal trimmers, *J Pathol Bacteriol* 51:277-285, 1940.

61. Gough J, James WRL, Wentworth JE: A comparison of the radiological and pathological changes in coal workers pneumoconiosis, *J Fac Radiol* 1:28-60, 1949.

62. Greaves IA: Rheumatoid "pneumoconiosis" (Caplan's syndrome) in an asbestos worker: a 17 years' follow-up, *Thorax* 34:404-405, 1979.

63. Green RA, Dimcheff DG: Massive bilateral upper lobe fibrosis secondary to asbestos exposure, *Chest* 65:52-55, 1974.

64. Greening RR, Heslep JH: The roentgenology of silicosis, *Semin Roentgenol* 2:265-275, 1967.

65. Gregor A, Parkes RW, duBois R, et al: Radiographic progression of asbestosis: preliminary report, *Ann NY Acad Sci* 330:147-156, 1979.

66. Gurney JW, Schroeder BA: Upper lobe lung disease: physiologic correlates, *Radiology* 167:359-366, 1988.

67. Gurwitz D, Kaltan M, Levison H, et al: Pulmonary function abnormalities in asymptomatic children after hydrocarbon pneumonitis, *Pediatrics* 62:789-794, 1978.

68. Hanke R, Kretzschmar R: Round atelectasis, *Semin Roentgenol* 15:174-182, 1980.

69. Hansell DM, Moskovic E: High resolution computed tomography in extrinsic allergic alveolitis, *Clin Radiol* 43:8-12, 1991.

70. Harris KM, McConnochie K, Adams H: The computed tomographic appearances in chronic berylliosis, *Clin Radiol* 47(1):26-31, 1993.

71. Heimbach DM, Waeckerle JF: Inhalation injuries, *Ann Emerg Med* 17:1316-1320, 1988.

72. Heitzman ER: *The lung: radiologic and pathologic correlations,* St Louis, 1984, Mosby.

73. Heitzman ER, Naeye RL, Markarian B: Roentgen pathological correlations in coal workers pneumoconiosis, *Ann NY Acad Sci* 200:510-526, 1972.

74. Heppleston AG: The pathological recognition and pathogenesis of emphysema and fibrocystic disease of the lung with special reference to coal workers, *Ann NY Acad Sci* 200:347-369, 1972.

75. Hillerdal G: Pleural plaques in a health survey material: frequency, development and exposure to asbestos, *Scand J Respir Dis* 59:257-263, 1978.

76. Hillerdal G: Pleural plaques and risk for cancer in the county of Uppsala, *Eur J Respir Dis* 61(suppl 107):111-118, 1980.

77. Hillerdal G: Asbestos exposure and upper lobe involvement, *AJR* 139:1163-1166, 1982.

78. Hillerdal G, Hemmingsson A: Pulmonary pseudotumors and asbestos, *Acta Radiol (Diagn)* 21:615-620, 1980.

79. Hillerdal G, Lindgren A: Pleural plaques: correlation of autopsy findings to radiographic findings and occupational history, *Eur J Respir Dis* 61:315-319, 1980.

80. Hilt B, Lien JT, Lund-Larsen PG, et al: Asbestos-related findings in chest radiographs of the male population of the country of Telemark, Norway — a cross-sectional study, *Scand J Work Environ Health* 12:567-573, 1986.

81. Hooper WF: Acute beryllium lung disease, *North Carolina Med J* 42:551-553, 1981.

82. Hunter TB, Whitehouse WH: Fresh water drowning: radiological aspects, *Radiology* 112:51-56, 1974.

83. Hurley JF, Burns J, Copland L, et al: Coal workers' simple pneumoconiosis and exposure to dust at 10 British coalmines, *Br J Ind Med* 39:120-127, 1982.

84. Huxtable KA, Bolande RP, Klaus M: Experimental furniture polish pneumonia in rats, *Pediatrics* 34:228-235, 1964.

85. International Labour Office: *Guidelines for the use of the ILO international classification of radiographs of pneumoconiosis,* International Labor Office Occupational Safety and Health Series No. 22 (Rev. 80), Geneva, Switzerland, 1980, The Office.

86. Jacob B, Bohlig H: Die roentgenologische komplikationen der lungen asbestose, *Fortschr Roentgenstr* 83:515-525, 1955.

87. Jacobsen M: New data on the relationship between simple pneumoconiosis and exposure to coal mine dust, *Chest* 78:408-410, 1980.

88. Jacobson GJ, Felson B, Pendergrass EP, et al: Eggshell calcifications in coal and metal miners, *Semin Roentgenol* 2:276-282, 1967.

89. Kangarloo H, Beachley MC, Ghahremani GG: The radiographic spectrum of pulmonary complications in burn victims, *AJR* 128:441-445, 1977.

90. Kannerstein M: Recent advances and perspectives relevant to the pathology of asbestos-related diseases in man. In Wagner JC, ed: *Biological effects of mineral fibers,* Lyon, France, 1980, International Agency for Research on Cancer, pp. 149-162.

91. Katz D, Kreel L: Computed tomography in pulmonary asbestosis, *Clin Radiol* 30:207-213, 1979.

92. Kennedy T, Rawlings W, Baser M, et al: Pneumoconiosis in Georgia kaolin workers, *Am Res Respir Dis* 127:215-220, 1983.

93. Kim IG, Brummitt WM, Humphry A, et al: Foreign body in the airway: a review of 202 cases, *Laryngoscope* 83:347, 1973.

94. Kinsella M, Muller NL, Vedal S, et al: Emphysema in silicosis: a comparison of smokers with non-smokers using pulmonary function testing and computed tomography, *Am Rev Respir Dis* 141:497-500, 1990.

95. Kipen HM, Lilis R, Suzuki Y, et al: Pulmonary histopathological evaluation, *Br J Indust Med* 44:96-100, 1987.

96. Kiviluoto R, Meurman LO, Hakama M: Pleural plaques and neoplasia in Finland, *Ann NY Acad Sci* 330:31-33, 1979.

97. Kleinerman J: The pathology of some familiar pneumoconioses, *Semin Roentgenol* 2:244-264, 1967.

98. Kotloff RM, Richman PS, Greenacre JK, et al: Chronic beryllium disease in a dental laboratory technician, *Am Rev Respir Dis* 147:205-207, 1993.

99. Kreel L: Computer tomography in the evaluation of pulmonary asbestosis, *Acta Radiol (Diagn)* 17:405-412, 1976.

100. Kretzschmar R: Über atelektatische pseudotumoren der lunge, *Fortschr Roengtenstr* 122:19-29, 1975.

101. Landay MJ, Christensen EE, Bynum LJ: Pulmonary manifestations of acute aspiration of gastric contents, *AJR* 131:587-592, 1978.

102. Lee MJ, O'Connell DJ: The plain chest radiograph after acute smoke inhalations, *Clin Radiol* 39:33-37, 1988.

103. Leigh J, Outhred KG, McKenzie HI, et al: Quantified pathology of emphysema, pneumoconiosis, and chronic bronchitis in coal workers, *Br J Ind Med* 40:258-263, 1983.

104. Lynch DA, Gamsu G, Ray CS, et al: Asbestos-related focal lung masses: manifestations on conventional and high-resolution CT scans, *Radiology* 169:603-607, 1988.

105. Lyons JP, Ryder RC, Campbell H, et al: Significance of irregular opacities in the radiology of coal workers pneumoconiosis, *Br J Ind Med* 31:36-44, 1974.

106. Lyons JP, Ryder R, Campbell H, et al: Pulmonary disability: coal workers pneumoconiosis, *Br Med J* 1:713-716, 1972.

107. McHugh K, Blaquiere RM: CT features of rounded atelectasis, *AJR* 153:257-260, 1989.

108. McLoud TC, Woods BO, Carrington CB, et al: Diffuse pleural thickening in an asbestos-exposed population: prevalence and causes, *AJR* 144:9-18, 1985.

109. Mendelson CL: The aspiration of stomach contents into the lungs during obstetric anesthesia, *Am J Obstet Gynecol* 52:191-205, 1946.

110. Mintzer RA, Cugell DW: The association of asbestos-induced pleural disease and rounded atelectasis, *Chest* 81:457-460, 1982.

111. Moncada R, Baker D, Kenny J, et al: Reversible unilateral pulmonary hypoperfusion secondary to acute check-valve obstruction to a main bronchus, *Radiology* 106:361-362, 1973.

112. Morgan WKC, Lapp NC: Respiratory disease in coal miners: state of the art, *Am Rev Respir Dis* 113:531-559, 1976.

113. Morrissey WL, Gould IA, Carrington CB, et al: Silo-fillers disease, *Respiration* 32:81-92, 1975.

114. Murata K, Itoh H, Todo G, et al: Centrilobular lesions of the lung: demonstration by high resolution CT and pathologic correlation, *Radiology* 161:641-645, 1986.

115. Naeye RL: Rank of coal and coal workers pneumoconiosis, *Am Rev Respir Dis* 103:350-355, 1971.

116. Naeye RL, Dellinger WS: Coal workers' pneumoconiosis: correlation of roentgenographic and post mortem findings, *JAMA* 220:223-227, 1972.

117. Nagelschmidt G, Rivers D, King EJ, et al: Dust and collagen content of lungs of coal workers with progressive massive fibrosis, *Br J Ind Med* 20:181-191, 1963.

118. Neeld EM, Limacher MC: Chemical pneumonitis after the intravenous injection of hydrocarbon, *Radiology* 126:36, 1978.

119. Newell DJ, Browne RC: Symptomatology and radiology in pneumoconiosis: a survey in the Durham coalfield, *J Fac Radiol* 7:20-28, 1955.

120. Oldham PD: Pneumoconiosis in Cornish china clay workers, *Br J Ind Med* 40:131-137, 1983.

121. Padley SPG, Hansell DM, Flower CDR, et al: Comparative occuracy of high resolution, computed tomography in the diagnosis of chronic diffuse infiltrative lung disease, *Clin Radiol* 44:222-226, 1991.

122. Oxman AD, Muir DCF, Shannon HS, et al: Occupational dust exposure and chronic obstructive pulmonary disease: a systematic overview of the evidence, *Am Rev Respir Dis* 148:38-48, 1993.

123. Parkes WR: *Occupational lung disorders*, ed 2, London, 1982, Butterworths.

124. Pearn J: Pathophysiology of drowning, *Med J Aust* 142:586-588, 1985.

125. Picado C, Roisin R, Sala H, et al: Diagnosis of asbestosis, clinical, radiological and lung function data in 42 patients, *Lung* 162:325-335, 1984.

126. Pratt PC: Role of silica in progressive massive fibrosis in coal workers pneumoconiosis, *Arch Environ Health* 16:734-737, 1968.

127. Prendergrass EP: Silicosis and a few of the other pneumoconioses: observations on certain aspects of the problem with emphasis in the role of the radiologist, *AJR* 80:1-41, 1958.

128. Putman CE, Loke J, Matthay RA, et al: Radiographic manifestations of acute smoke inhalation, *AJR* 129:865-870, 1977.

129. Putman CE, Tummillo AM, Myerson DA, et al: Drowning: another plunge, *AJR* 125:543-548, 1975.

130. Pyman C: Inhaled foreign bodies in childhood: a review of 230 cases, *Med J Aust* 1:62-68, 1971.

131. Ramirez J, Dowell AR: Silo-fillers disease: nitrogen dioxide-induced lung injury; longterm follow-up and review of the literature, *Ann Intern Med* 74:569-576, 1971.

132. Remy-Jardin M, Beuscart R, Sault MC, et al: Subpleural micronodules in diffuse infiltrative lung diseases: evaluation with thin-section CT, *Radiology* 177:133-139, 1990.

133. Remy-Jardin M, Degreef JM, Beuscart R, et al: Coal workers pneumoconiosis: CT assessment in exposed workers and correlation with radiographic findings, *Radiology* 177:363-371, 1990.

134. Remy-Jardin M, Remy J, Deffontaines C, et al: Assessment of diffuse infiltrative lung disease: comparison of conventional CT and high-resolution CT, *Radiology* 181:157-162, 1991.

135. Rimmer MJ, Dixon AK, Flower CDR, et al: Bleomycin lung: computed tomographic observations, *Br J Radiol* 58:1041-1045, 1985.

136. Rivers D, Wise ME, King ES, et al: Dust content, radiology, and pathology in simple pneumoconiosis of coal workers, *Br J Ind Med* 17:87-108, 1960.

137. Roche G, Parent J, Daumet P: Atelectasis parcellaires du lobe inferieur et du lobe moyen au cours du pneumothorax thérapeutique, *Rev Tuberc (Paris)* 20:87-93, 1956.

138. Rockoff SD, Kagan E, Schwartz A, et al: Visceral pleural thickening in asbestos exposure: the occurrence and implications of thickened interlobar fissures, *J Thorac Imag* 2:58-66, 1987.

139. Rockoff SD, Schwartz A: Roentgenographic underestimation of early asbestosis by International Labor Organization classification: analysis of data and probabilities, *Chest* 9:1088-1091, 1988.

140. Roggli VL, Shelbourne JD: Mineral pneumoconioses. In Dail DH, Hammer SP, eds: *Pulmonary pathology*, New York, 1987, Springer-Verlag, p 598.

141. Rossiter CE: Relation of lung dust content to radiological changes in coal workers, *Ann NY Acad Sci* 200:465-477, 1972.

142. Rothmann BG, Boeckman CR: Foreign bodies in the larynx and tracheobronchial tree in children, *Ann Otol Rhinol Laryngol* 89:434-442, 1980.

143. Rous V, Studeny J: Aetiology of pleural plaques, *Thorax* 25:270-284, 1970.

144. Rubino GF, Newhouse M, Murray R, et al: Radiologic changes after cessation of exposure among chrysotile asbestos miners in Italy, *Ann NY Acad Sci* 330:157-161, 1979.

145. Ruckley VA, Fernie JM, Chapman JS, et al: Comparison of radiographic appearances with associated pathology and lung dust content in a group of coal workers, *Br J Ind Med* 41:459-467, 1984.

146. Ruckley VA, Gould SJ, Chapman JS, et al: Emphysema and dust exposure in a group of coal workers, *Am Rev Respir Dis* 129:528-532, 1984.

147. Rudavsky AZ, Leonidas JC, Abramson AL: Lung scanning for the detection of endobronchial foreign bodies in infants and children, *Radiology* 108:629-633, 1973.

148. Ryder R, Lyons JP, Campbell H, et al: Emphysema in coal workers' pneumoconiosis, *Br Med J* 3:481-487, 1970.

149. Sampson C, Hansell DM: The prevalence of enlarged mediastinal lymph nodes in asbestos-exposed individuals: a CT study, *Clin Radiol* 45:340-342, 1992.

150. Sargent EN, Boswell WD, Ralls PW, et al: Subpleural fat pads in patients exposed to asbestos: distinction from non calcified pleural plaques, *Radiology* 152:273-277, 1984.

151. Schneider HJ, Felson B, Gonzalez LL: Rounded atelectasis, *AJR* 134:225-232, 1980.

152. Schwartz DA, Fuortes LJ, Galvin JR, et al: Asbestos-induced pleural fibrosis and impaired lung function, *Am Rev Respir Dis* 141:321-326, 1990.

153. Scott EG, Hunt WB: Silo-fillers disease, *Chest* 63:701-706, 1973.

154. Scully RE, Mark EJ, McNeely BV: Case records of the Massachusetts General Hospital Case 27-1982, *N Engl J Med* 307:104-112, 1982.

155. Seal RME: Current views on pathological aspects of asbestos (the unresolved questions and problems). In Wagner JC, ed: *Biological effects of mineral fibers,* vol 1, Lyon, France, 1980, International Agency for Research on Cancer, pp 217-235.

156. Seal RME, Cockcroft A, Kung I, et al: Central lymph node changes and progressive massive fibrosis in coal workers, *Thorax* 41:531-537, 1986.

157. Seaton A, Dick JA, Dodgson J, et al: Quartz and pneumoconiosis in coalminers, *Lancet* 2:1272-1275, 1981.

158. Seaton A, Legge JS, Henderson J, et al: Accelerated silicosis in Scottish stonemasons, *Lancet* 337:341-344, 1991.

159. Sebastien P, Parson X, Gaudichet A, et al: Asbestos retention in human respiratory tissues: comparative measurements in lung parenchyma and in parietal pleura. In Wagner JC, ed: *Biological effects of mineral fibers,* vol 1, Lyon, France, 1980, International Agency for Research on Cancer, pp 237-246.

160. Shaver CG, Riddell AR: Lung changes associated with the manufacture of alumina abrasive, *J Ind Hyg* 29:145-157, 1947.

161. Sider L, Holland EA, Davis TM, et al: Changes on radiographs of wives of workers exposed to asbestos, *Radiology* 164:723-726, 1987.

162. Sinner WN: Pleuroma—a cancer-mimicking atelectatic pseudotumor of the lung, *Fortschr Roentgenstr* 133:578-585, 1980.

163. Solomon A: The radiology of asbestos-related diseases with special reference to diffuse mesothelioma, *Semin Oncol* 8:290-301, 1981.

164. Sperber M, Mohan KK: Computer tomography—a reliable diagnostic modality in pulmonary asbestosis, *Comput Radiol* 8:125-132, 1984.

165. Sprince NL, Kazemi H, Hardy HL: Current (1975) problems of differentiating between beryllium disease and sarcoidosis, *Ann NY Acad Sci* 278:654-664, 1976.

166. Staples CA, Gamsu G, Ray CS, et al: High resolution computed tomography and lung function in asbestos-exposed workers with normal chest radiographs, *Am Rev Respir Dis* 139:1502-1508, 1989.

167. Stark P: Round atelectasis: another pulmonary pseudotumor, *Am Rev Respir Dis* 125:248-250, 1982.

168. Stephens M, Gibbs AR, Pooley FD, et al: Asbestos induced diffuse pleural fibrosis: pathology and mineralogy, *Thorax* 42:583-588, 1987.

169. Suratt PM, Winn WC Jr, Brody AR, et al: Acute silicosis in tombstone sandblasters, *Am Rev Respir Dis* 115:521-529, 1977.

170. Swensen SJ, Aughenbaugh GL, Douglas WW, et al: High-resolution CT of the lungs: findings in various pulmonary diseases, *AJR* 158:971-979, 1992.

171. Talcott JA, Thurber WA, Kantor AF, et al: Asbestos-associated diseases in a cohort of cigarette-filter workers, *N Engl J Med* 321:1220-1223, 1989.

172. Teixidor HS, Novick GS, Rubin E: Pulmonary complications in burn patients, *J Can Assoc Radiol* 34:264-270, 1983.

173. Teixidor HS, Rubin E, Novick GS, et al: Smoke inhalation: radiologic manifestations, *Radiology* 149:383-387, 1983.

174. Tellesson WG: Rheumatoid pneumoconiosis (Caplan's syndrome) in an asbestos worker, *Thorax* 16:372-377, 1961.

175. Thiringer G, Blomqvist N, Brolin I: Pleural plaques in chest x-rays of lung cancer patients and matched controls (preliminary results), *Eur J Respir Dis* 61(suppl 107):119-122, 1980.

176. Trapnell DH: Septal lines in pneumoconiosis, *Br J Radiol* 37:805-810, 1964.

177. Tylen U, Nilsson U: Computed tomography in pulmonary pseudotumors and their relation to asbestos exposure, *J Comput Assist Tomogr* 6:229-237, 1981.

178. Verschakelen JA, Demaerel P, Coolen J, et al: Rounded atelectasis of the lung: MR appearance, *AJR* 152:965-966, 1989.

179. Wain SL, Roggli VL, Foster WL: Parietal pleural plaques, asbestos bodies and neoplasia: a clinical, pathologic and roentgenographic correlation of 25 consecutive cases, *Chest* 86:707-713, 1984.

180. Walker AM, Loughlin JE, Friedlander ER, et al: Projections of asbestos-related disease 1980-2009, *J Occup Med* 25:409-425, 1983.

181. Webb RW, Cooper C, Gamsu G: Interlobar pleural plaque mimicking a lung nodule in a patient with asbestos exposure, *J Comput Assist Tomogr* 7:135-136, 1983.

182. Weill H, Hughes JM: Asbestos as a public health risk: disease and policy, *Ann Rev Public Health* 7:171-192, 1986.

183. Wells IP, Bhatt RCV, Flanagan M: Kaolinosis: a radiological review, *Clin Radiol* 36:579-582, 1985.

184. Wesenberg RL, Blumhagen JD: Assisted expiratory chest radiography: effective technique for the diagnosis of foreign body aspiration, *Radiology* 130:538-539, 1979.

185. Williams JL, Moller GA: Solitary mass in the lungs of coal miners, *AJR* 117:765-770, 1973.

186. Wunderlich P, Rupprecht E, Trefftz R, et al: Chest radiographs of near-drowned children, *Pediatr Radiol* 15:297-299, 1985.

187. Yoshimura H, Hatakeyama M, Otsuji H, et al: Pulmonary asbestosis: CT study of subpleural curvilinear shadow, *Radiology* 158:653-658, 1986.

188. Youngberg AS: Unilateral diffuse lung opacity, *Radiology* 123:277-281, 1977.

189. Ziskind M, Jones RN, Weill H: Silicosis: state of the art, *Am Rev Respir Dis* 113:647-665, 1976.

190. Zwemer FL, Pratt DS, May JJ: Silo-fillers disease in New York State, *Am Rev Respir Dis* 146:650-653, 1992.

11 Drug- and Radiation-Induced Lung Disease

PAUL DEE

DRUG-INDUCED LUNG DISEASE

At present some 40 commonly used drugs have been shown to affect the lungs adversely. Prominent among these are the cytotoxic drugs used in the treatment of cancer and hematologic malignancies. Since the toxic effects of busulfan were first described over 30 years ago,[25] approximately 20 cytotoxic agents have been found to cause lung damage. This finding is perhaps not surprising, considering that cancer chemotherapy is essentially a form of controlled cellular poisoning. Pulmonary toxicity caused by noncytotoxic drugs occurs less frequently and less predictably. There is a great deal of overlap both clinically and radiographically in the toxic effects of different drugs. However, the radiographic manifestations of drug-induced disease are entirely nonspecific. Only a limited number of radiographic patterns reflect the changes in drug-induced disease. Hence any particular basic pattern can result from numerous different pathologic processes. The chest radiograph is simply one factor in a diagnostic equation that includes the clinical features, the nature of the drug therapy, the responses to alterations in therapy, hematologic and biochemical data, microbiologic testing, biopsy results, and other factors. Although chest radiography is the mainstay of imaging of drug-induced pulmonary reactions, several authors have studied the use of computed tomography (CT).[46,54,73,78] It is apparent that CT, particularly high-resolution CT, can detect the pulmonary changes of drug-induced reactions at an earlier stage than chest radiography, and this may have practical significance in a patient with altered pulmonary function tests. CT can better categorize the type of pulmonary reaction.

461

Padley and associates,[73] for example, were able to identify fibrotic reactions of diffuse alveolar damage and distinguish them from the ground-glass opacities of hypersensitivity reactions. Amiodarone toxicity, however, appears to be the only condition in which CT can be definitive by virtue of the high CT density of amiodarone deposits.[47,48,68,76] CT is best reserved for the problem case in which, for example, metastatic disease is difficult to distinguish from a drug-induced reaction or the patient's symptoms and pulmonary function tests do not correlate with the chest radiograph.

A number of clinicopathologic syndromes have been identified and linked to different drugs:

Direct toxic action on lung tissue with pulmonary infiltration and fibrosis
Hypersensitivity reactions
Systemic lupus erythematosus
Drug-induced phospholipidoses
Pulmonary edema
Pulmonary vasculitis
Pulmonary hemorrhage
Pulmonary thromboembolism
Pulmonary calcification
Pleural effusions and fibrosis
Mediastinal and hilar lymphadenopathy
Pulmonary granulomas
Mediastinal lipomatosis

A grasp of these clinicopathologic syndromes and their possible underlying mechanisms helps in understanding the various radiographic manifestations of toxic lung disease.

Mechanisms of injury

DIRECT TOXIC ACTION ON LUNG TISSUE. The mechanisms of direct toxic action of drugs on the lung are complex and poorly understood.[13] The production of excessive reactive oxygen metabolites and a disturbance of the complex oxidant-antioxidant system may result in damage to cells and cell membranes. Alveolar macrophages, polymorphonuclear leukocytes, and lymphocytes may be damaged, resulting in the release of leukokines, lymphokines, and other humoral factors with chemotactic, cytotoxic, or immune system–modulating effects. The balance between collagenosis and collagenolysis may be altered, causing excess collagen deposition that leads to pulmonary fibrosis. The collagen itself may be disordered either by damage to the fibroblasts or by the action of anticollagen antibodies. Inflammatory cells release proteolytic enzymes, and a complex antiprotease system exists to combat the effects of these enzymes. Any inhibition of the antiprotease systems could lead to damage.

Histologic study shows swelling of the endothelial cells, fibrinous exudate in the interstitium and the alveoli, interstitial inflammatory cell infiltrate, and necrosis of type I alveolar epithelial cells.[102] Hyaline membranes may form. Later, dysplastic type II alveolar epithelial cells

proliferate, and depending on the extent of damage, fibroblast proliferation and collagen deposition also occur. The toxic effects cause both interstitial lung disease and, to a variable extent, an acinar filling process. These processes are variably reflected on the chest radiographs, depending on the extent of the reaction and the degree of permanent damage and fibrosis.

Direct toxic action on lung tissue usually takes some time to reach a clinically appreciable threshold, and the effects may not be manifest for weeks or months after treatment has begun. In many cases the effect is dose related, a relationship that is most apparent with the cytotoxic agents bleomycin, busulfan, and carmustine. The toxic effects may be enhanced by other factors such as increasing age, decreased renal function, radiation therapy, oxygen therapy, and other cytotoxic drug therapy.[13]

HYPERSENSITIVITY REACTIONS. The molecular size of drugs is too small to provoke an immune response, and it is therefore likely that they act as haptenes in combination with endogenous protein. The immune responses provoked are most commonly type I (immediate hypersensitivity reactions) or type III (immune complex reactions). The airways show bronchial constriction, mucous hypersecretion and inspissation, and mucosal edema with eosinophilic infiltration. The lung parenchyma may show patchy areas of edema and inflammatory reaction, with a preponderance of eosinophils in the cellular infiltrate.

Hypersensitivity reactions are usually immediate and may become clinically apparent within hours or days of beginning therapy with the offending drug. Predominant airway involvement causes an asthmalike syndrome, whereas pulmonary parenchymal involvement results in patchy eosinophilic infiltrates. These infiltrates are often fleeting, and eosinophilia may be present in the peripheral blood. Withdrawal of the offending drug and administration of corticosteroids usually results in prompt and complete clearing.

NEURAL OR HUMORAL MECHANISMS. Neurogenic noncardiac pulmonary edema is the most common neural response and is encountered particularly with certain central nervous system depressants. The pulmonary capillary permeability for proteins is altered either by a direct toxic action on the lung or by impulses emanating from the brainstem and hypothalamus.[24,92] Fluid exudes into the pulmonary interstitium and alveoli, and the result may be analogous to cardiogenic edema in the rapidity of onset and the radiographic features. However, not all cases of drug-induced pulmonary edema operate through this central neurogenic mechanism. A number of drugs cause water and salt retention, leading to fluid imbalances. A direct toxic action on the pulmonary capillary bed is also possible.[58]

Asthma may result from other, less conspicuous neurohumoral mechanisms. Certain drugs, for example, beta-adrenergic antagonists such as propranolol and parasympatheticomimetics such as neostigmine, cause asthma by directly affecting bronchial innervation. Aspirin may cause asthma by inhibiting prostaglandin synthesis.[33]

AUTOIMMUNE MECHANISMS. A number of drugs cause a systemic lupus erythematosus syndrome, presumably by triggering an autoimmune response. The pleural and pulmonary manifestations of the drug-induced syndrome are indistinguishable from those of the spontaneous form of the disease. Antinuclear factors are detectable in the serum and are found in many patients taking these drugs even in the absence of clinical or radiographic evidence of systemic lupus erythematosus.

VASCULITIS, THROMBOEMBOLISM, PULMONARY VASOSPASM, AND PULMONARY HEMORRHAGE. The association between pulmonary vasculitis and drugs is perhaps strongest with the sulfonamides, although the list of potential causative drugs is extensive. Pulmonary involvement is usually associated with and often overshadowed by systemic vasculitis, particularly involving the skin, kidneys, and liver. The result of the pulmonary vasculitis is patchy pulmonary infarction and hemorrhage that may cause acute interstitial infiltration or patchy airspace consolidation. The vasculitis may be an expression of a type III (immune complex) or a type IV (cell-mediated) hypersensitivity response.

Intravenous administration of illicit drugs may cause a granulomatous vasculitis with resultant pulmonary hypertension. The vasculitis in these cases is caused by contaminants or suspending agents such as talc, starch, or cellulose and is more like a foreign body reaction.[79] On occasion the granulomatous response is so extensive and severe as to resemble the progressive massive fibrosis seen in silicosis.[15]

Thromboembolism is particularly associated with the oral contraceptives and estrogens.[69] It is important to identify this group of patients because the individuals are young and otherwise healthy. They are at risk for secondary pulmonary arterial hypertension.

Oil embolism occurs to some extent in all properly conducted lymphangiography examinations. Only when patients have poor pulmonary reserve or when excessive amounts of the contrast medium are administered is there any potential for harm. A transient miliary nodular pattern, accompanied on occasion by slight fever and slight dyspnea on exertion, is the most that should be expected under normal circumstances.[57]

Pulmonary vasospasm appears to be rare. The best documented instance of this complication occurred in the 1960s when Aminorex, an over-the-counter appetite suppressant, was marketed in Europe. The pulmonary arteriolar vasospasm caused pulmonary arterial hypertension leading to cor pulmonale.[23]

Pulmonary hemorrhage is usually secondary to a disorder of the clotting mechanisms. In some cases, as in oxyphenbutazone- or quinidine-induced thrombocytopenia, the coagulopathy is unexpected and idiosyncratic. Most commonly, however, the hemorrhage is the result of

anticoagulant therapy and is therefore not entirely unexpected. In rare instances penicillamine causes a syndrome of pulmonary hemorrhage with or without renal failure, similar to Goodpasture's syndrome and idiopathic pulmonary hemosiderosis, respectively.[55] Penicillamine-induced pulmonary hemorrhage is presumed to be an immune complex disorder. The predominant effect of pulmonary hemorrhage is patchy airspace consolidation of variable severity, which is generally rapid in onset and clears fairly quickly. Hemoptysis and a falling hematocrit value may be the only clinical clues to the nature of the process.

DRUG-INDUCED PHOSPHOLIPIDOSES. The lungs have a number of metabolic functions other than respiration and acid-base balance. These include the inactivation of various endogenous amines such as norepinephrine, 5-hydroxytryptamine, serotonin, and some prostaglandins. Certain drugs are capable of entering and saturating these carrier mechanisms. Together with phospholipids, these drugs form complexes that are resistant to breakdown by phospholipases. The process results in an abnormal accumulation of phospholipids within the cells. A notable example of a drug-induced phospholipidosis is that caused by the antiarrhythmic drug amiodarone (see boxes on pp. 464 to 466).[32,43]

Radiographic features of adverse drug reactions in the lung

DIFFUSE ALVEOLAR DAMAGE. In the early stages of toxicity the chest radiograph may be normal even when gallium scanning, CT scanning, pulmonary function testing, or lung biopsies give direct or indirect evidence of diffuse alveolar damage. The radiographic shadows of diffuse alveolar damage are variably interstitial, alveolar, or mixed in type, and it is usually clear that the problem is a generalized pulmonary process (Figures 11-1 and 11-2). Segmental or lobar consolidations are not a feature of diffuse toxic lung damage. The shadowing tends to be more apparent in the lung bases. Pleural effusions are rarely found, except in some cases of procarbazine or methotrexate toxicity. However, such effusions might occur as part of a hypersensitivity response. On rare occasion, diffuse alveolar damage, caused for example by cytoxan, bleomycin, and methotrexate, results in single or multiple pulmonary masses or nodules, which are likely to cause diagnostic confusion with neoplasm in a patient being treated for a malignant process.[29]

Most cases of diffuse alveolar damage secondary to drugs develop in patients undergoing chemotherapy for various malignant processes, a group in whom diffuse pulmonary shadowing could develop from causes other than drug toxicity. These causes include lymphangitis carcinomatosa, leukemic or lymphomatous infiltration of the lung, opportunistic infections such as *Pneumocystis carinii* pneumonia, and pulmonary hemorrhage. The clinical circumstances, sequence of events, and radiographic appearances may provide circumstantial evidence

DRUGS CAUSING HYPERSENSITIVITY LUNG DISEASE

ANTIARTHRITIC

Aurothioglucose

ANTIASTHMATIC

Cromolyn sodium

ANTIBACTERIALS

Erythromycin
Nitrofurantoin
Paraaminosalicylic acid
Isoniazid
Penicillin
Sulfonamides

ANTIDEPRESSANT

Imipramine

ANTIHYPERTENSIVES

Mecamylamine
Hydralazine

CENTRAL NERVOUS SYSTEM STIMULANT

Methylphenidate

CYTOTOXIC AGENTS

Bleomycin
Methotrexate
Procarbazine
Azathioprine

HYPOGLYCEMIC AGENT

Chlorpropamide

MUSCLE RELAXANT

Dantrolene

CHELATING AGENT

Penicillamine

DRUGS CAUSING DIFFUSE ALVEOLAR DAMAGE

CYTOTOXIC AGENTS

Azathioprine
BCNU
Bleomycin
Busulfan
CCNU
Chlorambucil
Chlorozotocin
Cyclophosphamide
Cytosine arabinoside
Melphalan
6-Mercaptopurine
Methotrexate
Methyl CCNU
Mitomycin
Neocarzinostatin
VM 26
Vinblastine
Vindesine

NONCYTOTOXIC AGENTS

Antibacterial
Nitrofurantoin
Sulfasalazine
Antiarrhythmics
Amiodarone
Tocainide
Antimigraine
Methysergide
Antihypertensives
Hexamethonium
Mecamylamine
Pentolinium
Miscellaneous
Penicillamine
Gold salts
Amitriptyline
Oxygen

DRUGS CAUSING PULMONARY EDEMA

ANALGESICS

Acetylsalicylic acid
Codeine
Pentazocine

ANTIBACTERIAL

Nitrofurantoin

ANTIDEPRESSANTS

Amitryptyline
Doxepin
Desipramine
Imipramine

ANTIINFLAMMATORIES

Phenylbutazone
Oxyphenbutazone

BETA-ADRENERGIC AGONISTS

Ritodrine
Terbutaline

CYTOXIC AGENTS

Cyclophosphamide
Methotrexate
Cytosine arabinoside

DIURETICS

Hydrochlorothiazide

IMMUNE SUPPRESSANTS

Interleukin-2
OKT3

PHENOTHIAZINES

Chlorpromazine

SEDATIVES

Chlordiazepoxide
Ethchlorvynol

OPIATES

Heroin
Propoxyphene
Methadone

ORGANOPHOSPHATE INSECTICIDES

Parathion
Malathion

MISCELLANEOUS

Iodinated ionic radiographic contrast media
Dextran
Colchicine
Epinephrine

DRUGS THAT INDUCE SYSTEMIC LUPUS ERYTHEMATOSUS

ANTIBACTERIALS

Griseofulvin
Isoniazid
Nitrofurantoin
Paraaminosalicylic acid
Penicillin
Streptomycin
Sulfonamides

ANTICONVULSANTS

Carbamazepine
Ethosuximide
Methsuximide
Phenytoin
Primidone
Trimethadone

ANTIINFLAMMATORIES

Phenylbutazone
Oxyphenbutazone

CARDIOVASCULAR PREPARATIONS

Clofibrate
Digitalis
Hydralazine
Methyldopa
Procainamide
Propranolol
Reserpine
Quinidine

DIURETICS

Chlorthalidone
Thiazides

THYROID BLOCKERS

Thiouracil
Propylthiouracil

MISCELLANEOUS

Phenothiazines
Penicillamine
Methysergide
Gold salts
Levodopa

DRUGS ASSOCIATED WITH PULMONARY VASCULITIS

ANTIASTHMATICS

Cromolyn sodium

ANTIBACTERIALS

Sulfonamides
Penicillin

ANTICONVULSANTS

Phenytoin

ANTIINFLAMMATORIES

Phenylbutazone

CARDIOVASCULAR PREPARATIONS

Quinidine
Hydralazine

CYTOTOXIC AGENTS

Busulfan

THYROID BLOCKERS

Thiouracil
Propylthiouracil

TRANQUILIZERS

Phenothiazines

ILLICIT INTRAVENOUS DRUG USE (TALC)

DRUGS CAUSING PULMONARY HEMORRHAGE

Anticoagulants
Estrogens
Penicillamine
Quinidine
Oxyphenbutazone

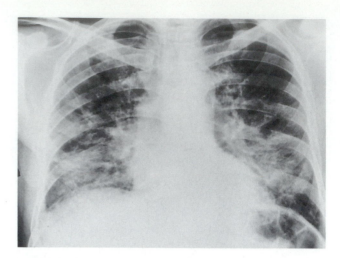

FIGURE 11-1
Diffuse alveolar damage resulting from bleomycin, showing basally predominant pulmonary infiltration.

that drug-induced diffuse alveolar damage is present. Recourse to lung biopsy may, however, be necessary on occasion. The radiographic appearances alone do not permit a firm diagnosis of diffuse alveolar damage.

HYPERSENSITIVITY REACTIONS. Hypersensitivity reactions are often apparent within hours or days of beginning treatment. Fever and peripheral eosinophilia are features of these reactions and provide useful diagnostic clues. Predominant involvement of the airways produces an asthmalike syndrome that lacks specific radiographic features. Parenchymal involvement may result in a condition similar to cryptogenic acute or chronic pulmonary eosinophilia (see p. 525). Focal patchy consolidations develop, often in the periphery of the lung (Figure 11-3). The extent of consolidation varies, and the distribution within the peripheral lung zones is random. The shadows represent an acinar filling process and are usually subsegmental in size (Figure 11-4). They tend to be fleeting — resolving in one area of the lung only to appear in another. Particularly following previous exposure the hypersensitivity reaction is hyperacute and is seen as pulmonary edema with interstitial or even alveolar densities (Figure 11-5). On other occasions the physician encounters a diffuse reticulonodular pattern, a reaction exemplified by the hypersensitivity response to methotrexate. The response to discontinuation of the offending drug is usually prompt. If rechallenge with the drug is attempted, the same hypersensitivity reaction may be expected. Only three cytotoxic agents, bleomycin, methotrexate, and procarbazine, are associated with the hypersensitivity reaction. With bleomycin, a hypersensitivity reaction occurs far less frequently than diffuse alveolar damage.

PULMONARY EDEMA. The edema resulting from the toxic effect of drugs is indistinguishable from cardiogenic edema both in radiographic appearance (see p. 409) and in rapidity of onset and clearing (Figures 11-6 and 11-7).

SYSTEMIC LUPUS ERYTHEMATOSUS. The systemic lupus erythematosus syndrome that results from the toxic effects of drugs does not differ in its pleural or pulmonary manifestations from the idiopathic form of the disease. Pleural effusions are by far the most common manifestation of this condition, and there may be a concomitant pericardial effusion (Figure 11-8). The fact that some of the most common drugs causing this condition are used in the treatment of cardiac disease may delay the realization that pleuropericardial effusions and interstitial lung disease are a complication of therapy rather than a manifestation of the primary disease. At least 90% of

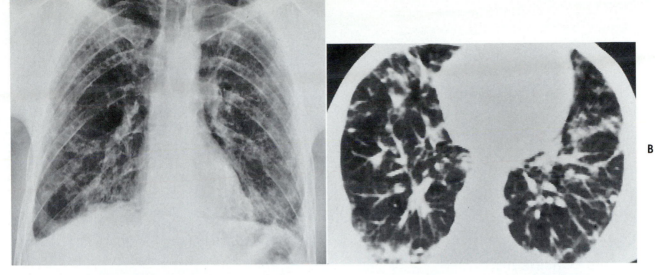

FIGURE 11-2
Diffuse alveolar damage resulting from bleomycin. **A,** Diffuse coarse pulmonary infiltration. **B,** Computed tomographic scan of the same patient showing scattered irregular parenchymal densities. (Courtesy Dr. Elizabeth Bellamy, London.)

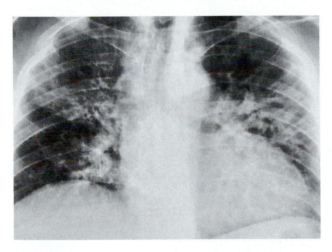

FIGURE 11-3
Hypersensitivity pneumonia (biopsy proven) secondary to administration of desipramine. Shadowing in this case is more central than is usual.

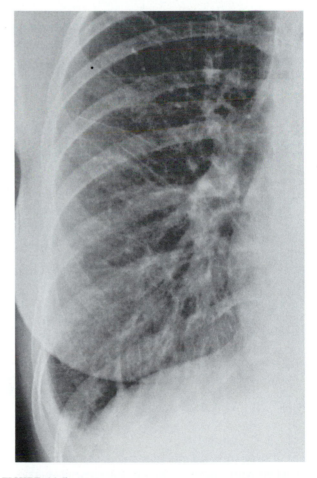

FIGURE 11-5
Hyperacute hypersensitivity reaction to nitrofurantoin showing interstitial edema and small pleural effusion. The patient, a young woman, developed dyspnea and tachypnea a few hours after a single dose of nitrofurantoin.

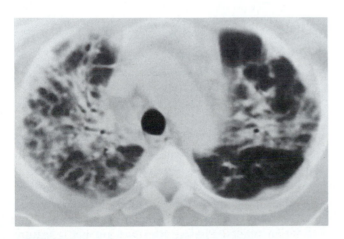

FIGURE 11-4
Computed tomographic scan of the patient in Figure 11-3. Peripheral infiltrates are seen in the right lung, whereas these are less pronounced in the left lung.

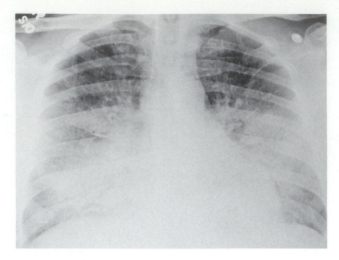

FIGURE 11-6
Pulmonary edema secondary to intravenous administration of cocaine. The patient, a young man, recovered promptly with only supportive therapy.

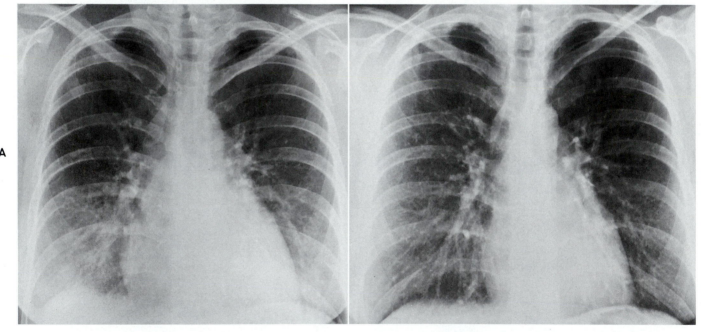

FIGURE 11-7
A, Fluid overload following induction of labor using pitocin. B, Prompt recovery occurred within 24 hours. Note change in size of the azygous vein.

cases of drug-induced systemic lupus erythematosus are associated with procainamide, hydralazine, isoniazid, or phenytoin. When parenchymal shadowing occurs, it is predominantly basal and interstitial. Actual parenchymal involvement is, however, a comparatively unusual manifestation of the systemic lupus erythematosus syndrome.

PULMONARY VASCULITIS. The radiographic findings in pulmonary vasculitis are variable and nonspecific.

Patchy subsegmental infiltrates with a random peripheral distribution may occur, a pattern similar to the hypersensitivity pattern except that fluctuations are not so marked. In other patients diffuse coarse streaky shadows may be seen that may appear interstitial in some patients and alveolar in others. Pleural effusions are not a feature. Cavitation may occur in areas of infarction caused by the vasculitis. The radiographic findings in this complication

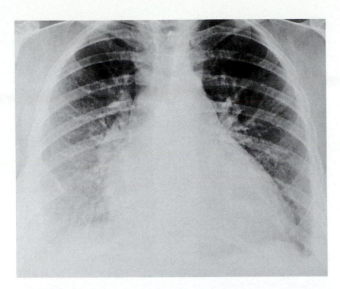

FIGURE 11-8
Procainamide-induced systemic lupus erythematosus showing pleuropericardial effusions.

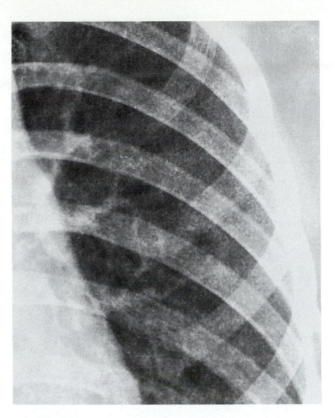

FIGURE 11-9
Oil embolization. Radiograph taken 24 hours following ethiodol lymphography shows fine diffuse granular infiltration of lung.

are probably the least specific of all adverse reactions to drugs. A diagnosis of pulmonary vasculitis is unlikely to be made without biopsy evidence of vasculitis in the lungs or other organ systems.

PULMONARY THROMBOEMBOLISM, OIL EMBOLISM. As previously indicated, some degree of oil embolism is to be expected during lymphangiography. For this reason patients with poor respiratory function should not undergo this form of examination. A very fine miliary nodular pattern may be detected on good-quality radiographs taken 24 to 48 hours following the administration of contrast medium (Figure 11-9). At the same time the patient may experience mild fever and slight shortness of breath on exertion. These clinical and radiographic findings are transient.

PULMONARY HEMORRHAGE. Pulmonary hemorrhage rarely occurs as a toxic reaction to drug therapy. It causes diffuse patchy alveolar shadowing, which may be extensive and severe. Depending on the rapidity and severity of the hemorrhage, there may be a fall in the hematocrit values, and hemoptysis is common. The radiographic findings are confined to the pulmonary parenchyma, and there are no associated pleural, hilar, or mediastinal abnormalities. Drug-induced pulmonary hemorrhage is likely to be an isolated event, and chronic lung sequelae, such as those in patients with idiopathic pulmonary hemosiderosis or Goodpasture's syndrome, are not to be expected. Radionuclide studies using Tc-99m-tagged red blood cells offer a method of diagnosing this condition.[104]

PULMONARY CALCIFICATION. The most frequent cause of pulmonary parenchymal calcification is hyperparathyroidism, but pulmonary calcification has also been found after prolonged vitamin D and calcium therapy and in the milk alkali syndrome. The calcification

is extremely fine and cannot usually be resolved into distinct microcalculi like those seen in pulmonary microlithiasis. The calcifications are generally patchy and produce cloudlike shadowing of unusually high radiographic density.

PLEURAL EFFUSIONS AND FIBROSIS. Pleural effusions most commonly occur in association with the systemic lupus erythematosus syndrome. In over 50% of patients with drug-induced systemic lupus erythematosus, pleural effusions develop at some stage of the illness. Effusions may be noted in hypersensitivity reactions to drugs, for example, nitrofurantoin, methotrexate, and procarbazine. The effusions associated with systemic lupus erythematosus and hypersensitivity reactions can be expected to resolve without trace. Methysergide, on the other hand, is associated with the development of pleural fibrosis as well as pleural fluid.[27] Irregular masses of pleural fibrosis may be interspersed with loculated pleural fluid, and there may be associated mediastinal fibrosis. Ergotamine and ergonovine maleate may produce similar effects.

HILAR AND MEDIASTINAL ADENOPATHY. The principal drugs causing hilar and mediastinal adenopathy are phenytoin and methotrexate. The adenopathy caused by methotrexate is part of the hypersensitivity reaction to this drug. Since methotrexate is used in the treatment of

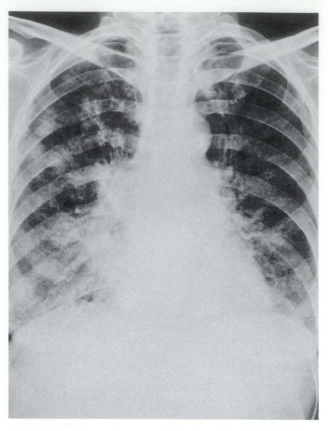

FIGURE 11-10
Chronic lipoid pneumonia in an elderly woman with a hiatal hernia and chronic constipation. The patient had used mineral oils for many years and also had esophageal reflux.

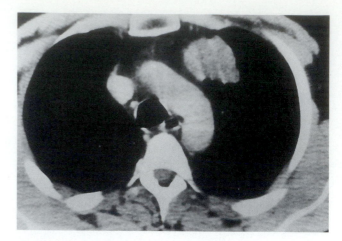

FIGURE 11-11
Computed tomographic scan of focal lipoid pneumonia. This mass so closely resembled pulmonary neoplasm that it was resected.

malignant processes, the possibility of mistaking the hypersensitivity reaction for tumoral adenopathy is real. Phenytoin-induced adenopathy is usually based on a hypersensitivity reaction. Phenytoin may, however, cause a pseudolymphoma syndrome with generalized adenopathy, fever, skin rashes, eosinophilia, and hepatosplenomegaly. Moreover, there is a slightly increased risk of the development of lymphoma in patients taking this drug. Angioimmunoblastic lymphadenopathy is another manifestation of the adverse effects of phenytoin on the hematologic system.

PULMONARY GRANULOMAS. Pulmonary granulomas are aggregations of pulmonary macrophages reacting to certain microorganisms, foreign particles, various drugs such as methotrexate and nitrofurantoin, or other stimuli as yet undefined. A fairly common form of granulomatous reaction is seen following chronic aspiration of mineral oils. These "paraffinomas" are usually seen as chronic bibasilar, often conglomerate, masses (Figures 11-10 and 11-11). Pulmonary granulomas may develop as a reaction to particulate suspending agents in intravenously administered oral drugs. Talc is the most commonly used filler for drugs, and since it is a silicate, it produces a granulomatous reaction.[86] Granulomatous angiitis may

result in pulmonary hypertension.[79] Alternatively, disseminated granulomatosis may be produced and can become radiographically visible as a diffuse interstitial pulmonary shadowing. More unusually, large conglomerate masses similar to the progressive massive fibrosis of classic silicosis develop in the upper lung zones.[15]

MEDIASTINAL LIPOMATOSIS. Corticosteroids may cause excessive fat deposition in the mediastinum, a finding rather grandiosely termed mediastinal lipomatosis. Widening of the mediastinum may be noted radiographically and may cause concern, particularly in patients being treated for malignant processes. Additional evidence of fat deposition may be seen as extrapleural fat thickening along the lateral chest walls or as increasingly prominent cardiac fat pads (Figure 11-12). CT readily determines the nature of the process but should scarcely be necessary.

Specific drugs and their adverse effects

Certain drugs are discussed in greater detail either because adverse effects are relatively common or serious or because the adverse effects have noteworthy features.

BLEOMYCIN. The cytotoxic antibiotic bleomycin is used in the treatment of squamous cell carcinoma, lymphoma, and testicular neoplasms. It is concentrated in the lung, which is therefore a primary target for adverse effects. Toxicity is related to the cumulative dose and significantly increases when doses exceed a total of 400 mg.[62] The incidence of overt pulmonary toxic side effects has varied from 4%[103] to 15%.[105] The frequency and severity of pulmonary toxicity increase with age, prior or concomitant radiation therapy, oxygen therapy, decreased renal function, or concomitant treatment with other chemotherapeutic agents.[105]

An acute hypersensitivity reaction to low doses of bleomycin can occur. However, diffuse alveolar damage is the most common and most significant toxic pulmo-

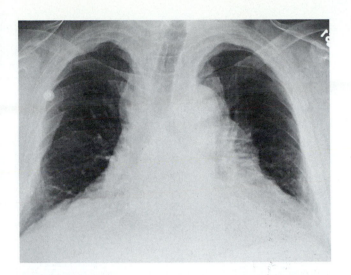

FIGURE 11-12
Medial lipomatosis in a patient receiving long-term steroid therapy. Note the extrapleural fat deposits along the lateral chest wall.

nary reaction. Bleomycin toxicity ordinarily becomes manifest within 3 months after therapy is begun. The chest radiograph may be normal despite decreased diffusing capacity, abnormal lung accumulation of gallium-67, increased CT attenuation by the lung, and abnormal pulmonary lavage or biopsy findings.[4,77] On the other hand, Wolkowicz and associates[105] found radiographic abnormalities in 40% of patients receiving an average dose of 555 mg. However, only 15% were symptomatic or had detectable pulmonary function abnormalities.[105] The initial radiographic changes are predominantly basal and reticulonodular in character (Figures 11-1 and 11-2). Progression of disease may result in conglomerate acinar shadowing. On occasion discrete pulmonary nodules simulating metastases may be seen.[11,29,84] The acute hypersensitivity reaction causes a relatively rapid appearance of patchy acinar shadowing with a random distribution, changes that resolve rapidly when therapy is discontinued. On the other hand, diffuse alveolar damage may be progressive and lead to irreversible pulmonary fibrosis. The earlier the toxic effects are detected, the greater is the likelihood of a favorable response to discontinuation of the drug. Hence strict surveillance of patients under treatment with bleomycin, as with all patients undergoing chemotherapy, is imperative.

BUSULFAN. Busulfan is used in the treatment of chronic myelogenous leukemia and was one of the earliest chemotherapeutic agents.[25] The reported incidence of toxic pulmonary changes ranges from 2% to 10%. Evidence of pulmonary toxicity may be detected within months of starting treatment, but some patients do not have toxic changes for several years. This variability makes the existence of a true dose relationship uncertain. The pulmonary changes are those of interstitial and

intraalveolar fibrosis with a predominantly reticular pattern on the chest radiograph.

METHOTREXATE. Methotrexate is used extensively in the treatment of hematologic and other malignancies and is also used to treat a number of benign conditions such as psoriasis. Pulmonary toxicity occurs in some 7% of cases according to the most reliable estimate available.[91] Methotrexate toxicity differs in certain respects from the toxicity induced by other cytotoxic drugs. The condition being treated appears to play a role in determining whether toxic reactions occur. For example, patients with acute lymphocytic leukemia have a relatively high incidence of toxic reactions to methotrexate compared with patients being treated for trophoblastic tumors or osteogenic sarcomas.[31] Methotrexate is also unusual in that a hypersensitivity response accompanied by pulmonary consolidations and peripheral eosinophilia is fairly frequent. Hilar and mediastinal adenopathy may also occur as part of the hypersensitivity reaction, a unique feature among the cytotoxic drugs. Pleural effusions may occur and may be associated with the development of acute pleuritis.[96] Intrathecal administration of methotrexate has been associated with the development of pulmonary edema.[5]

Despite these atypical effects, diffuse alveolar damage leading to restrictive lung disease remains the significant complication. Fibrosis occurs in an estimated 10% of patients with methotrexate-induced pulmonary toxicity.

The prognosis is generally favorable, with an overall mortality of approximately 1%. Corticosteroids may help in cases of hypersensitivity lung disease. In some cases pulmonary complications resolve despite continued use of the drug, and in other cases rechallenge does not cause a recurrence of toxic manifestations.

NITROFURANTOIN. Nitrofurantoin is an antiseptic agent that has been widely used in the treatment of urinary tract infections. Over 80% of cases of nitrofurantoin-induced pulmonary toxicity occur in women, largely because of their higher incidence of urinary tract infection.[36] The incidence of adverse reactions is probably not high; the large number of reported cases is more a reflection of the extensive use of the drug in the past.

The pulmonary reaction to nitrofurantoin may be divided into two distinct patterns, an acute form and a chronic form. The acute form, an acute hypersensitivity reaction (a lupus reaction occurs but is rare), is far more common, constituting some 90% of reactions.[36] Symptoms appear within 1 month of the beginning of nitrofurantoin therapy, or within 24 hours if the patient was previously sensitized. Symptoms include fever, chest pain, dyspnea, nonproductive cough, arthralgias, and rashes. Peripheral eosinophilia is common. Chest radiographs show basally predominant interstitial or mixed interstitial-alveolar shadowing. Pleural effusions occur fairly frequently and are usually small. Particularly in hyperacute presentations the pattern resembles cardiogenic edema, especially in the rapidity of its appearance

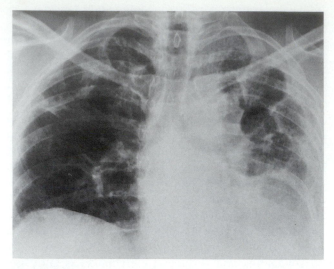

FIGURE 11-13
Chronic nitrofurantoin toxicity showing very coarse linear infiltrates with some lung volume reduction.

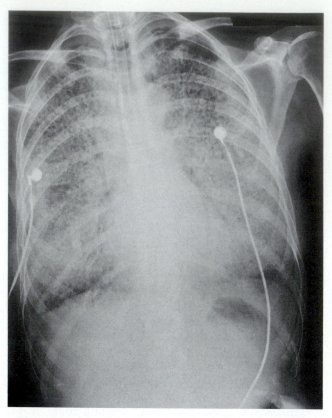

FIGURE 11-14
Pulmonary edema in a chronic aspirin abuser. Blood salicylate level exceeded 40 mg/dl.

(Figure 11-5). Response to withdrawal of the drug is prompt and almost invariably complete.

The chronic form of reaction develops only after some 6 months of nitrofurantoin therapy (Figure 11-13). In many instances the patient has had several years of therapy before manifesting a pulmonary toxic effect. The pulmonary reaction, a fibrosing alveolitis, is reflected on the chest radiograph as a chronic basally predominant interstitial pattern accompanied by a gradual reduction in lung volume. Improvement usually follows discontinuation of nitrofurantoin therapy, an important diagnostic feature. Depending on the duration and severity of the changes, resolution may not be complete, and approximately 10% of patients die.[36]

HYDROCHLOROTHIAZIDE. Adverse reactions to the widely used diuretic hydrochlorothiazide are extremely rare, and the drug is widely regarded as safe. Nevertheless, the acute onset of a form of pulmonary edema within hours of taking the drug is well described.[6] Hydrochlorothiazide is normally used in an older population group for the treatment of hypertension and heart disease. In such patients pulmonary edema is not unusual, and the diagnosis of an adverse drug reaction may not be established until rechallenge elicits the same reaction.

TRICYCLIC ANTIDEPRESSANTS. The widespread use of tricyclic antidepressants in a population group prone to attempt suicide probably explains why tricyclic antidepressant overdose is a common cause of admission to intensive care units. Pulmonary problems in these patients are overshadowed by the problems of coma, seizures, and cardiac arrhythmias. Apart from producing the nonspecific problems of aspiration pneumonia and atelectasis, the tricyclic antidepressants are known to cause interstitial pulmonary edema and adult respiratory distress syndrome.[83,97] The mechanism of edema produc-

tion is unknown, although it does not appear to be cardiac in origin. Pulmonary edema develops in approximately 10% of patients and is more likely to occur with severe overdoses. The great majority of patients recover quickly and are only transiently under intensive care. That 40% to 50% of patients have some chest radiographic abnormality while under intensive care is not surprising. Most abnormalities on chest radiographs are nonspecific airspace shadows and atelectasis.

SALICYLATES. Salicylates probably exert their adverse effects by inhibiting prostaglandin synthesis. In some patients this leads to bronchospasm. The other principal effect is an alteration in capillary permeability of the lungs, a process leading to noncardiogenic pulmonary edema (Figure 11-14). Salicylate-induced pulmonary edema generally occurs only with blood levels greater than 30 mg/dl and may be related to acute or chronic intoxication.[33] The radiographic features of salicylate-induced pulmonary edema are indistinguishable from those of cardiogenic edema. Increasing age and smoking are risk factors. Neurologic disturbances and proteinuria are frequently associated features and possibly indicate alterations in capillary permeability elsewhere. It is interesting therefore that a clinical presentation similar to toxic shock syndrome has been reported in chronic salicylate intoxication.[50] The extravascular fluid losses result in tachycardia, reduced systemic vascular resistance, hypotension, and multiple organ system failure, including adult respiratory distress syndrome.

MINERAL OIL ASPIRATION. Chronic aspiration of mineral oils or vegetable oils used as laxatives or lubricants is most common in elderly patients with swallowing disorders or hiatal hernias. The result is a granulomatous infiltration of the lung associated with fibrosis, which tends to be basal and may be localized or more generalized (Figures 11-11 and 11-12). In the early stages the chest radiograph shows alveolar consolidation, which may become confluent and masslike with the ensuing fibrosis. The changes may be extensive, and the resultant contraction of the lungs can be severe. An isolated area of chronic lipoid pneumonia is easily mistaken for a primary pulmonary neoplasm (Figure 11-12). The diagnosis can be difficult, since many patients fail to volunteer information about their use of mineral oils. Too often they regard the use of mineral oils as something normal and inconsequential. The diagnosis has been established by both CT examination and percutaneous needle aspiration.[101] With CT the areas of lipoid pneumonia may have a low attenuation comparable to fat.

GOLD SALTS. Gold salts used in the treatment of rheumatoid arthritis probably cause pulmonary toxicity in less than 1% of patients,[14] although much higher incidences have been reported. Pulmonary toxicity is overshadowed by the far more frequent complications of stomatitis and dermatitis. Pulmonary toxicity occurs within 3 months of beginning of therapy and usually develops subacutely. The most common reaction is hypersensitivity with a variable combination of diffuse reticulonodular and patchy alveolar densities.[20,98] Patients may have evidence of a hypersensitivity response in other systems, with fever, proteinuria, or a skin rash. Such manifestations of hypersensitivity may precede the pulmonary abnormalities and be associated with peripheral eosinophilia. Diffuse alveolar damage with fibrosis is also noted on occasion. A lupus reaction is exceptionally uncommon. The major diagnostic problem is that the disease under treatment, rheumatoid arthritis, may itself be associated with diffuse interstitial disease. However, the shadowing associated with gold-induced toxic reactions can in most instances be expected to resolve on cessation of therapy, particularly if steroid therapy is administered. Pulmonary disease related to gold therapy tends to be acute or subacute in onset, whereas pulmonary involvement in rheumatoid arthritis is more insidious and is inexorably progressive.

METHYSERGIDE. Methysergide, an ergot alkaloid, is interesting because it may be associated with a syndrome consisting of chronic pleural effusions accompanied by irregular pleural thickening.[27] Rounded atelectasis may also be associated. The syndrome becomes manifest 6 months to several years after therapy begins. Depending on the extent of the fibrosis a variable degree of regression

occurs after cessation of therapy. There does not appear to be any definite association with the endomyocardial, mediastinal, and retroperitoneal fibrosis that also occurs with methysergide therapy. Ergotamine tartrate, another ergot derivative, used in the treatment of migraine headaches, has also been incriminated in causing pleural effusions and fibrosis.[94]

BROMOCRIPTINE. Bromocriptine is an ergot alkaloid derivative used in the treatment of Parkinson's disease and prolactinemia. Bromocriptine is an extremely effective and valuable treatment for these conditions and cannot be readily abandoned or replaced. The chemical structure of bromocriptine is similar to that of methysergide, which may account for the occurrence of pleural effusions and fibrosis in a small minority of patients receiving bromocriptine therapy. Less than 5% of patients are affected, and all reported patients have been male.[44,60] Adverse effects appear to be confined to the pleura and adjacent lung. Symptoms and radiographic signs of effusion and pleural fibrosis usually take months or years to evolve. Slow resolution occurs after cessation of treatment, although it appears that the situation will stabilize if continuation of treatment is necessary.

INTERLEUKIN-2. Interleukin-2 is used in the treatment of disseminated malignancies, notably renal cell carcinoma and malignant melanoma. An extremely high incidence of toxicity is associated with interleukin-2 therapy; thoracic radiographic abnormalities are found in 50% to 80% of patients.[12,17,59,85] The basis for the clinical and radiographic findings appears to be a diffuse capillary leak syndrome caused by a toxic effect of interleukin-2 on the vascular endothelium.[81] The consequent depletion of intravascular volume may result in a clinical state analogous to the toxic shock syndrome, with diminished peripheral vascular resistance, hypotension, severe tachycardia, and decreased cardiac output. A direct myocardial toxic effect[71] may complicate matters and contribute to the pulmonary edema, but the pulmonary capillary wedge pressure usually remains normal.[26]

The onset of signs and symptoms of toxicity usually is closely related to the initiation of therapy. In the series reported by Saxon and co-workers[85] radiologic abnormalities developed within 4 days in 50% of patients, within 8 days in 75%, and beyond 8 days in only 25%. The radiologic findings are essentially those of diffuse interstitial or alveolar edema. Patients with diffuse alveolar edema may pass through phases of interstitial edema. Saxon and co-workers[85] found focal lobar or segmental consolidation in about one fourth of the patients in their series but imply that these focal consolidations may have resulted from nosocomial infection, an association also noted by Snydman and associates.[90] Pleural effusions occur in over 50% of patients, and this incidence may be underestimated. In contrast, pleural effusions are unusual in other pulmonary capillary leak syndromes such as neurogenic edema or adult respiratory distress syndrome. Presumably the effusions reflect the widespread systemic capillary leak. The signs of toxicity usually resolve completely within 2 weeks after cessation of therapy.[80] Although the incidence of toxicity is high, deaths attributable solely to interleukin-2 therapy are rare.

OKT3. OKT3 is a monoclonal antibody used in the treatment of acute rejection of allografts. OKT3 interacts with the T3 antigen of human T cells, thereby blocking the rejection reaction. OKT3 toxicity is manifested as acute pulmonary edema, usually occurring within hours of the commencement of therapy. Fluid is restricted before the administration of OKT3 to limit the toxic side effects.[72]

OXYGEN. Oxygen has significant toxic effects on the lungs particularly when administered in very high concentrations.[39] It is estimated that 100% inspired oxygen causes damage within 48 hours; lesser concentrations take a proportionally longer time. Patients receiving high levels of oxygen for extended periods almost invariably have significant pulmonary abnormalities from other causes, and it may be difficult or impossible to determine how much additional change can reasonably be attributed to the oxygen therapy.

Oxygen toxicity differs somewhat between the mature and the immature lung. In the mature lung the most significant damage occurs at alveolar level with endothelial cell and type I pneumocyte damage, fibrinous exudates with hyaline membranes, and proliferation of type II pneumocytes. This is the classic picture of diffuse alveolar damage, and its onset is rapid. As with diffuse alveolar damage from any cause, pulmonary fibrosis may ensue. Other effects of oxygen include damage to the terminal airways and inhibition of phagocytosis, resulting in a predisposition to infection.

The immature lung may show a more defined response clinically and radiographically, resulting in bronchopulmonary dysplasia (BPD), a fairly common sequel to the treatment of hyaline membrane disease (respiratory distress syndrome). The damage is more apparent in the terminal airways with epithelial cell necrosis and squamous metaplasia. Damage to the alveoli is less obvious but may in the long run prove more significant because lung growth and pulmonary vascular development may be impaired.

Premature infants, with birth weights less than 2000 g, are at high risk for hyaline membrane disease and subsequent BPD. Respiratory distress syndrome is, however, not a necessary precursor to the development of BPD. The major factors are pulmonary immaturity and assisted ventilation with supplemental oxygen. Thus initial radiographs are normal in perhaps as many as 50% of cases.[22] The evolution of BPD may not be recognized in the early stages because of preexisting pulmonary disease. Many of the features of BPD, such as hyperexpansion of the lungs, pulmonary interstitial emphysema, atelectasis, and pneumonia, also occur in other diffuse pulmonary diseases involving premature infants. The development of progressively coarse reticular infiltration

of the lung, irregular cystlike spaces, coarse stranding, and pulmonary hyperexpansion points to BPD (Figure 11-15). The changes become increasingly "fixed"; in other words, the basic radiographic pattern does not show any significant day-to-day variation other than changes related to varying radiographic technique or incidental complications such as atelectasis or barotrauma. The long-term prognosis for survivors is uncertain. Severe cases of BPD are usually fatal, but mild cases may be clinically and radiographically undetectable.

TALC. The illicit intravenous injection of crushed tablets carries the risk of talc granulomatosis in the lungs. Granulomatous vasculitis may be associated with the development of pulmonary hypertension. The radiographic features vary from normal through diffuse interstitial shadowing to the occasional development of conglomerate upper zone masses.[15,74,79,87] Signs of coexistent pulmonary hypertension may be present. Biopsy shows giant cell granulomas containing birefringent talc crystals together with a granulomatous arteritis.[86]

NITROSOUREAS (BCNU, CCNU). The nitrosoureas are used in the treatment of glioma, lymphoma, and multiple myeloma. There is a significant incidence of diffuse alveolar damage with nitrosourea therapy, particularly in large doses. The incidence may be as high as 30% with prolonged aggressive treatment.[1] The pulmonary changes are comparable to those found in cases of diffuse alveolar damage caused by other cytotoxic drugs. The only differences are that the chest radiograph is more likely to remain normal, despite other evidence of pulmonary toxic effects, and that these patients have an unexplained high incidence of pneumothorax.

Carmustine (BCNU) is slightly unusual in that it may be associated with effective cure of central nervous system tumors of children. Thus unusually prolonged follow-up is feasible. O'Driscoll and associates[70] and Taylor and co-workers[95] were able to reassess six young adults 13 to 17 years after treatment of central nervous system tumors. These patients had interstitial pulmonary fibrosis with a mainly upper zone peripheral distribution. The authors mentioned six delayed deaths from pulmonary fibrosis in their study group of 30 cases.

NARCOTICS. Overdoses of heroin, methadone, and propoxyphene are notoriously associated with pulmonary edema. Pulmonary edema develops in as many as one third of individuals exhibiting signs of opiate overdose.[89] The mechanism of pulmonary injury has not been elucidated, but possible mechanisms include direct effects on the central nervous system leading to neurogenic edema, hypoxemic or direct drug toxic effects on the alveolar-capillary membrane, allergic responses, and immunologic activation. The radiographic findings are the same as those seen with interstitial or alveolar edema from any other cause (Figure 11-6).

Intravenous drug abusers are careless about antiseptic and aseptic precautions, so that septic cardiopulmonary complications may be encountered in this group. The

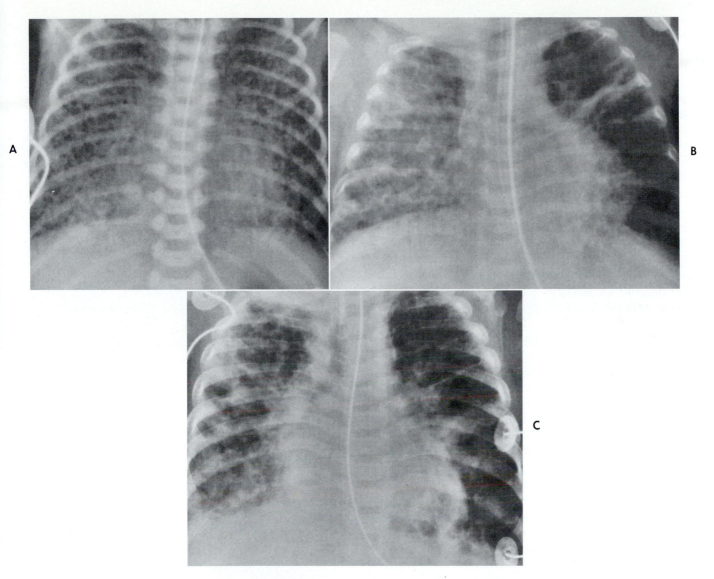

FIGURE 11-15
Bronchopulmonary dysplasia in an infant treated for hyaline membrane disease. **A,** At 10 days. **B,** At 3 months. **C,** At 7 months.

complications include endocarditis, particularly involving the tricuspid valve; multiple septic pulmonary emboli; and pulmonary mycotic aneurysms. As peripheral veins become used up, these desperate people may resort to direct injections into the subclavian and jugular veins, which may result in hematoma formation or mycotic or traumatic pseudoaneurysms involving the superior mediastinum. Other problems encountered include bronchopneumonia following aspiration during drug-induced stupor and hematogenous spread of infection to the musculoskeletal system. Thus septic arthritis involving the sternoclavicular joints or osteomyelitis of the thoracic spine may result in radiographic abnormalities on chest radiographs.

Cocaine hydrochloride, the acidic form of the drug, has

been used in the Western world as an illicit drug for decades. In this form the drug is either insufflated intranasally or injected intravenously. The advent of the alkaloid form of cocaine, "crack," has had a major impact on the drug scene. This form of cocaine can be smoked, producing a rapid, intense, but short-lived high. Crack is highly addictive. Apart from the central toxic effects common to illicit drugs, there are specific toxic effects of crack. Thus pneumothorax and pneumomediastinum may occur, possibly as a result of explosive coughing and straining.[19] Focal airspace disease and atelectasis may be encountered, which may be related to distal airway damage with poor mucociliary clearance or to a hypersensitivity reaction.[45] Pulmonary hemorrhage has been described, and hemoptysis is a relatively common symptom.[65] Pulmonary edema is well described in crack addicts, although the overall incidence is probably much lower than in intravenous drug abusers.[19,35] Cocaine is known to induce a range of cardiac problems, including dysrhythmias, myocarditis, endocarditis, and cardiomyopathy. Generally however, pulmonary edema related to crack is not cardiac in origin.

PENICILLAMINE. Penicillamine is used to treat lead poisoning, Wilson's disease, cystinuria, and, on occasion, connective tissue disorders such as rheumatoid arthritis. Penicillamine is not a commonly used drug, however, and pulmonary toxic effects are rare. This drug is a recognized cause of diffuse alveolar damage and hypersensitivity pneumonitis.[107] The primary reason for singling out penicillamine for special mention is that it may cause a hemorrhagic pneumonitis with acute glomerulonephritis clinically and radiographically indistinguishable from Goodpasture's syndrome.[93] In these cases the onset is acute, with the development of widespread patchy alveolar densities in the lungs. Renal dysfunction develops synchronously. In rare cases, penicillamine also causes an obliterative bronchiolitis.[64] The chest radiograph is usually normal in these cases.

AMIODARONE. The antidysrhythmic drug amiodarone is invaluable in the treatment of refractory cardiac rhythm disturbances. However, amiodarone therapy is associated with a relatively high (5%) incidence of pulmonary toxicity.[106] In 10% to 20% of these patients amiodarone toxicity is fatal. Amiodarone is concentrated in the lung and has a relatively long tissue half-life. This accounts for the slow appearance of pulmonary toxic effects (median interval 6 months) and the slow clearing following cessation of therapy (median interval 3 months).[28] Toxicity from amiodarone appears to be dose related and is much more common when doses greater than 400 mg/day are used.[42] The mechanisms by which amiodarone exerts its toxic effects are discussed on p. 463.

The most common initial symptom of amiodarone toxicity is dyspnea, and patients occasionally have pleuritic chest pain. Pulmonary function tests commonly show a decrease in carbon monoxide diffusing capacity.[42] The most common radiographic appearance is multiple peripheral areas of consolidation resembling those seen in patients with the hypersensitivity reaction (Figures 11-16 and 11-17). However, no evidence of eosinophilia is seen in either the blood or the tissues. The other notable radiographic manifestation is the development of diffuse interstitial shadowing leading to evidence of pulmonary fibrosis (Figure 11-18). Patchy alveolar consolidation frequently coexists with these interstitial changes. The signs resemble those of diffuse lung damage caused by drugs such as bleomycin or nitrofurantoin. Amiodarone may also cause pleural effusions or pleural thickening. Some reports have suggested that patients treated preoperatively with amiodarone have an increased risk of adult respiratory distress syndrome following cardiac surgery. A synergistic relationship to receiving supplemental oxy-

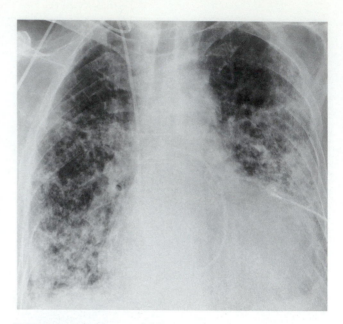

FIGURE 11-16
Amiodarone toxicity showing patchy alveolar infiltrates with peripheral and basal distribution.

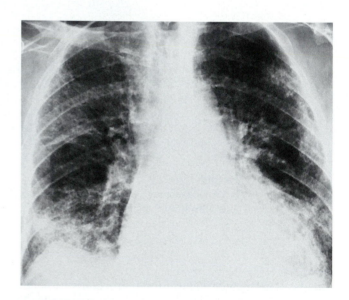

FIGURE 11-17
Amiodarone toxicity showing widespread peripheral and basal organized pulmonary infiltrates.

gen in the postoperative period has been suggested.[41,66]

Patients being treated with amiodarone have significant cardiac disease, and the changes of amiodarone toxicity may be difficult to distinguish from changes secondary to congestive cardiac failure. Lack of response to treatment of heart failure and lack of short-term fluctuations of the pulmonary abnormalities point toward amiodarone toxicity. Stringent monitoring of patients receiving amio-

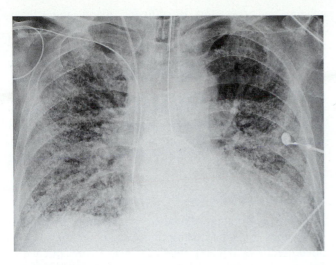

FIGURE 11-18
Amiodarone toxicity (biopsy proven). Diffuse mixed interstitial-alveolar infiltrates in the lungs. Pulmonary wedge pressure was within normal limits.

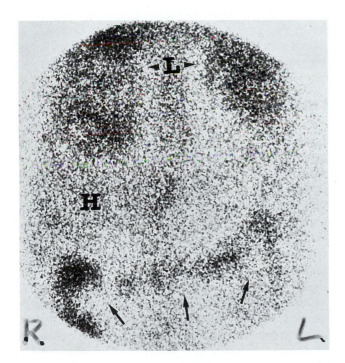

FIGURE 11-19
Gallium scan of the patient in Figure 11-18 shows markedly increased uptake in the lungs (L) relative to the liver (H). Arrow indicates the colon.

darone therapy is essential and should include routine follow-up chest radiographs. Any pulmonary toxicity should thereby be detected and reversed by cessation of the drug before fibrosis develops. There are indications that gallium scintigraphy is more sensitive than plain radiography in diagnosing amiodarone pulmonary toxic-

ity (Figure 11-19).[51,61,67] Certainly, gallium scintigraphy could be useful in distinguishing the interstitial pattern of cardiac edema from the interstitial pattern of amiodarone toxicity. Amiodarone contains 37% iodine by weight, and the concentration of amiodarone in the liver and lung may be sufficient to alter the CT density of these tissues.[47,48,68,76] CT may provide fairly definitive evidence of amiodarone toxicity if high-density pleuroparenchymal lesions are detected and there is increased liver or spleen CT attenuation. Other changes are nonspecific and include interstitial infiltrates, mixed interstitial and alveolar infiltrates, and isolated masses.

Amiodarone pulmonary toxicity is unusual in that it has a specific histologic feature, the accumulation of macrophages with a characteristic foamy cytoplasm in the alveolar spaces. However, such macrophages may be found in completely asymptomatic patients, with no evidence of pulmonary disease by any imaging modality. Therefore their presence may indicate no more than exposure to amiodarone.

DEFEROXAMINE. The chelating agent deferoxamine is used to treat overload of metals such as iron and aluminum, particularly in patients undergoing dialysis. In vivo the amount of free iron available for microbial growth is low. Some organisms have evolved mechanisms that enable them to compete for iron in the host, usually by secreting siderophores. Siderophores entrap iron and deliver it to the microorganism, enhancing its growth and virulence.[16] One such siderophore is deferoxamine. Although the growth of several microorganisms, for example, *Yersinia enterocolitica,* may be enhanced in this way, the most significant example is encountered with the zygomycetes. Mucormycosis is the opportunistic infection caused by members of this species. Dialysis patients, especially those receiving deferoxamine therapy, are at increased risk of mucormycosis in any of its clinical variants: rhinocerebellar, pulmonary, disseminated, and so on.[8]

EFFECTS OF RADIATION ON THE LUNG

Radiation therapy is widely used in the treatment of thoracic malignancies and lymphoma of the mediastinum. Normal tissues are inevitably included in the radiation field and are subject to damage. Radiation effects on the lung are commonly seen on chest radiographs, and abnormalities may also be noted in other structures such as the thoracic skeleton, pleura, or heart.

The severity and extent of damage to normal lung tissue depend on a number of factors[52]:

1. The volume of normal lung irradiated is related to field size. Lung damage does not occur outside the field of irradiation, which is purposely kept as small as adequate therapy permits. On average only one fourth to one third of a lung is included in the field, but on occasion very large tumors necessitate irradiation of much larger lung volumes. The administration of 3000 rads to all of both lungs will kill most individuals, whereas the same or even

higher doses administered to a portion of one lung may not even produce symptoms in many cases.

2. The total dose and the fractionation of that dose are of critical importance. The effect of a single large dose is more severe than the effect of the same dose divided into a series of fractions given over 2 to 3 weeks. There is of course no threshold at which deleterious effects become manifest, but they do become more apparent and inevitable with increasing total doses. With modern radiation therapy there are no significant differences in the effects of radiation from different sources, for example, from cobalt sources as opposed to linear accelerators.

3. Individual susceptibility to radiation is variable and at the same time is inexplicable and unpredictable. Clinical or radiographic evidence of radiation pneumonitis may develop in one patient but not in another receiving comparable treatment. The preexisting state of the lungs may also play a role in determining the full clinical effects of radiation. For example, a patient with severe chronic obstructive pulmonary disease and poor respiratory reserve may be severely affected by even a localized radiation pneumonitis resulting from this supposedly tolerable form of treatment.

4. Previous or concomitant therapy may influence the timing and the severity of the radiation changes. A second course of radiation therapy produces earlier and more severe changes than the first. Certain cytotoxic agents such as bleomycin heighten the effects of radiation.[49] Other agents, such as actinomycin D and adriamycin, that do not in themselves cause pulmonary toxicity accentuate the effects of radiation by a form of synergism.[9,56] Steroids dampen the effects of irradiation as they do in other inflammatory processes.[75]

Pathology

A knowledge of the underlying pathologic changes is useful in understanding the radiographic manifestations. A series of phases is recognized by pathologic, clinical, and radiographic criteria.[63] In the initial 24 to 48 hours the lymph follicles degenerate, the bronchial mucosa becomes hyperemic and edematous, and leukocytes infiltrate the bronchial wall. Ordinarily these changes are undetectable clinically or radiographically. In rare cases a central tumor may have narrowed the bronchial lumen so critically that the mucosal swelling and reaction produce clinically and radiographically detectable effects. This reaction subsides and a latent phase ensues. The phase of acute radiation pneumonitis develops some 1 to 6 months after the therapy. Histologic findings include thickening of the alveolar septa by edema and round cell infiltration, hyperplasia and desquamation of the alveolar lining cells, fibrinous alveolar exudation leading to hyaline membrane formation, endothelial cell damage with engorgement and thrombus formation, and evidence of arteritis. Depending on the severity of reaction a variable degree of interstitial and alveolar fibrosis is seen. A simultaneous reaction occurs in the bronchial mucosa, with hyperemia,

edema, and cessation of mucous gland and ciliary function. These changes peak and merge into a regenerative phase in which the exudates and edema disperse, the alveolar lining cells regenerate, and the capillary endothelial cells become normal. Fibrosis, however, progresses, consolidates, and contracts over the following weeks and months. In addition, there may be progressive sclerosis of the pulmonary vascular bed and bronchial structural damage. The latter changes may lead to bronchiectasis and altered perfusion of the affected portions of the lung.[88]

Clinical features

If any symptoms related to pulmonary irradiation occur, they are seen during the phase of acute radiation pneumonitis or develop much later as a consequence of fibrosis and lung contraction. The severity of symptoms depends on the extent and severity of the postirradiation changes and on the presence of underlying lung disease. The usual symptoms in the acute phase are dyspnea, cough, production of tenacious sputum, and sometimes fever and night sweats. These symptoms may persist for several weeks.

In the fibrotic phase the patient is usually asymptomatic. If the fibrosis is severe and extensive, however, the patient may be completely disabled. Cough, hemoptysis, dyspnea, orthopnea, clubbing of the fingers, and recurrent infections are all features of such cases.

Radiographic findings

On the chest radiograph the changes of radiation pneumonitis are generally confined to the field of irradiation (Figure 11-20). In some cases it may be necessary to correlate the chest radiograph with the radiation portals, particularly when tangential beams have been employed. The single most striking feature of radiation pneumonitis is the geometric shape of the resulting pulmonary shadowing. The line of demarcation between involved and noninvolved lung is usually linear, and normal anatomic boundaries such as fissures are crossed with seeming impunity. On a frontal radiograph of the chest the involved areas may be clearly delineated, but on the lateral radiograph the changes may extend fairly uniformly across the chest in the sagittal plane. To observers accustomed to using the lateral film for segmental or lobar localization, this seeming disregard for anatomic boundaries can be striking. Although the chest radiograph may suggest that the changes are confined to the field of radiation, CT and ^{67}Ga-citrate imaging may indicate evidence of disease in nonirradiated portions of the lungs.[38,40] The cause of changes outside the field of irradiation has been the subject of speculation. Suggested causes include blockage of lymphatic pathways, errors in dosimetry or placement of portals, scattered radiation, or radiation-induced hypersensitivity pneumonitis.[18]

The first change is a diffuse haze in the irradiated region with obscuring of the vascular outlines. Patchy

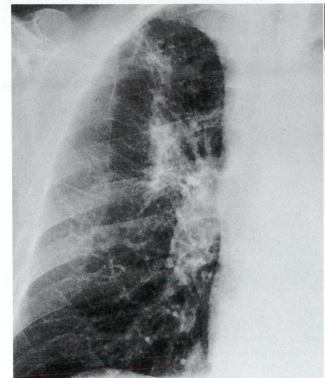

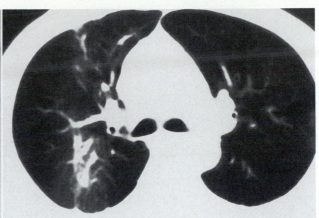

FIGURE 11-20
Changes resulting from irradiation of a bronchogenic carcinoma. **A,** Straight lateral margin to infiltration in right upper lobe. **B,** Corresponding computed tomographic scan shows that the infiltration extends sagittally across chest with same straight lateral margin.

consolidations appear, and these areas may coalesce into a nonanatomic but geometric area of pulmonary density (Figures 11-20 and 11-21). Pleural effusions are relatively uncommon.[2] Libshitz and Shuman[53] indicate that demonstrable radiographic changes usually appear at about 8 weeks after treatment with 4000 cGy delivered over 4 weeks. For each increment of 1000 cGy greater than 4000 cGy the changes appear about 1 week earlier. Bell and co-workers[3] have shown that CT and ventilation perfusion studies, particularly with single photon emission computed tomography (SPECT), are more sensitive than chest radiographs in detecting postirradiation changes in the lungs. This applies both to the field of irradiation and to the nonirradiated portions of the lungs. The superiority of CT for this purpose should occasion no surprise; CT is recognized as intrinsically more sensitive than chest radiographs in detecting pulmonary infiltrates, and the radiation effects on local perfusion of the lung may be profound as a result of radiation-induced vasculitis and vascular sclerosis.

The regenerative fibrotic phase develops almost imperceptibly from the phase of acute pneumonitis. With time the opacities become more linear or reticular, in other words, "more structured." Fibrous contraction condenses the shadows and distorts adjacent structures such as the hilar vessels (Figure 11-22). The fibrosis is often not severe, and the changes can easily be overlooked or attributed to granulomatous scarring. The experienced eye, however, instinctively picks up the alteration, such as the slight paramediastinal change that may be seen after mediastinal irradiation of patients with lymphoma.

The earliest radiographic changes appear 6 to 8 weeks after the beginning of radiation therapy, and the peak reaction occurs usually at 3 to 4 months. The ensuing fibrosis and contraction continue over a 12- to 18-month period and then become quiescent. Bronchiectasis may be present within the regions of fibrosis, but this change is usually undetectable on plain films. However, radiation damage to the lung is occasionally severe, and the resultant bronchiectasis may be apparent (Figure 11-23). Fortunately, with modern radiation therapy such damage is rare.

The CT findings following radiation therapy clearly reflect the described pathologic changes.[53] In the phase of acute radiation pneumonitis, patchy and increasingly confluent areas of increased attenuation appear in the irradiated field. The geographic distribution of the changes may be striking. Transition to the phase of regeneration and fibrosis is gradual. Fibrous stranding that merges smoothly with the pleura becomes apparent, and contraction can be recognized by the distortion of adjacent structures. Bronchiectasis within the contracted portion of lung may be readily apparent on CT (Figure 11-24). CT is more sensitive than plain radiographs in detecting postirradiation changes in the lungs, particularly in peripheral tangential radiation fields.[3] CT may also indicate shrinkage of vessels in lung peripheral to a central field of irradiation. This presumably is a reflection of diminished perfusion resulting from radiation-induced vascular sclerosis. Bell and associates,[3] using scintigraphy, were able to demonstrate significant perfusion abnormalities in lung beyond the field of irradiation. In

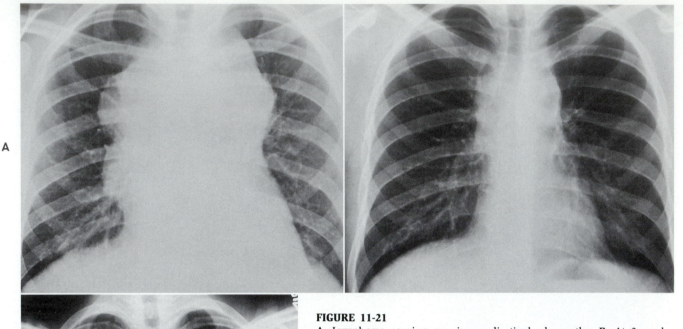

FIGURE 11-21
A, Lymphoma causing massive mediastinal adenopathy. **B,** At 2 weeks, considerable resolution of the adenopathy following irradiation. **C,** At 10 weeks, radiation pneumonitis in the necessarily wide field of irradiation.

general these changes outside the radiation field could not be detected on plain chest radiographs.

Less common manifestations of radiation damage are hyperlucency of a lung,[21,99] pleural effusions, and spontaneous pneumothorax.[7,82] Pulmonary hyperlucency presumably results from diminished pulmonary perfusion. Pleural effusions secondary to irradiation are usually coincident with the phase of acute radiation pneumonitis. In rare cases a second primary tumor such as an osteogenic sarcoma or a bronchial carcinoma may arise in the field of irradiation and may well be radiation induced.[34,37]

Differential diagnosis of radiation pneumonitis

The two major differential diagnoses to be considered in patients with radiation pneumonitis are infections and tumor recurrence. An infective pneumonitis is not usually confined by the radiotherapy ports and normally runs a less indolent course than radiation pneumonitis. Nevertheless, an area of radiation damage may become secondarily infected, and if it does, the diagnosis cannot be established radiographically. Tumor recurrence may be difficult to discern at the height of the postirradiation change, but as these changes stabilize and contraction develops, a focal enlargement should become increasingly apparent. A primary bronchial carcinoma may develop a lymphangitic pattern of spread initially confined to one lung or even one lobe. Lymphangitis carcinomatosa may initially cause diagnostic problems, but the inexorable worsening with the development of septal lines, effusions, and spread to the opposite lung will soon make the situation clear.

CT and magnetic resonance imaging (MRI) have been investigated as means of detecting tumor recurrence. CT, by detecting focal masses or cavitation, may provide some

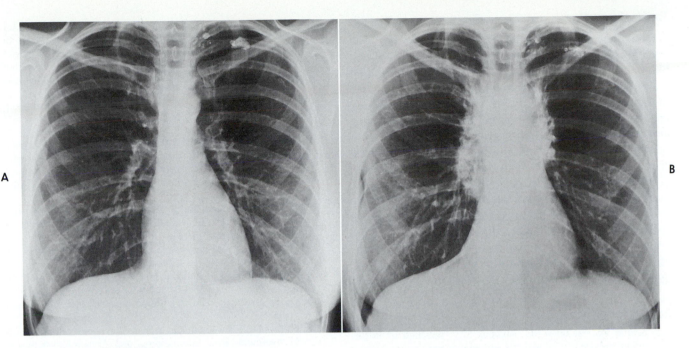

FIGURE 11-22
Radiographs taken, **A**, before and, **B**, approximately 4 months after mantle radiation therapy for Hodgkin's disease. Dense geometric infiltrates with evidence of fibrous contraction have developed in the radiation portals.

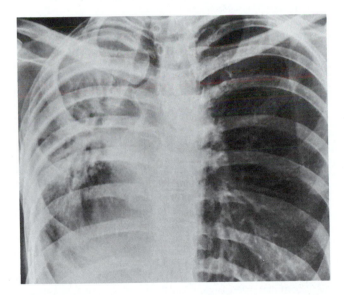

FIGURE 11-23
Severe radiation damage to the lungs of a 32-year-old woman irradiated several years previously for lymphoma.

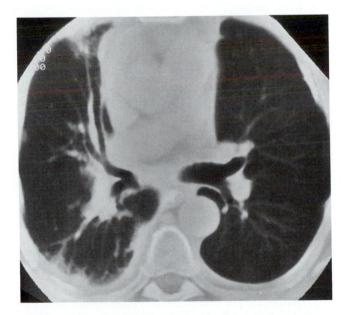

FIGURE 11-24
Computed tomographic scan demonstrating bronchiectasis in the field of previous irradiation.

evidence of recurrence. MRI is theoretically capable of differentiating tissue, but at the present time the practical results of MRI in postirradiation cases are inconclusive. Radiation fibrosis has low signal intensity on both T1- and T2-weighted sequences.[30] Tumors, on the other hand, have high signal intensity on T2-weighted sequences and can therefore be distinguished from pure fibrosis. However, acute radiation pneumonitis, second-ary infective pneumonitis, or hemorrhage may have signal intensities similar to tumor and therefore may be confused with recurrent disease. Enhancement with gadolinium-DTPA is not helpful in distinguishing between radiation fibrosis and tumor recurrence.[100] Magnetic resonance spectroscopy has been suggested as a possible solution but thus far has not evolved into a clinically accepted method.[10]

Radiation effects on other thoracic structures

Radiation may damage other thoracic structures, producing either radiographically visible manifestations or indirect effects on the lungs. Radiation-induced abnormalities in the bony thorax are most commonly seen after radiation therapy for carcinoma of the breast. The bones appear atrophic and osteoporotic, fractures are frequent and may fail to unite, and dystrophic calcifications may be seen in the adjacent soft tissues. Necrotic bone appears sclerotic. Radiation damage to the heart and the pericardium may cause enlargement of the cardiac silhouette and signs of pulmonary vascular congestion and edema. Pericardial effusion is the most common manifestation of radiation damage, but myocardial fibrosis and coronary artery damage may occur. Radiation damage to the esophagus may cause dysmotility, stricture formation, or fistula development, and chronic aspiration may ensue.

REFERENCES

1. Aronin PA, Mahaley MS, Rudnick SA: Prediction of BCNU pulmonary toxicity in patients with malignant gliomas, *N Engl J Med* 303:183-188, 1980.
2. Bachman AL, Macken K: Pleural effusions following supervoltage radiation for breast carcinoma, *Radiology* 72:699-709, 1959.
3. Bell J, McGivern D, Bullimore J, et al: Diagnostic imaging of post-irradiation changes in the chest, *Clin Radiol* 39:109-119, 1988.
4. Bellamy EA, Husband JE, Blaquiere RM, et al: Bleomycin related lung damage: CT evidence, *Radiology* 157:155-158, 1985.
5. Bernstein ML, Sobel DB, Wimmer RS: Non-cardiogenic pulmonary edema following injection of methotrexate into the cerebro-spinal fluid, *Cancer* 50:866-868, 1982.
6. Biron P, Dessureault J, Napke E: Acute allergic interstitial pneumonitis induced by hydrochlorothiazide, *Can Med Assoc J* 145:28-34, 1991.
7. Blane CE, Silberstein RJ, Sue JY: Radiation therapy and spontaneous pneumothorax, *J Can Assoc Radiol* 32:153-154, 1981.
8. Boelaert JR, Fenves AZ, Coburn JW: Deferoxamine therapy and mucormycosis in dialysis patients: report of an international registry, *Am J Kidney Dis* 18:660-667, 1991.
9. Cassaday JR, Richter MP, Piro AJ, et al: Radiation-adriamycin interactions; preliminary clinical observations, *Cancer* 36:946-949, 1974.
10. Charles HC, Baker ME, Hathorn JW, et al: Differentiation of radiation fibrosis from recurrent neoplasia: a role for 31P MR spectroscopy, *AJR* 164:67-68, 1990.
11. Cohen MB, Austin JHM, Smith-Vaniz A, et al: Nodular bleomycin toxicity, *Am J Clin Pathol* 92:101-104, 1989.
12. Conant EF, Fox KR, Miller WT: Pulmonary edema as a complication of interleukin-2 therapy, *AJR* 152:749-752, 1989.
13. Cooper JAD, White DA, Matthay RA: Drug induced pulmonary diseases. Part 1. Cytotoxic drugs, *Am Rev Respir Dis* 133:321-340, 1986.
14. Cooper JAD, White DA, Matthay RA: Drug-induced pulmonary disease. Part 2. Non cytotoxic drugs, *Am Rev Respir Dis* 133:488-505, 1986.
15. Crouch E, Chart A: Progressive massive fibrosis of the lung secondary to intravenous injection of talc: a pathologic and mineralogic analysis, *Am J Clin Pathol* 80:520-526, 1983.
16. Daly HL, Velazquez LA, Bradley SF, et al: Mucormycosis: association with deferoxamine therapy, *Am J Med* 87:468-471, 1989.
17. Davis SD, Berkmen YM, Wang JCL: Interleukin-2 therapy for advanced renal cell carcinoma: radiographic evaluation of response and complications, *Radiology* 177:127-131, 1990.
18. Davis SD, Yankelevitz DF, Henschke CI: Radiation effects on the lung: clinical features, pathology and imaging findings, *AJR* 159:1157-1164, 1992.
19. Eurman DW, Potash HI, Eyler WR, et al: Chest pain and dyspnea related to "crack" cocaine smoking: value of chest radiography, *Radiology* 172:459-462, 1989.
20. Evans RB, Ettensohn DB, Fawaz-Estrup F, et al: Gold lung: recent developments in pathogenesis, diagnosis and treatment, *Semin Arthritis Rheum* 16:196-205.
21. Farmer W, Ravin C, Schachter EN: Hyperlucent lung after radiation therapy, *Am Rev Respir Dis* 112:255-258, 1975.
22. Fitzgerald P, Donoghue V, Gorman W: Bronchopulmonary dysplasia: a radiographic and clinical review of 20 patients, *Br J Radiol* 63:444-447, 1990.
23. Follath F, Burkart F, Sehweizer W: Drug induced pulmonary hypertension? *Br Med J* 1:265-266, 1971.
24. Frand UI, Shim CS, Williams MK: Methadone induced pulmonary edema, *Intern Med* 76:975-979, 1972.
25. Galton DAG: Myleran in chronic myeloid leukemia, *Lancet* 1:208-213, 1953.
26. Gaynor ER, Vitek L, Sticklin L, et al: The hemodynamic effects of treatment with interleukin-2 and lymphokine-activated killer cells, *Ann Intern Med* 109:953-958, 1988.
27. Gefter WB, Epstein DM, Bonavita JA, et al: Pleural thickening caused by Sansert and Ergotrate in the treatment of migraine, *AJR* 135:375-377, 1980.
28. Gefter WB, Epstein DM, Pietra GG, et al: Lung disease caused by amiodarone, a new antiarrhythmic agent, *Radiology* 147:339-344, 1983.
29. Glasier CM, Siegel MJ: Multiple pulmonary nodules: unusual manifestation of bleomycin toxicity, *AJR* 137:155-156, 1981.
30. Glazer HS, Lee JKT, Levitt RG, et al: Radiation fibrosis: differentiation from recurrent tumor by MR imaging; work in progress, *Radiology* 156:721-726, 1985.
31. Gockerman JP: Drug-induced interstitial lung diseases, *Clin Chest Med* 3:521-536, 1982.
32. Heath MF, Costa-Jussa FR, Jacobs JM, et al: The induction of pulmonary phospholipidosis and the inhibition of lysosomal phospholipases by amiodarone, *Br J Exp Pathol* 66:391-397, 1985.
33. Heffner JE, Sahn SA: Salicylate induced pulmonary edema: clinical features and prognosis, *Ann Intern Med* 95:405-409, 1981.
34. Hill CA, North LB, Osborne BM: Bronchogenic carcinoma in breast carcinoma, *AJR* 140:259-264, 1983.
35. Hoffman CK, Goodman PC: Pulmonary edema in cocaine smokers, *Radiology* 172:463-465, 1989.
36. Holmberg L, Boman G: Pulmonary reactions to nitrofurantoin: 447 cases reported to the Swedish Adverse Drug Reaction Committee 1966-1976, *Eur J Respir Dis* 62:180-189, 1981.
37. Huvos AG, Woodward HQ, Cahan WB, et al: Post irradiation osteogenic sarcoma of bone and soft tissue: a clinico-pathologic study in 66 patients, *Cancer* 55:1244-1255, 1985.
38. Ikezoe J, Takashima S, Morimoto S, et al: CT appearance of acute radiation-induced injury in the lung, *AJR* 150:765-770, 1988.
39. Jackson RM: Review: pulmonary oxygen toxicity, *Chest* 86:900-905, 1985.
40. Kataoka M, Kawamura M, Veda N, et al: Diffuse gallium-67 uptake in radiation pneumonitis, *Clin Nucl Med* 10:707-711, 1990.
41. Kay GN, Epstein AE, Kirklin JK, et al: Fatal postoperative amiodarone pulmonary toxicity, *Am J Cardiol* 62:490-492, 1988.
42. Kennedy JI: Clinical aspects of amiodarone pulmonary toxicity, *Clin Chest Med* 11:119-129, 1990.

43. Kennedy JL, Myers JL, Plumb VJ, et al: Amiodarone pulmonary toxicity: clinical radiologic and pathologic correlations, *Arch Intern Med* 147:50-55, 1987.

44. Kinnunen E, Viljanen A: Pleuropulmonary involvement during bromocriptine treatment, *Chest* 94:1034-1036, 1988.

45. Kissner DG, Lawrence DW, Selis JE, et al: Crack lung: pulmonary disease caused by cocaine abuse, *Am Rev Respir Dis* 136:1250-1252, 1987.

46. Kuhlman JE: The role of chest computed tomography in the diagnosis of drug-related reactions, *J Thorac Imag* 6:52-61, 1991.

47. Kuhlman JE, Scatarige JC, Fishman EK, et al: CT demonstration of high attenuation pleural-parenchymal lesions due to amiodarone therapy, *J Comput Assist Tomogr* 11:160-162, 1987.

48. Kuhlman JE, Teigen C, Ren H, et al: Amiodarone pulmonary toxicity: CT findings in symptomatic patients, *Radiology* 177:121-125, 1990.

49. Lamoureux K: Increased clinically symptomatic pulmonary radiation reactions with adjuvant chemotherapy, *Cancer Chemother Res (Part 1)* 35:1322-1324, 1975.

50. Leatherman JW, Schmitz PG: Fever, hyperdynamic shock and multiple-system organ failure: a pseudo-sepsis syndrome associated with chronic salicylate intoxication, *Chest* 100:1391-1396, 1991.

51. Lecklitner ML, Johnson DR, Hughes JJ: Gallium-67 and pulmonary complications of amiodarone, *Clin Nucl Med* 13:826-827, 1988.

52. Libshitz HI: Thoracic radiotherapy changes. In Herman PG, ed: *Iatrogenic thoracic complications,* New York, 1983, Springer-Verlag, pp 141-160.

53. Libshitz HI, Shuman LS: Radiation-induced pulmonary change: CT findings, *J Comput Assist Tomogr* 8:15-19, 1984.

54. Lien HH, Brodahl U, Telhaug R, et al: Pulmonary changes at computed tomography in patients with testicular carcinoma treated with cis-platinum, vinblastine and bleomycin, *Acta Radiol (Diagn)* 26:507-510, 1985.

55. Louie S, Gamble CN, Cross CE: Penicillamine associated pulmonary hemorrhage, *J Rheumatol* 135:963-966, 1986.

56. Ma LD, Taylor GA, Wharam MD, et al: "Recall" pneumonitis: adriamycin potentiation of radiation pneumonitis in two children, *Radiology* 187:465-467, 1993.

57. MacDonald JS: Lymphography. In Ansell G, ed: *Complications in diagnostic radiology,* Oxford, Eng, 1976, Blackwell, pp 301-316.

58. MacLennan FM, Thomson MAR, Rankin R, et al: Fatal pulmonary oedema associated with the use of ritodrine in pregnancy: case report, *Br J Obstet Gynecol* 92:703-705, 1985.

59. Mann H, Ward JH, Samlowski WE: Vascular leak syndrome associated with interleukin-2: chest radiographic manifestations, *Radiology* 176:191-194, 1990.

60. McElvaney NG, Wilcox PG, Churg A, et al: Pleuropulmonary disease during bromocriptine treatment of Parkinson's disease, *Arch Intern Med* 148:2231-2236, 1988.

61. Moinuddin M, Rockett J: Gallium scintigraphy in the detection of amiodarone lung toxicity, *AJR* 147:607-609, 1986.

62. Moseley PL, Shasby DM, Brady M, et al: Lung parenchymal injury induced by bleomycin, *Am Rev Respir Dis* 130:1082-1086, 1984.

63. Moss WT, Brand WN, Battifora H: *Radiation oncology: rationale, technique, results,* ed 5, St Louis, 1979, Mosby, pp 253-288.

64. Murphy KC, Atkins CJ, Offer RC, et al: Obliterative bronchiolitis in two rheumatoid arthritis patients treated with penicillamine, *Arthritis Rheum* 24:557-560, 1981.

65. Murray RJ, Albin RJ, Mergner W, et al: Diffuse alveolar hemorrhage temporally related to cocaine smoking, *Chest* 93:427-429, 1988.

66. Nalos PC, Kass RM, Gang ES, et al: Life-threatening postoperative pulmonary complications in patients with previous amiodarone pulmonary toxicity undergoing cardiothoracic operations, *J Thorac Cardiovasc Surg* 93:904-912, 1987.

67. Nguyen BD, Isaacs GH, Alhakim N, et al: Ga-67 imaging of amiodarone pulmonary toxicity with pseudocavitary lesion, *Clin Nucl Med* 17:507-508, 1992.

68. Nicholson AA, Hayward C: The value of computed tomography in the diagnosis of amiodarone-induced pulmonary toxicity, *Clin Radiol* 40:564-567, 1989.

69. Oakley C, Somerville J: Oral contraceptives and progressive pulmonary vascular disease, *Lancet* 1:890-893, 1968.

70. O'Driscoll BR, Hastleton PS, Taylor PM, et al: Active lung fibrosis up to 17 years after chemotherapy with carmustine (BCNU) in childhood, *N Engl J Med* 323:378-382, 1990.

71. Ognibene FP, Rosenberg SA, Lotze M, et al: Interleukin-2 administration causes reversible hemodynamic changes and left ventricular dysfunction similar to those seen in septic shock, *Chest* 94:750-754, 1988.

72. Ortho Multicenter Transplant Study Group: A randomized clinical trial of OKT3 monoclonal antibody for acute rejection of cadaveric renal transplants, *N Engl J Med* 313:337-342, 1985.

73. Padley SPG, Adler B, Hansell DM, et al: High-resolution computed tomography of drug-induced lung disease, *Clin Radiol* 46:232-236, 1992.

74. Padley SPG, Adler BD, Staples CA, et al: Pulmonary talcosis: CT findings in three cases, *Radiology* 186:125-127, 1993.

75. Parris TM, Knight JG, Hess CE, et al: Severe radiation pneumonitis precipitated by withdrawal of steroids: a diagnostic and therapeutic dilemma, *AJR* 132:284-286, 1970.

76. Ren H, Kuhlman JE, Hruban RH, et al: CT-pathology correlation of amiodarone lung, *J Comput Assist Tomogr* 14:760-765, 1990.

77. Richman SD, Levenson SM, Bunn PA, et al: 67 Ga accumulation in pulmonary lesions associated with bleomycin toxicity, *Cancer* 36:1966-1972, 1975.

78. Rimmer MJ, Dixon AK, Flower CDR: Bleomycin lung: computed tomographic observations, *Br J Radiol* 58:1041-1045, 1985.

79. Robertson CH, Reynolds RC, Wilson JE: Pulmonary hypertension and foreign body granulomatosis in intravenous drug abusers, *Am J Med* 61:657-664, 1976.

80. Rosenberg SA, Lotze MT, Muul LM, et al: A progress report on the treatment of 157 patients with advanced cancer using lymphokine-activated killer cells and interleukin-2 or interleukin-2 alone, *N Engl J Med* 316:889-897, 1987.

81. Rosenstein M, Ettinghausen SE, Rosenberg SA: Extravasation of intravascular fluid mediated by the systemic administration of recombinant interleukin-2, *J Immunol* 137:1735-1742, 1986.

82. Rowinsky EK, Abeloff MD, Wharam MD: Spontaneous pneumothorax following thoracic irradiation, *Chest* 88:703-708, 1985.

83. Roy TM, Ossario MA, Cipolla LM, et al: Pulmonary complications after tricyclic antidepressant overdose, *Chest* 96:852-856, 1989.

84. Santrach PJ, Askin FB, Wells RJ, et al: Nodular form of bleomycin-related pulmonary injury in patients with osteogenic sarcoma, *Cancer* 64:806-811, 1989.

85. Saxon RR, Klein JS, Bar MH, et al: Pathogenesis of pulmonary edema during interleukin-2 therapy: correlation of chest radiographic and clinical findings in 54 patients, *AJR* 156:281-285, 1991.

86. Schwartz IS, Basken C: Pulmonary vascular talc granulomatosis, *JAMA* 256:2584, 1986.

87. Sieniewicz DJ, Nidecker AC: Conglomerate pulmonary disease: a form of talcosis in intravenous methadone abusers, *AJR* 135:697-702, 1980.

88. Slavin JD, Friedman NC, Spencer RP: Radiation effects on pulmonary ventilation and perfusion, *Clin Nucl Med* 18:81-82, 1993.

89. Smith WR, Wells ID, Glauser FL, et al: Immunologic abnormalities in heroin lung, *Chest* 68:651-653, 1975.

90. Snydman DR, Sullivan B, Gill M, et al: Nosocomial sepsis associated with interleukin-2, *Ann Intern Med* 112:102-107, 1990.

91. Sostman HD, Matthay RA, Putman CE, et al: Methotrexate-induced pneumonitis, *Medicine* 55:371-388, 1976.

92. Steinberg AD, Karliner JS: The clinical spectrum of heroin pulmonary edema, *Arch Intern Med* 122:122-127, 1968.

93. Sternbieb I, Bennett B, Scheinberg IH: D-Penicillamine induced Goodpasture's syndrome in Wilson's disease, *Ann Intern Med* 82:673-676, 1975.

94. Taal BG, Spierings ELH, Hilvering C: Pleuropulmonary fibrosis associated with chronic and excessive intake of ergotamine, *Thorax* 38:396-398, 1983.

95. Taylor PM, O'Driscoll BR, Galtamaneni HR, et al: Chronic lung fibrosis following carmustine (BCNO) chemotherapy: radiological features, *Clin Radiol* 44:299-301, 1991.

96. Urban C, Nisenberz A, Caparros B, et al: Chemical pleuritis as a cause of acute chest pain following high dose methotrexate treatment, *Cancer* 51:34-37, 1983.

97. Varnell RM, Godwin JD, Richardson ML, et al: Adult respiratory distress syndrome from overdose of tricyclic antidepressants, *Radiology* 170:667-670, 1989.

98. Weaver LT, Law JS: Lung changes after gold salts, *Br J Dis Chest* 72:247-250, 1978.

99. Wencel ML, Sitrin RG: Unilateral lung hyperlucency after mediastinal irradiation, *Am Res Respir Dis* 137:955-957, 1988.

100. Werthmuller WC, Schiebler ML, Whaley RA, et al: Gadolinium-DTPA enhancement of lung radiation fibrosis, *J Comput Assist Tomogr* 13:946-948, 1989.

101. Wheeler S, Stitik FP, Hutchins GM, et al: Diagnosis of lipoid pneumonia by computed tomography, *JAMA* 245:65-66, 1981.

102. Whimster WF, de Poitiers W: The lung. In Riddell RH, ed: *Pathology of drug induced and toxic diseases,* New York, 1982, Churchill Livingstone, pp 167-200.

103. White DA, Stover DE: Severe bleomycin-induced pneumonitis: clinical features and response to corticosteroids, *Chest* 86:723-728, 1984.

104. Winzelberg GG, Wholey MH, Jarmolowski CA, et al: Patients with hemoptysis examined by Tc-99m sulfur colloid and Tc-99m-labelled red blood cells: a preliminary appraisal, *Radiology* 153:523-526, 1984.

105. Wolkowicz J, Sturgeon J, Rawji M, et al: Bleomycin-induced pulmonary function abnormalities, *Chest* 101:97-101, 1992.

106. Wood DL, Osborn MJ, Rooke J, et al: Amiodarone pulmonary toxicity: report of two cases associated with rapidly progressive fatal adult respiratory distress syndrome after pulmonary angiography, *Mayo Clin Proc* 60:601-603, 1985.

107. Zitnik RJ, Cooper JAD: Pulmonary disease due to antirheumatic agents, *Clin Chest Med* 11:139-150, 1990.

12 Immunologic Diseases of the Lungs

ALAN G. WILSON

Diffuse interstitial pulmonary fibrosis
  Cryptogenic fibrosing alveolitis or idiopathic pulmonary fibrosis
  End-stage lung
Lung vasculitides
  Granulomatous vasculitis
    Wegener's granulomatosis
    Churg-Strauss syndrome
    Necrotizing sarcoidal angiitis
  Microscopic polyarteritis nodosa
  Hypersensitivity vasculitis
    Anaphylactoid purpura (Henoch-Schönlein purpura)
    Systemic urticarial vasculitis
    Essential mixed cryoglobulinemia
    Connective tissue disease and malignancy
    Nonspecific hypersensitivity vasculitis and disseminated leukocytoclastic vasculitis
  Giant cell vasculitis
    Systemic temporal arteritis
    Other giant cell arteritides
  Behçet's disease and Hughes-Stovin syndrome
  Polyangiitis overlap syndrome
Collagen vascular disease
  Rheumatoid arthritis
    Pleural disease
    Fibrosing alveolitis
    Intrapulmonary nodules
    Caplan's syndrome
    Pulmonary arteritis and hypertension
    Other associations
  Systemic lupus erythematosus
    Primary manifestations
      Pleuritis or pleural effusion
      (Acute) lupus pneumonitis
      Pulmonary hemorrhage
      Fibrosing alveolitis
      Diaphragm dysfunction
      Pulmonary arterial hypertension and vasculitis
      Rarities
    Secondary manifestations
      Atelectasis
      Pneumonia
      Pericarditis, myocarditis, and renal disease
    Drug-induced systemic lupus erythematosus
  Polymyositis and dermatomyositis
    Primary manifestations
      Interstitial lung disease

      Pulmonary arterial hypertension
      Diaphragmatic myositis
    Secondary manifestations
      Carcinoma lung and polymyositis and dermatomyositis
    Overlap syndrome
    Juvenile dermatomyositis and polymyositis
  Systemic sclerosis
    CREST syndrome (limited cutaneous systemic sclerosis)
    Overlap — systemic sclerosis syndrome
  Sjögren's syndrome
  Overlap syndromes and mixed connective tissue disease
  Relapsing polychondritis
Diffuse pulmonary (alveolar) hemorrhage
  Principal causes
    Anti–basement membrane antibody disease
    Connective tissue disorders, systemic vasculitides, "immune complex disease"
    Idiopathic glomerulonephritis
    Idiopathic (primary) pulmonary hemosiderosis
    Bleeding disorders
    Drugs and chemicals
  Radiology of diffuse pulmonary hemorrhage
  Differential diagnosis of alveolar hemorrhage
Eosinophilic lung disease
  Asthma
  Cryptogenic eosinophilic pneumonia
    Acute eosinophilic pneumonia
    Chronic eosinophilic pneumonia
  Allergic bronchopulmonary aspergillosis
  Drug-induced eosinophilic lung disease
  Tropical pulmonary eosinophilia
  Eosinophilic lung disease from other worm infestations
  Bronchocentric granulomatosis
  Hypereosinophilic syndrome
  Hyperimmunoglobulin E, recurrent-infection (Job's) syndrome
Extrinsic allergic alveolitis
  Organic dust toxic syndrome
Amyloidosis and amyloid deposition
  Systemic amyloidosis
    AL (light chain) amyloidosis
    Reactive systemic amyloidosis
    Radiographic changes in systemic amyloidosis
  Localized amyloidosis
    Tracheobronchial amyloidosis
    Parenchymal nodular amyloidosis
    Parenchymal alveolar septal disease

DIFFUSE INTERSTITIAL PULMONARY FIBROSIS

Diffuse interstitial pulmonary fibrosis (IPF) may follow acute or chronic insults to the lung. This discussion is concerned with chronic interstitial pneumonias (CIPs), particularly the idiopathic form.

CIPs are diffuse inflammatory processes that affect mainly the lung interstitium, namely the alveolar septa and the peribronchial and perivascular sheaths. A large variety of CIPs are recognized.[159,253,262,418,461] The most important are (1) cryptogenic fibrosing alveolitis (CFA) and idiopathic pulmonary fibrosis; (2) CIP associated with collagen vascular disorders, especially rheumatoid disease and systemic sclerosis[213]; (3) drug-related CIP, especially following use of cytotoxic agents and nitrofurantoin[289]; (4) postinfective CIP, particularly following viral,[517,593] mycoplasmal,[727] and chlamydial infections; (5) pneumoconioses, particularly from inhalation of asbestos, talc, beryllium, and tungsten carbide, the organic dusts that give extrinsic allergic alveolitis, and also CIP from inhalation of noxious gases[581]; (6) radiation pneumonitis; (7) chronic pulmonary edema; and (8) miscellaneous conditions, including genetic, metabolic, reactive, and inflammatory disorders.[169,702,789] Some authors extend this list to include granulomatous processes such as histiocytosis X and sarcoidosis.[345]

Regardless of the context, the pathology and pathogenesis are basically similar,[157,265] beginning with an injury. This injury may be attributed directly or indirectly to a toxic agent or may be mediated by immune complex deposition or recruitment of inflammatory cells. The result is an acute alveolitis that may be arrested at any stage or may go on to fibrosis with restructuring and destruction of air exchange units, airway distortion, and eventual development of an end-stage lung.[279,354] Therapy is directed at removal of the inciting agents, suppression of alveolitis, and palliation of complications. Every effort is made to suppress the alveolitis before it leads to irreversible fibrosis, and steroids are the therapeutic mainstay. Because of the importance of identifying reversible active alveolitis at a stage when only minor fibrosis is present, much effort has been spent in disease "staging." This is achieved by evaluating lung dysfunction and assessing the activity of the alveolitis, as indicated by the number, type, and activation of inflammatory cells.[158,159] In making these assessments, the physician considers the patient history, clinical signs, chest radiograph, respiratory function tests, and, most reliably, lung biopsy, which should ideally be an open biopsy. In addition, three other tests have been used to assess activity: gallium-67 scintiscanning,[158,159,467] bronchoalveolar lavage,[158,265,339] and high-resolution computed tomography (HRCT).[337,452,739,757]

Most of the chronic interstitial pneumonitides are considered as specific entities elsewhere; the discussion here is limited to the idiopathic variety and to end-stage lung.

Cryptogenic fibrosing alveolitis or idiopathic pulmonary fibrosis

CFA is a specific disorder characterized by a combination of clinical, physiologic, morphologic, lavage, and scintigraphic features.[158] Its terminology has been the cause of much confusion, and about 20 synonyms now exist.[265] In much of the literature the terms "usual interstitial pneumonia" and "desquamative interstitial pneumonia" have been used, although strictly speaking these are not specific to the idiopathic form. The term "Hamman-Rich syndrome" has been used to describe the acute, aggressive form of the disease,[326] although now this syndrome is considered a form of diffuse alveolar damage.[559] In the following discussion the term introduced by Scadding, "cryptogenic fibrosing alveolitis," is used.[465,659]

CFA is a disorder of unknown cause. A familial factor has been identified in a few patients,[51,400,702] and in one study the occurrence of eight cases in three generations was consistent with an autosomal dominant inheritance.[59] However, a well-established relationship exists with autoimmune conditions, particularly rheumatoid arthritis and other connective tissue disorders.[213] To classify such cases as cryptogenic might seem a contradiction in terms, but several major studies of CFA include such patients. A problem centers on deciding which patients to exclude, because some have an associated, full-blown collagen vascular disorder, whereas many others manifest only certain features, such as isolated arthropathy or Raynaud's syndrome. Such difficulties have led to such terms as "lone CFA." In the Brompton Hospital series of 220 patients, 70% had lone CFA and 30% had an additional polyarthritis or immunologic disorder. Of the latter group, about one third had rheumatoid arthritis and one third some other collagen vascular disease.[761] Recognized associations of CFA, other than collagen vascular disease, include chronic active hepatitis, primary biliary cirrhosis, ulcerative colitis, adult celiac disease, Sjögren's syndrome, Raynaud's phenomenon, thyroid disorders including Hashimoto's thyroiditis, renal tubular acidosis, pernicious anemia, and autoimmune hemolytic anemia.[490,699,759,761] An arthropathy that is not part of a recognized connective tissue disorder is fairly common.

Most theories concerning pathogenesis implicate injury to alveolar endothelial and epithelial cells by circulating or inhaled agents. Following this an immune response occurs with activated macrophages secreting factors that activate neutrophils and stimulate fibroblasts to produce collagen. A number of recent articles have considered pathogenesis.[118,202,685]

On pathologic examination of the lungs the distribution of the alveolitic process is characteristically patchy[104,158]; therefore histologic assessment requires open lung biopsy.[269] A definite diagnosis cannot be made from a transbronchial lung biopsy.[779] Histologic changes evolve from an inflammatory alveolitis to an interstitial fibrosis,[187] and finding the whole range of pathologic changes in the same patient within a small compass may be possible.[418] Early changes consist of infiltration of alveolar septa by inflammatory cells, made up mainly of lymphocytes and plasma cells with occasional polymorphonuclear leukocytes, eosinophils, and mast cells. Type II pneumocytes proliferate, and type I cells diminish. Intraalveolar cells, predominantly macrophages, also increase in number. Hyaline membranes are notable by their absence, which helps in differentiating these changes from those of diffuse alveolar damage. Later, interstitial inflammatory cells are replaced by fibrous tissue, with deposition of collagen in the septa and subsequent obliteration of capillaries. Alveoli coalesce and become restructured with the formation of cystlike airspaces, some of which are lined by bronchiolar epithelium that grows into alveoli. Focal lymphoid follicle hyperplasia and hyperplasia of smooth muscle are also present, particularly in relation to terminal bronchioles, accounting for the term "muscular cirrhosis," which appears in the older literature.[418] The final appearance is that of an end-stage lung.

A variant on the preceding pattern was described in 1965[463] and called "desquamative interstitial pneumonia" (DIP). It was distinguished from CFA (usual interstitial pneumonitis) by extensive filling of alveoli with desquamated cells, later shown to be largely macrophages[264]; striking uniformity of the histologic appearance; less interstitial component and fibrosis; the young age of the patients; a characteristic chest radiograph; and a better prognosis, being more responsive to steroids. A number of authors support the contention that DIP is a specific clinicopathologic entity,[104,270,418] but others regard it as merely representing an early phase of CFA.[149,662,751] On balance, this latter view seems reasonable, especially because some of the original features of DIP such as specific radiologic signs and better prognosis have been shown to be inconstant.[238,581] In addition, pathologic changes of DIP can coexist with those of typical CFA.[662]

Several large series of CFA have been described in detail.[104,158,469,708,761] The prevalence rate is about 3 to 5 patients per 100,000 population.[157] The patients are typically adults in their fifth or sixth decades, but the disorder has a wide age range and is even described in infants and children.[359] Most series have shown a slight male preponderance.[761] The most common initial symptoms are progressive exertional dyspnea and cough, which is usually nonproductive but in one series was productive in just over half of the patients.[761] Less common symptoms include nonspecific chest pain[469]; constitutional symptoms such as fever, weight loss, and fatigue[396]; and joint pains. Some patients date the onset to an influenza-like illness.[396] In a small proportion of patients CFA is detected because of an abnormal "routine radiograph." In one series 47% of patients had the disease found in this manner, an exceptionally high frequency for this form of presentation.[810] Late, fine inspiratory crackles at the lung bases are an almost universal finding,[761]

and two thirds to three fourths of the patients show clubbing of the fingers.[469,661,761,810] Occasionally, full-blown hypertrophic osteoarthropathy is seen.[469] In advanced disease cor pulmonale and cyanosis may develop.[396]

Changes in respiratory function tests[158,396,761] are those that might be expected from a diffuse interstitial process: reduced compliance and lung volumes, particularly vital capacity and total lung capacity with relative sparing of residual volume; altered small airway function; and hyperventilation and arterial desaturation, particularly on exercise. Reduction in diffusing capacity is a particularly early and characteristic change. Laboratory blood tests show raised erythrocyte sedimentation rate (ESR) and immunoglobulin levels in about one third of patients.[761] Overall more than one half of the patients have autoantibodies. Antinuclear antibody is present in 15% to 45% of patients, and rheumatoid factor is found in up to one third.[302,708,761,804]

As in other diffuse interstitial disease,[222,269] the lungs can be histologically affected despite a normal chest radiograph.[269,463,469] Patients with a normal chest radiograph may be symptomatic and have an abnormal diffusion capacity.[662] In other patients the radiographic appearance is abnormal before symptoms develop.[708]

A variety of radiographic changes have been described,* the most common of which are small irregular opacities (Figure 12-1), seen in about three fourths of patients, and less commonly small round opacities, seen in about one fifth. This reticulonodular shadowing may be basal (Figures 12-2 and 12-3) or may be more generally distributed (Figure 12-4), with a lower zone accentuation.[158] A peripheral accentuation is also a common feature (Figure 12-3) that is much more easily appreciated on computed tomography (CT) (Figure 12-5)[47,541] than on plain radiographs.[469] The shadowing is usually symmetric from side to side, but atypical distributions such as limitation to a lobe[158] or apex[158,469] may be seen. Another common pattern is hazy, ground-glass opacification (Figure 12-6), which may be diffuse or patchy and may contain an air bronchogram.[158] This pattern is seen in up to one third of patients.[104] At one time this pattern, particularly when confined to the lower zones, was thought to be characteristic of the DIP variant of CFA,[270,463] but this is no longer held to be true.[581] Septal lines are occasionally recorded.[158] Volume loss characterized by diaphragmatic elevation[158,661] is seen in 25% to 60% of cases,[104,112,535] and basal discoid atelectasis is occasionally seen secondary to elevation of the diaphragm.[238] The loss of volume may be basally predominant or generalized.[423] Although pleural opacity is recorded in some series,[112,187,761] it is generally not a feature of CFA and should raise the question of other conditions such as asbestosis,[423] rheumatoid disease, or systemic lupus erythematosus. Pneumothorax occurs

---

*References 104, 112, 158, 238, 469, 535, 712, 761.

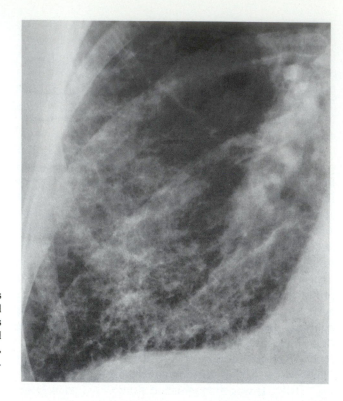

FIGURE 12-1
Cryptogenic fibrosing alveolitis. Localized view of right lung base shows widespread interstitial shadowing. Predominant opacities are small rounded, linear, and irregular shadows. Other, less profuse elements include small rounded transradiancies about 1 to 2 mm in diameter and a variety of thin line opacities, some resembling septal lines. In parts, shadowing has become confluent, taking on a ground-glass appearance. Characteristically shadowing overall is rather fine and uniform.

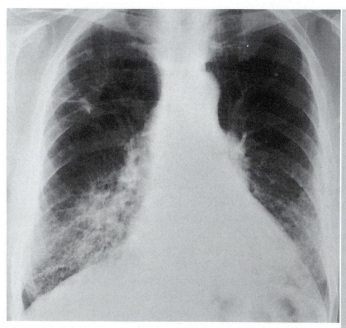

A

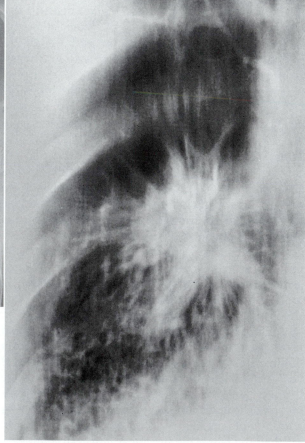

B

FIGURE 12-2
Cryptogenic fibrosing alveolitis. **A,** Posteroanterior chest radiograph. Note symmetric, basally predominant shadowing made up of small irregular and rounded opacities. Distribution is characteristic of fibrosing alveolitis. Just below the right hilum is an area of confluent shadowing 5 cm in diameter. **B,** Conventional tomogram of right lower zone shows 5 cm, star-shaped, spiculated opacity typical of bronchial carcinoma. Histologically lesion is squamous cell carcinoma.

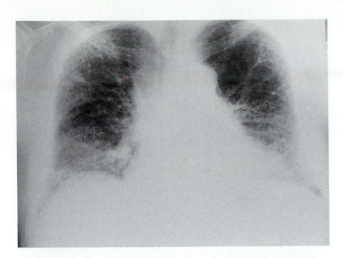

FIGURE 12-3
Cryptogenic fibrosing alveolitis. Note interstitial opacity with predominantly basal and peripheral distribution. Both of these patterns are characteristic. Opacity is reticulonodular with dominant reticular element. Cardiomegaly is caused by incidental ischemic heart disease.

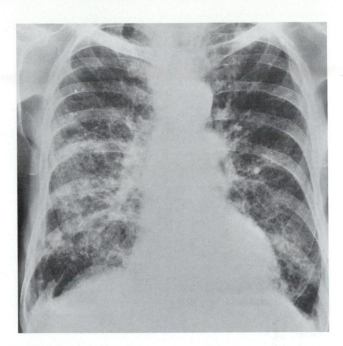

FIGURE 12-4
Cryptogenic fibrosing alveolitis. Bilateral changes are more severe on right than on left. Shadowing is a mixture of small rounded and irregular nodules generalized on right but basally predominant on left. Lung volume is slightly increased, a recognized but not common finding in fibrosing alveolitis.

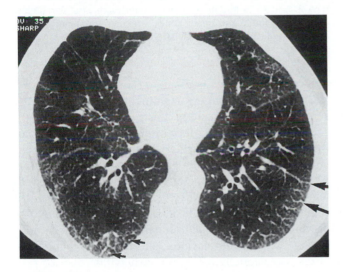

FIGURE 12-5
Cryptogenic fibrosing alveolitis (CFA) on high-resolution computed tomogram. Radiologic features in patient with biopsy-proven CFA are well recognized but less common than honeycombing and ground-glass opacity. Lesions are distributed in characteristic peripheral and posterolateral fashion. They consist of interlobular *(large arrows)* and intralobular septal thickening with prominent centrilobular structures *(small arrows).* Note also a ground-glass element.

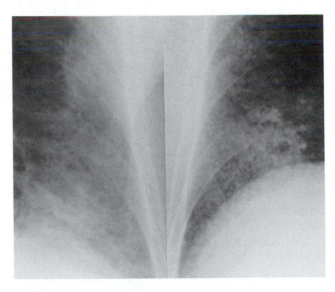

FIGURE 12-6
Cryptogenic fibrosing alveolitis in 65-year-old man. Localized views of same costophrenic angle region (one laterally inverted), on left at presentation and on right 30 months later. Initial opacity has ground-glass appearance, which is commonly seen in "active," early alveolitis. It evolves into predominantly small nodular (small rounded and small irregular) pattern with early small ring opacities.

occasionally and in one series was recorded in 4 of 45 patients.[469] Pneumomediastinum (Figure 12-7) is also a recognized complication that is probably more common than pneumothorax.[423] Ossific nodules recognized on pathologic study may in rare cases be seen radiologically.[507]

With progression of the alveolitis to fibrosis the initially fine shadowing becomes coarser[469] and small cystlike transradiancies appear (Figure 12-6). Initially these are

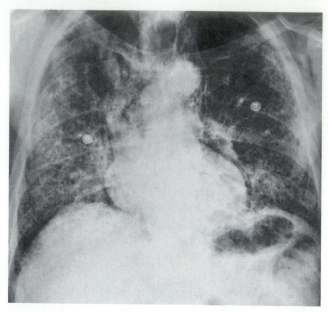

FIGURE 12-7
Pneumomediastinum and cryptogenic fibrosing alveolitis. Note long-standing fibrosing alveolitis with changes on right of aggregated, small, thick-walled ring opacities (honeycomb shadowing). Note also pneumomediastinum.

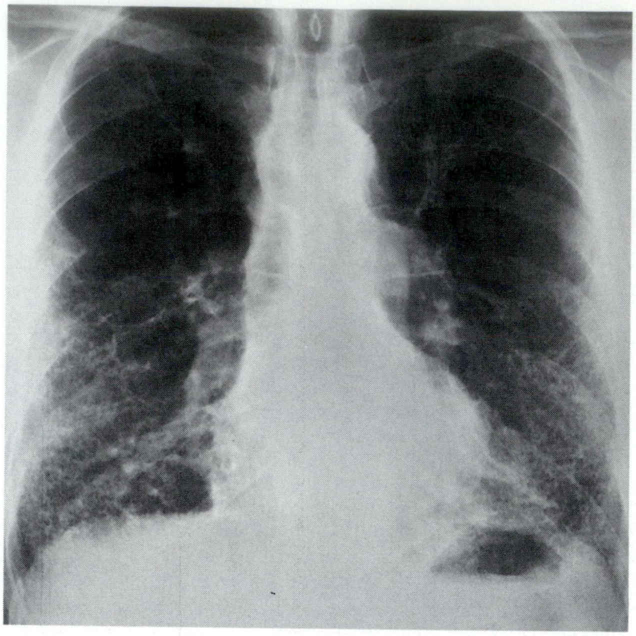

FIGURE 12-8
Radiograph of patient with cryptogenic fibrosing alveolitis shows typical changes in middle and lower zones with extensive bullous changes in middle and upper zones. Proximal pulmonary arteries are large, indicating pulmonary arterial hypertension.

just 2 mm or so in diameter, but later they increase in size until they correspond to the 5 to 7 mm ring opacities of honeycomb lung. In several series honeycomb opacities have been present in one third to one half of patients.[104,712] With gross fibrosis, larger cysts and bullae appear,[469] and despite the fibrosis lung volumes may increase (Figure 12-8). Commonly radiographic evidence of pulmonary arterial hypertension can be seen.

Attempts have been made to correlate chest radiographic findings with histology, respiratory function tests, symptoms, prognosis, and response to treatment. The literature on the subject is confusing; correlations are largely negative and often inconsistent. Thus, for example, profusion of opacities has been shown both to correlate[761] and not to correlate[712] with dyspnea. The only correlation that appears with any consistency is that coarse reticulation or honeycomb opacities indicate severe fibrosis.[158,469,809] Alveolar or ground-glass shadowing may correlate with mild fibrosis or marked cellularity.[158,463,661,662,804] However, this is not a universal finding, and other workers find no correlation between histologic features and the chest radiograph.[187,761] In an attempt to overcome the unreliability of the chest radiograph taken on its own, scoring systems that include other variables have been assessed.[784]

A number of reports have documented the CT and HRCT findings in CFA.* These studies have shown that for optimal evaluation HRCT must be used,[534] and this is

*References 46, 337, 534, 535, 549, 712, 718, 757.

particularly true in assessing ground-glass opacity.[535] HRCT is now the imaging examination of choice for CFA, being both more sensitive and more specific than the chest radiograph.[492,757] Two quite distinct types of opacity are found: those considered to represent active alveolitis, as exemplified by ground-glass opacity (Figure 12-9), and those characteristic of fibrosis, typified by honeycombing (Figure 12-10). Ground-glass opacity is commonly seen.[337,549] It is usually symmetric and may be distributed as a subpleural band (Figure 12-9); in a patchy and random fashion; or, least commonly, diffusely. Occasionally areas of consolidation may be seen with air bronchograms. Honeycomb opacity characteristically forms a peel immediately below the pleura with a posterolateral and lower zone distribution (Figure 12-11). In its early stages honeycomb opacity sometimes forms a band of reticulation just inset from the pleura from which it is separated by a narrow strip of normal lung.[718] In advanced disease cysts become widely dispersed throughout the lung parenchyma (Figure 12-12). The cystic airspaces range from 2 to 20 mm in diameter, and walls range from hairline to 2 mm in thickness. Honeycombing is usually bilaterally symmetric, but it can be localized and asymmetric.

Within areas of honeycombing the normal lung structure is totally destroyed, and apart from traction bronchiolectasis (Figure 12-11) and volume loss, other signs of fibrosis cannot be appreciated. However, in the adjacent lung other features of fibrosis may be detected: (1) irregular interfaces (Figures 12-5 and 12-10) between the

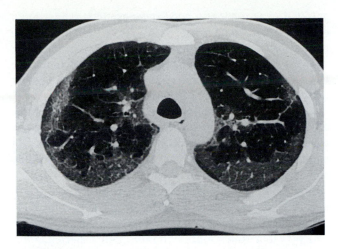

FIGURE 12-9
Cryptogenic fibrosing alveolitis on high-resolution computed tomogram. Predominant finding is posterolateral, subpleural band of ground-glass opacity. This appearance suggests "active," cellular alveolitis, which was confirmed by biopsy. Some pathologists would call histologic appearance "desquamative interstitial pneumonitis."

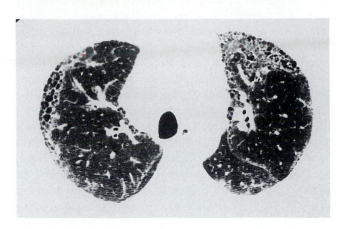

FIGURE 12-10
Cryptogenic fibrosing alveolitis (CFA) on high-resolution computed tomogram. Predominant change in patient is of small aggregated, peripheral ring opacities, typical of fibrotic stage of CFA. In anterior segment of left upper lobe note a mixed honeycomb and ground-glass pattern.

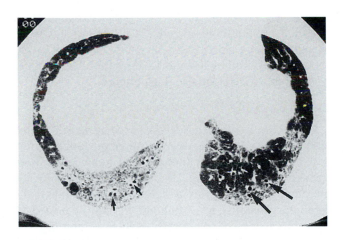

FIGURE 12-11
Cryptogenic fibrosing alveolitis on high-resolution computed tomogram. Small ring opacities indicated on right are small airways that can be identified by accompanying artery. Airways *(large arrows)* show changes of traction bronchiolectasis. They are closer to pleura than normal 3 cm limit and are dilated. Small rounded low-density features on right, in region of confluent opacity *(small arrows)*, are also airways.

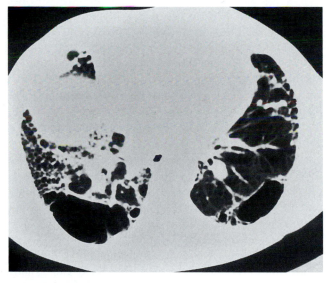

FIGURE 12-12
High-resolution thin-section computed tomography scan of long-standing cryptogenic fibrosing alveolitis. On right note mixture of honeycomb reticulation and larger ring opacities, probably bullae. The 6 cm round opacity anteriorly in right lung is a complicating adenocarcinoma.

lung and vessels, airways, and pleura. Pleural irregularity is often best seen against the mediastinum (Figure 12-10).[718] (2) Interlobular septal thickening (irregular) and intralobular interstitial thickening (Figure 12-5), manifest as fine reticulation. (3) Lobular distortion and traction bronchi(ol)ectasis (Figure 12-11), and (4) prominent centrilobular structures (Figure 12-5) are seen. Prominence is caused by scarring around arteries and airways. When airways are affected, their walls become

thickened and they are seen more peripherally than usual, less than 3 cm from the pleural surface (Figure 12-11). (5) Long irregular lines of scarring often extend inward from the pleural surface. (6) Subpleural linear opacity may be seen (Figure 12-10). This is most commonly relatively narrow and irregular. It lies within 1 cm of the pleural surface to which it is parallel.

In CFA the predominant histologic type predicts response to treatment and likely outcome. Cellular biopsies with accumulation of inflammatory cells in the interstitium and alveoli indicate the likelihood of a more favorable response to treatment and better prognosis than fibrotic biopsies.[104,761] Lung histologic findings also correlate with CT patterns, and scan findings can therefore be used to predict outcome and guide treatment. Ground-glass opacity is associated with the active alveolitic phase, with increase in inflammatory cells in the interstitium and alveoli, whereas reticulation (honeycomb opacity) indicates fibrosis.[337,452,535,739] Other evidence supports this association. Thus irregular linear opacities on HRCT, representing scarring, have been shown to evolve from ground-glass areas on previous scans.[739] Furthermore, the extent of ground-glass opacity before treatment has been shown to correlate with the degree of clinical and respiratory function improvement following steroid therapy.[452,535] More recent studies suggest that the predominance of ground-glass opacity compared with honeycombing is a more important predictor of favorable prognosis than is the absolute extent of ground-glass opacity per se.[793,794]

CT has a number of advantages over biopsy in evaluation of the activity of alveolitis: CT is noninvasive; it is repeatable; and since it is a global assessment, it is not subject to sampling error. This last point is an important consideration in CFA, in which lesions and types of lesions are often distributed in a patchy and random fashion. In view of the sensitivity and specificity of HRCT in CFA and the correlation of HRCT changes with histologic findings, the point has been reached when lung biopsy can probably be avoided in a significant number of patients with CFA.[757]

HRCT studies in CFA have unexpectedly shown that mild lymphadenopathy is common; it was present in 13 out of 14 patients in one series.[45] The bronchopulmonary, paratracheal, aortopulmonary, and anterior mediastinal sites were most commonly affected, with 1 to 7 sites involved in each patient.[45] HRCT also enables evaluation of coexisting disease such as emphysema.[798]

Gallium-67 is taken up in "active" CFA, and in most series about 70% of patients have had positive scintiscans. In one study the gallium index (a derivative of the area, intensity, and texture of uptake) correlated with the severity of the alveolitis as assessed by cellularity.[467] The gallium scintiscan is one of the investigations used to stage CFA, but it is not widely used and its place in management has yet to be clearly defined.

The prognosis in CFA is poor, with mean survival after presentation ranging from about 3 to 6 years.[104,707,761] Hidden within these figures, however, is a great variation, ranging in one series from 4 months to 20 years.[708] Progression of CFA can be slow or even come to a halt.[662] The possibility that some cases in which there is rapid progression to death represent diffuse alveolar damage (acute interstitial pneumonitis) rather than CFA should be considered.[418] Features that carry a good prognosis are an age of less than 40 years, a short history of symptoms

at initial examination, a good response to steroids, and a cellular biopsy with little in the way of fibrosis. The prognosis is probably the same in fibrosing alveolitis, whether it is cryptogenic or associated with a connective tissue disorder.[754,761] Some studies, however, suggest that the cryptogenic form progresses more rapidly.[5]

The chief treatment for CFA is steroids; occasionally other drugs such as penicillamine and cytotoxic agents are tried. Steroids are of some help, with 40% to 60% of patients experiencing subjective improvement and 20% showing objective improvement.[396,761]

About 50% of patients die of a cause directly related to the CFA, such as respiratory failure. The second most common cause of death is cardiovascular disease,[754] which is four times more common than expected.[708,761] The third most common cause of death is carcinoma of the lung, which develops 14 times more frequently in these patients than in the general population (Figure 12-2).[764] Its development is related to the CFA itself, apart from smoking, and no predicting factors for its development in the presence of CFA have been identified.[764] An analogous increase in the prevalence of bronchial carcinoma in lung fibrosis associated with systemic sclerosis is well recognized.[621] The prevalence of carcinoma in various series has ranged between 5% and 13%.[708,754,764] A review of 62 cases found squamous carcinomas in 35%, alveolar cell carcinomas in 27%, adenocarcinomas in 21%, and 11% undifferentiated.[256] This preponderance of adenocarcinoma, particularly alveolar cell, is not a universal finding, and in some series the pattern of cell types is no different from the usual experience.[764]

End-stage lung

Many diffuse diseases, such as fibrosing alveolitis, that predominantly affect the interstitium of the lung progress to a final nonspecific pathologic and radiologic pattern termed "end-stage lung."[279] The term describes the morphologic change only and does not imply functional respiratory insufficiency, although this may be present. A large number of conditions can evolve to produce this pattern.[279,345,368] These include fibrosing alveolitis, both cryptogenic and secondary to collagen vascular disorders; histiocytosis X; drug-induced interstitial pneumonitis; lymphocytic interstitial pneumonitis; extrinsic allergic alveolitis; inorganic dust inhalation, such as asbestosis and berylliosis; chronic granulomatous infections (fungal); sarcoidosis; lymphangioleiomyomatosis; and rarely pulmonary alveolar proteinosis.[376] End-stage lung is also recognized with chronic venous hypertension, with chronic gastric aspiration, and following various forms of diffuse alveolar damage, for example, from toxic inhalations, oxygen, infections, and radiation.[418]

The distal airspaces are restructured, remaining walls become thick and fibrotic, and airways are obliterated. This results in the macroscopic appearance of honeycomb lung in which multiple cysts are separated by dense interstitial fibrosis.[418] The chief pathologic find-

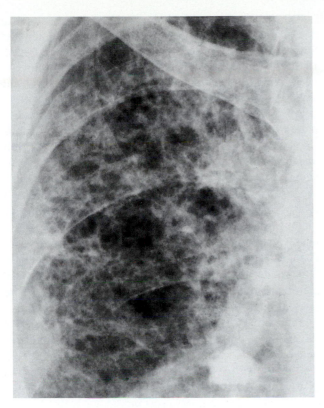

FIGURE 12-13
End-stage lung. Localized view, right middle and upper zones. Underlying process in this patient was cryptogenic fibrosing alveolitis. Much of the shadowing consists of 2 to 6 mm ring opacities, which in part have characteristics of honeycomb shadowing. Ring opacities like these are the hallmark of end-stage lung.

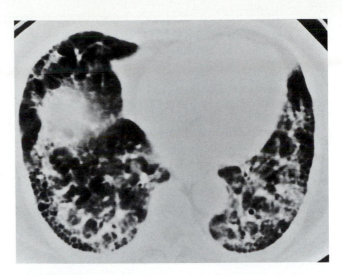

FIGURE 12-14
High-resolution thin-section computed tomography of end-stage lung. Primary process in this patient was fibrosing alveolitis associated with rheumatoid disease. Dominant element is 2 to 10 mm ring opacities separated by band densities of varying thickness produced by fibrosis.

ings[279,354,418] consist of septal thickening from cellular infiltration and fibrosis; septal dissolution leading to restructuring and coalescence of alveoli; bronchiolectasis and small airway obliteration; obstructive vascular changes and capillary obliteration; smooth muscle proliferation; proliferation of bronchiolar epithelium, which grows along alveolar ducts and alveoli; metaplastic and neoplastic change of bronchiolar epithelium; mesenchymal osseous metaplasia; and endogenous lipid pneumonitis. On gross examination the most characteristic feature of ESL is the presence of small cystic spaces, which gives the surface of the lung a bosselated appearance.[279] These cysts vary in size from 1 mm to 2 cm, but the typical size is on the order of 5 to 10 mm. Three mechanisms account for the formation of cysts: alveolar simplification secondary to septal dissolution, bronchiolectasis, and obstructive emphysema.

Just as the cysts are the most characteristic gross morphologic finding in pathologic specimens, so too are they the most characteristic radiologic feature. They appear as aggregated, small, ring opacities that are termed honeycomb shadows when they have a diameter of 5 to 10 mm with walls 1 to 2 mm thick (Figure 12-13).[258] There may be additional small rounded and irregular opacities, but these lack the specificity of honeycomb

opacities in the diagnosis of ESL. The radiologic changes are usually diffuse, bilateral, and asymmetric. Lung volume may be normal, increased, or decreased, depending on the mix of pathologic processes. Features of cor pulmonale are evident in advanced disease, and in long-standing cases small calcified nodules[507] may form as a result of metaplastic ossification.[615] Scar carcinoma is a recognized complication[514] and may appear radiologically as a mass or as consolidation. Multifocal carcinomas are described.[418] CT findings (Figure 12-14) consist of honeycombing, extensive cystic change with well-defined walls and conglomerate fibrosis. Interspersed with these features often are nonspecific findings that reflect the antecedent disorder.[604]

Although end-stage lung is a nonspecific appearance with a wide variety of causes, limiting the differential possibilities is often possible using plain radiographic features (see Chapter 5). Radiologic features that help in this way include the zonal distribution of changes, lung volume, pleural changes, and the presence or absence of adenopathy. Zonal distribution is particularly helpful in this regard.[258] CT findings may be used in a similar fashion and have been shown to have a specificity of 80% to 100% in histiocytosis X, silicosis, asbestosis, fibrosing alveolitis, extrinsic allergic alveolitis, and sarcoidosis.[604] Features with the highest diagnostic value are zonal distribution; relationship of changes to bronchovascular structures; and the presence or absence of diffuse cystic spaces, pleural opacity, and ground-glass opacity.[604]

LUNG VASCULITIDES

The vasculitides are a large and varied group of disorders characterized by inflammation and necrosis of

---

**CLASSIFICATION OF PULMONARY
VASCULITIDES**

Granulomatous vasculitis
  Wegener's granulomatosis
  Allergic granulomatosis and angiitis (Churg-Strauss
    syndrome)
  Necrotizing sarcoidal angiitis and granulomatosis
Microscopic polyarteritis nodosa
Hypersensitivity vasculitis
  Anaphylactoid purpura (Henoch-Schönlein)
  Systemic urticarial vasculitis
  Essential mixed cryoglobulinemia
  Vasculitis associated with connective tissue disease
  Vasculitis associated with malignancy
  Nonspecific hypersensitivity vasculitis
Giant cell vasculitis
  Systemic temporal arteritis
  Other giant cell arteritides
Behçet's disease and Hughes-Stovin syndrome
Polyangiitis overlap syndrome

---

blood vessels.[235] They may be localized to one organ or may be disseminated (systemic). Much evidence now indicates that immune complex deposition is of prime pathogenic importance in these disorders, with other mechanisms such as cell-mediated immunity making a contribution.[235,450]

Several schemes have been used to classify the systemic vasculitides, reflecting the fact that no one classification is entirely satisfactory. The classification used here is based on several recent reviews (see box above).[197,235,342,450,500] Note that the table does not include *classic* polyarteritis nodosa, since this vasculitis characteristically spares the lungs.[235,637] Several papers discuss the contentious relationship of classic polyarteritis nodosa, Churg-Strauss syndrome, and polyangiitis overlap syndrome.[197,235]

Granulomatous vasculitis

A pathologic characteristic of granulomatous vasculitis is the cellular infiltrate consisting predominantly of histiocytes (tissue macrophages).

Three vasculitic processes affecting the lungs can be considered granulomatous: Wegener's granulomatosis (WG), allergic granulomatosis and angiitis (Churg-Strauss syndrome), and necrotizing sarcoidal angiitis and granulomatosis.

WEGENER'S GRANULOMATOSIS. Wegener's granulomatosis was first described in the 1930s.[210] It has distinctive clinicopathologic features and can therefore be more easily recognized as a distinct entity than most of the other vasculitides.[235] Its cause is obscure, but accumulating evidence suggests that the entity is probably an immunologic reaction to a specific antigen and that immune complex formation plays an important role.[450]

WG is characterized pathologically by three features: a necrotizing granulomatous vasculitis of the upper and lower respiratory tracts, a disseminated small vessel vasculitis involving both arteries and veins, and a focal, necrotizing glomerulonephritis.[450] A limited form of the disease has been described as affecting the lung with or without upper respiratory disease but without renal or other systemic involvement.[105,372] In making the diagnosis of WG, having biopsy evidence of a mixed vasculitic and granulomatous process affecting both arteries and veins is important.[123] In practice the lung biopsy provides the most useful information. Renal changes are usually nonspecific, rarely showing either vasculitic or granulomatous lesions, and the specific lesions in the upper airways are often masked by the secondary infective changes. The wide range of pathologic findings in the lung in addition to parenchymal necrosis, vasculitis, and granulomatous inflammation has recently been reviewed.[749]

A set of four clinical criteria for making the diagnosis of WG has been proposed: an abnormal urine sediment (red blood cells or casts), an abnormal chest radiograph (consistent with WG), oral ulcers or nasal discharge, and granulomatous inflammation on biopsy. These criteria are 88% sensitive and 92% specific.[451]

Clinical features have recently been reviewed.[366] The mean age at presentation is in the fifth decade[13,140,236,366] with a wide range: 8 to 75 years in one series.[181] Sex incidence is equal or slightly male predominant. Onset is usually acute or subacute but may be indolent, and when the latter is combined with atypical features, diagnosis may be delayed for years.[198] Upper airway involvement with sinusitis, rhinitis, and otitis is the most common clinical feature at presentation, encountered twice as often as lung and systemic symptoms. Functional renal impairment is unusual at the time of diagnosis, occurring in only about 10% of patients.[236] Laboratory examination often shows a normochromic, normocytic anemia; leukocytosis; raised ESR; and the presence of rheumatoid factor.[236] More than 90% of patients with active multiorgan WG have a positive test for cytoplasmic antineutrophil cytoplasmic antibodies (cANCA).[366,704] With limited disease these figures fall to 60% to 70% and in remission to 30% to 40%. Positive tests are also seen in systemic necrotizing small vessel vasculitis (microscopic polyarteritis), rapidly progressive glomerulonephritis, and the Churg-Strauss syndrome.

During the course of the illness 85% to 90% of patients have lung involvement and all have lung or upper respiratory tract disease. A majority (85%) develop renal disease, and in about 50% of patients joint, ear, skin, and eye disorders become manifest with occasional involvement of the heart and nervous system.[236] In established WG, pulmonary or nonpulmonary infection may precipitate clinical relapse,[1] and in some series such infections have accounted for about 50% of relapses.[591] Untreated WG carries a poor prognosis, with death in about 5 months from renal failure.[210] The outlook, however, has been trans-

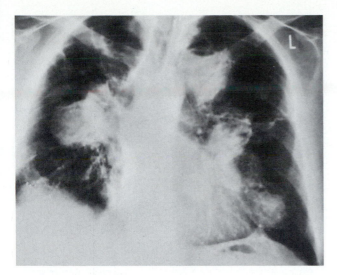

FIGURE 12-15
Wegener's granulomatosis. Note multiple, well-defined nodules ranging in size from 1 to 7 cm. Lesion in left upper zone has cavitated and contains small air-fluid level. *L*, Left. (Courtesy Dr. G.J. Hunter, London.)

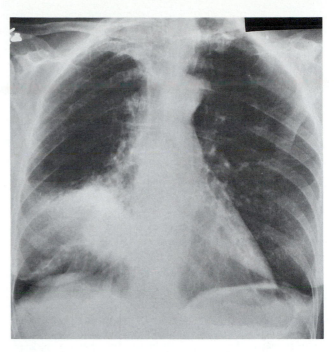

FIGURE 12-16
Wegener's granulomatosis. Main finding in this patient is 10 × 6 cm triangular opacity in right lower zone. It has features of consolidation.

formed by treatment with cyclophosphamide and steroids, which can induce and maintain remission in a high percentage of patients,[236] giving a 5-year survival in the order of 90% to 95%. In the recent National Institutes of Health review of 158 patients, 75% had complete remission, often taking a year or more, following which 50% had one or more relapses and almost all had serious morbidity from irreversible features of the disease or infection.[366] The lung localized form of WG is not uncommon with a frequency of 9% and 10% in two pulmonary series[13,140] and generally pursues an indolent course for years,[105] after which it commonly becomes systemic.

Radiographic changes in the lungs occur at presentation in about 75% of patients and are usually manifestations of the primary disease. In established disease the situation is more complicated and radiographic findings may be related to relapse or progression, a complication of management (drug toxicity, infection, neoplasm), or secondary to disease of a nonpulmonary organ (renal failure). The account that follows concentrates on primary manifestations. These may be accompanied by cough, hemoptysis, pain, or dyspnea, but these symptoms are often not a dominant finding. Not infrequently the patient has no chest symptoms.

The most characteristic pulmonary radiologic finding is discrete focal opacities that vary in character from nodular masses (Figure 12-15) to ill-defined areas of consolidation (Figure 12-16), either of which may cavitate. Nodular shadows are visible at presentation in the majority of patients (62% in one series).[233] In one fifth to one third of the patients nodules are single. In the remaining majority, nodules are multiple (Figure 12-15). Commonly 2 to 4 cm in diameter,[443] the nodules may range in size from 3 mm to 10 cm.[393,502] They are rounded or oval and may be well or poorly defined, sometimes becoming confluent.[502] They are usually less than 10 in number but occasionally are innumerable.[393] The nodules have no strong affinity for any one zone; some series have a preponderance of nodules in the middle and lower zones,[13,296] while others do not.[291] Nodules commonly resolve with or without treatment over a period of months. They may heal without residual abnormality, or they may leave a visible scar.[296]

Focal opacities with the features of pulmonary consolidation occur in about 30% of patients (Figure 12-16).[233] They may be single or multiple and vary from small heterogeneous patches[502] to homogeneous segmental or lobar consolidations.[140,233,291] Sometimes a mixed pattern of nodules and consolidation is seen, and the radiographic distinction between the two is not always clear.[296] New lung lesions during relapses often occur in areas affected in previous episodes, even though the radiographic appearance of the lesions may be different from that seen originally.[233]

Cavitation of the nodules (Figure 12-17) and consolidations is seen in approximately 40% of cases at initial examination.[233] Cavities may be unilocular or multilocular,[502] and the outer margins of their walls are more commonly irregular than smooth.[443] Wall width varies greatly. Typically it is thick, with an irregular or smooth inner margin, but when the cavities have been present for some time, the walls tend to become thinner.[233] Cavities may have air-fluid levels,[502] sometimes indicating secondary infection.[1,450]

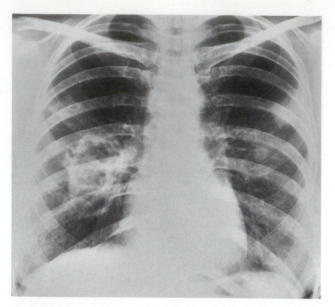

FIGURE 12-17
Wegener's granulomatosis. Multiple nodules with large (6 cm) cavitary lesion adjacent to right hilum. Its walls are thick and irregular on both aspects. (Courtesy Dr. G.J. Hunter, London.)

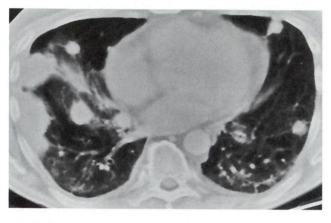

FIGURE 12-18
Wegener's granulomatosis. Computed tomography scan shows mixed radiologic lesions. There are several nodules, flame-shaped consolidation anteriorly on right, and confluent subpleural opacities, also on right.

CT studies have confirmed plain radiographic studies and added new observations,[436] including consolidations with air bronchograms (Figure 12-18), or pleurally based and wedgelike, resembling pulmonary infarcts (Figure 12-18). Nodules commonly (88%) have feeding vessels as described in pulmonary infarcts and metastases, and additional spiculation and pleural tags ascribed to fibrosis. Nodules may also have low-density (necrotic) centers,[140] and there is a single case report of widespread bronchovascular cuffing.[254]

Diffuse bilateral consolidation is likely to be caused by diffuse pulmonary hemorrhage,[448] which occurs both in

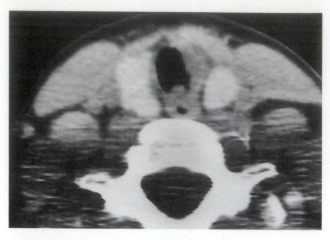

FIGURE 12-19
Wegener's granulomatosis. Computed tomography scan at level of thyroid shows irregular soft tissue thickening of tracheal wall, posteriorly and on left, which compromises lumen. (Courtesy Dr. S.C. Rankin, London.)

established disease[717] and at presentation.[140] In a series of 77 patients with respiratory WG, 8% presented with diffuse pulmonary hemorrhage.[140] In one patient, who was in respiratory failure at diagnosis, massive consolidation was caused by extensive WG tissue.[454]

Tracheal narrowing is an infrequent but important phenomenon in WG. It was present in 17 of 108 patients with WG in the Mayo Clinic series,[501] and all but one of these patients was female. All patients had nasal involvement, but only four (24%) had pulmonary disease. Hoarseness and stridor usually occurred with or just after the onset of nasal symptoms, although in a few patients the symptoms were delayed by several years. Half the patients needed tracheostomy.[501] Patients with isolated laryngotracheal disease are also described.[348]

Tracheal stenoses are subglottic and can be clearly imaged by conventional tomography, which demonstrates smooth or irregular circumferential stenoses about 3 to 4 cm long.[134, 501] CT shows abnormal soft tissue within the tracheal rings (Figure 12-19), which themselves may be abnormally thickened and calcified.[714] Stenotic lesions of the more distal airways, usually mainstem or lobar, are well recognized, and in one pulmonary series bronchial stenoses had a frequency of 18%.[140] They usually become manifest by causing distal collapse or consolidation of a lobe or lung.[232]

Pleural effusions in WG, some of which are quite large, have been reported with a prevalence ranging from 5% to 55%.[13,291,296,480] Some of these effusions were probably only indirectly related to the presence of WG, and in general pleural effusions are unusual. Pneumothorax[399] and hydropneumothorax are occasionally seen. In one case they were associated with cavitary lung disease and in another with a bronchopleural fistula, the track of which was lined by Wegner's granulomatosis tissue.[224,480] Pleural thickening and subpleural masses have also been reported.[221,480]

Occasional cases have been described with hilar and mediastinal adenopathy detected on chest radiography[1,291] or CT.[134,140]

CHURG-STRAUSS SYNDROME. The Churg-Strauss syndrome is a systemic necrotizing vasculitis that occurs in patients with asthma and is characterized by a marked peripheral eosinophilia. Pathologic study shows a necrotizing vasculitis associated with a prominent eosinophilic infiltrate together with vascular and extravascular granulomas. However, histologic diagnosis is not entirely satisfactory because pathologic areas may be distributed in a patchy fashion, and biopsies may not reveal key features such as granulomas.[487] A more clinical approach to diagnosis may be adopted, and a list of six diagnostic criteria has recently been proposed with an 85% sensitivity and 99.7% specificity when four of six criteria are positive.[487] The criteria are asthma, blood eosinophilia (more than 10% eosinophils), neuropathy, nonfixed pulmonary consolidations, paranasal sinus abnormality, and extravascular eosinophilia on biopsy.

The Churg-Strauss syndrome has a variety of synonyms including angiitis and allergic granulomatosis. It was first described in 1951,[125] and since then three major series have reported the clinical and postmortem features.[122,444,637] Patients with the syndrome are commonly middle aged; the mean age at onset is 38 years,[444] with a range of 15 to 69 years.[122] The sexes are equally affected. A significant number of patients are atopic.[444]

In many patients the disease evolves in three stages: asthmatic, eosinophilic, and vasculitic.

Asthma is the first manifestation in all patients and is accompanied in 70% of cases by allergic rhinitis.[122] There is on average a 3-year gap between the onset of asthma and the development of vasculitis,[444] but this interval has ranged from a few months to as long as 30 years. Occasionally the illness is so telescoped that asthma and vasculitis are simultaneous in onset.[122] A short interval is associated with a poor prognosis.[122] With the onset of the vasculitic phase the asthma may increase in severity[444] or may remit.[125]

An eosinophilic phase commonly follows the asthmatic prodrome. It is characterized by blood eosinophilia and eosinophilic infiltration of tissues, particularly the lungs and gastrointestinal tract. At this stage the disease may relapse and remit for years before transforming into the final vasculitic phase.[444]

Many different tissues and organs may be involved by the vasculitis, including the myocardium, pericardium, joints, and muscles. The skin may show palpable purpura, erythema, urticaria, or subcutaneous nodules. Vasculitic involvement of the nerves may result in a mononeuritis multiplex and in the gut may cause abdominal pain, diarrhea, or intestinal bleeding. The kidneys may show segmental glomerulonephritis similar to that in

WG; however, such renal involvement rarely causes significant clinical disease.[122] The vasculitic phase is accompanied by systemic symptoms such as weight loss and fever. The ESR is raised, and usually a marked leukocytosis is present with a striking eosinophilia, with an eosinophil count as high as 30×10^9/L. However, active vasculitis may occur without blood eosinophilia.[444] The serum IgE value is commonly raised.[122,444]

Changes on the chest radiograph in the Churg-Strauss syndrome can occur in the eosinophilic or vasculitic phases. The reported frequency of chest radiographic abnormalities varies between 27%[122] and 72%.[444] This variation appears to be related to the frequency of obtaining chest radiographs; the higher figure is probably a better reflection of the true frequency of radiographic abnormalities during the course of the disease. The most common findings are transient, multifocal, and nonsegmental consolidations that show no zonal predilection,[125,142,444] an appearance that, when combined with blood eosinophilia, sometimes fulfills the criteria for Löffler's syndrome (Figure 12-20, *A*) (see p. 526). Multifocal consolidation may take on the appearance of multiple fluffy nodules.[432] The pulmonary consolidation, however, can be unifocal[432] or may even have the pattern of chronic eosinophilic pneumonia (see p. 526).[131,437] Widespread symmetric consolidation is seen with diffuse pulmonary hemorrhage.[444] Cavitation is unusual,[176] and both large nodule formation and cavitation are much less common than in WG. Less common findings include a diffuse or basal interstitial pattern[122]; diffuse miliary nodulation[86,122,456]; and hilar and mediastinal adenopathy, either unilateral or bilateral.[432,456] In a large review of 154 cases pleural effusions (Figure 12-20) occurred in 29% of patients,[444] and in many the effusions were eosinophilic. A single case report with pathologic correlation described HRCT changes in a patient with interstitial opacity on a chest radiograph.[86] The main findings were enlargement with irregularity of outline of peripheral arteries and veins, peribronchial thickening, interlobular septal thickening, and patchy consolidation. These changes were caused by an eosinophilic inflammatory cell infiltrate, granuloma formation, and lymphatic dilatation.

Cardiac involvement causes cardiomegaly resulting from pericarditis or myocarditis, as well as signs of raised pulmonary venous pressure. These signs may complicate the primary pleuropulmonary changes on the radiograph (Figure 12-20).[175,639]

The radiographic abnormalities may or may not clear with treatment.[122] Churg-Strauss syndrome responds well to steroids, but a small proportion of patients require adjunctive immunosuppressive agents. The vasculitic phase in most treated patients lasts less than a year, and late relapses are uncommon.[444]

NECROTIZING SARCOIDAL ANGIITIS. Necrotizing sarcoidal angiitis was first described in 1973 by Liebow.[460] A problem posed then — whether the entity was sarcoidosis

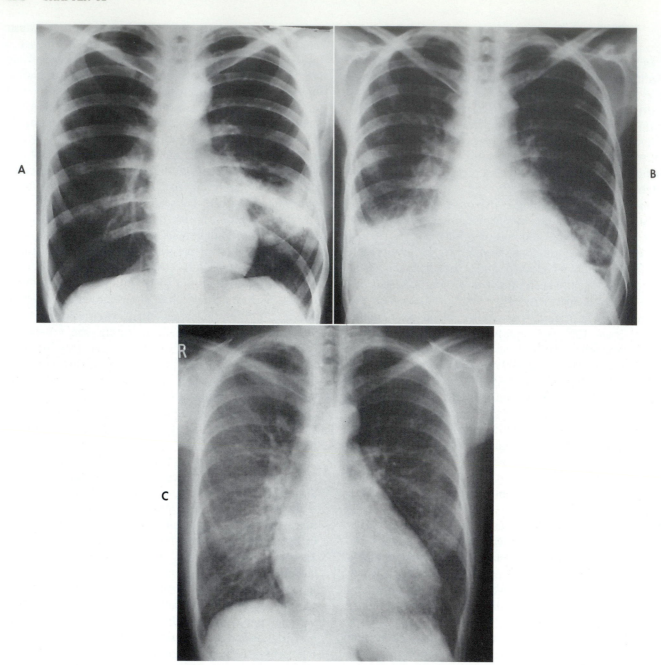

FIGURE 12-20
Churg-Strauss syndrome. Patient, 28-year-old asthmatic woman, had colitis followed by Löffler type of syndrome and blood eosinophilia (10.3×10^9/L). At this stage a few microaneurysms were demonstrated on hepatic and renal arteries. Within a year cardiomyopathy had developed. **A**, Chest radiograph during Löffler syndrome phase shows consolidation in left lower zone. This followed right upper zone consolidation. **B**, Six months later bilateral pleural effusions developed. **C**, One year later cardiomegaly has developed on basis of cardiomyopathy.

with necrosis of the granulomas and vessels, or a necrotizing vasculitis with a sarcoid reaction—remains unsettled. Some workers, however, consider that the case for its being a form of sarcoidosis is overwhelming.[123] The pathologic findings include many sarcoidlike granulomas with necrosis or hyalinization, sometimes associated with an intervening chronic inflammatory infiltrate; a vasculi-

tis of arteries and veins that is often granulomatous; and small airway obstruction by granulomas, which may cause an endogenous lipid pneumonia.[123,460]

Much of the information available on this condition comes from several series totaling about 80 cases.[123,433,649] The mean age at presentation is about 45 years (range 12 to 75 years), with a 2.5:1 predominance of female patients.[123,433,649] At the time of presentation between one fourth and two thirds of the patients are asymptomatic.[123,649] The remainder have systemic or respiratory symptoms (cough, chest pain, shortness of breath). Only a few patients have had extrapulmonary lesions that are consistent with sarcoidosis; the chief one is uveitis (9%).[123,433]

In general, necrotizing sarcoidal angiitis is a benign condition[266] that does not require treatment.[197] When treatment is indicated, steroids are used.

The most common radiologic pattern (about 75% of patients[123,460]) is bilateral nodules ranging up to about 4 cm in diameter.[262] Sometimes the nodules are small enough to be considered miliary.[124,460] The nodules show a predilection for the lower zones and occasionally cavitate.[249] When followed over years with repeat chest radiographs they may show a slow increase in size and number[124] and may become confluent.[197] Spontaneous disappearance of nodules has been recorded.[123] When unilateral the nodules are often solitary[124,249] and resemble a bronchial neoplasm.[716] Less common patterns include bilateral consolidations[124,460]; basal interstitial shadowing[433]; and pleural effusions, which are absent from most series but present in 54% in one study.[433] As with pleural effusions, the prevalence of hilar adenopathy has varied considerably from series to series, ranging from 8%[433] to 65%.[123]

Microscopic polyarteritis nodosa

Microscopic polyarteritis nodosa (MPN) is a systemic small vessel vasculitis accompanied by focal segmental necrotizing glomerulonephritis with no evidence of WG or conditions known to be associated with small vessel vasculitis.[658] In a series of 34 patients the male/female ratio was 2:1 with a mean age of 50 years (range 14 to 73 years).[658] Common clinical features were constitutional disorder, fever, arthralgia, myalgia, and purpura. All patients developed a focal segmental necrotizing glomerulonephritis, and 20% to 30% had gastrointestinal, ENT, or neurologic disorders. Diffuse pulmonary hemorrhage was present in one third of the patients and was manifest as airspace opacity (Figure 12-21).[341] The only other common radiologic findings were pleural effusion (15%) and pulmonary edema (6%). A high percentage of patients are cANCA positive[37] like those with WG, and some authors consider that MPN is best considered a WG variant.[464] Patients with MPN progressing to diffuse interstitial pulmonary fibrosis[538] and irreversible airflow obstruction[674] are described. Some of these patients had only a few of the multisystem features of MPN, and cANCA-positive patients are reported with isolated lung capillaritis and hemorrhage.[62]

Hypersensitivity vasculitis

The term "hypersensitivity vasculitis" refers to a heterogeneous group of clinical disorders with vasculitis of arterioles, capillaries, and venules. This group often

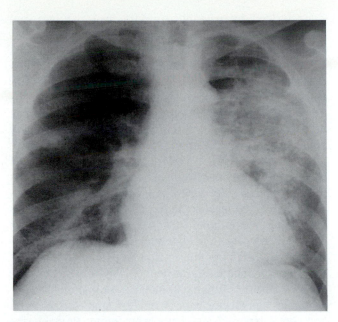

FIGURE 12-21
Microscopic polyarteritis nodosa. This 56-year-old man had diffuse pulmonary hemorrhage manifest as bilateral airspace opacity. He was positive for antineutrophil cytoplasmic antibodies, and renal biopsy showed necrotizing glomerulonephritis.

has a recognized precipitating agent,[235,285,450] including infectious organisms, particularly *Streptococcus*, *Mycobacterium*, viruses, or parasites; foreign proteins; chemicals; drugs[203]; and endogenous antigens, such as those associated with malignant neoplasms.[342] Immune complex formation plays an important role in the pathogenesis of hypersensitivity vasculitis.[235] Skin lesions, classically palpable purpura, tend to be a major finding in these disorders. Systemic involvement, notably of the kidneys, joints, gastrointestinal tract, lungs, and nervous system,[655] also occurs but is rarely life threatening.[342] It is usually self-limiting and responds to conservative treatment.[197]

Hypersensitivity vasculitis embraces a number of well-recognized syndromes, particularly anaphylactoid purpura, systemic urticarial vasculitis, and essential mixed cryoglobulinemia. Hypersensitivity vasculitis also occurs in collagen vascular diseases and may be cryptogenic.

ANAPHYLACTOID PURPURA (HENOCH-SCHÖNLEIN PURPURA). Although found primarily in children, anaphylactoid purpura occurs at any age and frequently follows an upper respiratory tract infection. The virus or bacterium responsible for this infection is the most common source of the inciting antigen. Other antigenic sources include varicella, *Yersinia*, food, drugs, and neoplasms.[353]

Immune complexes containing IgA are found in the walls of blood vessels and distinguish anaphylactoid purpura from other cutaneous vasculitides. The entity is characterized by palpable purpura over the legs and buttocks, abdominal pain, gastrointestinal bleeding, arthralgia, and in 10% to 25% of cases renal involvement with glomerulonephritis. Diagnostic criteria have been described.[520] The acute illness may be followed by one or more relapses occurring over weeks or months. The prognosis is generally good, although renal disease can progress to chronic renal failure and death. Pulmonary involvement is uncommon and probably occurs more often in adults than in children.[197] In one series of 64 adults, pulmonary involvement was seen in 6.25%,[152] but in several other large series lung involvement was absent altogether.[450] At least some of the 64 cases described by Cream and co-authors[152] would now be classified as micropolyarteritis. Consolidation, the most common finding on chest radiography,[152] is often patchy and multifocal[417] and occasionally transient.[397] Pleural effusions are also described.[152] When pathologic examination has been available, leukocytoclastic vasculitis and intraalveolar and septal hemorrhages have been found. Probably the majority of chest radiologic findings are related to alveolar hemorrhage, which can be a cause of death.[560]

SYSTEMIC URTICARIAL VASCULITIS. Systemic urticarial vasculitis is a syndrome most commonly seen in middle-aged women. It is characterized by chronic urticaria on the basis of a neutrophilic leukocytoclastic vasculitis variably accompanied by extradermal features, typically arthralgia, myalgia, and eye disorders. If multisystem involvement is severe, complement levels fall (hypocomplementemic urticarial vasculitis syndrome [HUVS]), and the disorder often closely resembles systemic lupus erythematosus.[24] In view of the latter an association between HUVS and recurrent pleural effusion is not unexpected.[430] Studies have described reversible[818] and fixed[671] airflow limitation in patients with HUVS. The Mayo Clinic series consisted of 16 patients, six of whom had chronic obstructive pulmonary disease (COPD), some at an early age, with hyperinflation and reduced peripheral vasculature on the chest radiograph.[671] The anatomic basis of this was unclear. It might have been caused by generalized emphysema. The authors considered that the lung disease was probably caused by the interaction of smoking and an immunologic process.[671]

ESSENTIAL MIXED CRYOGLOBULINEMIA. In essential mixed cryoglobulinemia (EMC) the vasculitis is usually of the leukocytoclastic type affecting small vessels, but it may also affect medium-sized arteries.[450] The cryoglobulinemia may be primary or secondary to a variety of disorders such as lymphoma, myeloma, collagen vascular disease, or infectious diseases. In the essential (primary) mixed form the cryoglobulin is an immune complex commonly made up of IgM rheumatoid factor directed against IgG, hence the term "mixed." EMC is associated with vasculitis, palpable purpura, nephritis, arthralgia, hepatosplenomegaly, and lymphadenopathy.[266] In a series of 23 patients with EMC a high prevalence of small airway disease and impaired gas exchange on respiratory

function testing was seen. Nearly 80% of patients had an abnormality on the chest radiograph, with a diffuse, finely nodular interstitial pattern.[57] The pathologic basis for this change is a matter of speculation.[266] A case associated with the adult respiratory distress syndrome has been reported.[709]

CONNECTIVE TISSUE DISEASE AND MALIGNANCY. Hypersensitivity vasculitis is a recognized finding in some connective tissue diseases and is discussed under the specific disorders. It also has an established association with various malignancies, particularly lymphoid and reticuloendothelial neoplasms.[235,511]

NONSPECIFIC HYPERSENSITIVITY VASCULITIS AND DISSEMINATED LEUKOCYTOCLASTIC VASCULITIS. These conditions are diagnosed by exclusion of hypersensitivity vasculitides, such as Henoch-Schönlein purpura, that have distinctive clinicopathologic features.[285] Presentation is usually with cutaneous lesions that are polymorphic but that early on are often typical palpable purpura. Systemic involvement may occur, with renal involvement the most frequent and serious. Other organs or systems that may be affected include the joints and the gastrointestinal, respiratory, and central and peripheral nervous systems. Although death may occur from renal involvement,[655] hypersensitivity vasculitis generally has a favorable outcome. Up to 25% of patients have pulmonary involvement,[450] but unfortunately descriptions of the radiologic changes have generally lacked detail, and histologic material from the lungs has been only rarely available. The radiologic patterns described include airspace opacity, which is often diffuse or perihilar[482,655] and probably represents diffuse pulmonary hemorrhage[801]; bilateral basal consolidations on the basis of a hemorrhagic alveolitis[266]; fleeting consolidations[197]; unspecified nodular shadows[655,801]; and linear interstitial opacities.[164]

Giant cell vasculitis

Giant cells are a recognized component of the cellular infiltrate of vasculitic processes and represent a nonspecific response to elastic tissue destruction. In two conditions, Takayasu arteritis (see p. 401) and temporal arteritis, the presence of giant cells is a prominent histologic feature.

SYSTEMIC TEMPORAL ARTERITIS. Although systemic temporal arteritis primarily affects branches of the carotid artery, it may also affect other arteries,[428,459,561] including the pulmonary. Cough and hoarseness responding to steroids are described in about 10% of patients.[445] Descriptions of radiologic changes in the chest are rare, which raises the question that such findings may be purely incidental. Described abnormalities include pleural effusion[634]; symmetric basal reticular opacity[415]; a diffuse interstitial pattern affecting the lower and upper zones, with bullae[266]; and multiple nodules up to 3 cm in diameter together with thick-walled cavities containing air-fluid levels.[68]

OTHER GIANT CELL ARTERITIDES. Patients are described with giant cell arteritis who do not fall into the classic clinicopathologic subgroups of Takayasu's or temporal arteritis. Some have had pulmonary involvement, including infarctive middle lobe consolidation with segmental pulmonary artery stenosis,[775] main pulmonary artery aneurysm,[179] and pulmonary capillaritis and hemorrhage.[690]

Behçet's disease and Hughes-Stovin syndrome

Behçet's disease is a rare, multisystem, chronic relapsing vasculitis considered to be secondary to immune complex deposition.[450] It is characterized by recurrent aphthous ulcerations of the mouth or genitalia together with erythema nodosum; various skin infections; and ocular lesions, notably uveitis, choroiditis, retinal vasculitis, and conjunctivitis. Almost half of the patients have arthropathy, and one fifth show thrombophlebitis and neurologic manifestations.[110] Lesser degrees of involvement are described in other organs, including the cardiac, renal, and gastrointestinal systems. A proposed set of diagnostic criteria consists of recurrent oral ulceration, recurrent genital ulceration, eye lesions (specified), skin lesions (specified), and positive pathergy test.[388] The diagnosis is considered positive if recurrent oral ulceration is present with two other criteria.

Histologic study of the affected vessels shows a leukocytoclastic vasculitis. Vasculitis leads to thrombosis, obstruction, aneurysm formation, and rupture of vessels. Arteries, capillaries, and veins of various sizes are affected.

Behçet's disease occurs about twice as frequently in men as in women and occurs most commonly in the third decade of life.[111] Although worldwide in distribution, it occurs particularly in the Mediterranean, the Middle East, and Japan. It is associated with HLA B5.

Pleuropulmonary involvement occurs in about 5% to 10% of patients,[172,227,610,687] predominantly males.[227,610] It is usually heralded by hemoptysis, fever, pleuritic pain, cough, or dyspnea. Hemoptysis is frequently a dominant and serious feature, and in a combined series it necessitated transfusion in 40% of patients and led to death in 30%.[610]

A variety of radiologic changes in the chest have been described.[90,110,172,211,314] These are best understood when correlated with the following pathologic findings: pulmonary hemorrhage from vessel rupture or vasculitis; pulmonary vessel occlusion, nearly always as a result of in situ thrombosis rather than embolism[110]; proximal pulmonary artery aneurysm; and collateralization from superior or inferior vena caval occlusion (Figure 12-22).

Consolidations are probably caused by hemorrhage (Figure 12-23). These may be focal, multifocal (unilateral or bilateral), or diffuse.[90,227,314,610] Sometimes they are fleeting.[110] Some of the consolidations may represent pulmonary infarcts, since some have cavitated.[314] Nodu-

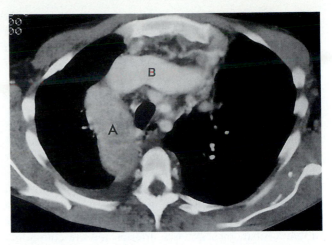

FIGURE 12-22
Behçet's syndrome. Contrast-enhanced computed tomogram just above carina shows, **A,** greatly dilated azygos vein and, **B,** left brachiocephalic vein and small mediastinal collaterals. Patient's current problem is heart failure secondary to cardiomyopathy. Venous dilatation reflects increased right heart pressures. Another important factor contributing to azygos vein dilatation is increased flow following inferior vena cava thrombosis.

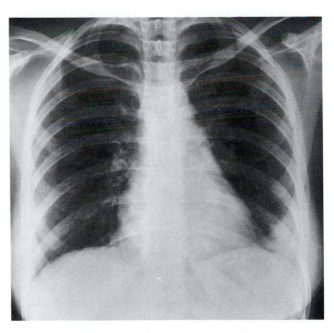

FIGURE 12-23
Chest radiograph in 27-year-old woman with known Behçet's syndrome and hemoptysis. Note area of consolidation in left costophrenic angle, probably caused by pulmonary hemorrhage or infarction. It cleared in 2 months without leaving a residuum.

lar shadows, usually several centimeters in diameter, have also been a common finding. Some have had the appearance of a focal consolidation rather than a mass, some cavitate, and a number have been subpleural in location.[314] The cavitary nodules are almost certainly pulmonary infarcts.[172] They usually resolve in 3 to 9 months.[314] Consolidation and large nodules have been demonstrated on CT.[227] Basal band shadows, possibly from infarcts, are also seen.[211,227]

Vascular occlusions may result in hypovascular areas on the plain chest radiograph[314] and ventilation-perfusion (V/Q) mismatch on radionuclide lung scanning.[227,284] The occlusions have been demonstrated angiographically and are predominantly of lobar or segmental arteries.[314] When widespread, the occlusions can cause radiographically detectable pulmonary arterial hypertension.[284] Pulmonary artery aneurysms may be visible on plain chest radiographs and CT.[227] They occur in main, lobar, or segmental arteries and are commonly bilateral[610] and proximal to an occlusion.[284] The aneurysms are demonstrable at angiography, although, on occasion, thrombus within the aneurysm itself may make them difficult to detect; CT scanning may have an advantage in this situation.[284] Limited data suggest that HRCT shows small vessel disease with an increased vascular size and irregular outline, narrowing, and cutoffs.[227] Resolution of occlusions and aneurysms has been demonstrated after therapy with steroids and heparin.[314]

Pleural effusions are sometimes present, and these may be serous or bloody. Most are probably secondary to pulmonary infarcts,[314] but some are hemothoraces resulting from rupture of blood vessels,[172] and a few have been chylothoraces secondary to superior vena cava and brachiocephalic vein thrombosis.[145] A cavitated infarct in Behçet's disease is a reported cause of a hydropneumothorax.[314]

The Hughes-Stovin syndrome[377] manifests some, but not all, of the features of Behçet's disease, and some consider it to be a variant.[450] It is even rarer than Behçet's disease. Most patients have been males in their second to fourth decades. The youngest was aged 12 years.[627] At least one reported description was of a female patient.[738] The major features are one or more segmental pulmonary artery aneurysms, pulmonary artery occlusions from emboli or thrombi, and systemic venous thrombi (limb veins, vena cava, cerebral sinuses). Common presentations are venous thromboses, fever, or hemoptysis; the last is caused by erosion of an aneurysm into an airway[806] and is the major cause of death. Radiologic features are similar to those of Behçet's disease.

Polyangiitis overlap syndrome

Polyangiitis overlap syndrome is characterized by a systemic vasculitis with features that overlap the well-defined vasculitic syndromes.[450] In one series of 11 patients pulmonary vasculitis was seen in 54%.[450] Pleuropulmonary radiologic findings are those to be expected from the component conditions. Several overlaps have been seen of the Churg-Strauss syndrome and polyarteritis nodosa; the evidence for the latter was the presence of

aneurysms of visceral vasculature. Some workers think that separating such patients from the Churg-Strauss syndrome does not serve any useful purpose.[197]

COLLAGEN VASCULAR DISEASE
Rheumatoid arthritis

Rheumatoid arthritis (RA) is a subacute or chronic inflammatory polyarthropathy of unknown cause that particularly affects peripheral joints. It is about three times more common in females than in males and usually has an insidious onset, pursuing a variable course that is typically one of relapse and remission. The diagnosis of RA is based on the presence of certain clinical and laboratory features.[18]

In addition to an arthropathy many patients have one or more extraarticular manifestations. These tend to be seen in subjects who are seropositive, particularly with high rheumatoid factor titers, and in patients with rheumatoid nodules.

The association of pulmonary disease and rheumatoid disease was suggested as early as 1948,[215] and although some large early surveys failed to confirm a positive relationship,[763] a number of positive associations are now generally accepted.* Definite and probable associations are listed (see box below).

PLEURAL DISEASE. Pleural involvement is probably the most common thoracic manifestation of rheumatoid disease.[647] At postmortem examination, pleural changes are seen in some 50% of cases,[647] and on the chest radiograph pleural thickening is seen in 20% of patients.[411] However, clinical pleural effusion is much less

---

*References 380, 381, 411, 686, 763, 814.

PLEUROPULMONARY LESIONS IN RHEUMATOID DISEASE

Pleural
    Pleuritis
    Effusion and thickening
    Empyema
    Bronchopleural fistula, pneumothorax
Fibrosing alveolitis
Parenchymal (necrobiotic) nodules
Caplan's syndrome
Pulmonary arteritis, hypertension
Other associations
    Bronchiolitis obliterans
    Follicular bronchiolitis
    Bronchiectasis
    Organizing pneumonia
    Upper zone fibrosis
    Bronchocentric granulomatosis
    Amyloidosis
    Drug-related changes
    Pulmonary neoplasm

common, with a 3.3% prevalence in one large series[777] and an annual incidence of effusion of about 1% in patients with rheumatoid disease.[412] Unlike rheumatoid disease in general, but in common with other pulmonary manifestations of the disease, pleural effusion shows a striking preponderance of male patients,[778] and some quite sizable series have recorded virtually no females.[102] Patients are usually middle aged, with a mean age of about 50 years.[778] The effusions in rheumatoid disease, unlike those in systemic lupus erythematosus, are commonly asymptomatic.[380]

Pleural effusions most commonly occur in the setting of established disease and may develop more than 20 years after its onset. They may, however, develop simultaneously with the onset of arthritis or predate the arthritis by several months.[102,778] In one series 4% of effusions developed several months before the arthritis and 20% developed simultaneously with the onset of joint disease.[777] The arthritis in established disease sometimes undergoes an exacerbation as the pleural effusion develops.[93,102,412] Effusions are positively associated with the presence of cutaneous nodules in some 50% of patients[102,778] and with pericarditis,[777] but not with the clinical or radiographic severity of the arthritis.[777] In about one third of patients other rheumatoid-related abnormalities on the chest radiograph are evident such as fibrosing alveolitis or parenchymal nodules.[778]

Effusions are most commonly small to moderate in size (Figure 12-24),[778] although they can be large.[73] About

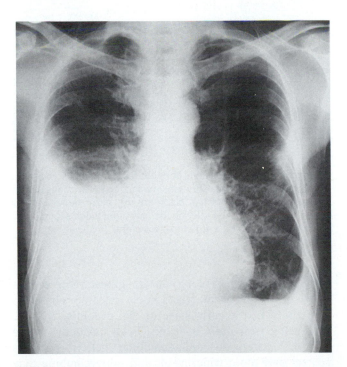

FIGURE 12-24
Pleural effusion in rheumatoid disease. Bilateral pleural effusions are present with mild changes of fibrosing alveolitis. Effusions were painless, and that on right had been present, more or less unchanged, for 5 months.

one fifth occur bilaterally.[778] Once formed the effusions behave in a variable fashion, and although some resolve within weeks, more characteristically they persist for months and indeed sometimes for several years.[778] Effusions may recur on the same or opposite side of the chest.[483] Once the effusion has cleared, it commonly leaves residual pleural thickening.[102,412] Fibrothorax and folded lung are recognized complications of rheumatoid pleural thickening[647] that may on occasion be severe enough to warrant decortication.[79,777]

The diagnosis may be strongly suspected or established by the findings in the pleural fluid[647,680,763] and sometimes by pleural biopsy that, although frequently nonspecific, may show rheumatoid nodules.[763] The pleural fluid is usually rich in protein and lymphocytes, pale yellow to yellow-green, and occasionally milky. Sometimes in the acute stage it is polymorph predominant and occasionally eosinophilic.[599] Its most characteristic features are its low sugar, low pH, and raised lactic dehydrogenase level. Rheumatoid factor is often present but is unfortunately a nonspecific finding.[680]

Rheumatoid patients are generally at risk from infection and may develop an empyema either de novo or on top of an established effusion.[186,407] There are isolated reports of pneumothorax and pyopneumothorax in rheumatoid disease,[483] some associated with diffuse pulmonary fibrosis and others with cavitary nodules and bronchopleural fistula.[153,170,186,681]

FIBROSING ALVEOLITIS. Diffuse interstitial pulmonary fibrosis (fibrosing alveolitis, interstitial pneumonitis) was first associated with RA by Ellman and Ball in 1948.[215] After the initial case reports, however, several large series failed to show an increased prevalence of IPF in rheumatoid disease.[19,708,728] Because overlooking uncommon associations is possible, unless very large numbers are used,[763] looking at the frequency of the common condition (RA) in series of the more uncommon disorder (IPF/fibrosing alveolitis) is useful. When looked at in this way, the prevalence is in the order of 10% to 20%.[190,761,763] In a large series of patients with RA, 8 of 516 patients (1.6%) had radiologic pulmonary fibrosis.[778] Abnormal respiratory function tests consistent with interstitial lung disease are much more common[635] with a 40% prevalence in one series.[257]

In the early stages an active alveolitis with interstitial thickening is evident as well as a lymphocyte- and plasma cell–rich infiltrate that is slowly replaced by interstitial fibrosis and eventually, in some, by an end-stage lung pattern.[418] Lymphoid aggregates with germinal centers are commonly seen, and although nonspecific they are very suggestive of rheumatoid lung. Sometimes the histologic appearance is that of a desquamative interstitial pneumonitis.[763]

Rheumatoid IPF is twice as common in men as in women[763]; the mean age at onset is about 50 years.[778] A possible relationship exists between alveolitis and alpha$_1$-antitrypsin genotype.[635] Most cases of alveolitis occurred

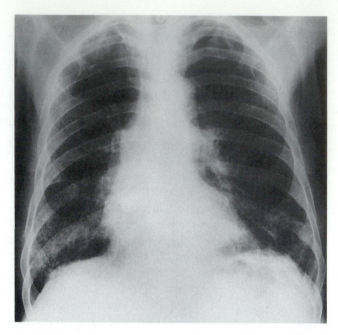

FIGURE 12-25
Fibrosing alveolitis in rheumatoid disease. Bilateral basal shadowing consists mainly of small irregular and rounded nodules. Appearances are indistinguishable from other varieties of fibrosing alveolitis.

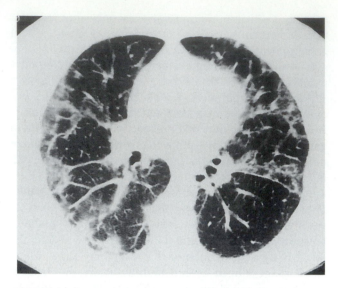

FIGURE 12-26
Rheumatoid arthritis, fibrosing alveolitis. High-resolution computed tomogram (CT) at mid left atrial level shows patchy subpleural ground-glass opacity and a little consolidation. Appearances are of active alveolitis that evolved over 3 years into honeycomb pattern on CT.

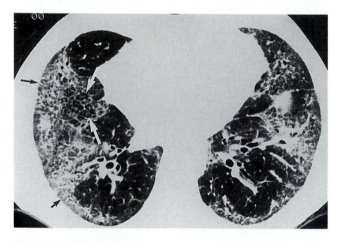

FIGURE 12-27
Rheumatoid arthritis, fibrosing alveolitis. High-resolution computed tomogram shows peripherally predominant complex changes with ground-glass opacity *(small black arrow),* early honeycombing *(large black arrow),* and interlobular and intralobular septal thickening with prominent centrilobular structures *(white arrows).*

after the onset of the arthritis, although about 15% to 30% occur before or coincident with the initial joint manifestations.[763,778] In general, no matter which develops first, the gap between the onset of the two conditions is not more than 5 years.[69,763] Respiratory symptoms can be absent despite radiologic changes,[582,778] but if present they consist chiefly of exertional dyspnea and cough. The severity and pattern of joint involvement do not differ from that seen generally in RA,[763,778] but an exacerbation of joint symptoms may occur with the onset of alveolitis.[69] The principal physical signs are basal crackles and finger clubbing. Generally stated, a high prevalence of associated subcutaneous nodules is seen,[380] but figures from various series vary considerably from 75%[748,778] to 15%.[763] Some think that the prevalence of subcutaneous nodules is no different from that seen in the general rheumatoid population.[598] Respiratory function tests usually show restriction with impaired carbon monoxide transfer and evidence of hypoxemia at rest or on exercise.[380,635] Serum rheumatoid factor is elevated in more than two thirds of patients with alveolitis.[748,763,778]

The chest radiograph shows changes that are indistinguishable from CFA (Figure 12-25) (see p. 487), namely, interstitial opacities. These are largely symmetric and basally predominant,[470] although they can involve all zones[763] and are occasionally midzone predominant.[778] A fine nodular pattern, either rounded (q) or irregular (t) opacities, is evident.[763] When the nodulation is very fine, a diffuse loss of transradiancy is seen, giving a ground-glass appearance.[470] These small opacities, at least ini-

tially, make the vascular shadows appear more prominent, although eventually vessels become obscured. Sometimes in the early stage of the alveolitis, airspace shadowing (soft fluffy opacities) is also evident (Figure 12-26).[69] Later, the reticulonodular pattern becomes coarser and more widespread, and honeycombing may appear.[470] Septal lines (Kerley A and B) are not features of rheumatoid alveolitis, although the occasional B line is seen.[470] As fibrosis advances, lung volume tends to be lost, a situation reflected in elevation of the diaphragm.[260] Pleural effusion or thickening may coexist with interstitial changes in about 5% to 15% of cases.[763,778] Cases have been described with interstitial shadowing accompanied by both pleural effusion and intrapulmonary nodules.[740]

CT and HRCT findings in interstitial disease associated with RA (Figures 12-26 and 12-27) are also generally considered indistinguishable from those of CFA.[47,242,712,715] However, comprehensive CT and histopathologic correlation in RA is lacking, and since lung biopsies in rheumatoid lung disease show a wide range of changes in addition to fibrosing alveolitis (lymphoid hyperplasia, cellular interstitial pneumonia, bronchiolitis obliterans, organizing pneumonia, and diffuse alveolar damage),[814] HRCT changes probably reflect more than just fibrosing alveolitis.

Alveolitis in rheumatoid disease probably carries as bad a prognosis as it does in the cryptogenic form,[763] although some authors think it is less severe.[380] In one series the mean duration of lung disease to death was 5 years, with a range of 1 to 17 years.[763] A subset of patients have a fulminant course, dying within months of the initial diagnosis.[477,603] Treatment with steroids or immunosuppressants helps a portion of the patients, at least in the short term.[477,763]

INTRAPULMONARY NODULES. The third well-recognized pleuropulmonary abnormality associated with rheumatoid disease is the intrapulmonary (necrobiotic) nodule. These nodules are pathologically identical to subcutaneous nodules[763] and consist of a necrotic center bounded by palisading histiocytes (epithelioid cells) surrounded by plasma cells and lymphocytes. Peripherally there may be a moderate, nonnecrotizing vasculitis.[418]

Intrapulmonary nodules are rare; two large series of 955 patients contained no examples,[19,582] and another contained only two cases in 516 patients.[778] Nodules, like pleural effusions and IPF, are more common in men than women, with about a twofold excess. Mean patient age at presentation is 51 years (range 24 to 64 years).[574] Nodules usually occur in patients with established disease but may occur with or before the onset of arthritis,[379,763] as did some 27% of nodules reported by Eraut and co-workers.[226] Should nodules predate arthritis, the gap is often less than a year,[226,599,660] but intervals of up to 11 years are also described.[226] Some patients with histologically proven nodules remain seronegative and never develop arthritis.[84,226]

Nodules are usually asymptomatic, but a cough or hemoptysis may be present, particularly if a lesion cavitates.[574] Occasionally symptoms result from infection,[85] bronchopleural fistula formation, or pneumothorax.[599] Discounting cases in which nodules predate arthritis, pulmonary necrobiotic nodules usually occur in the context of established and advanced disease,[260] and subcutaneous nodules are seen in 80%.[483,574,778] Serum rheumatoid factor is found in nearly 90% of patients with nodules,[483,574] although early on it may be absent or present in low titer.[574] Blood eosinophilia is reported in some cases.[599,691] Unless nodules are indolent or resolve,

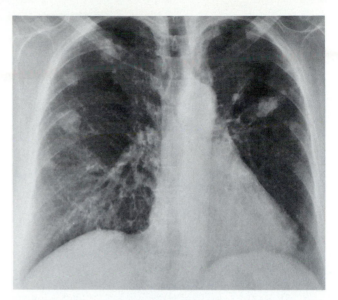

FIGURE 12-28
Parenchymal nodules in rheumatoid disease. Patient is 57-year-old woman with long-standing rheumatoid disease and subcutaneous nodules. Chest radiograph shows multiple 4 to 25 mm nodules distributed bilaterally in middle and upper zones. Nodules are relatively well-demarcated round, oval, or lobulated and had remained essentially unchanged for 6 months. Their distribution and indolent behavior are typical.

they are radiologically indistinguishable from pulmonary neoplasms and need histologic identification.[406] The nodules (Figure 12-28) are usually radiologically discrete, rounded or lobulated, and subpleural.[715] They may be single or, in about three fourths of patients, multiple,[778] sometimes coalescing (Figure 12-29)[715] and showing some middle and upper zone predilection.[226] They range in size from a few millimeters[778] to 7 cm (Figure 12-30). Occasionally when the nodules are small and widely disseminated, a miliary pattern is produced.[483] In about 50% of cases the nodules cavitate,[483,778] producing ring opacities often with relatively smooth thick walls (Figure 12-29).[260,470,483] Cavitation is more easily appreciated on CT (Figure 12-31).[715] Occasionally nodules calcify.[470,478] Subpleural nodules may erode through the pleura and cause a bronchopleural fistula and hydropneumothorax.[170,361,483] Rib erosion by a nodule is rare but has been described as giving an appearance that resembles an invasive carcinoma.[336] Pleural thickening or effusion is present in 40% to 50% of patients with intrapulmonary nodules.[483,778] Likewise, alveolitis and pulmonary nodules can coexist.[483] Nodular lesions may increase in size and number, resolve completely, or remain stable for many years[778]; at other times they wax and wane with the activity of subcutaneous nodules and arthritis.[531,599]

Small rheumatoid nodules are also described in the trachea[389,405] and pleura.

CAPLAN'S SYNDROME. The original description of Caplan's syndrome was of multiple, large (0.5 to 5 cm in diameter), round nodules seen on the chest radiographs

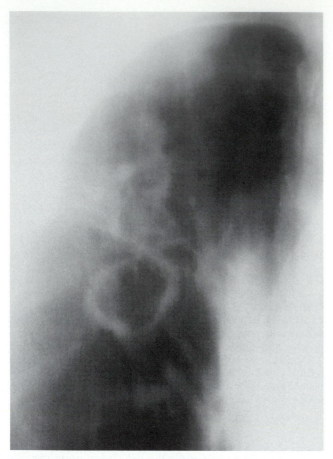

FIGURE 12-29
Parenchymal nodules in patient with rheumatoid disease. Linear tomogram of right upper zone shows cluster of nodules that have cavitated. Lowest nodule is 3 cm in diameter with wall that varies from 1 to 6 mm in thickness.

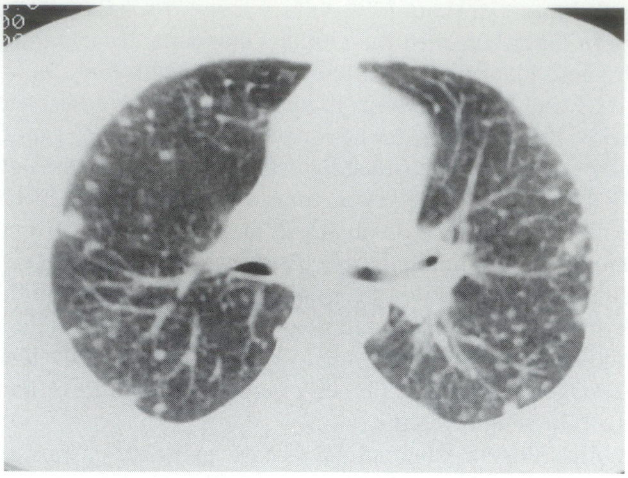

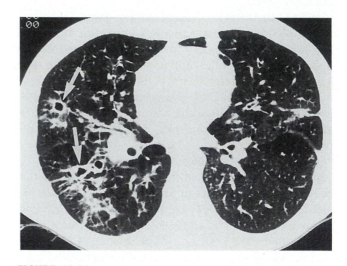

FIGURE 12-30
Nodular rheumatoid arthritis. Computed tomogram just below carina shows multiple nodules ranging from 2 to 12 mm. These nodules are smaller and more numerous than is usual. Patient had active arthritis with systemic symptoms and subcutaneous nodules.

FIGURE 12-31
Cavitary nodules in rheumatoid arthritis. High-resolution CT at midatrial level shows several thick-walled ring opacities (arrows) surrounded by irregular linear opacity consistent with scarring.

of coal miners with rheumatoid arthritis.[96] Radiographic evidence of simple coal miner's pneumoconiosis was often absent. Since that time the features of the syndrome have been extended to include individuals exposed to inorganic agents other than silica or coal, those with serologic but not clinical rheumatoid disease, and patients with radiologic patterns other than large nodules.[98] In affected patients clinical rheumatoid disease may occur before, with, or after the pulmonary changes.[96,515] Caplan's syndrome, based on broad criteria, has been described with exposure to asbestos,[530,623,737] aluminum,[409] dolomite,[16] silica,* and carbon.[783]

Caplan's nodules are pathologically similar to necrobiotic rheumatoid nodules: a necrotic center is surrounded by a cuff of cellular infiltrate consisting of macrophages and polymorphonuclear leukocytes, fibroblasts, and giant cells.[304] Some of the macrophages contain dust, and on macroscopic section these give the characteristic annular ring pattern that distinguishes Caplan's nodules from ordinary rheumatoid nodules. Fibroblasts adjacent to the

necrotic area show palisading, which is also a striking feature of subcutaneous rheumatoid nodules. Although the pathogenesis of Caplan's syndrome is not completely understood, the development of rheumatoid factor seems to be associated with a modified tissue response in coal dust–induced lung disease.[763]

The prevalence of Caplan's syndrome in a population of more than 21,000 miners in the United Kingdom, according to the broad criteria,[466] was about 2.5 cases per 1000 subjects without pneumoconiosis, and between 22 and 62 cases per 1000 subjects with pneumoconiosis. For an unexplained reason the prevalence in the United States

_____

*References 94, 97, 116, 163, 343, 608.

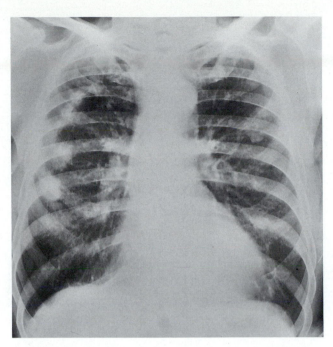

FIGURE 12-32
Rheumatoid disease with Caplan's syndrome. This 61-year-old coal miner has multiple peripheral nodules, mostly on right. They range between 1 and 2 cm in diameter. Changes of coal worker's pneumoconiosis are characteristically mild. (Courtesy Dr. P.M. Hacking, Newcastle upon Tyne, U.K.)

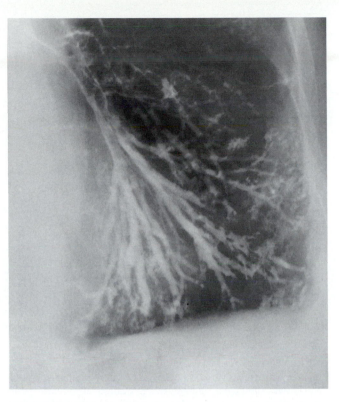

FIGURE 12-33
Rheumatoid disease with bronchiolitis obliterans. Patient was 56-year-old woman whose main complaint was progressive exertional dyspnea. Bronchogram of left lower lobe shows mild failure of airway tapering and striking lack of filling of small airways. Patient had not received penicillamine. Pleural thickening is also present.

appears to be low,[577] and no cases were found in a series of 100 Pennsylvania miners with RA.[41]

The classic radiologic finding in Caplan's syndrome is bilateral pulmonary nodules (Figure 12-32), usually 1 to 2 cm in diameter but ranging from 0.5 to 5 cm.[96] Nodules are typically situated at the junction of the outer and middle thirds of the lung and tend to appear in crops of lesions having a similar size and rate of growth.[515] Nodules are not necessarily bilateral, and in one series one fifth were unilateral.[466] Nodules tend to develop rapidly and grow over a period of months. Then they often remain stable or grow slowly for several years. Established nodules occasionally heal by fibrosis and give a stellate scarlike shadow. In East Midlands, United Kingdom, about 10% of coal miners with Caplan's syndrome developed calcification (7 of 55) or cavitation (4 of 55) of the nodules.[466] Radiologic changes of coal worker's pneumoconiosis may or may not be present and are not a striking feature. In the original series, in 45% of patients the radiographic changes of coal worker's pneumoconiosis were category I or less.[96]

Other radiographic findings are now included in the wider concept of Caplan's syndrome. The most common are 0.3 to 1 cm rounded opacities ranging from just a few confined to one lung zone to a "snowstorm" appearance,[98] and mixed nodular and irregular opacities with no background of simple pneumoconiosis.[98]

PULMONARY ARTERITIS AND HYPERTENSION.[774] Systemic vasculitis in rheumatoid disease is usually of the hypersensitivity type and affects chiefly the skin. The lung is rarely involved in rheumatoid vasculitis,[675] and only a few cases have been reported,[34,422,811] either with or without clinical evidence of a systemic vasculitis. Prognosis is poor, and most patients have died within 1 year of diagnosis.[811] In most of these cases the only radiographic finding has been enlargement of the heart and proximal pulmonary arteries. Although pulmonary arterial hypertension may be caused by vasculitis, it is much more likely to be caused by rheumatoid-associated fibrosing alveolitis.[763]

A few case reports of pulmonary consolidations are either proved[17] or assumed to be the result of vasculitis.[36,478] Diffuse pulmonary hemorrhage from vasculitis is also described.[449]

OTHER ASSOCIATIONS. An association between rheumatoid disease and bronchiolitis obliterans is recognized (Figure 12-33).[276,358,478,496] In at least half of these patients treatment with penicillamine or gold has been implicated,[223,537,554] but bronchiolitis obliterans also occurs in patients taking neither drug.[680] Clinically dyspnea and evidence of irreversible airflow obstruction are seen with a chest radiograph that either is normal or shows

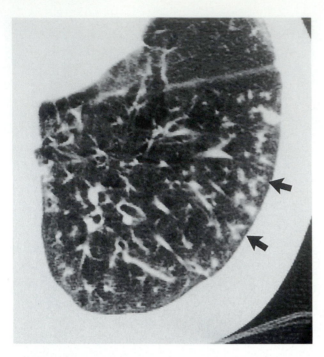

FIGURE 12-34
Rheumatoid arthritis with bronchiectasis. High-resolution computed tomography shows mild bronchiectatic changes at left base (mild airway dilatation), airways seen more peripherally than normal, and airway walls mildly thickened. Peripheral nodular and linear opacity, some of which branches *(arrow)*, probably represents bronchiolar impaction.

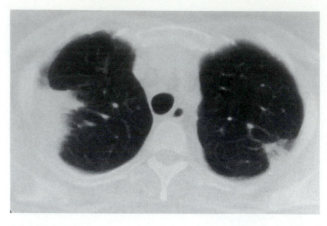

FIGURE 12-35
Rheumatoid arthritis with organizing pneumonia. Computed tomogram of upper lung in 55-year-old woman with rheumatoid arthritis who had pleuritic pain and systemic symptoms. The patient had about 10 pleurally based focal consolidations that on biopsy showed organizing pneumonia. Lesions resolved on steroid therapy with residual scarring.

hyperinflation with or without oligemic areas.

Lymphoid hyperplasia is an uncommon histologic manifestation of rheumatoid lung disease in which interstitial lymphoid follicles develop along lymphatic channels. This was the primary pattern in 5 of 40 open lung biopsies in patients with rheumatoid lung disease.[814] When this reaction is most marked along airways, the term "follicular bronch(iol)itis" is used.[814] Follicular bronchiolitis probably produces a reticulonodular pattern on the chest radiograph.[814]

Postmortem and clinical evidence suggests that bronchitis and bronchiectasis (Figure 12-34) are more frequent in patients with rheumatoid disease than in matched control subjects.[19,680,776] Thus in a controlled study bronchiectasis was 10 times more common in patients with rheumatoid disease than in control subjects with degenerative joint disease.[776] In another review of 13 patients with clinical bronchiectasis and rheumatoid disease, bronchiectasis developed after the onset of arthritis in more than half of the patients and hypogammaglobulinemia was present in a number of cases.[141]

A small number of cases of organizing pneumonia (bronchiolitis obliterans organizing pneumonia [BOOP]) have been described in patients with RA (Figure 12-35).[814]

About 10 patients with rheumatoid disease are reported

with apical fibrosis and cavitation giving rise to a radiologic appearance that resembles tuberculosis.[478,479,587,720,815] In some of these patients the pathologic finding reported has been confluent necrobiotic nodules.[815]

A handful of patients with rheumatoid disease have had biopsy-proven bronchocentric granulomatosis (see p. 538).[44,58,347] Radiologic findings were bilateral nodules and focal consolidations ranging from 2 to 15 cm, some of which were cavitated.

Various agents used in the treatment of rheumatoid arthritis can cause drug-related pulmonary toxicity.[820] Methotrexate- or gold-induced pneumonitis is not uncommon, complicating the interpretation is chest radiographs in rheumatoid disease.[680]

Some evidence points to an increased prevalence of lung neoplasm in patients with RA, but the relationship is controversial.[680]

Systemic lupus erythematosus

Systemic lupus erythematosus (SLE) is a multisystem collagen vascular disease characterized by widespread inflammatory changes, particularly in the vessels, serosa, and skin. A characteristic feature is production of autoantibody against a wide variety of cellular constituents, including nuclear material, particularly deoxyribonucleic acid (DNA). Because the manifestations of the disease are so variable, diagnostic criteria have been drawn up (see box on p. 509).[729] Should any four of the criteria be present simultaneously or serially during a period of observation, SLE can be diagnosed.

The prevalence of the various clinical manifestations in four series[120] was arthropathy, 85%; skin lesions, 80%; nephritis, 53%; pleurisy, 52%; neuropsychiatric disorders, 44%; lymphadenopathy, 43%; pericarditis, 39%; and

CRITERIA FOR DIAGNOSIS OF SYSTEMIC LUPUS ERYTHEMATOSUS

Malar rash
Discoid lupus erythematosus
Photosensitivity
Ulceration of mouth and oropharynx
Arthropathy (nonerosive, nondeforming)
Serositis
Renal disorder (proteinuria or cellular casts)
Neurologic disorder (epilepsy or psychosis)
Hematologic disorder (hemolytic anemia, leukopenia, lymphopenia, or thrombocytopenia)
Immunologic disorder (positive LE cell preparation, or antibody to native DNA or S_m nuclear antigen, or false-positive test for syphilis)
Antinuclear antibody

Modified from Tan EM, Cohen AS, Fries JF, et al: *Arthritis Rheum* 25:1271-1277, 1982.

THORACIC MANIFESTATIONS OF SYSTEMIC LUPUS ERYTHEMATOSUS

PRIMARY

Pleuritis, pleural effusion
Diffuse alveolar damage
(Acute) lupus pneumonitis
Pulmonary hemorrhage
Fibrosing alveolitis
Diaphragm dysfunction
Pulmonary arterial hypertension, vasculitis
Rarities
Lupus anticoagulant pulmonary embolism
Lymphocytic pneumonitis, pseudolymphoma
Bronchiolitis obliterans
Organizing pneumonia
Acute reversible hypoxemia

SECONDARY

Atelectasis
Pneumonia (simple, opportunistic)
Cardiac failure, pericarditis
Renal failure, nephrotic syndrome
Drug-induced changes

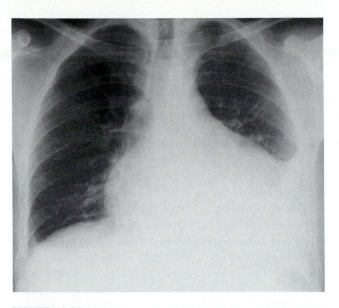

FIGURE 12-36
Systemic lupus erythematosus (SLE). Large heart was caused by pericardial effusion and was accompanied by bilateral pleural effusions, moderate on left, small on right. This combination of findings is characteristic of SLE.

reported prognosis has greatly improved over the years, in part because of better therapy, but also because subclinical cases have been included in the various studies. In two recent series the 5-year survival was 97% to 98% and 10-year survival was 89% to 93%.[315,595]

Thoracic involvement is common in SLE, and the lungs, pleura, heart, diaphragm, and intercostal muscles may all be affected.[758] Thoracic manifestations (see box at left) can be divided into primary changes or secondary complications, but this distinction is not always clear. Cardiac and pericardial disease have been recently reviewed[113] and will be only briefly considered here. The lungs and pleura are involved more frequently in SLE than in any other collagen vascular disease,[380,796] with 50% to 70% of patients developing pleuropulmonary manifestations in the course of the disease.[315,338,365,380,647] Only 5%, however, have such changes at presentation.[228,338,594]

PRIMARY MANIFESTATIONS

Pleuritis or pleural effusion. Pleuritis is found in 40% to 60% of patients with SLE.[201,228,338] It may be an initial feature[802] but occurs more commonly during an exacerbation of established disease.[380]

The pleuritis is dry 50% of the time,[457] but in the other 50% it is accompanied by a pleural effusion and sometimes by a pericardial effusion (Figure 12-36).[758] Aspirated pleural fluid is usually a clear exudate with white blood cells (granulocytes early and lymphocytes later) and normal levels of glucose; it often contains antinuclear antibodies.[297] The pleural effusions are usually small or moderate in size[297] but are on rare occasion large.[306]

mucosal ulceration, 15%. The illness characteristically shows relapses and remissions, with a tendency to progression and eventual multiorgan dysfunction.[120] Its overall prevalence rate is about 20 to 50 per 10^5 population, and it is 10 times more common in women as in men,[488] with an increased prevalence among relatives and blacks. It typically occurs during the childbearing period with a wide variety of manifestations, particularly those of joint, skin, and systemic disorders.[201] The

Unilateral and bilateral effusions are found with equal frequency.[297,732,802] Sometimes the pleural effusions resolve spontaneously, but many require treatment with steroids or immunosuppressive drugs. Clearing may be complete or incomplete, leaving minor pleural thickening.[82,802] Other causes of pleural effusion in SLE include nephrotic syndrome, cardiac and renal failure, pulmonary embolism, and pneumonia.[340,647] That primary pleural effusions in SLE are almost always painful[297,457] can be a helpful differentiating feature.

Pleural thickening[40] is a common finding at autopsy but is underreported as a radiologic finding in patients. It was, however, seen in 12% of patients in one series.[315] Pneumothorax is not a feature of pleuropulmonary SLE.

(Acute) lupus pneumonitis. Pathologic changes of diffuse alveolar damage (DAD) may be seen in SLE associated with two clinical entities that blur into each other: (acute) lupus pneumonitis and pulmonary hemorrhage. The alveolar damage is most likely mediated by immune complex deposition.[796] Histologic examination shows an acute, exudative stage with interstitial and intraalveolar edema, intraalveolar hemorrhage, hyaline membrane formation, and sloughing of alveolar lining cells. The later, organizing stage is characterized by alveolar lining cell proliferation and interstitial and, to a lesser extent, intraalveolar fibrosis.[418] The presence of immunoglobulin and complement may be shown by immunofluorescence.

Acute lupus pneumonitis is an unusual life-threatening condition characterized by acute onset of fever, cough, tachypnea, and radiologic consolidation. Clinically it resembles pneumonia, pulmonary infarction, and hemorrhage and is a diagnosis of exclusion. Rarely it is a presenting feature of SLE,[493] and an increased postpartum prevalence has been noted.[796] The true prevalence is uncertain and probably on the order of 4% (range of 1% to 12%).[201,228,315,457,493] In a selected group of 30 patients seen in a tertiary center with pleuropulmonary SLE, about one fifth had probable acute pneumonitis.[369]

The chest radiograph most commonly shows one or more areas of consolidation, usually bilateral and basal, but sometimes unilateral.[315,457,493] A mixed alveolar and interstitial pattern with nodules has also been described.[457] The consolidations are often accompanied by pleural effusions[493] and are sometimes migratory.[392] Cavitation is rare and suggests pneumonia or infarction rather than lupus pneumonitis. Some patients respond dramatically to steroids,[380] with complete or partial clearance, but others have needed additional cyclophosphamide.[796] Residual radiographic shadowing often has an interstitial pattern[493] and may be accompanied by a diffusion defect and restrictive abnormality on lung function testing.

Pulmonary hemorrhage. Pulmonary hemorrhage is common in the lungs at postmortem examination of patients with SLE[518] but is not often recognized clinically. Lung hemorrhage ranges from a mild, chronic subclinical

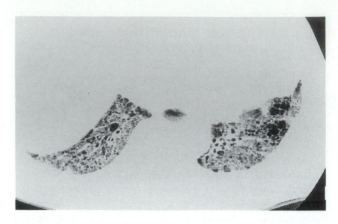

FIGURE 12-37
Systemic lupus erythematosus. Long-standing basally predominant changes consistent with fibrosing alveolitis with ground-glass opacity, honeycombing, bronchiolectasis, and cysts.

process to one that is acute and life threatening.[796] In a series of more than 400 patients with SLE at the National Institutes of Health, the prevalence of acute hemorrhage was only about 1.5%.[99] Very rarely it is the mode of presentation of SLE.[88] Acute pulmonary hemorrhage carries a 70% mortality[448] and is an important diagnosis to make because urgent treatment is needed.[756] The pathologic findings are diffuse alveolar damage with predominant alveolar hemorrhage. Some patients have additional capillaritis.[418] Clinical manifestations of acute hemorrhage include a rapid onset of severe dyspnea, fever, and hemoptysis, with crepitations on auscultation. Pulmonary hemorrhage is typically accompanied by signs of active disease elsewhere, fever, arthropathy, and nephritis.[208] Helpful clinical pointers include hemoptysis and a fall in blood hemoglobin level. Confirmation can be obtained by finding hemosiderin-laden macrophages in the sputum[272] or a rise in carbon monoxide uptake in the lung.[230]

The radiographic appearances are nonspecific. They resemble those of Goodpasture's syndrome (see p. 523) and consist of airspace opacity that is usually bilateral and diffuse. This results in a variety of patterns: multiple acinar nodules; homogeneous, ill-defined, coalescent, patchy shadows; ground-glass opacity; and lobar or segmental consolidations with air bronchograms.[208,563] The opacities usually clear within days.[592] Magnetic resonance findings (intermediate signal on proton density and low signal on T2-weighted images) are characteristic and may have differential diagnostic value.[371]

Fibrosing alveolitis. Fibrosing alveolitis (Figure 12-37) is generally regarded as an unusual manifestation of SLE.[380] However, chronic interstitial infiltrates were present in just over one third of cases in four autopsy series.[518] In some clinical series diffuse interstitial fibrosis has been notable by its absence.[260] Nevertheless, four patients with pleuropulmonary SLE in a selected group of 30 had radiographic evidence of fibrosing alveolitis

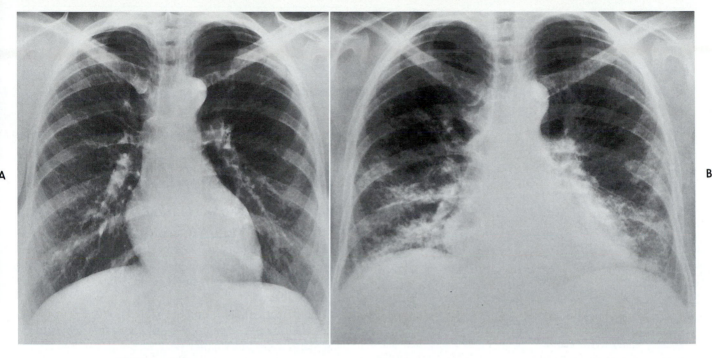

FIGURE 12-38
Systemic lupus erythematosus (SLE) in 35-year-old woman. **A**, Normal posteroanterior chest radiograph predating symptoms. **B**, Four years later SLE with progressive exertional dyspnea had developed. Chest radiograph now shows bilateral basal reticulonodular and ground-glass opacities consistent with fibrosing alveolitis. Diaphragm has become elevated. This could be related to decreased lung compliance subsequent to alveolitis or to diaphragmatic myopathy.

(confirmed by biopsy in two),[369] and in an unselected series of outpatients with SLE a 3% prevalence of pulmonary fibrosis was judged radiologically.[214] A number of patients with chronic fibrosis have had preceding acute pneumonitis.[373,493] In general, fibrosis pursues an insidious course, but exceptions are not uncommon, and it may cause death.[790]

Diaphragm dysfunction. Diaphragm dysfunction in SLE may be manifest as elevation of one or both hemidiaphragms (Figure 12-38) and is a cause of dyspnea. Bilateral elevation is a common finding and in some series has been the most common radiologic pleuropulmonary abnormality in SLE, seen in as many as 18% of patients.[315] In the presence of interstitial lung disease it is even more common at 8 of 14 (57%).[790] As the diaphragm rises, the lungs lose volume; hence the term "shrinking lungs,"[365] a finding first noted in 1954.[216,338,756] The loss of lung volume was initially ascribed to reduction in lung compliance, but it has recently been shown to be caused by diaphragmatic weakness[281] presumed to be caused by a myopathy[283,484] for which there is some pathologic evidence.[642] Pleuritic pain with splinting is an uncommon contributory factor.[283] Steroid treatment has given inconsistent results.[592,796]

Pulmonary arterial hypertension and vasculitis. A variety of changes are described pathologically in the pulmonary vessels.[237,418] Chronic lesions consist of intimal thickening, medial hypertrophy, and periadventitial

fibrosis. Acute lesions of vasculitis and fibrinoid necrosis are generally regarded as unusual,[340] but a frequency of up to 20% in SLE[237,319] has been recorded in some autopsy series. Pulmonary arterial hypertension is uncommon,[758] with many reports consisting of small numbers of cases.[23,435,592] Some cases of pulmonary arterial hypertension have been associated with the presence of lupus anticoagulant, which predisposes to thrombosis and may be pathogenetically important.[23] About 10 cases have been indistinguishable from primary pulmonary hypertension,[796] while others have had interstitial lung disease[586] or features of mixed connective tissue disease.[758]

Rarities. A number of case reports have recorded rare associations with SLE: (1) pulmonary embolism[54] in patients with SLE who have circulating lupus anticoagulant; this antibody is also associated with livedo reticularis, recurrent abortion, and labile hypertension; (2) lymphocytic interstitial pneumonitis and pseudolymphoma[592,816]; (3) obliterative bronchiolitis[796]; (4) organizing pneumonia[418]; and (5) acute reversible hypoxemia, accompanied by a normal chest radiograph and ascribed to possible white blood cell aggregation.[2]

SECONDARY MANIFESTATIONS

Atelectasis. Elevation of the diaphragm with resultant lower zone underinflation may be associated with basal line or band shadows that are usually horizontal, several

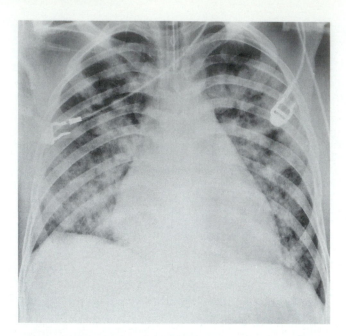

FIGURE 12-39
Systemic lupus erythematosus (SLE). Chest radiograph shows diffuse patchy airspace shadowing consistent with edema in patient with acute nephritic syndrome secondary to SLE.

millimeters wide, and up to 5 cm long. These shadows are often transient and most likely represent discoid or plate atelectasis,* although some could be caused by pulmonary infarcts.[758] Postmortem evidence suggests that pulmonary infarcts are uncommon, and in two large autopsy series of 138 patients with SLE they are not recorded.[340,518]

Pneumonia. Pneumonia is probably the single most common pleuropulmonary abnormality in SLE,[380] occurring in about 50% of patients.[319,340,518] Most cases are simple bacterial pneumonias, including tuberculosis,[239] but some are opportunistic infections.[340] The latter are an increasingly important cause of death.[349,796] The responsible organisms that have been recorded include *Candida, Cytomegalovirus, Legionella, Pneumocystis, Cryptococcus, Aspergillus,* and *Nocardia.†* Cavitary lesions, which are uncommon in SLE, are most often the result of infections.[301,607,788]

Pericarditis, myocarditis, and renal disease. Twenty to thirty percent of all SLE patients have pericarditis at some time.[113] A reliable figure for myocarditis is not available but is probably on the order of 8%.[201,228] Myocarditis, however, rarely gives rise to cardiac failure. Renal failure and the nephrotic syndrome may cause pulmonary edema (Figure 12-39) and pleural effusion. The pleural effusions, unlike those from lupus pleuritis, are pain free.

DRUG-INDUCED SYSTEMIC LUPUS ERYTHEMATO-SUS. This is considered in the section on drug-induced lung disease.

---

*References 260, 305, 315, 369, 457, 732, 790.
†References 99, 340, 349, 457, 518, 758.

CLASSIFICATION OF POLYMYOSITIS AND DERMATOMYOSITIS
Primary, idiopathic polymyositis
Primary, idiopathic dermatomyositis

Polymyositis or dermatomyositis in association with:
  Neoplasia
  Other collagen vascular disorders (overlap syndrome)

Polymyositis or dermatomyositis of childhood

Data from Bohan A. Peter JB: *N Engl J Med* 292:344-347, 403-407, 1975.

Polymyositis and dermatomyositis

Polymyositis (PM) and dermatomyositis (DM) are diffuse inflammatory myopathies of striated muscle. In addition, DM has characteristic skin changes. Several subgroups are identified, and these may be classified as in the box above.[55]

Female patients outnumber male about 2:1,[380] and in most the diseases develop at between 40 and 60 years of age, with a second smaller peak in the 5- to 15-year-old group.[55] Clinical presentation may be with an acute, subacute, or chronic illness[375] characterized by a progressive, symmetric weakness of the girdle and neck muscles. In the acute disease, muscle pain and tenderness are common, and pharyngeal and respiratory symptoms may also be present.[375] In DM, additional and characteristic skin changes are present: heliotrope periorbital rash and violaceous or red papular rash over bony prominences. Associated findings, particularly in the subacute form, include systemic symptoms, arthropathy, dysphagia, pulmonary disease, and cardiac disease.[92,672] Five major diagnostic criteria have been suggested, and all should be present to make a definite diagnosis of DM or, if the skin changes are not present, of PM.[55] These criteria are listed in the box on p. 513.

Pulmonary involvement is quite common in PM and DM and may occur in up to 50% of patients.[184] It is an important determinant of the clinical course and contributes directly to death in about 10% of patients.[184]

The chest manifestations of PM and DM take on a variety of forms: features that are primary to the disease, namely interstitial lung disease and, rarely, isolated pulmonary arterial hypertension or diaphragmatic myopathy; features that are secondary to muscular dysfunction, namely respiratory failure, aspiration pneumonia, simple pneumonia, underinflation, and atelectasis; drug-related changes, including opportunistic infection; changes of heart failure; and predisposing conditions, namely lung carcinoma.

PRIMARY MANIFESTATIONS

Interstitial lung disease. This was first described in DM in 1956 by Mills and Matthews.[519] It is now a well-recognized association[747] that occurs in 5% to 10% of patients (Figure 12-40).[184,261,652] It has been reported slightly more commonly with PM than with DM[92] and has

CRITERIA FOR DIAGNOSIS OF
POLYMYOSITIS AND DERMATOMYOSITIS

Proximal muscle weakness (symmetric, present weeks
or months)
Muscle biopsy (necrobiotic and inflammatory change)
Raised serum creatine phosphokinase
Characteristic electromyograph
Characteristic skin rash

Data from Bohan A, Peter JB: *N Engl J Med* 292:344-347, 403-407, 1975.

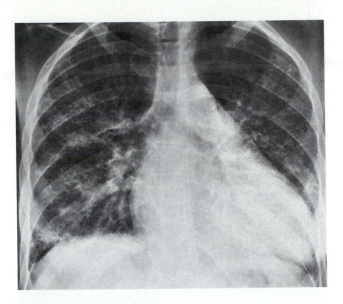

FIGURE 12-40
Dermatomyositis. Radiograph of 21-year-old woman with dermatomyositis shows large heart secondary to myocarditis and diffuse reticulonodular shadowing with apical sparing caused by fibrosing alveolitis.

a controversial association with the presence of Jo1 antibody.[101] Interstitial lung disease (ILD) tends to be accompanied by joint involvement,[669] and as with ILD in other collagen vascular disease, pulmonary change on the chest radiograph can be the first clinical manifestation, preceding the skin rash or myositis.[205,558,669] The usual pattern, however, is for the fibrosis to follow soon after the onset of muscle weakness. Biopsy and respiratory function tests are more sensitive than the chest radiograph in the detection of ILD, and histologic involvement is possible when the plain radiograph shows a normal-appearing lung.[184] The clinical manifestations vary greatly. At one extreme is an acute, rapidly fatal illness resistant to therapy,[241,261,672,673] in which the muscle disease can be masked by respiratory involvement. At the other is a benign, indolent, and asymptomatic form.[261,703] Generally the pneumonitis of PM and DM is more steroid responsive than that of systemic sclerosis.[380] About half the patients respond with lessening of dyspnea, clearing of the chest radiograph, and improvement in lung function tests.[184,673]

Pathologic findings are varied and include fibrosing alveolitis,[442,672,734] diffuse alveolar damage,[734] organizing pneumonitis (BOOP),[673,734] and vasculitis.[442] Radiologic changes commonly consist of symmetric, basally predominant reticulonodular shadowing.[261,673] The more acute cases may show areas of airspace opacities[261] or even widespread ground-glass shadowing superimposed on a reticulonodular background.[184] Some evidence suggests that the alveolar pattern indicates an organizing pneumonia and alveolar desquamation in addition to the interstitial pneumonitis.[673] Alveolar opacities tend to occur early in the course of lung disease and are more likely to be steroid responsive. In time, pulmonary shadowing can progress to involve the whole lung (Figure 12-40), and small circular transradiancies may form (honeycombing),[382,652,673] giving the appearance of end-stage lung. Although pleural inflammatory changes and fibrosis together with small effusions are commonly found on pathologic study,[673] they have not been described radiologically. The same applies to multifocal dystrophic pulmonary ossification, which has been demonstrated pathologically[673] but not radiographically. Adenocarcinoma secondary to scarring has not been recorded in PM or DM alveolitis.[184]

Pulmonary arterial hypertension. Pulmonary arterial hypertension produces large main and proximal pulmonary arteries on the chest radiograph. Such hypertension may be seen as a complication of alveolitis (Figure 12-40),[205] hypoventilation,[250] or vasculitis.[83] Some cases resemble primary pulmonary hypertension.[672]

Diaphragmatic myositis. When the diaphragm becomes involved in the myositis,[665] functional and radiographic changes are produced similar to those seen with the diaphragmatic myopathy of SLE. Characteristically the myopathy produces bilateral hemidiaphragm elevation, reduced lung volume, and discoid basal atelectasis.[184,665]

SECONDARY MANIFESTATIONS. Aspiration pneumonia is probably the most common finding on chest radiographs in PM and DM. In one series nearly one third of patients had radiographic evidence of pneumonia at some stage, and half of these cases were thought to be caused by aspiration.[184] Aspiration is caused by cough impairment, pharyngeal dysfunction, and general weakness of body movements. Pharyngeal dysfunction is probably the most important factor, and most patients who aspirate are dysphagic.[184] Since PM and DM affect striated muscle, the upper esophagus and pharynx are selectively involved. These structures are normally closed at rest, but in PM and DM they are hypotonic and often contain air on plain radiographs. A barium swallow demonstrates vallecular and pyriform pooling, defective bolus propulsion, defective pharyngeal emptying, nasopharyngeal reflux, and tracheal aspiration.[321,512,557]

Other pneumonias may arise from compromised defenses secondary to muscle weakness and impaired cough.[71,184] Some pneumonias are opportunistic.[442]

Respiratory muscle weakness coupled with stiff lungs

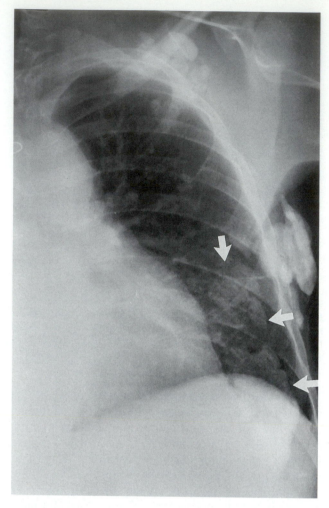

FIGURE 12-41
Dermatomyositis. A 23-year-old man who had childhood dermato-myositis and also has cardiomyopathy. Note extensive soft tissue calcification in chest wall, some seen en face *(white arrows)* and some tangentially.

and increased chest wall compliance produces small-volume lungs with diaphragmatic elevation and atelecta-sis, which is often basilar and discoid.[71,184] Marked weakness of respiratory muscles occasionally produces hypercapnic respiratory failure necessitating mechanical ventilation.[184]

CARCINOMA LUNG AND POLYMYOSITIS AND DER-MATOMYOSITIS. There is a twofold to sevenfold increase in the frequency of malignant disease in PM and DM,[31,692] especially in older patients. The average preva-lence in various series is 21% for PM and 15% for DM.[622] The carcinomas recorded roughly parallel their frequency in the general population.[622] PM or DM may precede, accompany, or follow the carcinoma. One series found equal numbers in each group,[92] although others have found only 10% of cases to be synchronous.[31] Using Callen's data to estimate,[91] in about 1% to 2% of cases the chest radiograph will show a previously unrecognized lung carcinoma at the time of diagnosis of DM, and the

chance of a preceding or subsequent lung carcinoma is similar.

OVERLAP SYNDROME. Overlap of PM and DM with other collagen vascular disorders occurs in 20% to 40% of patients.[101] It occurs more commonly with PM than DM and shows a strong female predilection.[101] Overlap is most common with systemic sclerosis but is also seen with SLE, RA, and Sjögren's syndrome.[56] The chest radiograph reflects this admixture.

JUVENILE DERMATOMYOSITIS AND POLYMYOSITIS. Juvenile dermatomyositis and polymyositis differ from the adult forms in a number of ways.[572,800] In children, DM occurs much more frequently (10 to 20 times) than PM, calcinosis is common, and widespread vasculitis is a feature, although it does not appear to cause pulmonary complications. A diffuse interstitial pulmonary fibrosis similar to that seen in adults is described.[576] One third of patients have soft tissue calcification, particularly over pressure points.[572] When calcinosis affects the chest wall (Figure 12-41), it is detectable on the chest radiograph and may occasionally be a striking finding.

SYSTEMIC SCLEROSIS

Systemic sclerosis (SS) is a generalized connective tissue disorder characterized by tightening, induration, and thickening of the skin (scleroderma); Raynaud's phenomenon and other vascular abnormalities; muscu-loskeletal manifestations; and visceral involvement, espe-cially of the gastrointestinal tract, lungs, heart, and kidneys.[630] The diagnosis can be made with a high degree of certainty if the single major criterion of proximal scleroderma is present (proximal to metacarpophalangeal joints) or if there are two or more minor criteria (sclerodactyly, pitting scars, or loss of substance of the fingertips, or bilateral basal pulmonary fibrosis).[489]

The pathogenesis is complex and not completely understood.[455,568,693] Pathologic study of the lungs shows two types of change that are independent of each other[812]: an interstitial fibrosis indistinguishable from cryptogenic fibrosing alveolitis and vascular changes in small vessels (intimal proliferation, medial hypertrophy, and myxoma-tous change).[418] At postmortem examination the lungs are abnormal in more than 80% of cases.[168] Interstitial fibrosis affects all lobes but is particularly marked peripherally and in lower zones.[418,786] Pleural fibrosis and adhesions are common, as well as subpleural cysts.[213] Severe cases show extensive parenchymal de-struction with the development of honeycomb lung[418] and bronchiolectasis.[786]

SS has a 3:1 female to male distribution and develops most commonly in the third to fifth decades of life, although a wide range exists from the teens upward.[489] The most common presentation is with Raynaud's phe-nomenon, which occurs in about 80% to 90% of cases and may precede skin changes by several years. Other early manifestations include tendinitis, arthralgia, and arthri-tis. Treatment has little to offer,[380] and prognosis is

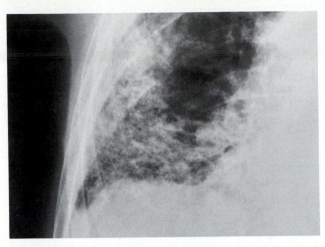

FIGURE 12-42
Systemic sclerosis with fibrosing alveolitis. Localized view of right lower zone in patient with systemic sclerosis shows fine reticulonodular opacities with basal and peripheral distribution characteristic of fibrosing alveolitis.

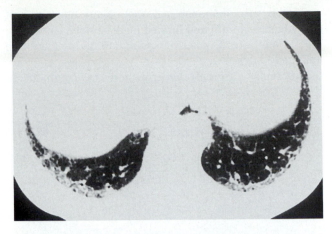

FIGURE 12-43
Systemic sclerosis on computed tomogram of lung bases. Early changes of fibrosing alveolitis with typical distribution. Patient had no respiratory symptoms, and chest radiograph was normal.

variable depending on the degree of visceral involvement, particularly of the heart, kidneys, and lungs.[505] The 5-year survival is on the order of 70%,[453] and pulmonary disease has now replaced renal disease as the major cause of death.[20,453]

Less than 1% of patients initially have respiratory symptoms,[568] and just a few of these will have yet to develop sclerodermatous changes.[472] However, in established disease respiratory symptoms are common, with dyspnea in more than 60% and less commonly cough and pleuritic pain. Dyspnea may be caused by lung fibrosis or pulmonary arterial hypertension.[693] Respiratory function tests are commonly (80% to 90%) abnormal in SS, but the defects are often mild.[568] The main abnormalities are a reduced carbon monoxide diffusion and a restrictive defect with hypoxemia and airflow obstruction in some.[325,568] A poor correlation exists between respiratory function tests and radiologic findings,[713] and as with other lung fibroses the interstitial fibrosis of SS can be present even though the chest radiograph appears normal.[786] Respiratory disease usually pursues an indolent and progressive course and adversely affects survival.[20]

Generally the chest radiograph is abnormal in about 25% to 50% of patients with established disease,[325] although the range in various series is from 10% to 80%.[20,731] Very occasionally chest radiographic changes consistent with fibrosis predate the onset of scleroderma.[472] The most common radiologic abnormality is interstitial fibrosis (Figure 12-42), which causes a symmetric, diffuse, basally predominant reticulonodular pattern[294,786] that typically starts with very fine reticulation and progresses to coarser reticulation with nodules. Sometimes the nodular shadowing is so fine that it has a ground-glass appearance.[22] Recognized variants of distribution include unilateral[785] and total lung involve-

ment.[731] Cystic lesions commonly develop in the areas of fibrosis and range in size from 1 to 30 mm.[325,785] Sometimes they are aggregated and have the appearance of honeycombing. Occasionally the cysts are quite large, more than 5 cm in diameter.[66] Presumably the rupture of such cysts accounts for the occasional pneumothorax seen in SS.[294,394] Gross fibrosis can cause airway distortion and bronchiectasis.[22,66] Interstitial fibrosis is associated with an increased uptake of gallium-67 in the lungs.[267] Loss of lung volume often occurs and is probably caused by reduced compliance that is associated with fibrosis. Such volume loss is manifest by elevation of the diaphragm. However, diaphragmatic muscle atrophy and replacement fibrosis have also been demonstrated, and weakness may be an additional factor contributing to elevation.[383] Pleural thickening, inflammation, adhesions, and effusion are recorded post mortem in about 50% to 80% of cases.[168,786] On radiologic study, however, pleural changes are infrequent and relatively minor.

HRCT findings in SS have been described in a number of papers.* CT may be abnormal despite a normal chest radiograph.[335,670] Changes, other than in advanced disease, tend to occur caudad and posterolaterally (Figure 12-43).[617,670] The reporting of various abnormalities has shown some inconsistency among series. The main findings have been ground-glass opacity (Figure 12-44); honeycombing, particularly subpleurally with traction bronchiolectasis and subpleural cysts (1 to 3 cm in diameter); lines of various types, such as septal, subpleural, and long (nonseptal) parenchymal lines (Figure 12-44); and micronodulation, particularly beneath the pleura but also within lobules.[617,670] Correlation between CT and biopsies has shown that ground-glass changes are more commonly associated with a cellular biopsy than are honeycomb opacities.[792]

---

*References 274, 335, 535, 616, 617, 670, 782, 792.

CT has also demonstrated that about one third of patients have a mild and limited mediastinal adenopathy; only 4 out of 21 positive cases had more than two enlarged nodes.[274]

Pulmonary arterial hypertension is common in

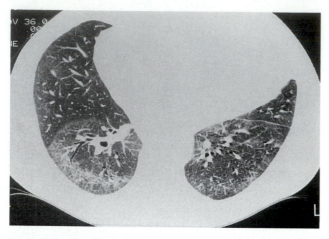

FIGURE 12-44
Systemic sclerosis with fibrosing alveolitis. High-resolution computed tomogram in patient with shortness of breath caused by intrinsic lung disease and cardiomyopathy. In right lower lobe note band of abnormal opacity inset 10 to 15 mm from pleural surface consisting of intralobular and interlobular septal thickening with ground-glass opacity that throws airways into prominence. Volume of right lower lobe is reduced. Similar milder changes are present on left.

SS[213,645] and occurs independently of lung fibrosis (Figure 12-45).[750,812] It occurs in one third to one half of patients, particularly in anticentromere antibody (ACA)–positive patients with the CREST syndrome (limited cutaneous systemic sclerosis).[722,768,812] Its presence may be signaled by an isolated reduction in diffusing capacity.[722,768] Pulmonary arterial hypertension can cause enlargement of the main and proximal pulmonary arteries and lead to cor pulmonale with cardiomegaly[325]; however, normal pulmonary arteries do not exclude the diagnosis.[768]

Generally an increased prevalence of lung carcinoma (Figure 12-46) is seen in SS,[20] although not all studies agree.[206] Data with regard to the histologic type of neoplasm are also inconsistent. Particularly high prevalences of alveolar cell carcinoma and adenocarcinoma are described,[325] but in contrast some series have no cases of alveolar cell carcinoma.[640]

Pneumonia is a recognized complication of SS and in some cases may be an aspiration pneumonia related to esophageal dysfunction.[564,693] Most authors consider that aspiration does not play a significant part in the pathogenesis of basal fibrotic changes.[785] This view has recently been questioned.[404] Infection is a serious complication of advanced SS, and it, rather than respiratory failure, is the main cause of respiratory deaths.[568]

Two extrapulmonary features of SS may be seen on the chest radiograph: posterolateral superior rib erosion[723] and esophageal dilatation. Superior rib erosion is not

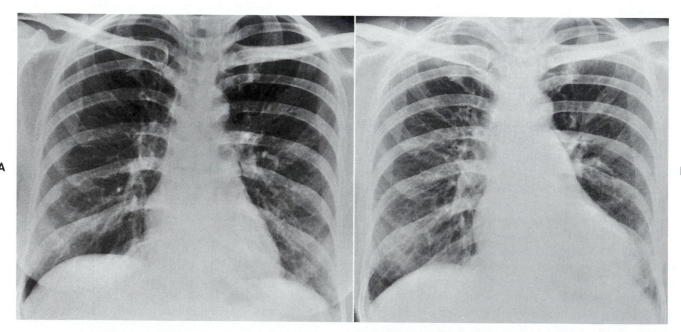

A   B

FIGURE 12-45
Systemic sclerosis with pulmonary arterial hypertension in patient who developed progressive exertional dyspnea in 5-year interval between radiographs **A** and **B**. Enlarged heart and prominent main pulmonary artery result from pulmonary arterial hypertension. Mean pulmonary artery pressure at time of radiograph **B** was 55 mm Hg. Because pulmonary vascular changes and hypertension occur independent of alveolitis, absence of fibrosis on chest radiograph is not surprising.

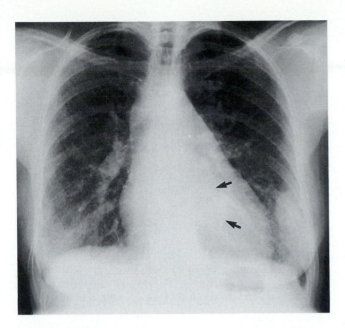

FIGURE 12-46

Systemic sclerosis with fibrosing alveolitis and carcinoma in 56-year-old woman with long history of systemic sclerosis. Fibrosing alveolitis manifest by fine bibasilar and peripheral interstitial opacity developed 10 years before this radiograph and 2 years before a mass developed in left lower zone, later followed by mediastinal adenopathy *(arrows)*. Histologic examination showed mass to be adenocarcinoma. Evidence of pulmonary arterial hypertension can be seen, which can also be seen in systemic sclerosis without fibrosing alveolitis.

specific for SS, since it has been seen in other collagen vascular diseases.[657,731] A 10% to 20% prevalence rate is reported in SS.[324,657]

Clinical disease of the esophagus occurs in more than one half of cases and is present pathologically in three fourths.[168] The esophagus becomes functionally abnormal and fibrosed, ending up as a dilated, air-filled tube that may be detected on the lateral chest radiograph.[188,324] It does not contain an air-fluid level, since the dilatation is not associated with obstruction.[485] An air esophagogram is found in many other conditions.[605]

CREST syndrome (limited cutaneous systemic sclerosis)

CREST is an acronym for calcinosis, Raynaud's phenomenon, esophagus, sclerodactyly, and telangiectasia, stressing the major features and organ involvement of this form of SS.[666,803] Selection bias in various series makes prevalence difficult to assess, but it is probably similar to that of classic SS.[20,631] The majority of patients are older women with a long history of Raynaud's phenomenon and swollen fingers.[20,631] More than 50% of patients have ACA, which is an unusual finding in SS.[20] The CREST syndrome also differs from SS in that life expectancy is greater, and the disease is quite often mild and slowly progressive.[631] Systemic involvement such as that of the kidney is less.[263] However, the CREST syndrome is by no

means benign, and there are several reports of severe pulmonary hypertension and deaths from cor pulmonale,[263,651,722] with an overall prevalence of pulmonary hypertension of about 10%.[651,813] In addition, although several smaller series suggest a lower prevalence of interstitial lung disease ranging up to 11%,[263,731,770] in a recent large series of 88 CREST patients the prevalence of lung involvement was similar to that in SS, with 72% having abnormal respiratory function tests and 33% having radiologic pulmonary fibrosis.[567]

Overlap — systemic sclerosis syndrome

This is the other major clinical variant of SS, constituting 10% to 27% of all cases of SS.[489,731,752] Overlap occurs with one or more connective tissue disorders, namely SLE, rheumatoid disease, and dermatomyositis. Pleuropulmonary involvement is more common than in classic SS, with radiologic fibrosis in 25% to 65%[489,731,752,753] and pleural effusions in 15% to 36%.[200,731]

SJÖGREN'S SYNDROME

Sjögren's syndrome (sicca syndrome, SjS) is an autoimmune disorder characterized by dry eyes (keratoconjunctivitis sicca) and dry mouth (xerostomia). The syndrome is often, but not invariably, accompanied by features of one or more of the connective tissue diseases. The pathologic hallmark of SjS is widespread tissue infiltration by immunoglobulin-producing lymphocytes. This infiltration particularly affects various exocrine glands (lacrimal, salivary, airway mucous glands) causing enlargement and later atrophy with impairment of secretion. The diagnosis is established by the demonstration of reduced tear secretion (Schirmer's test), a filamentary or punctate keratitis, and biopsy evidence of focal lymphocytic and plasma cell infiltration of an exocrine gland (most conveniently a labial salivary gland).[323]

The syndrome is divided into primary and secondary forms according to the presence or absence of an associated collagen vascular disease. The most commonly associated collagen vascular disease is RA, but SjS may also be seen with systemic sclerosis, SLE, and polymyositis. Various autoimmune disorders occur with both primary and secondary forms and include chronic active hepatitis, primary biliary cirrhosis, Hashimoto's thyroiditis, myasthenia gravis, and celiac disease. Primary SjS differs from the secondary form in that exocrine function is more severely disturbed and extraglandular manifestations are frequent.[390] These extraglandular features include renal tubular disorders, such as renal tubular acidosis; myopathy and peripheral neuropathy, and central nervous system disorders[11]; vascular disorders, including Raynaud's phenomenon, vasculitis, and purpura; and nonerosive polyarthropathy. Finally, both types of SjS may develop into a lymphoproliferative disorder including pseudolymphoma and frank lymphoma.

Most patients have a polyclonal gammopathy, especially of IgG and IgM. Ninety percent have rheumatoid

PLEUROPULMONARY MANIFESTATIONS OF
SJÖGREN'S SYNDROME

AS SEEN IN COLLAGEN VASCULAR DISEASE

Pleural thickening, effusion
Fibrosing alveolitis
Discoid basal atelectasis
Vasculitis
Pulmonary arterial hypertension
Diaphragm weakness

AIRWAY DRYNESS/OBSTRUCTION; RECURRENT INFECTION

Xerotrachea
Atelectasis
Bronchitis
Pneumonia
Bronchiectasis

LYMPHOPROLIFERATIVE

Lymphocytic airway infiltration
Lymphocytic interstitial pneumonitis
Focal polyclonal lymphoproliferation
Malignant lymphoma
Amyloidosis

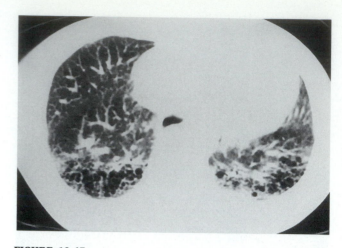

FIGURE 12-47
Fibrosing alveolitis in 65-year-old woman with Sjögren's syndrome secondary to rheumatoid disease. Posterobasal computed tomogram shows changes that are consistent with fibrosing alveolitis.

factor, and 70% have antinuclear antibody. Organ-specific autoantibodies are also common, and the antibodies to extractable nuclear antigens (SS-A, SS-B) are relatively specific and sensitive for primary SjS.[730]

Sjögren's syndrome is typically a disease of middle-aged women; only 10% of patients are male. The various pleuropulmonary manifestations of SjS fall into three major groups (see box above). These manifestations give rise to symptoms of hoarseness (dry larynx), cough (xerotrachea), pleuritic pain, and exertional dyspnea. Recurrent infections, particularly bronchitis and pneumonia, are common,[53,684] although some recent series suggest that this may no longer be so.[139] Factors considered to predispose to airway infections are complex and include mucus hyposecretion, which leads to dry airways[53] and lymphocytic infiltration of small airway walls, causing obstruction.[547] Obstructive, restrictive, and diffusion abnormalities are found on respiratory function tests, with different abnormalities predominating in different series.[231,547,569,678]

The prevalence of pleuropulmonary involvement is difficult to assess. With symptoms and the radiologic signs together, the prevalence is probably about 30%, with a range of 9% to 75%.[53,719,730] When assessed by respiratory function tests, the prevalence of respiratory involvement is higher.[30,138,547,569,773] Somewhat surprisingly, the prevalence of pleuropulmonary abnormalities is about the same in primary and secondary SjS.[30,53,575,678,773] Xerotrachea,[137] recurrent tracheobronchitis, recurrent pneumonia, and interstitial lung disease

(Figure 12-47) are the most common problems, each occurring in one third or more of those with chest involvement. Pleuritis with or without effusion and pleural thickening occur in about one tenth of the patients, while most of the other manifestations (listed in the box at left) have a prevalence of 5% or less.

A number of the manifestations, particularly fibrosing alveolitis and lymphocytic interstitial pneumonitis, give rise to basally predominant nodular or reticulonodular shadowing.[678,719] In general the chest radiograph is not specific enough to distinguish among these processes. However, the combination of airspace shadowing[346] and an interstitial pattern suggests lymphocytic interstitial pneumonitis.[410] Fibrosing alveolitis can occur in both primary and secondary SjS.[231,416] Interstitial lung disease of various and often obscure types is the most common pulmonary finding in most series, and such patients are often asymptomatic.[139] Mediastinal lymph nodes are not enlarged in uncomplicated SjS.[15] Enlargement of mediastinal lymph nodes or a multifocal large nodular or alveolar pattern suggests the development of pseudolymphoma[231,547,719] or malignant lymphoma.[231,719] In SjS there is a twofold increase in malignancy in general and a 44-fold increase in malignant lymphoma (Figure 12-48). This finding applies to both primary and secondary SjS.[390] Lymphomas tend to occur in patients with extraglandular abnormalities.[730]

OVERLAP SYNDROMES AND MIXED CONNECTIVE TISSUE DISEASE

Some patients have an illness with the characteristic features of more than one connective tissue disorder. These patients are said to have an overlap syndrome or undifferentiated connective tissue disorder. The thoracic manifestations in these cases are those of the various connective tissue disorders that make up the overlap, and

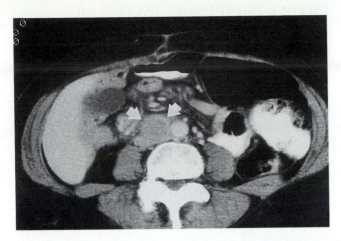

FIGURE 12-48
Lymphoma with Sjögren's syndrome in same patient as in Figure 12-47. Abdominal computed tomography shows paraaortic mass (*arrows*), determined on biopsy to be non-Hodgkin's lymphoma.

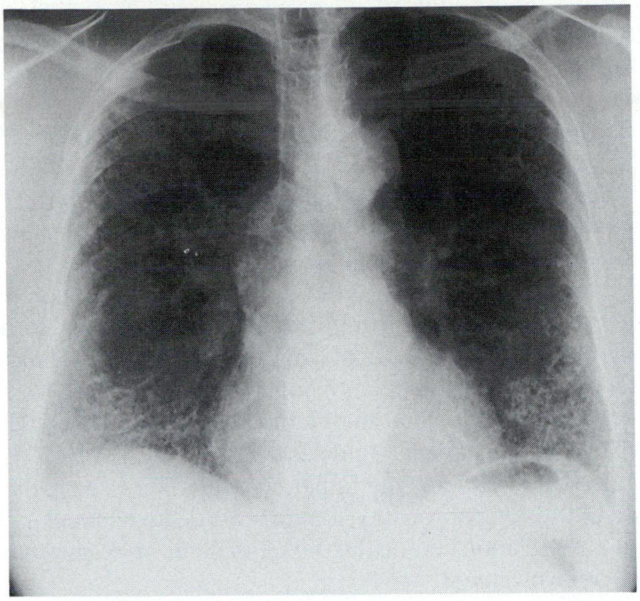

FIGURE 12-49
Mixed connective tissue disease with fibrosing alveolitis. Patient is 48-year-old woman with 15-year history of arthropathy who over the years has had features of both rheumatoid arthritis and systemic lupus erythematosus. Currently she has polyarthropathy with myositis and positive extractable nuclear antigen (ENA) titer. Radiologic changes are consistent with fibrosing alveolitis, but patient is only minimally dyspneic.

they are discussed under individual connective tissue disorders.

Mixed connective tissue disease is an overlap syndrome that is a distinct clinicopathologic entity,[682] although not everyone agrees with this view.[614] The principal characteristics are the presence of features of SLE, SS, DM, or PM, occurring together or evolving sequentially during observation, and antibodies to an extractable nuclear antigen (RNP).[682] Suggested clinical criteria for the diagnosis are positive anti-RNP plus three or more clinical features, including hand edema, synovitis, myositis, Raynaud's phenomenon, and acrosclerosis.[9] Those with initially limited disease tend to show more overlap as time goes on,[724] and there is a tendency to transform eventually into SS.[548] Eighty to ninety percent of the patients have been women[42] with an average age of 37 years (range 4 to 80).[600] Its prevalence is approximately the same as that of SS,[600] and its overall prognosis is like that of SLE and better than that of SS.

The pulmonary findings have recently been reviewed.[600] The prevalence of chest disease ranges in various series between 25% and 80% with the upper figures probably the closer estimate.[180,333,601,724] Many affected patients are unaware of respiratory disease.[600] In two series chest radiographs were abnormal in 30%[724] and 63%[333] of cases. The 30% figure represents changes on the initial chest radiograph only and undoubtedly underestimates the long-term chest involvement. The pulmonary abnormalities resemble those seen in SLE, SS, and PM or DM.[380] Thus pleural thickening and pleural and pericardial effusions have been described,* as has steroid-sensitive pneumonitis, manifested as fleeting basal consolidations.[42] However, the most frequent pleuropulmonary finding has been small irregular interstitial

*References 322, 333, 555, 600, 695, 724.

opacities most prevalent in the lower half of the lungs (Figure 12-49).[4,601,724] Histologically, these changes are caused by fibrosing alveolitis,[797] and the radiologic picture is entirely consistent with this finding. The other common finding has been pulmonary arterial hypertension,[4,724,797] which may produce characteristic radiographic changes but which also occurs with a normal chest radiograph. The changes of pulmonary arterial hypertension may or may not be accompanied by a fibrosing alveolitis pattern.[42] Other reported associations include pulmonary vasculitis,[797] pulmonary embolism,[408] diffuse pulmonary hemorrhage,[656] and hypoventilatory respiratory failure.[486] There is a high prevalence (74%) of esophageal abnormality, which can lead to aspiration pneumonia.[724] A patient has been described with mediastinal adenopathy that was nonspecific on biopsy.[322]

Although early reports suggest that the pulmonary changes respond well to steroids,[333] not all studies bear this out.[797]

RELAPSING POLYCHONDRITIS

Relapsing polychondritis is a rare disease of unknown cause characterized by recurrent inflammatory episodes that affect various cartilaginous structures, particularly the pinna, nose, and airways. Other features include nonerosive inflammatory polyarthritis, arteritis of medium to large vessels, and recurrent inflammation of the eyes and inner ears.[495] The mean age of onset is the fifth decade,[495] although all age groups may be affected. Most patients have been white,[191] and the overall sex incidence is equal,[495] although patients with serious airway involvement are more commonly (3:1) female.[220] About 30% of patients have an associated "autoimmune" disease,[204] most commonly RA[495] or a systemic vasculitis.[516] The diagnosis is based on characteristic combinations of clinical features,[204,495,516] since the pathology is nonspecific.

Pathologically, this disease is characterized by a loss of glycosaminoglycans from cartilage, chondrolysis with fibrous tissue replacement, and surrounding inflammatory change. Cartilage antibodies have been detected[209] and are probably important in the pathogenesis, although the exact mechanism is unclear.[204]

In half of patients the initial manifestation is auricular chondritis or arthropathy, and in most of the remainder it is nasal chondritis, ocular inflammation, or respiratory tract involvement.[495,516]

About 20% of patients initially have respiratory symptoms,[220] and eventually one third to one half of the patients have respiratory tract involvement,[114,495] manifested by laryngeal tenderness, hoarseness, dyspnea, and stridor or wheeze. Disease of the respiratory tract is a serious development, since it may be immediately life threatening and in the long term is associated with a bad prognosis.[516] Airway involvement causes narrowing, primarily of the larynx or trachea, but the major bronchi,[119,154] including segmental ones, can also be involved.[173,220] However, significant disease beyond the main bronchi is unlikely.[282] Stenoses are usually single and localized,[495] but they can be multiple.[523] Thus tracheal narrowing is typically subglottic, smooth, and up to several centimeters long[426] but can involve the whole trachea.[119] CT shows wall thickening, expansion and calcification of cartilage, and luminal narrowing.[108,384,508] The tracheal lumen may take on a polygonal configuration.[290,384] Furthermore, stenoses may be fixed or variable. In this latter instance, increased wall compliance predisposes to dynamic collapse.[282,545] The dynamic behavior of stenoses can be investigated by flow volume loops,[220,523] with fluoroscopy and cineradiography,[282] or with dynamic CT.[290] Airflow obstruction in lobar and segmental airways can lead to pulmonary oligemia and air trapping,[154] atelectasis,[523] obstructive pneumonitis, or bronchiectasis.[173]

Cardiovascular involvement is recorded in 24% of patients,[495] and some of the described lesions such as aortic and mitral regurgitation and aortic aneurysm may produce changes on a chest radiograph.

The mainstay of treatment is systemic steroids, and tracheostomy may be necessary. The outcome is variable, and the course may be rapidly fatal or indolent with about a 75% 5-year survival.[516] The frequency of respiratory involvement as a cause of death has been 50% or more in some series[191,495] but was only 10% in a recent major series.[516]

DIFFUSE PULMONARY (ALVEOLAR) HEMORRHAGE

Bleeding into the lung parenchyma is common in a wide variety of disorders, but in this chapter the discussion is limited to conditions in which bleeding is diffuse or multifocal and contributes significantly to the radiologic changes. A triad of features suggests diffuse pulmonary hemorrhage (DPH): hemoptysis, anemia, and airspace opacities on the chest radiograph.[67] Sometimes bleeding is covert and hemoptysis is absent.[701] The diagnosis is often missed, at least initially, particularly when hemoptysis is not present.[75] The pulmonary features of all DPH syndromes are the same, and chest radiographs are generally not helpful in distinguishing among them.[448]

There have been a number of recent reviews,* and the classification given in the box below has been drawn from a combination of these sources. DPH may also be seen in conditions other than those listed,[447,533,749] including mitral stenosis, venoocclusive disease,[135] infectious hemorrhagic necrotizing pneumonias such as leptospirosis,[385] fat embolism, bone marrow transplant,[805] and hemorrhagic pulmonary edema of renal failure. These disorders can usually be differentiated taking into account clinical setting, extrapulmonary involvement, serology, and renal biopsy.[447]

Principal causes

ANTI–BASEMENT MEMBRANE ANTIBODY DISEASE. Anti–basement membrane antibody (ABMA) disease is the most common cause of DPH. Sixty to eighty percent of patients with ABMA disease have alveolar hemorrhage and glomerulonephritis (Goodpasture's syndrome), and most of the rest have glomerulonephritis only. A few

---

*References 10, 67, 447, 448, 528, 533, 742, 762.

CAUSES OF DIFFUSE PULMONARY HEMORRHAGE

Anti–basement membrane antibody disease (Goodpasture's syndrome)
Connective tissue disorder, systemic vasculitis, "immune complex disease"
  Systemic lupus erythematosus
  Systemic necrotizing vasculitis
  Wegener's granulomatosis
  Microscopic polyarteritis nodosa
  Henoch-Schönlein disease
  Rheumatoid disease
  Mixed connective tissue disease
Idiopathic glomerulonephritis
Idiopathic pulmonary hemosiderosis
Bleeding disorders
Drugs, chemicals[355]

patients with ABMA disease have alveolar hemorrhage and no kidney disease, but this is very unusual.

In 1919 Goodpasture described a patient who had fatal pulmonary hemorrhage and glomerulonephritis 6 weeks after an attack of influenza.[298] In 1958 Stanton and Tange[711] were the first to use the term "Goodpasture's syndrome" to describe the combination of pulmonary hemorrhage and glomerulonephritis. With a clearer understanding of the pathogenesis, researchers have given the term a restricted meaning that defines a syndrome with DPM, glomerulonephritis, and anti–glomerular basement antibodies in the serum, lung, or kidney.[742]

Goodpasture's syndrome is essentially a disease of young white men. In one major review the median age at onset was 21 years (range 16 to 61 years), with 90%

males and 51 of 52 white.[43] The entity has been occasionally reported in children.[570] The clinical presentation is usually with respiratory symptoms: hemoptysis (80%), dyspnea (72%), and cough,[735] and the patients are usually found to have an iron-deficient anemia (93%) and an abnormal chest radiograph (80%) (Figure 12-50). Either at the time of presentation or in the ensuing weeks or months, urinalysis findings and renal function become abnormal. Occasionally renal failure takes years to develop.[664] In one series 55% of patients were anemic on admission and about 80% had proteinuria or hematuria.[735] Rarely the order of events is reversed, with pulmonary hemorrhage following a nephritic presentation.[67] Demonstrating the presence of anti–glomerular basement antibodies in the serum is both a sensitive and

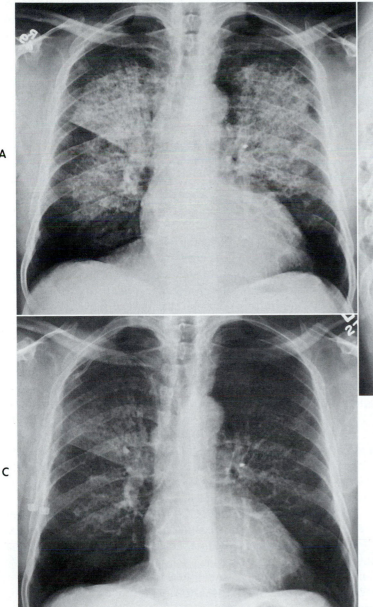
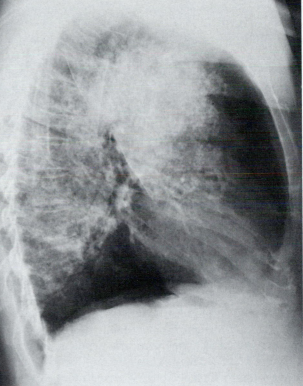

FIGURE 12-50
Goodpasture's syndrome. **A,** Radiograph shows bilateral perihilar consolidation, some of which is sharply marginated by minor fissure. Note bilateral air bronchogram. Apex and base are spared by airspace shadowing, which is caused by intraalveolar blood. **B,** Lateral view of same patient. Note holdup of consolidation by oblique fissure and peripheral acinar nodules. **C,** One week later, considerable although incomplete resolution of consolidation. Typically pulmonary hemorrhage clears in a matter of days.

a specific indicator of the disease and establishes the diagnosis.[448] However, generally the level of serum antibody and the severity of the disease do not correlate.[67]

Renal biopsy shows evidence of subacute proliferative glomerulonephritis with linear IgG deposition in the glomeruli. Lung biopsy is not usually performed, but if it were, it would show blood and hemosiderin-laden macrophages in the alveoli and in the interstitium and linear immunofluorescence along alveolar septa. In addition, sometimes septal thickening or fibrosis together with linear deposits of IgG on the alveolar capillary membranes is evident.[418,528] Therapy, apart from supportive measures, is directed at removing anti–basement membrane antibody by plasmapheresis and stopping its production with steroids and immunosuppressives.[613] In the past the reported prognosis was poor, with about half the patients dying of pulmonary complications and almost all the rest dying of renal disease.[43] An occasional patient went into remission and recovered.[677] In one major series 96% died, with a mean survival of 15 weeks.[43] The prognosis is better now with improved treatment and because milder cases are included in the various series.[67]

CONNECTIVE TISSUE DISORDERS, SYSTEMIC VASCULITIDES, "IMMUNE COMPLEX DISEASE." Many collagen vascular disorders and systemic vasculitides are occasionally associated with DPH, with or uncommonly without a glomerulonephritis. Many, and possibly all, are immune complex mediated, although hard evidence is lacking with some of the entities. The association is most commonly seen with SLE and systemic necrotizing vasculitides of the polyarteritis nodosa type.[67]

DPH is well documented in patients with SLE[563] usually occurring in the context of established disease with extrapulmonary features including glomerulonephritis.[447] Rarely is DPH the initial feature.[88,208] It has many shared features with lupus pneumonitis, including probable pathogenesis, and it carries a poor prognosis, with 70% of the patients dying within a few days.[448]

DPH is well recognized in systemic necrotizing vasculitides, including microvascular polyarteritis nodosa.[387,448,578,743] There is usually multisystem involvement together with a necrotizing glomerulonephritis with or without immune deposits on biopsy. On histologic study the lung shows a capillaritis.[482]

DPH is also seen in WG (see p. 496).[148]

Isolated examples of DPH are reported with rheumatoid disease, SS,[413] mixed connective tissue disease, Henoch-Schönlein syndrome (hypersensitivity vasculitis),[560] immune complex glomerulonephritis, and essential mixed cryoglobulinemia.[67,447,448] A case of microangiopathic hemolytic anemia and pulmonary vasculitis is also recorded.[528]

IDIOPATHIC GLOMERULONEPHRITIS. Idiopathic glomerulonephritis is diagnosed when crescentic glomerulonephritis occurs without linear immunofluorescence or vasculitis. Two varieties, one with granular immunofluorescence (immune complex deposition) and one

without,[449] may be associated with DPH. The former includes conditions listed in the previous paragraph,[39] while the latter is not an uncommon (19% in one series) cause of pulmonary hemorrhage with glomerulonephritis.[448]

IDIOPATHIC (PRIMARY) PULMONARY HEMOSIDEROSIS. Idiopathic pulmonary hemosiderosis (IPH) is a disorder of unknown etiology characterized by episodic alveolar hemorrhage that eventually leads to lung fibrosis.[762] Multisystem involvement and, in particular, glomerulonephritis are not features. An association with celiac disease[117,571] and dermatitis herpetiformis[550] is recognized. Light microscopic changes are the same as those of Goodpasture's syndrome, namely alveolar hemorrhage; hemosiderin-laden macrophages in the alveoli and, to a lesser extent, in the interstitium; and mild interstitial thickening. Late in the disease, alveolar septal fibrosis develops.[67] Some workers describe ultrastructural abnormalities of the capillary basement membranes,[193] and others have described a capillaritis. Immunofluorescent staining is negative.

Unlike Goodpasture's syndrome, IPH is a disease of childhood. The onset is typically from 1 to 7 years of age with one fifth of patients first having symptoms in the late teens and twenties.[701] It is the most common DPH syndrome in childhood.[528] The sex incidence in children is equal, but adults have a twofold preponderance in males. Episodic cough, hemoptysis, and the signs and symptoms of anemia (tiredness, pallor, failure to gain weight) are present. The magnitude of hemoptysis varies greatly. In some it is absent altogether, leading to diagnostic difficulties; in others it is massive enough to cause death.[316] Bleeding into the lungs is evidenced by consolidation on the chest radiograph (Figure 12-51) and the presence of iron-deficiency anemia, with low iron stores. With recurrent bleeding, pulmonary hemosiderosis and fibrosis develop, and most of those who survive several years are chronically dyspneic, anemic, and underweight.[701] Although some patients have been followed for 20 years, whether the disease ever permanently remits is unclear. The outcome is variable. In one series of 68 patients followed for 5 years, 29% died, 25% had active disease, 18% had inactive disease but chronic symptoms, and 28% were well.[701] Some of the deaths were caused by pulmonary arterial hypertension and cor pulmonale. Treatment is supportive. Steroids and immunosuppressive drugs may be used, but there is no clear evidence that they help. Formerly splenectomy was performed, but it is no longer recommended.

BLEEDING DISORDERS. DPH is an unusual complication of the various coagulopathies. It has been recorded with thrombocytopenia,[247,293,573,696] particularly in the context of leukemia,[10,52] anticoagulation,[246] coronary thrombolysis,[542] and diffuse intravascular coagulation.[626]

DRUGS AND CHEMICALS. A number of exogenous agents are recorded as causing alveolar hemorrhage (see Chapter 11).

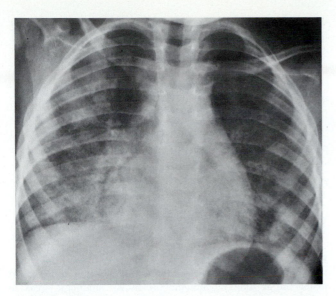

FIGURE 12-51
Primary pulmonary hemosiderosis. Patient is 2½-year-old boy who had low-grade fever, cough, and hemoptysis. Chest radiograph at time of presentation shows multiple, bilateral, focal consolidations.

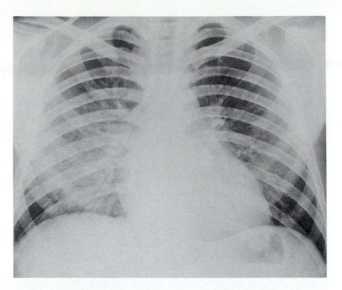

FIGURE 12-52
Goodpasture's syndrome. Homogeneous perihilar shadowing on right extends into middle and lower zones. On left note subtle ground-glass opacification in middle and lower zones. (Courtesy Professor A.N. Adam, London.)

Radiology of diffuse pulmonary hemorrhage

The radiographic changes of acute alveolar hemorrhage are the same regardless of etiology and consist of airspace consolidation. In some of the conditions under consideration, particularly primary pulmonary hemosiderosis, the bleeding tends to be recurrent over a long time, and in these cases persistent interstitial changes may develop, reflecting interstitial fibrosis. When acute bleeding is superimposed on chronic changes, a mixed alveolar and interstitial pattern is produced.

The consolidation ranges from acinar shadows (Figure 12-50)[70,698] through patchy airspace consolidation[43,698] to widespread confluent consolidation with air bronchograms (Figure 12-50).[65] At other times the consolidation is migratory[10] or ground glass.[65,70,117] The consolidation can be widespread or show a perihilar (Figure 12-52)[533] or middle to lower zone predominance[10,65] and tends to be more pronounced centrally. The costophrenic angles and apices are usually spared.[698] The consolidation clears within 2 to 3 days (Figure 12-50),[65] either completely or partially, to leave a linear or reticular pattern,[726,741] occasionally with septal (Kerley B) lines[357] or a ground-glass haziness.[65] Sometimes these two patterns are mixed.[70,726] In any event, this interstitial shadowing is also transient and clears completely 10 to 12 days after the beginning of the episode. Two cases of hilar adenopathy have been reported.[80,189] Pleural effusions are not uncommon, but most, if not all, are likely to be secondary phenomena related to infection and fluid overload.[65]

With repeated bleeding episodes, seen typically in primary pulmonary hemosiderosis, the interstitial shadowing fails to clear completely and the patient may be left with a permanent, fine reticulonodular (Figure 12-53)[701]

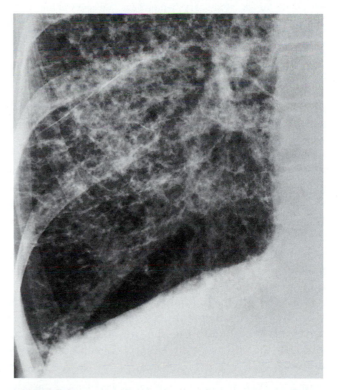

FIGURE 12-53
Primary pulmonary hemosiderosis. Localized view of right lung base. Reticulonodular shadowing with pronounced linear element of interstitial lines including septal (Kerley B) lines. Primary pulmonary hemosiderosis was diagnosed 30 years before current radiograph, and the patient had been intermittently symptomatic over intervening years. Changes are permanent and are caused largely by fibrosis.

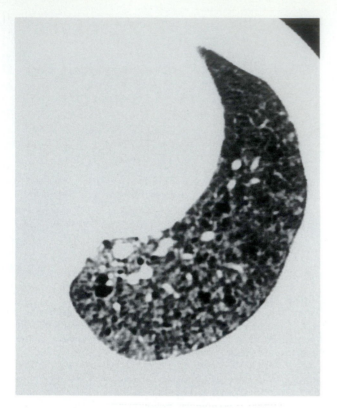

FIGURE 12-54
Idiopathic diffuse pulmonary hemorrhage, subacute phase. High-resolution computed tomogram shows widely distributed 1 to 2 mm nodules characteristic of subacute phase of pulmonary hemorrhage.

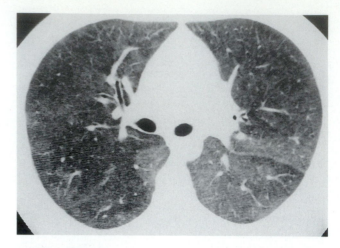

FIGURE 12-55
Idiopathic pulmonary hemosiderosis. High-resolution computed tomogram at time of presentation shows multifocal areas of ground-glass opacity, in some places sharply marginated from adjacent normal lung. Findings are characteristic of acute diffuse alveolar hemorrhage.

or nodular (2 to 3 mm) opacity[117] that tends to increase in profusion with each acute episode. New bleeding episodes superimposed on permanent shadowing give a mixed alveolar-interstitial pattern.

The radiographic changes corresponded with HRCT findings in a series of six patients scanned largely in the subacute phase of pulmonary hemorrhage. In this series the striking abnormality was multiple, 1 to 3 mm nodules (Figure 12-54) distributed in a uniform fashion, commonly with a patchy ground-glass opacity (Figure 12-55) (4 of 6 patients) and interlobular septal thickening (4 of 6 patients).[117] In the acute phase CT shows consolidation[533] or ground-glass opacity.[117]

Note that diffuse pulmonary bleeding can be present when the chest radiograph appears normal.[64,230] In one series this was found to be the case in 22% of bleeding episodes in patients with DPH of Goodpasture's syndrome.[64]

Differential diagnosis of alveolar hemorrhage

Hemoptysis, iron-deficiency anemia, and a sudden fall in the hematocrit of more than 2 g without bleeding elsewhere[65] are obvious pointers to the diagnosis of DPH. Because alveolar hemorrhage occurs distal to the muco-ciliary escalator, hemoptysis may be absent. Additionally, blood brought up on the escalator may be swallowed and produce a misleading positive stool blood test. Hemosiderin-laden macrophages in sputum, gastric washings, or alveolar lavage[199] indicate bleeding within the recent past but can also be found with pulmonary edema.[65]

Radiologic signs, unfortunately, are not particularly helpful in distinguishing between DPH and various other causes of consolidation. The interpretation of the chest radiograph is made particularly difficult by the fact that fluid overload and infection — the two major differential diagnoses — are well-recognized precipitators of DPH in Goodpasture's syndrome[65] and may coexist with hemorrhage.

The most specific and useful test for DPH in clinical practice is detection of increased carbon monoxide uptake by the blood sequestered in the lungs. This can be demonstrated by cyclotron produced $C^{15}O$,[230] or more conveniently, by the single-breath carbon monoxide uptake (Kco) test, with a 40% rise considered positive.[64]

Radionuclide scintiscans using sulfur colloid or labeled red blood cells have been used in the diagnosis[130] but have not gained wide acceptance.

Recent reports suggest that magnetic resonance findings may be relatively specific for DPH. In vitro studies with blood instilled into the lung initially demonstrate long T1 and T2 times that fall rapidly within 24 hours and thereafter remain short.[374] This finding has been confirmed in two patients, one imaged 3 days and the other an indeterminate time after bleeding in whom hemorrhage appeared as an intermediate signal on T1 and proton density images and as low signal on T2 images.[371,741]

The possibility that consolidation is the result of DPH should always be considered, particularly in the presence of hemoptysis, iron-deficient anemia, glomerulonephritis, or a systemic vasculitis. The Kco test is probably the most useful investigation to confirm or exclude the diagnosis. The chest radiograph and Kco provide the best means of monitoring progress.[64] The specific cause is usually determined by clinical assessment, serologic studies, and biopsy of the kidney or other extrapulmonary organs; lung biopsy is needed only when no extrapulmonary features are present and when anti–glomerular basement membrane antibodies are absent.[448]

EOSINOPHILIC LUNG DISEASE

The term "pulmonary eosinophilia" was introduced in 1952 to describe a group of diseases "in which pulmonary infiltration on the radiograph is accompanied by blood eosinophilia but in which pneumonia, hydatid disease of the lung, Hodgkin's disease, and sarcoidosis can be excluded."[155] Later authors widened this concept,[127] using the term "eosinophilic lung disease" to include all disorders associated with blood and/or tissue eosinophilia that affect major airways and lung parenchyma.[260] Note that a blood eosinophilia is not necessary to make a diagnosis of eosinophilic lung disease. The widely used term "pulmonary infiltration with eosinophilia" (PIE) is synonymous with the term "pulmonary eosinophilia."

Eosinophils are granulocytes that develop in the bone marrow and are carried in the blood to those epithelia that are exposed to the external environment, particularly the respiratory, gastrointestinal, and genitourinary mucosa. Only one eosinophil is in the blood compartment for every 100 in the marrow and in the tissues, and therefore not surprisingly eosinophilic tissue lesions are not necessarily accompanied by blood eosinophilia.[663] Blood eosinophil counts normally vary between 0.05 and 0.35×10^9/L and show diurnal variation, with counts high in the night and low in the morning.[275] Eosinophilia is generally taken to mean an eosinophil count of more than 0.4×10^9/L, although some set the level at 0.5×10^9/L. Eosinophils contain a range of enzymes that account for their ability to damage parasitic worms and cells including those of humans, and to modulate mast cell–dependent reactions such as immediate hypersensitivity.

Various classifications of eosinophilic lung states have been proposed,* but none has proved entirely satisfactory. The classification used here (see box at right) is based on that of Schatz and co-workers.[663] The conditions considered in detail in the text are only those in which tissue or blood eosinophilia is a major feature. The possible causes in a patient under investigation can usually be significantly reduced by taking into account a few key historical, clinical, and laboratory findings, notably work exposure, ethnic background, travel in endemic areas, and a history of asthma, atopy, and any medication. Useful information from first-line investigations include the magnitude of blood eosinophilia, skin

---

*References 127, 155, 275, 309, 462, 583, 663, 705.

CLASSIFICATION OF EOSINOPHILIC LUNG DISEASE

Pulmonary conditions in which tissue and blood eosinophilia are pathogenically important
  Asthma
  Cryptogenic eosinophilic lung
    Acute eosinophilic pneumonia (Löffler's syndrome)
    Chronic eosinophilic pneumonia
  Allergic bronchopulmonary aspergillosis
  Drug-induced disease
  Parasitic disease
    Tropical pulmonary eosinophilia
    Other worms
  Vasculitic and granulomatous disease
    Churg-Strauss syndrome
    Bronchocentric granulomatosis
  Hypereosinophilic syndrome
  Hyperimmunoglobulin E syndrome
Pulmonary conditions with occasional, or minor, tissue, or blood eosinophilia
  Infections
    Bacterial (*Brucella, Mycobacterium*)
    Chlamydia
    Viral (adenovirus)
    Protozoal (*Pneumocystis*)
    Fungal (*Coccidioides, Histoplasma*)
  Neoplasms[437]
    Bronchogenic carcinoma,[344] bronchial carcinoid
    Metastases
    Irradiated neoplasms
    Lymphoma (Hodgkin's and non-Hodgkin's, lymphomatoid granulomatosis)
  "Immunologic" conditions
    Wegener's granulomatosis
    Rheumatoid disease
    Extrinsic allergic alveolitis
    Sarcoidosis
  Miscellaneous
    Hemodialysis[527]
Pulmonary conditions with coincidental blood eosinophilia

Data from Schatz M, Wasserman S, Patterson R: *Arch Intern Med* 142:1515-1519, 1982.

---

sensitivity, total serum IgE, serum *Aspergillus* precipitins, and stool examination for cysts, ova, and parasites.

Asthma

Patients with asthma often have a mild to moderate eosinophilia.[474] The radiology of asthma is discussed elsewhere (p. 842). In addition, asthma is often a prominent symptom in a number of specific eosinophilic lung states such as allergic bronchopulmonary aspergillosis and the Churg-Strauss syndrome.

Cryptogenic eosinophilic pneumonia

Cryptogenic eosinophilic pneumonia is commonly and usefully divided into two subgroups: acute (Löffler's syndrome) or chronic, depending on whether the condition lasts more or less than 1 month.[155] The 1 month dividing line is arbitrary and not universally applied, so that the acute or chronic distinction is not always clear, particularly since steroids have been used for treatment. However, the division is useful clinically, since the majority of chronic cryptogenic eosinophilic pneumonias form a relatively homogeneous group.

ACUTE EOSINOPHILIC PNEUMONIA. Synonyms for acute eosinophilic pneumonia include simple pulmonary eosinophilia and Löffler's syndrome.[471] The characteristic features of the syndrome are blood eosinophilia, absence of or mild symptoms and signs (cough, fever, dyspnea), one or more nonsegmental pulmonary consolidations that are transitory or migratory, and spontaneous clearing of consolidations. Originally opacities were described as disappearing within 6 to 12 days,[471] but this interval is now generally extended to a month.[155]

Löffler's syndrome may be idiopathic (cryptogenic) or may result from a variety of inciting agents, particularly drugs (p. 535), parasites (pp. 536 to 538), and miscellaneous agents such as nickel carbonyl.[725]

On pathologic study, eosinophilic pneumonia shows edema and an eosinophilic infiltrate in both alveoli and interstitium. The radiographic finding is one or more fairly homogeneous, nonsegmental consolidations that can be small or so large as to occupy much of a lobe. They are transitory and may disappear from one area while appearing in another. They have a tendency to be peripherally located. Pleural effusions, mediastinal adenopathy, and cavitation are not described.

Recently there have been a number of reports of acute eosinophilic pneumonia differing from Löffler's syndrome in that the patients have been significantly symptomatic and in respiratory failure. Eosinophilia is prominent on bronchoalveolar lavage but usually absent in the peripheral blood. Radiologic studies show bilateral alveolar opacities but in addition unspecified interstitial opacity, including septal lines in one patient and small pleural effusions in others.[12,27] The cause in these patients is obscure, but they have responded rapidly to steroids.

CHRONIC EOSINOPHILIC PNEUMONIA. Chronic eosinophilic pneumonia (CEP) is a cryptogenic form of eosinophilic lung disease with consistent and characteristic clinicopathologic features. Pathologically, eosinophil-rich exudate is evident in alveoli and interstitium.[103,760] Angiitis is mild, fibrosis sparse, and necrosis very rare.[103]

Since the condition was first identified in 1969,[103] several series have been published.* The disease often develops in middle life, but prevalence remains high from the third to seventh decades,[401] with a range of 7 to 77

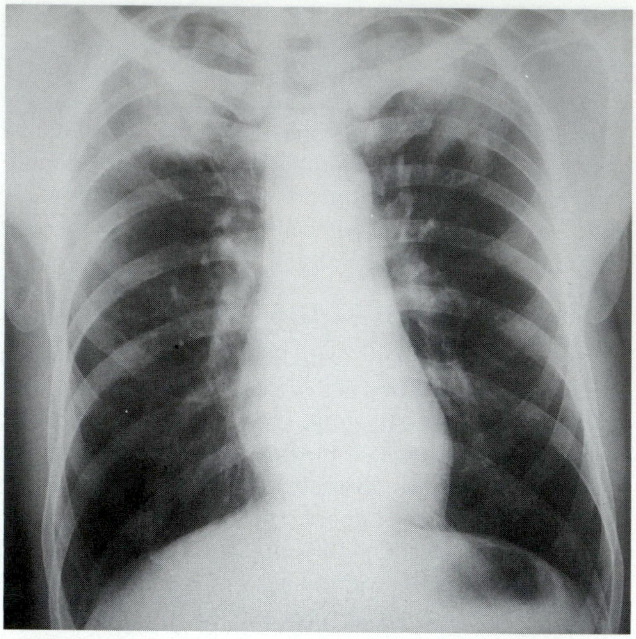

---

*References 255, 268, 401, 462, 498, 760.

FIGURE 12-56
Chronic eosinophilic pneumonia. Chest radiograph is of 52-year-old man who when first examined had 2-month fever, weight loss, and cough. He had blood eosinophilia (2×10^9/L) and had had nasal polypectomies in the past. Radiographic findings of bilateral apical consolidation coupled with history was considered very suggestive of tuberculosis, and patient was inappropriately treated for 1 month despite lack of firm evidence.

years. Women outnumber men by 2 to 1.[401] Fifty percent of patients are atopic, 40% are asthmatic, and 5% to 10% have allergic rhinitis and nasal polyps.[401] Asthma can antedate the condition by many years[462] or can develop with the onset of CEP. The symptoms are often highly characteristic and range from mild to severe. Typical symptoms are dyspnea; cough with mucoid sputum; wheeze; malaise; marked weight loss (8 to 12 kg); high fever, particularly in the evenings; and drenching night sweats. Occasional symptoms include chest pain and hemoptysis. Not surprisingly therefore patients are often believed initially to have tuberculosis, an impression that may be reinforced by the chest radiograph. Blood eosinophilia is common, but not universal, occurring in nearly 90% of patients[401] and ranging from mild to marked.[760] Sputum eosinophilia occurs in less than 50% of patients.[401] Total white blood cell count and the ESR are raised. Serum IgE, which is normal or only minimally elevated,[760] is a particularly helpful finding, allowing distinction from such conditions as allergic bronchopulmonary aspergillosis and tropical and parasitic pulmonary eosinophilias, in which serum IgE levels are significantly elevated. However, in a number of recent reports IgE levels have been significantly raised.[295]

Many patients with chronic eosinophilic pneumonia have a characteristic radiologic pattern that is virtually

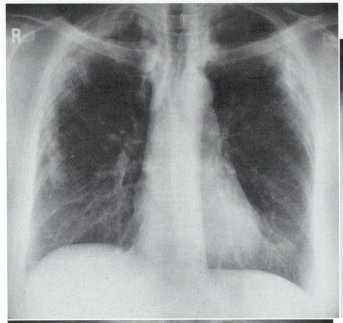

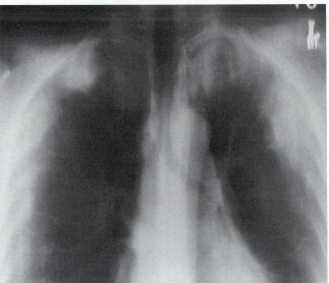

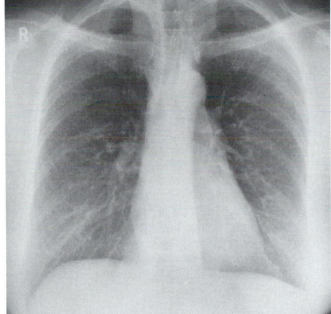

FIGURE 12-57

Chronic eosinophilic pneumonia (CEP). Radiographs are of 65-year-old woman with 1-month fever, night sweats, cough, and weight loss. Patient did not have asthma but had blood eosinophilia (1.6 × 10⁹/L). **A,** Posteroanterior radiograph shows bilateral, confluent, peripheral shadowing that lines chest wall in middle and upper zones. It is consistent with nonsegmental consolidation. **B,** Anteroposterior tomogram confirms peripheral distribution of shadowing, which is characteristic of CEP. **C,** Radiograph 2 weeks after **A** shows complete resolution following steroid therapy.

pathognomonic. At its most classic the pattern seen in two thirds of patients[401] consists of peripheral, nonsegmental, homogeneous consolidations sometimes with an air bronchogram (Figures 12-56 and 12-57).[562] These opacities lie against the chest wall and may surround the lung or occupy just one or two zones. In one series the zonal distribution was 46% upper, 40% middle, and 14% lower.[498] About 50% of patients have bilateral shadowing that may cloak the upper and outer aspects of the lung in a characteristic fashion.[155,268] Opacities may appear in one lung to be followed by others on the opposite side, or they may disappear spontaneously. They are rarely truly migratory, usually coming and going in the same place. Although this last feature has been stressed as a charac-

teristic finding,[268,498] it is not unique and is also a feature of allergic bronchopulmonary aspergillosis. Some 30% of patients with CEP do not show the classic peripheral pattern described here (Figure 12-58).[255,268,498,760] The consolidations may even be perihilar in distribution.[498] A common pattern is mixed peripheral and central consolidations (Figure 12-59)[498] that may even progress to opacify one lung totally.[760] Isolated lesions in the upper zone may closely mimic those of tuberculosis. Other features that are occasionally seen include pleural effusions (2% to 4%),[107] cavitation (5%),[401] and the occasional case of mediastinal lymphadenopathy best appreciated on CT.[121,494,562,817]

Limited CT studies confirm the chest radiographic findings (Figure 12-60), showing strikingly peripheral, multifocal consolidations with a few areas of subsegmental and focal consolidation.[494] Sometimes the consolidation is platelike and parallel to the chest wall but inset and may even cross fissures.[562]

The disease occasionally remits spontaneously[268]; however, treatment is usually required. CEP is remarkably sensitive to steroid therapy. Rapid clearing is usually seen within a few days, considerable resolution in about

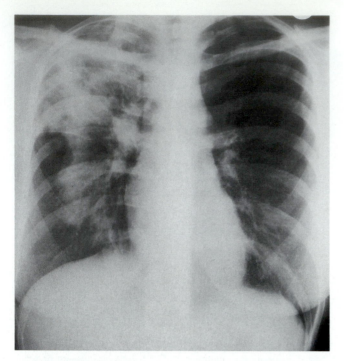

FIGURE 12-58
Chronic eosinophilic pneumonia. A 35-year-old woman with 6-week history of cough, fever, and 3 kg weight loss. Extensive right-sided consolidation is present. Unilateral distribution is less common than bilateral but well recognized. Zonal distribution is characteristic as is bandlike consolidation lying parallel to chest wall in midzone.

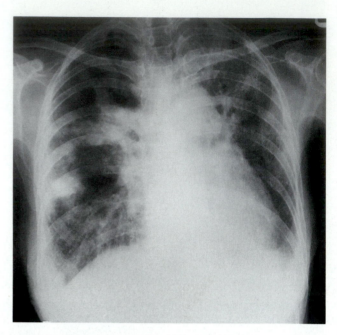

FIGURE 12-59
Chronic eosinophilic pneumonia (CEP). Radiograph shows mixed peripheral and central, multifocal consolidation. This is recognized pattern but less common than one shown in Figure 12-57. Both costophrenic angles are blunted in this patient. On right, blunting is almost certainly result of peripheral consolidation, but on left a small pleural effusion cannot be excluded. Pleural effusions are very unusual in CEP.

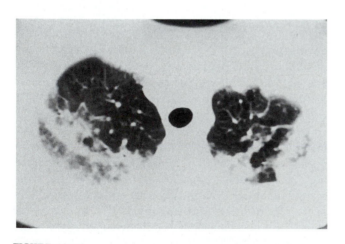

FIGURE 12-60
Chronic eosinophilic pneumonia. A 23-year-old woman was seen in emergency department 6 days before with findings thought to be consistent with infective pneumonia. Chest radiograph was similar to that of patient in Figure 12-57, and computed tomography confirmed peripheral and apical nature of consolidation.

a week, and complete clearing by 1 month.[103] In fact some authors recommend a therapeutic trial of steroids in previously well patients with classic clinicoradiologic features.[401] Resolution is usually complete but may occur by way of unusual and highly characteristic bandlike shadows, parallel to the chest wall (Figure 12-61).[268,401] Relapse is common; in a review of 62 patients 21% relapsed during reduction of steroid dose and 58% after discontinuation.[401] The majority of patients need long-term low-dose steroids,[543] and late-onset asthma develops in a proportion.[268] In rare instances patients who initially have all the features of CEP go on to develop a diffuse vasculitis.[131,268]

Allergic bronchopulmonary aspergillosis

Allergic bronchopulmonary aspergillosis (ABPA) is almost certainly the most common cause of eosinophilic lung disease in developed countries. It accounted for 78% of the patients in a series of 143 in the United Kingdom who were admitted to a tertiary referral center with a diagnosis of pulmonary eosinophilia.[497] First described in 1952,[362] the disease is characterized by asthma, radiographic pulmonary shadows, blood eosinophilia, and evidence of allergy to antigens of *Aspergillus* species. Its importance lies in the fact that recurrent acute episodes cause progressive lung damage that can be controlled by steroid administration.[646]

In ABPA a hypersensitivity reaction develops to *Aspergillus* species that grow as a mycelial plug in proximal airways, usually the second- or third-order bronchi.[277] Tissue invasion is either absent[288] or very limited.[313] The

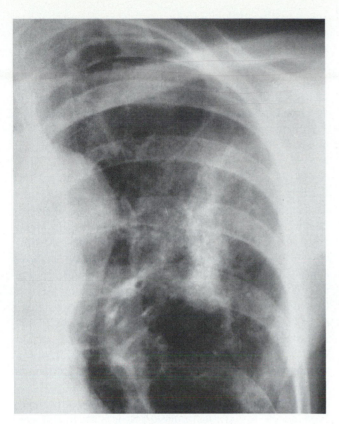

FIGURE 12-61
Chronic eosinophilic pneumonia (CEP). Local view of left middle and upper zone. Partial resolution of classic peripheral consolidation has resulted in band opacity parallel to chest wall. Such a finding on an interval chest radiograph is highly suggestive of CEP.

factors that favor the initial airway colonization by *Aspergillus* are unclear[288] but are probably related in some way to the almost universal presence of asthma and atopy in affected patients. Certainly, once the fungus gains a foothold, local damage will promote further colonization. *Aspergillus* fungi are worldwide in distribution and ubiquitous. In more than 90% of patients the species involved is *Aspergillus fumigatus*, but occasionally other species are implicated, including *A. flavus, A. niger, A. nidulans*,[288] *A. terreus*,[441] *A. oryzae*,[8] and *A. ochraceus*.[552] In addition, there are isolated case reports of an ABPA-like syndrome caused by fungi other than *Aspergillus* spp., including *Candida albicans*[7] and at least six other genera.[744]

Patients characteristically have evidence of both a type I and a type III Gell and Coombs immune reaction,[638] possibly an element of a type IV reaction, and complement activation.[312] The type I reaction is manifest by bronchospasm and is associated with blood eosinophilia and IgE production that results in high specific and nonspecific serum levels. The type III reaction causes tissue damage leading to pulmonary shadowing and is associated with serum precipitins (IgG). Because antigen production is localized to the mycelial plug in the proximal airway, tissue damage tends to be greatest in this region, giving rise to the characteristic proximal bronchiectasis.

Typically ABPA occurs in atopic patients with long-standing asthma. A few patients have been predisposed by cystic fibrosis,[446] and in some, particularly older ones, asthma develops concurrently with the first attack of ABPA.[497] Although unusual, the disease is well recognized in nonasthmatics.[286,497] Overall the condition has a slight female preponderance.[277,350,497,588] It may occur at any age, but 20 to 40 years is typical. However, it may develop into the sixties,[481,588] and at the other extreme cases are described in children less than 2 years old.[386] The length of the interval between the onset of asthma and ABPA is inversely related to the age at onset of asthma. McCarthy and co-workers found that with asthma beginning before 10 years of age the average gap was 24 years, but with late-onset asthma (30 years of age or more) the mean gap was only 3.5 years.[499] Late-onset asthma was associated with more frequent attacks of ABPA and greater lung damage.[499]

ABPA runs a relapsing and remitting course. Acute attacks are characterized by wheeze, dyspnea, and a cough that is often productive and associated with minor hemoptysis. Systemic symptoms such as fever, malaise, and weight loss are common. About 50% of patients have pleuritic pain, and about the same percentage give a history of coughing up sputum plugs.[497] These contain fungal mycelia and are important pointers to the diagnosis.[497] Plugs are about 1 to 2 cm long, firm, friable, and pelletlike.[497] An abnormal chest radiograph, blood eosinophilia, and an immediate skin reaction to *Aspergillus* antigens are characteristic of the acute phase. Eosinophilia is usually mild to moderate, with 74% of patients having eosinophil counts between 1 and 3 × 10⁹/L.[497] The eosinophil level may be depressed by steroid treatment. Serum precipitins against *Aspergillus* antigens are detected in 90% to 100% of patients in the acute phase, particularly if the serum is concentrated.[350,497,638] However, this test is nonspecific in that up to 25% of patients with extrinsic asthma have a positive precipitin test.[364] Both nonspecific and *Aspergillus* antigen-specific IgE are greatly raised, perhaps 20 times normal.[638] As with the finding of precipitins, elevation of IgE per se is not diagnostic of ABPA and increases that are usually smaller may be found in simple asthma.

Criteria for the diagnosis of ABPA vary from study to study. They have changed with time as knowledge about the disease has become more sophisticated; even now no universally accepted diagnostic criteria are available. Rosenberg and co-workers[638] have set out the following major and minor criteria and suggest that if the first six of the major criteria are satisfied, the diagnosis of ABPA can be made with reasonable certainty. The presence of central bronchiectasis makes the diagnosis certain.[638]

Table 12-1   Radiographic findings in allergic bronchopulmonary aspergillosis (% = prevalence of finding)

Major	Minor
Acute (transient)	
Consolidation (80%)	Parallel line shadows
Mucoid impaction (bronchocele) (30%)	Ring shadows
Atelectasis (20%)	Small nodules
	Pleural effusion
Chronic (permanent)	
Overinflation (50%)	Pleural thickening
Tubular shadows (75%)	Mycetoma
Ring shadows (60%)	Small nodules
Vascular deficiency (30%)	Line shadows
Labor shrinkage (40%)	

Greenberger[311] recommends in addition measuring *A. fumigatus*–specific IgE or IgA to make the diagnosis more certain in patients without bronchiectasis.

Major criteria for ABPA are (1) asthma, (2) blood eosinophilia, (3) immediate skin reactivity to *Aspergillus* antigen, (4) precipitin antibodies to *Aspergillus* antigen, (5) raised serum IgE, (6) history of radiographic pulmonary opacities, and (7) central bronchiectasis. Minor criteria for ABPA include *A. fumigatus* in sputum, history of expectorating brown plugs, and late skin reactivity to *Aspergillus* antigen.

A great variety of radiologic changes are found in ABPA.* Consideration of the underlying disease processes makes the bewildering range of radiologic findings easier to understand and remember. In the acute stage mycelial plugging occurs in segmental airways and an intense local inflammatory response leads to bronchial wall thickening. Airway obstruction variously causes distal collapse, a mucoid impaction pattern, or consolidation. Judging by clinical features and response to treatment, secondary infection is probably an important aspect of some consolidations.[350] In the chronic phase, plugs have disappeared, leaving damaged and bronchiectatic airways, while the more distal changes have healed, often with a major fibrotic element.

The radiologic changes are best considered either acute and transient or chronic and permanent (Table 12-1).[499]

Transient changes are listed in Table 12-1. Despite some discrepancies between series, no doubt consolidations are the most common type of opacity (Figures 12-62 and 12-63). They range from massive and homogeneous (occupying a whole lobe), to smaller and subsegmental, to even smaller (in the order of 1 cm). The smaller shadows are more common. Consolidations show little if

*References 277, 292, 350, 468, 481, 499, 522, 588, 819.

any zonal predilection and are often multiple. Larger shadows are often triangular, pointing to the hilum with a segmental or lobar configuration, as might be expected of a process based on airway obstruction (Figure 12-62). This appearance contrasts with the nonsegmental consolidations seen in other eosinophilic states. Cavitation is described in the larger consolidations; the frequency was 3% in one series[588] but a surprising 14% and 21% in others.[277,499] The cause of cavitation is largely speculative. In some cases it is undoubtedly caused by bronchiectasis, and in others it may be secondary to cavitary bacterial infection. Although consolidations are regarded as transient, they can last 6 weeks or more. Recently Phelan and Kerr[588] described some patients with apparently permanent consolidation. When consolidations clear, they often leave residual ring and line shadows consistent with bronchiectasis. Such bronchiectasis creates favorable conditions for fungal recolonization, a finding that explains why 25% to 50% of consolidations recur later in the same area. It is notable that 20% to 30% of patients with radiographic consolidation are asymptomatic,[481,646] and ABPA is one of those conditions in which gross radiographic changes may be accompanied by minor symptoms.[499]

The second most common acute change is probably bronchocele formation (mucoid impaction). In this condition an airway becomes obstructed and distended by retained secretions. At the same time the subtended lung remains aerated by collateral air drift, allowing visualization of the impacted airway, which contrasts with the surrounding air-containing lung. Bronchoceles take on a wide variety of shapes depending on the extent and degree of airway filling. The basic opacity is a linear, sharply demarcated, branched or unbranched, bandlike shadow that points to the hilum (Figure 12-64), the so-called toothpaste shadow, which is a band about 2 to 3 cm long and 5 to 8 mm wide. Variants include V-shaped, inverted V-shaped, and Y-shaped opacities. Sometimes bronchoceles are more rounded than linear and simulate a mass (if single) or a cluster of masses (if multiple, the "bunch of grapes" pattern). Similarly rounded opacities are produced by linear bronchoceles seen end on. Impacted airways are usually proximal (typically segmental). They are often inseparable from the hilum and may simulate lymphadenopathy[522] or a mass. Another variant is produced by distal bronchiectatic airways that, when impacted, give a band shadow with a club-shaped end, the so-called gloved finger shadow. Bronchoceles show a strong upper zone predilection (Figure 12-65).[481] They disappear once their contents have been coughed up, leaving ring or parallel line shadows (Figure 12-66). Like consolidations in ABPA they may recur at the same site. Occasionally they persist for many months; they are recorded as remaining for at least 18 months.

The third major acute manifestation of ABPA is atelectasis (Figure 12-67), which ranges in frequency from 3%[481] to 46%.[277] It may be subsegmental, segmental, or

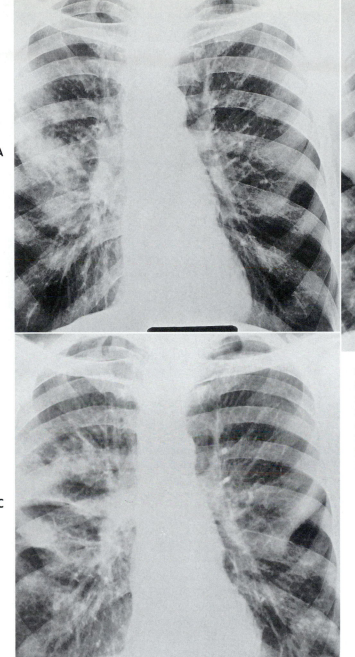

A

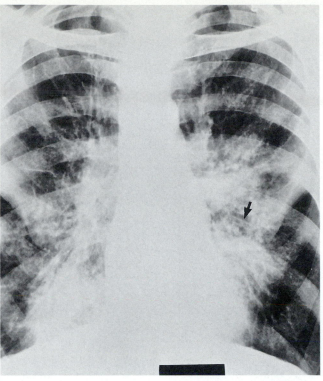

B

C

FIGURE 12-62
Consolidation in allergic bronchopulmonary aspergillosis. Three radiographs (**A to C**) taken at approximately yearly intervals show recurring, multifocal bilateral consolidations. A number of opacities suggest segmental/subsegmental consolidation. Some of the opacities contain air bronchograms. Remote from consolidations are parallel and single line shadows consistent with bronchial wall thickening (*arrow* in **B**).

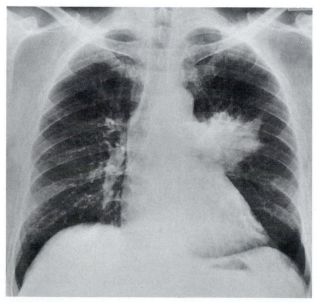

FIGURE 12-63
Consolidation in allergic bronchopulmonary aspergillosis simulating mass lesion.

lobar or even affect a whole lung.[48,468,588] Collapse is of course a complication of asthma per se.[370] Like consolidations and mucoid impaction, collapse has a tendency to recur in the same area.

A variety of less important acute opacities have been described. One is parallel line shadows from bronchial wall thickening, presumably from inflammation and edema (Figure 12-62). McCarthy and co-workers[499] distinguish between two types of parallel line shadows: tubular opacities, in which the walls are inappropriately wide apart, consistent with bronchiectasis, and tram-line

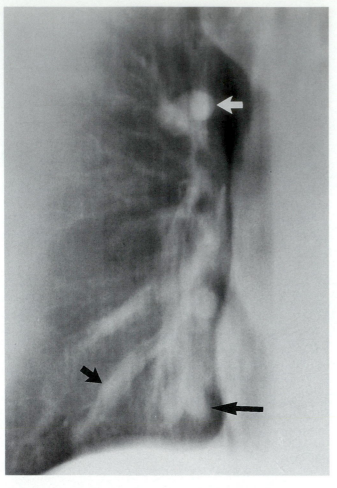

FIGURE 12-64
Bronchocele in allergic bronchopulmonary aspergillosis. Whole-lung tomogram demonstrates variety of shapes adopted by bronchoceles. Most common is bandlike opacity pointing to hilum — toothpaste shadow *(short black arrow)*. Other variants include Y-shaped *(long black arrow)* and rounded opacities *(white arrow)*. It is unusual to find so many bronchoceles in allergic aspergillosis, and their lower zone predominance is also unusual.

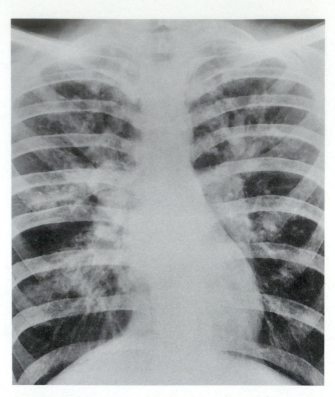

FIGURE 12-65
Bronchoceles in allergic bronchopulmonary aspergillosis. Bronchoceles are in the middle and upper zones, more typical distribution than that shown in Figure 12-64. In left upper zone are several fingerlike bronchoceles; a number on right are clustered and rounded, overlying hilum and giving it a lobulated appearance.

opacities, in which wall separation is consistent with a normal airway caliber. Parallel line shadows are most commonly seen in patients less than 15 years old, an age group in which asthma alone may be associated with such changes. Occasionally, thick-walled ring shadows (walls 3 to 5 mm wide, rings 2 to 3 cm diameter) are seen divorced from consolidation.[499] Their pathologic basis is obscure. Small, ill-defined, rounded or irregular opacities (miliary opacities) are described as both transient and permanent shadows. They may represent granulomas formed as a result of an extrinsic allergic alveolitis. Pleural effusion has been noted in a few reports.[481,536]

Permanent changes (Table 12-1) are important because they indicate irreversible lung damage and may be the only clues that an asthmatic person has ABPA when in remission. Before a discussion of permanent changes, bronchographic findings should be considered. Although bronchographic studies are no longer performed, findings from such studies are informative and clarify chest radiographic appearances. A majority of patients with ABPA have abnormal bronchograms[499,522,638] with some exceptions.[320] Findings consist of nonspecific cylindrical and cystic bronchiectasis together with a highly characteristic proximal bronchiectasis affecting lobar and first- and second-order segmental bronchi (Figure 12-68). Beyond the proximal bronchiectasis more distal airways remain normal and patent and are not affected by bronchiolitis obliterans. The latter is a common finding in other forms of bronchiectasis.[638] Most authors consider proximal bronchiectasis to be highly specific for ABPA,[509] but its sensitivity in early cases is open to question,[165] and Greenberger, using sophisticated serologic tests to diagnose ABPA in 531 patients with asthma, found nearly equal numbers with and without central bronchiectasis.[311] CT has replaced bronchography in the assessment of bronchiectasis, and findings in ABPA consist principally of proximal and nonproximal bronchiectasis and bronchial wall thickening (Figure 12-69).[165,544] In one study about 50% of predominantly upper bronchiectatic lobes showed a characteristic proximal pattern of bronchiectasis.[165] There is a single case report of high-attenuation mucus plugs in bronchiectatic airways on

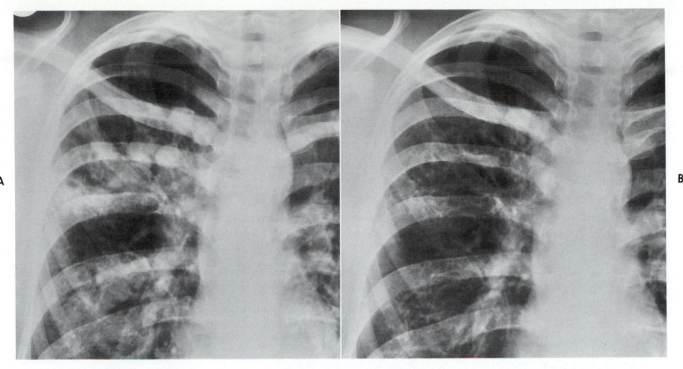

FIGURE 12-66
Bronchoceles in allergic bronchopulmonary aspergillosis. **A,** Local view of right upper and middle zones shows multiple rounded bronchoceles. **B,** When these clear, they leave collection of delicate curvilinear and ring opacities, which are walls of bronchiectatic airways. Such opacities close to hilum in middle and upper zones are a characteristic interval finding in allergic aspergillosis.

enhanced CT in a patient with acute ABPA.[307]

Persistent radiologic changes are a direct or indirect result of bronchiectasis. Abnormally dilated airways may be seen, particularly in perihilar regions and upper zones, as tubular and ring shadows (Figure 12-66). Tubular shadows are parallel line shadows in which the lines, representing bronchial walls, are more widely separated than would be expected for airways of normal caliber, implying that they must be bronchiectatic. They are bilateral and more common in the upper zone. When filled with secretions, the dilated airways produce bronchoceles, and the transformation of bronchoceles into tubular shadows and back again is common on serial radiographs. Frequently only small segments of one wall of an airway are seen, giving rise to single-line opacities rather than tubular shadows. Thin-walled ring shadows 1 to 2 cm in diameter commonly represent bronchiectatic airways seen end on, although some represent bullae or another form of abnormal airspace. When filled wholly or in part with secretions, end-on bronchiectatic airways appear as nodules or ring shadows with air-fluid levels. Occasionally aggregations of ring shadows between 0.5 and 1 cm in diameter appear as honeycombing.

Bronchiectatic airways are also detected by their secondary effects. The reduced ventilation of lung distal to bronchiectasis is reflected in a reduction in vascularity.

Parenchymal scarring commonly follows bronchiectasis and is manifest as line shadows and lobar shrinkage (Figure 12-70). Mirroring the distribution of bronchiectasis, these features have a strong upper zone predilection, with 78% so distributed in one series.[499] Such lobar shrinkage is accompanied by a variety of ring and linear opacities. Lower lobe shrinkage, although described, is unusual.[588] Although chronic lobar shrinkage is seen often, the overall lung volume is frequently increased, reflecting airflow limitation, emphysema, and bulla formation. Between 30% and 40% of patients in one series showed overinflation.[588] Pleural thickening is not a major feature, having a prevalence of 18% in the same series.

Mycetomas may form in the bronchiectatic cavities. In one series of 111 patients with ABPA, eight had mycetomas, predominantly midzonal.[499] Since midzone mycetomas are unusual in other conditions, workers have suggested that a mycetoma found in this position should raise the possibility of underlying ABPA.[499] Patients with ABPA and mycetoma might be expected to be particularly symptomatic because of their immune status coupled with massive antigen production, but this does not appear to be so. However, an ABPA type of syndrome has been recorded as resulting from a mycetoma lodged in a tuberculous cavity.[212]

In summary, a chest radiograph of an asthmatic patient

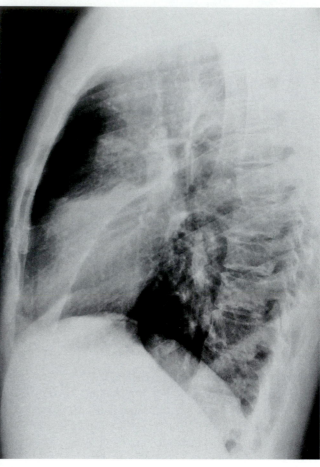

FIGURE 12-67
Atelectasis in allergic bronchopulmonary aspergillosis. **A** and **B**, Patient presented with lingular consolidation associated with minor volume loss, and then went on to develop complete collapse of upper lobe (**C**).

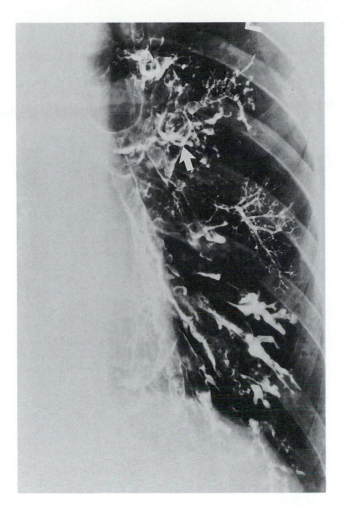

FIGURE 12-68
Bronchiectasis in allergic bronchopulmonary aspergillosis. In left lower zone bronchogram shows nonspecific cylindrical bronchiectasis. In left upper zone, however, is proximal cystic bronchiectasis *(arrow)* with preserved distal branches. This is highly characteristic finding in allergic bronchopulmonary aspergillosis.

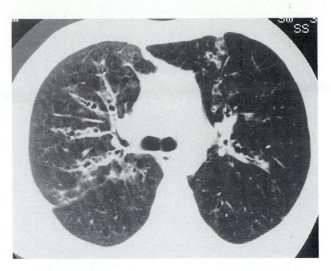

FIGURE 12-69
Allergic bronchopulmonary aspergillosis. Computed tomography at level of carina shows varicose bronchiectasis affecting segmental and subsegmental airways. Absence of more distal bronchiectasis is characteristic.

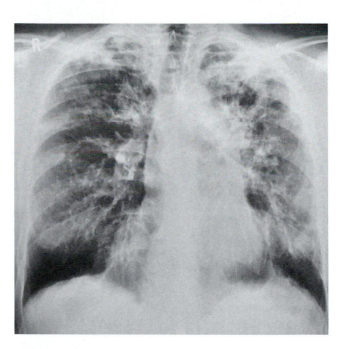

FIGURE 12-70
Fibrosis in allergic bronchopulmonary aspergillosis (ABPA). Bilateral middle and upper zone fibrosis following multiple acute attacks of ABPA. Upper zone shadowing is complex mixture of linear, ring, nodular, and conglomerate opacities, reflecting diverse underlying pathologic condition including bronchiectasis, scarring, and bulla formation.

showing consolidation, collapse, upper zone fibrosis, or, particularly, mucoid impaction should prompt consideration of ABPA, as should the more subtle changes of perihilar and upper zone bronchiectasis.

Drug-induced eosinophilic lung disease

A large number of drugs can produce pulmonary opacities together with blood eosinophilia; these are listed in the box on p. 536. In some patients an associated rash and pyrexia develop. These can provide a helpful clue to the nature of the radiologic shadowing. A variety of chest radiographic patterns are produced:

1. Airspace consolidation (Figure 12-71), which may be localized or diffuse. In some instances the pattern is that of Löffler's syndrome. Drugs that are particularly associated with a consolidative pattern include penicillin, sulfonamides, paraaminosalicylic acid, chlorpropamide, nitrofurantoin, methotrexate, carbamazepine, mephenesin, imipramine, trimipramine, and hydrochlorothiazide.

2. Hilar lymphadenopathy. This is recorded with the antiepileptic drugs phenytoin and trimethadione.[532]

3. Pleural effusions. These are occasionally seen with nitrofurantoin (see Chapter 15).

DRUGS ASSOCIATED WITH EOSINOPHILIC LUNG DISEASE

ANTIBIOTICS

Ampicillin[144]
Capreomycin[705]
Isoniazid[144,705]
Nitrofurantoin[144,532,663,705]
Paraaminosalicylic acid[144,532,663,705]
Penicillin[144,532,663,705]
Rifampicin[705]
Sulfonamides[144,532,663,705]
Tetracycline[663]
Pyrimethamine[38]

ANALGESICS AND ANTIINFLAMMATORY DRUGS

Aspirin[663,705]
Gold[532]
Naproxen[539]
Ibuprofen[299]

CYTOTOXICS

Azathioprine[143]
Bleomycin[143,705]
Methotrexate[143,532,663,705]
Procarbazine[143]

SULFONYLUREAS

Chlorpropamide[144,532,663]
Tolazamide[60]
Tolbutamide[705]

NEUROPSYCHIATRIC DRUGS

Carbamazepine[144,162,663,705]
Chlorpromazine[663]
Dantrolene[144]
Imipramine[144,663]
Mephenesin[144,663,705]
Phenytoin[144]
Trimethadione[532]

MISCELLANEOUS DRUGS

Beclomethasone[663]
Clofibrate[352]
Cromoglycate[663]
Cocaine[556]
Hydralazine[144]
Methylphenidate[144,663]
Penicillamine[171]
L-Tryptophan

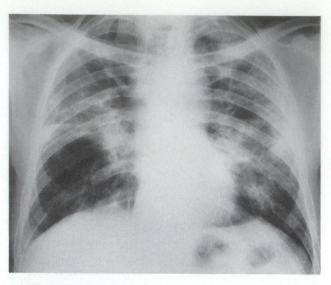

FIGURE 12-71
Drug-related eosinophilic lung disease. Multifocal nonsegmental consolidations in 66-year-old man who developed a nonproductive cough and dyspnea after starting nonsteroidal antiinflammatory drug (naproxen). There was blood eosinophilia (6.4 × 10^9/L). Opacities cleared after naproxen was discontinued and systemic steroids were begun. (Courtesy Dr. J.D. Stevenson, Poole, Dorset, U.K.)

5. Other patterns. Patterns other than those described and that are not easy to classify are recorded with a number of drugs such as penicillamine.[171]

A distinctive syndrome associated with L-tryptophan ingestion has recently been described (L-tryptophan eosinophilia myalgia syndrome). Principal features include peripheral eosinophilia, myopathy, peripheral neuropathy, eosinophilic fasciitis, and respiratory disorder. The respiratory changes are characterized radiologically as bilateral, often basally predominant opacity with mixed alveolar and interstitial features, and pleural effusions.[420,721,733] Chronic interstitial pneumonitis, tissue eosinophilia, and vasculitis are evident.[733]

Tropical pulmonary eosinophilia

Tropical pulmonary eosinophilia is a specific systemic disease caused by hypersensitivity to microfilariae, the early larval forms of various filarial nematodes, the most important of which are *Brugia malayi* and *Wuchereria bancrofti*.[566,765] Tropical pulmonary eosinophilia is found in all parts of the world where filariasis is endemic, particularly the Indian subcontinent, Southeast Asia, the South Pacific, North Africa, and South America. It occurs chiefly in the indigenous residents (particularly in the Indian subcontinent)[194,356] and is rare in visitors unless they have resided in the area for many months.[546] In nonendemic areas the disease is seen in immigrants and, because of persistence of the parasite in the host, may develop as long as 3 years after he or she returns from an endemic area.[166] Occurrence is extremely rare in whites.[424]

4. Reticulonodular shadowing. A fibrosing alveolitis type of pattern is produced in particular by nitrofurantoin and methotrexate (see Chapter 11). With nitrofurantoin the chronic interstitial pattern is associated with a blood eosinophilia in about 40% of patients.[144] Other drugs that produce an interstitial pattern include gold[532] and clofibrate.[352]

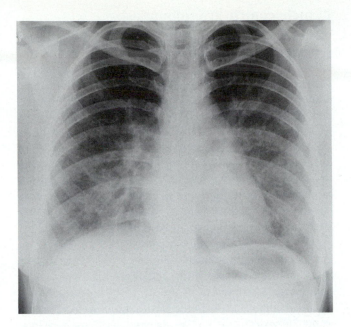

FIGURE 12-72
Tropical pulmonary eosinophilia. Chest radiograph in 32-year-old patient living in United Kingdom who was ethnically Indian and who had returned 4 months before from extended visit to South India. Initial symptoms were cough, wheezing, and systemic upset. Changes are in middle and lower zone and consist of fine linear opacities with haziness and blurring of vessels and in parts a ground-glass appearance.

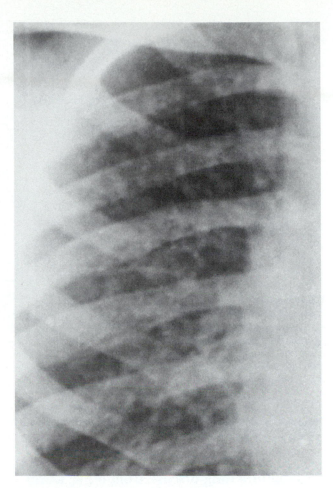

FIGURE 12-73
Tropical pulmonary eosinophilia. Principal finding in this patient was 2 to 3 mm nodulation distributed throughout lungs but more marked on right side. (Courtesy Professor C.J.F. Spry, London.)

The disease is more common in males, in some series by as much as 4:1,[706] but this is not a universal finding.[424] The usual age at presentation is between 5 and 40 years,[706] although the range can be larger. In one series of 350 it varied from 1.5 to 74 years.[356] The principal features of the illness are a systemic disturbance marked by fatigue, weight loss, and low-grade fever together with respiratory symptoms. The main respiratory symptoms are chronic cough, which is particularly troublesome at night and may be productive of mucoid or mucopurulent sputum with occasional hemoptysis, dyspnea, and wheeze. Even without treatment, symptoms tend to remit after several weeks or months only to recur later.[546] On auscultation of the patient's chest, crackles and wheezes are heard. Hepatosplenomegaly and nodal enlargement are rarely seen except in children.[706] There is gross eosinophilia (eosinophil count more than 3×10^9/L and, characteristically, between 5 and 60×10^9/L). IgE levels are greatly elevated, usually more than 1000 units/ml, with a high titer of antifilarial antibody.

Several reports have described the radiologic findings in the chest.[28,33,356,424,602] The chest radiograph has a normal appearance in 2% to 13% of cases. The most common abnormalities, seen in one third to two thirds of patients, are fine linear opacities distributed diffusely and symmetrically, accompanied by hilar haziness and an accentuation or blurring of vessels (Figure 12-72). Some authors describe a basal preponderance,[424] and others stress a general loss in transradiancy accompanying the diffuse shadowing.[356] Small nodules are a slightly less common finding, seen in about 30% to 50% of patients (Figure 12-73). The nodules range in size from 1 to 5 mm and may occur alone or with the linear opacities previously described.[424] Although generally bilateral and symmetric, nodulation may be asymmetric or even unilateral.[602] Other patterns are much less common and consist of areas of consolidation that are generally small and single. They can, however, be large,[398] multifocal,[33,424] or even cavitary.[391] Diffuse ground-glass opacification[33] and small pleural effusions[602] are also described. Many accounts describe bilateral hilar enlargement or prominence.[28,33,356,602] Enlargement is almost always mild and has been ascribed to vessels rather than nodes,[356] although pathologic evidence of slight hilar adenopathy was seen in one study.[787]

Tropical pulmonary eosinophilia characteristically responds rapidly to diethylcarbamazine therapy, and this is an important diagnostic criterion. In about 20% of

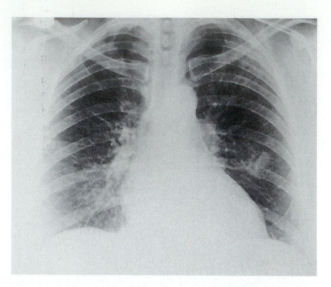

FIGURE 12-74
Eosinophilic lung disease following worm infestation. This 52-year-old woman had buttock rash caused by cutaneous larva migrans (*Ancylostoma braziliense*) acquired on vacation in West Indies. She had blood eosinophilia and dry cough. Chest radiograph shows two areas of consolidation: one in left midzone and the other peripherally in left upper zone. Both cleared in 2 weeks.

patients, however, long-term outcome is unsatisfactory because of persisting alveolitis or reinfection, and chronic interstitial fibrosis develops in some patients.[566,765]

Eosinophilic lung disease from other worm infestations

The larval stages of a number of worms other than filarial nematodes pass through the lung and may in the process induce an allergic response. It most commonly takes the form of Löffler's syndrome with transient, migratory, nonsegmental areas of consolidation associated with blood eosinophilia (Figure 12-74).[612] Nearly all the worms that cause this response are nematodes: *Ascaris lumbricoides*,[35,278] *Ascaris suum*,[589] *Strongyloides stercoralis*,[612] *Toxocara canis*,[807,633] *Toxocara cati*,[612] *Ancylostoma braziliense*,[87] *Ancylostoma duodenale, Necator americanus*,[260] *Trichuris trichiura*,[155] *Taenia saginata*,[155] *Echinococcus alveolaris*,[155] and *Schistosoma* spp.[177] In at least some of these infestations the pulmonary reaction is probably not related to local larvae but rather is a remote response to a soluble antigen.[87] Thus in 26 patients with eosinophilic lung disease from *A. braziliense* (Figure 12-74), larvae could not be demonstrated in the sputum.[807] Some idea of the possible frequency of eosinophilic lung disease caused by nematode infestations may be gained from the last authors, who found lung shadowing in 34% of 76 patients with cutaneous larva migrans (hookworm infestation).

Radiologic patterns other than Löffler's syndrome rarely occur but include isolated eosinophilic pleural effusion.[429]

Bronchocentric granulomatosis

First described by Liebow in 1973, bronchocentric granulomatosis[460] differs from other lung granulomatoses, such as Wegener's, in that it is localized to the lung and centered around airways (bronchocentric) rather than vessels (angiocentric). Small airways and bronchioles are filled and replaced by cellular debris and necrotic granulomas surrounded by palisaded epithelioid cells. In asthmatic patients the cellular infiltrate is made up largely of eosinophils, whereas in nonasthmatic persons the plasma cell is dominant.[419] Large airways may show bronchocele formation, and distal lung is often consolidated by an eosinophilic or obstructive pneumonitis. Vasculitic changes appear to be minor and incidental.

Only three series of patients with bronchocentric granulomatosis have been recorded,[419,434,650] representing a total of 55 cases; however, there have been many additional case reports.

The incidence peaks in the forties, but a wide age range (9 to 76 years) exists. The disease develops earlier in asthmatic patients (mean age 22 years) than in nonasthmatic ones (mean age 50 years).[419] The incidence in both sexes is equal. In the combined series 16 (29%) of the 55 patients have been asthmatic, and some patients have had associated disorders, although the significance of this observation is unclear. These disorders include rheumatoid disease,[44] ankylosing spondylitis,[632] glomerulonephritis,[781] and echinococcosis.[178] Symptoms may be absent or minor and when present are not particularly characteristic. They consist of fever, cough, chest pain, wheeze, and hemoptysis. About 50% of patients have had blood eosinophilia, a finding that appears to be limited to asthmatic patients.[419,434]

Two major radiologic patterns are seen: consolidations or masslike lesions.[419,434,629,650] Consolidations may be lobar or sublobar and may be accompanied by volume loss (Figure 12-75). They are thought to represent either eosinophilic or obstructive pneumonitis.[419] They tend to be more common in the upper zones[419,629] and are unilateral in about 75% of patients. Sublobar consolidation was the most common finding (16 of 22) in one large series.[419] Masslike lesions are commonly solitary but can be multiple. They are considered to represent a mass of necrotic tissue with surrounding granulomatous or organizing pneumonitis. They vary in size from 2 to 15 cm[44] and are often not well defined. Occasionally they cavitate.[44,419] Less common radiologic patterns include mucoid impaction (Figure 12-76)[129,419] and reticulonodular opacities. On occasion the reticulonodular shadowing has evolved from antecedent consolidation.

Evidence shows that bronchocentric granulomatosis in asthmatic patients is different etiologically from that in persons without asthma. In many asthmatic patients histologic, serologic, and microbiologic evidence shows that bronchocentric granulomatosis is caused by *Aspergillus* and forms part of the spectrum of allergic broncho-

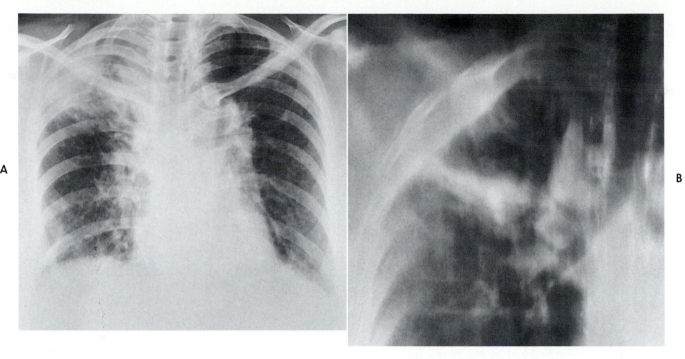

FIGURE 12-75
Bronchocentric granulomatosis. This 52-year-old woman presented with weight loss and cough. **A,** Chest radiograph shows right upper zone consolidation with some volume loss and scattered linear and nodular opacities in left upper zone, these latter changes being ascribed to old granulomatous disease. Patient was treated with antituberculous therapy without established diagnosis. **B,** Localized tomogram of right upper zone 1 month later. Consolidation has been replaced by thick-walled, 5 cm diameter cavity. Following right upper lobectomy, asthma and blood eosinophilia developed. Hyphae of *Aspergillus* were found in pathologic specimen.

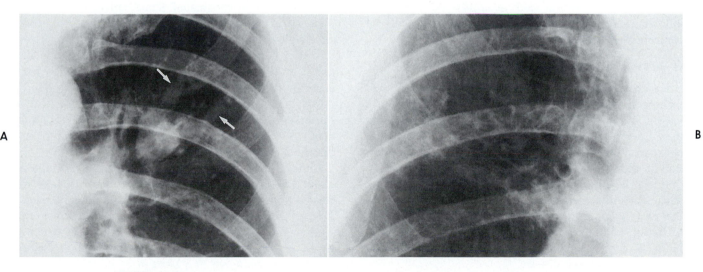

FIGURE 12-76
Bronchocentric granulomatosis. **A,** Localized view of left middle zone in 50-year-old woman shows 2 × 3 cm lobulated well-demarcated masslike lesion with two fingerlike projections *(arrows)* that strongly suggest a bronchocele. **B,** Localized view of right midzone shows thin curvilinear and ring opacities caused by bronchiectasis resulting from allergic aspergillosis. (Courtesy Dr. J.D. Stevenson, Poole, Dorset, U.K.)

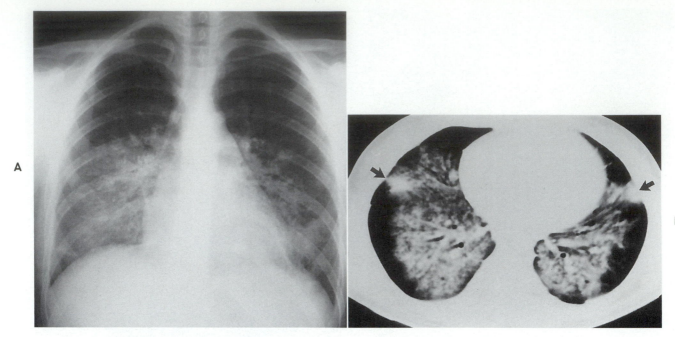

FIGURE 12-77

Hypereosinophilic syndrome. This 35-year-old man had 6-week history of malaise and increasing shortness of breath and on examination was found to be in heart failure. Peripheral blood eosinophil count was grossly raised at 38 × 10⁹/L. **A,** Chest radiograph shows borderline large heart and diffuse consolidative opacity in middle and lower zones consistent with edema. **B,** Computed tomogram confirms and also shows two focal consolidations *(arrows)* that could represent infarcts (unproven).

pulmonary aspergillosis.[328,418] Sensitivity to other fungi such as *Candida* spp. may also be possible.[419] In non-asthmatic persons the cause is generally obscure, although recently cases associated with tuberculosis and a variety of fungi have been reported.[418]

The prognosis is good. Lesions may clear spontaneously or with steroids and generally do not recur following surgical removal. Recurrences can usually be controlled with steroid treatment.

Hypereosinophilic syndrome

Hypereosinophilic syndrome is a rarely encountered, heterogenous group of disorders characterized by prolonged and marked eosinophilia (a blood count of more than 1.5 × 10⁹/L for more than 6 months); no recognizable cause for the eosinophilia, such as parasitic infestation or allergy; and signs or symptoms of organ dysfunction.[126] The illness varies from mild to fatal, involving particularly the cardiovascular and nervous systems. In the past it has gone under a variety of other names, including Löffler's syndrome with cardiac involvement, Löffler's fibroplastic endocarditis, and disseminated eosinophilic collagen disease.[225]

There is widespread tissue infiltration with mature eosinophils that cause tissue damage,[234] particularly endocardial damage leading to endocardial fibrosis, restrictive cardiomyopathy, and thrombosis. Almost all patients have been men, typically young or middle-aged

adults with progressive cardiopulmonary symptoms, skin rash, or myalgia together with systemic symptoms such as weight loss, weakness, fatigue, and fever. The peripheral blood shows a marked eosinophilia, often in the order of 30% to 70% of the total white blood cell count (10 to 50 × 10⁹/L). Some of the eosinophils are degranulated and vacuolated. Some patients have a mild increase in IgE. The organ systems most commonly affected are the nervous and cardiovascular systems and the skin. Cardiovascular involvement is usually the dominant feature and is a major cause of morbidity, with signs of restrictive cardiomyopathy and pump failure, mitral and tricuspid regurgitation, and endocardial thrombosis. The thrombosis leads to systemic emboli in about 5% of patients[579] or pulmonary emboli if the thrombus is on the right side.[234]

Clinical pulmonary involvement has been recorded in about 40% of patients.[126,234] In most, these findings are related to heart failure[225] and include pulmonary edema (Figure 12-77) and pleural effusions.[126] Because the cardiomyopathy is restrictive in type, any accompanying cardiomegaly is often mild.[579] Pulmonary emboli (Figure 12-78) were recorded in 5 (9%) of 57 patients reviewed from the literature.[126] Other, less common pulmonary manifestations include transient consolidations, which are presumably eosinophilic pneumonias and diffuse interstitial fibrosis.[126,579]

Before the use of steroids and cytotoxic drugs the

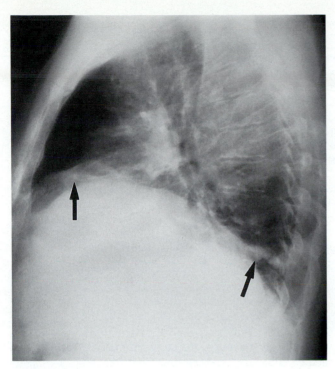

FIGURE 12-78
Hypereosinophilic syndrome. Basal band opacities *(arrows)* in patient with hypereosinophilic syndrome (peripheral eosinophil count $23 \times 10^9/L$) were considered clinically to be caused by pulmonary infarcts.

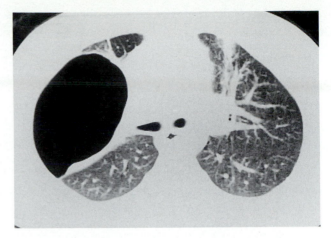

FIGURE 12-79
Hyperimmunoglobulin E, recurrent-infection syndrome. Computed tomogram of 3½-year-old boy with a past history of sinusitis and three episodes of pneumonia. Patient had eczematous dermatitis and dysmorphic facies. Large airspace occupies much of right upper lobe that had developed from previous infective consolidation. Cysts are most common interval changes on chest radiographs in this condition.

prognosis was poor, with a 25% 2-year survival rate.[126] This figure has now improved considerably, and the 3-year mortality rate is down to 4%.[580]

Hyperimmunoglobulin E, recurrent infection (Job's) syndrome

Job's syndrome is a rare primary immunodeficiency disorder that was first described in 1966[174] and is characterized by recurrent bacterial infections of the lungs, sinuses, and skin dating from birth or early childhood and a more than 10-fold elevation of serum IgE.[192] The immunologic derangement is complex and only partly understood.[510] Recurrent bronchitis and pneumonia are major features, often caused by *Staphylococcus aureus,* although other bacteria and fungi may also be responsible. Commonly an eczematous dermatitis, mucocutaneous candidiasis, recurrent furunculosis, and cutaneous cold abscesses may be present. Lack of the usual systemic and local inflammatory findings with the abscesses is a striking feature, particularly because most are caused by *S. aureus.* Other features include dysmorphism with retarded growth and coarse facies and osteoporosis.[427] A mild or mild to moderate eosinophila occurs in 77% to 100% of patients.[192,510] Occasionally eosinophilia is marked.[81] Radiologic findings in the chest have been well described[510] and consist of recurrent infective consolidations beginning before 3 years of age

and cyst formation. All patients in the series of Merten and co-workers,[510] in which the average age was 18 years, had lung cysts (Figure 12-79). Some cysts disappeared after a few years while others were recurrent or persistent. About one third of cysts were multiple and could be very large, occupying much of a hemithorax; their walls were usually smooth but varied in thickness. The pathogenesis of these cysts is not definitely established. Some are probably pneumatoceles, and others arise in a cavitating consolidation. In a number of cases, however, their development could not be related to an infective episode.[510] Other pulmonary findings include empyema, bronchopleural fistula,[427] bronchiectasis,[458,510] and pneumothorax.[251,458] Eighty percent in Merten's series had chronic sinusitis.[510]

EXTRINSIC ALLERGIC ALVEOLITIS

Extrinsic allergic alveolitis (EAA) is a disorder in which repeated inhalation of particulate organic antigens causes a predominantly immunologic response in the air-exchange units of the lung. This condition has several synonyms, the most common of which is hypersensitivity pneumonitis.

A large number of causal antigens have already been identified, including microorganisms (bacteria, fungi, thermophilic actinomycetes, amebas), animal and plant proteins, drugs, and some low–molecular weight chemicals.[244,654] Thermophilic actinomycetes are particularly important agents. They are widely distributed bacteria with morphologic features of fungi that thrive in the high temperatures (45° to 60° C) commonly found in decomposing vegetable matter.[620]

Table 12-2   Major causes of extrinsic allergic alveolitis

Disease	Source of antigen	Antigen	Reference
Farmer's lung	Moldy hay	Thermophilic actinomycetes (*Faeni rectivirgula, Thermoactinomyces vulgaris*)	Cadhan[89] Campbell[95] Dickie and Rankin[185] Emanuel et al.[217] Hapke et al.[329]
Bagassosis	Moldy sugar cane	*T. sacchari*	Hargreave et al.[331]
Mushroom worker's lung	Mushroom compost	Thermophilic actinomycetes, mushroom spores	Bringhurst et al.[76] Sakula[648] Jackson and Welch[395]
Ventilation pneumonitis	Dust or mist	*T. vulgaris, T. thalpophilus,* amebas, thermotolerant bacteria	Banaszak et al.[29] Medical Research Council[504] Stankus and Salvaggio[710] Kohler et al.[431]
Maltworker's lung	Moldy barley	*Aspergillus clavatus, F. rectivirgula*	Riddle et al.[624]
Bird fancier's (breeder's) lung	Droppings and feathers	Avian protein	Reed et al.[611] Hargreave et al.[332]

Agents that cause EAA are particulates[653] small enough (1 to 5 μm) that they can enter and be retained in the gas exchange units of the lung, especially the alveoli. To induce disease, the exposure has to be heavy, either short and intense or prolonged and low grade. With one or two exceptions, for example, exposure to pet birds or to agents from humidifiers, such exposures are found only in association with specific occupations or hobbies.

The most important and common disorders are listed in Table 12-2 together with the inciting agents and antigens. Many less common disorders not included in the table are recognized, including hard metal lung disease (cobalt),[160,161] Japanese summer-type hypersensitivity pneumonitis,[14] suberosis from moldy cork dust,[590] maple bark disease,[218] wood pulp worker's disease,[689] sauna taker's disease,[513] sequoiosis,[133] cheese washer's lung,[183] dry rot lung,[553] grain or wheat weevil lung,[475] animal handler's lung,[106] Pauli's reagent "alveolitis,"[229] fish meal worker's lung,[25] mollusk shell hypersensivity pneumonitis,[565] diisocyanate alveolitis,[115] phthalic anhydride hypersensitivity pneumonitis,[244] pyrethrum alveolitis,[100] *Bacillus subtilis* alveolitis,[403] drugs (amiodarone pneumonitis),[771] *A. fumigatus* alveolitis,[772] and coffee worker's lung.[769] More comprehensive lists are available in the literature.[259,577,620,628,697]

The immunopathogenesis is complicated and not completely worked out. Antigen inhalation probably leads to precipitin antibody formation and T cell sensitization in all exposed individuals, but EAA develops in only some. The pathologic changes are probably mediated by both type III (immune complex, Arthus-type) and type IV (cell-mediated, delayed-type) reactions. Other mechanisms, such as complement activation by the alternative pathway, probably play a part. Several reviews discuss the pathogenesis in detail.*

Histologic changes are conventionally classified into acute, subacute, and chronic, but the so-called acute changes are occurring days or weeks into the illness.[620] Early an interstitial pneumonitis starts near terminal bronchioles and extends intraparenchymally. The septa develop a mononuclear cell infiltrate with lymphocytes and histiocytes. Alveolar spaces may be filled by alveolar epithelial proliferation or fluid, which can be serous, hemorrhagic, or exudative.[32,217,367] Bronchiolitis is common and in some cases obstructive.[217,676] Vasculitis is also described,[32] but it is not a dominant feature. These acute changes are more common in the lower zones.[676] In the subacute phase, noncaseating, loose, histiocytic granulomas appear at about 3 weeks and may last up to 1 year.[676] The interstitial pneumonitis persists as does the alveolar inflammatory exudate.[619] With the development of the chronic phase, granulomas disappear and fibrosis ensues, affecting particularly the upper zones.[259] This results in honeycomb and cystic changes with air-containing spaces varying in size between 1 mm and several centimeters.[676] Some of these airspaces represent irregular emphysema secondary to peribronchial scarring. Eventually changes of pulmonary arterial hypertension and cor pulmonale may occur.[217,676] Pleural fibrosis is seen in about 50% of patients[367] but is not a major feature.

The age and sex patterns in the various types of EAA simply reflect differing opportunities for exposure. Bird fancier's lung, for example, when caused by budgerigars (parakeets) occurs typically in women over 65 years of age. When caused by pigeons it is seen in men under 45 years.[618] Another feature of EAA is the relatively low attack rate: many people develop immune reactions to recognized antigens, yet fail to develop overt lung disease.[620]

Farmer's lung shows regional variations in prevalence and also seasonal fluctuations, occurring particularly in

---

*References 244, 577, 620, 628, 653, 654.

late autumn, winter, and early spring.[577] Absolute prevalence rates are difficult to assess and compare, varying widely among series.[636] It would seem that, for both farmer's lung and bird fancier's lung caused by budgerigars, the prevalence rate in exposed individuals is about 2% to 4% (lying between 0.5% and 7.5%), making bird fancier's lung 10 times more common than farmer's lung in the United Kingdom.[351]

Three types of illness are recognized: acute, subacute, and chronic, and each is associated with a variable mixture of respiratory and constitutional symptoms.[244,329] The acute form occurs commonly in those with bird fancier's lung caused by pigeons and typically follows loft cleaning. Acute illness is seen in only about one third of patients with farmer's lung.[584] The acute illness develops 4 to 8 hours after heavy exposure to the antigen and consists of dry cough, chest tightness, dyspnea, wheeze, fever, chills, malaise, and occasionally hemoptysis. These symptoms are often mistakenly diagnosed as a viral or bacterial illness unless suspicions of EAA are aroused by repeated episodes. With repeated episodes anorexia and weight loss are common.[244] Spontaneous recovery follows separation from the agent, with substantial improvement in 1 to 2 days. Recovery is usually complete by 7 to 10 days. Physical examination of the patient in the acute phase usually reveals fine to medium basal crackles.[329] Tachypnea and central cyanosis with restlessness and apprehension are found in the more severe cases.[577] Leukocytosis is common during the acute illness, and respiratory function tests show restrictive and obstructive abnormalities.

The subacute syndrome consists of acute episodes superimposed on a background of deteriorating respiratory function. The chronic form is dominated by progressive shortness of breath and is a common mode of presentation in farmer's lung and in bird fancier's lung related to the budgerigar.[259] It is associated with continual low-grade exposure that if allowed to persist causes irreversible lung damage. It may be accompanied by constitutional symptoms such as malaise and weight loss. Physical signs in the chronic form are usually not striking. Serum precipitins have long been regarded as the hallmark of extrinsic allergic alveolitis,[259] but like asbestos-related pleural plaques, they are indicators of exposure and not necessarily of disease. Thus 40% of pigeon breeders clinically free of EAA had tests positive for serum precipitin antibody.[245] Positive serum precipitin tests are also present in disease-free farmers[795] and even in the community at large. The reverse situation is also possible, with definite disease but a negative serum precipitin test, especially when the disease is at the more advanced, fibrotic end of the spectrum.[310,584,679] Nevertheless, about 90% of patients have detectable serum precipitin values at the time of diagnosis, particularly if the last exposure was in the preceding weeks or months. In a series of patients with farmer's lung, all the acute cases and 53% of chronic cases had positive serum precipitins and the precipitins remained for about 2 or 3 years.[329]

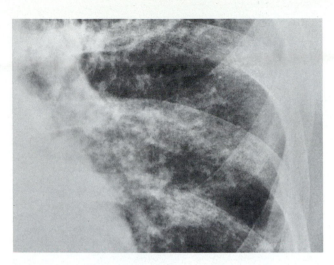

FIGURE 12-80
Acute farmer's lung. Localized view of left midzone shows diffuse shadowing consisting predominantly of small nodules up to 2 mm in diameter.

The diagnosis of EAA is usually based on the characteristic clinical symptoms and signs, together with evidence of exposure and improvement following withdrawal. Supportive evidence is provided by a late reaction to intracutaneous antigen, compatible radiologic findings and respiratory function tests, and the presence of precipitins in the blood. However, none of these tests is pathognomonic. A more specific test is bronchial provocation with the suspect antigen, although this is not commonly performed and can be dangerous.[243] Histologic changes are never diagnostic except for a few types of allergic alveolitis in which organic particles can be identified, for instance, bagassosis and maple bark disease. On histologic study the principal differential diagnoses are granulomatous infections, sarcoidosis, and interstitial pneumonitis (usual and lymphocytic).[418]

The chest radiographic changes are the same regardless of the provocative agent,[766] but evidence for this is incomplete. In the acute stage the chest radiograph is occasionally normal,[21,330] or it may be interpreted as normal because the findings are subtle.[577] The radiograph may also be normal later,[363] even in patients with abnormal diffusing capacity[525,755] and biopsy-proven granulomas.[521,609]

The most common radiographic finding in the acute or subacute stage is small pulmonary nodules (Figure 12-80), usually 1 to 3 mm,[140,521] but ranging up to 5 mm.[217,329] These opacities may be so small and profuse that they give a ground-glass appearance (Figure 12-81).[525] The nodules may be discrete and sharply defined[329] or ill defined.[822] They are almost always bilateral; in one series of 132 patients only 2% of the nodules were unilateral.[618] Opacities are most commonly found in all lung zones,[330,767] but may show a middle to lower zone

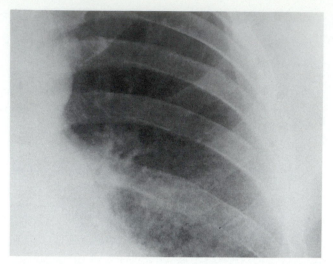

FIGURE 12-81
Acute farmer's lung. Localized view of left midzone shows diffusely distributed micronodulation summating to give ground-glass appearance best seen inferolaterally. (Courtesy Dr. R.B. Pickford, Abergavenny, Gwent, U.K.)

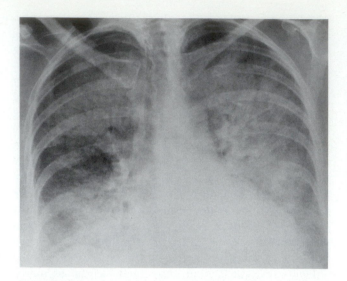

FIGURE 12-82
Acute farmer's lung. Gross changes in 55-year-old woman who was exposed during grain grinding. Widespread, diffuse consolidation with air bronchogram is evident. Focal consolidation is recognized finding in extrinsic allergic alveolitis, but such marked airspace shadowing is unusual.

preponderance, sparing the apices,[217] or a middle to upper zone predominance, sparing the periphery at the bases.[140,521] They appear just a few hours after exposure[63] and clear in several weeks[521] or months.[329] They can, however, persist indefinitely and become part of the chronic changes.[329] Occasionally, nodules in the 4 to 8 mm range are seen,[330] but these are far less common. Focal patchy consolidations develop in some 10% to 25% of patients (Figure 12-82).[140,217,330,618,767] Sometimes the interstitial pattern takes on a more linear appearance in the acute stage with accentuation of bronchovascular structures[525,767,822] and the occasional septal B line.[329,330] Pleural changes are not a feature of EAA,[577] although the minor fissure may become thickened.[330] Nodal enlargement has been reported on only a handful of occasions and has been described with mushroom worker's lung,[648] bird fancier's lung,[822] and farmer's lung.[32,259]

Chronic changes reflect healing by fibrosis and may occur after one or more acute attacks[525] or may develop insidiously in relation to chronic low-grade antigen exposure, as for example with bird fancier's lung related to budgerigars (Figure 12-83).[330] The characteristic radiologic changes in the chronic stage are of a scarring process with loss of lung volume,[259] which has a marked (85%) upper lobe predominance (Figures 12-84 and 12-85).[330] The principal opacities are reticular or reticulonodular, sometimes with a definite honeycomb pattern.[72,330] Larger ring shadows, 1 to 4 cm in diameter, are due to bullae, blebs, cysts, or bronchiectasis. Line shadows secondary to scarring are common, particularly in the upper zones.[329] Parallel line shadows are caused by bronchiectasis or simple bronchial wall thickening and in the latter case are often transient.[330] Other changes that

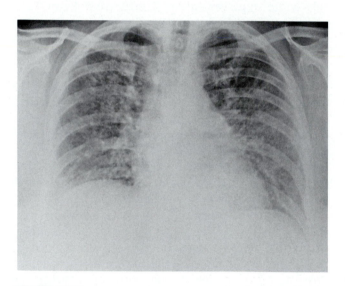

FIGURE 12-83
Chronic bird fancier's lung. Patient was exposed to budgerigar (parakeet) for many years. Basic shadowing consists of irregular 2 to 4 mm nodules with reticulation and linear element. Appearances were essentially stable, but unusual in that they are equally distributed in all zones.

are sometimes seen in the chronic stage include persisting small nodules,[329] massive opacities,[330] and evidence of cor pulmonale.[329] Pneumothorax is recorded in the fibrotic stage but is uncommon.[217]

High-resolution CT findings have been reported on a little fewer than 100 patients with EAA. In most studies patients have been in the subacute[6,327,476] or chronic[3] phase, and data on the acute phase are limited. In one other study patients were mixed.[694]

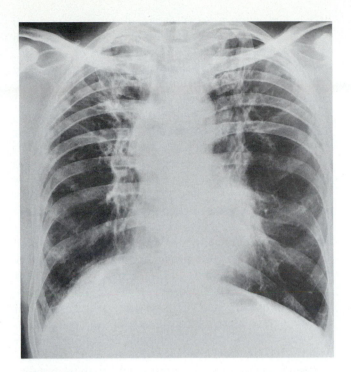

FIGURE 12-84
Chronic farmer's lung. Patient had recurrent acute episodes of allergic alveolitis over 15-year period. He then discontinued farming, and this radiograph was taken 10 years later. It shows linear scarlike shadows in both upper zones together with volume loss in upper zones. Upper zone distribution of scarring is typical of extrinsic allergic alveolitis. (Courtesy Dr. R.B. Pickford, Abergavenny, Gwent, U.K.)

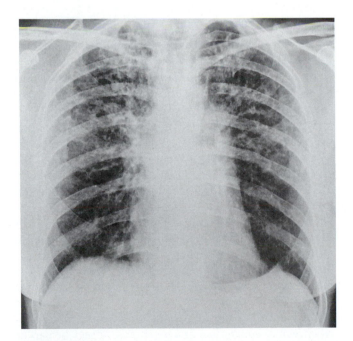

FIGURE 12-85
Chronic bird fancier's lung. Alveolitis in this patient resulted from exposure to budgerigars (parakeets). Fixed middle and upper zone changes exist with upper lobe volume loss. Shadowing is reticulonodular, with predominant reticular-linear element, producing many ring shadows.

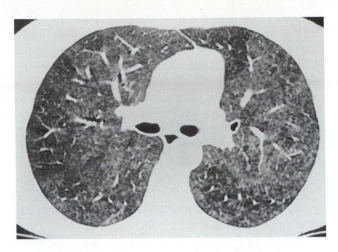

FIGURE 12-86
Extrinsic allergic alveolitis (pigeon fancier's lung). High-resolution computed tomogram showing subacute phase with extensive ground-glass opacity, sparing some regions (especially peripherally on right). Airways in involved regions become more obvious.

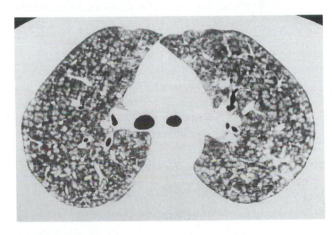

FIGURE 12-87
Extrinsic allergic alveolitis. Diagnosis in 43-year-old man with 2- to 3-month history of exertional dyspnea was made by open lung biopsy. No definite inciting agent was identified, and diagnosis therefore cannot be regarded as definitely established. However, computed tomographic findings of widespread, evenly distributed 2 to 4 mm nodules are entirely consistent with allergic alveolitis.

In the subacute phase the majority of patients have diffuse ground-glass opacity and small nodulation on HRCT. Ground-glass opacity (Figure 12-86) (sometimes described as a slight increase in lung density)[6] is diffuse, often affecting all zones but with a middle or lower zone predominance. It may be a subtle finding; two reports (18 patients) do not record it as a sign in EAA.[476,492] It causes airways to appear prominent (Figure 12-86),[6,327] and this may be a more obvious finding than the ground-glass opacity itself. The pathologic basis of ground-glass opacity is unclear,[694] although in one pathologic and radiologic study it was considered to be caused by interstitial inflammatory infiltration.[49] Nodules (Figure 12-87) are rounded, about 2 to 4 mm in diameter, and widespread. They show no predilection for a central or peripheral distribution in the lung,[327] but within the lobule they tend to be centrally placed.[6,476] Bronchovascular interfaces remain sharp.[6] Other findings are described, but these are less frequent or less pronounced. They include patchy airspace consolidation with the occasional acinar nodule; reticulation,[327,492] which is more a feature of the chronic phase; minor interlobular septal thickening [327]; and focal pleural thickening.[327] Studies comparing the chest radiograph and HRCT showed that the latter is more sensitive, particularly in detecting ground-glass opacity, and that the HRCT can show abnormalities in the presence of a normal chest radiograph.[6,327,694]

Chronic HRCT changes consist of coarse, irregular, linear opacities with parenchymal distortion.[3] These scars are either midzonal or widely scattered and may be peribronchovascular, subpleural, or randomly distributed. Honeycombing is common as are the changes (small nodules and ground-glass opacity) associated with the subacute stage.[3,694]

The prognosis of EAA is variable. After a single attack the patient usually recovers completely,[577] although there are exceptions.[32,525] With continuing exposure, chronic changes are likely to supervene and become permanent despite cessation of exposure. In a series of 143 patients with bird fancier's lung, all of whom were treated by avoidance of bird contact and 22% of whom were treated with steroids, only 50% showed radiologic improvement and a significant increase in vital capacity. The death rate from farmer's lung disease in two series of 141 and 24 patients was 9% and 17%, respectively.[72,217]

Organic dust toxic syndrome

Massive exposure to organic dusts from hay, grain, and other agricultural products can cause a delayed (several hours) influenza-like syndrome with or without respiratory symptoms unaccompanied by hypersensitivity and with no long-term sequelae.[196] This syndrome was originally described as mycotoxicosis,[219] but currently endotoxins rather than mycotoxins are thought to be etiologically important and the term "organic dust toxic syndrome" is preferred. Bronchoalveolar lavage has demonstrated a neutrophil alveolitis in some patients. Radiologic changes are usually absent, although in Emanuel and associates' original series,[219] 50% had bilateral, basally predominant radiologic changes described as interstitial or reticulonodular.

AMYLOIDOSIS AND AMYLOID DEPOSITION

In amyloidosis there is an abnormal extracellular deposition of amyloid, an autologous fibrillar protein material that histochemically binds with congo red, giving a green birefringence in polarized light. This pathognomonic staining property is caused by the unique structure of amyloid.

Amyloid is deposited in a number of conditions and as part of the aging process. Organ dysfunction occurs if enough amyloid material accumulates. The deposition may be generalized when it occurs as part of a systemic disease, or it may be localized to a single organ. Local deposition within an organ may itself be diffuse or focal. Localized disease never becomes generalized.

Amyloid is produced from one of a number of circulating or locally produced protein precursors when their structure or concentration becomes abnormal.[585] Important proteins are (1) AL (amyloid light chain), which is derived from monoclonal immunoglobulin light chain, is manufactured by plasma cells, and is found in various plasma cell dyscrasias, including primary amyloidosis, a disease now classified as an immunocyte dyscrasia with a monoclonal gammopathy; (2) AA (amyloid A), an alphaglobulin that is an acute-phase reactant in inflammatory or infective conditions, found in secondary amyloidosis (reactive systemic amyloidosis); (3) prealbumin in hereditary syndromes; and (4) beta$_2$-microglobulin with chronic hemodialysis. A classification of the major clinical forms of amyloidosis and amyloid deposition together with the type of chest involvement is given in Table 12-3.

Some cases of amyloidosis do not fit comfortably into the scheme presented in Table 12-3, and no classification is entirely satisfactory. Difficulties most commonly occur with the so-called localized disease that, although not systemic, is in many instances clearly not limited to a single organ. This occurs for example in the chest, where lung or airway disease can be accompanied by mediastinal and cervical adenopathy.[182,271]

Systemic amyloidosis

Respiratory involvement is an unimportant part of systemic amyloidosis, and clinical and radiologic findings in the chest are usually incidental or secondary to a complication such as heart failure. Should primary chest involvement occur, it takes the form of interstitial parenchymal disease or lymphadenopathy.

AL (LIGHT CHAIN) AMYLOIDOSIS. AL amyloidosis has two main subtypes: one associated with a monoclonal gammopathy (formerly primary amyloidosis) and the other associated with myelomatosis. They are virtually identical in their clinical manifestations, except that the prognosis of amyloidosis associated with myeloma is worse (5-month versus 13-month mean survival).[439] In AL amyloidosis, infiltration with amyloid material affects mesenchymal tissues and to a lesser extent the kidney, liver, and spleen. AL amyloidosis has a 2:1 male predominance with a mean age at presentation of about 60 years.[280,287]

The clinical features of AL amyloidosis may be nonspecific, such as weight loss and weakness, or may be part of one or more classic disorders. The frequency of such disorders at diagnosis[439] is nephrotic syndrome, 32%; carpal tunnel syndrome, 24%; restrictive cardiomyopathy, 23%; peripheral neuropathy, 17%; orthostatic hypotension, 14%; and occasionally macroglossia, purpura, pap-

Table 12-3 Major clinical forms of amyloidosis and amyloid deposition with type of respiratory involvement

Major subdivision	Clinicopathologic entity	Chest involvement
Systemic amyloidosis	Immunocyte dyscrasia amyloidosis (AL amyloidosis) 　Amyloidosis with monoclonal gammopathy 　　(formerly primary systemic amyloidosis) 　Plasma cell myeloma 　Waldenström's macroglobulinemia 　Others	Diffuse parenchymal (usually 　subclinical) ± lymph nodes
	Reactive systemic amyloidosis (AA amyloidosis, 　formerly secondary amyloidosis)	Diffuse parenchymal (subclinical)
	Heredofamilial amyloidosis 　Neuropathic 　Nephropathic 　Cardiomyopathic	Diffuse parenchymal (in some)
	Senile systemic amyloidosis 　(formerly senile cardiac amyloidosis)	Diffuse parenchymal
	Hemodialysis associated	—
Localized amyloidosis	Lung	Tracheobronchial 　Parenchymal 　　Nodular 　　Diffuse 　± Lymph nodes
	Senile (heart, joints)	—
	Cerebral amyloid angiopathy	—
	Endocrine	Metastatic medullary carcinoma of 　thyroid[128]
	Skin, bladder, larynx, eye	—

Modified from Papys MB: *Q J Med* 67:283-298, 1988.

ular skin rash, and arthropathy. About 80% of patients have proteinuria. Electrophoresis of serum shows a protein spike in 40% and, on immunoelectrophoresis, a monoclonal protein in 68%. When urine and blood test results are combined, 89% of patients have a monoclonal protein.[439] The diagnosis is made by rectal biopsy, which shows the abnormality in approximately 75% of affected patients.[439] Bone marrow aspiration is positive for the disease in only 30% of patients, but it does allow assessment of plasma cells for the presence of possible myelomatosis. If both rectal biopsy and bone marrow aspiration are negative, biopsy of a suspect organ should be performed.

The median survival in a series of 153 patients with AL amyloidosis was 12 months, with fewer than 20% alive at 5 years.[280] Heart failure was associated with a particularly bad prognosis.

Involvement of the lungs on pathologic examination is common in AL amyloidosis, with a prevalence range between 70% and 92%,[78,109,132,700,780] but it is rarely of clinical importance. For example, in a major clinical review of 229 patients with AL amyloid, no mention is made of the lung being clinically affected,[439] while in a later report just 2 patients of 153 had diffuse interstitial pulmonary involvement.[280] Reports of significant lung involvement occur mostly in individual case reports or in small selected series.* In one such series 5 of 12 patients with "primary amyloidosis" showed radiographic and pathologic evidence of diffuse alveolar septal amyloidosis, and in one patient it contributed to death[109] as it did in another small series.[147] A further point is that cardiac amyloidosis commonly accompanies lung involvement,[700] and it is well recognized that both the clinical and radiologic signs of pulmonary amyloid infiltration can be obscured by heart failure.[147,597,700,780] In the appropriate context, persistent radiologic changes despite adequate treatment of heart failure should raise the possibility of amyloid infiltration of the lungs.[360] Isolated massive mediastinal deposition of amyloid, presumably in nodes, has been described in myeloma-related AL amyloidosis.[402]

Light chains that are not polymerized into amyloid can be set down in the lungs in systemic light chain deposition disease. Light chains accumulate in the lung interstitium or airways, sometimes producing a miliary pattern on the chest radiograph.[425]

REACTIVE SYSTEMIC AMYLOIDOSIS. Reactive systemic amyloidosis (secondary or AA amyloidosis) is usually secondary to chronic infective or inflammatory processes.[438] Rare cryptogenic cases are described.[596] The

---

*References 77, 147, 156, 414, 625, 780.

most common cause now is probably rheumatoid arthritis,[78] in which the prevalence of amyloidosis is usually quoted as 10%, although this figure is likely too high.[808] Other causes include tuberculosis, leprosy, osteomyelitis, bronchiectasis, chronically infected decubitus ulcers, ankylosing spondylitis, regional enteritis, and some malignancies such as Hodgkin's disease and renal cell carcinoma.[287,438] The organs most commonly affected by amyloid deposition are the kidneys, liver, spleen, and adrenal glands. The first manifestation is usually renal disease (proteinuria, nephrotic syndrome, hypertension) or hepatosplenomegaly. Renal failure is the most common cause of death. The prevalence of lung involvement pathologically varies considerably in various series. Two give a prevalence rate of 1% to 5%,[700,780] whereas in others the prevalence has been very high, approaching 100%.[109,808] These discrepancies are probably unimportant because the involvement is usually diffuse within the lung and not severe enough to cause functional or radiologic changes. Exceptions, however, were seen in one series of 24 patients, in which 16% had marked amyloid deposition at pathologic study.[78] There have also been a few reports of significant clinical lung involvement.[109,526,596] The distribution of amyloid deposition (alveolar septal versus perivascular) differs from patient to patient and affects the type of pathophysiologic disturbance. Predominant perivascular deposits can give pulmonary arterial hypertension.[688]

RADIOGRAPHIC CHANGES IN SYSTEMIC AMYLOIDOSIS. The chest radiograph is normal in the majority of patients with generalized amyloidosis and lung involvement,[318] even when the lung involvement is severe enough to cause major pulmonary dysfunction.[156] When abnormalities are seen, the findings are those of an interstitial process reflecting the predominantly septal and perivascular nature of amyloid deposition.[700] The radiographic appearances in the AA and AL forms are probably similar, but descriptions in AA amyloidosis are rare.[596] The usual findings are a diffuse micronodular, reticulonodular, or linear pattern with accentuated bronchovascular markings.* Parenchymal changes are usually diffuse and symmetric, but they can be segmental.[77] In time the nodular shadowing may become conglomerate or calcify.[780]

Pleural effusions in amyloidosis are usually caused by heart failure secondary to myocardial infiltration.[109,780] However, amyloid involvement of the pleura is seen pathologically[440,668] and probably occasionally causes effusion.[421,643,799]

CT descriptions are few[308,596] and show 2 to 4 mm nodules (some calcified) and a reticular or linear network from interlobular septal thickening (Figure 12-88).

Hilar and mediastinal nodal enlargement is not described in AA amyloidosis but is occasionally seen in AL amyloidosis, either as the sole radiologic finding in the chest,[61,77,317,799] or with parenchymal micronodula-

---

*References 77, 147, 414, 529, 625, 780, 799.

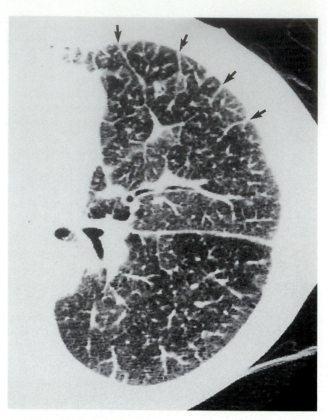

FIGURE 12-88
Alveolar septal amyloidosis. Patient was in heart failure when initially examined and was found to have cardiac amyloidosis and diffuse alveolar septal involvement (biopsy proven). Other organs were not involved, and patient fits best into senile systemic amyloidosis pattern. On high-resolution computed tomogram, principal finding is interlobular septal thickening (arrows). Minor features are intralobular septal thickening and mild prominence of some centrilobular structures.

tion.[780,792] Both mediastinal and hilar nodes may be involved, often massively, giving a pattern that may resemble sarcoidosis.[799] Nodal calcification is common (Figure 12-89).[683,799] The pattern of calcification is usually described as coarse or nonspecific; it may occasionally be of the eggshell type.[317] Nodal enlargement has also been described in AL amyloidosis associated with multiple myeloma[506] and Waldenström's macroglobulinemia.[109,317]

When AA amyloidosis is secondary to inflammatory lung disease, the chest radiograph will show major abnormalities, for example, changes of cystic fibrosis or bronchiectasis.[78,109,318] Heart failure is common in AL amyloidosis, and interstitial opacity resulting from raised pulmonary venous pressure may obscure pulmonary lesions of amyloid infiltration.[109,414]

Localized amyloidosis.

Localized amyloidosis may affect either the lung parenchyma or the airways (Table 12-4). These structures are usually involved independently,[147] but very occasionally both are affected together.[736] A few cases are also

Table 12-4 Localized forms of lower respiratory tract amyloidosis with relative percentage prevalence

Classification	Prevalence (%)	Form
Tracheobronchial	45	Multifocal submucosal plaques
	8	Tumorlike masses
Parenchymal	44	Nodular
		Solitary
		Multiple
	4	Diffuse alveolar septal

Modified from Thompson PJ, Citron KM: *Thorax* 38:84-87, 1983.

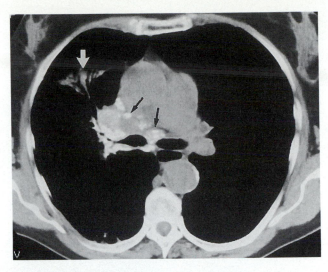

FIGURE 12-89
Nodal and airway amyloidosis. A 56-year-old woman had history of hemoptysis. Computed tomogram shows calcified nodal mass (*black arrows*). In addition, right upper lobar airway and its segmental branches were irregularly narrowed by submucosal amyloid tissue. This caused obstructive pneumonitis (*white arrow*). This combination of isolated nodal and airway disease is uncommon. Airway narrowing was successfully treated with laser therapy.

recorded in which isolated amyloidosis of mediastinal nodes is present.

TRACHEOBRONCHIAL AMYLOIDOSIS. Amyloid may occur in the airways as focal or diffuse submucosal deposits[745]; both are considered together here. The mean age of patients in a large review was 53 years, with a range of 16 to 76 years.[303] Twice as many men as women experience the disease.[643] Affected patients are often symptomatic[318] for several years before they seek treatment,[606] an indication that the disease progresses relatively slowly.

The major symptoms are cough, dyspnea, hemoptysis, stridor, and hoarseness.[606,643] A number of patients are believed to have asthma initially,[74,540] and recurrent pulmonary infections are common.[643]

Airway amyloid is more commonly diffuse than focal.[378,745] When diffuse, it can involve the trachea and mainstem bronchus and the lobar and proximal segmental bronchi, together or in part. This involvement can be demonstrated by bronchoscopy or by conventional[540] or computed tomography (Figure 12-89),[273] showing multiple concentric or eccentric strictures and mural nodulation. Local as opposed to diffuse lesions give rise to endobronchial masses that are radiologically indistinguishable from bronchial neoplasm.[150,745] With either type of lesion the chest radiograph may be normal[540] or show one of a number of obstructive features, most commonly collapse, which is seen in more than 50% of patients.[643] Other manifestations include recurrent infective consolidations and obstructive hyperinflation.[195] A few patients have had hilar or mediastinal masses on plain chest radiography, definitely[167] or possibly representing nodal enlargement.[503,551,667]

If treatment is required, the amyloid deposits may be removed by intermittent bronchoscopic resection[252] or laser photoresection.[74] Prognosis is not good, and lesions tend to recur 6 to 12 months after treatment.[643] In one review of 39 patients 21 were well at 4 to 6 years but 18 died, 12 from respiratory causes.[643]

PARENCHYMAL NODULAR AMYLOIDOSIS. This form of organ-limited amyloidosis produces one or more parenchymal nodules. Although about as common as tracheobronchial amyloidosis, it is still a rare condition,

with only 55 reports in a recent literature review.[745] Reviews of previous cases have appeared at regular intervals.[248,440,643,644,791] The pathologic changes have been summarized by Saab and co-workers.[644] Amyloid nodules are discrete and often subpleural, puckering the adjacent pleura to which they may be adherent. They are firm, sometimes well demarcated but not encapsulated, and waxy when sectioned. On microscopic study lung tissue is replaced by acellular amyloid surrounded peripherally by a low-grade inflammatory infiltrate containing giant cells. Calcification, cartilage formation, and ossification within the tumor are common. Bronchioles, alveolar septa, and blood vessels in the region of the tumor often contain amyloid as well.

The mean age at presentation in several series is 68 years,[248,440,644] with the youngest patient 38 years old[136]; sex incidence has been equal. Unless the disease is extensive, the patients are usually asymptomatic, with only occasional reports of cough and hemoptysis.[745] The nodules may be single (Figure 12-90) or multiple (Figure 12-91). In some series both patterns have been equally prevalent,[643] whereas in others multiple nodules have been predominant.[248] When tumors are multiple, the numbers vary from two to innumerable, with two thirds bilateral and one third unilateral.[248] Lobar predilection is absent.[643,644] Characteristically nodules are sharp and round,[318] but they may also be oval, lobulated (Figure 12-90),[360] irregular,[150,799] or ill defined.[360] Generally, in any one patient the nodules vary in size and shape. Some authors stress that a radiograph with multiple nodules of various shapes should raise the possibility of amyloidosis.

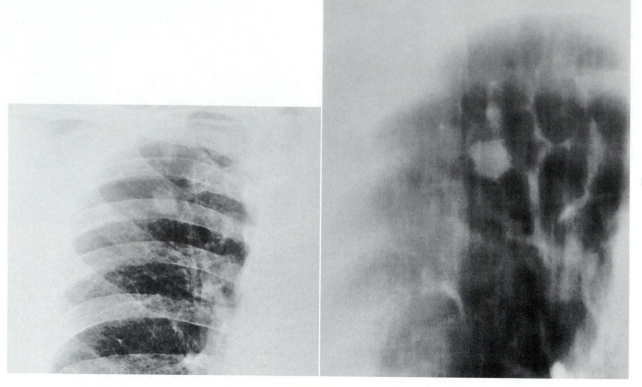

FIGURE 12-90

Parenchymal nodular amyloidosis. **A,** Posteroanterior chest radiograph of this asymptomatic 72-year-old man shows isolated 1.5 cm nodule in right upper zone. **B,** On tomography nodule is shown to be slightly lobulated, sharply marginated, and homogeneous.

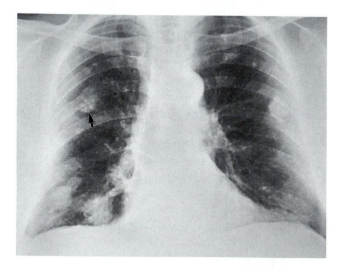

FIGURE 12-91

Parenchymal nodular amyloidosis. A 55-year-old man had ischemic chest pain and was found to have multiple, bilateral pulmonary nodules ranging from 0.5 to 3.0 cm. Several are calcified in irregular nodular fashion best seen in indicated nodule *(arrow)*. (Courtesy Dr. M.G. Britton, Chertsey, Surrey, U.K.)

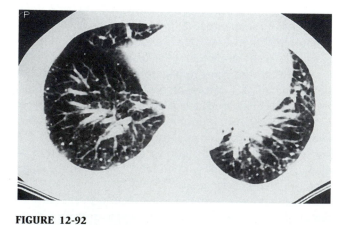

FIGURE 12-92

Micronodular amyloidosis. This 60-year-old man had lung-limited amyloidosis characterized mainly by multiple small (1 to 4 mm) nodules, some of which were calcified.

Nodules are commonly 0.5 to 5 cm in diameter but range from micronodular[240,360] to massive — up to 15 cm in diameter. Calcification (Figure 12-91) is common in both small[318,644] and large nodules; in the latter it is variously described as irregular, cloudy, flocculent, or stippled. It may occur centrally or throughout the nodule.[248,318,360] Calcification is detected in approximately 30% to 50% of cases,[643,736] depending on the method of assessment. Although calcification may be seen on the plain radiograph,[318,791] standard tomography and CT are more sensitive.[26,182,736] Calcification is clearly a helpful finding that may suggest the nature of such lesions.[360] Although cavitation was described in 11% of cases in one review series,[643] this is probably an overestimate.[151,791] It seems generally to be a rare complication.[318] Occasionally the nodules are locally confluent and mimic consolidation, an appearance that in the upper zone can be mistaken for tuberculosis.[524] The nodules tend to behave in an indolent fashion, growing slowly and sometimes remaining stable over several years.[736] In rare cases they grow rapidly, over months, behaving like a neoplasm.[248] In a few cases additional mediastinal lymphadenopathy has been described.[26,77,440,491,746]

The diagnosis is usually established by thoracotomy or percutaneous needle biopsy.[50] In patients with only one or a few nodules, the prognosis is excellent. Recurrence after removal of a nodule, although recorded, is extremely rare.[207] Very occasionally the disease is so widespread that it contributes to[240] or causes[440] death.

PARENCHYMAL ALVEOLAR SEPTAL DISEASE. Although alveolar septal deposition of amyloid is typical of systemic amyloidosis, it is occasionally found in disease that appears to be limited to the lung.[378,643,821] Unlike patients with the systemic disorder, most patients have had symptoms and deaths are recorded.[821] On pathologic study amyloid deposition in the interstitium may be diffuse or micronodular.[378] The radiologic pattern is of an interstitial process with fine linear or reticulonodular shadowing that can become confluent. Other patients have a diffuse micronodular pattern (Figure 12-92) that is sometimes accompanied by larger nodules, and this type may be considered one end of the spectrum of parenchymal nodular amyloidosis.[77,240,300,360] These patients are often symptomatic. Alveolar septal, micronodular lung-limited amyloid, and nodular parenchymal amyloidosis thus merge into one another and may be regarded as a continuum.

REFERENCES

1. Aberle DR, Gamsu G, Lynch D: Thoracic manifestations of Wegener granulomatosis: diagnosis and course, *Radiology* 174:703-709, 1990.
2. Abramson SB, Dobro J, Eberle MA, et al: Acute reversible hypoxemia in systemic lupus erythematosus, *Ann Intern Med* 114:941-947, 1991.
3. Adler BD, Padley SPG, Müller NL, et al: Chronic hypersensitivity pneumonitis: high-resolution CT and radiographic features in 16 patients, *Radiology* 185:91-95, 1992.
4. Agia GA, Reddy VC, Maltby J, et al: Pulmonary involvement in mixed connective tissue disease, *Am Rev Respir Dis* 121(suppl 4):105, 1980.
5. Agusti C, Xaubert A, Roca J, et al: Interstitial pulmonary fibrosis with and without associated collagen vascular disease: results of a two year follow up, *Thorax* 47:1035-1040, 1992.
6. Akira M, Kita N, Higashihara T, et al: Summer-type hypersensitivity pneumonitis: comparison of high-resolution CT and plain radiographic findings, *AJR* 158:1223-1228, 1992.
7. Akiyama K, Mathison DA, Riker JB, et al: Allergic bronchopulmonary candidiasis, *Chest* 85:699-701, 1984.
8. Akiyama K, Takizawa H, Suzuki M, et al: Allergic bronchopulmonary aspergillosis due to *Aspergillus oryzae*, *Chest* 91:285-286, 1987.
9. Alarcon-Segovia D, Cardiel MH: Comparison between three diagnostic criteria for mixed connective tissue disease: study of 593 patients, *J Rheumatol* 16:328-334, 1989.
10. Albelda SM, Gefter WB, Epstein DM, et al: Diffuse pulmonary hemorrhage: a review and classification, *Radiology* 154:289-297, 1985.
11. Alexander EL, Provost TT, Stevens MB, et al: Neurologic complications of primary Sjogren's syndrome, *Medicine* 61:247-257, 1982.
12. Allen JN, Pacht ER, Gadek JE, et al: Acute eosinophilic pneumonia as a reversible cause of noninfectious respiratory failure, *N Engl J Med* 321:569-574, 1989.
13. Anderson G, Coles ET, Crane M, et al: Wegener's granuloma: a series of 265 British cases seen between 1975 and 1985; a report by a sub-committee of the British Thoracic Society Research Committee, *Q J Med* 83:427-438, 1992.
14. Ando M, Arima K, Yoneda R, et al: Japanese summer-type hypersensitivity pneumonitis, *Am Rev Respir Dis* 144:765-769, 1991.
15. Andonopoulos AP, Karadanas AH, Drosos AA: CT evaluation of mediastinal lymph nodes in primary Sjögren syndrome, *J Comput Assist Tomogr* 12:199-201, 1988.
16. Anttila S, Sutinen S, Paakko P, et al: Rheumatoid pneumoconiosis in a dolomite worker: a light and electron microscopic, and X-ray microanalytical study, *Br J Dis Chest* 78:195-200, 1984.
17. Armstrong JG, Steele RH: Localised pulmonary arteritis in rheumatoid disease, *Thorax* 37:313-314, 1982.
18. Arnett FC, Edworthy SM, Bloch DA, et al: The American Rheumatism Association 1987 revised criteria for the classification of rheumatoid arthritis, *Arthritis Rheum* 31:315-324, 1988.
19. Aronoff A, Bywaters EGL, Fearnley GR: Lung lesions in rheumatoid arthritis, *Br Med J* 2:228-232, 1955.
20. Arroliga AC, Podell DN, Matthay RA: Pulmonary manifestations of scleroderma, *J Thorac Imag* 7:30-45, 1992.
21. Arshad M, Braun SR, Sunderrajan EV: Severe hypoxemia in farmer's lung disease with normal findings on chest roentgenogram, *Chest* 91:274-275, 1987.
22. Ashba JK, Ghanem MH: The lungs in systemic sclerosis, *Dis Chest* 47:52-64, 1965.
23. Asherson RA, Mackworth-Young CG, Boey ML, et al: Pulmonary hypertension in systemic lupus erythematosus, *Br Med J* 287:1024-1025, 1983.
24. Asherson RA, Sontheimer R: Urticarial vasculitis and syndromes in association with connective tissue diseases, *Ann Rheum Dis* 50:743-744, 1991.
25. Avila R: Extrinsic allergic alveolitis in workers exposed to fish meal and poultry, *Clin Allergy* 1:343-346, 1971.
26. Ayuso MC, Gilabert R, Bombi JA, et al: CT appearance of localized pulmonary amyloidosis, *J Comput Assist Tomogr* 11:197-199, 1987.
27. Badesch DB, King TE, Schwartz MI: Acute eosinophilic pneumonia: a hypersensitivity phenomenon? *Am Rev Respir Dis* 139:249-252, 1989.

28. Ball JD: Tropical pulmonary eosinophilia, *Trans R Soc Trop Med Hyg* 44:237-258, 1950.

29. Banaszak EF, Thiede WH, Fink JN: Hypersensitivity pneumonitis due to contamination of an air conditioner, *N Engl J Med* 283:271-276, 1970.

30. Bariffi F, Pesci A, Bertorelli G, et al: Pulmonary involvement in Sjögren's syndrome, *Respiration* 46:82-87, 1984.

31. Barnes BE: Dermatomyositis and malignancy: a review of the literature, *Ann Intern Med* 84:68-76, 1976.

32. Barrowcliff DF, Arblaster PG: Farmer's lung: a study of an early acute fatal case, *Thorax* 23:490-500, 1968.

33. Basu SP: X-ray appearances in the lung fields in tropical eosinophilia, *Indian Med Gaz* 89:212-217, 1954.

34. Baydur A, Mongan ES, Slager UT: Acute respiratory failure and pulmonary arteritis without parenchymal involvement: demonstration in a patient with rheumatoid arthritis, *Chest* 75:518-520, 1979.

35. Bean WJ: Recognition of ascariasis by routine chest or abdomen roentgenograms, *AJR* 94:379-384, 1965.

36. Beck ER, Hoffbrand BI: Acute lung changes in rheumatoid arthritis, *Ann Rheum Dis* 25:459-462, 1966.

37. Beer DJ: ANCAs aweigh, *Am Rev Respir Dis* 146:1128-1130, 1992.

38. Begbie S, Burgess KR: Maloprim-induced pulmonary eosinophilia, *Chest* 103:305-306, 1993.

39. Beirne GJ, Kopp WL, Zimmerman SW: Goodpasture's syndrome: dissociation from antibodies to glomerular basement membrane, *Arch Intern Med* 132:261-263, 1973.

40. Bell R, Lawrence DS: Chronic pleurisy in systemic lupus erythematosus treated with pleurectomy, *Br J Dis Chest* 73:314-316, 1979.

41. Benedek TG, Zawadzki ZA, Medsger TA: Serum immunoglobulins, rheumatoid factor and pneumoconiosis in coal miners with rheumatoid arthritis, *Arthritis Rheum* 19:731-736, 1976.

42. Bennett RM, O'Connell DJ: Mixed connective tissue disease: a clinicopathologic study of 20 cases, *Semin Arthritis Rheum* 10:25-51, 1980.

43. Benoit FL, Rulon DB, Theil GB, et al: Goodpasture's syndrome, *Am J Med* 37:424-444, 1964.

44. Berendsen HH, Hofstee N, Kapsenberg PD, et al: Bronchocentric granulomatosis associated with seropositive polyarthritis, *Thorax* 40:396-397, 1985.

45. Bergin C, Castellino RA: Mediastinal lymph node enlargement on CT scans in patients with usual interstitial pneumonitis, *AJR* 154:251-254, 1990.

46. Bergin CJ, Müller NL: CT in the diagnosis of interstitial lung disease, *AJR* 145:505-510, 1985.

47. Bergin CJ, Müller NL: CT of interstitial lung disease: a diagnostic approach, *AJR* 148:9-15, 1987.

48. Berkin KE, Vernon DRH, Kerr JW: Lung collapse caused by allergic bronchopulmonary aspergillosis in non-asthmatic patients, *Br Med J* 285:552-553, 1982.

49. Bessis L, Callard P, Gotheil C, et al: High-resolution CT of parenchymal lung disease: precise correlation with histologic findings, *Radiographics* 12:45-58, 1992.

50. Bierny J-P: Multinodular primary amyloidosis of the lung: diagnosis by needle biopsy, *AJR* 131:1082-1083, 1978.

51. Bitterman PB, Crystal RG: Is there a fibrotic gene? *Chest* 78:549-550, 1980.

52. Blank N, Castellino RA, Shah V: Radiographic aspects of pulmonary infection in patients with altered immunity, *Radiol Clin North Am* 11:175-190, 1973.

53. Bloch KJ, Buchanan WW, Wohl MJ, et al: Sjögren's syndrome: a clinical, pathological and serological study of sixty-two cases, *Medicine* 44:187-231, 1965.

54. Boey ML, Colaco CB, Gharavi AE, et al: Thrombosis in systemic lupus erythematosus: striking association with the presence of circulating lupus anticoagulant, *Br Med J* 287:1021-1023, 1983.

55. Bohan A, Peter JB: Polymyositis and dermatomyositis, *N Engl J Med* 292:344-347, 403-407, 1975.

56. Bohan A, Peter JB, Bowman RL, et al: A computer-assisted analysis of 153 patients with polymyositis and dermatomyositis, *Medicine* 56:255-286, 1977.

57. Bombardieri S, Paoletti P, Ferri C, et al: Lung involvement in essential mixed cryoglobulinemia, *Am J Med* 66:748-756, 1979.

58. Bonafede RP, Benatar SR: Bronchocentric granulomatosis and rheumatoid arthritis, *Br J Dis Chest* 81:197-201, 1987.

59. Bonanni PP, Frymoyer JW, Jacox RF: A family study of idiopathic pulmonary fibrosis, *Am J Med* 39:411-421, 1965.

60. Bondi E, Slater S: Tolazamide-induced chronic eosinophilic pneumonia, *Chest* 80:652, 1981.

61. Borge MA, Parker LA, Mauro MA: Amyloidosis: CT appearance of calcified, enlarged periaortic lymph nodes, *J Comput Assist Tomogr* 15:855-857, 1991.

62. Bosch X, Font J, Mirapeix E, et al: Antimyeloperoxidase autoantibody–associated necrotizing alveolar capillaritis, *Am Rev Respir Dis* 146:1326-1329, 1992.

63. Bowey RR: Bird fancier's lung, *Australas Radiol* 18:292-296, 1974.

64. Bowley NB, Hughes JMB, Steiner RE: The chest x-ray in pulmonary capillary haemorrhage: correlation with carbon monoxide uptake, *Clin Radiol* 30:413-417, 1979.

65. Bowley NB, Steiner RE, Chin WS: The chest x-ray in antiglomerular basement membrane antibody disease (Goodpasture's syndrome), *Clin Radiol* 30:419-429, 1979.

66. Boyd JA, Patrick SI, Reeves RJ: Roentgen changes observed in generalized scleroderma, *Arch Intern Med* 94:248-258, 1954.

67. Bradley JD: The pulmonary hemorrhage syndromes, *Clin Chest Med* 3:593-605, 1982.

68. Bradley JD, Pinals RS, Blumenfeld HB, et al: Giant cell arteritis with pulmonary nodules, *Am J Med* 77:135-140, 1984.

69. Brannan HM, Good CA, Divertie MB, et al: Pulmonary disease associated with rheumatoid arthritis, *JAMA* 189:914-918, 1964.

70. Brannan HM, McCaughey WTE, Good CA: The roentgenographic appearance of pulmonary hemorrhage associated with glomerulonephritis, *AJR* 90:83-88, 1963.

71. Braun NMT, Arora NS, Rochester DF: Respiratory muscle and pulmonary function in polymyositis and other proximal myopathies, *Thorax* 38:616-623, 1983.

72. Braun SR, doPico GA, Tsiatis A, et al: Farmer's lung disease: long-term clinical and physiologic outcome, *Am Rev Respir Dis* 119:185-191, 1979.

73. Brennan SR, Daly JJ: Large pleural effusions in rheumatoid arthritis, *Br J Dis Chest* 73:133-140, 1979.

74. Breuer R, Simpson GT, Rubinow A, et al: Tracheobronchial amyloidosis: treatment by carbon dioxide laser photoresection, *Thorax* 40:870-871, 1985.

75. Briggs WA, Johnson JP, Teichman S, et al: Antiglomerular basement membrane antibody–mediated glomerulonephritis and Goodpasture's syndrome, *Medicine* 58:348-361, 1979.

76. Bringhurst LS, Byrne RN, Gershon-Cohen J: Respiratory disease of mushroom workers: farmer's lung, *JAMA* 171:15-18, 1959.

77. Brown J: Primary amyloidosis, *Clin Radiol* 15:358-367, 1964.

78. Browning MJ, Banks RA, Tribe CR, et al: Ten years' experience of an amyloid clinic — a clinicopathological survey, *Q J Med* 54:213-227, 1985.

79. Brunk JR, Drash EC, Swineford O: Rheumatoid pleuritis successfully treated with decortication: report of a case and review of the literature, *Am J Med Sci* 251:545-551, 1966.

80. Bruwer AJ, Kennedy RLJ, Edwards JE: Recurrent pulmonary hemorrhage with hemosiderosis: so-called idiopathic pulmonary hemosiderosis, *AJR* 76:98-107, 1956.

81. Buckley RH, Wray BB, Belmaker EZ: Extreme hyperimmunoglobulinemia E and undue susceptibility to infection, *Pediatrics* 49:59-70, 1972.

82. Bulgrin JG, Dubois EL, Jacobson G: Chest roentgenographic changes in systemic lupus erythematosus, *Radiology* 74:42-48, 1960.

83. Bunch TW, Tancredi RG, Lie JT: Pulmonary hypertension in polymyositis, *Chest* 79:105-107, 1981.

84. Burke GW, Carrington CB, Grinnan R: Pulmonary nodules and rheumatoid factor in the absence of arthritis, *Chest* 72:538-540, 1977.

85. Burrows FGO: Pulmonary nodules in rheumatoid disease: a report of two cases, *Br J Radiol* 40:256-261, 1967.

86. Buschman DL, Waldron JA, King TE: Churg-Strauss pulmonary vasculitis: high-resolution computed tomography scanning and pathologic findings, *Am Rev Respir Dis* 142:458-461, 1990.

87. Butland RJA, Coulson IH: Pulmonary eosinophilia associated with cutaneous larva migrans, *Thorax* 40:76-77, 1985.

88. Byrd RB, Trunk G: Systemic lupus erythematosus presenting as pulmonary hemosiderosis, *Chest* 64:128-129, 1973.

89. Cadhan FT: Asthma due to grain rusts, *JAMA* 83:27, 1924.

90. Cadman EC, Lundberg WB, Mitchell MS: Pulmonary manifestations in Behcet syndrome, *Arch Intern Med* 136:944-947, 1976.

91. Callen JP: Myositis and malignancy, *Clin Rheum Dis* 10:117-130, 1984.

92. Callen JP: Dermatomyositis — an update 1985, *Semin Dermatol* 4:114-125, 1985.

93. Campbell GD, Ferrington E: Rheumatoid pleuritis with effusion, *Dis Chest* 53:521-527, 1968.

94. Campbell JA: A case of Caplan's syndrome in a boiler-scaler, *Thorax* 13:177-180, 1958.

95. Campbell JM: Acute symptoms following work with hay, *Br Med J* 2:1143-1144, 1932.

96. Caplan A: Certain unusual radiological appearances in the chest of coal-miners suffering from rheumatoid arthritis, *Thorax* 8:29-37, 1953.

97. Caplan A, Cowen EDH, Gough J: Rheumatoid pneumoconiosis in a foundry worker, *Thorax* 13:181-184, 1958.

98. Caplan A, Payne RB, Withey JL: A broader concept of Caplan's syndrome related to rheumatoid factors, *Thorax* 17:205-212, 1962.

99. Carette S, Macher AM, Nussbaum A, et al: Severe, acute pulmonary disease in patients with systemic lupus erythematosus: ten years of experience at the National Institutes of Health, *Semin Arthritis Rheum* 14:52-59, 1984.

100. Carlson JE, Villaveces JW: Hypersensitivity pneumonitis due to pyrethrum, *JAMA* 237:1718-1719, 1977.

101. Caro I: Dermatomyositis as a systemic disease, *Med Clin North Am* 73:1181-1192, 1989.

102. Carr DT, Mayne JG: Pleurisy with effusion in rheumatoid arthritis, with reference to the low concentration of glucose in pleural fluid, *Am Rev Respir Dis* 85:345-350, 1962.

103. Carrington CB, Addington WW, Goff AM, et al: Chronic eosinophilic pneumonia, *N Engl J Med* 280:788-798, 1969.

104. Carrington CB, Gaensler EA, Coutu RE, et al: Natural history and treated course of usual and desquamative interstitial pneumonia, *N Engl J Med* 298:801-809, 1978.

105. Carrington CB, Liebow AA: Limited forms of angiitis and granulomatosis of Wegener's type, *Am J Med* 41:497-527, 1966.

106. Carroll KB, Pepys J, Longbottom JL, et al: Extrinsic allergic alveolitis due to rat serum proteins, *Clin Allergy* 5:443-456, 1975.

107. Case record of the Massachusetts General Hospital (Case 39-1981), *N Engl J Med* 305:748-756, 1981.

108. Casselman JW, Lemahieu SF, Peene P, et al: Polychondritis affecting the laryngeal cartilages: CT findings, *AJR* 150:355-356, 1988.

109. Celli BR, Rubinow A, Cohen AS: Patterns of pulmonary involvement in systemic amyloidosis, *Chest* 74:543-547, 1978.

110. Chajek T, Fainaru M: Behcet's disease: report of 41 cases and a review of the literature, *Medicine* 54:179-196, 1975.

111. Chamberlain MA: Behcet's syndrome in 32 patients in Yorkshire, *Ann Rheum Dis* 36:491-499, 1977.

112. Chandler PW, Shin MS, Friedman SE, et al: Radiographic manifestations of bronchiolitis obliterans with organizing pneumonia vs usual interstitial pneumonia, *AJR* 147:899-906, 1986.

113. Chang RW: Cardiac manifestations of SLE, *Clin Rheum Dis* 8:197-206, 1982.

114. Chang-Miller A, Okamura M, Torres VE, et al: Renal involvement in relapsing polychondritis, *Medicine* 66:202-217, 1987.

115. Charles J, Bernstein A, Jones B, et al: Hypersensitivity pneumonitis after exposure to isocyanates, *Thorax* 31:127-136, 1976.

116. Chatgidakis CB, Theron CP: Rheumatoid pneumoconiosis (Caplan's syndrome): a discussion of the disease and a report of a case in a European Witwatersrand goldminer, *Arch Environ Health* 2:397-408, 1961.

117. Cheah FK, Sheppard MN, Hansell DM: Computed tomography of diffuse pulmonary haemorrhage with pathological correlation, *Clin Radiol* 48:89-93, 1993.

118. Cherniack RM, Crystal RG, Kalica AR: Current concepts in idiopathic pulmonary fibrosis: a road map for the future, *Am Rev Respir Dis* 143:680-683, 1991.

119. Choplin RH, Wehunt WD, Theros EG: Diffuse lesions of the trachea, *Semin Roentgenol* 18:38-50, 1983.

120. Christian CL: Systemic lupus erythematosus: clinical manifestations and prognosis, *Arthritis Rheum* 25:887-888, 1982.

121. Christoforidis AJ, Molnar W: Eosinophilic pneumonia: report of two cases with pulmonary biopsy, *JAMA* 173:157-161, 1960.

122. Chumbley LC, Harrison EG, DeRemee RA: Allergic granulomatosis and angiitis (Churg-Strauss syndrome): report and analysis of 30 cases, *Mayo Clin Proc* 52:477-484, 1977.

123. Churg A: Pulmonary angiitis and granulomatosis revisited, *Hum Pathol* 14:868-883, 1983.

124. Churg A, Carrington CB, Gupta R: Necrotizing sarcoid granulomatosis, *Chest* 76:406-413, 1979.

125. Churg J, Strauss L: Allergic granulomatosis, allergic angiitis and periarteritis nodosa, *Am J Pathol* 27:277-301, 1951.

126. Chusid MJ, Dale DS, West BC, et al: The hypereosinophilic syndrome: analysis of fourteen cases with review of the literature, *Medicine* 54:1-27, 1975.

127. Citro LA, Gordon ME, Miller WT: Eosinophilic lung disease (or how to slice P.I.E.), *AJR* 117:787-797, 1973.

128. Clague JE, Pearson MG, Sharma A, et al: Medullary carcinoma of the thyroid presenting as multifocal bronchial carcinoid tumour, *Thorax* 46:67-68, 1991.

129. Clee MD, Lamb D, Urbaniak SJ, et al: Progressive bronchocentric granulomatosis: case report, *Thorax* 37:947-949, 1982.

130. Coel MN, Druger G: Radionuclide detection of the site of hemoptysis, *Chest* 81:242-243, 1982.

131. Cogen FC, Mayock RL, Zweiman B: Chronic eosinophilic pneumonia followed by polyarteritis nodosa complicating the course of bronchial asthma, *J Allergy Clin Immunol* 60:377-382, 1977.

132. Cohen AS: Amyloidosis, *N Engl J Med* 277:522-530, 1967.

133. Cohen HI, Merigan TC, Kosek JC, et al: Sequoiosis, *Am J Med* 43:785-794, 1967.

134. Cohen MI, Gore RM, August CZ, et al: Tracheal and bronchial stenosis associated with mediastinal adenopathy in Wegener's granulomatosis: CT findings, *J Comput Assist Tomogr* 8:327-329, 1984.

135. Cohn RC, Wong R, Spohn WA, et al: Death due to diffuse alveolar hemorrhage in a child with pulmonary venoocclusive disease, *Chest* 100:1456-1458, 1991.

136. Condon RE, Pinkham RD, Hames GH: Primary isolated nodular pulmonary amyloidosis: report of a case, *J Thorac Cardiovasc Surg* 48:498-505, 1964.

137. Constantopoulos SH, Drosos AA, Maddison PJ, et al: Xerotrachea and interstitial lung disease in primary Sjögren's syndrome, *Respiration* 46:310-314, 1984.

138. Constantopoulos SH, Papadimitriou CS, Moutsopoulos HM: Respiratory manifestations in primary Sjögren's syndrome, *Chest* 88:226-229, 1985.

139. Constantopoulos SH, Tsianos EV, Moutsopoulos HM: Pulmonary and gastrointestinal manifestations of Sjögren's syndrome, *Rheum Dis Clin North Am* 18:617-635, 1992.

140. Cook PG, Wells IP, McGavin CR: The distribution of pulmonary shadowing in farmer's lung, *Clin Radiol* 39:21-27, 1988.

141. Cooke NT, Bamji AN, Banks RA, et al: Rheumatoid arthritis and chronic suppurative lung disease, *Thorax* 36:229-230, 1981.

142. Cooper BJ, Bacal E, Patterson R: Allergic angiitis and granulomatosis: prolonged remission induced by combined prednisone-azathioprine therapy, *Arch Intern Med* 138:367-371, 1978.

143. Cooper JAD, White DA, Matthay RA: Drug-induced pulmonary disease. 1. Cytotoxic drugs, *Am Rev Respir Dis* 133:321-340, 1986.

144. Cooper JAD, White DA, Matthay RA: Drug-induced pulmonary disease. 2. Noncytotoxic drugs, *Am Rev Respir Dis* 133:488-505, 1986.

145. Çöplü L, Emri S, Selçuk ZT, et al: Life threatening chylous pleural and pericardial effusion in a patient with Behçet's syndrome, *Thorax* 47:64-65, 1992.

146. Çöplü L, Emri S, Selçuk ZT, et al: Life-threatening chylous pleural and pericardial effusion in a patient with Behçet's syndrome, *Thorax* 47:64-65, 1992.

147. Cordier JF, Loire R, Brune J: Amyloidosis of the lower respiratory tract: clinical and pathologic features in a series of 21 patients, *Chest* 90:827-831, 1986.

148. Cordier JF, Valeyre D, Guillevin L, et al: Pulmonary Wegener's granulomatosis: a clinical and imaging study of 77 cases, *Chest* 97:906-912, 1990.

149. Corrin B, Price AB: Electron microscopic studies on desquamative interstitial pneumonia associated with asbestos, *Thorax* 27:324-331, 1972.

150. Cotton RE, Jackson JW: Localized amyloid "tumours" of the lung simulating malignant neoplasms, *Thorax* 19:97-103, 1964.

151. Craver WL: Solitary amyloid tumour of the lung, *J Thorac Cardiovasc Surg* 49:860-867, 1965.

152. Cream JJ, Gumpel JM, Peachey RDG: Schonlein-Henoch purpura in the adult, *Q J Med* 39:461-484, 1970.

153. Crisp AJ, Armstrong RD, Grahame R, et al: Rheumatoid lung disease, pneumothorax, and eosinophilia, *Ann Rheum Dis* 41:137-140, 1982.

154. Crockford MP, Kerr IH: Relapsing polychondritis, *Clin Radiol* 39:386-390, 1988.

155. Crofton JW, Livingstone JL, Oswald NC, et al: Pulmonary eosinophilia, *Thorax* 7:1-35, 1952.

156. Crosbie WA, Lewis ML, Ramsay ID, et al: Pulmonary amyloidosis with impaired gas transfer, *Thorax* 27:625-630, 1972.

157. Crystal RG, Bitterman PB, Rennard SI, et al: Interstitial lung disease of unknown cause: disorders characterized by chronic inflammation of the lower respiratory tract, *N Engl J Med* 310:154-166, 235-244, 1984.

158. Crystal RG, Fulmer JD, Roberts WC, et al: Idiopathic pulmonary fibrosis: clinical, histologic, radiographic, physiologic, scintigraphic, cytologic and biochemical aspects, *Ann Intern Med* 85:769-788, 1976.

159. Crystal RG, Gadek JF, Ferrans VJ, et al: Interstitial lung disease: current concepts of pathogenesis, staging and therapy, *Am J Med* 70:542-568, 1981.

160. Cugell DW: The hard metal diseases, *Clin Chest Med* 13:269-279, 1992.

161. Cugell DW, Morgan WKC, Perkins DG, et al: The respiratory effects of cobalt, *Arch Intern Med* 150:177-183, 1990.

162. Cullinan SA, Bower GC: Acute pulmonary hypersensitivity to carbamazepine, *Chest* 68:580-581, 1975.

163. Cunningham CDB, Hugh AE: Pneumoconiosis in women, *Clin Radiol* 24:491-493, 1973.

164. Cupps TR, Springer RM, Fauci AS: Chronic, recurrent small-vessel cutaneous vasculitis, *JAMA* 247:1994-1998, 1982.

165. Currie DC, Goldman JM, Cole PJ, et al: Comparison of narrow section computed tomography and plain chest radiography in chronic allergic bronchopulmonary aspergillosis, *Clin Radiol* 38:593-596, 1987.

166. Dalrymple W: Tropical eosinophilia: report of two cases occurring more than a year after departure from India, *N Engl J Med* 252:585-586, 1955.

167. Dalton HR, Featherstone T, Athanasou N: Organ limited amyloidosis with lymphadenopathy, *Postgrad Med J* 68:47-50, 1992.

168. D'Angelo WA, Fries JF, Masi AT, et al: Pathologic observations in systemic sclerosis (scleroderma), *Am J Med* 46:428-440, 1969.

169. Davies BH, Tuddenham EGD: Familial pulmonary fibrosis associated with oculocutaneous albinism and platelet function defect, *Q J Med* 45:219-232, 1976.

170. Davies D: Pyopneumothorax in rheumatoid lung disease, *Thorax* 21:230-235, 1966.

171. Davies D, Lloyd Jones JK: Pulmonary eosinophilia caused by penicillamine, *Thorax* 35:957-958, 1980.

172. Davies JD: Behcet's syndrome with haemoptysis and pulmonary lesions, *J Pathol* 109:351-356, 1973.

173. Davis SD, Berkmen YM, King T: Peripheral bronchial involvement in relapsing polychondritis: demonstration by thin-section CT, *AJR* 153:953-954, 1989.

174. Davis SD, Schaller J, Wedgwood RJ: Job's syndrome: recurrent, "cold," staphylococcal abscesses, *Lancet* 1:1013-1015, 1966.

175. Davison AG, Thompson PJ, Davies J, et al: Prominent pericardial and myocardial lesions in the Churg-Strauss syndrome (allergic granulomatosis and angiitis), *Thorax* 38:793-795, 1983.

176. Degesys GE, Mintzer RA, Vrla RF: Allergic granulomatosis: Churg-Strauss syndrome, *AJR* 135:1281-1282, 1980.

177. deLeon EP, deTavera MP: Pulmonary schistosomiasis in the Philippines, *Dis Chest* 53:154-161, 1968.

178. Den Hertog RW, Wagenaar SS, Westermann CJJ: Bronchocentric granulomatosis and pulmonary echinococcosis, *Am Rev Respir Dis* 126:344-347, 1982.

179. Dennison AR, Watkins RM, Gunning AJ: Simultaneous aortic and pulmonary artery aneurysms due to giant cell arteritis, *Thorax* 40:156-157, 1985.

180. Derderian SS, Tellis CJ, Abbrecht PH, et al: Pulmonary involvement in mixed connective tissue disease, *Chest* 88:45-48, 1985.

181. DeRemee RA, Weiland LH, McDonald TJ: Respiratory vasculitis, *Mayo Clin Proc* 55:492-498, 1980.

182. Desai RA, Mahajan VK, Benjamin S, et al: Pulmonary amyloidoma and hilar adenopathy, *Chest* 76:170-173, 1979.

183. DeWeek AL, Gutersohn J, Butikofer E: La maladie des laveurs de fromage ("Kasenwacherkrankheit"): une forme particuliere du syndrome du poumon du fermir, *Schweiz Med Wochenschr* 99:872-876, 1969.

184. Dickey BF, Myers AR: Pulmonary disease in polymyositis/dermatomyositis, *Semin Arthritis Rheum* 14:60-76, 1984.

185. Dickie HA, Rankin J: Farmer's lung — an acute granulomatous interstitial pneumonia occurring in agricultural workers, *JAMA* 167:1069-1076, 1958.

186. Dieppe PA: Empyema in rheumatoid arthritis, *Ann Rheum Dis* 34:181-185, 1975.

187. Dill J, Ghose T, Landrigan P, et al: Cryptogenic fibrosing alveolitis, *Chest* 67:411-416, 1975.

188. Dinsmore RE, Goodman D, Dreyfuss JR: The air esophagogram: a sign of scleroderma involving the esophagus, *Radiology* 87:348-349, 1966.

189. Ditto WR, Ognibene AJ: Idiopathic pulmonary hemosiderosis without anemia: report of two cases, *Arch Intern Med* 114:490-493, 1964.

190. Doctor L, Snider GL: Diffuse interstitial pulmonary fibrosis associated with arthritis, *Am Rev Respir Dis* 85:413-422, 1962.

191. Dolan DL, Lemmon GB, Teitelbaum SL: Relapsing polychondritis: analytical literature review and studies on pathogenesis, *Am J Med* 41:285-299, 1966.

192. Donabedian H, Gallin JI: The hyperimmunoglobulin E recurrent-infection (Job's) syndrome, *Medicine* 62:195-208, 1983.

193. Donald KJ, Edwards RL, McEvoy JDS: Alveolar capillary basement membrane lesions in Goodpasture's syndrome and idiopathic pulmonary hemosiderosis, *Am J Med* 59:642-649, 1975.

194. Donohugh DL: Tropical eosinophilia: an etiologic inquiry, *N Engl J Med* 269:1357-1364, 1963.

195. Dood AR, Manan JD: Primary diffuse amyloidosis of the respiratory tract, *Arch Pathol* 67:39-42, 1959.

196. do Pico GA: Hazardous exposure and lung disease among farm workers, *Clin Chest Med* 13:311-328, 1992.

197. Dreisin RB: Pulmonary vasculitis, *Clin Chest Med* 3:607-618, 1982.

198. Dreisin RB: New perspectives in Wegener's granulomatosis, *Thorax* 48:97-99, 1993.

199. Drew WL, Finley TN, Golde DW: Diagnostic lavage and occult pulmonary hemorrhage in thrombocytopenic immunocompromised patients, *Am Rev Respir Dis* 116:215-221, 1977.

200. Dubois EL, Chandor S, Friou GJ: Progressive systemic sclerosis (PSS) and localized scleroderma (morphea) with positive LE cell test and unusual systemic manifestations compatible with systemic lupus erythematosus (SLE), *Medicine* 50:199-222, 1971.

201. Dubois EL, Tuffanelli DL: Clinical manifestations of systemic lupus erythematosus: computer analysis of 520 cases, *JAMA* 190:104-111, 1964.

202. du Bois RM: Advances in our understanding of the pathogenesis of fibrotic lung disease, *Respir Med* 84:185-187, 1990.

203. Dubost JJ, Souteyrand P, Sauvezie B: Drug-induced vasculitides, *Baillieres Clin Rheumatol* 5:119-138, 1991.

204. Duke OL: Relapsing polychondritis, *Br J Rheumatol* 27:423-425, 1988.

205. Duncan PE, Griffin JP, Garcia A, et al: Fibrosing alveolitis in polymyositis: a review of histologically confirmed cases, *Am J Med* 57:621-626, 1974.

206. Duncan SC, Winkelmann RK: Cancer and scleroderma, *Arch Dermatol* 115:950-955, 1979.

207. Dyke PC, Demaray MJ, Delavan JW, et al: Pulmonary amyloidoma, *Am J Clin Pathol* 61:301-305, 1974.

208. Eagen JW, Memoli VA, Roberts JL, et al: Pulmonary hemorrhage in systemic lupus erythematosus, *Medicine* 57:545-560, 1978.

209. Ebringer R, Rook G, Swana GT, et al: Autoantibodies to cartilage and type II collagen in relapsing polychondritis and other rheumatic disease, *Ann Rheum Dis* 40:473-479, 1981.

210. Edwards CW: Vasculitis and granulomatosis of the respiratory tract (editorial), *Thorax* 37:81-87, 1982.

211. Efthimiou J, Johnston C, Spiro SG, et al: Pulmonary disease in Behçet's syndrome, *Q J Med* 58:259-280, 1986.

212. Ein ME, Wallace RJ, Williams TW: Allergic bronchopulmonary aspergillosis–like syndrome consequent to aspergilloma, *Am Rev Respir Dis* 119:811-820, 1979.

213. Eisenberg H: The interstitial lung diseases associated with the collagen-vascular disorders, *Clin Chest Med* 3:565-578, 1982.

214. Eisenberg H, Dubois EL, Sherwin RP, et al: Diffuse interstitial lung disease in systemic lupus erythematosus, *Ann Intern Med* 79:37-45, 1973.

215. Ellman P, Ball RE: "Rheumatoid disease" with joint and pulmonary manifestations, *Br Med J* 2:816-820, 1948.

216. Ellman P, Cudkowicz L: Pulmonary manifestations in the diffuse collagen diseases, *Thorax* 9:46-57, 1954.

217. Emanuel DA, Wenzel FJ, Bowerman CI, et al: Farmer's lung: clinical, pathologic and immunologic study of twenty-four patients, *Am J Med* 37:392-401, 1964.

218. Emanuel DA, Wenzel FJ, Lawton BR: Pneumonitis due to *Cryptostroma corticale* (maple bark disease), *N Engl J Med* 274:1413-1418, 1966.

219. Emanuel DA, Wenzel FJ, Lawton BR: Pulmonary mycotoxicosis, *Chest* 67:293-297, 1975.

220. Eng J, Sabanathan S: Airway complications in relapsing polychondritis, *Ann Thorac Surg* 51:686-692, 1991.

221. England DM, Unger JM: Roentgenogram of the month: pleural-based mass in an elderly man with arthralgias, *Chest* 91:603-604, 1987.

222. Epler GR, McLoud TC, Gaensler EA, et al: Normal chest roentgenograms in chronic diffuse infiltrative lung disease, *N Engl J Med* 298:934-939, 1978.

223. Epler GR, Snider GL, Gaensler EA, et al: Bronchiolitis and bronchitis in connective tissue disease: a possible relationship to the use of penicillamine, *JAMA* 242:528-532, 1979.

224. Epstein DM, Gefter WB, Miller WT, et al: Spontaneous pneumothorax: an uncommon manifestation of Wegener granulomatosis, *Radiology* 135:327-328, 1980.

225. Epstein DM, Taormina V, Gefter WB, et al: The hypereosinophilic syndrome, *Radiology* 140:59-62, 1981.

226. Eraut D, Evans J, Caplin M: Pulmonary necrobiotic nodules without rheumatoid arthritis, *Br J Dis Chest* 72:301-306, 1978.

227. Erkan F, Cavdar T: Pulmonary vasculitis in Behçet's disease, *Am Rev Respir Dis* 146:232-239, 1992.

228. Estes D, Christian CL: The natural history of systemic lupus erythematosus by prospective analysis, *Medicine* 50:85-95, 1971.

229. Evans WV, Seaton A: Hypersensitivity pneumonitis in a technician using Pauli's reagent, *Thorax* 34:767-770, 1979.

230. Ewan PW, Jones HA, Rhodes CG, et al: Detection of intrapulmonary hemorrhage with carbon monoxide uptake: application in Goodpasture's syndrome, *N Engl J Med* 295:1391-1396, 1976.

231. Fairfax AJ, Haslam PL, Pavia D, et al: Pulmonary disorders associated with Sjögren's syndrome, *Q J Med* 50:279-295, 1981.

232. Farrelly C, Foster DR: Atypical presentation of Wegener's granulomatosis, *Br J Radiol* 53:721-722, 1980.

233. Farrelly CA: Wegener's granulomatosis: a radiological review of the pulmonary manifestations at initial presentation and during relapse, *Clin Radiol* 33:545-551, 1982.

234. Fauci AS, Harley JB, Roberts WC, et al: The idiopathic hypereosinophilic syndrome: clinical, pathophysiologic, and therapeutic considerations, *Ann Intern Med* 97:78-92, 1982.

235. Fauci AS, Haynes BF, Katz P: The spectrum of vasculitis: clinical, pathologic, immunologic, and therapeutic considerations, *Ann Intern Med* 89:660-676, 1978.

236. Fauci AS, Haynes BF, Katz P, et al: Wegener's granulomatosis: prospective clinical and therapeutic experience with 85 patients for 21 years, *Ann Intern Med* 98:76-85, 1983.

237. Fayemi AO: Pulmonary vascular disease in systemic lupus erythematosus, *Am J Clin Pathol* 65:284-290, 1976.

238. Feigin DS, Friedman PJ: Chest radiography in desquamative interstitial pneumonitis: a review of 37 patients, *AJR* 134:91-99, 1980.

239. Feng PH, Tan TH: Tuberculosis in patients with systemic lupus erythematosus, *Ann Rheum Dis* 41:11-14, 1982.

240. Fenoglio C, Pascal RR: Nodular amyloidosis of the lungs, *Arch Pathol* 90:577-582, 1970.

241. Fergusson RJ, Davidson NM, Nuki G, et al: Dermatomyositis and rapidly progressive fibrosing alveolitis, *Thorax* 38:71-72, 1983.

242. Fewins HE, McGowan I, Whitehouse GH, et al: High definition computed tomography in rheumatoid arthritis associated pulmonary disease, *Br J Rheumatol* 30:214-216, 1991.

243. Fink J: The use of bronchoprovocation in the diagnosis of hypersensitivity pneumonitis, *J Allergy Clin Immunol* 64:590-591, 1979.

244. Fink JN: Hypersensitivity pneumonitis, *Clin Chest Med* 13:303-309, 1992.

245. Fink JN, Schlueter DP, Sosman AJ, et al: Clinical survey of pigeon breeders, *Chest* 62:277-281, 1972.

246. Finley TN, Aronow A, Cosentino AM: Occult pulmonary hemorrhage in anticoagulated patients, *Am Rev Respir Dis* 112:23-29, 1975.

247. Fireman Z, Yust I, Abramov AL: Lethal occult pulmonary hemorrhage in drug-induced thrombocytopenia, *Chest* 79:358-359, 1981.

248. Firestone FN, Joison J: Amyloidosis: a cause of primary tumors of the lung, *J Thorac Cardiovasc Surg* 51:292-299, 1966.

249. Fisher MR, Christ ML, Bernstein JR: Necrotizing sarcoid-like granulomatosis: radiologic-pathologic correlation, *J Can Assoc Radiol* 35:313-315, 1984.

250. Fishman AP: Chronic cor pulmonale, *Am Rev Respir Dis* 114:775-794, 1976.

251. Fitch SJ, Magill HL, Herrod HG, et al: Hyperimmunoglobinemia E syndrome: pulmonary imaging considerations, *Pediatr Radiol* 16:285-288, 1986.

252. Flemming AFS, Fairfax AJ, Arnold AG, et al: Treatment of endobronchial amyloidosis by intermittent bronchoscopic resection, *Br J Dis Chest* 74:183-188, 1980.

253. Flint A: The interstitial lung diseases: a pathologist's view, *Clin Chest Med* 3:491-502, 1982.

254. Foo SS, Weisbrod GL, Herman SJ, et al: Wegener's granulomatosis presenting on CT with atypical bronchovasocentric distribution, *J Comput Assist Tomogr* 14:1004-1006, 1990.

255. Fox B, Seed WA: Chronic eosinophilic pneumonia, *Thorax* 35:570-580, 1980.

256. Fraire AE, Greenberg SD: Carcinoma and diffuse interstitial fibrosis of lung, *Cancer* 31:1078-1086, 1973.

257. Franks T, Weg JG, Harkelroad LE, et al: Pulmonary dysfunction in rheumatoid disease, *Chest* 63:27-34, 1973.

258. Fraser RG: The radiology of interstitial lung disease, *Clin Chest Med* 3:475-484, 1982.

259. Fraser RG, Pare JAP: Extrinsic allergic alveolitis, *Semin Roentgenol* 10:31-42, 1975.

260. Fraser RG, Pare JAP, Pare PD: *Diagnosis of diseases of the chest*, vol 2, ed 3, Philadelphia, 1989, WB Saunders.

261. Frazier AR, Miller RD: Interstitial pneumonitis in association with polymyositis and dermatomyositis, *Chest* 65:403-407, 1974.

262. Friedman PJ: Idiopathic and autoimmune type III-like reactions: interstitial fibrosis, vasculitis, and granulomatosis, *Semin Roentgenol* 10:43-51, 1975.

263. Fritzler MJ, Kinsella TD: The CREST syndrome: a distinct serological entity with anticentromere antibodies, *Am J Med* 69:520-526, 1980.

264. Fromm GB, Dunn LJ, Harris JO: Desquamative interstitial pneumonitis: characterization of free intraalveolar cells, *Chest* 77:552-554, 1980.

265. Fulmer JD: An introduction to the interstitial lung diseases, *Clin Chest Med* 3:457-473, 1982.

266. Fulmer JD, Kaltreider HB: The pulmonary vasculitides, *Chest* 82:615-624, 1982.

267. Furst D, Davis J, Clements P, et al: Abnormalities of pulmonary vascular dynamics and inflammation in early progressive systemic sclerosis, *Arthritis Rheum* 14:1403-1408, 1981.

268. Gaensler EA, Carrington CB: Peripheral opacities in chronic eosinophilic pneumonia: the photographic negative of pulmonary edema, *AJR* 128:1-13, 1977.

269. Gaensler EA, Carrington CB: Open biopsy for chronic diffuse infiltrative lung disease: clinical, roentgenographic, and physiological correlations in 502 patients, *Ann Thorac Surg* 30:411-426, 1980.

270. Gaensler EA, Goff AM, Prowse CM: Desquamative interstitial pneumonia, *N Engl J Med* 274:113-128, 1966.

271. Gallegos FG, Canelas JLC: Hilar enlargement in amyloidosis, *N Engl J Med* 291:531, 1974.

272. Gamsu G, Webb WR: Pulmonary hemorrhage in systemic lupus erythematosus, *J Can Assoc Radiol* 29:66-68, 1978.

273. Gamsu G, Webb WR: Computed tomography of the trachea and mainstem bronchi, *Semin Roentgenol* 18:51-60, 1983.

274. Garber SJ, Wells AU, duBois RM, et al: Enlarged mediastinal lymph nodes in the fibrosing alveolitis of systemic sclerosis, *Br J Radiol* 66:983-986, 1992.

275. Geddes DM: Pulmonary eosinophilia, *J R Coll Phys Lond* 20:139-145, 1986.

276. Geddes DM, Corrin B, Brewerton DA, et al: Progressive airway obliteration in adults and its association with rheumatoid disease, *Q J Med* 46:427-444, 1977.

277. Gefter WB, Epstein DM, Miller WT: Allergic bronchopulmonary aspergillosis: less common patterns, *Radiology* 140:307-312, 1981.

278. Gelpi AP, Mustafa A: *Ascaris*-pneumonia, *Am J Med* 44:377-389, 1968.

279. Genereux GP: The end-stage lung: pathogenesis, pathology and radiology, *Radiology* 116:279-289, 1975.

280. Gertz MA, Kyle RA: Primary systemic amyloidosis — a diagnostic primer, *Mayo Clin Proc* 64:1505-1519, 1989.

281. Gibson GJ: Diaphragmatic paresis: pathophysiology, clinical features, and investigation, *Thorax* 44:960-970, 1989.

282. Gibson GJ, Davis P: Respiratory complications of relapsing polychondritis, *Thorax* 29:726-731, 1974.

283. Gibson GJ, Edmonds JP, Hughes GRV: Diaphragm function and lung involvement in systemic lupus erythematosus, *Am J Med* 63:926-932, 1977.

284. Gibson RN, Morgan SH, Krausz T, et al: Pulmonary artery aneurysms in Behcet's disease, *Br J Radiol* 58:79-82, 1985.

285. Gilliam JN, Smiley JD: Cutaneous necrotizing vasculitis and related disorders, *Ann Allergy* 37:328-339, 1976.

286. Glancy JJ, Elder JL, McAleer R: Allergic bronchopulmonary fungal disease without clinical asthma, *Thorax* 36:345-349, 1981.

287. Glenner GG: Amyloid deposits and amyloidosis: the β fibrilloses, *N Engl J Med* 302:1283-1292, 1333-1343, 1980.

288. Glimp RA, Bayer AS: Fungal pneumonias. 3. Allergic bronchopulmonary aspergillosis, *Chest* 80:85-94, 1981.

289. Gockerman JP: Drug-induced interstitial lung diseases, *Clin Chest Med* 3:521-536, 1982.

290. Goddard P, Cook P, Laszlo G, et al: Relapsing polychondritis: report of an unusual case and a review of the literature, *Br J Radiol* 64:1064-1067, 1991.

291. Gohel VK, Dalinka MK, Israel HL, et al: The radiological manifestations of Wegener's granulomatosis, *Br J Radiol* 46:427-432, 1973.

292. Goldberg B: Radiological appearances in pulmonary aspergillosis, *Clin Radiol* 13:106-114, 1962.

293. Golde DW, Drew WL, Klein HZ, et al: Occult pulmonary haemorrhage in leukaemia, *Br Med J* 2:166-168, 1975.

294. Gondos B: Roentgen manifestations in progressive systemic sclerosis (diffuse scleroderma), *AJR* 84:235-247, 1960.

295. Gonzalez EB, Hayes D, Weedn VW: Chronic eosinophilic pneumonia (Carrington's) with increased serum IgE levels: a distinct subset? *Arch Intern Med* 148:2622-2624, 1988.

296. Gonzalez L, Van Ordstrand HS: Wegener's granulomatosis, *Radiology* 107:295-300, 1973.

297. Good JT, King TE, Antony VB, et al: Lupus pleuritis: clinical features and pleural fluid characteristics with special reference to pleural fluid antinuclear antibodies, *Chest* 84:714-718, 1983.

298. Goodpasture EW: The significance of certain pulmonary lesions in relation to the etiology of influenza, *Am J Med Sci* 158:863-870, 1919.

299. Goodwin SD, Glenny RW: Nonsteroidal anti-inflammatory drug–associated pulmonary infiltrates with eosinophilia, *Arch Intern Med* 152:1521-1524, 1992.

300. Gordonson JS, Sargent N, Jacobson G: Roentgenographic manifestations of pulmonary amyloidosis, *J Can Assoc Radiol* 23:269-272, 1972.

301. Gorevic PD, Katler EI, Agus B: Pulmonary nocardiosis: occurrence in men with systemic lupus erythematosus, *Arch Intern Med* 140:361-363, 1980.

302. Gottlieb AJ, Spiera H, Teirstein AS, et al: Serologic factors in idiopathic diffuse interstitial pulmonary fibrosis, *Am J Med* 39:405-410, 1965.

303. Gottlieb LS, Gold WM: Primary tracheobronchial amyloidosis, *Am Rev Respir Dis* 105:425-429, 1972.

304. Gough J, Rivers D, Seal RME: Pathological studies of modified pneumoconiosis in coal-miners with rheumatoid arthritis (Caplan's syndrome), *Thorax* 10:9-18, 1955.

305. Gould DM, Daves ML: Roentgenologic findings in systemic lupus erythematosus: an analysis of 100 cases, *J Chron Dis* 2:136-145, 1955.

306. Gould DM, Daves ML: A review of roentgen findings in systemic lupus erythematosus (SLE), *Am J Med Sci* 235:596-610, 1958.

307. Goyal R, White CS, Templeton PA, et al: High attenuation mucous plugs in allergic bronchopulmonary aspergillosis: CT appearance, *J Comput Assist Tomogr* 16:649-650, 1992.

308. Graham CM, Stern EJ, Finkbeiner WE, et al: High-resolution CT appearance of diffuse alveolar septal amyloidosis, *AJR* 158:265-267, 1992.

309. Grant IWB: Bronchopulmonary eosinophilia, *Hosp Update* 8:491-501, 1982.

310. Grant IWB, Blyth W, Wardrop VE, et al: Prevalence of farmer's lung in Scotland: a pilot survey, *Br Med J* 1:530-534, 1972.

311. Greenberger PA: Allergic bronchopulmonary aspergillosis and fungoses, *Clin Chest Med* 9:599-608, 1988.

312. Greenberger PA, Patterson R: Allergic bronchopulmonary aspergillosis, *Chest* 91(suppl):165s-171s, 1987.

313. Greene R: Pulmonary aspergillosis: three distinct entities or a spectrum of disease, *Radiology* 140:527-530, 1981.

314. Grenier P, Bletry O, Cornud F, et al: Pulmonary involvement in Behcet disease, *AJR* 137:565-569, 1981.

315. Grigor R, Edmonds J, Lewkonia R, et al: Systemic lupus erythematosus: a prospective analysis, *Ann Rheum Dis* 37:121-128, 1978.

316. Grill C, Szogi S, Bogren H: Fulminant idiopathic pulmonary haemosiderosis, *Acta Med Scand* 171:329-334, 1962.

317. Gross BH: Radiographic manifestations of lymph node involvement in amyloidosis, *Radiology* 138:11-14, 1981.

318. Gross BH, Felson B, Birnberg FA: The respiratory tract in amyloidosis and the plasma cell dyscrasias, *Semin Roentgenol* 21:113-127, 1986.

319. Gross M, Esterly JR, Earle RH: Pulmonary alterations in systemic lupus erythematosus, *Am Rev Respir Dis* 105:572-577, 1972.

320. Groves TS, Fink JN, Patterson R, et al: A familial occurrence of allergic bronchopulmonary aspergillosis, *Ann Intern Med* 91:378-382, 1979.

321. Grunebaum M, Salinger H: Radiologic findings in polymyositis-dermatomyositis involving the pharynx and upper oesophagus, *Clin Radiol* 22:97-100, 1971.

322. Guit GL, Shaw PC, Ehrlich J, et al: Mediastinal lymphadenopathy and pulmonary arterial hypertension in mixed connective tissue disease, *Radiology* 154:305-306, 1985.

323. Gumpel JM: Sjogren's syndrome, *Br Med J* 285:1598, 1982.

324. Gurtte KF, Erbe W, Kreysel HW, et al: Roentgenologic internal observations of the chest in progressive scleroderma, *Fortschr Geb Roentgenstr Nuklearmed* 126:97-101, 1977.

325. Guttadauria M, Ellman H, Kaplan D: Progressive systemic sclerosis: pulmonary involvement, *Clin Rheum Dis* 5:151-166, 1979.

326. Hamman L, Rich AR: Acute diffuse interstitial fibrosis of the lungs, *Bull Johns Hopkins Hosp* 74:177-212, 1944.

327. Hansell DM, Moskovic E: High-resolution computed tomography in extrinsic allergic alveolitis, *Clin Radiol* 43:8-12, 1991.

328. Hanson G, Flod N, Wells I, et al: Bronchocentric granulomatosis: a complication of allergic bronchopulmonary aspergillosis, *J Allergy Clin Immunol* 59:83-90, 1977.

329. Hapke EJ, Seal RME, Thomas GO, et al: Farmer's lung: a clinical, radiographic, functional, and serological correlation of acute and chronic stages, *Thorax* 23:451-468, 1968.

330. Hargreave F, Hinson KF, Reid L, et al: The radiological appearances of allergic alveolitis due to bird sensitivity (bird fancier's lung), *Clin Radiol* 23:1-10, 1972.

331. Hargreave FE, Pepys J, Holford-Strevens V: Bagassosis, *Lancet* 1:619-620, 1968.

332. Hargreave FE, Pepys J, Longbottom JL, et al: Bird breeder's (fancier's) lung, *Lancet* 1:445-449, 1966.

333. Harmon C, Wolfe F, Lillard S, et al: Pulmonary involvement in mixed connective tissue disease (MCTD), *Arthritis Rheum* 19:801, 1976.

334. Harrison NK, Glanville AR, Strickland B, et al: Pulmonary involvement in systemic sclerosis: the detection of early changes by thin section CT scan, bronchoalveolar lavage and 99mTc-DPTA clearance, *Respir Med* 83:403-414, 1989.

335. Harrison NK, Myers AR, Corrin B, et al: Structural features of interstitial lung disease in systemic sclerosis, *Am Rev Respir Dis* 144:706-713, 1991.

336. Hart FD: Complicated rheumatoid disease, *Br Med J* 2:131-135, 1966.

337. Hartman TE, Primack SL, Swensen SJ, et al: Desquamative interstitial pneumonia: thin-section CT findings in 22 patients, *Radiology* 187:787-790, 1993.

338. Harvey AM, Shulman LE, Tumulty PA, et al: Systemic lupus erythematosus: review of the literature and clinical analysis of 138 cases, *Medicine* 33:291-437, 1954.

339. Haslam PL, Turton CWG, Lukoszek A, et al: Bronchoalveolar lavage fluid cell counts in cryptogenic fibrosing alveolitis and their relation to therapy, *Thorax* 35:328-339, 1980.

340. Haupt HM, Moore GW, Hutchins GM: The lung in systemic lupus erythematosus: analysis of the pathologic changes in 120 patients, *Am J Med* 71:791-798, 1981.

341. Haworth SJ, Savage COS, Carr D, et al: Pulmonary haemorrhage complicating Wegener's granulomatosis and microscopic polyarteritis, *Br Med J* 290:1775-1778, 1985.

342. Haynes BF, Allen NB, Fauci AS: Diagnostic and therapeutic approach to the patient with vasculitis, *Med Clin North Am* 70:355-368, 1986.

343. Hayes DS, Posner E: A case of Caplan's syndrome in a roof tile maker, *Tubercle* 41:143-145, 1960.

344. Healy TM: Eosinophilia in bronchogenic carcinoma, *N Engl J Med* 291:794, 1974.

345. Heitzman ER: *The lung: radiologic-pathologic correlations*, St Louis, 1984, Mosby.

346. Heitzman ER, Markarian B, DeLise CT: Lymphoproliferative disorders of the thorax, *Semin Roentgenol* 10:73-81, 1975.

347. Hellems SO, Kanner RE, Renzetti AD: Bronchocentric granulomatosis associated with rheumatoid arthritis, *Chest* 83:831-832, 1983.

348. Hellman D, Laing T, Petri M, et al: Wegener's granulomatosis: isolated involvement of the trachea and larynx, *Ann Rheum Dis* 46:628-631, 1987.

349. Hellman DB, Petri M, Whiting-O'Keefe Q: Fatal infections in systemic lupus erythematosus: the role of opportunistic organisms, *Medicine* 66:341-348, 1987.

350. Henderson AH: Allergic aspergillosis: review of 32 cases, *Thorax* 23:501-512, 1968.

351. Hendrick DJ, Faux JA, Marshall R: Budgerigar-fancier's lung: the commonest variety of allergic alveolitis in Britain, *Br Med J* 2:81-84, 1978.

352. Hendrickson RM, Simpson F: Clofibrate and eosinophilic pneumonia, *JAMA* 247:3082, 1982.

353. Heng MCY: Henoch-Schonlein purpura, *Br J Dermatol* 112:235-240, 1985.

354. Heppleston AG: The pathology of honeycomb lung, *Thorax* 11:77-93, 1956.

355. Herbert FA, Orford R: Pulmonary hemorrhage and edema due to inhalation of resins containing trimellitic anhydride, *Chest* 76:546-551, 1979.

356. Herlinger H: Pulmonary changes in tropical eosinophilia, *Br J Radiol* 36:889-901, 1963.

357. Herman PG, Balikian JP, Seltzer SE, et al: The pulmonary-renal syndrome, *AJR* 130:1141-1148, 1978.

358. Herzog CA, Miller RR, Hoidal JR: Bronchiolitis and rheumatoid arthritis, *Am Rev Respir Dis* 124:636-639, 1981.

359. Hewitt CJ, Hull D, Keeling JW: Fibrosing alveolitis in infancy and childhood, *Arch Dis Child* 52:22-37, 1977.

360. Himmelfarb E, Wells S, Rabinowitz JG: The radiologic spectrum of cardiopulmonary amyloidosis, *Chest* 72:327-332, 1977.

361. Hindle W, Yates DAH: Pyopneumothorax complicating rheumatoid lung disease, *Ann Rheum Dis* 24:57-60, 1965.

362. Hinson KFW, Moon AJ, Plummer NS: Broncho-pulmonary aspergillosis, *Thorax* 7:317, 1952.

363. Hodgson M, Parkinson D, Karpf M: Chest X-rays in hypersensitivity pneumonitis: meta-analysis of a secular trend, *Am J Ind Med* 16:45-53, 1989.

364. Hoehne JH, Reed CE, Dickie HA: Allergic bronchopulmonary aspergillosis is not rare, *Chest* 63:177-181, 1973.

365. Hoffbrand BI, Beck ER: "Unexplained" dyspnoea and shrinking lungs in systemic lupus erythematosus, *Br Med J* 1:1273-1277, 1965.

366. Hoffman GS, Kerr GS, Leavitt RY, et al: Wegener's granulomatosis: an analysis of 158 patients, *Ann Intern Med* 116:488-498, 1992.

367. Hogg JC: The histologic appearance of farmer's lung, *Chest* 81:133-134, 1982.

368. Hogg JC: Chronic interstitial lung disease of unknown cause: a new classification based on pathogenesis, *AJR* 156:225-233, 1991.

369. Holgate ST, Glass DN, Haslam P, et al: Respiratory involvement in systemic lupus erythematosus: a clinical and immunological study, *Clin Exp Immunol* 24:385-395, 1976.

370. Hopkirk JAC, Stark JE: Unilateral pulmonary collapse in asthmatics, *Thorax* 33:207-210, 1978.

371. Hsu BY, Edwards DK, Trambert MA: Pulmonary hemorrhage complicating systemic lupus erythematosus: role of MR imaging in diagnosis, *AJR* 158:519-520, 1992.

372. Hsu JT: Limited form of Wegener's granulomatosis, *Chest* 70:384-385, 1976.

373. Huang C-T, Hennigar GR, Lyons HA: Pulmonary dysfunction in systemic lupus erythematosus, *N Engl J Med* 272:288-293, 1965.

374. Huber DJ, Kobzik L, Solorzano C, et al: Nuclear magnetic resonance spectroscopy of acute and evolving hemorrhage: an in vitro study, *Invest Radiol* 22:632-637, 1987.

375. Hudgson P: Polymyositis and dermatomyositis in adults, *Clin Rheum Dis* 10:85-93, 1984.

376. Hudson AR, Halprin GM, Miller JA, et al: Pulmonary interstitial fibrosis following alveolar proteinosis, *Chest* 65:700-702, 1974.

377. Hughes JP, Stovin PG: Segmental pulmonary artery aneurysms with peripheral venous thrombosis, *Br J Dis Chest* 53:19-27, 1959.

378. Hui AN, Koss MN, Hochholzer L, et al: Amyloidosis presenting in the lower respiratory tract, *Arch Pathol Lab Med* 110:212-218, 1986.

379. Hull S, Mathews JA: Pulmonary necrobiotic nodules as a presenting feature of rheumatoid arthritis, *Ann Rheum Dis* 41:21-24, 1982.

380. Hunninghake GW, Fauci AS: Pulmonary involvement in the collagen vascular diseases, *Am Rev Respir Dis* 119:471-503, 1979.

381. Hurd ER: Extraarticular manifestations of rheumatoid arthritis, *Semin Arthritis Rheum* 8:151-176, 1979.

382. Hyun BH, Diggs CI, Toone EC: Dermatomyositis with cystic fibrosis (honeycombing) of the lung, *Dis Chest* 42:449-453, 1962.

383. Iliffe GD, Pettigrew NM: Hypoventilatory respiratory failure in generalised scleroderma, *Br Med J* 286:337-338, 1983.

384. Im JG, Chung JW, Han SK, et al: CT manifestations of tracheobronchial involvement in relapsing polychondritis, *J Comput Assist Tomogr* 12:792-793, 1988.

385. Im JG, Yeon KM, Han MC, et al: Leptospirosis of the lung: radiographic findings in 58 patients, *AJR* 152:955-959, 1989.

386. Imbeau SA, Cohen M, Reed CE: Allergic bronchopulmonary aspergillosis in infants, *Am J Dis Child* 131:1127-1130, 1977.

387. Imoto EM, Lombard CM, Sachs DPL: Pulmonary capillaritis and hemorrhage: a clue to the diagnosis of systemic necrotizing vasculitis, *Chest* 96:927-928, 1989.

388. International Study Group for Behçet's Disease: Evaluation of diagnostic ("classification") criteria in Behçet's disease—towards internationally agreed criteria, *Br J Rheumatol* 31:299-308, 1992.

389. Ip MSM, Wong MP, Wong KL: Rheumatoid nodules in the trachea, *Chest* 103:301-303, 1993.

390. Isenberg D, Crisp A: Sjögren's syndrome, *Hosp Update* 11:273-283, 1985.

391. Islam N, Haq AWMN: Eosinophilic lung abscess—a new entity, *Br Med J* 1:1810-1811, 1962.

392. Israel HL: The pulmonary manifestations of disseminated lupus erythematosus, *Am J Med Sci* 226:387-392, 1953.

393. Israel HL, Patchefsky AS, Saldana MJ: Wegener's granulomatosis, lymphomatoid granulomatosis and benign lymphocytic angiitis and granulomatosis of lung, *Ann Intern Med* 87:691-699, 1977.

394. Israel MS, Harley BJS: Spontaneous pneumothorax in scleroderma, *Thorax* 11:113-118, 1956.

395. Jackson E, Welch KMA: Mushroom worker's lung, *Thorax* 25:25-30, 1970.

396. Jackson LK: Idiopathic pulmonary fibrosis, *Clin Chest Med* 3:579-592, 1982.

397. Jacome AF: Pulmonary hemorrhage and death complicating anaphylactoid purpura, *South Med J* 60:1003-1004, 1967.

398. Jain VK, Beniwal OP: Unusual presentation of tropical pulmonary eosinophilia, *Thorax* 39:634-635, 1984.

399. Jaspan T, Davison AM, Walker WC: Spontaneous pneumothorax in Wegener's granulomatosis, *Thorax* 37:774-775, 1982.

400. Javaheri S, Lederer DH, Pella JA, et al: Idiopathic pulmonary fibrosis in monozygotic twins: the importance of genetic predisposition, *Chest* 78:591-594, 1980.

401. Jederlinic PJ, Sicilian L, Gaensler EA: Chronic eosinophilic pneumonia: a report of 19 cases and a review of the literature, *Medicine* 67:154-162, 1988.

402. Jenkins MCF, Potter M: Calcified pseudotumoural mediastinal amyloidosis, *Thorax* 46:686-687, 1991.

403. Johnson CL, Bernstein IL, Gallagher JS, et al: Familial hypersensitivity pneumonitis induced by *Bacillus subtilis*, *Am Rev Respir Dis* 122:339-348, 1980.

404. Johnson DA, Drane WE, Curran J, et al: Pulmonary disease in progressive systemic sclerosis: a complication of gastroesophageal reflux and occult aspiration? *Arch Intern Med* 149:589-593, 1989.

405. Johnson TS, White P, Weiss ST, et al: Endobronchial necrobiotic nodule antedating rheumatoid arthritis, *Chest* 82:199-200, 1982.

406. Jolles H, Moseley PL, Peterson MW: Nodular pulmonary opacities in patients with rheumatoid arthritis: a diagnostic dilemma, *Chest* 96:1022-1025, 1989.

407. Jones FL, Blodgett RC: Empyema in rheumatoid pleuropulmonary disease, *Ann Intern Med* 74:665-671, 1971.

408. Jones MB, Osterholm RK, Wilson RB, et al: Fatal pulmonary hypertension and resolving immune-complex glomerulonephritis in mixed connective tissue disease: a case report and review of the literature, *Am J Med* 65:855-863, 1978.

409. Jordan JW: Pulmonary fibrosis in a worker using an aluminum powder, *Br J Ind Med* 18:21-23, 1961.

410. Julsrud PR, Brown LR, Li CY, et al: Pulmonary processes of mature-appearing lymphocytes: pseudolymphoma, well-differentiated lymphocytic lymphoma, and lymphocytic interstitial pneumonitis, *Radiology* 127:289-296, 1978.

411. Jurik AG, Davidsen D, Graudal H: Prevalence of pulmonary involvement in rheumatoid arthritis and its relationship to some characteristics of the patients, *Scand J Rheumatol* 11:217-224, 1982.

412. Jurik AG, Graudal H: Pleurisy in rheumatoid arthritis, *Scand J Rheumatol* 12:75-80, 1983.

413. Kallenbach J, Prinsloo I, Zwi S: Progressive systemic sclerosis complicated by diffuse pulmonary haemorrhage, *Thorax* 32:767-770, 1977.

414. Kanada DJ, Sharma OP: Long-term survival with diffuse interstitial pulmonary amyloidosis, *Am J Med* 67:879-882, 1979.

415. Karam GH, Fulmer JD: Giant cell arteritis presenting as interstitial lung disease, *Chest* 82:781-784, 1982.

416. Karlish AJ: Lung changes in Sjögren's syndrome, *Proc R Soc Med* 62:1042-1043, 1969.

417. Kathuria S, Chejfec G: Fatal pulmonary Henoch-Schonlein syndrome, *Chest* 82:654-656, 1982.

418. Katzenstein A-LA, Askin FB: *Surgical pathology of non-neoplastic lung disease*, ed 2, Philadelphia, 1990, WB Saunders.

419. Katzenstein A-L, Liebow AA, Friedman PJ: Bronchocentric granulomatosis, mucoid impaction, and hypersensitivity reactions to fungi, *Am Rev Respir Dis* 111:497-537, 1975.

420. Kaufman LD, Seidman RJ, Gruber BL: L-Tryptophan associated eosinophilic perimyositis, neuritis and fasciitis: a clinicopathologic and laboratory study of 25 patients, *Medicine* 69:187-199, 1990.

421. Kavuru MS, Adamo JP, Ahmad M, et al: Amyloidosis and pleural disease, *Chest* 98:20-23, 1990.

422. Kay JM, Banik S: Unexplained pulmonary hypertension with pulmonary arteritis in rheumatoid disease, *Br J Dis Chest* 71:53-59, 1977.

423. Kerr IH: Interstitial lung disease: the role of the radiologist, *Clin Radiol* 35:1-7, 1984.

424. Khoo FY, Danaraj TJ: The roentgenographic appearance of eosinophilic lung (tropical eosinophilia), *AJR* 83:251-259, 1960.

425. Kijner CH, Yousem SA: Systemic light chain deposition disease presenting as multiple pulmonary nodules: a case report and review of the literature, *Am J Surg Pathol* 12:405-413, 1988.

426. Kilman WJ: Narrowing of the airway in relapsing polychondritis, *Radiology* 126:373-376, 1978.

427. Kirchner SG, Sivit CJ, Wright PF: Hyperimmunoglobulinemia E syndrome: association with osteoporosis and recurrent fractures, *Radiology* 156:362, 1985.

428. Klein RG, Hunder GG, Stanson AW, et al: Large artery involvement in giant cell (temporal) arteritis, *Ann Intern Med* 83:806-812, 1975.

429. Klion AD, Eisenstein EM, Smirniotopoulos TT, et al: Pulmonary involvement in loiasis, *Am Rev Respir Dis* 145:961-963, 1992.

430. Knobler H, Admon D, Leibovici V, et al: Urticarial vasculitis and recurrent pleural effusion: a systemic manifestation of urticarial vasculitis, *Dermatologica* 172:120-122, 1986.

431. Kohler PF, Gross G, Salvaggio J, et al: Humidifer lung: hypersensitivity pneumonitis related to thermotolerant bacterial aerosols, *Chest* 69:294-296, 1976.

432. Koss MN, Antonovych T, Hochholzer L: Allergic granulomatosis (Churg-Strauss syndrome): pulmonary and renal morphologic findings, *Am J Surg Pathol* 5:21-28, 1981.

433. Koss MN, Hochholzer L, Feigin DS, et al: Necrotizing sarcoid-like granulomatosis: clinical, pathologic, and immunopathologic findings, *Hum Pathol* 11(suppl):510-519, 1980.

434. Koss MN, Robinson RG, Hochholzer L: Bronchocentric granulomatosis, *Hum Pathol* 12:632-638, 1981.

435. Kramer N, Perez H: Pulmonary hypertension in systemic lupus erythematosus: report of four cases and review of the literature, *Semin Arthritis Rheum* 11:177-181, 1981.

436. Kuhlman JE, Hruban RH, Fishman EK: Wegener's granulomatosis: CT features of parenchymal lung disease, *J Comput Assist Tomogr* 15:948-952, 1991.

437. Kus J, Bergin C, Miller R, et al: Lymphocyte subpopulations in allergic granulomatosis and angiitis (Churg-Strauss syndrome), *Chest* 87:826-827, 1985.

438. Kyle RA, Bayrd ED: Amyloidosis: review of 236 cases, *Medicine* 54:271-299, 1975.

439. Kyle RA, Greipp PR: Amyloidosis (AL): clinical and laboratory features in 229 cases, *Mayo Clin Proc* 58:665-683, 1983.

440. Laden SA, Cohen ML, Harley RA: Nodular pulmonary amyloidosis with extrapulmonary involvement, *Hum Pathol* 15:594-597, 1984.

441. Laham MN, Carpeneter JL: *Aspergillus terreus*, a pathogen capable of causing infective endocarditis, pulmonary mycetoma, and allergic bronchopulmonary aspergillosis, *Am Rev Respir Dis* 125:769-772, 1982.

442. Lakhanpal S, Lie JT, Conn DL, et al: Pulmonary disease in polymyositis/dermatomyositis: a clinicopathological analysis of 65 autopsy cases, *Ann Rheum Dis* 46:23-29, 1987.

443. Landman S, Burgener F: Pulmonary manifestations in Wegener's granulomatosis, *AJR* 122:750-757, 1974.

444. Lanham JG, Elkon KB, Pusey CD, et al: Systemic vasculitis with asthma and eosinophilia: a clinical approach to the Churg-Strauss syndrome, *Medicine* 63:65-81, 1984.

445. Larson TS, Hall S, Hepper NGG, et al: Respiratory tract symptoms as a clue to giant cell arteritis, *Ann Intern Med* 101:594-597, 1984.

446. Laufer P, Fink JN, Bruns WT, et al: Allergic bronchopulmonary aspergillosis in cystic fibrosis, *J Allergy Clin Immunol* 73:44-48, 1984.

447. Leatherman JW: Immune alveolar hemorrhage, *Chest* 91:891-897, 1987.

448. Leatherman JW, Davies SF, Hoidal JR: Alveolar hemorrhage syndromes: diffuse microvascular lung hemorrhage in immune and idiopathic disorders, *Medicine* 63:343-361, 1984.

449. Leatherman JW, Sibley RK, Davies SF: Diffuse intrapulmonary hemorrhage and glomerulonephritis unrelated to anti–glomerular basement membrane antibody, *Am J Med* 72:401-410, 1982.

450. Leavitt RY, Fauci AS: Pulmonary vasculitis, *Am Rev Respir Dis* 134:149-166, 1986.

451. Leavitt RY, Fauci AS, Bloch DA, et al: The American College of Rheumatology 1990 criteria for the classification of Wegner's granulomatosis, *Arthritis Rheum* 33:1101-1107, 1990.

452. Lee JS, Im JG, Ahn JM, et al: Fibrosing alveolitis: prognostic implication of ground-glass attenuation at high-resolution CT, *Radiology* 184:451-454, 1992.

453. Lee P, Longevitz P, Alderdice CA, et al: Mortality in systemic sclerosis (scleroderma), *Q J Med* 82:139-148, 1992.

454. Lenclud C, De Vuyst P, Dupont E, et al: Wegener's granulomatosis presenting as acute respiratory failure with anti-neutrophil-cytoplasm antibodies, *Chest* 96:345-347, 1989.

455. LeRoy EC: A brief overview of the pathogenesis of scleroderma (systemic sclerosis), *Ann Rheum Dis* 51:286-288, 1992.

456. Levin DC: Pulmonary abnormalities in the necrotizing vasculitides and their rapid response to steroids, *Radiology* 97:521-526, 1970.

457. Levin DC: Proper interpretation of pulmonary roentgen changes in systemic lupus erythematosus, *AJR* 111:510-517, 1971.

458. L'Huillier J-P, Thoreux P-H, Delaval P, et al: The hyperimmunoglobulinaemia E and recurrent infections syndrome in an adult, *Thorax* 45:707-708, 1990.

459. Lie JT: Disseminated visceral giant cell arteritis, *Am J Clin Pathol* 69:299-305, 1978.

460. Liebow AA: The J. Burns Amberson Lecture — pulmonary angiitis and granulomatosis, *Am Rev Respir Dis* 108:1-18, 1973.

461. Liebow AA, Carrington CB: The interstitial pneumonias. In Simon M, Potchen EJ, LeMay M, eds: *Frontiers of pulmonary radiology*, New York, 1969, Grune & Stratton, pp 102-141.

462. Liebow AA, Carrington CB: The eosinophilic pneumonias, *Medicine* 48:251-285, 1969.

463. Liebow AA, Steer A, Billingsley JG: Desquamative interstitial pneumonia, *Am J Med* 39:369-404, 1965.

464. Lightfoot RW: Churg-Strauss syndrome and polyarteritis nodosa, *Curr Opin Rheum* 3:3-7, 1991.

465. Lillington GA: Ban the boomerang, *Chest* 80:122, 1981.

466. Lindars DC, Davies D: Rheumatoid pneumoconiosis: a study in colliery populations in the East Midlands coalfield, *Thorax* 22:525-532, 1967.

467. Line BR, Fulmer JD, Reynolds HY, et al: Gallium 67 citrate scanning in the staging of idiopathic pulmonary fibrosis: correlation with physiologic and morphological features and bronchoalveolar lavage, *Am Rev Respir Dis* 118:355-365, 1978.

468. Lipinski JK, Wisbrod GL, Sanders DE: Unusual manifestations of pulmonary aspergillosis, *J Can Assoc Radiol* 29:216-220, 1978.

469. Livingstone JL, Lewis JG, Reid L, et al: Diffuse interstitial pulmonary fibrosis: a clinical, radiological and pathological study based on 45 patients, *Q J Med* 33:71-103, 1964.

470. Locke GB: Rheumatoid lung, *Clin Radiol* 14:43-53, 1963.

471. Löffler W: Zur Differential-Diagnose der Lungen Infiltreerunger: III Uber fluchtige Succedan — Infiltrate (mit Eosinophilia), *Beitr Klin Tuberk* 79:368-392, 1932.

472. Lomeo RM, Cornella RJ, Schabel SI, et al: Progressive systemic sclerosis sine scleroderma presenting as pulmonary interstitial fibrosis, *Am J Med* 87:525-527, 1989.

473. Lowe D, Jorizzo J, Hutt MSR: Tumour-associated eosinophilia: a review, *J Clin Pathol* 34:1343-1348, 1981.

474. Luksza AR, Jones DK: Comparison of whole-blood eosinophil counts in extrinsic asthmatics with acute and chronic asthma, *Br Med J* 285:1229-1231, 1982.

475. Lunn JA, Hughes DTD: Pulmonary hypersensitivity to the grain weevil, *Br J Ind Med* 24:158-161, 1967.

476. Lynch DA, Rose CS, Way D, et al: Hypersensitivity pneumonitis: sensitivity of high-resolution CT in a population-based study, *AJR* 159:469-472, 1992.

477. Lynch JP, Hunninghake GW: Pulmonary complications of collagen vascular disease, *Annu Rev Med* 43:17-35, 1992.

478. MacFarlane JD, Dieppe PA, Rigden BG, et al: Pulmonary and pleural lesions in rheumatoid disease, *Br J Dis Chest* 72:288-300, 1978.

479. MacFarlane JD, Franken CK, Van Leeuwen AWFM: Progressive cavitating pulmonary changes in rheumatoid arthritis: a case report, *Ann Rheum Dis* 43:98-101, 1984.

480. Maguire R, Fauci AS, Doppman JL, et al: Unusual radiographic features of Wegener's granulomatosis, *AJR* 130:233-238, 1978.

481. Malo JL, Pepys J, Simon G: Studies in chronic allergic bronchopulmonary aspergillosis: 2 radiological findings, *Thorax* 32:262-268, 1977.

482. Mark EJ, Ramirez JF: Pulmonary capillaritis and hemorrhage in patients with systemic vasculitis, *Arch Pathol Lab Med* 109:413-418, 1985.

483. Martel W, Abell MR, Mikkelsen WM, et al: Pulmonary and pleural lesions in rheumatoid disease, *Radiology* 90:641-653, 1968.

484. Martens J, Demedts M, Vanmeenen MT, et al: Respiratory muscle dysfunction in systemic lupus erythematosus, *Chest* 84:170-175, 1983.

485. Martinez LO: Air in the esophagus as a sign of scleroderma, *J Can Assoc Radiol* 25:234-237, 1974.

486. Martyn JB, Wong MJ, Huang SHK: Pulmonary and neuromuscular complications of mixed connective tissue disease: a report and review of the literature, *J Rheumatol* 15:703-705, 1988.

487. Masi AT, Hunder GG, Lie JT, et al: The American College of Rheumatology 1990 criteria for the classification of Churg-Strauss syndrome allergic granulomatosis and angiitis, *Arthritis Rheum* 33:1094-1100, 1990.

488. Masi AT, Kaslow RA: Sex effects in systemic lupus erythematosus, *Arthritis Rheum* 21:480-484, 1978.

489. Masi AT, Rodnan GP, Medsger TA, et al: Preliminary criteria for the classification of systemic sclerosis (scleroderma), *Arthritis Rheum* 23:581-590, 1980.

490. Mason AMS, McIllmurray MB, Golding PL, et al: Fibrosing alveolitis associated with renal tubular acidosis, *Br Med J* 4:596-599, 1970.

491. Mata JM, Caceres J, Senac JP, et al: General case of the day, *Radiographics* 11:716-718, 1991.

492. Mathieson JR, Mayo JR, Staples CA, et al: Chronic diffuse infiltrative lung disease: comparison of diagnostic accuracy of CT and chest radiography, *Radiology* 171:111-116, 1989.

493. Matthay RA, Schwarz MI, Petty TL, et al: Pulmonary manifestations of systemic lupus erythematosus: review of twelve cases of acute lupus pneumonitis, *Medicine* 54:397-409, 1974.

494. Mayo JR, Müller NL, Road J, et al: Chronic eosinophilic pneumonia: CT findings in six cases, *AJR* 153:727-730, 1989.

495. McAdam LP, O'Hanlan MA, Bluestone R, et al: Relapsing polychondritis: prospective study of 23 patients and a review of the literature, *Medicine* 55:193-215, 1976.

496. McCann BG, Hart GJ, Stokes TC, et al: Obliterative bronchiolitis and upper-zone pulmonary consolidation in rheumatoid arthritis, *Thorax* 38:73-74, 1983.

497. McCarthy DS, Pepys J: Allergic bronchopulmonary aspergillosis: clinical immunology. 1. Clinical features, *Clin Allergy* 1:261-286, 1971.

498. McCarthy DS, Pepys J: Cryptogenic pulmonary eosinophilias, *Clin Allergy* 3:339-351, 1973.

499. McCarthy DS, Simon G, Hargreave FE: The radiological appearances in allergic broncho-pulmonary aspergillosis, *Clin Radiol* 21:366-375, 1970.

500. McCluskey RT, Fienberg R: Vasculitis in primary vasculitides, granulomatoses, and connective tissue diseases, *Hum Pathol* 14:305-315, 1983.

501. McDonald TJ, Neel HB, DeRemee RA: Wegener's granulomatosis of the subglottis and the upper portion of the trachea, *Ann Otol Rhinol Laryngol* 91:588-592, 1982.

502. McGregor MBB, Sandler G: Wegener's granulomatosis: a clinical and radiological survey, *Br J Radiol* 37:430-439, 1964.

503. McGurk FM: Primary bronchial amyloidosis, *Br J Radiol* 41:795-797, 1968.

504. Medical Research Council Symposium: Humidifier fever, *Thorax* 32:653-663, 1977.

505. Medsger TA, Masi AT: Survival with scleroderma. II. A life-table analysis of clinical and demographic factors in 358 male US veteran patients, *J Chronic Dis* 26:647-660, 1973.

506. Melato M, Antonutto G, Falconieri G, et al: Massive amyloidosis of mediastinal lymph nodes in a patient with multiple myeloma, *Thorax* 38:151-152, 1983.

507. Mendeloff J: Disseminated nodular pulmonary ossification in the Hamman-Rich lung, *Am Rev Respir Dis* 103:269-274, 1971.

508. Mendelson DS, Som PM, Crane R, et al: Relapsing polychondritis studied by computed tomography, *Radiology* 157:489-490, 1985.

509. Mendelson EB, Fisher MR, Mintzer RA, et al: Roentgenographic and clinical staging of allergic bronchopulmonary aspergillosis, *Chest* 87:334-339, 1985.

510. Merten DF, Buckley RH, Pratt PC, et al: Hyperimmunoglobulinemia E syndrome: radiographic observations, *Radiology* 132:71-78, 1979.

511. Mertz LE, Conn DL: Vasculitis associated with malignancy, *Curr Opin Rheum* 4:39-46, 1992.

512. Metheny JA: Dermatomyositis: a vocal and swallowing disease entity, *Laryngoscope* 88:147-161, 1978.

513. Metzger WJ, Patterson R, Fink J, et al: Sauna-taker's disease, *JAMA* 236:2209-2211, 1976.

514. Meyer EC, Liebow AA: Relationship of interstitial pneumonia honeycombing and atypical epithelial proliferation to cancer of the lung, *Cancer* 18:322-351, 1965.

515. Miall WE, Caplan A, Cochrane AL, et al: An epidemiological study of rheumatoid arthritis associated with characteristic chest x-ray appearances in coal workers, *Br Med J* 2:1231-1236, 1953.

516. Michet CJ, McKenna CH, Luthra HS, et al: Relapsing polychondritis: survival and predictive role of early disease manifestations, *Ann Intern Med* 104:74-78, 1986.

517. Millar JW: Infectious mononucleosis and fibrosing alveolitis, *Br Med J* 1:612, 1977.

518. Miller LR, Greenberg SD, McLarty JW: Lupus lung, *Chest* 88:265-269, 1985.

519. Mills ES, Mathews WH: Interstitial pneumonitis in dermatomyositis, *JAMA* 160:1467-1470, 1956.

520. Mills JA, Michel BA, Bloch DA, et al: The American College of Rheumatology 1990 criteria for the classification of Henoch-Schönlein purpura, *Arthritis Rheum* 33:1114-1121, 1990.

521. Mindell HJ: Roentgen findings in farmer's lung, *Radiology* 97:341-346, 1970.

522. Mintzer RA, Rogers LF, Kruglik GD, et al: The spectrum of radiologic findings in allergic bronchopulmonary aspergillosis, *Radiology* 127:301-307, 1978.

523. Mohsenifar Z, Tashkin DP, Carson SA, et al: Pulmonary function in patients with relapsing polychondritis, *Chest* 81:711-717, 1982.

524. Moldow RE, Bearman S, Edelman MH: Pulmonary amyloidosis simulating tuberculosis, *Am Rev Respir Dis* 105:114-117, 1972.

525. Monkare S, Ikonen M, Haahtela T: Radiologic findings in farmer's lung: prognosis and correlation to lung function, *Chest* 87:460-466, 1985.

526. Monreal FA: Pulmonary amyloidosis: ultrastructural study of early alveolar septal deposits, *Hum Pathol* 15:388-390, 1984.

527. Montoltu J, Lopez-Pedret J, Andreu L, et al: Eosinophilia in patients undergoing dialysis, *Br Med J* 282:2098, 1981.

528. Morgan PGM, Turner-Warwick M: Pulmonary haemosiderosis and pulmonary haemorrhage, *Br J Dis Chest* 75:225-242, 1981.

529. Morgan RA, Ring NJ, Marshall AJ: Pulmonary alveolar-septal amyloidosis — an unusual radiographic presentation, *Respir Med* 86:345-347, 1992.

530. Morgan WKC: Rheumatoid pneumoconiosis in association with asbestosis, *Thorax* 19:433-435, 1964.

531. Morgan WKC, Wolfel DA: The lungs and pleura in rheumatoid arthritis, *AJR* 98:334-342, 1966.

532. Morrison DA, Goldman AL: Radiographic patterns of drug-induced lung disease, *Radiology* 131:299-304, 1979.

533. Müller NL, Miller RR: Diffuse pulmonary hemorrhage, *Radiol Clin North Am* 29:965-971, 1991.

534. Müller NL, Miller RR, Webb WR, et al: Fibrosing alveolitis: CT-pathologic correlation, *Radiology* 160:585-588, 1986.

535. Müller NL, Staples CA, Miller RR, et al: Disease activity in idiopathic pulmonary fibrosis: CT and pathologic correlation, *Radiology* 165:731-734, 1987.

536. Murphy D, Lane DJ: Pleural effusion in allergic bronchopulmonary aspergillosis: two case reports, *Br J Dis Chest* 75:91-95, 1981.

537. Murphy KC, Atkins CJ, Offer RC, et al: Obliterative bronchiolitis in two rheumatoid arthritis patients treated with penicillamine, *Arthritis Rheum* 24:557-560, 1981.

538. Nada AK, Torres VE, Ryu JH, et al: Pulmonary fibrosis as an unusual clinical manifestation of a pulmonary-renal vasculitis in elderly patients, *Mayo Clin Proc* 65:847-856, 1990.

539. Nader DA, Schillaci RF: Pulmonary infiltrates with eosinophilia due to naproxen, *Chest* 83:280-282, 1983.

540. Naef AP, Savary M, Schmid de Gruneck JM, et al: Amyloid pseudotumor treated by tracheal resection, *Ann Thorac Surg* 23:578-581, 1977.

541. Nakata H, Kimoto T, Nakayama T, et al: Diffuse peripheral lung disease: evaluation by high-resolution computed tomography, *Radiology* 157:181-185, 1985.

542. Nathan PE, Torres AV, Smith AJ, et al: Spontaneous pulmonary hemorrhage following coronary thrombolysis, *Chest* 101:1150-1152, 1992.

543. Naughton M, Fahy J, Fitzgerald MX: Chronic eosinophilic pneumonia: a long-term follow-up of 12 patients, *Chest* 103:162-165, 1993.

544. Neeld DA, Goodman LR, Gurney JW, et al: Computerized tomography in the evaluation of allergic bronchopulmonary aspergillosis, *Am Rev Respir Dis* 142:1200-1205, 1990.

545. Neilly JB, Winter JH, Stevenson RD: Progressive tracheobronchial polychondritis: need for early diagnosis, *Thorax* 40:78-79, 1985.

546. Neva FA, Ottesen EA: Tropical (filarial) eosinophilia, *N Engl J Med* 298:1129-1131, 1978.

547. Newball HH, Brahim SA: Chronic obstructive airway disease in patients with Sjögren's syndrome, *Am Rev Respir Dis* 115:295-304, 1977.

548. Nimelstein SH, Brody S, McShane D, et al: Mixed connective tissue disease: a subsequent evaluation of the original 25 patients, *Medicine* 59:239-248, 1980.

549. Nishimura K, Kitaichi M, Izumi T, et al: Usual interstitial pneumonia: histologic correlation with high-resolution CT, *Radiology* 182:337-342, 1992.

550. Nomura S, Kanoh T: Association of idiopathic pulmonary haemosiderosis with IgA monoclonal gammopathy, *Thorax* 42:696-697, 1987.

551. Noring O, Paaby H: Diffuse amyloidosis in the lower air passages, *Acta Pathol Microbiol Scand* 31:470-475, 1952.

552. Novey HS, Wells ID: Allergic bronchopulmonary aspergillosis caused by *Aspergillus ochraceus*, *Am J Clin Pathol* 70:840-843, 1978.

553. O'Brien IM, Bull J, Creamer B, et al: Asthma and extrinsic allergic alveolitis due to *Merulius lacrymans*, *Clin Allergy* 8:535-542, 1978.

554. O'Duffy JD, Luthra HS, Unni KK, et al: Bronchiolitis in a rheumatoid arthritis patient receiving auranofin, *Arthritis Rheum* 29:556-559, 1986.

555. Oetgen WJ, Mutter ML, Lawless OJ, et al: Cardiac abnormalities in mixed connective tissue disease, *Chest* 83:185-188, 1983.

556. Oh PI, Balter MS: Cocaine induced eosinophilic lung disease, *Thorax* 47:478-479, 1992.

557. O'Hara JM, Szemes G, Lowman RM: The esophageal lesions in dermatomyositis: a correlation of radiologic and pathologic findings, *Radiology* 89:27-31, 1967.

558. Olsen GN, Swenson EW: Polymyositis and interstitial lung disease, *Am Rev Respir Dis* 105:611-617, 1972.

559. Olson J, Colby TV, Elliott CG: Hamman-Rich syndrome revisited, *Mayo Clin Proc* 65:1538-1548, 1990.

560. Olson JC, Kelly KJ, Pan CG, et al: Pulmonary disease with hemorrhage in Henoch-Schoenlein purpura, *Pediatrics* 89:1177-1181, 1992.

561. O'Niell WM, Hammar SP, Bloomer HA: Giant cell arteritis with visceral angiitis, *Arch Intern Med* 136:1157-1160, 1976.

562. Onitsuka H, Onitsuka S, Yokomizo Y, et al: Computed tomography of chronic eosinophilic pneumonia, *J Comput Assist Tomogr* 7:1092-1094, 1983.

563. Onomuro K, Nakata H, Tanaka Y, et al: Pulmonary hemorrhage in patients with systemic lupus erythematosus, *J Thorac Imag* 6:57-61, 1991.

564. Opie LH: The pulmonary manifestations of generalised scleroderma (progressive systemic sclerosis), *Dis Chest* 28:665-680, 1955.

565. Orriols R, Manresa J-M, Aliaga J-L, et al: Mollusk shell hypersensitivity pneumonitis, *Ann Intern Med* 113:80-81, 1990.

566. Ottesen EA, Nutman TB: Tropical pulmonary eosinophilia, *Annu Rev Med* 43:417-424, 1992.

567. Owens GR, Fino GJ, Herbert DL, et al: Pulmonary function in progressive systemic sclerosis: comparison of CREST syndrome variant with diffuse scleroderma, *Chest* 84:546-550, 1983.

568. Owens GR, Follansbee WP: Cardiopulmonary manifestations of systemic sclerosis, *Chest* 91:118-127, 1987.

569. Oxholm P, Bundgaard A, Birk Masden E, et al: Pulmonary function in patients with primary Sjögren's syndrome, *Rheumatol Int* 2:179-181, 1982.

570. Ozsoylu S, Hisconmex G, Berkel I, et al: Goodpasture's syndrome: pulmonary haemosiderosis with nephritis, *Clin Pediatr* 15:358-360, 1976.

571. Pacheco A, Casanova C, Fogue L, et al: Long-term clinical follow-up of adult idiopathic pulmonary hemosiderosis and celiac disease, *Chest* 99:1525-1526, 1991.

572. Pachman LM, Maryjowski MC: Juvenile dermatomyositis and polymyositis, *Clin Rheum Dis* 10:95-115, 1984.

573. Palmer PES, Finley TN, Drew WL, et al: Radiographic aspects of occult pulmonary haemorrhage, *Clin Radiol* 29:139-143, 1978.

574. Panettiere F, Chandler BF, Libcke JH: Pulmonary cavitation in rheumatoid disease, *Am Rev Respir Dis* 97:89-95, 1968.

575. Papathanasiou MP, Constantopoulos SH, Tsampoulas C, et al: Reappraisal of respiratory abnormalities in primary and secondary Sjögren's syndrome: a controlled study, *Chest* 90:370-374, 1986.

576. Park S, Nyhan WL: Fatal pulmonary involvement in dermatomyositis, *Am J Dis Child* 129:723-726, 1975.

577. Parkes WR: *Occupational lung disorders*, ed 2, London, 1982, Butterworths.

578. Parkin TW, Rusted IE, Burchell HB, et al: Hemorrhagic and interstitial pneumonitis with nephritis, *Am J Med* 18:220-236, 1955.

579. Parrillo JE, Borer JS, Herisy WL, et al: The cardiovascular manifestations of the hypereosinophilic syndrome: prospective study of 26 patients, with review of the literature, *Am J Med* 67:572-582, 1979.

580. Parrillo JE, Fauci AS, Wolff SM: Therapy of the hypereosinophilic syndrome, *Ann Intern Med* 89:167-172, 1978.

581. Patchefsky AS, Israel HL, Hoch WS, et al: Desquamative interstitial pneumonia: relationship to interstitial fibrosis, *Thorax* 28:680-693, 1973.

582. Patterson CD, Harville WE, Pierce JA: Rheumatoid lung disease, *Ann Intern Med* 62:685-697, 1965.

583. Patterson R, Irons JS, Kelly JF, et al: Pulmonary infiltrates with eosinophilia, *J Allergy Clin Immunol* 53:245-255, 1974.

584. Pepys J: Pulmonary hypersensitivity disease due to inhaled organic antigens (editorial), *Ann Intern Med* 64:943-948, 1966.

585. Pepys MB: Amyloidosis: some recent developments, *Q J Med* 67:283-298, 1988.

586. Perez HD, Kramer N: Pulmonary hypertension in systemic lupus erythematosus: report of four cases and review of the literature, *Semin Arthritis Rheum* 11:177-181, 1981.

587. Petrie GR, Bloomfield P, Grant IWB, et al: Upper lobe fibrosis and cavitation in rheumatoid disease, *Br J Dis Chest* 74:263-267, 1980.

588. Phelan MS, Kerr IH: Allergic broncho-pulmonary aspergillosis: the radiological appearance during long-term follow-up, *Clin Radiol* 35:385-392, 1984.

589. Phills JA, Harrold AJ, Whiteman GV, et al: Pulmonary infiltrates, asthma, and eosinophilia due to *Ascaris suum* infestation in man, *N Engl J Med* 286:965-970, 1972.

590. Pimentel JC, Avila R: Respiratory disease in cork workers ("suberosis"), *Thorax* 28:409-423, 1973.

591. Pinching AJ, Rees AJ, Pussell BA, et al: Relapses in Wegener's granulomatosis: the role of infection, *Br Med J* 281:836-838, 1980.

592. Pines A, Kaplinsky N, Olchovsky D, et al: Pleuropulmonary manifestations of systemic lupus erythematosus: clinical features of its subgroups, *Chest* 88:129-135, 1985.

593. Pinsker KL, Schneyer B, Becker N, et al: Usual interstitial pneumonia following Texas A2 influenza infection, *Chest* 80:123-126, 1981.

594. Pisetsky DS: Systemic lupus erythematosus, *Med Clin North Am* 70:337-353, 1986.

595. Pistiner M, Wallace DJ, Nessim S, et al: Lupus erythematosus in the 1980s: a survey of 570 patients, *Semin Arthritis Rheum* 21:56-64, 1991.

596. Planes C, Kleinknecht D, Brauner M, et al: Diffuse interstitial lung disease due to AA amyloidosis, *Thorax* 47:323-324, 1992.

597. Poh SC, Tjia TS, Seah HC: Primary diffuse alveolar septal amyloidosis, *Thorax* 30:186-191, 1975.

598. Popper MS, Bogdonoff ML, Hughes RL: Interstitial rheumatoid lung disease, *Chest* 62:243-249, 1972.

599. Portner MM, Gracie WA: Rheumatoid lung disease with cavitary nodules, pneumothorax and eosinophilia, *N Engl J Med* 275:697-700, 1966.

600. Prakash UBS: Lungs in mixed connective tissue disease, *J Thorac Imag* 7:55-61, 1992.

601. Prakash UBS, Luthra HS, Divertie MB: Intrathoracic manifestations in mixed connective tissue disease, *Mayo Clin Proc* 60:813-821, 1985.

602. Prasad M, Bhargava SK, Tewari SG, et al: Radiological changes in tropical pulmonary eosinophilia, *Ind J Radiol* 33:25-31, 1979.

603. Pratt DS, Schwartz MI, May JJ, et al: Rapidly fatal pulmonary fibrosis: the accelerated variant of interstitial pneumonitis, *Thorax* 34:587-593, 1979.

604. Primack SL, Hartman TE, Hansell DM, et al: End-stage lung disease: CT findings in 61 patients, *Radiology* 189:681-686, 1993.

605. Proto AV, Lane EJ: Air in the esophagus: a frequent radiographic finding, *AJR* 129:433-440, 1977.

606. Prowse CB: Amyloidosis of the lower respiratory tract, *Thorax* 13:308-320, 1958.

607. Purnell DC, Baggenstoss AH, Olsen AM: Pulmonary lesions in disseminated lupus erythematosus, *Ann Intern Med* 42:619-628, 1955.

608. Ramirez-R J, Lopez-Majano V, Schultze G: Caplan's syndrome: a clinicopathologic study, *Am J Med* 37:643-652, 1964.

609. Rankin J, Jaeschke WH, Callies QC, et al: Farmer's lung: physiopathologic features of the acute interstitial granulomatous pneumonitis of agricultural workers, *Ann Intern Med* 57:606-626, 1962.

610. Raz I, Okon E, Chajek-Shaul T: Pulmonary manifestations in Behçet's syndrome, *Chest* 95:585-589, 1989.

611. Reed CE, Sosman A, Barbee RA: Pigeon-breeders' lung, *JAMA* 193:261-265, 1965.

612. Reeder MM, Palmer PES: Acute tropical pneumonias, *Semin Roentgenol* 15:35-49, 1980.

613. Rees AJ: Pulmonary injury caused by antibasement membrane antibodies, *Semin Respir Med* 5:264-272, 1984.

614. Reichlin M: Problems in differentiating SLE and mixed connective-tissue disease, *N Engl J Med* 295:1194-1195, 1976.

615. Reingold IM, Mizunoue GS: Idiopathic disseminated pulmonary ossification, *Dis Chest* 40:543-546, 1961.

616. Remy-Jardin M, Beuscart R, Sault MC, et al: Subpleural micronodules in diffuse infiltrative lung diseases: evaluation with thin-section CT scans, *Radiology* 177:133-139, 1990.

617. Remy-Jardin M, Remy J, Wallaert B, et al: Pulmonary involvement in progressive systemic sclerosis: sequential evaluation with CT, pulmonary function tests, and bronchoalveolar lavage, *Radiology* 188:499-506, 1993.

618. Research Committee of the British Thoracic Society: A national survey of bird fanciers' lung: including its possible association with jejunal villous atrophy, *Br J Dis Chest* 78:75-87, 1984.

619. Reyes CN, Wenzel FJ, Lawton BR, et al: The pulmonary pathology of farmer's lung disease, *Chest* 81:142-146, 1982.

620. Reynolds HY: Hypersensitivity pneumonitis, *Clin Chest Med* 3:503-519, 1982.

621. Richards RL, Milne JA: Cancer of the lung in progressive systemic sclerosis, *Thorax* 13:238-245, 1958.

622. Richardson JB, Callen JP: Dermatomyositis and malignancy, *Med Clin North Am* 73:1211-1220, 1989.

623. Richards AG, Barrett GM: Rheumatoid lung changes associated with asbestosis, *Thorax* 13:185-193, 1958.

624. Riddle HFV, Channell S, Blyth W, et al: Allergic alveolitis in a maltworker, *Thorax* 23:271-280, 1968.

625. Road JD, Jacques J, Sparling JR: Diffuse alveolar septal amyloidosis presenting with recurrent hemoptysis and medial dissection of pulmonary arteries, *Am Rev Respir Dis* 132:1368-1370, 1985.

626. Robboy SJ, Minna JD, Colman RW, et al: Pulmonary hemorrhage syndrome as a manifestation of disseminated intravascular coagulation: analysis of ten cases, *Chest* 63:718-721, 1973.

627. Roberts DH, Jimenez JF, Golladay ES: Multiple pulmonary artery aneurysms and peripheral venous thromboses—the Hughes-Stovin syndrome, *Pediatr Radiol* 12:214-216, 1982.

628. Roberts RC, Moore VL: Immunopathogenesis of hypersensitivity pneumonitis, *Am Rev Respir Dis* 116:1075-1090, 1977.

629. Robinson RG, Wehunt WD, Tsou E, et al: Bronchocentric granulomatosis: roentgenographic manifestations, *Am Rev Respir Dis* 125:751-756, 1982.

630. Rodnan GP. In McCarthy DJ, ed: *Progressive systemic sclerosis (scleroderma), arthritis and allied conditions*, ed 9, Philadelphia, 1979, Lea & Febiger, pp 762-809.

631. Rodnan GP, Jablonska S, Medsger TA: Classification and nomenclature of progressive systemic sclerosis (scleroderma), *Clin Rheum Dis* 5:5-13, 1979.

632. Rohatgi PK, Turrisi BC: Bronchocentric granulomatosis and ankylosing spondylitis, *Thorax* 39:317-318, 1984.

633. Roig J, Romeu J, Riera C, et al: Acute eosinophilic pneumonia due to toxocariasis with bronchoalveolar lavage findings, *Chest* 102:294-296, 1992.

634. Romero S, Vela P, Padilla I, et al: Pleural effusion as manifestation of temporal arteritis, *Thorax* 47:398-399, 1992.

635. Roschmann RA, Rothenberg RJ: Pulmonary fibrosis in rheumatoid arthritis: a review of clinical features and therapy, *Semin Arthritis Rheum* 16:174-185, 1987.

636. Rose C, King TE: Controversies in hypersensitivity pneumonitis, *Am Rev Respir Dis* 145:1-2, 1992.

637. Rose GA, Spencer H: Polyarteritis nodosa, *Q J Med* 26:43-81, 1957.

638. Rosenberg M, Patterson R, Mintzer R, et al: Clinical and immunologic criteria for the diagnosis of allergic bronchopulmonary aspergillosis, *Ann Intern Med* 86:405-414, 1977.

639. Rosenberg TF, Medsger TA, DeCicco FA, et al: Allergic granulomatous angiitis (Churg-Strauss syndrome), *J Allergy Clin Immunol* 55:56-67, 1975.

640. Roumm AD, Medsger TA: Cancer and systemic sclerosis: an epidemiologic study, *Arthritis Rheum* 28:1336-1340, 1985.

641. Rubin GD, Edwards DK, Reicher MA, et al: Diagnosis of pulmonary hemosiderosis by MR imaging, *AJR* 152:573-574, 1989.

642. Rubin LA, Urowitz MB: Shrinking lung syndrome in SLE—a clinical pathologic study, *J Rheumatol* 10:973-976, 1983.

643. Rubinow A, Celli BR, Cohen AS, et al: Localized amyloidosis of the lower respiratory tract, *Am Rev Respir Dis* 118:603-611, 1978.

644. Saab SB, Burke J, Hopeman A, et al: Primary pulmonary amyloidosis, *J Thorac Cardiovasc Surg* 67:301-307, 1974.

645. Sackner MA, Akgun N, Kimbel P, et al: The pathophysiology of scleroderma involving the heart and respiratory system, *Ann Intern Med* 60:611-630, 1964.

646. Safirstein BH, D'Souza MF, Simon G, et al: Five-year follow-up of allergic bronchopulmonary aspergillosis, *Am Rev Respir Dis* 108:450-459, 1973.

647. Sahn SA: Immunologic disease of the pleura, *Clin Chest Med* 6:83-102, 1985.

648. Sakula A: Mushroom-worker's lung, *Br Med J* 3:708-710, 1967.

649. Saldana MJ: Necrotizing sarcoid granulomatosis: clinicopathologic observations in 24 patients, *Lab Invest* 38:364, 1978.

650. Saldana MJ: Bronchocentric granulomatosis: clinicopathologic observations in 17 patients, *Lab Invest* 40:281-282, 1979.

651. Salerni R, Rodnan GP, Leon DF, et al: Pulmonary hypertension in the CREST syndrome variant of progressive systemic sclerosis (scleroderma), *Ann Intern Med* 86:394-399, 1977.

652. Salmeron G, Greenberg SD, Lidsky MD: Polymyositis and diffuse interstitial lung disease: a review of the pulmonary histopathologic findings, *Arch Intern Med* 141:1005-1010, 1981.

653. Salvaggio JE, deShazo RD: Pathogenesis of hypersensitivity pneumonitis, *Chest* 89(suppl):190S-193S, 1986.

654. Salvaggio JE, Karr RM: Hypersensitivity pneumonitis: state of the art, *Chest* 75(suppl 2):270-274, 1979.

655. Sams WM, Thorne EG, Small P, et al: Leukocytoclastic vasculitis, *Arch Dermatol* 112:219-226, 1976.

656. Sanchez-Guerrero J, Cesarman G, Alarcon-Segovia D: Massive pulmonary hemorrhage in mixed connective tissue disease, *J Rheumatol* 16:1132-1134, 1989.

657. Sargent EN, Turner AF, Jacobson G: Superior marginal rib defects: an etiologic classification, *AJR* 106:491-505, 1969.

658. Savage COS, Winearls CG, Evans DJ, et al: Microscopic polyarteritis: presentation, pathology and prognosis, *Q J Med* 56:467-483, 1985.

659. Scadding JG: Fibrosing alveolitis, *Br Med J* 2:686, 1964.

660. Scadding JG: The lung in rheumatoid arthritis, *Proc R Soc Med* 62:227-238, 1969.

661. Scadding JG: Diffuse pulmonary alveolar fibrosis, *Thorax* 29:271-281, 1974.

662. Scaddding JG, Hinson KFW: Diffuse fibrosing alveolitis (diffuse interstitial fibrosis of the lungs): correlation of histology at biopsy with prognosis, *Thorax* 22:291-304, 1967.

663. Schatz M, Wasserman S, Patterson R: The eosinophil and the lung, *Arch Intern Med* 142:1515-1519, 1982.

664. Scheer RL, Grossman MA: Immune aspects of the glomerulonephritis associated with pulmonary hemorrhage, *Ann Intern Med* 60:1009-1021, 1964.

665. Schiavi EA, Roncoroni AJ, Puy RJM: Isolated bilateral diaphragmatic paresis with interstitial lung disease: an unusual presentation of dermatomyositis, *Am Rev Respir Dis* 129:337-339, 1984.

666. Schimke RN, Kirkpatrick CH, Delp MH: Calcinosis, Raynaud's phenomenon, sclerodactyly, and telangiectasia, *Arch Intern Med* 119:365-370, 1964.

667. Schmidt HW, McDonald JR, Clagett OT: Amyloid tumours of the lower respiratory tract and mediastinum, *Ann Otol Rhinol Laryngol* 62:880-893, 1953.

668. Schuller H, Bolin H, Linder E, et al: Tumor-forming amyloidosis of the lower respiratory system, *Dis Chest* 42:58-67, 1962.

669. Schumacher HR, Schimmer B, Gordon GV, et al: Articular manifestations of polymyositis and dermatomyositis, *Am J Med* 67:287-292, 1979.

670. Schurawitzki H, Stiglbauer R, Graninger W, et al: Interstitial lung disease in progressive systemic sclerosis: high-resolution CT versus radiography, *Radiology* 176:755-759, 1990.

671. Schwartz HR, McDuffie FC, Black LF, et al: Hypocomplementemic urticarial vasculitis: association with chronic obstructive pulmonary disease, *Mayo Clin Proc* 57:231-238, 1982.

672. Schwartz MI: Pulmonary and cardiac manifestations of polymyositis-dermatomyositis, *J Thorac Imag* 7:46-54, 1992.

673. Schwartz MI, Matthay RA, Sahn SA, et al: Interstitial lung disease in polymyositis and dermatomyositis: analysis of six cases and review of the literature, *Medicine* 55:89-104, 1976.

674. Schwartz MI, Mortenson RL, Colby TV, et al: Pulmonary capillaritis: the association with progressive irreversible airflow limitation and hyperinflation, *Am Rev Respir Dis* 148:507-511, 1993.

675. Scott DCI, Bacon PA, Tribe CR: Systemic rheumatoid vasculitis: a clinical and laboratory study of 50 cases, *Medicine* 60:288-297, 1981.

676. Seal RME, Hapke EJ, Thomas GO, et al: The pathology of the acute and chronic stages of farmer's lung, *Thorax* 23:469-489, 1968.

677. Seaton A, Meland JM, Lapp NL: Remission in Goodpasture's syndrome: report of two patients treated by immunosuppression and review of the literature, *Thorax* 26:683-688, 1971.

678. Segal I, Fink G, Machtey I, et al: Pulmonary function abnormalities in Sjögren's syndrome and the sicca complex, *Thorax* 36:286-289, 1981.

679. Sennekamp J, Niese D, Stroehmann I, et al: Pigeon breeder's lung lacking detectable antibodies, *Clin Allergy* 8:305-310, 1978.

680. Shannon TM, Gale ME: Noncardiac manifestations of rheumatoid arthritis in the thorax, *J Thorac Imag* 7:19-29, 1992.

681. Sharma SS, Reynolds PMG: Broncho-pleural fistula complicating rheumatoid lung disease, *Postgrad Med J* 58:187-189, 1982.

682. Sharp GC, Irvin WS, Tan EM, et al: Mixed connective tissue disease — an apparently distinct rheumatic disease syndrome associated with a specific antibody to an extractable nuclear antigen (ENA), *Am J Med* 52:148-159, 1972.

683. Shaw P, Grossman R, Fernandes BJ: Nodular mediastinal amyloidosis, *Hum Pathol* 15:1183-1185, 1984.

684. Shearn MA: Sjögren's syndrome, *Med Clin North Am* 61:271-282, 1977.

685. Sheppard MN, Harrison NK: Lung injury, inflammatory mediators, and fibroblast activation in fibrosing alveolitis, *Thorax* 47:1064-1074, 1992.

686. Shiel WC, Prete PE: Pleuropulmonary manifestations of rheumatoid arthritis, *Semin Arthritis Rheum* 13:235-243, 1984.

687. Shimizu T, Ehrlich GE, Inaba G, et al: Behçet disease (Behçet syndrome), *Semin Arthritis Rheum* 3:223-260, 1976.

688. Shiue S-T, McNally DP: Pulmonary hypertension from prominent vascular involvement in diffuse amyloidosis, *Arch Intern Med* 148:687-689, 1988.

689. Shlueter DP, Fink JN, Hensley GT: Wood-pulp workers' disease: a hypersensitivity pneumonitis caused by *Alternaria*, *Ann Intern Med* 77:907-914, 1972.

690. Sieber SC, Cuello B, Gelfman NA, et al: Pulmonary capillaritis and glomerulonephritis in an antineutrophil cytoplasmic antibody−positive patient with prior granulomatous aortitis, *Arch Pathol Lab Med* 114:1223-1226, 1990.

691. Sieniewicz DJ, Martin JR: Cavitating rheumatoid nodules in the lungs: follow-up report, *J Can Assoc Radiol* 18:401-403, 1967.

692. Sigurgeirsson B, Lindelöf B, Edhag O, et al: Risk of cancer in patients with dermatomyositis or polymyositis: a population-based study, *N Engl J Med* 326:363-367, 1992.

693. Silver RM, Miller KS: Lung involvement via systemic sclerosis, *Rheum Dis Clin North Am* 16:199-216, 1990.

694. Silver SF, Müller NL, Miller RR, et al: Hypersensitivity pneumonitis: evaluation with CT, *Radiology* 173:441-445, 1989.

695. Silver TM, Farber SJ, Bole GG, et al: Radiological features of mixed connective tissue disease and scleroderma−systemic lupus erythematosus overlap, *Radiology* 120:269-275, 1976.

696. Singer C, Armstrong D, Rosen PP, et al: Diffuse pulmonary infiltrates in immunosupressed patients: prospective study of 80 cases, *Am J Med* 66:110-120, 1979.

697. Slavin RG, Avioli LV: The Jewish Hospital of St. Louis Therapeutic Grand Rounds. 14. Hypersensitivity pneumonitis, *Arch Intern Med* 136:352-356, 1976.

698. Slonim L: Goodpasture's syndrome and its radiological features, *Aust J Radiol* 13:164-172, 1969.

699. Smith MJL, Benson MK, Strickland ID: Coeliac disease and diffuse interstitial lung disease, *Lancet* 1:473-475, 1971.

700. Smith RRL, Hutchins GM, Moore GW, et al: Type and distribution of pulmonary parenchymal and vascular amyloid: correlation with cardiac amyloidosis, *Am J Med* 66:96-104, 1979.

701. Soergel KH, Sommers SC: Idiopathic pulmonary hemosiderosis and related syndromes, *Am J Med* 32:499-511, 1962.

702. Solliday NH, Williams JA, Gaensler EA, et al: Familial chronic interstitial pneumonia, *Am Rev Respir Dis* 108:193-204, 1973.

703. Songcharoen S, Raju SF, Pennebaker JB: Interstitial lung disease in polymyositis and dermatomyositis, *J Rheumatol* 7:353-360, 1980.

704. Specks U, Deremee RA: Granulomatous vasculitis, Wegener's granulomatosis, and Churg-Strauss syndrome, *Rheum Dis Clin North Am* 16:377-397, 1990.

705. Spry CJ: Lung diseases associated with eosinophils. In Goetzl EJ, Kay AB, editors: *Current perspectives in allergy*, vol 1, Edinburgh, 1983, Churchill Livingstone, pp 67-77.

706. Spry CJF, Kumaraswami V: Tropical eosinophilia, *Semin Haematol* 19:107-115, 1982.

707. Stack BHR, Choo-Kang YFJ, Heard BE: The prognosis of cryptogenic fibrosing alveolitis, *Thorax* 27:535-542, 1972.

708. Stack BHR, Grant IWB, Irvine WJ, et al: Idiopathic diffuse interstitial lung disease, *Am Rev Respir Dis* 92:939-948, 1965.

709. Stagg MP, Lauber J, Michalski JP: Mixed essential cryoglobulinemia and adult respiratory distress syndrome: a case report, *Am J Med* 87:445-448, 1989.

710. Stankus RP, Salvaggio JE: Hypersensitivity pneumonitis, *Clin Chest Med* 4:55-62, 1983.

711. Stanton MC, Tange JD: Goodpasture's syndrome (pulmonary haemorrhage associated with glomerulonephritis), *Aust Ann Med* 7:132-144, 1958.

712. Staples CA, Müller NL, Vedal S, et al: Usual interstitial pneumonia: correlation of CT with clinical, functional and radiologic findings, *Radiology* 162:377-381, 1987.

713. Steen VD, Owens GR, Fino GJ, et al: Pulmonary involvement in systemic sclerosis (scleroderma), *Arthritis Rheum* 28:759-767, 1985.

714. Stein MG, Gamsu G, Webb WR, et al: Computed tomography of diffuse tracheal stenosis in Wegener granulomatosis, *J Comput Assist Tomogr* 10:868-870, 1986.

715. Steinberg DL, Webb WR: CT appearances of rheumatoid lung disease, *J Comput Assist Tomogr* 8:881-884, 1984.

716. Stephen JG, Baimbridge MV, Corrin B, et al: Necrotizing "sarcoidal" angiitis and granulomatosis of the lung, *Thorax* 31:356-360, 1976.

717. Stokes TC, McCann BG, Rees RT, et al: Acute fulminating intrapulmonary haemorrhage in Wegener's granulomatosis, *Thorax* 37:315-316, 1982.

718. Strickland B, Strickland NH: Value of high definition, narrow section computed tomography in fibrosing alveolitis, *Clin Radiol* 39:589-594, 1988.

719. Strimlan CV, Rosenow EC, Divertie MB, et al: Pulmonary manifestations of Sjögren's syndrome, *Chest* 70:354-361, 1976.

720. Strohl KP, Feldman NT, Ingram RH: Apical fibrobullous disease with rheumatoid arthritis, *Chest* 75:739-741, 1979.

721. Strumpf IJ, Drucker RD, Anders KH, et al: Acute eosinophilic pulmonary disease associated with the ingestion of l-tryptophan-containing products, *Chest* 99:8-13, 1991.

722. Stupi AM, Steen VD, Owens GR, et al: Pulmonary hypertension in the CREST syndrome variant of systemic sclerosis, *Arthritis Rheum* 29:515-524, 1986.

723. Subbarao K, Jacobson HG: Systemic disorders affecting the thoracic cage, *Radiol Clin North Am* 22:497-517, 1984.

724. Sullivan WD, Hurst DJ, Harmon CE, et al: A prospective evaluation emphasizing pulmonary involvement in patients with mixed connective tissue disease, *Medicine* 63:92-107, 1984.

725. Sunderman FW, Sunderman FW: Loffler's syndrome associated with nickel sensitivity, *Arch Intern Med* 107:405-408, 1961.

726. Sybers RG, Sybers JL, Dickie HA, et al: Roentgenographic aspects of hemorrhagic pulmonary-renal disease (Goodpasture's syndrome), *AJR* 94:674-680, 1965.

727. Tablan OC, Reyes MP: Chronic interstitial pulmonary fibrosis following *Mycoplasma pneumoniae* pneumonia, *Am J Med* 79:268-270, 1985.

728. Talbott JA, Calkins E: Pulmonary involvement in rheumatoid arthritis, *JAMA* 189:911-913, 1964.

729. Tan EM, Cohen AS, Fries JF, et al: The 1982 revised criteria for the classification of systemic lupus erythematosus, *Arthritis Rheum* 25:1271-1277, 1982.

730. Tanoue LT: Pulmonary involvement in collagen vascular disease: a review of the pulmonary manifestations of the Marfan syndrome, ankylosing spondylitis, Sjögren's syndrome, and relapsing polychondritis, *J Thorac Imag* 7:62-77, 1992.

731. Taormina VJ, Miller WT, Gefter WB, et al: Progressive systemic sclerosis subgroups: variable pulmonary features, *AJR* 137:277-285, 1981.

732. Taylor TL, Ostrum H: The roentgenologic evaluation of systemic lupus erythematosus, *AJR* 82:95-107, 1959.

733. Tazelaar HD, Myers JL, Drage CW, et al: Pulmonary disease associated with l-tryptophan-induced eosinophilic myalgia syndrome: clinical and pathologic features, *Chest* 97:1032-1036, 1990.

734. Tazelaar HD, Viggiano RW, Pickersgill J, et al: Interstitial lung disease in polymyositis and dermatomyositis, *Am Rev Respir Dis* 141:727-733, 1990.

735. Teague CA, Doak PB, Simpson IJ, et al: Goodpasture's syndrome: an analysis of 29 cases, *Kidney Int* 13:492-504, 1978.

736. Teixidor HS, Bachman AL: Multiple amyloid tumors of the lung, *AJR* 111:525-529, 1971.

737. Tellesson WG: Rheumatoid pneumoconiosis (Caplan's syndrome) in an asbestos worker, *Thorax* 16:372-377, 1961.

738. Teplick JG, Haskin ME, Nedwich A: The Hughes-Stovin syndrome, *Radiology* 113:607-608, 1974.

739. Terrif BA, Kwan SY, Chan-Yeung MM, et al: Fibrosing alveolitis: chest radiography and CT as predictors of clinical and functional impairment at follow-up in 26 patients, *Radiology* 184:445-449, 1992.

740. Thadani U: Rheumatoid lung disease with pulmonary fibrosis, necrobiotic nodules and pleural effusion, *Br J Dis Chest* 67:146-152, 1973.

741. Theros EG, Reeder MM, Eckert JF: An exercise in radiologic-pathologic correlation, *Radiology* 90:784-791, 1968.

742. Thomas HM, Irwin RS: Classification of diffuse intrapulmonary hemorrhage, *Chest* 68:483-484, 1975.

743. Thomashow BM, Felton CP, Navarro C: Diffuse intrapulmonary hemorrhage, renal failure and a systemic vasculitis, *Am J Med* 68:299-304, 1980.

744. Thompson PJ: Allergic bronchopulmonary fungal disease, *Postgrad Med J* 64(suppl 4):96-102, 1988.

745. Thompson PJ, Citron KM: Amyloid and the lower respiratory tract, *Thorax* 38:84-87, 1983.

746. Thompson PJ, Jewkes J, Corrin B, et al: Primary bronchopulmonary amyloid tumour with massive hilar lymphadenopathy, *Thorax* 38:153-154, 1983.

747. Thompson PL, MacKay IR: Fibrosing alveolitis and polymyositis, *Thorax* 25:504-507, 1970.

748. Tomasi TB, Fudenberg HH, Finby N: Possible relationship of rheumatoid factors and pulmonary disease, *Am J Med* 33:243-248, 1962.

749. Travis WD, Hoffman GS, Leavitt RY, et al: Surgical pathology of the lung in Wegener's granulomatosis: review of 87 open lung biopsies from 67 patients, *Am J Surg Pathol* 15:315-333, 1991.

750. Trell E, Lindstrom C: Pulmonary hypertension in systemic sclerosis, *Ann Rheum Dis* 30:390-400, 1971.

751. Tubbs RR, Benjamin SP, Reich NF, et al: Desquamative interstitial pneumonitis — cellular phase of fibrosing alveolitis, *Chest* 72:159-166, 1977.

752. Tuffanelli DL, Winkelmann RK: Systemic scleroderma, *Arch Dermatol* 84:359-371, 1961.

753. Tuffanelli DL, Winkelmann RK: Scleroderma and its relationship to the "collagenoses": dermatomyositis, lupus erythematosus, rheumatoid arthritis and Sjögren's syndrome, *Am J Med Sci* 243:133-146, 1962.

754. Tukiainen P, Taskinen E, Holsti P, et al: Prognosis of cryptogenic fibrosing alveolitis, *Thorax* 38:349-355, 1983.

755. Tukiainen P, Taskinen E, Korhola O, et al: Farmer's lung: needle biopsy findings and pulmonary function, *Eur J Respir Dis* 61:3-11, 1980.

756. Tumulty PA: The clinical course of systemic lupus erythematosus, *JAMA* 156:947-953, 1954.

757. Tung KT, Wells AU, Rubens MB, et al: Accuracy of the typical computed tomographic appearance of fibrosing alveolitis, *Thorax* 48:334-338, 1993.

758. Turner-Stokes L, Turner-Warwick M: Intrathoracic manifestations of SLE, *Clin Rheum Dis* 8:229-242, 1982.

759. Turner-Warwick M: Fibrosing alveolitis and chronic liver disease, *Q J Med* 37:133-149, 1968.

760. Turner-Warwick M, Assem ESK, Lockwood M: Cryptogenic pulmonary eosinophilia, *Clin Allergy* 6:135-145, 1976.

761. Turner-Warwick M, Burrows B, Johnson A: Cryptogenic fibrosing alveolitis: clinical features and their influence on survival, *Thorax* 35:171-180, 1980.

762. Turner-Warwick M, Dewar A: Pulmonary haemorrhage and pulmonary haemosiderosis, *Clin Radiol* 33:361-370, 1982.

763. Turner-Warwick M, Evans RC: Pulmonary manifestations of rheumatoid disease, *Clin Rheum Dis* 3:549-564, 1977.

764. Turner-Warwick M, Lebowitz M, Burrows B, et al: Cryptogenic fibrosing alveolitis and lung cancer, *Thorax* 35:496-499, 1980.

765. Udwadia FE: Tropical eosinophilia: a review, *Respir Med* 87:17-21, 1993.

766. Unger GF, Scanlon GT, Fink JN, et al: A radiologic approach to hypersensitivity pneumonias, *Radiol Clin North Am* 11:339-356, 1973.

767. Unger J DeB, Fink JN, Unger GF: Pigeon breeder's disease: a review of the roentgenographic pulmonary findings, *AJR* 90:683-687, 1968.

768. Ungerer RG, Tashkin DP, Furst D, et al: Prevalence and clinical correlates of pulmonary arterial hypertension in progressive systemic sclerosis, *Am J Med* 75:65-74, 1983.

769. Van Toorn DW: Coffee worker's lung: a new example of extrinsic allergic alveolitis, *Thorax* 25:399-405, 1970.

770. Velayos EE, Masi AT, Stevens MB, et al: The "CREST" syndrome: comparison with systemic sclerosis (scleroderma), *Arch Intern Med* 139:1240-1244, 1979.

771. Venet A, Caubarrere I, Bonan G: Five cases of immune-mediated amiodarone pneumonitis, *Lancet* 1:962-963, 1984.

772. Vincken W, Roels P: Hypersensitivity pneumonitis due to *Aspergillus fumigatus* in compost, *Thorax* 39:74-75, 1984.

773. Vitali C, Tavoni A, Viegi G, et al: Lung involvement in Sjögren's syndrome: a comparison between patients with primary and with secondary syndrome, *Ann Rheum Dis* 44:455-461, 1985.

774. Vollertsen RS, Conn DL: Vasculitis asssociated with rheumatoid arthritis, *Rheum Dis Clin North Am* 16:445-461, 1990.

775. Wagenaar SSC, Westermann CJJ, Corrin B: Giant cell arteritis limited to large elastic pulmonary arteries, *Thorax* 36:876-877, 1981.

776. Walker WC: Pulmonary infections and rheumatoid arthritis, *Q J Med* 36:239-251, 1967.

777. Walker WC, Wright V: Rheumatoid pleuritis, *Ann Rheum Dis* 26:467-474, 1967.

778. Walker WC, Wright V: Pulmonary lesions and rheumatoid arthritis, *Medicine* 47:501-520, 1968.

779. Wall CP, Gaensler EA, Carrington CB, et al: Comparison of transbronchial and open biopsies in chronic infiltrative lung diseases, *Am Rev Respir Dis* 123:280-285, 1981.

780. Wang CC, Robbins LL: Amyloid disease: its roentgen manifestations, *Radiology* 66:489-501, 1956.

781. Warren J, Pitchenik AE, Saldana MJ: Bronchocentric granulomatosis with glomerulonephritis, *Chest* 87:832-834, 1985.

782. Warrick JH, Bhalla M, Schabel SI, et al: High resolution computed tomography in early scleroderma lung disease, *J Rheumatol* 18:1520-1528, 1991.

783. Watson AJ, Black J, Doig AT, et al: Pneumoconiosis in carbon electrode makers, *Br J Ind Med* 16:274-285, 1959.

784. Watters LC, King TE, Schwartz JA, et al: A clinical, radiographic, and physiologic scoring system for the longitudinal assessment of patients with idiopathic pulmonary fibrosis, *Am Rev Respir Dis* 133:97-103, 1986.

785. Weaver AL, Divertie MB, Titus JL: The lung in scleroderma, *Mayo Clin Proc* 42:754-766, 1967.

786. Weaver AL, Divertie MB, Titus JL: Pulmonary scleroderma, *Dis Chest* 54:490-498, 1968.

787. Webb JKG, Job CK, Gault EW: Tropical eosinophilia: demonstration of microfilariae in lung, liver, and lymph-nodes, *Lancet* 1:835-842, 1960.

788. Webb WR, Gamsu G: Cavitary pulmonary nodules with systemic lupus erythematosus: differential diagnosis, *AJR* 136:27-31, 1981.

789. Webb WR, Goodman PC: Fibrosing alveolitis in patients with neurofibromatosis, *Radiology* 122:289-293, 1977.

790. Weinrib L, Sharma OP, Quismorio FP: A long-term study of interstitial lung disease in systemic lupus erythematosus, *Semin Arthritis Rheum* 20:48-56, 1990.

791. Weiss L: Isolated multiple nodular pulmonary amyloidosis, *Am J Clin Pathol* 33:318-329, 1960.

792. Wells AU, Hansell DM, Corrin B, et al: High resolution computed tomography as a predictor of lung histology in systemic sclerosis, *Thorax* 47:738-742, 1992.

793. Wells AU, Hansell DM, Rubens MB, et al: The predictive value of appearances on thin-section computed tomography in fibrosing alveolitis, *Am Rev Respir Dis* 148:1076-1082, 1993.

794. Wells AU, Rubens MB, du Bois RM, et al: Serial CT in fibrosing alveolitis: prognostic significance of the initial pattern, *AJR* 161:1159-1165, 1993.

795. Wenzel FJ, Gray RL, Roberts RC, et al: Serologic studies in farmer's lung, *Am Rev Respir Dis* 109:464-468, 1974.

796. Wiedemann HP, Matthay RA: Pulmonary manifestations of systemic lupus erythematosus, *J Thorac Imag* 7:1-18, 1992.

797. Wiener-Kronish JP, Solinger AM, Warnock ML, et al: Severe pulmonary involvement in mixed connective tissue disease, *Am Rev Respir Dis* 124:499-503, 1981.

798. Wiggins J, Strickland B, Turner-Warwick M: Combined cryptogenic fibrosing alveolitis and emphysema: the value of high resolution computed tomography in assessment, *Respir Med* 84:365-369, 1990.

799. Wilson SR, Sanders DE, Delarue NC: Intrathoracic manifestations of amyloid disease, *Radiology* 120:283-289, 1976.

800. Winkelmann RK: Dermatomyositis in childhood, *Clin Rheum Dis* 8:353-368, 1982.

801. Winkelmann RK, Ditto WB: Cutaneous and visceral syndromes of necrotizing or "allergic" angiitis: a study of 38 cases, *Medicine* 43:59-89, 1964.

802. Winslow WA, Ploss LN, Loitman B: Pleuritis in systemic lupus erythematosus: its importance as an early manifestation in diagnosis, *Ann Intern Med* 49:70-88, 1958.

803. Winterbauer RH: Multiple telangiectasia, Raynaud's phenomenon, sclerodactyly, and subcutaneous calcinosis: a syndrome mimicking hereditary hemorrhagic telangiectasia, *Bull Johns Hopkins Hosp* 114:361-383, 1964.

804. Winterbauer RH, Hammar SP, Hallman KO, et al: Diffuse interstitial pneumonitis: clinicopathologic correlations in 20 patients treated with prednisone/azathioprine, *Am J Med* 65:661-672, 1978.

805. Witte RJ, Gurney JW, Robbins RA, et al: Diffuse pulmonary alveolar hemorrhage after bone marrow transplantation: radiographic findings in 39 patients, *AJR* 157:461-464, 1991.

806. Wolpert SM, Kahn PC, Farbman K: The radiology of the Hughes-Stovin syndrome, *AJR* 112:383-388, 1971.

807. Wright DO, Gold EM: Loeffler's syndrome associated with creeping eruption (cutaneous helminthiasis), *Arch Intern Med* 78:303-312, 1946.

808. Wright JR, Calkins E: Clinical-pathologic differentiation of common amyloid syndromes, *Medicine* 60:429-448, 1981.

809. Wright PH, Buxton-Thomas M, Kreel L, et al: Cryptogenic fibrosing alveolitis: pattern of disease in the lung, *Thorax* 39:857-861, 1984.

810. Wright PH, Heard BE, Steel SJ, et al: Cryptogenic fibrosing alveolitis: assessment by graded trephine lung biopsy histology compared with clinical, radiographic and physiologic features, *Br J Dis Chest* 75:61-70, 1981.

811. Young ID, Ford SE, Ford PM: The association of pulmonary hypertension with rheumatoid arthritis, *J Rheumatol* 16:1266-1269, 1989.

812. Young RH, Mark GJ: Pulmonary vascular changes in scleroderma, *Am J Med* 64:998-1004, 1978.

813. Yousem SA: The pulmonary pathologic manifestations of the CREST syndrome, *Hum Pathol* 21:467-474, 1990.

814. Yousem SA, Colby TV, Carrington CB: Lung biopsy in rheumatoid arthritis, *Am Rev Respir Dis* 131:770-777, 1985.

815. Yue CC, Park CH, Kushner I: Apical fibrocavitary lesions of the lung in rheumatoid arthritis: report of two cases and review of the literature, *Am J Med* 81:741-746, 1986.

816. Yum MN, Ziegler JR, Walker PD, et al: Pseudolymphoma of the lung in a patient with systemic lupus erythematosus, *Am J Med* 66:172-176, 1979.

817. Zaki I, Wears R, Parnell A, et al: Case report: mediastinal lymphadenopathy in eosinophilic pneumonia, *Clin Radiol* 48:61-62, 1993.

818. Zeiss CR, Burch FX, Marder RJ, et al: A hypocomplementemic vasculitic urticarial syndrome: report of four new cases and definition of the disease, *Am J Med* 68:867-875, 1980.

819. Zimmerman RA, Miller WT: Pulmonary aspergillosis, *AJR* 109:505-515, 1970.

820. Zitnik RJ, Cooper JAD: Pulmonary disease due to antirheumatic agents, *Clin Chest Med* 11:139-150, 1990.

821. Zundel WE, Prior AP: An amyloid lung, *Thorax* 26:357-363, 1971.

822. Zylak CJ, Dyck DR, Warren P, et al: Hypersensitive lung disease due to avian antigens, *Radiology* 114:45-49, 1975.

13 Pulmonary Diseases of Unknown Origin and Miscellaneous Lung Disorders

ALAN G. WILSON

SARCOIDOSIS

Sarcoidosis is a common systemic disease characterized by widespread development of noncaseating epithelioid cell granulomas that eventually either resolve or convert into fibrous tissue. Although the cause and pathogenesis of sarcoidosis are obscure, it is likely to be the result of an immunologically mediated response to one or more unidentified and possibly inhaled agents. Various agents have been suggested, including *Mycobacterium* species (either alone or with viruses), pollen, and inorganic dusts,[367] but no one theory has gained widespread acceptance.

Pathology and clinical features

It is now generally accepted that granuloma formation in the lung is preceded by a mononuclear alveolitis,[306] in which monocytes, macrophages, and lymphocytes accumulate.[77] Early loose granulomas evolve into mature ones that consist of a tightly packed central collection of epithelioid cells, macrophages, and multinucleate giant cells surrounded by lymphocytes, monocytes, and fibroblasts.[367] Morphologic evidence suggests that all three cellular elements in the center of granulomas are secre-

tory and that the surrounding lymphocytes are activated T cells. Necrosis is rare and when it does occur is minimal and confined to the center of granulomas.[107] Granulomas are distributed along lymphatic pathways and are characteristically found along bronchovascular bundles, interlobular septa, and pleura.[177,251] Granulomas remain stable for months or years, and then, in about 80% of cases, resolve completely. In the remaining 20% the granulomas become obliterated by centripetal fibrosis that may develop into extensive interstitial fibrosis, with destruction of lung architecture and the eventual production of an end-stage lung.

Sarcoid granulomas are nonspecific and resemble those in many other granulomatous processes[161] except granulomas resulting from tuberculosis, in which some caseous necrosis usually is seen. Sarcoid granulomas are found in all organs and tissues, although some, like the adrenal gland, are not commonly involved.[219] The generalized nature of the sarcoid response is an important feature that distinguishes sarcoidosis from various local sarcoidlike responses associated with neoplastic conditions.[123]

Incidence rates for sarcoidosis vary greatly from country to country and depend, among other factors, on race, the sophistication of medical care, and use of screening programs. Quoted figures are on the order of 1 to 10 cases per 100,000 population per year, but this is almost certainly an underestimate because many cases remain subclinical.[198] Sarcoidosis occurs with about 10 times greater frequency in blacks than in whites.[19,94,219,314] About 1% to 3% of patients with sarcoidosis have a family history of the disease.[219,316,333] The HLA type does not influence susceptibility, but it does have some effect on prognosis.[112] A number of conditions have been suggested as showing an association with sarcoidosis; the relationship is best established for tuberculosis.[206,318,346] In a series of 425 patients with sarcoidosis, tuberculosis immediately preceded sarcoidosis in 1.6% and sarcoidosis developed into overt tuberculosis in 1.9%.[317]

Presentation is most common between 20 and 40 years of age,[156,185,219] but the age range is wide, even including the first year of life[140] and the eighth decade.[219] Whites have a more or less equal sex incidence or slight female preponderance, whereas blacks have a definite twofold to threefold excess in females.[108,156,185,219,303]

The mode of presentation varies greatly among series, depending particularly on racial mix and the use of screening radiography. In white-dominated series, presentation as an incidental radiographic finding is common and may occur in 40% to 50% of cases.[162,302] Respiratory illness (21%), erythema nodosum (16%), ocular symptoms (7%), and other skin lesions (4%)[162] represent the other common presentations. In predominantly black series, respiratory and systemic symptoms such as fatigue, malaise, weakness, weight loss, and fever are most common.[330] A striking difference between blacks and whites at presentation is the frequency of erythema nodosum. This finding is uncommon in blacks but very common in whites, particularly in the United Kingdom, where 30% to 40% of patients present with the condition[94,146,162,234] often as part of the erythema nodosum/febrile arthralgia syndrome, with or without uveitis.[316] In general the disease in blacks is later in onset, involves peripheral nodes, skin, and eyes, and is more likely to become chronic and disseminated. The prognosis is worse in blacks than in whites.*

Findings on investigation

Laboratory investigations may show anemia, leukopenia, or a raised erythrocyte sedimentation rate. A significant blood eosinophilia is seen in up to one fourth of patients.[219] Both hypercalcemia and hypercalciuria are recorded and may become prominent features.[367] The former is often transient and occurs in 10% to 20% of patients.[161,219,340] Hypercalcemia can cause metastatic calcification and renal failure.[185] Hypercalciuria is two to three times more common than hypercalcemia.[232,234] Disordered calcium homeostasis is caused by synthesis of

1,25-dihydroxyvitamin D by activated sarcoid macrophages and is rapidly responsive to steroids.[313]

Serum levels of angiotensin-converting enzyme (ACE) are raised in about 50% to 60% of patients because of its production by activated macrophages.[203,204] Serum ACE levels correlate with the activity of clinical disease as a whole[302] but not convincingly with the degree and activity of pulmonary disease.[322,367] The presence of raised levels of serum ACE is not specific for sarcoidosis, and the false-positive rate is approximately 10%.[330]

Various immunologic derangements are seen with sarcoidosis. Cutaneous anergy is well recognized. About two thirds of patients have a negative tuberculin test, and in many of the remainder it is only weakly positive.[162,219,330] Cutaneous anergy is probably related to the relative abundance of suppressor T cells in the peripheral blood following sequestration of helper T cells in active sarcoid lesions. Activated helper T cells stimulate nonspecific antibody production by B cells,[367] producing a whole range of antibodies[161] and resulting in hypergammaglobulinemia[367] in about 50% of patients, particularly in blacks.[162] In the acute disease about half of the patients have circulating immune complexes, the presence of which correlates with various clinical features such as erythema nodosum.[286]

Bronchoalveolar lavage (BAL) provides information concerning the type of alveolitis and the degree of activity.[77] In active sarcoidosis BAL shows an increase in T lymphocytes (particularly activated helper cells)[77,330] and to a lesser extent macrophages. The usefulness of BAL to predict outcome and to monitor treatment, however, is still debated.[367]

Another investigation that has been used during the last decade in much the same way as BAL is gallium scintigraphy.[205] Forty-eight hours after intravenous administration of gallium citrate, normally a little uptake is seen in bone but none in the lung or mediastinum. However, in sarcoidosis both lung and mediastinal (nodal) uptake is seen.[139,155,223] What cells take up the agent is still not exactly clear. Some studies suggest activated macrophages,[262] while other workers on indirect evidence suggest activated T lymphocytes.[77] Irrespective of which cell is involved, it seems possible that gallium uptake may reflect the degree of "activity" of the sarcoid process. Unfortunately, there is no consensus regarding the criteria of activity and no clear-cut way of using gallium scanning has emerged; its clinical value therefore remains undefined.[12,16,296] Respiratory function tests are commonly deranged in sarcoidosis with the following results: a decrease in total lung capacity, a reduced diffusing capacity, a restrictive defect of ventilatory capacity, reduced compliance, and, in advanced disease, abnormal airway function.[199,318,380] A loose relationship exists between respiratory function tests and chest radiographic changes.[380] The mean values for respiratory function tests correlate well with the radiographic stage, becoming worse from stage I to stage III.[237]

---

*References 18, 19, 94, 146, 159, 363.

However, individual exceptions to this correlation are common. For example, several studies have shown that about 50% of patients in stage I have a diffusion defect.[147,331,380] Also, respiratory function tests can give results in the normal range in stage II and III disease.[147] Discrepancies between radiographs and function are most likely to arise when patients are treated with steroids, which commonly improve function in the face of an unchanging chest radiograph.[380]

Diagnosis and prognosis

A firm diagnosis of sarcoidosis can be made with consistent clinicoradiologic findings and histologic evidence of widespread noncaseating epithelioid cell granulomas in more than one organ or a positive Kveim skin test. In clinical practice the organs most commonly sampled are lymph nodes, liver, and lung. In sarcoidosis, even though the chest radiograph shows adenopathy with clear lungs, on pathologic study the lung is diffusely infiltrated with granulomas.[305] Lung biopsies are usually performed by means of a fiberoptic bronchoscope, and, provided that enough tissue samples are obtained,[114] positive rates for the test are in the order of 90%.[190,242,299,361]

A large number of conditions can produce granulomatous lesions,[161] and if the diagnosis of sarcoidosis rests on histologic appearances, these other conditions must be excluded as far as possible by history, special histologic stains, and microbiologic culture. Establishing the widespread nature of the granulomatous process is also important, since local sarcoidlike reactions can be produced by a number of primary processes, including lymphoma and carcinoma.[106,123] A common everyday practice is to accept a diagnosis of sarcoidosis without biopsy, provided that clinical, laboratory, and radiologic features are typical, particularly when they correspond to a classic syndrome such as erythema nodosum, arthropathy, and bilateral hilar adenopathy. When the clinical diagnosis is less firmly based, histologic proof, either from biopsy or a Kveim test, is mandatory.

The Kveim test[255] is based on the fact that in sarcoidosis the intracutaneous injection of a saline suspension of human sarcoid tissue leads to the development of a granulomatous nodule within 4 to 6 weeks. About two thirds to three fourths of tests are positive in the first 2 years after symptoms appear, with the positive rate decreasing with time[337] and with the development of stage II disease.[33,176,337] About a 2% false-positive rate is seen, especially in Crohn's disease.

Of all organs the lung is the most commonly involved in sarcoidosis and accounts for most of the morbidity and mortality.[367] When death occurs from sarcoidosis, it is most commonly related to pulmonary involvement: cor pulmonale, hemorrhage, mycetoma, and respiratory failure. In two series of 85 sarcoid-related deaths, 67% resulted from pulmonary involvement.[148,167] In several large series, overall mortality ranged between 2.2% and 7.6%.*

Staging of sarcoidosis

Sarcoidosis is commonly staged according to its appearance on the chest radiograph. Several different classifications have been proposed. DeRemee[87] recently reviewed the subject and recommended the following:

Stage 0 — clear chest radiograph
Stage I — node enlargement only
Stage II — node enlargement and parenchymal shadowing
Stage III — parenchymal shadowing alone

The objection to this system is that it does not permit a distinction between transient (nonfibrotic) and fixed (fibrotic) parenchymal opacity. Several other systems in use attempt to overcome this problem. DeRemee maintains, and we agree, that the distinction between fibrotic and nonfibrotic shadowing cannot be reliably made based on radiologic criteria.[87] Another objection is that the term "stage" suggests a temporal evolution from stage 0 to a higher stage, which almost certainly does not happen in every patient. For example, stage 0 is a common late finding, and cases are seen in which it seems unlikely that stage III was preceded by a stage I or II. Nevertheless, patients commonly pass sequentially from stage I to III, and the term is so hallowed by use that it is unlikely to be changed.

At the time of presentation the percentages of patients at each stage are stage 0, 5% to 15%; stage I, 45% to 65%; stage II, 30% to 40%; and stage III, 10% to 15%. The stage at presentation is generally considered to correlate with prognosis[337]; it therefore provides a useful method for characterizing patient groups in studies and a guide to clinical management. In the worldwide series of 3679 patients,[162] 65% of stage I patients showed resolution of the chest radiographic findings. The corresponding figures for stages II and III were 49% and 20%, respectively. Not all workers, however, agree on a correlation between outcome and stage.[152]

Chest radiology

The chest radiograph is abnormal at some point in 90% to 95% of patients with sarcoidosis.[219] About 5% to 15% of patients have a clear chest radiograph when examined initially,† but pulmonary granulomas can be demonstrated on biopsy in these patients despite the absence of radiologic change.[224,294]

Lymph nodes

Lymphadenopathy is the most common intrathoracic manifestation of sarcoidosis, occurring in 75% to 80% of

---

*References 96, 148, 162, 219, 338, 346.
†References 156, 161, 162, 185, 219, 234.

patients at some point in their illness.[162,185,338] Pulmonary shadowing as a result of sarcoidosis that antedates adenopathy is extremely rare[25,102,206,230] and as a working rule can be discounted. Possibly less rare, but still extremely unusual, is thoracic adenopathy that develops after documented involvement of extrathoracic sites such as eyes and skin.[96,211,248,303]

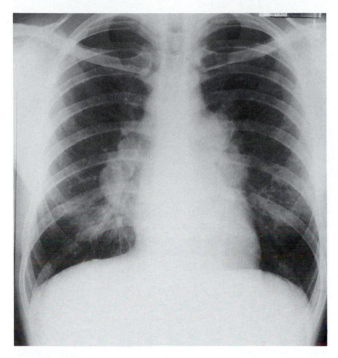

FIGURE 13-1
Sarcoidosis showing characteristic lymphadenopathy. Hilar nodes are symmetrically enlarged, with involvement of both proximal tracheobronchial and more distal bronchopulmonary nodes. Right paratracheal and aortopulmonary nodes are mildly affected.

Symmetric, bilateral hilar adenopathy with some form of paratracheal adenopathy is the classic pattern in sarcoidosis (Figure 13-1). In one series of 150 patients with sarcoidosis and an abnormal chest radiograph, about 30% had bilateral hilar lymphadenopathy (BHL) alone, 30% had BHL with right paratracheal adenopathy, and 30% had BHL with bilateral paratracheal adenopathy.[186] This series and earlier ones probably underestimate the prevalence of left paratracheal adenopathy, which is not as easy to detect as right-sided adenopathy.[26] The lowest part of the left paratracheal chain, the aortopulmonary (ductus) nodes, have only recently received attention, and these are seen to be enlarged in most patients,[386] producing a characteristic local convexity in the aortopulmonary window (Figure 13-2).[15] Isolated paratracheal or isolated aortopulmonary adenopathy has rarely been recorded in sarcoidosis.[15,298]

Bilateral hilar adenopathy is common to all of these major patterns and is the most characteristic aspect of nodal enlargement in sarcoidosis. The degree of hilar node enlargement ranges from barely detectable to massive, in which case nodes may reach halfway to the chest wall (Figure 13-3). The outer margins of the hila are usually lobulated[341] and well demarcated except when there is adjacent parenchymal shadowing.[287,318] Both the more proximal tracheobronchial and the more distal bronchopulmonary nodes are involved in sarcoidosis, and enlargement of the latter is characteristic.[341]

These more peripheral nodes may have lung or lower lobe bronchus on their medial aspect, and thus when enlarged they typically have a clearly demarcated inner border (Figure 13-3).[341] Symmetry is an important diagnostic feature of the hilar adenopathy associated with sarcoidosis because symmetric adenopathy is unusual in the major diagnostic alternatives such as lymphoma,

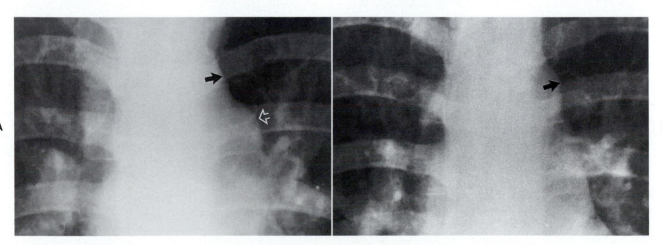

A   B

FIGURE 13-2
Sarcoidosis of aortopulmonary nodes. Local view of midmediastinum and hilar regions. **A,** Local convexity *(open arrow)* below the aortic knob *(closed arrow)* is caused by aortopulmonary nodal enlargement. **B,** Same patient 8 months later; convexity below aortic knob *(arrow)* has disappeared and has been replaced by shadow of normal main pulmonary artery.

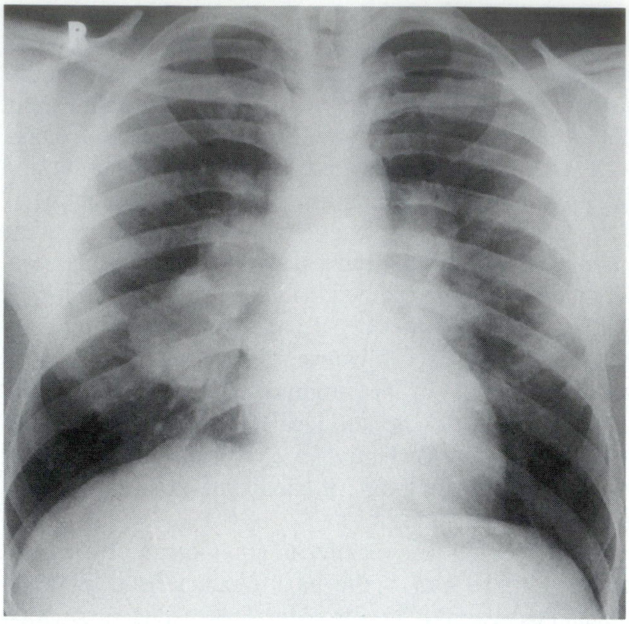

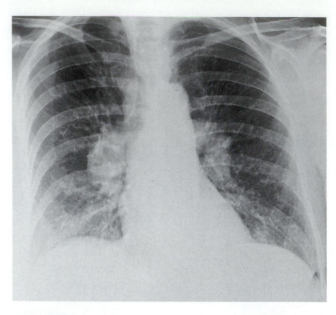

FIGURE 13-3
Sarcoidosis. Hilar adenopathy is more massive than in Figure 13-1 and reaches halfway to chest wall. Bronchopulmonary nodes are markedly enlarged and clearly demarcated medially. Lower aspect of right hilum presents "squared-off" appearance.

FIGURE 13-4
Chronic lymphatic leukemia. Symmetric bilateral hilar and right paratracheal adenopathy simulates sarcoidosis. Adenopathy in tuberculosis, histoplasmosis, and lymphoma is usually asymmetric, but in leukemia, metastatic disease, and silicosis, symmetric nodal enlargement is well recognized.

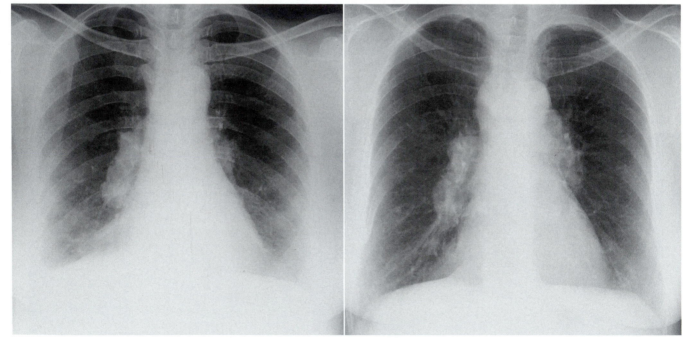

FIGURE 13-5
Sarcoidosis, essentially unilateral adenopathy. **A,** Patient with pronounced right tracheobronchial and bronchopulmonary adenopathy with probable minimal left hilar adenopathy. **B,** Six months later note marked symmetric hilar lymphadenopathy with enlarged aortopulmonary and right paratracheal nodes.

tuberculosis, and metastatic disease (Figure 13-4). Sometimes the adenopathy appears more marked on the right on a frontal radiograph simply because the right hilum normally stands more proud than the left[207] and because left paratracheal nodes are more difficult to identify. Tomography can clarify this situation.[108] In about 3% of patients the asymmetry is real and striking, even to the extent that the adenopathy may be considered unilateral (Figure 13-5).[163,186,287,303] In one series of 135 patients an exceptionally high proportion of patients (9.6%) showing true unilateral hilar adenopathy was recorded[96] and a surprising 29% in 21 patients aged 50 years or more with adenopathy.[70] Unilateral hilar adenopathy is about twice as common on the right as on the left and can occur either alone or with right paratracheal adenopathy.[96,348]

Other nodes in the chest may be involved with a recorded frequency that reflects the imaging modality used and the diligence with which they are sought. In general, involvement of these other nodal groups accompanies the more classic adenopathy, and the degree of enlargement is usually modest. Anterior mediastinal nodes are difficult to appreciate on plain radiographs, but CT scanning shows involvement in 25% to 66% of patients (Figure 13-6; see also Figure 13-13).[133,345,386] Isolated anterior mediastinal adenopathy is rare[53,225,287,369] and should strongly suggest a diagnosis other than sarcoidosis, particularly lymphoma.

Subcarinal adenopathy (Figure 13-7) occasionally may be marked and can cause airway compression[25] or dysphagia.[358] The prevalence of subcarinal adenopathy in a study not using CT was 21%,[15] but with CT (Figure 13-8) the figures are in the order of 50%.[133,386] Involvement of subcarinal nodes in the absence of hilar adenopathy is rare but has been recorded.[175]

Posterior mediastinal adenopathy (Figures 13-9 and 13-10) is one of the least common patterns in sarcoidosis, ranging in frequency from 2% to 20%.[15,319,345] Only one case report exists of sarcoidosis presenting with isolated posterior mediastinal adenopathy.[194]

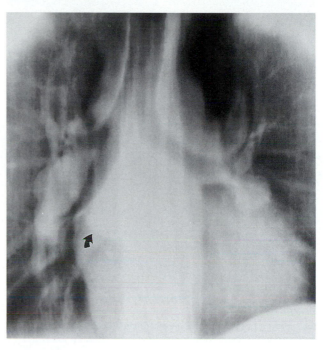

FIGURE 13-7
Sarcoidosis of subcarinal nodes. Anteroposterior tomogram of mediastinum shows subcarinal adenopathy. This deviates azygoesophageal interface *(arrow)* to right to meet intermediate stem bronchus distally. Note also bilateral hilar adenopathy.

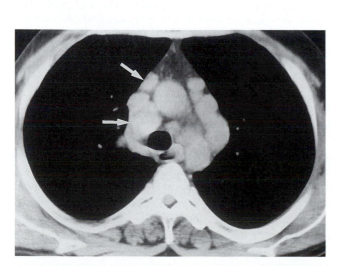

FIGURE 13-6
Sarcoidosis, mediastinal adenopathy on computed tomogram. Note numerous lymph nodes both in front of and behind superior vena cava *(arrows)*, in aortopulmonary window, and in paraaortic position.

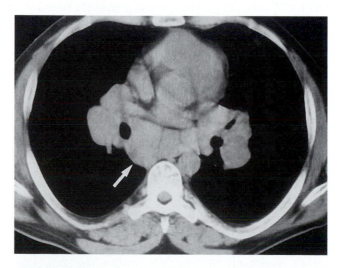

FIGURE 13-8
Sarcoidosis of subcarinal nodes. Computed tomogram 2 cm below carina shows massive subcarinal adenopathy *(arrow)*. Note also massive, symmetric hilar adenopathy.

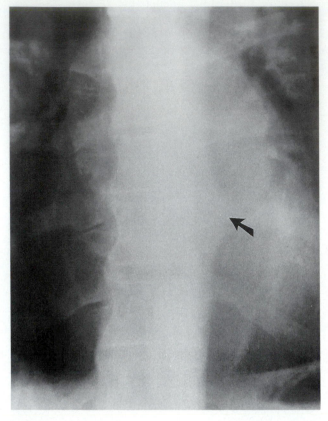

FIGURE 13-9
Sarcoidosis of posterior mediastinal nodes. Localized view of lower mediastinum is taken from high-kilovoltage chest radiograph. Local convexity *(arrow)* of paraaortic interface is caused by posterior mediastinal, paraaortic node enlargement.

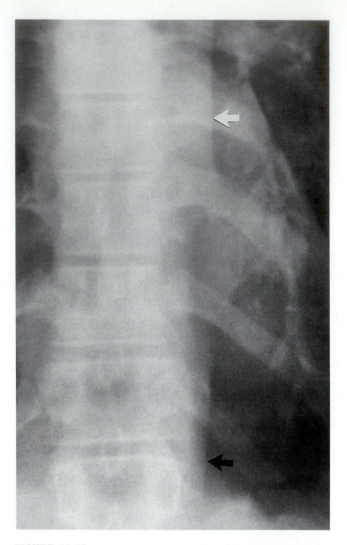

FIGURE 13-10
Sarcoidosis of posterior mediastinal nodes. Localized view of lower mediastinum taken from high-kilovoltage chest radiograph. As in Figure 13-9 posterior mediastinal adenopathy is present, but here loss of paraaortic interface *(arrows)* over 5 cm segment is most striking finding.

Most mediastinal nodes are at their maximum size when first seen; they decrease in size over the next 3 to 6 months so that two thirds are no longer visible after 1 year[341]; and very few are visible after 2 years.[163,318] In one review only 6% persisted at 2 years, and most of these were smaller than when first examined.[318] If nodes persist for 2 years, they commonly remain unchanged for many years,[158,341] and probably indefinitely. Given this fact and the commonness of sarcoidosis, the possibility that mediastinal lymphadenopathy is caused by sarcoidosis must always be considered even in the context of malignant disease.[269,276]

Of patients with stage I disease at initial examination, about 60% go on to complete resolution,[96,161,303,316,341] the figure being higher in those with erythema nodosum and arthropathy.[318] In the remaining 30% to 40% of patients presenting with adenopathy, parenchymal shadowing develops,[318,341] usually within the first year, although longer intervals are not uncommon[341] and gaps of 10 years or more are recorded.[158] The adenopathy has commonly begun to decrease in size at the time that parenchymal shadowing appears,[185,318,341] a feature that can be helpful in distinguishing sarcoidosis from lymphoma or carcinoma in which the nodes would be expected to remain stable or to enlarge.[96]

Fluctuation of nodal enlargement during intermittent steroid therapy is well recognized (Figure 13-11),[350] but once the nodes have completely resolved radiologically they probably will not enlarge again spontaneously. Such a train of events should raise the possibility of malignant adenopathy.[41] Only about 10 cases of nodal recurrence are reported, and these spanned periods of up to 20 years.[210] Nodal recurrence developed either alone[207,350] or with other features of sarcoidosis.[357] Recurrences may be multiple, and as many as three or four episodes have been recorded.[316] Different nodal groups may be involved in separate episodes, as in one patient in whom first one hilum and then the other was involved.[179,287]

Sarcoid nodes may calcify (Figures 13-12 and 13-13);

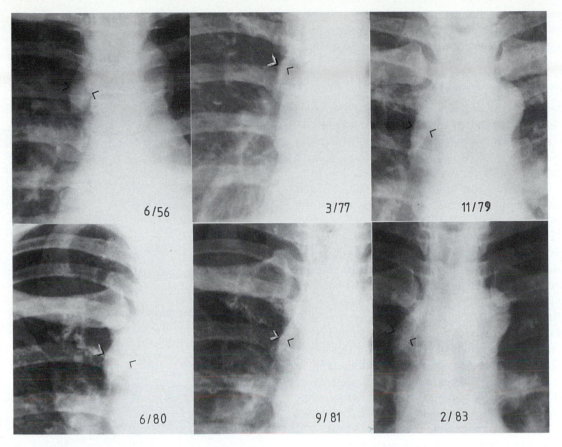

FIGURE 13-11

Sarcoidosis, nodal recurrence. Localized view of the right paratracheal region shows azygos node *(arrowheads)*. Initial adenopathy in 1956 was result of tuberculosis. Subsequent adenopathy has been associated with sarcoidosis and has fluctuated in degree in relation to steroid therapy.

FIGURE 13-12

Sarcoidosis, nodal calcification. Local view of middle and lower mediastinum shows extensive calcification affecting hilar, paratracheal, subcarinal, posterior mediastinal, and anterior mediastinal lymph nodes.

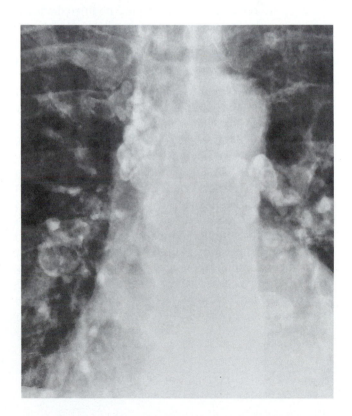

the frequency is related to duration of disease and period of observation.[298] In short-term studies using chest radiography, nodal calcification is seen in about 1% to 3% of cases,[157,185,316,329] but in a longer term study of 111 patients observed for 10 years or more the prevalence was 20%.[153] A prevalence of 40% is recorded on CT.[259] Calcification is thought to develop only in diseased nodes, occurring in a dystrophic fashion in fibrous tissue. Its occurrence appears unrelated to either hypercalcemia or coincident tuberculosis. Most descriptions are of paratracheal and hilar involvement, but any nodal group may be involved.[26] The morphology of the calcification is generally variable and nonspecific when seen radiographically. However, in a number of patients peripheral, eggshell calcification develops (Figure 13-13).[26,125,225,287,316] This is of diagnostic value because its occurrence is largely limited to sarcoidosis and silicosis.[125] Spontaneous resolution of eggshell calcification has been seen in a single report.[316]

Parenchymal sarcoidosis

Parenchymal shadowing is seen at the time of presentation in approximately half of the patients with sarcoidosis.* In addition, about one third of patients presenting with stage I disease go on to develop parenchymal opacity with a frequency that shows a marked variation from series to series, ranging from 10% to 43%.† Such parenchymal shadowing frequently develops within the year and is usually accompanied, at least to some degree, by nodal regression.

Parenchymal shadowing in sarcoidosis is customarily divided into prefibrotic and fibrotic.[316] This distinction is often not clear, and a more practical division between reversible and irreversible shadowing is used here.

REVERSIBLE CHANGES. Reversible changes consist of three patterns: reticulonodular opacities, ill-defined opacities with the characteristics of consolidation (alveolar), and large nodules. These patterns can occur alone or in varying combinations.[186] They may resolve partially or completely, or they may progress to an irreversible, fibrotic pattern. The approximate frequency of the various forms of parenchymal shadowing is reticulonodular, 75% to 90%; "alveolar," 10% to 20%; and large nodular, 2%.

(Reticulo)nodular opacities. Small rounded or irregular opacities constitute by far the most frequent pulmonary pattern and are seen in some 75% to 90% of patients with parenchymal shadowing.[96,152,224,316,342] Reticulonodular opacities are more common than pure nodular shadows. In an attempt to characterize these opacities, a number of workers have used the pneumoconiosis classification of the International Labor Office/University of Cincinnati (ILO/UC; see Chapter 10), extending it to include x, y, and z opacities to denote small rounded opacities from which irregular linear tentacles arise.[51,224] In the study by McLoud and co-workers,[224] 35% of opacities were classified as "xyz," 33% as "pqr," and 19% as "stu." The nodules range in size from just under 1 mm to over 5 mm, with most 2 to 4 mm (Figures 13-14 to 13-17) in diameter.[152,186,316] Very small nodules, 1 mm or less in diameter, when aggregated may take on a ground-glass appearance.[96] In addition to discrete interstitial abnormalities such as nodules, more diffuse changes occur and are seen on radiographs as bronchial wall thickening, air bronchograms, and subpleural and fissural thickening (Figure 13-16).[285] Some suggest that these latter findings might give a better idea of "activity" in sarcoidosis than reticulonodular opacities, and their presence certainly correlates quite well with "disease activity" indicated by

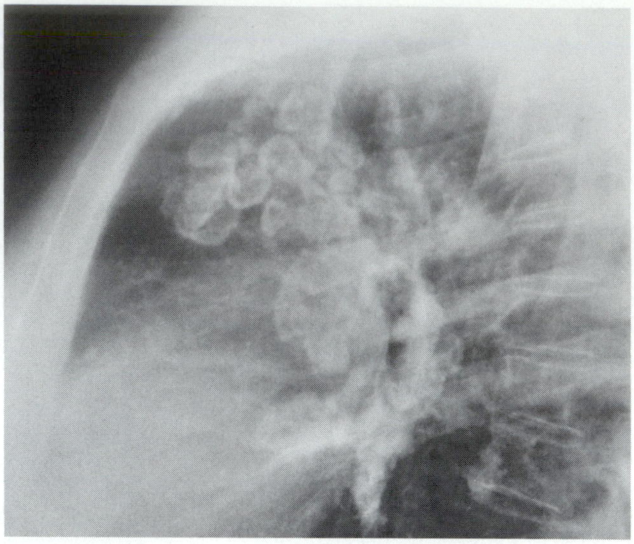

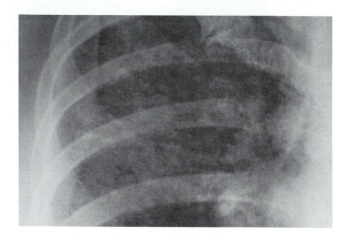

FIGURE 13-13
Sarcoidosis, nodal calcification. Lateral view of upper chest shows extensive nodal calcification, much of which has eggshell pattern. Many nodes are in anterior mediastinum.

FIGURE 13-14
Parenchymal sarcoidosis. Localized view of right upper zone shows profuse and evenly distributed multiple small nodules about 1 mm or less in diameter.

gallium scanning.[285] Sometimes parenchymal changes, which may themselves be quite mild, silhouette the outer aspect of the hilum and blur it, giving rise to the so-called hilar haze sign.[287]

The reticulonodular shadows are usually bilaterally symmetric (Figures 13-16 and 13-17), with about 15% showing significant asymmetry.[316] In exceptional cases parenchymal changes are strictly unilateral. In three series this pattern was seen in fewer than 1% of the cases.[96,156,237] Unilateral change however, was recorded in 8% in one recent series.[152] Unilateral parenchymal disease is usually, but not exclusively, of the (reticulo)nodular type and may occur with or without adenopathy.[86,131,230,298,316]

*References 96, 156, 162, 186, 219, 224, 234, 303, 342.
†References 96, 161, 303, 318, 342, 346.

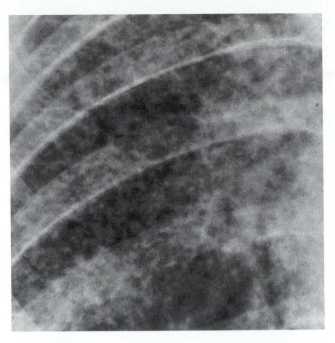

FIGURE 13-15
Parenchymal sarcoidosis. Localized view of right middle zone shows profuse nodules, larger than in Figure 13-14. These nodules are of a size more typically seen in sarcoidosis, ranging from 2 to 4 mm. Some nodules are rounded; others, irregular.

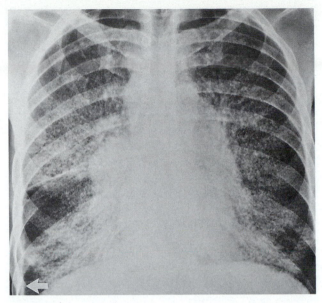

FIGURE 13-16
Parenchymal and nodal sarcoidosis. Diffuse fine reticulonodular opacities affect all zones in symmetric fashion, sparing apices. Minor fissure is thickened, and there is subpleural thickening ("laminar effusion") *(arrow)* in right lower zone laterally. These latter findings are feature of acute, active sarcoidosis.

Opacities tend to occur in all zones, often showing a middle zone or middle and upper predominance (Figure 13-17).[316,342] Isolated lower zone involvement is seen in less than 4% of patients.[152,342] Occasionally a strictly upper zone distribution[152] may resemble tuberculosis.[362]

Calcification within the lung in parenchymal sarcoidosis is rarely reported. It developed in 5 of 136 patients in one series followed for at least 5 years[315] and in 3 of 111 cases followed for 10 or more years.[154] However, other granulomatous causes, such as tuberculosis, cannot be excluded in these patients.

"Alveolar" opacities. In some 10% to 20% of patients with sarcoidosis, opacities with consolidative (airspace) features develop. These opacities form a spectrum ranging from ill-defined, irregular shadows of nondescript shape (Figure 13-18) to those that are focal, nodular, and quite well defined (Figure 13-19). In the past, many authors regarded these latter nodules as a separate entity, so-called large nodular sarcoidosis, and although this is an artificial distinction,[298] it is maintained here because it makes consideration of the literature easier. The pathologic basis for alveolar shadowing in sarcoidosis is loss of alveolar air and increase in soft tissue. This loss can be produced by a purely interstitial process if it compresses and obliterates alveoli, or it can be seen with an alveolar process that directly replaces alveolar air by inflammatory cells. In sarcoidosis evidence suggests that both interstitial compression[108,287,293] and alveolar filling[287] play a part. Histologic study may show the alveoli to be filled

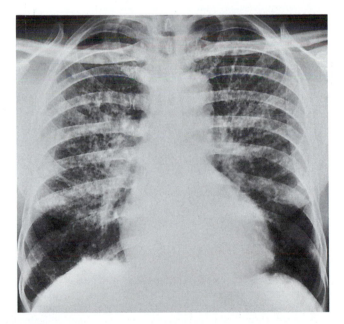

FIGURE 13-17
Parenchymal sarcoidosis. Adenopathy has subsided, leaving predominantly middle and upper zone, 2 to 4 mm reticulonodular opacities.

with macrophages[311] or granulomas.[287,336] In some cases the pathogenesis appears to be airway occlusion by granulomas, causing obstructive pneumonitis.[293]

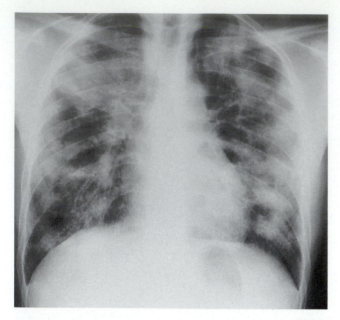

FIGURE 13-18
Alveolar sarcoidosis. Bilateral multifocal opacities have radiographic features of consolidation (airspace opacity). Adenopathy usually but not invariably accompanies alveolar sarcoidosis. Here right paratracheal, right hilar, and aortopulmonary nodes are enlarged. Some areas of consolidation have small marginal nodules—a finding of diagnostic value.

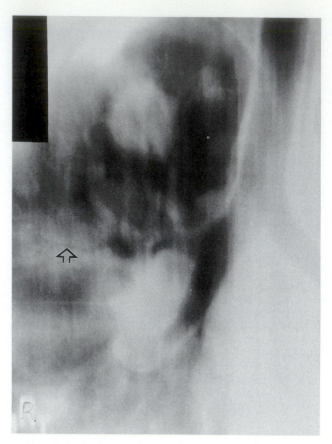

FIGURE 13-19
Large nodular and alveolar sarcoidosis. Tomogram of right middle and upper zone in patient with coexisting large nodular and alveolar sarcoidosis. In right upper zone is unusually well-defined 3 cm nodule. Below it and just above minor fissure ill-defined opacity approximately 2.5 × 4 cm is seen. This opacity has features that suggest consolidation, including air bronchogram (arrow). In addition note right hilar nodes and thickening of minor fissure.

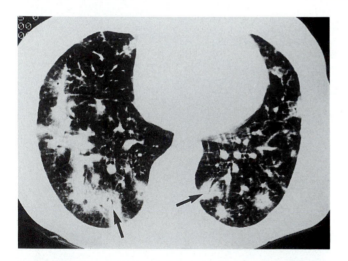

FIGURE 13-20
Alveolar sarcoidosis on high-resolution computed tomography. Note multiple airspace nodules 1 to 2 cm in diameter. On right side, confluent airspace opacity has formed subpleural band mimicking cryptogenic eosinophilic pneumonia. Opacities have ill-defined margins and contain air bronchograms (arrows).

Alveolar sarcoidosis has a prevalence rate of about 10% to 20%, but the range is 4% to 27%.* The typical appearance is of bilateral, multifocal, poorly defined opacities,[25,186] ranging in size from about 1 to 10 cm (Figure 13-18).[287] These opacities can occur anywhere,

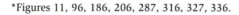

*Figures 11, 96, 186, 206, 287, 316, 327, 336.

but they show a predilection for the peripheral midzone,[11,287,336] sparing the costophrenic angles.[11] The peripheral distribution is particularly well seen with computed tomography (CT) (Figure 13-20).[133,386] An air bronchogram is commonly present (Figures 13-19 and 13-20).[11,25,186] At the edge the lesions often break up into a nodular pattern that may be very fine, creating an appearance of acinar rosettes.[388] Reticulonodular opacities are also present in about two thirds of these patients,[11,186] and their detection provides a helpful clue when the principal radiographic finding is disseminated multifocal consolidations of obscure origin (Figure 13-18). Another helpful pointer is mediastinal adenopathy, which is an even more common accompaniment, occurring in more than 80% of cases (Figure 13-19).[11,186] Kirks and co-workers[185,186] point out that all of their patients with alveolar sarcoidosis had mediastinal adenopathy or reticulonodular shadowing or both.

Recognized variants of the alveolar pattern include unilateral distribution,[206] upper zone distribution simu-

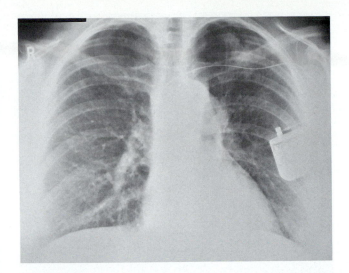

FIGURE 13-21
Alveolar sarcoidosis. Localized alveolar sarcoidosis in left upper zone with ipsilateral hilar adenopathy. This unusual pattern raised possibility of tuberculosis or bronchial carcinoma. Diagnosis in this case was proved at thoracotomy. Patient has pacemaker for complete heart block, possibly result of cardiac sarcoidosis, but this is unproved.

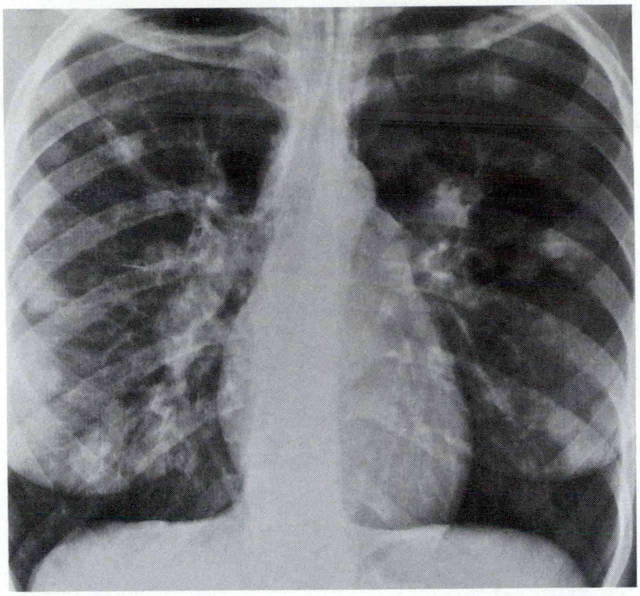

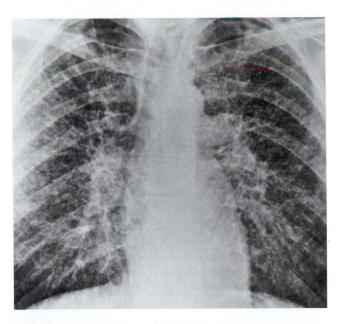

FIGURE 13-22
Large nodular sarcoidosis. Note multiple, relatively well-defined nodules ranging from 1 to 3 cm. In addition, mild bilateral hilar and right paratracheal adenopathy is evident. Nodal enlargement is almost universal finding in large nodular sarcoidosis.

lating tuberculosis (Figure 13-21),[131] or a peripheral pattern that resembles cryptogenic eosinophilic pneumonia (Figure 13-20). In one series of 64 patients, 9% showed a pronounced peripheral distribution, some with an alveolar and some with a reticulonodular pattern.[115] Sharma[327] describes two confusing cases in which the peripheral alveolar pattern was accompanied by blood eosinophilia, yet lung biopsy showed noncaseating granulomas consistent with sarcoidosis. Peripheral consolidation is usually accompanied by nodal enlargement, but exceptions are recorded.[170] Some authors have stressed the good prognosis and tendency for rapid clearing with alveolar sarcoidosis; in one report the opacity cleared in 21 of 22 patients with or without steroids,[11] and in another clearing occurred in 66% of patients within 9 months.[336] Not all authors agree; in the San Francisco series of 150 patients clearing occurred in only 31%.[186] The rapidity of change in some cases suggests that some clearing may result from resolution of obstructive pneumonitis.[293]

Large nodular sarcoidosis. Focal opacities with the radiologic features of large nodules are an uncommon but well-recognized finding in sarcoidosis, and when the various series are combined, a 2.4% prevalence rate (35 of 1449 cases) is seen.* The nodules are usually bilateral and multiple, ranging in size from 0.5 to 5 cm (Figures 13-22 and 13-26).[102,298] They can occur in any zone, but as with alveolar sarcoid a slight midzone predilection is evident.[102] The margins of the nodules are occasionally sharp[327,298] but are much more often ill defined and hazy.[11] Some nodules go on to coalesce.[327] They may

FIGURE 13-23
Parenchymal sarcoidosis. Note mild adenopathy and mild hilar elevation. Parenchymal shadowing is reticulonodular with pronounced linear element that suggests development of scarring. Uniformity of changes in all zones is unusual.

contain an air bronchogram,[316] a feature particularly well seen at CT.[37,133] Most are accompanied by mediastinal adenopathy, but a few cases are recorded in which adenopathy was absent.[102,271,332]

The nodules behave unpredictably over time and may

---

*References 11, 186, 206, 303, 316, 332.

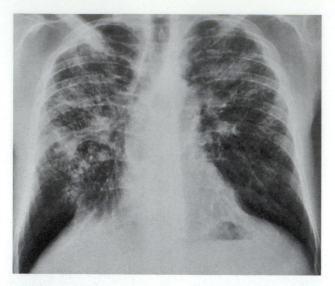

FIGURE 13-24
Sarcoidosis and fibrosis. Although some nodular shadowing is seen, predominant opacities are linear. Shadowing is maximal in middle and upper zones. Areas of confluent shadowing probably represent conglomerate fibrosis. Hila are elevated, and overexpanded lower zones are transradiant.

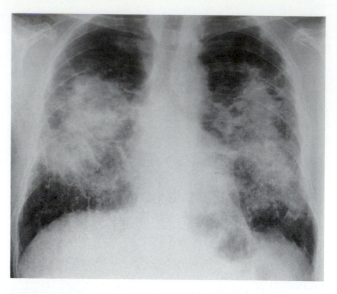

FIGURE 13-25
Sarcoidosis and massive fibrosis. Occasionally, sarcoid fibrosis forms large, conglomerate masses resembling that seen in progressive massive fibrosis. Here opacities are more caudad than usual.

remain static for years[332] or show partial[102] or complete regression.[332] Scattered reports tell of a single large sarcoid nodule.* In such cases the radiologic appearances strongly suggest bronchial carcinoma.

Primary cavitation is rarely seen in either alveolar or large nodular sarcoidosis. It probably occurs because of ischemic necrosis in conglomerate granulomas. Only about 10 cases are recorded.† Cavitation can be an early or late manifestion and may even be the presenting feature.[169] Cavities can be single or multiple and may occur with or without adenopathy. The walls of the cavity have a variable appearance: thick or thin, and smooth or irregular. Sarcoid cavities may resolve either with or without steroids.[298] Although cavitation is usually benign, fatal hemoptysis has been recorded.[93]

IRREVERSIBLE CHANGES. Sarcoid granulomas may resolve completely, or they may heal by fibrosis (Figure 13-23). Such fibrosis ranges from the minor and radiologically undetectable[342] to the gross, with scarlike shadowing and distortion on the chest radiograph. Gross fibrosis is present on the initial chest radiograph in about 5% to 25% of patients.[108,186,342] In addition, gross fibrosis develops in 10% to 15% of patients who when first examined have stage 0 to II disease.[25,96,342] The fibrosis usually takes years to develop,[25] with a range in one series of 2 to 14 years.[342]

The radiologic changes of gross fibrosis in sarcoidosis are fairly characteristic. Some authors consider them to be

almost pathognomonic.[318] The findings classically consist of permanent, coarse, linear opacities radiating laterally from the hilum into adjacent upper and middle zones (Figure 13-24).[287] On lateral view these changes can be seen to predominate in the lower part of the upper lobes.[318]

Predominant scarring remote from the middle to upper zone is unusual.[318] For example, in one series only 4% of patients had fibrosis, which was most marked in the lower zone.[342] Coincident with the development of scarring, the extreme upper and lower zones tend to become transradiant (Figure 13-24). In the upper zones this transradiancy is the result of cyst and bulla formation, whereas in the lower zones it is more commonly the result of compensatory hyperinflation following upper zone volume loss. The hila are generally pulled upward and outward, and vessels and fissures are distorted.[96,186] The fibrosis is occasionally so pronounced that it gives rise to massive parahilar opacities in the middle and upper zones that resemble those seen in progressive massive fibrosis (Figures 13-25 and 13-26).[133,318,342] At the other extreme, minor localized linear scarring may be the only finding.[186] Cor pulmonale may supervene in the fibrotic stage[10,219,221,316,346] and may be radiologically recognizable.

Ring opacities are particularly common in the upper zones in gross fibrosis.[108] Many are thin walled and caused by bronchiectasis[133,342] or bullae (Figure 13-27).[108,345] Ring opacities are occasionally thick walled when caused by an infected bulla, abscess, tuberculous cavity, or necrosis within a mass of conglomerate fibrosis.[108,287,316] A few cases of "vanishing lung" with

---

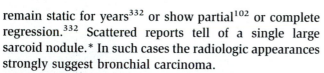

*References 61, 70, 266, 280, 298, 316.
†References 28, 132, 169, 219, 301, 364.

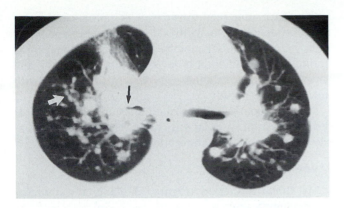

FIGURE 13-26
Sarcoidosis and massive fibrosis. Computed tomography demonstrates massive perihilar opacity caused by fibrosis surrounded by nodular sarcoid with nodules ranging from 3 to 15 mm. On right some nodules show characteristic bronchovascular distribution *(white arrow)*. Right upper lobar airway *(black arrow)* is grossly narrowed as it enters fibrotic mass.

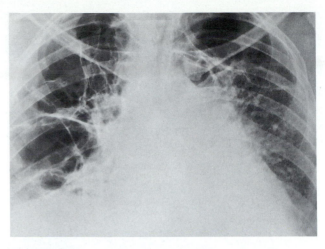

FIGURE 13-27
Sarcoidosis and fibrosis. Most of right lung and left apex are replaced by large cystic spaces.

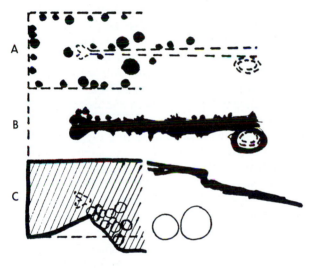

FIGURE 13-28
Sarcoidosis on high-resolution computed tomogram. Three peripheral pulmonary lobules with centrilobular artery and accompanying airway are shown. **A** and **B** represent common and **C** less common changes. **A**, Nodules 1 to 5 mm with predominant distribution along bronchovascular structures, interlobular septa, and visceral pleura. **B**, Irregular bronchovascular interfaces, wide bronchovascular structures, thick airway walls, acinar nodules with air bronchograms, and prominent centrilobular structures. **C**, Interlobular septal thickening; ground-glass opacity; lobular distortion; long irregular scars; honeycombing, cyst, and bulla formation.

marked emphysema and bulla formation are reported.[236,273]

Computed tomography and sarcoidosis

Three major studies have described the CT and high-resolution CT (HRCT) changes in sarcoidosis (Figure 13-28),[37,209,251] and a large number of others contain

important information.* The most common and almost universal finding is small, 1 to 5 mm nodules, usually with irregular margins (Figure 13-29). These tend to be distributed in a characteristic fashion that reflects the location of lymphatic vessels: along bronchovascular margins (Figures 13-26 and 13-29), along interlobular septa, subpleurally (including fissural pleura; Figure 13-30), and in the center of lobules. This is a nonspecific pattern of distribution shared, for example, by lymphangitis carcinomatosa.[257] Nodules abutting interfaces make the normally sharp borders of vessels, airways, pleura, and septa irregular and beaded (Figures 13-29 and 13-30). The overall number of nodules varies greatly, ranging from marked total lung involvement (often upper and middle zone predominant)[37] to a scanty, focal distribution.[209] In some areas they may be so numerous as to become confluent.[37] Slightly larger nodules (up to 10 mm) are less commonly seen, and one study describes cavitation,[37] but this is a rare finding. Focal opacities of 1 cm or more in diameter may be caused by localized areas of consolidation, such as alveolar sarcoid, characterized by ill-defined margins and an air bronchogram (Figure 13-30), or by conglomerate fibrosis, typically seen in the middle and upper zones and accompanied by marked volume loss and bronchovascular distortion.

Other CT signs include irregular bronchovascular interfaces (Figure 13-29) caused by adjacent nodules (see earlier discussion) and scarring. This causes bronchovascular structures to look bigger and more prominent, and it irregularly thickens airway walls.[209] By the same mechanism centrilobular core structures enlarge.[21,22] Septal lines are seen in about 50% of cases, but they are not profuse. Deep interlobular septal thickening forming polygonal structures is less common.[21,251,37] Ground-

---

*References 21-23, 39, 218, 249, 252, 257, 259.

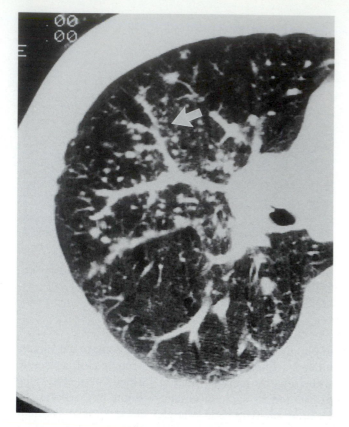

FIGURE 13-29
Sarcoidosis on high-resolution computed tomogram. Principal finding is 1 to 5 mm irregular nodules. In places these have pronounced peribronchovascular distribution *(arrow)*—very characteristic feature of sarcoidosis. Bronchovascular structures are widened, and interfaces with lung are irregular. Sarcoid nodules are often widespread, but more restricted distribution as seen here is not uncommon. Interlobular septal thickening is scarcely detectable.

glass opacity is also seen in about 50% of studies; it is patchy, may have a lobular distribution, and may sometimes represent active alveolitis, clearing on follow-up scans[209] and correlating with ^{67}Ga scintiscans.[22] This, however, is not always the case because ground-glass opacity may remain unchanged on follow-up CT.[39,259] A number of signs are caused by scarring: lobular distortion, found in about 50% of patients[37,39,251,259] (such distortion is absent in lymphangitis carcinomatosa and a useful discriminating sign); long, irregular, linear opacities; traction bronchiectasis; honeycombing and cyst or bulla formation; and crowding and posterior displacement of central bronchovascular structures.[37]

A number of studies have looked at the change in various opacities on follow-up scans,[37,39,209,259] shedding light on possible pathologies underlying CT signs. Results are not entirely consistent but in general show nodules and consolidation to be impermanent and lines, cysts, honeycombing, and distortion to be permanent. Unexpectedly, ground-glass opacity (see earlier discussion) behaved in an inconsistent fashion. A number of other

studies have attempted to correlate symptoms and respiratory function data with CT, giving discrepant results.[22,37,209,252] HRCT may be abnormal in the face of a normal chest radiograph in sarcoidosis,[209,251,252] and patients may have sarcoidosis proved by lung biopsy with a normal HRCT study.[209,251]

MRI can identify mediastinal nodes and allows a clear distinction from vascular structures. The T2 signal intensity of enlarged nodes shows no characteristic pattern.[227]

Mycetoma

Mycetoma formation (Figure 13-31) is a well-recognized complication of stage III cystic sarcoidosis.[120,382] Indeed, sarcoidosis is probably the second most common predisposing condition after tuberculosis.[298] This is particularly so in the United States, where the large black population results in more cases of sarcoidosis that progress to gross fibrobullous disease.[154] In a series of mycetomas reported from Philadelphia, 45% were in patients with sarcoidosis,[201] whereas in a series of 26 patients in the United Kingdom only 15% were in patients with sarcoidosis.[297] The frequency of mycetoma in sarcoidosis varies from series to series and ranges between 1% and 10% depending on racial mix of the patients and method of detection.* In the subset of sarcoid patients with stage III fibrocystic disease the proportion of patients harboring a mycetoma can be about 50%.[287,382]

Hemoptysis is the most common and worrisome symptom and may be life threatening.[151,166,174,382] In one small series of patients with sarcoidosis and mycetoma, major hemoptysis occurred every 5 years and minor hemoptysis every 2.5 years.[174] Of 46 deaths from sarcoidosis in one study, 6.5% were mycetoma related.[167] Steroid treatment does not seem to predispose to mycetoma formation.[382]

The radiologic features of mycetoma are discussed in Chapter 6. In sarcoidosis, mycetoma formation is worth consideration when any sort of new shadowing, particularly masslike lesions or pleural thickening, develops in patients with grade III fibrocystic disease.[201] Mycetomas are confined virtually to the upper lobes and are commonly bilateral, in 50% of cases in one series.[174] Serum precipitins against *Aspergillus* spp. are almost always strongly positive. CT scanning is the most sensitive imaging modality.[40,297]

Pulmonary and systemic vein involvement

Although mediastinal adenopathy is often massive, it rarely causes compression of great veins with subsequent superior vena cava syndrome, a fact that has been ascribed to the lack of perinodal fibrosis in sarcoidosis.[298] A handful of cases are described, some of which presented with superior vena caval obstruction and others in which it punctuates the course of established disease.[35,183,247] A single case of innominate vein obstruc-

---

*References 108, 174, 186, 287, 316, 382.

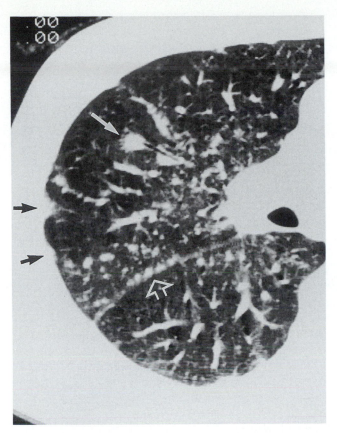

FIGURE 13-30

Sarcoidosis on high-resolution computed tomography. Dominant pattern is nodulation. Subpleural nodules are present in relation to visceral pleura, both peripherally *(black arrows)* and along thickened major fissue *(open arrow)*. Larger acinar nodule is present *(white arrow)* with air bronchogram.

tion that produced a large exudative effusion is recorded.[164] The rarity of superior vena cava syndrome with sarcoidosis is such that other causes of obstruction should be sought.[53,289]

In a recent report, granulomatous involvement of small pulmonary veins caused obliteration and resultant pulmonary arterial hypertension. The chest radiograph showed dilated proximal pulmonary arteries and a basal "interstitial pattern" resembling venoocclusive disease.[143]

Pulmonary artery involvement

Large vessel involvement is rare in sarcoidosis[321] and is usually the result of compression by large nodes.[100,117,141,180,377] Typically the lobar divisions, particularly the upper lobe vessels, are involved, and pulmonary arterial hypertension is usually absent. Perfusion scans show corresponding large defects.[133,377] A few cases are reported in which stenosis of major pulmonary arteries is attributed to sarcoid-induced scarring,[10,80,133,323] and in a single reported case multiple stenoses caused pulmonary arterial hypertension.[80]

Small vessel involvement by granulomas is common and is usually accompanied by widespread parenchymal disease.[51,307] Granulomas can lead to vessel narrowing, but not usually vascular necrosis or thrombosis. These changes probably account for patchy perfusion defects found on scintigraphy[267,335] and for pulmonary arterial hypertension.

Pulmonary artery hypertension in sarcoidosis may be caused by granulomatous vasculitis,[52,83,248,343] by fibrobullous disease,[10,356] or rarely by large vessel disease.[133]

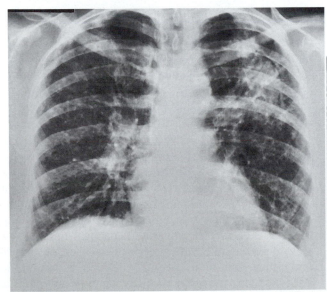

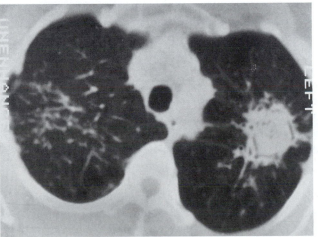

A

B

FIGURE 13-31

Sarcoidosis and mycetoma. **A,** Chest radiograph reveals diffusely distributed low-profusion linear and small nodular densities. In left mid-upper zone two masslike opacities are evident. Lower mass has peripheral air crescent. **B,** Computed tomography scan through lower mass demonstrates unequivocal, heterogeneous intracavitary body resulting from mycetoma.

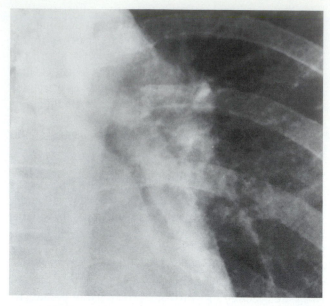

FIGURE 13-32
Airway sarcoidosis. Local view of left hilar region. Note mild narrowing of left lower lobar airway, probably result of extrinsic nodal compression. Such compression does not usually cause significant bronchial narrowing.

Airway involvement

Sarcoidosis can affect the trachea, bronchi, or bronchioles. Tracheal involvement is rare[36] and in the few reported cases has been associated with laryngeal involvement.[318] Both the proximal and distal trachea may be involved, and the stenosis can be smooth,[88,137] irregular and nodular,[187] or even masslike.[376]

The bronchi may be narrowed by external nodal compression (Figure 13-32), extrinsic scarring, or mural granulomas and fibrosis. Generally intrinsic mural disease is considered to be the most important mechanism.[298] Despite the sometimes massive enlargment of nodes in sarcoidosis, lymphadenopathy on its own is a rare cause of symptomatic airway narrowing.[228,248] Occasional examples are, however, recorded, particularly affecting the middle lobe.[89,256,358] The middle lobar airway seems to be particularly at risk because it is relatively long and narrow and is surrounded by lymph nodes.[118] The general lack of effect of sarcoid nodes on airways has been ascribed to the fact that node capsules remain intact so that scarring and fixation are rare. In addition, nodes do not erode into airways.[298]

Thus significant and symptomatic large airway narrowing is caused chiefly by mural granulomas and fibrosis (Figures 13-26 and 13-33). Although stenoses occur most commonly in well-established disease,[318] often with pulmonary fibrosis, they have been recorded early in the course of sarcoidosis and with stage 0 radiographic disease.[130,270] The frequency of large airway narrowing is about 5% (range 2.5% to 9%).[270,318,342] Patients present with either wheeze, stridor, and airflow limitation[130,378]

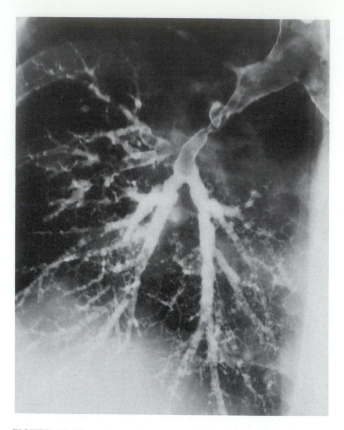

FIGURE 13-33
Airway sarcoidosis. Right bronchogram shows gross cicatricial narrowing of right upper lobar and intermediate stem bronchi. (From Hadfield JW, Page RL, Flower CDR, et al: *Thorax* 37:443-447, 1982.)

or episodes of lobar or segmental collapse and consolidation.[63,145] Collapse is a well-recognized but uncommon manifestation of sarcoidosis, occurring in about 1% of cases.[96,108,186,287,303] Any lobe may be affected, most commonly the middle (Figure 13-34).[118,167,298,303] Collapse of a whole lung has been recorded.[167]

Although the middle lobe is the most common to collapse, stenoses are distributed throughout the lung and show no particular lobar or segmental predilection. The stenoses may be single[270,318] or multiple[63,130,145,270] and most commonly affect mainstem, lobar, or proximal segmental divisions (Figure 13-33). At bronchoscopy, depending on the stage of the disease, the mucosa may be granular and hyperemic or even frankly inflamed and edematous.[172] Granulomas may even give rise to a local obstructing endobronchial mass.[70,75] Later, when healing by fibrosis occurs, the mucosa may appear normal.[130] In view of the variable pathogenesis of stenoses, not surprisingly they and their secondary effects show variable behavior, clearing spontaneously or with steroid treatment[167,256] or remaining unchanged.[270]

Airflow obstruction is common in sarcoidosis.[32,199,238,328] Evidence suggests that this is usually the result of small airway obstruction, presumably on the basis of granulomatous distortion,[328] and increased air-

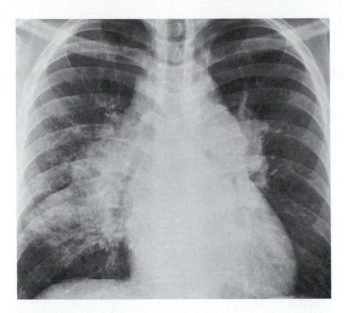

FIGURE 13-34
Airway sarcoidosis. Massive bilateral hilar and mediastinal adenopathy associated with collapse and consolidation of right middle lobe. Middle lobe is the most frequently collapsed lobe in sarcoidosis. Low-profusion, small nodular shadowing is present in right lung as well.

flow resistance can be demonstrated even in stage I disease.[331]

Obstructive bronchiectasis as a result of endobronchial sarcoidosis is considered rare,[298] although in the context of gross fibrobullous disease it is often difficult to be sure of the exact pathogenesis of bronchiectatic change. Only a few cases have been described.[133,298]

Pleural sarcoidosis

In sarcoidosis, granulomas may be found on both the visceral and parietal pleura. These pleural granulomas commonly cause no signs or symptoms.[79] On rare occasion, however, they may be associated with a dry pleurisy[111] or a pleural effusion that is usually painless[14] but may be painful.[168] These effusions are classically lymphocyte-rich exudates that in nearly one fifth of cases are sanguineous or serosanguineous.[263]

In 1870 cases of sarcoidosis taken from major series in the world literature, 55 had pleural effusions, giving a prevalence of 1.9%.* Effusions may be present initially,[237] but more often they develop during the course of established disease, a few months to 16 years after onset.[62] Sarcoid effusions are usually seen in the context of extensive pulmonary disease[379] or multisystem involvement.[62] However, pleural effusions with stage I disease are recorded,[186,326] and in rare cases patients have had an otherwise normal chest radiograph.[14,233] About one third of the effusions are bilateral,[62] and while they are usually small, large effusions have been de-

scribed.[27,173,263,373] The effusions resolve spontaneously in weeks or months and are almost invariably gone by 6 months.[206] Resolution is usually complete, but about 20% of patients are left with residual pleural thickening.[287,379]

In general, pleural effusion is a relatively minor and incidental finding in the course of sarcoidosis. However, because it is an atypical feature, it may prove a diagnostic puzzle. Several authors stress the importance of excluding other causes, particularly tuberculosis, which may occur concurrently.[96,189]

Bone involvement

Bone involvement that is detectable on the chest radiograph is rare; only about 20 cases are reported. The spine is the most common site, and the sternum is the least common. Spinal sarcoidosis is characterized by multiple lower dorsal destructive lesions, often with vertebral body collapse.[298] A few cases have simulated infective spondylitis,[354] and entirely sclerotic lesions are described.[387] The chest radiograph does not necessarily show changes of nonosseous sarcoidosis, and in one review two of eight cases were of this type.[42] Rib lesions have been recorded in five cases[298] and have been lytic or permeative in most cases, one presenting as a rib fracture.[128] One patient had sclerotic lesions.[387] The one reported sternal lesion was lytic and was part of widespread spine and rib involvement.[354]

Bone sarcoidosis, particularly of the hands, has a highly characteristic appearance, and its demonstration is of great diagnostic value in a patient with suspected chest sarcoidosis.[351] The likelihood of bone lesions at the time when sarcoidosis presents, which is the time when the diagnosis is most likely to be in doubt, is probably on the order of 1% to 2%.[207]

PULMONARY HISTIOCYTOSIS X (LANGERHANS' CELL HISTIOCYTOSIS, EOSINOPHILIC GRANULOMA OF LUNG)

Histiocytosis X (HX) is a granulomatous disorder of unknown cause characterized by the presence within the granulomas of a histiocyte, the Langerhans' cell, which has specific histochemical and electron microscopic features.* The Langerhans' cell is an antigen-presenting cell, and in HX for obscure reasons it becomes activated in an uncontrolled way, initiating an immune response.[54]

HX is a disease spectrum, with lung involvement seen either in infancy, as part of a serious multisystem disorder (Letterer-Siwe disease), or in (young) adults, as part of a more indolent disorder involving one organ system (single-site eosinophilic granuloma) or at most a few (multifocal eosinophilic granuloma, Hand-Schuller-Christian disease). The first description of pulmonary histiocytosis X (PHX) was in 1951.[99]

Pathologic examination† shows the typical pulmonary

*References 62, 96, 108, 186, 219, 237, 287, 303, 379.

*References 101, 109, 134, 213, 272, 344.
†References 6, 68, 109, 177, 213, 284.

lesion, a stellate interstitial nodule that is usually a few millimeters in size but ranges from 1 to 15 mm and lies most commonly in the walls of small airways. The nodules are granulomas containing histiocytes and a variable number of eosinophils, plasma cells, and lymphocytes. Some of the histiocytes show ultrastructural features of the antigen-presenting Langerhans' cell (histiocytosis X cell). The granulomas may encroach on airways and vessels and obstruct them. With time, fibrous replacement of the nodule occurs from the center outward. Sometimes the alveoli adjacent to the granulomas are filled with macrophages and desquamated alveolar lining cells. The appearances therefore may resemble desquamative interstitial pneumonia and lead to a mistaken diagnosis on limited biopsy. Scarring, if gross, eventually leads to the appearance of end-stage lung with honeycombing.

No good data on the prevalence of PHX are available, but it is clearly considerably lower than that of sarcoidosis, possibly by a factor of 20.[288] In the past, PHX was regarded as a male-predominant disease, but it is now considered equally prevalent in both sexes.[68,109,195,200,375] The disease may be milder in women. A very high proportion of patients, around 95%, give a history of cigarette smoking.[213] Its prevalence in blacks is low.[213] In most patients symptoms appear in the third or fourth decade, but the age spread is wide, from the teens to over 60 years. A small number of lung-limited cases have been reported in prepubertal children.[2] The patient may present with pulmonary or systemic symptoms or an asymptomatic radiographic abnormality. In one series of 100 patients, 23% were asymptomatic and their disease was detected radiographically, 31% had systemic symptoms, and 72% had pulmonary symptoms.[109] Systemic complaints usually coexist with pulmonary ones.[9,109] The most common complaints are cough, dyspnea, chest pain (nonspecific, pleuritic, or bony), and fever.[109] Pneumothorax is a classic manifestation of PHX (Figure 13-35). The frequency of pneumothorax as the initial manifestation may be as high as 14%.[195] Pneumothoraces occur in 6% to 25% of patients at some time during the course of the illness.[68,200] They are commonly recurrent, may be bilateral, and are sometimes fatal.[109] Respiratory function tests show great variation from subject to subject.[213] The usual pattern is restriction, reduced carbon monoxide diffusion, and in 20% to 50% evidence of airflow obstruction and small airway disease.[9,109,284] Diagnosis of PHX can be made on transbronchial lung biopsy, but since specific lesions are focal and widespread, they can easily be missed.[68] The diagnosis has been made by finding the characteristic histiocytosis X cells in bronchoalveolar lavage material,[9] although some doubt the specificity of this finding.[284] If these methods fail, open lung biopsy should be considered. Blood eosinophilia is rarely found in patients with PHX.[284]

In many cases PHX progresses through identifiable stages, from symptomatic disease to a stage of abnormal radiographic and functional findings to a period of

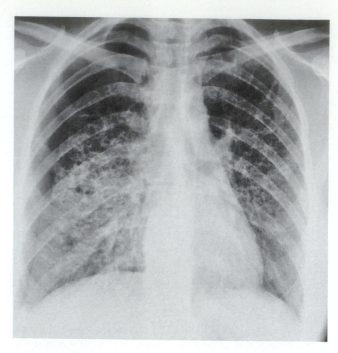

FIGURE 13-35
Histiocytosis X. Chest radiograph of 21-year-old woman with right pneumothorax. Bilateral changes can be seen throughout both lungs, mainly ring and linear opacities.

waning activity to partial or complete resolution. Evidence suggests that the prognosis is currently better than suggested by early series.[109] A high rate of spontaneous remission and a low rate of morbidity are seen.[284] Mortality is also low, probably on the order of 2% to 6%.[213] Some evidence shows that young adult men probably have a more severe form of the disease, and other adverse prognostic factors have been identified.[9,109] PHX developing in adulthood does not usually go on to disseminated disease. However, bone involvement accompanying pulmonary disease is recognized in 4% to 13% of adult patients.[109,200] Diabetes insipidus occurs in approximately the same number.

The characteristic radiographic appearance in PHX* consists of a diffuse, symmetric, reticulonodular pattern or, less commonly, a solely nodular pattern (Figure 13-36). The shadowing has a slight middle and upper zone predominance,[109,200,246] although some series show a middle to lower zone accentuation.[195] At any one time all zones tend to be affected, but in one fifth of cases in one series only half the lung was involved.[195] Isolated reports describe lung opacity that is initially unilateral.[4,200,260] The nodules are characteristically ill defined[4] and vary in size from 1 to 15 mm, generally averaging about 5 mm (Figure 13-36).[195] The nodules are usually innumerable, but occasionally they are sufficiently few in

---

*References 4, 109, 195, 200, 260, 375.

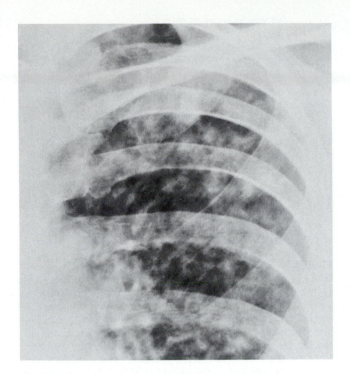

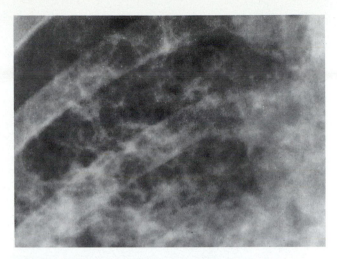

FIGURE 13-37
Histiocytosis X. Localized view of right middle zone shows multiple small ring shadows. Many of these are in 5 to 8 mm range and could be described as honeycomb opacities. Pneumothorax was present.

FIGURE 13-36
Histiocytosis X. Localized view of left middle and upper zone at presentation. Shadowing consists chiefly of ill-defined 3 to 8 mm nodules. Also minor linear element to shadowing is evident.

number to be countable.[109] Large nodules uncommonly mimic metastases,[260] and in rare cases the initial radiographic opacity shows the pattern of airspace consolidation.[260,375] Although necrosis and cavitation in nodules are not uncommonly seen on pathologic study[9] and CT,[246] they are unusual on the chest radiograph, being seen rarely in the larger nodules.[64,265] Beginning early, a linear or reticular element usually accompanies the nodulation (Figure 13-36) and was present in 94% of cases in one series.[195] With time this element tends to become dominant. Airspaces develop, and some areas show honeycomb opacities,[9] a feature that is more typical of PHX than of any other disorder (Figure 13-37). In addition, larger airspaces of up to 5 cm (cysts, blebs, and bullae) may form (Figure 13-38).[200,375] They have a predilection for the middle and upper zones and for the periphery.[9,109] Probably because of the development of these abnormal airspaces, lung volume does not decrease with time. If anything the reverse occurs,[195] and in one series one third of cases showed a definite increase in lung volume radiologically (Figure 13-38).[109] This progression to fibrobullous disease is by no means inevitable, and Lacronique and co-workers[195] found that on radiologic examination about one third cleared (Figure 13-39), one third remained stable, and one third deteriorated. In other series the outcome has been even more favorable.[109]

HRCT changes have been described in two series.[38,246] The principal findings are cysts and nodules, often in

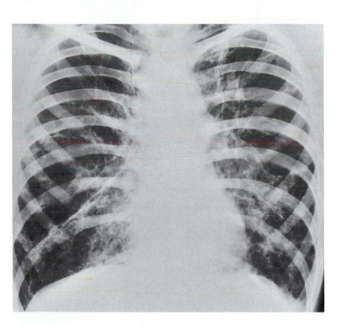

FIGURE 13-38
Histiocytosis X. "Vanishing lungs." Progression to gross lung destruction in this patient, with much of both lungs replaced by avascular bullae and other airspaces.

combination, giving a characteristic appearance (Figure 13-40). When only one type of lesion is present, it is more commonly cyst than nodule. Cysts are seen in the majority of patients (Figure 13-41) and range in diameter from 1 to 30 mm or more. Small cysts (less 10 mm) are more common than bigger cysts (10 to 20 mm), and bullae (more than 20 mm) are the least common. Walls are usually hairline, although in a few patients they are several millimeters thick. Some cysts have bizarre shapes, and others are completely or incompletely septated.

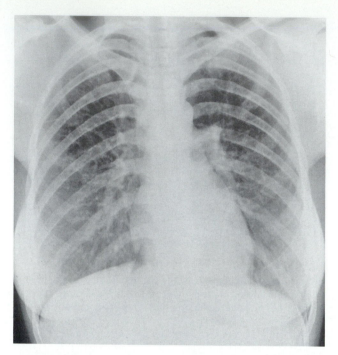

FIGURE 13-39
Histiocytosis X. Same patient as in Figure 13-35. This radiograph, obtained 14 months after image in Figure 13-35, shows almost complete resolution of parenchymal opacities.

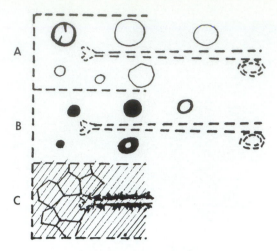

FIGURE 13-40
Histiocytosis X on high-resolution computed tomogram. Three peripheral pulmonary lobules with centrilobular artery and accompanying airway are shown. **A** and **B** represent common and **C** less common changes. **A**, Cysts, varying in size from 2 to 30 mm. Walls are well defined, usually of hairline thickness but occasionally thicker. Some cysts are not rounded, and others are septated. **B**, Nodules, 1 to 10 mm diameter, some cavitated with thick walls, showing no particular distribution within lobule. **C**, Interface irregularity, ground-glass opacity, and reticulation.

Nodules, the other major lesions (Figure 13-42), are typically 1 to 5 mm in diameter with a significant proportion (50% in one series) 5 to 10 mm and a few more than 10 mm. Nodular margins tend to be indistinct, and some are cavitated with a relatively thick wall. Lung between nodules may be strikingly normal.[246] Other signs (interface irregularity, ground-glass opacity, and reticulation) occasionally may be seen. Cysts and nodules are usually diffusely distributed with a middle and upper zone predominance, but occasionally they are confined to the upper zones.[38] On axial sections no characteristic pattern of distribution is seen. When CT changes are correlated with length of history,[38] the findings suggest a progression from nodules to cavitary nodules and to cysts, with end-stage disease showing great destruction and resembling generalized emphysema (Figure 13-43).[246]

Pleural effusion is extremely uncommon. A few cases have been reported, and in two the effusion was probably secondary to bone involvement.[126,274] Mediastinal and hilar node enlargement is likewise uncommon, with occasional reports,[34] some of which have been histologically unconfirmed.[109,217,246] In a single case report, an endobronchial mass caused lung collapse.[268] Of the 10% or so of patients with bone involvement, possibly one fifth have rib involvement that is detectable on the chest radiograph.

NEUROCUTANEOUS SYNDROMES (PHAKOMATOSES)

Five conditions are included in the neurocutaneous syndromes: neurofibromatosis, tuberous sclerosis, ataxia

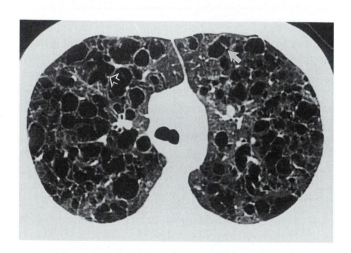

FIGURE 13-41
Histiocystosis X, cystic changes on high-resolution computed tomogram. Multiple cysts with hairline walls ranging in size from 3 to 20 mm. Some cysts are bizarre shape (*open arrow*) and others septated (*closed arrow*).

telangiectasia, Sturge-Weber syndrome, and von Hippel-Lindau syndrome. In these conditions aberrant development of neuroectodermal tissue causes neurologic abnormalities associated with skin and eye lesions. In some cases there are additional mesodermal and endodermal abnormalities.[5]

Neurofibromatosis and tuberous sclerosis are considered in this section. Pulmonary lymphangiomyomatosis is also discussed here because, although it is not a

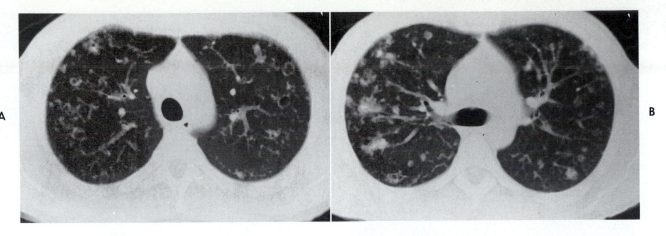

FIGURE 13-42
Histiocytosis X, acute phase. Computed tomograms of same patient were taken, **A**, at and, **B**, just above carina, showing virtually pathognomonic combination of nodules and small ring opacities. Nodules range in size from 3 to 20 mm with majority being about 5 mm diameter. A few are well defined, but most have hazy margin. Ring opacities vary from nodules with pinpoint central lucency through small rings with relatively thick walls to larger lesions that are cystlike. Nodules evolve into cysts with time. (Courtesy Dr. N. Strickland, London.)

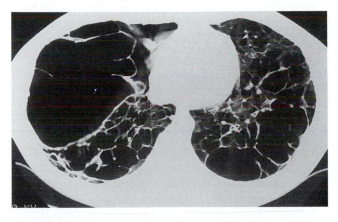

FIGURE 13-43
Histiocytosis X, end-stage disease. High-resolution computed tomography shows destroyed lung replaced by cystic airspaces.

neurocutaneous disorder, it has many features in common with pulmonary tuberous sclerosis.

Neurofibromatosis type I

Neurofibromatosis type I (von Recklinghausen's disease) is an autosomal dominant neurocutaneous syndrome (neurocristopathy) with a prevalence rate of about 1 per 3000 births,[295] one half being mutations. No sex or racial predominance has been found. The principal features are café au lait spots, peripheral nerve tumors (neurofibromas and schwannomas) that particularly affect the skin (fibroma molluscum), and Lisch nodules (pigmented hamartomas of the iris). However, a multitude of other features exist, and virtually any organ can be affected.[188] A set of diagnostic criteria has been proposed.[254]

Neurofibromatosis has a variety of manifestations in the chest (Table 13-1).

CHEST WALL INVOLVEMENT. Cutaneous tumors, especially if they are polypoid, appear as nodules on the chest radiograph. If they are peripheral and unequivocally cutaneous in position, they establish the diagnosis of neurofibromatosis. If, however, they are projected over the lungs, they may resemble intrapulmonary nodules (Figure 13-44). It should not be assumed that because some nodules are unequivocally cutaneous they all are[320]; to do so means the risk of missing a primary or secondary pulmonary neoplasm. The latter consideration is particularly important, since in about 5% of patients with generalized neurofibromatosis, neurofibrosarcomas develop (Figure 13-44),[278] often metastasizing to the lungs.[193]

A neural tumor arising from intercostal nerves away from the spine, if large enough, will give rise to the signs of an extrapleural soft tissue mass,[103] possibly with pressure remodeling (notching) of adjacent upper or lower rib borders. The resulting well-marginated defect is usually relatively wide and shallow compared with the notches seen in coarctation of the aorta. A primary defect in bone formation may also give rise to rib notching,[188] as well as the characteristic "twisted ribbon" deformity.[56,150] Another described pattern of rib abnormality is altered architecture with cyst formation.[308]

Bony thoracic abnormality, particularly kyphoscoliosis, is common (Figure 13-45), and although a prevalence of about 10% is usually quoted for kyphoscoliosis,[150] some recent series have recorded it in up to 60% of patients.[56] Kyphosis occurs only in the presence of scoliosis.[144] Although the appearance of the scoliosis may be nonspecific, some patterns are characteristic, in particular low thoracic, short-segment, angular scolioses involving five

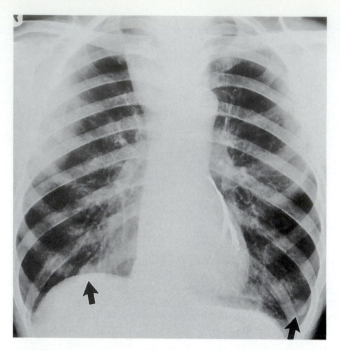

FIGURE 13-44
Neurofibromatosis. Superior mediastinal mass is result of neurofibrosarcoma. Skin nodules (fibroma molluscum) are projected over lungs (arrows) and simulate intrapulmonary nodules. Aspirated barium lies in left bronchial tree. (Courtesy N.L. Wright, London.)

Table 13-1   Thoracic lesions of neurofibromatosis

Location	Lesion
Chest wall	
Skin	Cutaneous tumors (fibroma molluscum)
Nerves	Intercostal nerve tumors
Spine	Kyphoscoliosis, vertebral body modeling abnormality
Ribs	Modeling and architecture abnormality, notching
Mediastinum	
Middle	Neural tumor
Posterior	Lateral meningocele, neural tumor, pheochromocytoma
Lungs	Interstitial fibrosis, airway tumors

vertebrae or fewer in the primary curve.[144,150,231] Vertebral lesions include the following modeling and developmental abnormalities: vertebral body scalloping (posterior, lateral, or anterior)[312]; hypoplastic or pressure remodeled pedicles, particularly mesial flattening; intervertebral foramen enlargement; and transverse process hypoplasia. The most common and best known of these abnormalities is posterior vertebral scalloping, which is typically sharply marginated and smooth and extends over several segments.[55,231] It is usually associated with, and probably causally related to, dural ectasia, although it will occasionally result from pressure by a tumor or simply be caused by developmental hypoplasia.

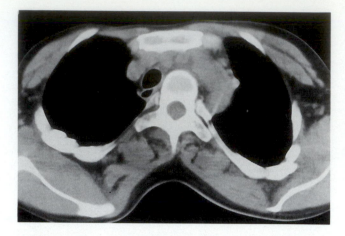

FIGURE 13-45
Neurofibromatosis, skeletal deformity. Gross skeletal deformity with marked reduction of anteroposterior chest diameter. This distorted normal upper mediastinal envelope, and gave an appearance on chest radiograph that suggested nonexistent mediastinal mass.

MEDIASTINAL MASSES. Posterior mediastinal masses are usually caused by neural tumor (neurofibroma or neurilemmoma and their malignant counterparts) or a lateral thoracic meningocele. Lateral thoracic meningoceles are produced by protrusion of dura and arachnoid through an exit foramen, and the majority occur at the apex of a scoliosis on its convex aspect, particularly between T3 and T7.[188] Right-sided lesions predominate, and about 10% are multiple.[235] They are often, but not invariably, associated with vertebral scalloping, pedicle thinning, and expansion of intervertebral foramina.[235] Affected patients are commonly middle aged (30 to 60 years old) and more often than not asymptomatic.[235] Some consider that lateral thoracic meningoceles are the most common posterior mediastinal mass in neurofibromatosis,[188] but this is not borne out in all series.[56] The radiologic features of lateral thoracic meningocele are discussed in Chapter 16.

Neural tumors are usually benign and cause well-demarcated, rounded paraspinal masses (discussed in detail in the section on posterior mediastinal masses). Neural tumors can become malignant with a transformation rate that is probably on the order of 5%.[5]

The third type of associated posterior mediastinal mass is the pheochromocytoma, with a 1% prevalence in neurofibromatosis.[188] It should be considered a possible explanation for hypertension in neurofibromatosis.

Two types of middle mediastinal masses are recognized in neurofibromatosis: one localized and the other diffuse. Discrete masses are the result of solitary neurofibromas, neurilemmomas, or their malignant counterparts affecting the vagus or phrenic nerves (Figure 13-44). They are more commonly left sided and usually asymptomatic, but they may cause hoarseness if the recurrent laryngeal nerve is affected.[78] Diffuse masses often involve adjacent mediastinal compartments, extending down from the thoracic inlet to the hilar level, and may be bilateral. They

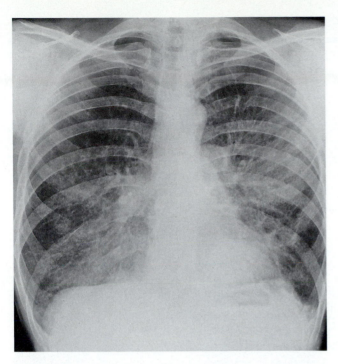

FIGURE 13-46
Neurofibromatosis. Note diffuse interstitial shadowing, predominantly fine and linear. In transradiant right upper zone, vessels are stretched and reduced in number because of bullae. Overall lung volume is increased. Combination of interstitial opacities with bullae and hyperexpanded lungs is characteristic but not pathognomonic of neurofibromatosis.

are the result of plexiform neurofibromas, normal nerve elements bizarrely arranged in a network of fusiform swellings that often infiltrate and incorporate adjacent fat and muscle.[5] On CT they appear as low-attenuation masses, often in all compartments of the upper mediastinum, surrounding vessels in an infiltrative fashion.[30] Although usually slow growing and asymptomatic, they can cause tracheal and bronchial compression.[59]

LUNG INVOLVEMENT. Parenchymal lung involvement in neurofibromatosis takes the form of a fibrosing alveolitis that was first recognized in 1963.[84] Its prevalence increases with age; the youngest patient recorded was 28 years old.[277] The prevalence rate in adults with neurofibromatosis is about 20%,[215,374] with probably no sex difference. Lung involvement in neurofibromatosis is rather benign, in contrast to tuberous sclerosis, and symptoms are often mild, although some patients have progressed to respiratory failure and cor pulmonale.[308] Respiratory function tests show a mixed obstructive and restrictive pattern with impaired diffusion.[374]

The radiologic findings are interstitial opacity and bullous disease. Interstitial shadowing is initially finely linear, with or without a nodular element, and is usually basally predominant. Septal (Kerley B) lines are sometimes present.[374] In time the linear element becomes more marked and widespread (Figure 13-46), and honeycomb opacity may develop.[374] The other principal findings are thin-walled bullae (Figure 13-46),[24,215,216,374] largely middle to upper zonal, often asymmetric, and sometimes large (occupying at least one lung zone). Bullae are sometimes an isolated radiologic finding,[215] but lung biopsy in these circumstances always shows an occult alveolitis.[374]

Rarely a neurofibroma or neurilemmoma produces a parenchymal mass that appears as a peripheral well-demarcated, lobulated nodule.[212] Just as rarely these lesions may arise endobronchially and cause obstructive bronchiectasis.[374] A patient is also described in whom there were multiple 2 mm intramural schwannomas involving the airways of a single lung subsegment.[371]

Tuberous sclerosis

Like neurofibromatosis, although only half as common, tuberous sclerosis is an autosomal dominant[45] neurocutaneous syndrome with an equal sex incidence. About half of the cases are hereditary and the rest sporadic, arising as a result of mutation.[104] The clinical expression is variable and often incomplete, giving rise to formes frustes, which make defining the condition for diagnostic purposes difficult.

The classic clinical features make up a triad of mental retardation, epilepsy, and dermal angiofibromas (adenoma sebaceum). However, only about one third of patients with tuberous sclerosis have all features of this classic triad.[17] Additional major manifestations include other skin lesions (ungual fibromas, shagreen patches, achromic patches), cerebral and paraventricular hamartomas, renal angiomyolipomas, retinal phakomas, bone lesions including calvarial sclerosis, and rhabdomyomas of the heart. The diagnostic criteria used by some workers are the presence of one or more of the following: adenoma sebaceum; retinal phakomas; mental retardation or epilepsy, plus a close relative with adenoma sebaceum or retinal phakomas; and mental retardation, epilepsy, and intracranial calcifications.[196] Other authors have used less stringent criteria.[104] CT scanning has proved particularly useful in the detection of the highly prevalent intracranial calcifications[104] and renal angiomyolipomas and cysts.[243] The prognosis is poor, with 75% of patients dying by age 20.[226]

Pulmonary involvement is distinctly unusual and occurs in about 1% of cases.[92,202] Given the low prevalence of tuberous sclerosis in the population (6 to 7 cases per million persons),[119] only a handful of pulmonary tuberous sclerosis patients are in either the United States or the United Kingdom at any one time. Considerable clinical, radiologic, and pathologic similarities exist between pulmonary involvement in tuberous sclerosis and that found in lymphangiomyomatosis (Table 13-2), some of which are touched on here.

On pathologic study the lungs in tuberous sclerosis show perivascular smooth muscle proliferation and small adenomatoid nodules, both of which probably contribute to the reticulonodular pattern seen radiologically. Proliferating smooth muscle spreads into the walls of airspaces,

Table 13-2   Comparison of lymphangioleiomyomatosis and pulmonary tuberous sclerosis

Factor	Lymphangioleiomyomatosis	Pulmonary tuberous sclerosis
Familial	No	Commonly
Female sex	All	85%
Age	Reproductive	Reproductive
Adenoma sebaceum	No	85%
Epilepsy	No	20%
Intelligence (IQ)	Normal	Low (46%)
Dyspnea	Yes	Yes
Pneumothorax	Yes	Yes
Chylous pleural effusions, ascites	Yes	Rare
Hemoptysis	Yes	Yes
Chest radiograph	Interstitial opacities, cysts, pleural effusion	Interstitial opacities, cysts
Renal angiomyolipoma	Occasional	60%

bronchioles, arterioles, and venules and causes obstruction of these structures. Venular obstruction accounts for hemoptysis, and airway obstruction causes the focal emphysema, cyst or bulla formation, and air trapping that may lead to pneumothorax. The smooth muscle proliferation in tuberous sclerosis tends to spare lymphatics[74,353] and probably accounts for the rarity of lymphatic complications such as chylothorax. Some workers, however, have found smooth muscle proliferation in pulmonary lymphatics and in lymph nodes.[372] The adenomatoid proliferations are a few millimeters in diameter and are scattered throughout the lung.[202]

The clinical features of patients with pulmonary tuberous sclerosis[92] differ from those of tuberous sclerosis in general. The patients are older, the mean age of presentation with respiratory symptoms being 34 years of age; predominantly women (85%); and with a lower prevalence of mental retardation (46%) and epilepsy (20%). However, most patients have adenoma sebaceum,[136] and 60% have renal angiomyolipomas. Once respiratory symptoms develop, they tend to dominate the clinical picture, with progressive dyspnea; recurrent pneumothoraces (in 50%); and less seriously, cough and hemoptysis. Eighty-five percent of patients die within 5 years from either cor pulmonale (59%) or pneumothorax (41%).[92]

The radiologic findings in the chest consist of an interstitial process with symmetric nodular, reticular, or reticulonodular opacities. The nodules are small, about 1 to 2 mm,[122,202] and are often overshadowed by a more dominant, linear element (Figure 13-47).[202] The changes may be diffuse or basally predominant.[122]

With progression of the disease the linear and reticular element becomes more marked and honeycomb and cystic changes may develop.[122,202,226] The cystic shadows tend to be less than 1 cm. Large cysts are uncommon.[226] HRCT findings are the same as those in lymphangioleiomyomatosis.[197]

Unlike most other interstitial processes the lung volume tends to be increased because of small airway obstruction, focal emphysema, air trapping,[352] and cyst formation. Respiratory function tests support this obser-

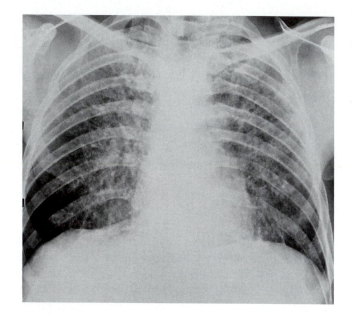

FIGURE 13-47
Tuberous sclerosis. Note diffuse interstitial pulmonary shadowing consisting of small irregular and rounded opacities with predominantly linear element. Although lung volume is commonly increased, it is not so in this patient.

vation and show airflow obstruction, increased static compliance, and increased total lung volume, together with impaired carbon monoxide diffusion.[202]

Pneumothorax is common,[136] frequently recurrent, and sometimes bilateral.[122] Late in the disease, pulmonary arterial hypertension and cor pulmonale may be present. In contrast to lymphangioleiomyomatosis, pleural effusions are uncommon in tuberous sclerosis. However, chylous effusions have been reported.[208,372] Bone changes are described and may be visible on the chest radiograph, notably an expanded dense rib resembling fibrous dysplasia or Paget's disease.[5]

LYMPHANGIO(LEIO)MYOMATOSIS

Although not a neurocutaneous disorder, lymphangio(leio)myomatosis (LAM) shares many pulmonary fea-

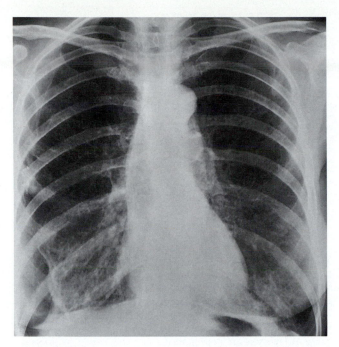

FIGURE 13-48
Lymphangiomyomatosis. Note basally predominant diffuse interstitial shadowing, chiefly fine and linear. Upper zones are transradiant because of bulla formation, and lung volume is increased. Right pneumothorax is present, a common presenting feature.

tures with pulmonary tuberous sclerosis (PTS). It differs from PTS in that it is not heredofamilial and lacks many of the neuroectodermal features of PTS such as adenoma sebaceum, epilepsy, and mental retardation. Furthermore, some findings, such as chylothorax, that are unusual in PTS are common in LAM. The features of LAM and PTS are compared in Table 13-2.

There have been several major reviews of LAM.[50,74,339]

The pathologic changes in the chest in LAM are similar to those in PTS in that both show smooth muscle proliferation. However, the muscle proliferation in LAM differs from that in PTS in two major ways: it is primarily perilymphatic, with later spread to involve airways, airspaces, and vessels; and it can affect pulmonary, mediastinal, and retroperitoneal lymph nodes.[192,353] In one series of patients with LAM, 69% had mediastinal and 53% had retroperitoneal node involvement.[339] Lymphatic involvement is a major feature in LAM but a minor one in PTS; hence chylothorax (and chyloperitoneum) are major features of LAM but unusual in PTS. Interstitial fibrosis is typically not found in LAM.[192] Some workers view LAM and PTS as different entities on histologic and other grounds,[353] while others consider the question unresolved.[74] One of the reasons for holding the latter view is that overlap cases occur. Thus renal angiomyolipomas, a characteristic finding in tuberous sclerosis, may occur in cases that according to all other criteria are cases of LAM.[74,229,245] In addition, both chylothorax[43,208] and lymph node involvement are recorded in PTS.[171] The issue is even more complicated because other patients have been identified

who have chylothorax or chyloperitoneum and lymph node involvement (mediastinal and retroperitoneal), which are typical findings of LAM, but whose lungs are normal.[339] Such patients have been reported to develop lung disease many years later.[339]

All patients are female and almost all are of childbearing age (mean age 30 years), except for a few postmenopausal patients on hormone replacement.[360] The initial manifestation is progressive dyspnea, pneumothorax, chylothorax, or hemoptysis. Pneumothoraces as an initial event are common, occurring in 53% of patients in one series,[360] and often recur (Figure 13-48).[50] The overall prevalence of pneumothorax in the 67 cases reported up to 1977 was 39.3%[50] and more recently was 81% in 32 patients.[360] Chylous pleural effusions in LAM are a recognized presenting feature and were the initial event in 7% of patients in one series.[74] Effusions occurred at some time or other during the course of the disease in 75% of 67 cases.[50] Effusions may be unilateral or bilateral and are typically large, recurrent,[339] and chylous.[192] Hemoptysis occurs in 40% of cases[50] and is occasionally the initial feature.[360] Chylous ascites is not uncommon (25% of one series[74]) and is often accompanied by a pleural effusion.[339] Some unusual manifestations noted in the review by Silverstein and co-workers[339] included chylopericardium, chyluria, and chyloptysis. In a group of seven patients delayed pulmonary parenchymal changes developed up to 5 years after the recognition of lymph node involvement or chylous effusion.[339] Respiratory function tests usually show airflow obstruction, increased total lung capacity, increased compliance, and impaired diffusion.[50]

As with other interstitial processes, the chest radiograph may appear normal despite histologically proven disease. This finding has been demonstrated in patients with pneumothorax in whom a pleurectomy and lung biopsy were performed.[50] The earliest radiographic signs of lung disease consist of fine nodular, reticular, or reticulonodular opacities (Figure 13-49).[74] These changes are symmetric; they may be generalized[240] or sometimes basally predominant, at least initially.[339] With time the reticular pattern, which may be very delicate and sharp,[74] tends to become coarser and more irregular. Some of the linear elements have features of septal (Kerley B) lines and may be transient.[50,240] Cysts, bullae,[240] and honeycomb opacity can develop, the last having thinner walls than the usual honeycomb shadows.[50] During this stage lung volumes commonly increase.[197] The combination of interstitial shadowing and increasing lung volume is characteristic of LAM, unlike the progressive loss in volume that accompanies most other interstitial lung disorders (Figures 13-48 and 13-49).[50] In advanced disease the proximal pulmonary arteries enlarge with the development of cor pulmonale (see Figure 13-52).[74]

Interstitial changes have a characteristic appearance on HRCT (Figure 13-50).* The principal findings are multi-

---

*References 1, 23, 197, 250, 292, 334, 365.

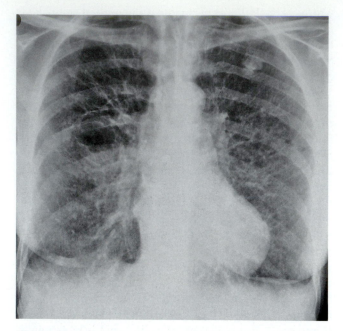

FIGURE 13-49
Lymphangiomyomatosis. Note diffuse fine reticulonodular shadowing with predominant linear pattern. Lung volume is increased, and thin-walled ring shadows in right middle and upper zones are evident. Combination of interstitial shadowing and increased lung volume is characteristic of lymphangiomyomatosis. Calcified opacity in left upper zone is incidental granuloma.

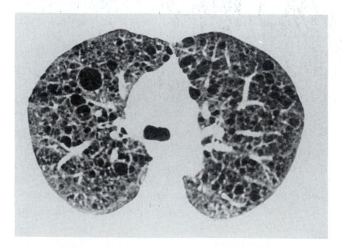

FIGURE 13-51
Lymphangioleiomyomatosis. High-resolution computed tomogram shows multiple thin-walled cysts distributed in essentially uniform fashion in otherwise normal lung. Cysts range in size from 2 to 30 mm and have thin (about 1 mm) well-defined walls.

ple, thin-walled cysts distributed in a uniform fashion in otherwise essentially normal lung (Figure 13-51). Cysts are clearly demarcated by a thin even wall (1 to 2 mm thick) and are usually rounded, although larger ones are occasionally polygonal or bizarrely shaped, sometimes suggesting coalescence.[197] The size of cysts ranges from 2 to 50 mm, with many in the 5 to 15 mm range. Cyst size

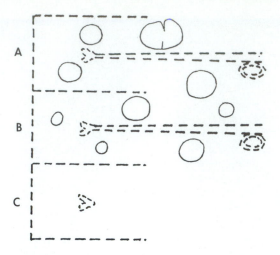

FIGURE 13-50
Lymphangioleiomyomatosis on high-resolution computed tomograms. Three peripheral pulmonary lobules with centrilobular artery and accompanying airway. A and B represent common changes. A and B, Multiple thin-walled cysts distributed in uniform fashion with intervening normal lung. Most cysts have diameters in 5 to 15 mm range. A few cysts are nonrounded.

increases as the disease becomes more widespread.[250] In general, cysts show no preferential distribution of any type, although two studies record relative apical sparing.[1,292] HRCT is more sensitive at detecting cysts than CT or chest radiographs, and the latter may be normal despite abnormalities in HRCT.[197,250,334] Furthermore, a case is reported with a normal HRCT but a positive biopsy.[250]

Chylous pleural effusions occur in some 75% of cases (Figure 13-52).[50] They may be unilateral or bilateral[240] and are typically large and recurrent.[339] Pleural effusion and pneumothorax may coexist.[240] On pathologic grounds[245] lymphadenopathy might be expected as a radiologic finding, but it is recorded only occasionally on chest radiography.[240,334] However, in a recent CT series of eight patients, 50% had mediastinal nodes. If this proves to be a repeatable observation, it will be a useful differentiating feature from pulmonary HX, which resembles LAM on CT.

Early reports suggested a poor prognosis.[74,339] The prognosis has, however, improved following the introduction of antiestrogen therapy (progesterone administration or oophorectomy),[95] and in a recent series 78% of patients were still alive 8.5 years after the onset of disease.[360] Early diagnosis is important. Although LAM is a rarity, it should be considered in women of childbearing age with chylous effusion or repeated pneumothoraces, particularly with airflow obstruction and disproportionately poor gas exchange together with large-volume lungs and interstitial opacity on the chest radiograph.[50]

ANKYLOSING SPONDYLITIS

Ankylosing spondylitis (AS) is a seronegative spondyloarthritis that affects primarily the axial skeleton, caus-

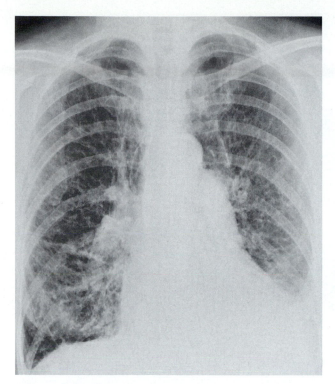

FIGURE 13-52
Lymphangiomyomatosis. Note diffuse reticulonodular interstitial shadowing. Pleural effusion at left base proved to be chylous, and there had been right chylous effusion 4 years before. Proximal pulmonary arteries are large, indicating presence of pulmonary artery hypertension, a recognized complication of lymphangiomyomatosis.

ing pain and progressive stiffness of the spine. The peripheral joints are involved in 35% of patients.[47] Extraarticular features may develop; these include anterior uveitis (up to 25%), aortic regurgitation (up to 10% in long-standing cases),[121] cardiac conduction defects,[20] and constitutional symptoms. The prognosis is variable. Some patients do not progress beyond sacroiliitis, whereas others develop progressive, widespread disease leading in particular to complete fusion of the axial joints and across the intervertebral disks of the spine.

Pleuropulmonary involvement has a late onset and is usually asymptomatic.[309] Two types exist: chest wall restriction and upper lobe fibrobullous disease.[149]

Restrictive disease is caused by fusion of costovertebral and costotransverse joints. Changes in lung function are surprisingly small because the chest becomes fixed at a high resting volume, allowing the diaphragm to make a greater contribution than usual to inspiration.[149] Apical hypoventilation, which might have been expected under these circumstances, is not present.[275] Generally, total lung capacity and vital capacity are mildly or moderately reduced while functional residual capacity and residual volume are normal or slightly increased.[149,359] This contrasts with the marked impairment of respiratory function seen in kyphoscoliosis.[359]

Upper zone "fibrobullous" disease was first recorded in

1941,[91] but its recognition as an extraarticular manifestation of AS had to wait more than 20 years for the paper by Campbell and MacDonald in 1965.[48] The phenomenon is rare; its frequency, based on a review of 2080 patients at the Mayo Clinic, is 1.25%.[309] A strong male predilection exists, with just 3 women out of a total of 160 patients in one review.[142] The pathologic findings are nonspecific and consist of fibrosis and a chronic inflammatory cell infiltrate, often lymphocytic, with elastic fragmentation, collagen degeneration, dilated bronchi, thin-walled bullae, and cavities.[165,383]

The radiologic changes* consist of nodular and linear shadowing or pleural thickening that begins in the lung apices. The early changes are usually symmetric but may be asymmetric (one third in one series).[82] After a while the opacity tends to become bilateral and symmetric and the nodules and pleural thickening become more pronounced and confluent. After a further interval, often several years,[48] one or more rounded transradiancies appear in most cases.[82,309,383] The transradiancies are usually multiple; they may be small or large and have thin or thick walls. These apical changes usually progress slowly,[82] but they can remain stable for many years. At this stage the process is essentially one of fibrosis; the hila become elevated, producing an appearance that mimics tuberculosis (Figure 13-53). Apical fibrosis is usually seen only in patients who have marked spinal involvement[57] and long-standing ankylosing spondylitis, 15 to 20 years on average.[82,309,383] A few cases are recorded in which the lung changes apparently developed within a few years of the onset of AS.[48,309] Patients are also recorded in whom a diagnosis of AS was made retrospectively after chest disease developed.[142]

The cavities that develop within the fibrotic lung may be colonized by a variety of fungi and nontuberculous mycobacteria,[31,149,309,359] most commonly *Aspergillus fumigatus*.[82] Colonization rates with *Aspergillus* have varied between 19%[309] and 50% to 60%.[48,82] Hemoptysis is common in patients with mycetoma and may be life threatening. Surgical removal is often attended by complications.[31,149,359]

By the time the pulmonary changes are visible, the skeletal manifestations of AS[90] are usually obvious on posteroanterior and lateral chest radiographs. The findings that are most easily seen in frontal view are ossification of costotransverse joints (particularly the first), vertebral syndesmophytes, and interspinous ossification. The diagnosis of AS is, however, generally more easily made from a lateral radiograph (Figure 13-53, *B*). The principal changes detected in this projection are kyphosis, syndesmophytes (particularly at the D9 to D12 level), and squared or barrel-shaped vertebral bodies. The manubriosternal joint is frequently eroded or fused.[325]

Pleural effusions and pleural thickening remote from the lung apex[182] have been seen in association with AS,

---

*References 48, 57, 82, 142, 165, 309, 383.

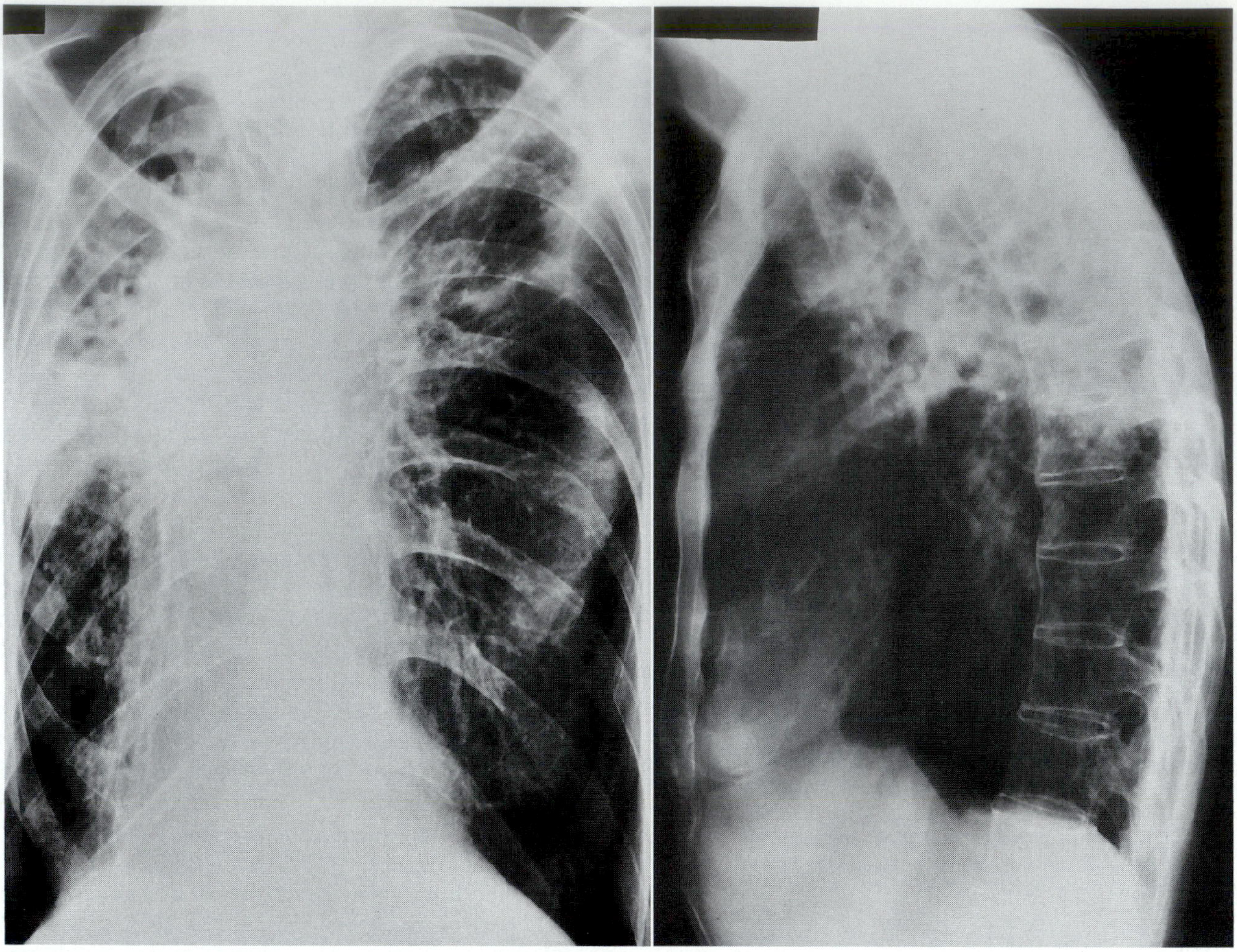

FIGURE 13-53
Ankylosing spondylitis. **A,** Posteroanterior chest radiograph with bilateral but grossly asymmetric apical changes. Note marked upper zone volume loss and many ring shadows. **B,** Lateral radiograph of same patient demonstrating spinal fusion.

but the prevalence is so low (only 3 of the 2080 cases in the Mayo Clinic series)[309] that they are almost certainly chance findings. The pneumothorax rate, however, is significantly increased, with a prevalence of about 8%.[309]

PULMONARY ALVEOLAR PROTEINOSIS

Pulmonary alveolar proteinosis (PAP) is a rare disorder characterized pathologically by filling of the alveoli with a lipid-rich, proteinaceous material (positive to periodic acid–Schiff stain), while the lung interstitium remains relatively normal.[177] It probably represents a nonspecific response of the type II pneumocyte, the alveolar macrophage, or both to a variety of injuries.[281] Although a history of exposure to dust or chemicals is common in some series,[81,222] a definite relationship has been established only in acute silicosis,[138] particularly caused by sand blasting.[355] Other associations that seem to be etiologically important, at least in some cases, are with hematologic malignancies (lymphoma and leukemia)[49]

and immunologic abnormalities, particularly in children. In one review 30% of children with PAP had thymic alymphoplasia.[69] The alveolar material is partly phospholipid derived from type II pneumocytes and resembles surfactant. The rest is cellular debris and protein from plasma. Whether phospholipid accumulation is the result of overproduction (proliferation and desquamation of type II pneumocytes), reduced clearance (defective macrophage function), or both is not clear.[281] The exact mechanism probably varies with the cause.

PAP is most common in adults, particularly between 30 to 50 years of age, although cases are seen in children, including in the first year of life.[81] Sixty to eighty percent of patients are male.[81,281] Children with this disorder are usually compromised hosts, and the disease is progressive and often fatal, whereas adults generally have no underlying disorder. In about one fifth of cases the onset is acute, with fever, weight loss, and dyspnea, either with or without a superadded opportunistic infection.[81] Most of

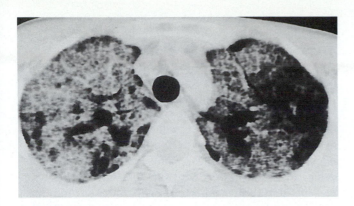

FIGURE 13-54
Pulmonary alveolar proteinosis. Computed tomogram demonstrates geographic nature of much of consolidation. Medially in right lung, air bronchogram is present. High-density reticulation is result of septal edema. (Courtesy Dr. C. Murch and the Royal College of Radiologists, London.)

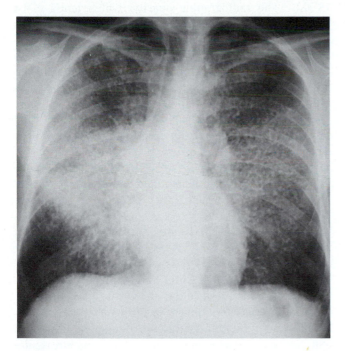

FIGURE 13-55
Pulmonary alveolar proteinosis. Note diffuse bilateral airspace opacity with perihilar predominance. Confluent opacity breaks up at margins into nodular pattern (2 to 3 mm) that is smaller than that of acinar nodules. In some areas, opacity could be described as ground glass.

the other cases have an insidious onset with progressive dyspnea and cough. Other early features include pleuritic chest pain, hemoptysis,[281] and pneumothorax.[81] Occasionally the disease is discovered by chest radiography in asymptomatic individuals.[310] The clinical signs consist of crepitations and sometimes hypoxemia, and clubbing. PAP is one of the conditions in which the radiologic signs are often striking even when the symptoms and clinical signs are mild.[3] Respiratory function tests show a restric-

tive defect with hypoxemia and impaired diffusion.[281] The diagnosis is established by bronchoalveolar lavage or transbronchial lung biopsy.

The main radiologic finding is airspace shadowing, since the pathologic changes are almost entirely the result of alveolar filling. In some cases, however, mild interstitial fibrosis and septal cellular infiltration and edema are present (Figure 13-54),[81,239,304,310] and probably account for occasional "interstitial" features on the chest radiograph. The classic radiologic finding is bilateral symmetric airspace opacity, particularly in a perihilar or hilar and basal distribution (Figure 13-55).[81,290,304] This shadowing often has a fine granularity. At other times the pattern consists of rather coarse (5 mm), ill-defined acinar nodules, perhaps in part confluent (Figure 13-55).[220] The nodules may be particularly obvious toward the edge of confluent areas of consolidation,[310] and at times the shadowing may even be reticulonodular.[220,239,281,310] Although usually symmetric, the consolidation can be asymmetric,[310] unilateral,[281,304] or lobar.[49,303] Sometimes the consolidation is basally predominant,[49] peripheral rather than central,[3] and multifocal rather than diffuse.[281] Simultaneous evolution and regression, producing a shifting pattern similar to that found in the eosinophilic lung states, has been described.[279] Occasional features include septal (Kerley B) lines[281,290] and small rounded transradiancies,[283,290] probably produced by obstructive overinflation of distal respiratory units, partly blocked by proteinaceous material. Rupture of a subpleural cyst has given rise to a pneumothorax.[3] Obstruction may also give rise to areas of collapse.[281,283,290]

CT and HRCT changes are characterized by a marked reticular pattern superimposed on ground-glass airspace opacity (Figures 13-54 and 13-56).[116,258] Involved areas are surrounded by normal lung and have a sharp, geographic margin reflecting lobular boundaries. Imaging changes show no characteristic distribution. Other airspace opacities that may be found include acinar nodules, limited air bronchograms, and areas of consolidation where the density of the opacity obscures underlying vessels. In the last instance the possibility of additional infective consolidation should be considered. The reticular pattern is confined largely to the areas of airspace opacity and resembles crazy paving. Intersecting lines probably represent interlobular and intralobular septal thickening. The striking reticulation contrasts with histologic data indicating only mild septal edema and cellular infiltration.[81,239,304,310]

Because of the functional macrophage impairment, complicating infections by pathogenic bacteria[290] or opportunistic bacterial, fungal, and viral[49] agents are common. In one review[13] 15% of 160 patients had such infections, and they were a major cause of death[81] before therapeutic lavage was introduced.[281] *Nocardia* is particularly prevalent.[49,81,310] Radiologic pointers to such an opportunistic infection include the development of focal consolidation, cavitation, and pleural effusion.[81]

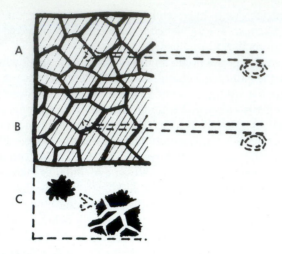

FIGURE 13-56
Pulmonary alveolar proteinosis on high-resolution computed tomogram. Three peripheral pulmonary lobules with centrilobular artery and accompanying airway. **A** and **B** represent common and **C** less common changes. **A** and **B**, Ground-glass opacity with superimposed "crazy paving" reticulation caused by intralobular and interlobular thickening. **C**, Acinar nodules, localized consolidation with air bronchogram.

PAP clears spontaneously in 25% of patients[81,281] but in the remainder needs to be treated with saline lung lavage.[291] Lavage has virtually eliminated mortality[300] and results in complete remission in 75% of patients.[281] When patients are treated with lavage, the chest radiograph is used to decide which side should be treated and to detect any complications.[110]

PULMONARY ALVEOLAR MICROLITHIASIS

Pulmonary alveolar microlithiasis was first described in 1918.[135] It is a rare disorder, with 225 cases recorded in the world literature.[370] Its cause is unknown, and it is one of the conditions in which gross radiographic changes are present in the face of minor clinical symptoms.

Alveolar microlithiasis is characterized pathologically by the accumulation of numerous, largely intraalveolar calcified bodies (calcispherites or microliths). Microliths have a mean diameter of about 200 μm[58] and contain calcium phosphate.[177] Dystrophic ossification occasionally develops around microliths.[58] There have been rare descriptions of extrapulmonary microliths.[66,324] Alveolar walls are commonly normal,[282] but later in the disease interstitial fibrosis may develop together with bullae and blebs.[324,347]

Although alveolar microlithiasis occurs worldwide, nearly one fourth of recorded patients are from Turkey.[370] About 40% of cases are sporadic, while the remainder show a strong familial association,[46] for practical purposes restricted to siblings and consistent with an autosomal recessive transmission. Sex incidence is approximately equal.[282] The disease is commonly first detected in the third and fourth decades,[282] but the range is large, with the disorder recorded in neonates[46] and in an 80-year-old woman.[324]

In three of four major series 60% to 80% of patients have been symptomless at the time of diagnosis.[214,282,347] The exception is a Turkish series in which 80% were symptomatic.[370] Later in the course of the disease cough may appear, and in a small proportion of patients hemoptysis, clubbing, hypertrophic osteoarthropathy,[370] pneumothorax, dyspnea, and cor pulmonale develop.[282,347] Respiratory function tests have been abnormal in about one third of reported cases and most commonly show a restrictive defect or a decreased carbon monoxide diffusing capacity.[282]

The chest radiograph is characteristic,[347] with innumerable, widespread, pinpoint nodules of calcific density (Figure 13-57). Nodules are less than 1 mm in diameter, but they may summate in areas to give a ground-glass or more coarsely nodular (up to 5 mm) pattern (Figure 13-58).[7] The radiographic opacity, which tends to be greatest at the bases, is generally diffuse but sometimes shows subpleural[7,347] and peribronchovascular accentuation.[7] In gross disease the radiographic opacity is so great that anatomic landmarks become completely obscured. Thus the heart may "vanish"[7] or even appear as a transradiant area on a penetrated radiograph (Figure 13-59). Pleural fissures can appear thickened,[7,368] and septal lines are occasionally seen.[7,241] Bullae and blebs develop with late fibrosis,[282,324,347] and these are particularly well seen on CT.[58,381] Such blebs and bullae probably predispose patients to pneumothorax and pneumomediastinum, which are recognized complications.[324,381]

CT data on microlithiasis are limited to nine cases (four seen on HRCT).[58,65,191,381] Alveolar calcification is either micronodular or ground glass with posterobasal predominance. The occasional 5 mm nodule presumably represents dystrophic ossification seen histopathologically. Calcification may be uniform or may show some macroscopic structure with accentuation along pleural margins and fissures, interlobular septa, and bronchovascular bundles,[65,381] explaining the coarsely linear nodulation, reticulation, and septal lines occasionally seen on the chest radiograph.[7,241] All CT studies showed airspaces (blebs or bullae) either apically[381] or throughout the lung.[65] In one study a striking subpleural peel of paraseptal emphysema was seen.[191]

Very few patients with microlithiasis are recorded in whom a preceding normal chest radiograph has been documented.[184,366] The micronodular opacities in microlithiasis usually appear from the beginning to be of calcific density. A few patients, however, have been described with nodulation that was initially of soft tissue density and that later became definitely calcific.[184] Bone-seeking agents such as technetium-99m diphosphonate are taken up by microliths, and this may be shown scintigraphically.[44]

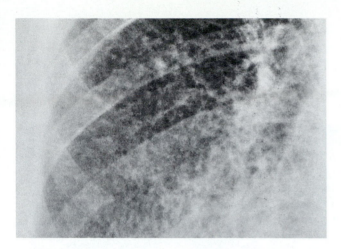

FIGURE 13-57
Alveolar microlithiasis. Localized view of right midzone shows basic element of shadowing: high-density nodules less than 1 mm in diameter. (Courtesy Dr. O. Heldaas, Konigsberg, Norway.)

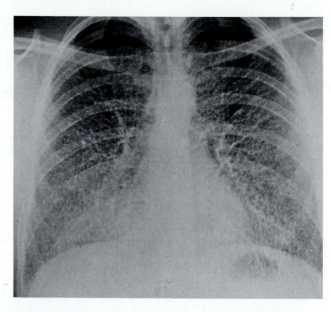

FIGURE 13-58
Alveolar microlithiasis. Opacities are distributed symmetrically throughout both lungs, sparing apices. Although basic opacity is high-density nodule less than 1 mm in diameter, as shown here, summation tends to produce larger nodules several millimeters in diameter. (Courtesy Dr. O. Heldaas, Konigsberg, Norway.)

The prognosis is variable. Many patients remain a symptomatic with stable chest radiographs for many years.[44] Others, sometimes after many years of stability, go on to experience pulmonary fibrosis or cor pulmonale and ultimately die of the disease.[58,324,347]

CRYPTOGENIC ORGANIZING PNEUMONIA

Cryptogenic organizing pneumonia (COP) is a clinico-pathologic entity of unknown cause characterized by a clinical disorder with systemic symptoms, cough, and dyspnea; patchy, peripheral airspace opacity on the chest radiograph; and on pathologic examination, granulation tissue plugs in alveoli, alveolar ducts, and occasionally small airways. COP is synonymous with idiopathic bronchiolitis obliterans organizing pneumonia (BOOP), and currently there is no consensus as to the preferred term.[73,97] BOOP is not to be confused with bronchiolitis obliterans per se, which is a quite separate entity.

The recognition of COP as a distinct clinicopathologic entity came with three reports in the early to middle 1980s,[85,98,124] although there had been sporadic earlier descriptions. The pathologic hallmark of COP is patchy cellular fibrosis that predominantly involves airspaces (alveoli, alveolar ducts, and less commonly distal bronchioles). The fibroblasts are embedded in a myxoid matrix with a variable infiltrate of lymphocytes, macrophages, plasma cells, and neutrophils[177] and form characteristic polypoidal masses (bourgeons conjonctifs or Masson bodies).[72] Other pathologic findings include alveolar accumulation of foamy macrophages and a mild, chronic interstitial inflammation. The histologic diagnosis can be made by transbronchial biopsy,[8] but open lung biopsy[67] or percutaneous cutting needle biopsy[129] is preferred.

A striking clinical similarity has been seen among cases of COP reported from various centers.[76,85,98,181,385] Mean

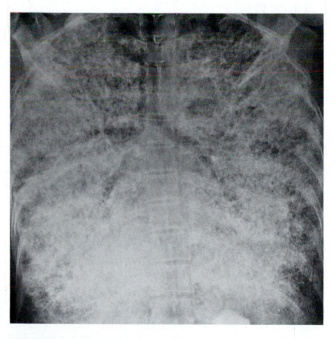

FIGURE 13-59
Alveolar microlithiasis. Gross disease. Mediastinum appears less dense radiographically than lungs.

patient age is 55 to 60 years (range 20 to 80 years),[181] and sex incidence is equal. Up to 50% of patients give a history of an influenza-like prodrome followed by a short illness of about 3 months characterized by cough (persistent and nonproductive), exertional dyspnea, malaise, fever, and

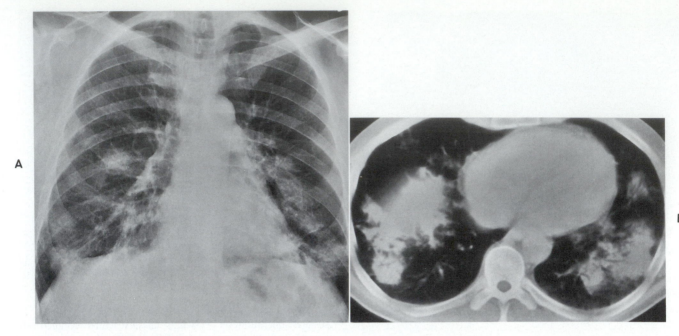

FIGURE 13-60
Cryptogenic organizing pneumonia. Patient is 55-year-old man who had viral-like syndrome during previous 3 months and complained of increasing tiredness and dyspnea. **A,** Posteroanterior radiograph. **B,** Computed tomogram (CT) through lung bases (obtained at time when diagnosis was not known) shows multiple, nonspecific areas of consolidation, some of which have nodular configuration. Air bronchograms are striking on CT. Diagnosis was established at open lung biopsy.

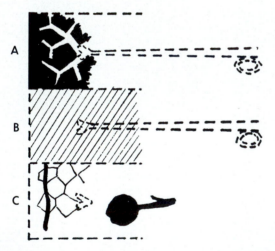

FIGURE 13-61
Cryptogenic organizing pneumonia, high-resolution computed tomography. Three peripheral pulmonary lobules with centrilobular artery and accompanying airway. **A** and **B** represent common and **C** less common changes. **A,** Peripheral consolidation with air bronchogram. **B,** Ground-glass opacity often with lobular configuration. **C,** Peripheral reticulation, subpleural lines, and nodules (sometimes with "feeder" vessel).

weight loss. Less common complaints include pleuritic pain[29,129] and hemoptysis.[71,129] On clinical examination of the lungs, fine, dry crepitations occur in 70% to 90% of patients; clubbing is rare.[76] The erythrocyte sedimentation rate is invariably raised and may be very high.[244]

Respiratory function tests show a restrictive abnormality, commonly with a diffusion defect and hypoxemia at rest or on exertion. Bronchoalveolar lavage is lymphocytic and nonspecific,[261] although some authors think it has diagnostic features.[76]

The radiologic hallmark of COP is bilateral, patchy consolidation (Figure 13-60). Consolidation is nonsegmental and commonly 2 to 6 cm in diameter. It occurs in all zones but shows a basal predominance (upper/mid/lower of approximately 1:1:3).[76,160] Consolidation may contain an air bronchogram[85] and sometimes has a ground-glass appearance.[8,29] On CT it has a strikingly peripheral distribution, and sometimes this is also a feature of the chest radiograph.[8,129] Consolidation tends to migrate and come and go even without treatment[85,129,160,244] and may rarely cavitate.[71,105] Ten to fifty percent of patients have other radiologic findings either isolated or accompanying typical consolidation: 1 to 2 cm ill-defined nodules,[29,129,253] smaller nodules ranging from 1 to 10 mm,[71,127,253] and a reticulonodular or fine linear pattern.[60,98,160] Pleural effusions occur occasionally with an overall frequency of less than 5%.[29,244]

A limited number of studies have looked at the CT and HRCT appearances of COP.[29,129,253,264] The main findings are focal consolidations, predominantly subpleural with air bronchograms (Figures 13-60 and 13-61). Consolidations are bilateral and asymmetric, ranging from about 1.5 cm in diameter to segmental size. In addition, ground-glass opacity is seen on HRCT, often with a lobular distribution.[264] Other findings include 1 to 10 mm well-defined nodules, sometimes predominantly along bronchovascular bundles[253]; peripheral reticulation and subpleural lines[29]; peripheral opacities, which are large nodular or masslike and sometimes have "feeder" airways or vessels[29]; and bronchial wall thickening and dilatation on HRCT.[253]

COP may resolve spontaneously[98,385] but usually needs treatment with steroids. With therapy clinical and radiographic signs clear in the majority of patients in days or weeks, but some are left with persistent disease and a small number die.[178] About one third of patients relapse on withdrawal of treatment.[98]

Pathologic changes in COP are nonspecific, and similar changes are seen in a wide range of disorders.[67,177,384] In most of these conditions the clinical and radiologic findings allow an easy distinction. However, in some disorders the clinicoradiologic features are identical to those of COP except for an identifiable precipitating condition. Identified disorders[113] are infections, including AIDS; most connective tissue disorders; drug toxicity (gold, amiodarone, cephalosporin, acebutalol, sulfasalazine, mesalazine); and other conditions, including thyroiditis[385] and ulcerative colitis. A seasonal variety has been identified.[349]

REFERENCES

1. Aberle DR, Hansell DM, Brown K, et al: Lymphangiomyomatosis: CT, chest radiographic and functional correlations, *Radiology* 176:381-387, 1990.
2. Aggarwal S, Arora NK, Koyyana R, et al: Interstitial lung disease in a young child, *Chest* 96:389-390, 1989.
3. Anton HC, Gray B: Pulmonary alveolar proteinosis presenting with pneumothorax, *Clin Radiol* 18:428-431, 1967.
4. Arnett NL, Schulz DM: Primary pulmonary eosinophilic granuloma, *Radiology* 69:224-230, 1957.
5. Aughenbaugh GL: Thoracic manifestations of neurocutaneous diseases, *Radiol Clin North Am* 22:741-756, 1984.
6. Auld D: Pathology of eosinophilic granuloma of the lung, *Arch Pathol Lab Med* 63:113-131, 1957.
7. Balikian JP, Fuleihan FJD, Nucho CN: Pulmonary alveolar microlithiasis: report of five cases with special reference to roentgen manifestations, *AJR* 103:509-518, 1968.
8. Bartter T, Irwin RS, Nash G, et al: Idiopathic bronchiolitis obliterans organizing pneumonia with peripheral infiltrates on chest roentgenogram, *Arch Intern Med* 149:273-279, 1989.
9. Basset F, Corrin B, Spencer H, et al: Pulmonary histiocytosis X, *Am Rev Respir Dis* 118:811-820, 1978.
10. Battesti JP, Georges R, Basset F, et al: Chronic cor pulmonale in pulmonary sarcoidosis, *Thorax* 33:76-84, 1978.
11. Battesti JP, Saumon G, Valeyre D, et al: Pulmonary sarcoidosis with an alveolar radiographic pattern, *Thorax* 37:448-452, 1982.
12. Baughman RP: Sarcoidosis: usual and unusual manifestations, *Chest* 94:165-170, 1988.
13. Bedrossian CWM, Luna MA, Conklin RH, et al: Alveolar proteinosis as a consequence of immunosuppression: a hypothesis based on clinical and pathologic observation, *Hum Pathol* 11(suppl):527-535, 1980.
14. Beekman JF, Zimmet SM, Chun BK, et al: Spectrum of pleural involvement in sarcoidosis, *Arch Intern Med* 136:323-330, 1976.
15. Bein ME, Putman CE, McLoud TC, et al: A reevaluation of intrathoracic lymphadenopathy in sarcoidosis, *AJR* 131:409-415, 1978.
16. Bekerman C, Szidon JP, Pinsky S: The role of gallium-67 in the clinical evaluation of sarcoidosis, *Semin Roentgenol* 20:400-409, 1985.
17. Bell DG, King BF, Hattery RR, et al: Imaging characteristics of tuberous sclerosis, *AJR* 156:1081-1086, 1991.
18. Benatar SR: Sarcoidosis in South Africa: a comparative study in whites, blacks and coloureds, *S Afr Med J* 52:602-606, 1977.
19. Benatar SR: A comparative study of sarcoidosis in white, black and coloured South Africans. In Williams WJ, Davies BH, eds: *Eighth International Conference on Sarcoidosis and Other Granulomatous Diseases*, Cardiff, Wales, 1980, Alpha Omega, pp 508-513.
20. Bergfeldt L: HLA B27-associated rheumatic diseases with severe cardiac bradyarrhythmias, *Am J Med* 75:210-215, 1983.
21. Bergin C, Roggli V, Coblentz C, et al: The secondary pulmonary lobule: normal and abnormal CT appearances, *AJR* 151:21-25, 1988.
22. Bergin CJ, Bell DY, Coblentz CL, et al: Sarcoidosis: correlation of pulmonary parenchymal pattern at CT with results of pulmonary function tests, *Radiology* 171:619-624, 1989.
23. Bergin CJ, Coblentz CL, Chiles C, et al: Chronic lung diseases: specific diagnosis by using CT, *AJR* 152:1183-1188, 1989.
24. Bergin CJ, Muller NL: CT in the diagnosis of interstitial lung disease, *AJR* 145:505-510, 1985.
25. Berkmen YM: Radiologic aspects of intrathoracic sarcoidosis, *Semin Roentgenol* 20:356-375, 1985.
26. Berkmen YM, Javors BR: Anterior mediastinal lymphadenopathy in sarcoidosis, *AJR* 127:983-987, 1976.
27. Berte SJ, Pfotenhauer MA: Massive pleural effusion in sarcoidosis, *Am Rev Respir Dis* 86:261-264, 1962.
28. Bistrong HW, Tenney RD, Sheffer AL: Asymptomatic cavitary sarcoidosis, *JAMA* 213:1030-1032, 1970.
29. Bouchardy LM, Kuhlman JE, Ball WC, et al: CT findings in bronchiolitis obliterans organizing pneumonia (BOOP) with radiographic, clinical, and histologic correlation, *J Comput Assist Tomogr* 17:352-357, 1993.
30. Bourgouin PM, Shepard J-A O, Moore EH, et al: Plexiform neurofibromatosis of the mediastinum: CT appearance, *AJR* 151:461-463, 1988.
31. Boushea DK, Sundstrom WR: The pleuropulmonary manifestations of ankylosing spondylitis, *Semin Arthritis Rheum* 18:277-281, 1989.
32. Bower JS, Dantzker DR: Airway obstruction in sarcoidosis, *Am Rev Respir Dis* 115(suppl 4):91, 1977.
33. Bradstreet CMP, Dighero MW, Mitchell DN: The Kveim test: analysis of results of tests using K 19 materials. In Williams WJ, Davies BH, eds: *Eighth International Conference on Sarcoidosis and Other Granulomatous Diseases*, Cardiff, Wales, 1980, Alpha Omega, pp 674-677.
34. Brambilla E, Fontaine E, Pison CM, et al: Pulmonary histiocytosis X with mediastinal lymph node involvement, *Am Rev Respir Dis* 142:1216-1218, 1990.
35. Brandstetter RD, Hansen DE, Jarowski CI, et al: Superior vena cava syndrome as the initial clinical manifestation of sarcoidosis, *Heart Lung* 10:101-104, 1981.
36. Brandstetter RD, Messina MS, Sprince NL, et al: Tracheal stenosis due to sarcoidosis, *Chest* 80:656, 1981.
37. Brauner MW, Grenier P, Mompoint D, et al: Pulmonary sarcoidosis: evaluation with high-resolution CT, *Radiology* 172:467-471, 1989.
38. Brauner MW, Grenier P, Mouelhi MM, et al: Pulmonary histiocytosis X: evaluation with high-resolution CT, *Radiology* 172:255-258, 1989.
39. Brauner MW, Lenoir S, Grenier P, et al: Pulmonary sarcoidosis: CT assessment of lesion reversibility, *Radiology* 182:349-354, 1992.

40. Breuer R, Baigelman W, Pugatch RD: Occult mycetoma, *J Comput Assist Tomogr* 6:166-168, 1982.

41. Brincker H, Wilbek E: The incidence of malignant tumours in patients with respiratory sarcoidosis, *Br J Cancer* 29:247-251, 1974.

42. Brodey PA, Pripstein S, Strange G, et al: Vertebral sarcoidosis: a case report and review of the literature, *AJR* 126:900-902, 1976.

43. Broughton RBK: Pulmonary tuberous sclerosis presenting with pleural effusion, *Br Med J* 1:477-478, 1970.

44. Brown ML, Swee RG, Olson RJ, et al: Pulmonary uptake of 99mTc diphosphonate in alveolar microlithiasis, *AJR* 131:703-704, 1978.

45. Bundey S, Evans K: Tuberous sclerosis: a genetic study, *J Neurol Neurosurg Psychiatry* 32:591-603, 1969.

46. Caffrey PR, Altman RS: Pulmonary alveolar microlithiasis occurring in premature twins, *J Pediatr* 66:758-763, 1965.

47. Calin A: Ankylosing spondylitis, *Clin Rheum Dis* 11:41-60, 1985.

48. Campbell AH, MacDonald CB: Upper lobe fibrosis associated with ankylosing spondylitis, *Br J Dis Chest* 59:90-101, 1965.

49. Carnovale R, Zornoza J, Goldman AM, et al: Pulmonary alveolar proteinosis: its association with hematologic malignancy and lymphoma, *Radiology* 122:303-306, 1977.

50. Carrington CB, Cugell DW, Gaensler EA, et al: Lymphangioleiomyomatosis: physiologic-pathologic-radiologic correlations, *Am Rev Respir Dis* 116:977-995, 1977.

51. Carrington CB, Gaensler EA, Mikus JP, et al: Structure and function in sarcoidosis, *Ann NY Acad Sci* 278:265-283, 1976.

52. Case records of the Massachusetts General Hospital: case 51-1974, *N Engl J Med* 291:1402-1408, 1974.

53. Case records of the Massachusetts General Hospital: case 11-1984, *N Engl J Med* 310:708-716, 1984.

54. Case records of the Massachusetts General Hospital: case 40-1985, *N Engl J Med* 313:874-883, 1985.

55. Casselman ES, Mandell GA: Vertebral scalloping in neurofibromatosis, *Radiology* 131:89-94, 1979.

56. Casselman ES, Miller WT, Lin SR, et al: Von Recklinghausen's disease: incidence of roentgenographic findings with a clinical review of the literature, *CRC Crit Rev Diagn Imag* 9:387-419, 1977.

57. Chakera TMH, Howarth FH, Kendall MJ, et al: The chest radiograph in ankylosing spondylitis, *Clin Radiol* 26:455-460, 1975.

58. Chalmers AG, Wyatt J, Robinson PJ: Computed tomographic and pathological findings in pulmonary alveolar microlithiasis, *Br J Radiol* 59:408-411, 1986.

59. Chalmers AH, Armstrong P: Plexiform mediastinal neurofibromas: a report of two cases, *Br J Radiol* 50:215-217, 1977.

60. Chandler PW, Shin MS, Friedman SE, et al: Radiographic manifestations of bronchiolitis obliterans with organizing pneumonia vs usual interstitial pneumonia, *AJR* 147:899-906, 1986.

61. Chrisholm JC, Lang GR: Solitary circumscribed pulmonary nodule: an unusual manifestation of sarcoidosis, *Arch Intern Med* 118:376-378, 1966.

62. Chusid EL, Siltzbach LE: Sarcoidosis of the pleura, *Ann Intern Med* 81:190-194, 1974.

63. Citron KM, Scadding JG: Stenosing non-caseating tuberculosis (sarcoidosis) of the bronchi, *Thorax* 12:10-17, 1957.

64. Clark RL, Margulies SI, Mulholland JH: Histiocytosis X: a fatal case with unusual pulmonary manifestations, *Radiology* 95:631-632, 1970.

65. Cluzel P, Grenier P, Bernadac P, et al: Pulmonary alveolar microlithiasis: CT findings, *J Comput Assist Tomogr* 15:938-942, 1991.

66. Coetzee T: Pulmonary alveolar microlithiasis with involvement of the sympathetic nervous system and gonads, *Thorax* 25:637-642, 1970.

67. Colby TV: Pathologic aspects of bronchiolitis obliterans organizing pneumonia, *Chest* 102(suppl):38S-43S, 1992.

68. Colby TV, Lombard C: Histiocytosis X in the lung, *Hum Pathol* 14:847-856, 1983.

69. Colon AR, Lawrence RD, Mills SD: Childhood pulmonary alveolar proteinosis (PAP): report of a case and review of the literature, *Am J Dis Child* 121:481-485, 1971.

70. Conant EF, Glickstein MF, Mahar P, et al: Pulmonary sarcoidosis in the older patient: conventional radiographic features, *Radiology* 169:315-319, 1988.

71. Cordier J-F, Loire R, Brune J: Idiopathic bronchiolitis obliterans organizing pneumonia: definition of characteristic clinical profiles in a series of 16 patients, *Chest* 96:999-1004, 1989.

72. Corrin B: Systemic pathology. Vol 5. *The lungs*, ed 3, Edinburgh, 1990, Churchill Livingstone.

73. Corrin B: Bronchiolitis obliterans organizing pneumonia: a British view, *Chest* 102(suppl):7S, 1992.

74. Corrin B, Liebow AA, Friedman PJ: Pulmonary lymphangiomyomatosis, *Am J Pathol* 79:348-382, 1975.

75. Corsello BF, Lohaus GH, Funahashi A: Endobronchial mass lesion due to sarcoidosis: complete resolution with corticosteroids, *Thorax* 38:157-158, 1983.

76. Costabel U, Teschler MD, Schoenfeld B, et al: BOOP in Europe, *Chest* 102(suppl):14S-20S, 1992.

77. Crystal RG, Roberts WC, Hunninghake GW, et al: Pulmonary sarcoidosis: a disease characterized and perpetuated by activated lung T-lymphocytes, *Ann Intern Med* 94:73-94, 1981.

78. Dabir RR, Piccione W, Kittle CF: Intrathoracic tumors of the vagus nerve, *Ann Thorac Surg* 50:494-497, 1990.

79. Da Costa JL, Chiang SC: Pleural sarcoidosis, *Singapore Med J* 6:224-226, 1975.

80. Damuth TE, Bower JS, Cho K, et al: Major pulmonary artery stenosis causing pulmonary hypertension in sarcoidosis, *Chest* 78:888-891, 1980.

81. Davidson JM, MacLeod WM: Pulmonary alveolar proteinosis, *Br J Dis Chest* 63:13-28, 1969.

82. Davies D: Ankylosing spondylitis and lung fibrosis, *Q J Med* 41:395-417, 1972.

83. Davies J, Nellen M, Goodwin JF: Reversible pulmonary hypertension in sarcoidosis, *Postgrad Med J* 58:282-285, 1982.

84. Davies PDB: Diffuse pulmonary involvement in von Recklinghausen's disease: a new syndrome, *Thorax* 18:198, 1963.

85. Davison AG, Heard BE, McAllister WAC, et al: Cryptogenic organizing pneumonitis, *Q J Med* 52:382-394, 1983.

86. Demicco WA, Fanburg BL: Sarcoidosis presenting as a lobar or unilateral lung infiltrate, *Clin Radiol* 33:663-669, 1982.

87. DeRemee RA: The roentgenographic staging of sarcoidosis, *Chest* 83:128-133, 1983.

88. Di Benedetto R, Lefrak S: Systemic sarcoidosis with severe involvement of the upper respiratory tract, *Am Rev Respir Dis* 102:801-807, 1970.

89. Di Benedetto RJ, Ribaudo C: Bronchopulmonary sarcoidosis, *Am Rev Respir Dis* 94:952-955, 1966.

90. Dihlmann W: Current radiodiagnostic concept of ankylosing spondylitis, *Skeletal Radiol* 4:179-188, 1979.

91. Dunham CL, Kautz FG: Spondylarthritis ankylopoietica: review and report of 20 cases, *Am J Med Sci* 201:232-250, 1941.

92. Dwyer JM, Hickie JB, Garvan J: Pulmonary tuberous sclerosis: report of three patients and a review of the literature, *Q J Med* 40:115-125, 1971.

93. Edelman RR, Johnson TS, Jhaveri HS, et al: Fatal hemoptysis resulting from erosion of a pulmonary artery in cavitary sarcoidosis, *AJR* 145:37-38, 1985.

94. Edmondstone WM, Wilson AG: Sarcoidosis in Caucasians, blacks and Asians in London, *Br J Dis Chest* 79:27-36, 1985.

95. Eliasson AH, Phillips YY, Tenholder MF: Treatment of lymphangioleiomyomatosis: a meta-analysis, *Chest* 196:1352-1355, 1989.

96. Ellis K, Renthal G: Pulmonary sarcoidosis: roentgenographic observations on course of disease, *AJR* 88:1070-1083, 1962.

97. Epler GR: Bronchiolitis obliterans organizing pneumonia: definition and clinical features, *Chest* 102(suppl):2S-6S, 1992.

98. Epler GR, Colby TV, McLoud TC, et al: Bronchiolitis obliterans organizing pneumonia, *N Engl J Med* 312:152-158, 1985.

99. Farinacci CJ, Jeffrey HC, Lackey RW: Eosinophilic granuloma of lung: report of two cases, *US Armed Forces Med J* 2:1085-1093, 1951.

100. Faunce HF, Ramsay GC, Sy W: Protracted yet variable major pulmonary artery compression in sarcoidosis, *Radiology* 119:313-314, 1976.

101. Favara BE: Langerhans' cell histiocytosis pathobiology and pathogenesis, *Semin Oncol* 18:3-7, 1991.

102. Felson B: Uncommon roentgen patterns of pulmonary sarcoidosis, *Dis Chest* 34:357-367, 1958.

103. Felson B: The extra pleural space, *Semin Roentgenol* 12:327-333, 1977.

104. Fleury P, de Groot WP, Delleman JW, et al: Tuberous sclerosis: the incidence of sporadic cases versus familial cases, *Brain Dev* 2:107-117, 1980.

105. Flowers JR, Clunie G, Burke M, et al: Bronchiolitis obliterans organizing pneumonia: the clinical and radiological features of seven cases and a review of the literature, *Clin Radiol* 45:371-377, 1992.

106. Fossa SD, Abeler V, Marton PF, et al: Sarcoid reaction of hilar and paratracheal lymph nodes in patients treated for testicular cancer, *Cancer* 56:2212-2216, 1985.

107. Freiman DG: The pathology of sarcoidosis, *Semin Roentgenol* 20:327-339, 1985.

108. Freundlich IM, Libshitz HI, Glassman LM, et al: Sarcoidosis: typical and atypical thoracic manifestations and complications, *Clin Radiol* 21:376-383, 1970.

109. Friedman PJ, Liebow AA, Sokoloff J: Eosinophilic granuloma of lung: clinical aspects of primary pulmonary histiocytosis in the adult, *Medicine* 60:385-396, 1981.

110. Gale ME, Karlinsky JB, Robins AG: Bronchopulmonary lavage in pulmonary alveolar proteinosis: chest radiograph observations, *AJR* 146:981-985, 1986.

111. Gardiner IT, Uff JS: Acute pleurisy in sarcoidosis, *Thorax* 33:124-127, 1978.

112. Gardner J, Kennedy HG, Hamblin A, et al: HLA associations in sarcoidosis: a study of two ethnic groups, *Thorax* 39:19-22, 1984.

113. Geddes DM: BOOP & COP, *Thorax* 46:545-547, 1991.

114. Gilman MJ, Wang KP: Transbronchial lung biopsy in sarcoidosis: an approach to determine the optimal number of biopsies, *Am Rev Respir Dis* 122:721-724, 1980.

115. Glazer HS, Levitt RG, Shackelford GD: Peripheral pulmonary infiltrates in sarcoidosis, *Chest* 86:741-744, 1984.

116. Godwin JD, Müller NL, Takasugi JE: Pulmonary alveolar proteinosis: CT findings, *Radiology* 169:609-613, 1988.

117. Goffman TE, Bloom RL, Dvorak VC: Acute dyspnea in a young woman taking birth control pills, *JAMA* 251:1465-1466, 1984.

118. Goldenberg GJ, Greenspan RH: Middle-lobe atelectasis due to endobronchial sarcoidosis with hypercalcemia and renal impairment, *N Engl J Med* 262:1112-1116, 1960.

119. Gomez MR: *Tuberous sclerosis*, New York, 1979, Raven Press.

120. Gorske KJ, Fleming RJ: Mycetoma formation in cavitary pulmonary sarcoidosis, *Radiology* 95:279-285, 1970.

121. Graham DC, Smythe HA: The carditis and aortitis of ankylosing spondylitis, *Bull Rheum Dis* 9:171-174, 1958.

122. Green GJ: The radiology of tuberose sclerosis, *Clin Radiol* 19:135-147, 1968.

123. Gregorie HB, Othersen HB, Moore MP: The significance of sarcoid-like lesions in association with malignant neoplasms, *Am J Surg* 104:577-586, 1962.

124. Grinblat J, Mechlis S, Lewitus Z: Organizing pneumonia–like process: an unusual observation in steroid responsive cases with features of chronic interstitial pneumonia, *Chest* 80:259-263, 1981.

125. Gross BH, Schneider HJ, Proto AV: Eggshell calcification of lymph nodes: an update, *AJR* 135:1265-1268, 1980.

126. Guardia J, Pedreira JD, Esteban R, et al: Early pleural effusion in histiocytosis X, *Arch Intern Med* 139:934-936, 1979.

127. Guerry-Force ML, Müller NL, Wright JL, et al: A comparison of bronchiolitis obliterans with organizing pneumonia, usual interstitial pneumonia, and small airways disease, *Am Rev Respir Dis* 135:705-712, 1987.

128. Guildford WB, Mentz WM, Kopelman HA, et al: Sarcoidosis presenting as a rib fracture, *AJR* 139:608-609, 1982.

129. Haddock JAA, Hansell DM: The radiology and terminology of cryptogenic organizing pneumonia, *Br J Radiol* 65:674-680, 1992.

130. Hadfield JW, Page RL, Flower CDR, et al: Localised airway narrowing in sarcoidosis, *Thorax* 37:443-447, 1982.

131. Hafermann DR, Solomon DA, Byrd RB: Sarcoidosis initially occurring as apical infiltrate and pleural reaction, *Chest* 73:413-414, 1978.

132. Hamilton R, Petty TL, Haiby G: Cavitary sarcoidosis of the lung, *Arch Intern Med* 116:428-430, 1965.

133. Hamper UM, Fishman EK, Khouri NF, et al: Typical and atypical CT manifestations of pulmonary sarcoidosis, *J Comput Assist Tomogr* 10:928-936, 1986.

134. Hance AJ, Cadranel J, Soler P, et al: Pulmonary and extra pulmonary Langerhans' cell granulomatosis (histiocytosis X), *Semin Respir Med* 9:349-368, 1988.

135. Harbitz F: Extensive calcification of the lungs as a distinct disease, *Arch Intern Med* 21:139-146, 1918.

136. Harris JO, Waltuck BL, Swenson EW: The pathophysiology of the lungs in tuberous sclerosis: a case report and literature review, *Am Rev Respir Dis* 100:379-387, 1969.

137. Henry DA, Cho SR: Tracheal stenosis in sarcoidosis, *South Med J* 76:1323-1324, 1983.

138. Heppleston AG, Wright NA, Stewart JA: Experimental alveolar lipo-proteinosis following the inhalation of silica, *J Pathol* 101:293-307, 1970.

139. Heshiki A, Schatz SL, McKusick KA, et al: Gallium 67 citrate scanning in patients with pulmonary sarcoidosis, *AJR* 122:744-749, 1974.

140. Hetherington S: Sarcoidosis in young children, *Am J Dis Child* 136:13-15, 1982.

141. Hietala S, Stinnett RG, Faunce HF: Pulmonary artery narrowing in sarcoidosis, *JAMA* 237:572-573, 1977.

142. Hillerdal G: Ankylosing spondylitis lung disease — an under-diagnosed entity? *Eur J Respir Dis* 64:437-441, 1983.

143. Hoffstein V, Ranganathan N, Mullen JBM: Sarcoidosis simulating pulmonary veno-occlusive disease, *Am Rev Respir Dis* 134:809-811, 1986.

144. Holt JF: Neurofibromatosis in children, *AJR* 130:615-639, 1978.

145. Honey M, Jepson E: Multiple bronchostenoses due to sarcoidosis: report of two cases, *Br Med J* 2:1330-1334, 1957.

146. Honeybourne D: Ethnic differences in the clinical features of sarcoidosis in South-East London, *Br J Dis Chest* 74:63-69, 1980.

147. Huang CT, Heurich AE, Rosen Y, et al: Pulmonary sarcoidosis: a radiographic, functional and pathological correlation. In Williams WJ, Davies BH, eds: *Eighth International Conference on Sarcoidosis and Other Granulomatous Diseases*, Cardiff, Wales, 1980, Alpha Omega, pp 368-377.

148. Huang CT, Heurich AE, Sutton AL, et al: Mortality in sarcoidosis. In Williams WJ, Davies BH, eds: *Eighth International Conference on Sarcoidosis and Other Granulomatous Diseases*. Cardiff, Wales, 1980, Alpha Omega, pp 522-526.

149. Hunninghake GW, Fauci AS: Pulmonary involvement in the collagen vascular diseases, *Am Rev Respir Dis* 119:471-503, 1979.

150. Hunt JC, Pugh DG: Skeletal lesions in neurofibromatosis, *Radiology* 76:1-20, 1961.

151. Israel HL: Experience with the treatment of aspergillosis complicating sarcoidosis. In *Proceedings of the Sixth International Conference on Sarcoidosis 1972*, Baltimore, 1974, University Park Press.

152. Israel HL, Karlin P, Menduke H, et al: Factors affecting outcome of sarcoidosis: influence of race, extrathoracic involvement, and initial radiologic lung lesion, *Ann NY Acad Sci* 465:609-617, 1986.

153. Israel HL, Lenchner G, Steiner RM: Late development of mediastinal calcification in sarcoidosis, *Am Rev Respir Dis* 124:302-305, 1981.

154. Israel HL, Lenchner GS, Atkinson GW: Sarcoidosis and aspergilloma: the role of surgery, *Chest* 82:430-432, 1982.

155. Israel HL, Park CH, Mansfield CM: Gallium scanning in sarcoidosis, *Ann NY Acad Sci* 278:514-516, 1976.

156. Israel HL, Sones M: Sarcoidosis: clinical observation on one hundred sixty cases, *Arch Intern Med* 102:766-776, 1958.

157. Israel HL, Sones M, Roy RL, et al: The occurrence of intrathoracic calcification in sarcoidosis, *Am Rev Respir Dis* 84:1-11, 1961.

158. Israel HL, Sperber M, Steiner RM: Course of chronic hilar sarcoidosis in relation to markers of granulomatous activity, *Invest Radiol* 18:1-15, 1983.

159. Israel HL, Washburne JD: Characteristics of sarcoidosis in black and white patients: analysis of 162 recent cases. In Williams WJ, Davies BH, eds: *Eighth International Conference on Sarcoidosis and Other Granulomatous Diseases*, Cardiff, Wales, 1980, Alpha Omega, pp 497-507.

160. Izumi T, Kitaichi M, Nishimura K, et al: Bronchiolitis obliterans organizing pneumonia: clinical features and differential diagnosis, *Chest* 102:715-719, 1992.

161. James DG, Carstairs LS: Pulmonary sarcoidosis, *Hosp Update* 8:1022-1030, 1982.

162. James DG, Neville E, Siltzbach LE, et al: A worldwide review of sarcoidosis, *Ann NY Acad Sci* 278:321-335, 1976.

163. James DG, Williams WJ: *Sarcoidosis and other granulomatous disorders*, Philadelphia, 1985, WB Saunders.

164. Javaheri S, Hales CA: Sarcoidosis: a cause of innominate vein obstruction and massive pleural effusion, *Lung* 157:81-85, 1980.

165. Jessamine AG: Upper lung lobe fibrosis in ankylosing spondylitis, *Can Med Assoc J* 98:25-29, 1968.

166. Johns CJ: Management of hemoptysis with pulmonary fungus balls in sarcoidosis, *Chest* 82:400-401, 1982.

167. Johns CJ, MacGregor MI, Zachary JB, et al: Chronic sarcoidosis: outcome, unusual features and complications. In Williams WJ, Davies BH, eds: *Eighth International Conference on Sarcoidosis and Other Granulomatous Diseases*, Cardiff, Wales, 1980, Alpha Omega, pp 558-566.

168. Johnson NM, Martin NDT, McNicol MW: Sarcoidosis presenting with pleurisy and bilateral pleural effusions, *Postgrad Med J* 56:266-267, 1980.

169. Jones DK, Dent RG, Rimmer MJ, et al: Thin-walled ring shadows in early pulmonary sarcoidosis, *Clin Radiol* 35:307-310, 1984.

170. Judson MA, Ghent S, Close TP: Sarcoidosis manifested as peripheral pulmonary infiltrates, *AJR* 160:1359-1360, 1993.

171. Kaku T, Toyoshima S, Enjoji M: Tuberous sclerosis with pulmonary and lymph node involvement: relationship to lymphangiomyomatosis, *Acta Pathol Jpn* 33:395-401, 1983.

172. Kalbian VV: Bronchial involvement in pulmonary sarcoidosis, *Thorax* 12:18-23, 1957.

173. Kanada DJ, Scott D, Sharma OP: Unusual presentations of pleural sarcoidosis, *Br J Dis Chest* 74:203-205, 1980.

174. Kaplan J, Johns CJ: Mycetomas in pulmonary sarcoidosis: nonsurgical management, *Johns Hopkins Med J* 145:157-161, 1979.

175. Karasick SR: Atypical thoracic lymphadenopathy in sarcoidosis, *AJR* 133:928-929, 1979.

176. Kataria YP, Sharma OM, Israel H, et al: Kveim antigen CRI. In Williams WJ, Davies BH, eds: *Eighth International Conference on Sarcoidosis and Other Granulomatous Diseases*, Cardiff, Wales, 1980, Alpha Omega, pp 660-667.

177. Katzenstein AA, Askin FB: *Surgical pathology of non-neoplastic lung disease*, ed 2, Philadelphia, 1990, WB Saunders.

178. Katzenstein AA, Myers JL, Prophet DW, et al: Bronchiolitis obliterans and usual interstitial pneumonia, *Am J Surg Pathol* 10:373-381, 1986.

179. Kent DC: Recurrent unilateral hilar adenopathy in sarcoidosis, *Am Rev Respir Dis* 91:272-276, 1965.

180. Khan MM, Gill DS, McConkey B: Myopathy and external pulmonary artery compression caused by sarcoidosis, *Thorax* 36:703-704, 1981.

181. King TE, Mortenson RL: Cryptogenic organizing pneumonitis: the North American experience, *Chest* 102(suppl):8S-13S, 1992.

182. Kinnear WJM, Shneerson JM: Acute pleural effusions in inactive ankylosing spondylitis, *Thorax* 40:150-151, 1985.

183. Kinney EL, Murthy R, Ascunce G, et al: Sarcoidosis: rare cause of superior vena caval obstruction, *Pa Med* 83:31, 1980.

184. Kino T, Kohara Y, Tsuji S: Pulmonary alveolar microlithiasis: a report of two young sisters, *Am Rev Respir Dis* 105:105-110, 1972.

185. Kirks DR, Greenspan RH: Sarcoid, *Radiol Clin North Am* 11:279-294, 1973.

186. Kirks DR, McCormick VD, Greenspan RH: Pulmonary sarcoidosis: roentgenologic analysis of 150 patients, *AJR* 117:777-786, 1973.

187. Kirschner BS, Hollinger PH: Laryngeal obstruction in childhood sarcoidosis, *J Pediatr* 88:263-265, 1976.

188. Klatte EC, Franken EA, Smith JA: The radiographic spectrum in neurofibromatosis, *Semin Roentgenol* 11:17-33, 1976.

189. Knox AJ, Wardman AG, Page RL: Tuberculous pleural effusion occurring during corticosteroid treatment of sarcoidosis, *Thorax* 41:651, 1986.

190. Koerner SK, Sakowitz AJ, Appelman RI, et al: Transbronchial lung biopsy for the diagnosis of sarcoidosis, *N Engl J Med* 293:268-270, 1975.

191. Korn MA, Schurawitzki H, Klepetko W, et al: Pulmonary alveolar microlithiasis: findings on high-resolution CT, *AJR* 158:981-982, 1992.

192. Kruglik GD, Reed JC, Daroca PJ: RPC from the AFIP, *Radiology* 120:583-588, 1976.

193. Kumar AJ, Kuhajda FP, Martinez CR, et al: Computed tomography of extra cranial nerve sheath tumours with pathological correlation, *J Comput Assist Tomogr* 7:857-865, 1983.

194. Kutty CPK, Varkey B: Sarcoidosis presenting with posterior mediastinal lymphadenopathy, *Postgrad Med* 71:64-66, 1982.

195. Lacronique J, Roth C, Battesti J-P, et al: Chest radiological features of pulmonary histiocytosis X: a report based on 50 adult cases, *Thorax* 37:104-109, 1982.

196. Lagos JC, Gomez MR: Tuberous sclerosis: reappraisal of a clinical entity, *Mayo Clin Proc* 42:26-49, 1967.

197. Lenoir S, Grenier P, Brauner MW, et al: Pulmonary lymphangiomyomatosis and tuberous sclerosis: comparison of radiographic and thin-section CT findings, *Radiology* 175:329-334, 1990.

198. Levinsky L, Cummiskey J, Romer FK, et al: Sarcoidosis in Europe: a cooperative study, *Ann NY Acad Sci* 278:335-346, 1976.

199. Levinson RS, Metzger LF, Stanley NN, et al: Airway function in sarcoidosis, *Am J Med* 62:51-59, 1977.

200. Lewis JG: Eosinophilic granuloma and its variants with special reference to lung involvement, *Q J Med* 33:337-359, 1964.

201. Libshitz HI, Atkinson GW, Israel HL: Pleural thickening as a manifestation of *Aspergillus* superinfection, *AJR* 120:883-886, 1974.

202. Lie JT, Miller RD, Williams DE: Cystic disease of the lungs in tuberous sclerosis: clinicopathologic correlation, including body plethysmographic lung function tests, *Mayo Clin Proc* 55:547-553, 1980.

203. Lieberman J: Elevation of serum angiotensin converting enzyme (ACE) level in sarcoidosis, *Am J Med* 59:365-372, 1975.

204. Lieberman J, Nosal A, Schlessner LA, et al: Serum angiotensin-converting enzyme for diagnosis and therapeutic evaluation of sarcoidosis, *Am Rev Respir Dis* 120:329-335, 1979.

205. Line BR, Hunninghake GW, Keogh BA, et al: Gallium-67 scanning to stage the alveolitis of sarcoidosis: correlation with clinical studies, pulmonary function studies, and bronchoalveolar lavage, *Am Rev Respir Dis* 123:440-446, 1981.

206. Littner MR, Schachter EN, Putman CE, et al: The clinical assessment of roentgenographically atypical pulmonary sarcoidosis, *Am J Med* 62:361-368, 1977.

207. Lofgren S: Primary pulmonary sarcoidosis, *Acta Med Scand* 145:424-431, 465-474, 1953.

208. Luna CM, Gene R, Jolly EC, et al: Pulmonary lymphangiomyomatosis associated with tuberous sclerosis, *Chest* 88:473-475, 1985.

209. Lynch DA, Webb WR, Gamsu G, et al: Computed tomography in pulmonary sarcoidosis, *J Comput Assist Tomogr* 13:405-410, 1989.

210. MacFarlane JT: Recurrent erythema nodosum and pulmonary sarcoidosis, *Postgrad Med J* 57:525, 1981.

211. MacPherson P: A survey of erythema nodosum in a rural community between 1954 and 1968, *Tubercle* 51:324-327, 1970.

212. Madewell JE, Feigin DS: Benign tumors of the lung, *Semin Roentgenol* 12:175-186, 1977.

213. Marcy TW, Reynolds HY: Pulmonary histiocytosis X, *Lung* 163:129-150, 1985.

214. Mascie-Taylor BH, Wardman AG, Madden CA, et al: A case of alveolar microlithiasis: observation over 22 years and recovery of material by lavage, *Thorax* 40:952-953, 1985.

215. Massaro D, Katz S: Fibrosing alveolitis: its occurrence, roentgenographic and pathologic features in von Recklinghausen's neurofibromatosis, *Am Rev Respir Dis* 93:934-942, 1966.

216. Massaro D, Katz S, Matthews MJ, et al: Von Recklinghausen's neurofibromatosis associated with cystic lung disease, *Am J Med* 38:233-240, 1965.

217. Masson RG, Tedeschi LG: Pulmonary eosinophilic granuloma with hilar adenopathy simulating sarcoidosis, *Chest* 73:682-683, 1978.

218. Mathieson JR, Mayo JR, Staples CA, et al: Chronic diffuse infiltrative lung disease: comparison of diagnostic accuracy of CT and chest radiography, *Radiology* 171:111-116, 1989.

219. Mayock RL, Bertrand P, Morrison CE, et al: Manifestations of sarcoidosis: analysis of 145 patients, with a review of nine series selected from the literature, *Am J Med* 35:67-89, 1963.

220. McCook TA, Kirks DR, Merten DF, et al: Pulmonary alveolar proteinosis in children, *AJR* 137:1023-1027, 1981.

221. McCort JJ, Pare PJ: Pulmonary fibrosis and cor pulmonale in sarcoidosis, *Radiology* 62:496-504, 1954.

222. McEuen DD, Abraham JL: Particulate concentrations in pulmonary alveolar proteinosis, *Environ Res* 17:334-339, 1978.

223. McKusick KA, Soin JS, Ghiladi A, et al: Gallium 67 accumulation in pulmonary sarcoidosis, *JAMA* 223:688, 1973.

224. McLoud TC, Epler GR, Gaensler EA, et al: A radiographic classification for sarcoidosis: physiologic correlation, *Invest Radiol* 17:129-138, 1982.

225. McLoud TC, Putman CE, Pascual R: Eggshell calcification with systemic sarcoidosis, *Chest* 66:515-517, 1974.

226. Medley BE, McLeod RA, Houser OW: Tuberous sclerosis, *Semin Roentgenol* 11:35-54, 1976.

227. Mendelson DS, Gray CE, Teirstein AS: Magnetic resonance findings in sarcoidosis of the thorax, *Magn Reson Imaging* 10:523-529, 1992.

228. Mendelson DS, Norton K, Cohen BA, et al: Bronchial compression: an unusual manifestation of sarcoidosis, *J Comput Assist Tomogr* 7:892-894, 1983.

229. Merchant RN, Pearson MG, Rankin RN, et al: Computerized tomography in the diagnosis of lymphangioleiomyomatosis, *Am Rev Respir Dis* 131:295-297, 1985.

230. Mesbahi SJ, Davies P: Unilateral pulmonary changes in the chest x-ray in sarcoidosis, *Clin Radiol* 32:283-287, 1981.

231. Meszaros WT, Guzzo F, Schorsch H: Neurofibromatosis, *AJR* 98:557-569, 1966.

232. Meyrier A, Valeyre D, Bouillon R, et al: Resorptive versus absorptive hypercalciuria in sarcoidosis, *Q J Med* 54:269-281, 1985.

233. Mikhail JR, Lovell D, McGhee KJ, et al: Sarcoidosis presenting with a pleural effusion, *Tubercle* 57:226-228, 1976.

234. Mikhail JR, Mitchell DN, Sutherland I, et al: Sarcoidosis presenting in a district general hospital. In Williams WJ, Davies BH eds: *Eighth International Conference on Sarcoidosis and Other Granulomatous Diseases*, Cardiff, Wales, 1980, Alpha Omega, pp 532-536.

235. Miles J, Pennybacker J, Sheldon P: Intrathoracic meningocele: its development and association with neurofibromatosis, *J Neurol Neurosurg Psychiatry* 32:99-110, 1969.

236. Miller A: The vanishing lung syndrome associated with pulmonary sarcoidosis, *Br J Dis Chest* 75:209-214, 1981.

237. Miller A, Einstein K, Thornton J, et al: Physiologic classification and staging of intrathoracic sarcoidosis. In Williams WJ, Davies BH, eds: *Eighth International Congress on Sarcoidosis and Other Granulomatous Diseases*, Cardiff, Wales, 1980, Alpha Omega, pp 331-336.

238. Miller A, Teirstein AS, Jackler I, et al: Airway function in chronic pulmonary sarcoidosis with fibrosis, *Am Rev Respir Dis* 109:179-189, 1974.

239. Miller PA, Ravin CE, Walker Smith GJ, et al: Pulmonary alveolar proteinosis with interstitial involvement, *AJR* 137:1069-1071, 1981.

240. Miller WT, Cornog JL, Sullivan MA: Lymphangiomyomatosis: a clinical-roentgenologic-pathologic syndrome, *AJR* 111:565-572, 1971.

241. Miro JM, Moreno A, Coca A, et al: Pulmonary alveolar microlithiasis with an unusual radiological pattern, *Br J Dis Chest* 76:91-96, 1982.

242. Mitchell DM, Mitchell DN, Collins JV, et al: Transbronchial lung biopsy through fibre optic bronchoscope in diagnosis of sarcoidosis, *Br Med J* 280:679-681, 1980.

243. Mitnick JS, Bosniak MA, Hilton S, et al: Cystic renal disease in tuberous sclerosis, *Radiology* 147:85-87, 1983.

244. Miyagawa Y, Nagata N, Shigematsu N: Clinicopathological study of migratory lung infiltrates, *Thorax* 46:233-238, 1991.

245. Monteforte WJ, Kohnen PW: Angiomyolipomas in a case of lymphangiomyomatosis syndrome: relationships to tuberous sclerosis, *Cancer* 34:317-321, 1974.

246. Moore ADA, Godwin JD, Müller NL, et al: Pulmonary histiocytosis X: comparison of radiographic and CT findings, *Radiology* 172:249-254, 1989.

247. Morgans WE, Al-Jilahawi AN, Mbatha PB: Superior vena caval obstruction caused by sarcoidosis, *Thorax* 35:397-398, 1980.

248. Moyer JH, Ackerman AJ: Sarcoidosis: a clinical and roentgenological study of twenty-eight cases, *Am Rev Tuberc* 61:299-322, 1950.

249. Müller NL: Differential diagnosis of chronic diffuse infiltrative lung disease on high-resolution computed tomography, *Semin Roentgenol* 26:132-142, 1991.

250. Müller NL, Chiles C, Kullnig P: Pulmonary lymphangiomyomatosis: correlation of CT with radiographic and functional findings, *Radiology* 175:335-339, 1990.

251. Müller NL, Kullnig P, Miller RR: The CT findings of pulmonary sarcoidosis: analysis of 25 patients, *AJR* 152:1179-1182, 1989.

252. Müller NL, Mawson JB, Mathieson JR, et al: Sarcoidosis: correlation of extent of disease at CT with clinical, functional, and radiographic findings, *Radiology* 171:613-618, 1989.

253. Müller NL, Staples CA, Miller RR: Bronchiolitis obliterans organizing pneumonia: CT features in 14 patients, *AJR* 154:983-987, 1990.

254. Mulvihill JJ: Neurofibromatosis 1 (Recklinghausen disease) and neurofibromatosis 2 (bilateral acoustic neurofibromatosis): an update, *Ann Intern Med* 113:39-52, 1990.

255. Munro CS, Mitchell DN: The Kveim response: still useful, still a puzzle, *Thorax* 42:321-331, 1987.

256. Munt PW: Middle lobe atelectasis in sarcoidosis: report of a case with prompt resolution concomitant with corticosteroid administration, *Am Rev Respir Dis* 108:357-360, 1973.

257. Murata K, Khan A, Herman PG: Pulmonary parenchymal disease: evaluation with high-resolution CT, *Radiology* 170:629-635, 1989.

258. Murch CR, Carr DH: Computed tomography appearances of pulmonary alveolar proteinosis, *Clin Radiol* 40:240-243, 1989.

259. Murdoch J, Müller NL: Pulmonary sarcoidosis: changes on follow-up CT examination, *AJR* 159:473-477, 1992.

260. Nadeau PJ, Ellis FH, Harrison EG, et al: Primary pulmonary histiocytosis X, *Dis Chest* 37:325-339, 1960.

261. Nagai S, Aung H, Tanaka S, et al: Bronchoalveolar lavage cell findings in patients with BOOP and related diseases, *Chest* 102(suppl):32S-37S, 1992.

262. Nakano I, Tsuneta Y, Terai T, et al: Clinical significance of bronchoalveolar lavage, Ga scintigraphy and serum angiotensin converting enzyme activity in granulomatous lung disease, *Jpn J Thorac Dis* 21:615-621, 1983.

263. Nicholls AJ, Friend JAR, Legge JS: Sarcoid pleural effusion: three cases and review of the literature, *Thorax* 35:277-281, 1980.

264. Nishimura K, Itoh H: High-resolution computed tomographic features of bronchiolitis obliterans organizing pneumonia, *Chest* 120(suppl):26S-31S, 1992.

265. Noble RH, Williams AJ: Multiple cavitating pulmonary nodules due to eosinophilic granuloma, *Clin Notes Respir Dis* 21:10-12, 1982.

266. Nutting S, Carr I, Cole FM, et al: Solitary pulmonary nodules due to sarcoidosis, *Can J Surg* 22:584-586, 1979.

267. O'Brien LE, Forsman PJ, Wiltse HE: Early onset sarcoidosis with pulmonary function abnormalities, *Chest* 65:472-474, 1974.

268. O'Donnell AE, Tsou E, Awh C: Endobronchial eosinophilic granuloma: a rare cause of total lung atelectasis, *Am Rev Respir Dis* 136:1478-1480, 1987.

269. Olliff JFC, Eeles R, Williams MP: Mimics of metastases from testicular tumours, *Clin Radiol* 41:395-399, 1990.

270. Olsson T, Bjornstad-Pettersen H, Stjernberg NL: Bronchostenosis due to sarcoidosis, *Chest* 75:663-666, 1979.

271. Onal E, Lopata M, Lourenco RV: Nodular pulmonary sarcoidosis: clinical, roentgenographic, and physiologic course in five patients, *Chest* 72:296-300, 1977.

272. Osband ME, Pochedly C, eds: Histiocytosis-X, *Haematol Oncol Clin North Am* 1:1-165, 1987.

273. Packe GE, Ayres JG, Citron KM, et al: Large lung bullae in sarcoidosis, *Thorax* 41:792-797, 1986.

274. Pappas CA, Rheinlander HF, Stadecker MJ: Pleural effusion as a complication of solitary eosinophilic granuloma of the rib, *Hum Pathol* 11:675-677, 1980.

275. Parkin A, Robinson PJ, Hickling P, et al: Regional lung ventilation in ankylosing spondylitis, *Br J Radiol* 55:833-836, 1982.

276. Parr MJA, Williams MV: Sarcoidosis mimicking metastatic testicular tumour, *Br J Radiol* 61:516-518, 1988.

277. Patchefsky AS, Atkinson WG, Hoch WS, et al: Interstitial pulmonary fibrosis and von Recklinghausen's disease: an ultrastructural and immunofluorescent study, *Chest* 64:459-464, 1973.

278. Patel YD, Moorhouse HT: Neurofibrosarcomas in neurofibromatosis: role of CT scanning and angiography, *Clin Radiol* 33:555-560, 1982.

279. Phillips WJE, Constance TJ: Pulmonary alveolar proteinosis, *Med J Aust* 2:357-359, 1963.

280. Pinsker KL: Solitary pulmonary nodule in sarcoidosis, *JAMA* 240:1379-1380, 1978.

281. Prakash UBS, Barham SS, Carpenter HA, et al: Pulmonary alveolar phospholipoproteinosis: experience with 34 cases and a review, *Mayo Clin Proc* 62:499-518, 1987.

282. Prakash UBS, Barham SS, Rosenow EC, et al: Pulmonary alveolar microlithiasis: a review including ultrastructural and pulmonary function studies, *Mayo Clin Proc* 58:290-300, 1983.

283. Preger L: Pulmonary alveolar proteinosis, *Radiology* 92:1291-1295, 1969.

284. Prophet D: Primary pulmonary histiocytosis X, *Clin Chest Med* 3:643-653, 1982.

285. Putman CE, Hoeck B: Reassessing the standard chest radiograph for intraparenchymal activity, *Ann NY Acad Sci* 465:595-608, 1986.

286. Quismorio FP, Sharma OP, Chandor S: Immunopathological studies on the cutaneous lesions in sarcoidosis, *Br J Dermatol* 97:635-642, 1977.

287. Rabinowitz JG, Ulreich S, Soriano C: The usual unusual manifestations of sarcoidosis and the "hilar haze" — a new diagnostic aid, *AJR* 120:821-831, 1974.

288. Radenbach KL, Brandt HL, Freise CG, et al: Special diagnostic and therapeutic aspects of pulmonary histocytosis X — twelve cases from 1969 to 1975 (author's translation), *Z Erkr Atmungsorgane* 147:26-40, 1977.

289. Radke JR, Kaplan H, Conway WA: The significance of superior vena cava syndrome developing in a patient with sarcoidosis, *Radiology* 134:311-312, 1980.

290. Ramirez-RJ: Pulmonary alveolar proteinosis: roentgenologic analysis, *AJR* 92:571-577, 1964.

291. Ramirez-RJ: Bronchopulmonary lavage: new techniques and observations, *Dis Chest* 50:581-588, 1966.

292. Rappaport DC, Weisbrod GL, Herman SJ, et al: Pulmonary lymphangioleiomyomatosis: high-resolution CT findings in four cases, *AJR* 152:961-964, 1989.

293. Reed JC, Madewell JE: The air bronchogram in interstitial disease of the lungs, *Radiology* 116:1-9, 1975.

294. Reid L, Lorriman G: Lung biopsy in sarcoidosis, *Br J Dis Chest* 54:321-334, 1960.

295. Riccardi VM: Von Recklinghausen neurofibromatosis, *N Engl J Med* 305:1617-1627, 1981.

296. Rizzato G, Blasi A: A European survey on the usefulness of 67Ga lung scans in assessing sarcoidosis: experience in 14 research centres in seven different countries, *Ann NY Acad Sci* 465:463-478, 1986.

297. Roberts CM, Citron KM, Strickland B: Intrathoracic aspergilloma: role of CT in diagnosis and treatment, *Radiology* 165:123-128, 1987.

298. Rockoff SD, Rohatgi PK: Unusual manifestations of thoracic sarcoidosis, *AJR* 144:513-528, 1985.

299. Roethe RA, Fuller PB, Byrd RB, et al: Transbronchoscopic lung biopsy in sarcoidosis: optimal number and sites for diagnosis, *Chest* 77:400-402, 1980.

300. Rogers RM, Levin DC, Gray BA, et al: Physiologic effects of bronchopulmonary lavage in alveolar proteinosis, *Am Rev Respir Dis* 118:255-264, 1978.

301. Rohatgi PK, Schwab LE: Primary acute pulmonary cavitation in sarcoidosis, *AJR* 134:1199-1203, 1980.

302. Rohrback MS, DeRemee RA: Pulmonary sarcoidosis and serum angiotensin-converting enzyme, *Mayo Clin Proc* 57:64-66, 1982.

303. Romer FK: Presentation of sarcoidosis and outcome of pulmonary changes, *Dan Med Bull* 29:27-32, 1982.

304. Rosen SH, Castleman B, Liebow AA: Pulmonary alveolar proteinosis, *N Engl J Med* 258:1123-1142, 1958.

305. Rosen Y, Amorosa JK, Moon S, et al: Occurrence of lung granulomas in patients with stage I sarcoidosis, *AJR* 129:1083-1085, 1977.

306. Rosen Y, Athanassiades TJ, Moon S, et al: Nongranulomatous interstitial pneumonitis in sarcoidosis: relationship to the development of epithelioid granulomas, *Chest* 74:122-125, 1978.

307. Rosen Y, Moon S, Huang C, et al: Granulomatous pulmonary angiitis in sarcoidosis, *Arch Pathol Lab Med* 101:170-174, 1977.

308. Rosenberg DM: Inherited forms of interstitial lung disease, *Clin Chest Med* 3:635-641, 1982.

309. Rosenow EC, Strimlan CV, Muhm JR, et al: Pleuropulmonary manifestations of ankylosing spondylitis, *Mayo Clin Proc* 52:641-649, 1977.

310. Rubin E, Weisbrod GL, Sanders DE: Pulmonary alveolar proteinosis: relationship to silicosis and pulmonary infection, *Radiology* 135:35-41, 1980.

311. Sahn SA, Schwarz MI, Lakshminarayan S: Sarcoidosis: the significance of an acinar pattern on chest roentgenogram, *Chest* 65:684-687, 1974.

312. Salerno NR, Edeiken J: Vertebral scalloping in neurofibromatosis, *Radiology* 97:509-510, 1970.

313. Sandler LM, Winearls CG, Fraher LJ, et al: Studies of the hypercalcaemia of sarcoidosis, *Q J Med* 53:165-180, 1984.

314. Sartwell PE: Racial differences in sarcoidosis, *Ann NY Acad Sci* 278:368-370, 1976.

315. Scadding JG: Calcification in sarcoidosis, *Tubercle* 42:121-135, 1961.

316. Scadding JG: *Sarcoidosis,* London, 1967, Eyre & Spottiswoode.

317. Scadding JG: Further observations on sarcoidosis associated with *M. tuberculosis* infection. In *Proceedings of the 5th International Conference on Sarcoidosis, 1969,* Prague, 1971, pp 89-92.

318. Scadding JG, Mitchell DN: *Sarcoidosis,* ed 2, London, 1985, Chapman & Hall.

319. Schabel SI, Foote GA, McKee KA: Posterior lymphadenopathy in sarcoidosis, *Radiology* 129:591-593, 1978.

320. Schabel SI, Schmidt GE, Vujic I: Overlooked pulmonary malignancy in neuro-fibromatosis, *J Can Assoc Radiol* 31:135-136, 1980.

321. Schermuly W, Behrend H: Die Angiographie de Lung ensarkoidose, *Radiologie* 8:116-123, 1968.

322. Schoenberger CI, Line BR, Keogh BA, et al: Lung inflammation in sarcoidosis: comparison of serum angiotensin-converting enzyme levels with bronchoalveolar lavage and gallium-67 scanning assessment of the T lymphocyte alveolitis, *Thorax* 37:19-25, 1982.

323. Schowengerdt CG, Suyemoto R, Main FB: Granulomatous and fibrous mediastinitis, *J Thorac Cardiovasc Surg* 57:365-379, 1969.

324. Sears MR, Chang AR, Taylor AJ: Pulmonary alveolar microlithiasis, *Thorax* 26:704-711, 1971.

325. Sebes JI, Salazar JE: The manubriosternal joint in rheumatoid disease, *AJR* 140:117-121, 1983.

326. Selroos O: Exudative pleurisy and sarcoidosis, *Br J Dis Chest* 60:191-196, 1966.

327. Sharma OP: Sarcoidosis: unusual pulmonary manifestations, *Postgrad Med J* 61:67-73, 1977.

328. Sharma OP: Airway obstruction in sarcoidosis, *Chest* 73:6-7, 1978.

329. Sharma OP: Unusual manifestations of pulmonary sarcoidosis: a radiographic panorama. In Williams WJ, Davies BH, eds: *Eighth International Conference on Sarcoidosis and Other Granulomatous Diseases,* Cardiff, Wales, 1980, Alpha Omega, pp 378-385.

330. Sharma OP: Sarcoidosis: clinical, laboratory, and immunologic aspects, *Semin Roentgenol* 20:340-355, 1985.

331. Sharma OP, Colp C, Williams MH: Pulmonary function studies in patients with bilateral sarcoidosis of hilar lymph nodes, *Arch Intern Med* 117:436-439, 1966.

332. Sharma OP, Hewlett R, Gordonson J: Nodular sarcoidosis: an unusual radiographic appearance, *Chest* 64:189-192, 1973.

333. Sharma OP, Neville E, Walker AN, et al: Familial sarcoidosis: a possible genetic influence, *Ann NY Acad Sci* 278:386-400, 1976.

334. Sherrier RH, Chiles C, Roggli V: Pulmonary lymphangioleiomyomatosis: CT findings, *AJR* 153:937-940, 1989.

335. Shibel EM, Tisi GM, Moser KM: Pulmonary photoscan-roentgenographic comparisons in sarcoidosis, *AJR* 106:770-777, 1969.

336. Shigematsu N, Emori K, Matsuba K, et al: Clinicopathologic characteristics of pulmonary acinar sarcoidosis, *Chest* 73:186-188, 1978.

337. Siltzbach LE: The Kveim test in sarcoidosis: a study of 750 patients, *JAMA* 178:476-482, 1961.

338. Siltzbach LE, James DG, Neville E, et al: Course and prognosis of sarcoidosis around the world, *Am J Med* 57:847-852, 1974.

339. Silverstein EF, Ellis K, Wolff M, et al: Pulmonary lymphangiomyomatosis, *AJR* 120:832-850, 1974.

340. Singer FR, Adams JS: Abnormal calcium homeostasis in sarcoidosis, *N Engl J Med* 315:755-757, 1986.

341. Smellie H, Hoyle C: The hilar lymph-nodes in sarcoidosis with special reference to prognosis, *Lancet* 2:66-70, 1957.

342. Smellie H, Hoyle C: The natural history of pulmonary sarcoidosis, *Q J Med* 29:539-559, 1960.

343. Smith LJ, Lawrence JB, Katzenstein AA: Vascular sarcoidosis: a rare cause of pulmonary hypertension, *Am J Med Sci* 285:38-44, 1983.

344. Soler P, Kambouchner M, Valeyre D, et al: Pulmonary Langerhans' cell granulomatosis (histiocytosis X), *Annu Rev Med* 43:105-115, 1992.

345. Solomon A, Kreel L, McNicol M, et al: Computed tomography in pulmonary sarcoidosis, *J Comput Assist Tomogr* 3:754-758, 1979.

346. Sones M, Israel HL: Course and prognosis of sarcoidosis, *Am J Med* 29:84-93, 1960.

347. Sosman MC, Dodd GD, Jones WD, et al: The familial occurrence of pulmonary alveolar microlithiasis, *AJR* 77:947-1012, 1957.

348. Spann RW, Rosenow EC, DeRemee RA, et al: Unilateral hilar or paratracheal adenopathy in sarcoidosis: a study of 38 cases, *Thorax* 26:296-299, 1971.

349. Spiteri MA, Klenerman P, Sheppard M: Seasonal cryptogenic organising pneumonia with intrahepatic cholestasis: a new clinical entity, *Thorax* 46:313p, 1991.

350. Steiger V, Fanburg BL: Recurrence of thoracic lymphadenopathy in sarcoidosis, *N Engl J Med* 314:1512, 1986.

351. Stein GN, Israel HL, Sones M: A roentgenographic study of skeletal lesions in sarcoidosis, *Arch Intern Med* 97:532-536, 1956.

352. Stern EJ, Webb WR, Golden JA, et al: Cystic lung disease associated with eosinophilic granuloma and tuberous sclerosis: air trapping at dynamic ultrafast high-resolution CT, *Radiology* 182:325-329, 1992.

353. Stovin PGI, Lum LC, Flower CDR, et al: The lungs in lymphangiomyomatosis and in tuberous sclerosis, *Thorax* 30:497-509, 1975.

354. Stump D, Spock A, Grossman H: Vertebral sarcoidosis in adolescents, *Radiology* 121:153-155, 1976.

355. Suratt PM, Winn WC, Brody AR, et al: Acute silicosis in tombstone sandblasters, *Am Rev Respir Dis* 115:521-529, 1977.

356. Svanborg N: Studies on the cardiopulmonary function in sarcoidosis, *Acta Med Scand* 170(suppl):366, 1961.

357. Symmons DPM, Woods KL: Recurrent sarcoidosis, *Thorax* 35:879, 1980.

358. Talbot FJ, Katz S, Matthews MJ: Bronchopulmonary sarcoidosis: some unusual manifestations and the serious complications thereof, *Am J Med* 26:340-355, 1959.

359. Tanoue LT: Pulmonary involvement in collagen vascular disease: a review of the pulmonary manifestations of the Marfan syndrome, ankylosing spondylitis, Sjögren's syndrome and relapsing polychondritis, *J Thorac Imag* 7:62-77, 1992.

360. Taylor JR, Ryu J, Colby TV, et al: Lymphangioleiomyomatosis: clinical course in 32 patients, *N Engl J Med* 323:1254-1260, 1990.

361. Teirstein AS, Chuang M, Miller A, et al: Flexible-bronchoscope biopsy of lung and bronchial wall in intrathoracic sarcoidosis, *Ann NY Acad Sci* 278:522-527, 1976.

362. Teirstein AS, Siltzbach LE: Sarcoidosis of the upper lung fields simulating pulmonary tuberculosis, *Chest* 64:303-308, 1973.

363. Teirstein AS, Siltzbach LE, Berger H: Patterns of sarcoidosis in three population groups in New York City, *Ann NY Acad Sci* 278:371-376, 1976.

364. Tellis CJ, Putnam JS: Cavitation in large multinodular pulmonary disease: a rare manifestation of sarcoidosis, *Chest* 71:792-793, 1977.

365. Templeton PA, McLoud TC, Muller NL, et al: Pulmonary lymphangioleiomyomatosis: CT and pathologic findings, *J Comput Assist Tomogr* 13:54-57, 1989.

366. Thind GS, Bhatia JL: Pulmonary alveolar microlithiasis, *Br J Dis Chest* 72:151-154, 1978.

367. Thomas PD, Hunninghake GW: Current concepts of the pathogenesis of sarcoidosis, *Am Rev Respir Dis* 135:747-760, 1987.

368. Thurairajasingam S, Dharmasena BD, Kasthuriratna T: Pulmonary alveolar microlithiasis, *Australas Radiol* 19:175-180, 1975.

369. Tsou E, Romano MC, Kerwin DM, et al: Sarcoidosis of anterior mediastinal nodes, pancreas, and uterine cervix: three unusual sites in the same patient, *Am Rev Respir Dis* 122:333-338, 1980.

370. Ucan ES, Keyf AI, Aydilek R, et al: Pulmonary alveolar microlithiasis: review of Turkish reports, *Thorax* 48:171-173, 1993.

371. Unger PD, Geller SA, Anderson PJ: Pulmonary lesions in a patient with neurofibromatosis, *Arch Pathol Lab Med* 108:654-657, 1984.

372. Valensi QJ: Pulmonary lymphangiomyoma, a probable forme fruste of tuberous sclerosis, *Am Rev Respir Dis* 108:1411-1415, 1973.

373. Watts R, Thompson JR, Jasuja ML: Sarcoidosis presenting with massive pleural effusion, *IMJ* 163:57-58, 1983.

374. Webb WR, Goodman PC: Fibrosing alveolitis in patients with neurofibromatosis, *Radiology* 122:289-293, 1977.

375. Weber WN, Margolin FR, Nielsen SL: Pulmonary histiocytosis X: a review of 18 patients with reports of 6 cases, *AJR* 107:280-289, 1969.

376. Weisman RA, Canalis RF, Powell WJ: Laryngeal sarcoidosis with airway obstruction, *Ann Otol Rhinol Laryngol* 89:58-61, 1980.

377. Westcott JL, deGraff AC: Sarcoidosis, hilar adenopathy and pulmonary artery narrowing, *Radiology* 108:585-586, 1973.

378. Westcott JL, Noehren TH: Bronchial stenosis in chronic sarcoidosis, *Chest* 63:893-897, 1973.

379. Wilen SB, Rabinowitz JG, Ulreich S, et al: Pleural involvement in sarcoidosis, *Am J Med* 57:200-209, 1974.

380. Winterbauer RH, Hutchinson JF: Use of pulmonary function tests in the management of sarcoidosis, *Chest* 78:640-647, 1980.

381. Winzelberg GG, Boller M, Sachs M, et al: CT evaluation of pulmonary alveolar microlithiasis, *J Comput Assist Tomogr* 8:1029-1031, 1984.

382. Wollschlager C, Khan F: Aspergillomas complicating sarcoidosis: a prospective study in 100 patients, *Chest* 86:585-588, 1984.

383. Wolson AH, Rohwedder JJ: Upper lobe fibrosis in ankylosing spondylitis, *AJR* 124:466-471, 1975.

384. Wright JL, Cagle P, Churg A, et al: Diseases of the small airways, *Am Rev Respir Dis* 146:240-262, 1992.

385. Yamamoto M, Yasutaka I, Kitaichi M, et al: Clinical features of BOOP in Japan, *Chest* 102(suppl):21S-25S, 1992.

386. Yotsumoto H, Hachiya J, Furuie T, et al: An estimation of computed tomography in detecting the intrathoracic changes of sarcoidosis. In Williams WJ, Davies BH, eds: *Eighth International Conference on Sarcoidosis and Other Granulomatous Diseases*, Cardiff, Wales, 1980, Alpha Omega, pp 386-393.

387. Young DA, Laman ML: Radiodense skeletal lesions in Boeck's sarcoid, *AJR* 114:553-558, 1972.

388. Ziskind MM, Weill H, Payzant AR: The recognition and significance of acinus-filling processes of the lung, *Am Rev Respir Dis* 87:551-559, 1963.

14 Congenital Disorders of the Lungs and Airways

PAUL DEE

Tracheoesophageal fistula
Bronchogenic cyst
Tracheomalacia
Tracheal bronchus and other abnormal bronchial branching
  patterns
Bronchial atresia
Congenital lobar emphysema
Absence (agenesis, aplasia) of the lungs or lobes of the lungs
Scimitar syndrome (hypogenetic lung syndrome, venolobar syn-
  drome)
Pulmonary hypoplasia and Potter's syndrome (oligohydramnios
  tetrad)

Unilateral primary pulmonary hypoplasia
Pulmonary sequestration
Pulmonary arteriovenous fistulas
Congenital lymphangiectasis
Congenital cystic adenomatoid malformation of the lung
Cystic fibrosis of the pancreas (mucoviscidosis)
Congenital diaphragmatic abnormalities
  Congenital diaphragmatic hernia
  Accessory diaphragm
  Morgagni hernia
  Bochdalek hernia

It is apparent from common clinical experience that congenital or developmental lesions of the lungs are neither as frequent nor, in general, as significant as their counterparts in the heart. Objective evidence from autopsy series supports this impression. For example, in a detailed analysis of over 2000 autopsies Sotelo-Avila and Skanklin[137] showed that some form of major or minor congenital malformation occurred in 46% of cases. Of these, 30% were cardiovascular, 10% urinary, and only 3% respiratory.

Classification of congenital lesions of the lungs and airways is difficult because the embryogenesis of specific pulmonary malformations is often obscure. Classification is further complicated by associated congenital heart disease, which can lead to difficulty in deciding whether a particular malformation should be categorized as a lung lesion or as a cardiovascular anomaly. In this chapter, for example, unilateral pulmonary artery aplasia and the scimitar syndrome are included with pulmonary lesions, whereas the various forms of pulmonary atresia and anomalous pulmonary venous return are excluded.

The box on p. 610 is therefore just one of many arbitrary classifications. The conditions discussed in this or other chapters are given in italics while the less common or frankly rare conditions are only referenced. Although some of the conditions are not present at birth, they are nevertheless developmental in origin. Because the lungs continue to form for an extended time after birth, deleterious factors operating postnatally can affect

their development, as in the Swyer-James syndrome and congenital bronchiectasis.

TRACHEOESOPHAGEAL FISTULA

Most tracheoesophageal fistulas are associated with esophageal atresia and appear in the neonatal period. They are not discussed further. In rare instances the so-called H-type tracheoesophageal fistula may not be detected until adult life even though symptoms may have been present from infancy.[139] The H-type fistula connects the adjacent trachea and esophagus, the fistula forming the transverse bar of the H (Figure 14-1). This type of fistula constitutes approximately 2% to 4% of all tracheoesophageal fistulas.[67,161] There is a relatively high incidence of other congenital abnormalities in association with tracheoesophageal fistulas,[5] and this association may provide a clue to the presence of an H-type fistula. An extensive literature describes the differing patterns of associated anomalies.[85] These patterns have been designated by a series of acronyms: the VATER complex (vertebral, anal, tracheoesophageal, and renal), the VACTEL complex (vertebral, anal, cardiac, tracheoesophageal, and limb), and the ARTICLE ± V complex (anal, renal, tracheal, intestinal, cardiac, limb, and esophageal ± vertebral). Other congenital pulmonary lesions such as pulmonary hypoplasia, tracheal stenosis, and pulmonary sequestration occur in approximately 2% of patients with these complexes.[156]

The symptoms are recurrent aspiration including par-

CLASSIFICATION OF DEVELOPMENTAL LESIONS OF THE LUNGS

ABNORMALITIES OF SEPARATION FROM THE FOREGUT

Tracheoesophageal fistula
Bronchobiliary fistula[133]
Bronchogenic cyst
Tracheal diverticulum[69]
Bronchopulmonary foregut malformation[61]

ABNORMAL DEVELOPMENT OF THE BRANCHING OUTGROWTH FROM THE FOREGUT

Tracheal agenesis[160]
Tracheal stenosis[19]
Tracheal abnormalities in skeletal dysplasias[86]
Tracheomalacia and tracheobronchomegaly (Mounier-Kuhn syndrome) (see p. 822)
Bronchial isomerism syndromes[85]
Tracheal bronchus, abnormal bronchial branching patterns
Bridging bronchus
Bronchial atresia
Bronchial stenosis[23]
Bronchomalacia[93]
Bronchiectasis
Congenital lobar emphysema
Absence (agenesis, aplasia) of the lungs or lobes of the lungs
Horseshoe lung
Ectopia of the lungs[29]
Scimitar syndrome
Emphysema[68]
Hypoplasia of the lungs
Potter's syndrome (oligohydramnios tetrad)

ABNORMALITIES OF THE PULMONARY VASCULATURE

Congenital pulmonary lymphangiectasis
Scimitar syndrome

Pulmonary arteriovenous fistula
Tracheobronchial narrowing caused by extrinsic vascular pressure — pulmonary sling, congenital absence of the pulmonary valves, vascular rings, etc.[90]
Pulmonary isomerism syndromes[85]
Pulmonary artery aplasia
Peripheral pulmonary stenosis[51]

ABNORMALITIES RELATED TO A LOCAL OR SYSTEMIC BIOCHEMICAL OR CELLULAR DEFECT

Pulmonary microlithiasis (see pp. 598-599)
Immotile cilia syndrome (see p. 835)
Alpha$_1$-antitrypsin deficiency (see p. 854)
Fibrocystic disease (mucoviscidosis)
Chronic granulomatous disease (see p. 256)

ABNORMALITIES FORMING A COMPONENT OF A SYSTEMIC FAMILIAL OR NONFAMILIAL DISEASE PROCESS

Hereditary telangiectasia
Pulmonary lymphangiomyomatosis (see pp. 592-594)
Potter's syndrome (oligohydramnios tetrad)
Yellow nail syndrome (see p. 680)

FAMILIAL ABNORMALITIES OF THE LUNGS

Familial primary pulmonary hypertension[129]
Familial spontaneous pneumothorax[88]
Familial fibrocystic pulmonary dysplasia[82]
Familial pulmonary fibrosis[71]

ECTOPIC OR HAMARTOMATOUS DEVELOPMENT; HYPERPLASIAS

Congenital cystic adenomatoid malformation
Intrapulmonary and extrapulmonary sequestration
Hamartomas of lung
Interstitial masses, hemangioma, thyroid[70]
Focal muscular hyperplasia of the trachea[9]

---

oxysmal coughing, feeding difficulties, and recurrent pneumonias. The pulmonary consolidations seen on the chest radiograph reflect the extent and severity of the aspiration. Excessive air may pass through the fistula into the esophagus and on into the gut. In infants with an H-type fistula an air esophagogram may be noted on the chest radiographs and there may be unusual degrees of gaseous distention of the bowel.[155] Diagnosing the condition by contrast studies of the esophagus can be difficult because the fistula may be relatively small and aspiration through it may be intermittent.[7] The patient should be examined in the prone position, with lateral fluoroscopy and video recording. It is advantageous to inject the contrast medium through a feeding tube while it is withdrawn along the length of the esophagus. In problem cases thin barium suspensions or nonionic water-soluble contrast media are useful. The purpose of these measures is to encourage the contrast medium to enter the fistula.[147] In some cases repeating the contrast studies on more than one occasion may be necessary to establish the diagnosis.[28] This clearly requires a high degree of suspicion and a dedication to proving the diagnosis.

BRONCHOGENIC CYST

Bronchogenic cysts (synonym bronchial cysts) are uncommon, usually isolated lesions representing a cystic reduplication of the tracheobronchial tree. They have a fibrous capsule, often containing cartilage, are lined with respiratory epithelium, and contain mucoid material that may be remarkably viscid. Most bronchogenic cysts arise in the mediastinum or hilar regions; a few arise within the lung parenchyma. In three large series, each including at

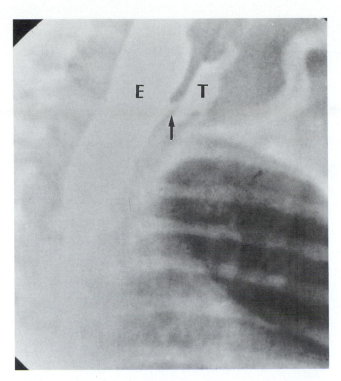

FIGURE 14-1
H-type tracheoesophageal fistula in an infant. Arrow indicates fistula between esophagus *(E)* and trachea *(T)*.

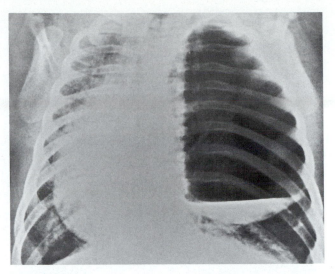

FIGURE 14-2
Huge expansile bronchogenic cystic in an infant. Note marked mediastinal shift and fluid in bottom of cyst (compare with congenital lobar emphysema). (Courtesy Dr. Harold Jacobson, New York.)

least 75 patients, bronchogenic cysts were described as mediastinal in 86%,[123] 77%,[142] and 65%.[35] In rare instances bronchogenic cysts develop in ectopic locations such as the cervical, infradiaphragmatic, pericardial, and paravertebral regions.[120] Some pulmonary bronchogenic cysts have a systemic arterial supply and therefore may represent a form of pulmonary sequestration[17,18]; surgeons need to consider the possibility of a systemic arterial supply in cases requiring resection.[32] Bronchial cysts have a certain plasticity; they partially displace and partially mold around normal anatomic structures, features that may to some extent account for the paucity of pressure effects.

The clinical features are variable. Infants may have respiratory distress caused by pressure effects on the tracheobronchial tree.[40] In such cases the chest radiograph may show hyperexpansion of an entire lung as a result of a ball valve mechanism or collapse of a lobe or an entire lung.[164] A mediastinal mass may be visible but may be masked by the thymus. Feeding difficulties caused by pressure effects on the esophagus, or effects on the venous return resulting in edema,[3,106] are less commonly seen. Many older children and adults are asymptomatic, and the lesions are detected on routine chest radiographs,[80] usually before the fourth decade.[128] St-Georges, Deslauriers, and Duranceau[142] found that 70% of a series of 86 patients had some form of chest symptom at the time of surgery; the symptoms included chest pain in 55% of symptomatic patients, cough in 50%, dyspnea in 40%,

fever in 30%, and purulent sputum in 20%. Complications related to the bulk of the cysts are relatively uncommon, except in infants, despite the central location.[75] On rare occasion a bronchogenic cyst undergoes a rapid increase in size caused by hemorrhage, infection, or distention with air (Figure 14-2). In these cases the compressive effects may cause a surgical emergency.[40,164] There is a single case report of a peripheral bronchogenic cyst manifested as a pneumothorax.[100] Occasionally patients complain of dysphagia, and there have been isolated reports of pulmonary artery obstruction.[162,172] The more rigid tracheobronchial tree does not appear to be subject to compression.

On plain chest radiograph, most bronchogenic cysts are seen as a well-defined, solitary mass in the mediastinum or hilum (Figure 14-3); approximately 10% show a lobular outline on plain film.[123] They are usually found in close proximity to the major airways, and therefore one of the surfaces of the cyst contacts the trachea or central bronchi. The single most frequent site is immediately adjacent to the lower trachea or proximal mainstem bronchi. Anterior and posterior mediastinal cysts remote from the airways are occasionally encountered.[14,112] As the cysts grow, they displace the adjacent lung and esophagus, but the central airways, except in very young children, are usually displaced little, if at all. Calcification, either rim calcification or milk of calcium within the cyst, has been described[11,123,171] but is unusual. The cysts are stable in size except when complicated by infection. Air may enter a cyst,[11,123] frequently a complication of infection of the cyst contents (Figure 14-4). If the cyst contains air or an air-fluid level, the smooth thin wall and the central location of the cavity should indicate its nature and permit distinction from primary abscess formation.

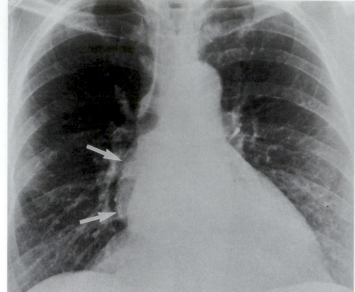
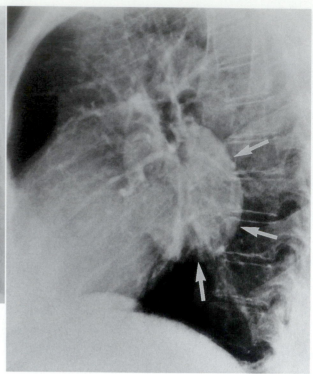

FIGURE 14-3
Large central bronchogenic cyst in an asymptomatic adult. **A,** Posteroanterior view. **B,** Lateral view.

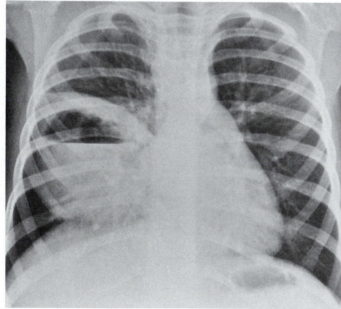
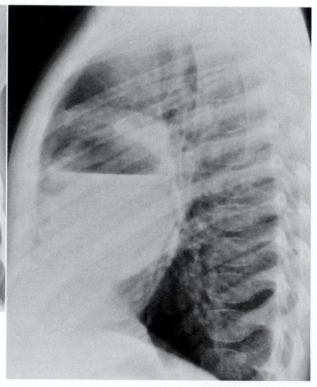

FIGURE 14-4
Infected bronchogenic cyst in a child. Cyst wall is considerably thickened by inflammation. **A,** Posteroanterior view. **B,** Lateral view.

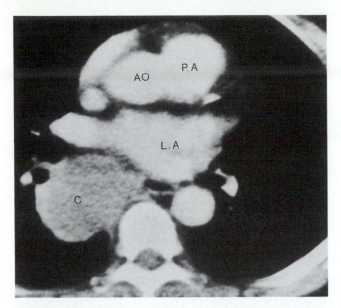

FIGURE 14-5
Bronchogenic cyst demonstrated by computed tomography (CT). *C,* Cyst; *P.A.,* pulmonary artery; *A.O.,* aorta; *L.A.,* left atrium. Note that cyst has CT density comparable to that of paraspinal muscles.

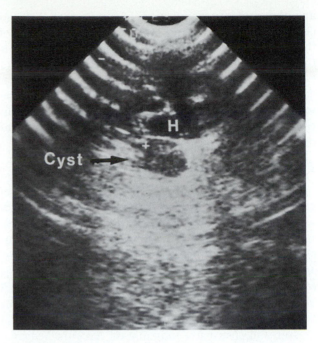

FIGURE 14-6
Frame from real-time ultrasound scan of a bronchogenic cyst *(arrow)*. Ribs produce linear echoes. Heart chambers *(H)* are echolucent. Lung is echo reflective. Note that the cyst contains diffuse internal echoes.

Barium swallow examination shows smooth extrinsic displacement of the esophagus by the cyst in at least half the cases. Typically the cyst invaginates between the airways and the esophagus.

CT is now the standard technique for evaluating bronchogenic cysts (Figure 14-5), revealing thin-walled cystic masses molded to the adjacent bronchovascular structures. The molding of the cyst may cause one margin of the cyst to have a pointed configuration.[33] The wall is smooth on both its inner and its outer margins and in uncomplicated masses is only a few millimeters thick. Many bronchogenic cysts have a CT density close to that of water, that is, -10 to $+10$ Hounsfield units (HU). Most are unilocular, but they can be multilocular.[171] The CT diagnosis of bronchogenic cyst can be accepted with confidence if the following criteria are met: a well-defined mass with a smooth or lobular outline, a uniformly thin wall, and contents of uniform CT density within a range of -10 to $+10$ HU. In some cases the CT densities are higher, often equaling soft tissue density but sometimes substantially higher (cysts with CT numbers as high as 120 HU have been reported). Such high CT densities presumably reflect a high proteinaceous content of the cyst, a feature that can be due to infection or, in the case of the very high-density lesions, to hemorrhage.[103,109] On rare occasion a bronchogenic cyst contains milk of calcium, resulting in extremely high CT density.[174] Curvilinear calcification in the cyst wall is particularly well demonstrated at CT.

Ultrasound has been used to diagnose mediastinal bronchogenic cysts in children when the lesion can be approached without the beam traversing the lung (Figure 14-6). In two cases described by Ries and associates[127] one lesion was clearly cystic whereas the second was an echogenic solid-appearing mass.

In a number of centers magnetic resonance imaging (MRI) has been used in the diagnosis of bronchogenic cysts.* MRI does not appear to have any special advantages over CT for defining the morphology of the mass. The magnetic resonance signal intensities fall into three broad categories. (1) Uniform low T1, high T2 intensities are similar to water. (2) Uniform high T1, high T2 intensities[4,108,115,148] presumably result from a high protein content or the presence of blood or cholesterol within the cyst. This pattern, although suggestive of a bronchogenic cyst, was found in only one case out of seven by Naidich and associates.[108] It may also be seen with certain intrathoracic neoplasms having a relatively high nuclear/cytoplasmic ratio, such as ganglioneuromas, pheochromocytomas, carcinoid tumors, and germ cell tumors, in hematomas, and in lesions with extensive hemorrhage. (3) Nonuniform or variable intensities are caused by complications such as hemorrhage.[108] In one patient with an uncomplicated bronchogenic cyst, MRI showed a fluid-fluid level, presumably a result of layering of proteinaceous debris.[92]

The diagnosis of bronchogenic cyst can be confirmed nonoperatively by needle aspiration of the contents[134]

---

*References 4, 15, 92, 98, 108, 115.

and the subsequent injection of contrast medium to demonstrate the smoothness and thickness of the wall of the cyst. Transthoracic aspiration under CT control[46] is the simplest technique, but it may prove more effective to pass the needle transbronchoscopically or via an esophagoscope. The cyst fluid can be examined to exclude malignant cells, and a confirmed diagnosis of bronchogenic cyst may in appropriate clinical circumstances obviate the need for operative removal.[169]

TRACHEOMALACIA

The term "tracheomalacia" implies an abnormal degree of compliance of the trachea, which tends to narrow when subjected to unusually negative intratracheal pressures during inspiration or unusually positive extratracheal pressures during expiration. Wittenborg, Gyepes, and Crocker[170] have demonstrated that in most instances collapse of the trachea is a normal response to abnormal pressures; that is, it is caused by localized tracheal or laryngeal obstruction in infants or abnormal external pressures in obstructive lung disease. True tracheomalacia secondary to defects in the supporting cartilaginous structures is rare[86] and is usually associated with more severe congenital malformations. For example, tracheomalacia resulting in tracheobronchial narrowing may be associated with a pulmonary artery sling. The sling is formed by an aberrant left pulmonary artery that arises from a normally positioned right pulmonary artery. The left pulmonary artery hooks around the right side of the trachea and traverses the mediastinum between the trachea and the esophagus to reach the left lung. Pulmonary sling is associated with dysplasia and narrowing of the carinal region.

TRACHEAL BRONCHUS AND OTHER ABNORMAL BRONCHIAL BRANCHING PATTERNS

In general, the bronchial branching pattern is remarkably uniform. Major variations in bronchial branching are rare. Bronchography and bronchoscopy are the usual methods of diagnosing such anomalies during life. Atwell[2] analyzed 1200 bronchograms and found only 23 showing an extra major bronchial branch (Figure 14-7) and 4 showing absence of a major bronchial branch. Minor bronchial branch anomalies were, however, fairly common, occurring in 104 cases including 88 cases of double-stem superior segment bronchi to the lower lobes. These figures suggest that virtually 90% of the population have the standard textbook pattern of division. Most anomalous divisions have no clinical significance, although they may be confusing to the bronchoscopist searching for landmarks. Mangiulea and Stingha[97] suggest that the accessory cardiac bronchus increases liability to infection (Figure 14-9), and Remy and co-workers[125] found focal emphysema, presumably secondary to pulmonary artery compression, in left apicoposterior segments that arose more proximally from the left main bronchus.

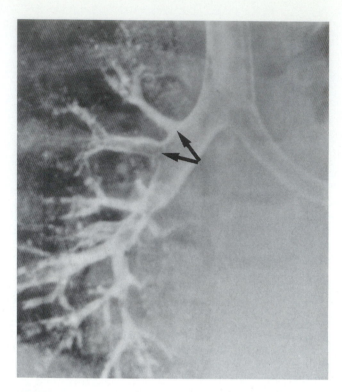

FIGURE 14-7
Bronchographic demonstration of double-stem right upper lobe bronchus in an infant.

Isolated cases of the so-called bridging bronchus have been described.[55,138] In this condition the right lower lobe bronchus has arisen from the left main bronchus and crossed or bridged the mediastinum to reach the right lung. The condition is difficult to explain on the basis of current theories of lung embryology.

BRONCHIAL ATRESIA

Bronchial atresia is a rare and benign condition producing a characteristic triad of radiographic findings:

1. A localized central mass density representing mucoid impaction in the bronchus distal to the focal atresia of the segmental bronchus. The mass density is rounded or ovoid and does not have the branching configuration often associated with acquired bronchoceles (Figure 14-9).

2. Emphysema of the affected segment of lung. Since the central bronchus is atretic, aeration of the lung presumably occurs through collateral air drift.

3. Hypoperfusion of the affected segment as indicated by a paucity of vessels in that segment (Figure 14-10). The hypoperfusion is presumed to reflect hypoplasia of the segmental vessels resulting from hypoxia in that segment.

Meng and colleagues[104] reviewed 36 cases of bronchial atresia and found 24 with involvement of the left upper lobe and 7 with involvement of the right upper lobe. In the affected upper lobes it is almost invariably the apical or apicoposterior segments that are involved. Tederlinic and co-workers[152] reported four cases of bronchial atresia

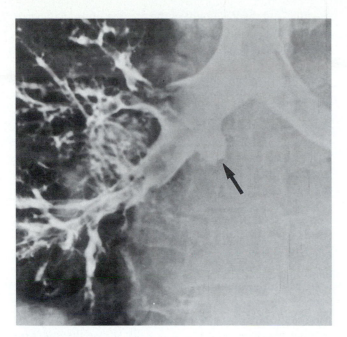

FIGURE 14-8
Bronchographic demonstration of an accessory cardiac bronchus *(arrow)* largely occluded by secretions.

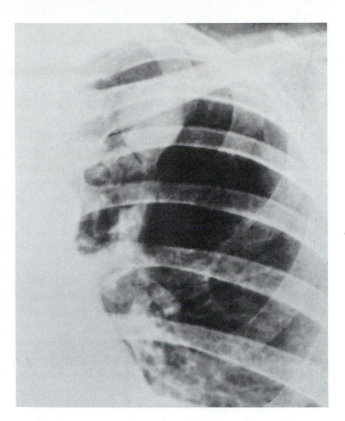

FIGURE 14-9
Bronchial atresia producing an ovoid upper lobe mass representing a mucocele. Note the hyperlucent lung surrounding the mucocele and the paucity of lung vessels in this region.

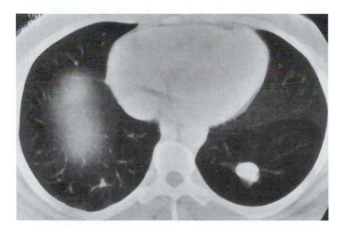

FIGURE 14-10
Computed tomography scan of bronchial atresia involving the left lower lobe. Mucocele is surrounded by hyperlucent lung with a paucity of vessels.

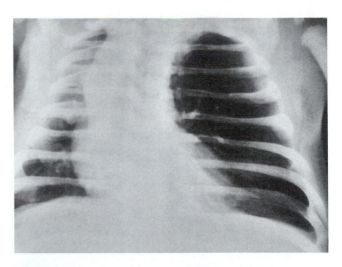

FIGURE 14-11
Congenital lobar emphysema involving the left upper lobe. Note the marked mediastinal shift and atelectasis of the lower lobe.

and showed that lower lobe involvement could occur, as illustrated in Figure 14-10. CT scanning more clearly demonstrates the surrounding emphysema and hypoperfusion. The clinical significance of the condition is minimal. Its importance is that the dilated mucus-filled bronchus distal to the atresia may be misdiagnosed as a neoplasm or other significant lesion.

CONGENITAL LOBAR EMPHYSEMA

Some form of aplasia, hypoplasia, or dysplasia of bronchial supporting structures is postulated as the primary cause of congenital lobar emphysema,[146] although the precise cause of the obstruction has been difficult to determine in resected specimens. The congenital nature of the condition has never been unequivocally established even though the circumstantial evidence is strong. There is a definite association with congenital heart disease.[62] An interesting infrequent form of the condition, in which the lobe is filled with fluid, is thought to be the result of amniotic fluid trapped behind an obstructed bronchus.[42]

In most cases congenital lobar emphysema is manifested in the neonatal period with respiratory distress, which may be life threatening. In as many as 25% of cases, however, presentation is delayed until after the first month of life.

The classic and by far the most common radiographic appearance is hyperexpansion of an isolated lobe in one lung, usually an upper or middle lobe (Figure 14-11). Remarkably, the lower lobes are involved in only about 2% of cases. Involvement of more than one lobe is equally exceptional. The expanded lobe may cause compression atelectasis of the rest of the lung accompanied by displacement of the heart, mediastinum, and diaphragm. The main differential diagnoses include localized pneumothorax and an expanding lung cyst. Careful study of the x-ray films should reveal the presence of blood vessels within the expanded lobes in cases of lobar emphysema. Pulmonary interstitial emphysema, an acquired condition most commonly seen in babies receiving positive-pressure ventilation, may affect a single lobe and closely resemble congenital lobar emphysema radiographically. The conditions differ clinically, however, in that interstitial emphysema usually occurs in children who are already receiving mechanical ventilation because of previously known diffuse lung disease. Mucus obstruction of a bronchus occasionally leads to obstructive overinflation, which can be radiographically identical to congenital lobar emphysema. Bronchoscopy to exclude a mucus plug is therefore performed before surgical resection of an overexpanded lobe.

Congenital lobar emphysema may first appear in a form with a fluid-filled lobe and the same tendency to expand as in the classic form.[42] On radiographic examination the fluid-filled form is seen as an expansile mass of soft tissue density (Figure 14-12). Compression of the remainder of the lung and displacement of the mediastinum may occur exactly as with the more usual hyperinflated form. The entrapped fluid drains, and conversion to the more conventional form of lobar emphysema ensues. On rare occasion a transitional phase between the fluid-filled and the air-filled forms may be encountered.[1] In this transitory phase there are linear interstitial markings resembling septal lines in the hyperexpanded lobe. These disappear, presumably as fluid drains or is absorbed.

The diagnosis of congenital lobar emphysema usually is readily made on the basis of the clinical and plain radiographic findings. CT scanning and ventilation-perfusion scintigraphy have, however, been used in the evaluation of such cases (Figure 14-13).[78,99,113,116] The main justification for such studies is to resolve doubts about possible alternative diagnoses such as primary pulmonary hypoplasia or scimitar syndrome. The findings at scintigraphy have been uniformly abnormal but vary in the extent to which ventilation or perfusion has been reduced. CT scanning simply confirms the presence of lobar emphysema and graphically shows the effect on adjacent structures.

Resection of the affected lobe may be necessary; if not, a policy of nonintervention with close radiographic observation is adopted in the hope that the condition will resolve.[130] Kennedy and co-workers[78] followed up a group of 12 patients treated conservatively for up to 12 years. They found a steady gradual improvement in all cases paralleled by a relative decrease in the lobar hyperexpansion on serial radiographs. Some cases were followed up with ventilation-perfusion scintigraphy, which generally showed a parallel improvement in function, with ventilation usually improving more than perfusion.

Congenital lobar emphysema is a true lobar emphy-

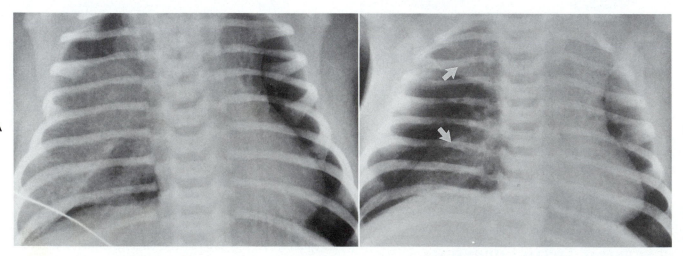

FIGURE 14-12
Congenital lobar emphysema involving the middle lobe. **A,** Fluid-filled at birth. **B,** Several hours later. Hyperexpanded middle lobe compressing the previously expanded upper and lower lobes *(arrows)*.

sema thought to result from some form of bronchial obstruction. A clinically identical but pathologically distinct condition, the polyalveolar lobe, has been identified.[22,65,151] In this condition the airways and the vascular supply to the involved lobe are normal. The lobe contains some three to five times the normal number of alveoli for the patient's age. The result is a relatively large lobe that may have all of the compressive effects seen with congenital lobar emphysema. This giant lobe is not emphysematous. However, in practical clinical terms the condition is indistinguishable from true lobar emphysema.

ABSENCE (AGENESIS, APLASIA) OF THE LUNGS OR LOBES OF THE LUNGS

Unilateral absence of a lung or a lobe is a rare congenital abnormality that in itself may cause surprisingly few clinical problems.[76,96] Indeed, absence of a lung may be encountered de novo in an adult who has had no symptoms referable to the chest (Figure 14-14). However, the condition is frequently associated with other congenital abnormalities, particularly as one of several associations with tracheoesophageal fistulas. Nearly 10% of patients with tracheobronchial malformations have unilateral pulmonary agenesis. Interestingly, agenesis of the

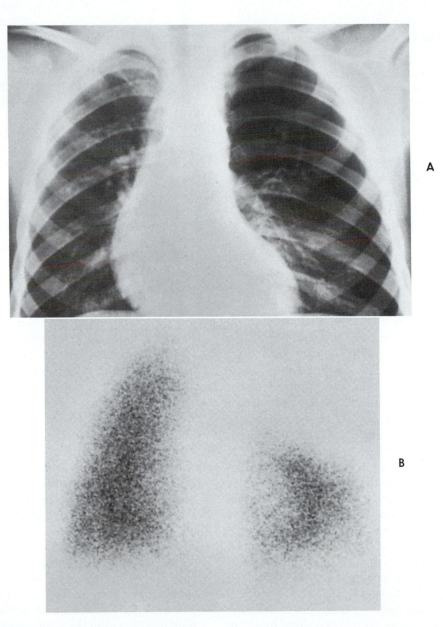

FIGURE 14-13
A, Posteroanterior radiograph. B, Radionuclide scan in a 4-year-old boy with surgically proven congenital lobar emphysema of the left upper lobe.

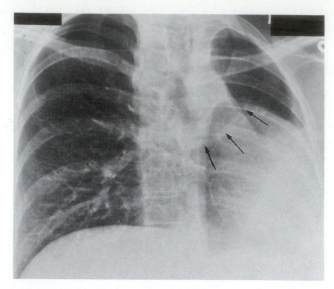

FIGURE 14-14
Routine radiograph in an asymptomatic male reveals aplasia of the left lung. Right upper lobe vessels *(arrows)* course to the left apex with the heart positioned posteriorly in the left side of chest.

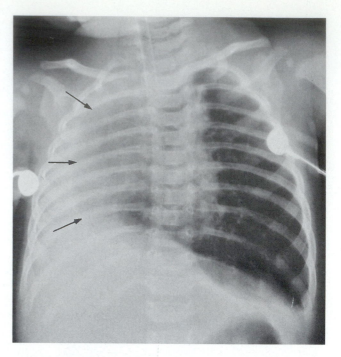

FIGURE 14-15
Agenesis of right lung in an infant, showing shift of the heart into the right side of the chest, elevation of the right hemidiaphragm, and herniation of the left lung *(arrows)*.

right lung appears to be strongly associated with esophageal atresia,[10,16] whereas in cases of isolated tracheoesophageal fistula without esophageal atresia the left lung is predominantly affected.[96] Absence of a lobe of a lung is less common and simulates pulmonary hypoplasia.

As might be expected, the finding in absence of a lung is absence of aeration of the lung on that side. Volume loss is manifested by elevation of the ipsilateral hemidiaphragm and shift of the mediastinum toward the abnormal side with herniation of the opposite lung anteriorly (Figure 14-15). The principal differential diagnosis is acquired total lung collapse, and further investigation with tomography, bronchography, or angiography may be necessary to make the distinction. The ipsilateral pulmonary artery is absent, and the bronchus to the affected lung or lobe is either absent (agenesis) or rudimentary (aplasia).[45] In isolated absence of a lobe there is compensatory expansion of the remaining lobe or lobes with consequent distortion of the bronchovascular structures. The compensatory expansion is never complete, and lung volume is reduced on the affected side. As in diffuse pulmonary hypoplasia, areolar tissue and fat may occupy the anterior part of the affected hemithorax and may compensate for the volume loss in the underlying lung. The chest radiographic findings in congenital absence of a lobe are indistinguishable from those of generalized pulmonary hypoplasia and are discussed under that heading. Bronchography identifies absence of a lobe by demonstrating agenesis or aplasia of the lobar bronchus with an otherwise normal bronchial tree.[45] In pulmonary hypoplasia, on the other hand, the number of lobes is appropriate but the bronchial tree is stunted and deformed.

In an infant with associated congenital abnormalities the diagnosis of absence of a lung may be more readily apparent than in an adult but the clinical significance of the lesion is likely to be overshadowed by the other abnormalities.

Isolated aplasia of a pulmonary artery produces few if any clinical problems other than difficulty in interpreting the chest radiograph. The volume of the affected lung is normal or slightly reduced, but the pulmonary vasculature is remarkably diminished (Figures 14-16 and 14-17). The vasculature in the normal lung may appear correspondingly plethoric because the entire cardiac output is shunted through that lung. The abnormal perfusion of the lungs presumably contributes to a relative hyperlucency of the affected lung. Radioisotope ventilation-perfusion scanning readily demonstrates the total absence of perfusion and the normal ventilation of the lung. CT scanning clearly shows the absence of a pulmonary artery and interestingly may also demonstrate evidence of systemic to pulmonary arterial collateral vessels.[57] CT scanning should obviate the need for angiography. Acquired conditions may, however, closely mimic aplasia of a pulmonary artery, but the Swyer-James syndrome (see p. 839) should have demonstrably abnormal ventilation of the affected lung. Fibrosing mediastinitis is sometimes indistinguishable radiographically from unilateral pulmonary artery aplasia. There may be strong clinical pointers in favor of fibrosing mediastinitis, including a tendency for the patient's condition to worsen. Further studies such as

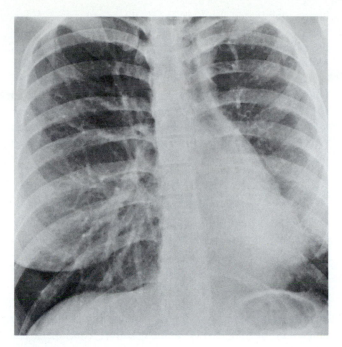

FIGURE 14-16
Routine chest radiograph in an asymptomatic male with aplasia of the left pulmonary artery. Aortic arch is right sided.

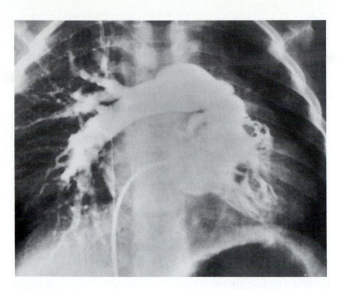

FIGURE 14-17
Right ventricular angiogram in an infant with aplasia of the left pulmonary artery. Left lung was normally ventilated.

angiography or ventilation-perfusion scanning usually indicate bilateral pulmonary vascular abnormalities.

SCIMITAR SYNDROME (HYPOGENETIC LUNG SYNDROME, VENOLOBAR SYNDROME)

The alternative designation for scimitar syndrome, "hypogenetic lung syndrome," emphasizes that this anomaly is not simply a variant of partial anomalous pulmonary venous return but a more widespread malformation. The condition is confined to the right lung. The lung is hypoplastic, with underdevelopment of both the bronchial tree and the vascular structures.[43,110] The bronchial tree on the involved side is stunted, and the arterial supply to the lungs may derive in much greater proportion than normal from systemic arteries. The pulmonary arteries are correspondingly hypoplastic. The syndrome derives its name from the anomalous pulmonary vein that descends vertically in the lung before curving medially to enter the inferior vena cava above or below the diaphragm. The vein broadens as it curves downward, resulting in a scimitar configuration (Figure 14-18).

Approximately 25% of patients have associated congenital heart disease, most commonly septal defects.[54] Such cases are more likely to appear in infancy or childhood, and the outcome depends on the type and severity of the cardiac abnormality. The scimitar syndrome, when isolated, is compatible with a normal life.[39] Patients occasionally have symptoms from associated bronchiectasis

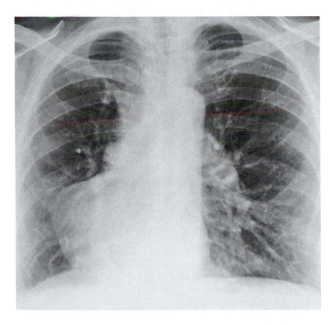

FIGURE 14-18
Scimitar syndrome. Note the dextropositioned heart, stunted pulmonary vascular pattern in the right lung, and the scimitar vein coursing behind the heart toward the inferior vena cava.

and tracheal diverticula. Other associated anomalies include eventration or Bochdalek hernia involving the right hemidiaphragm, accessory right hemidiaphragm, and horseshoe lung (see later discussion).

The anomalously draining vein is readily visible on chest radiographs in both the frontal and the lateral projections. The associated features of reduced lung volume with consequent dextroposition of the heart and the abnormal bronchovascular pattern in the right hilum

CONDITIONS ASSOCIATED WITH HYPOPLASIA OF THE LUNG

PRESSURE EFFECT ON THE DEVELOPING LUNG

Pulmonary sequestration
Cystic adenomatoid malformation of the lung
Diaphragmatic hernia
Diaphragmatic eventration
Chylothorax
Hydrops fetalis
Ascites or abdominal mass

RESTRICTIVE ABNORMALITIES OF THE THORACIC CAGE

Asphyxiating thoracic dystrophy
Achondroplasia
Thanatophoric dwarfism
Ellis-van Creveld syndrome
Osteogenesis imperfecta

OLIGOHYDRAMNIOS

Decreased urine output
    Renal agenesis
    Bladder outlet obstruction
Amniotic fluid leak

CONDITIONS ASSOCIATED WITH REDUCED OR ABSENT FETAL RESPIRATORY MOVEMENT

Central nervous system lesions
    Anencephaly
    Arnold-Chiari malformation
Pena-Shokeir syndrome[117]
Phrenic nerve agenesis
Congenital myotonic dystrophy

DECREASED PULMONARY VASCULAR PERFUSION

Bilateral
    Ebstein's anomaly
    Hypoplastic right heart syndrome
    Pulmonary stenosis
Unilateral
    Pulmonary artery agenesis
    Scimitar syndrome
Chromosomal abnormalities
    Trisomy 13, 18, and 21

---

better delineated and tracheal diverticula and bronchiectasis are readily detected. CT may also demonstrate the presence of horseshoe lung, a rare associated abnormality.[39]

Horseshoe lung is an uncommon malformation in which the right and left lungs are fused inferiorly by an isthmus of lung tissue crossing the posterior mediastinum.[41,49,50,59,150] Horseshoe lung occurring without the scimitar syndrome is often associated with other lethal malformations.

PULMONARY HYPOPLASIA AND POTTER'S SYNDROME (OLIGOHYDRAMNIOS TETRAD)

Bilateral primary pulmonary hypoplasia becomes manifest early in the neonatal period. Radiographs reveal small-volume but otherwise clear lungs with a bell-shaped thorax, indicating disproportion between the size of the thorax and the abdomen.[149] Pneumothoraces are frequent.

Pulmonary hypoplasia is more frequently secondary to other fetal developmental abnormalities. The box at left gives an outline of known associations with pulmonary hypoplasia. Pulmonary hypoplasia is found in approximately 10% of neonatal autopsies and in 50% of those with congenital anomalies. The mechanisms causing the pulmonary hypoplasia are a matter of debate. The fetal lung communicates freely with the amniotic sac, and the fetus is known to exhibit breathing movements in utero. Thus entry of amniotic fluid into the lungs probably occurs. The fetal lung itself produces fluid as evidenced by the expansile buildup of fluid behind a bronchial obstruction. The presence of lung fluid and respiratory movement appears to play a role in normal lung development. Decreased or absent respiratory movement in utero caused by central nervous system anomalies may be associated with pulmonary hypoplasia.[114] Decreased vascular perfusion of the fetal lung in Ebstein's anomaly, hypoplastic right heart syndrome, or pulmonary stenosis may impair fetal lung fluid production and be associated with hypoplasia. The most striking example of the influence of fluid on pulmonary embryogenesis is found in Potter's syndrome (oligohydramnios tetrad).[119] The oligohydramnios in these infants is the result of an abnormality in the development of the urinary tract, most commonly renal agenesis (Figure 14-19). The full tetrad comprises (1) the underlying renal abnormality that causes the oligohydramnios, (2) abnormal facies resulting from pressure effects in utero, (3) abnormal laxity of the skin, and (4) pulmonary hypoplasia.[47] There is debate as to whether the pulmonary hypoplasia results from a reduction in the amount of amniotic fluid actually within the developing lung or whether it is secondary to external pressure effects on the developing thorax. Clearly both factors could operate together.

More commonly pulmonary hypoplasia is secondary to any condition that by a mass effect stunts the growth of the lung or lungs in utero. A classic example is the

---

are usually present, and if so the diagnosis of hypogenetic lung syndrome may be made with total confidence. Partial anomalous pulmonary venous return to the inferior vena cava, right atrium, or coronary sinus may occur without pulmonary hypoplasia, particularly in association with intracardiac lesions such as an atrial septal defect. The key distinguishing feature in these cases is the absence of radiographic evidence of pulmonary hypoplasia.

CT provides a noninvasive method of confirming the diagnosis of the scimitar syndrome.[135] It has the additional advantage that the tracheobronchial anomalies are

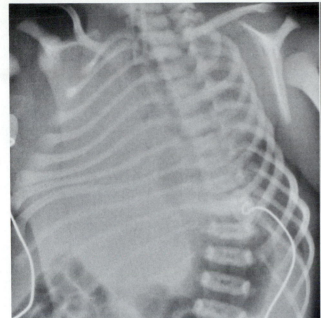

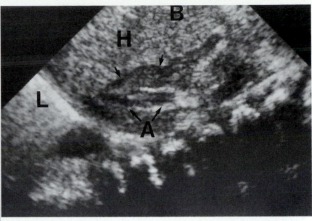

FIGURE 14-19
A, Radiograph of a neonate with Potter's syndrome. Note the largely airless lungs and the pressure deformities of ribs. B, Ultrasound scan shows liver *(H)*, adrenal gland *(A)*, solid lung *(L)*, and renal agenesis.

pulmonary hypoplasia that may result from a congenital diaphragmatic hernia. The underlying lung exhibits varying degrees of hypoplasia depending on the size of the hernia and the period during which pressure effects on the lung were operative. The basic problem in these cases is lack of space for growth and development of the lung. The extent of the hypoplasia may be a critical determinant of survival following repair of the hernia.

Although the extent of secondary pulmonary hypoplasia may be a critical factor in determining survival — for example, after the repair of a diaphragmatic hernia — the radiograph does not give a reliable indication of the possible outcome.[132] Failure of the lung to expand following relief of the pressure effects is clearly ominous. The radiographs demonstrate the disproportion in size between the thorax and the abdomen. Rib crowding and deformity may give an indication of intrauterine pressure effects as in Potter's syndrome. Respiratory distress is common, and the patients are often intubated. Pneumothoraces often complicate the clinical course.

UNILATERAL PRIMARY PULMONARY HYPOPLASIA

Unilateral primary pulmonary hypoplasia without accompanying scimitar syndrome is rare. Associated anomalies may be present in other body systems and may ultimately determine the outcome. The patients may be asymptomatic or have recurrent episodes of wheezing and pneumonia. Primary unilateral pulmonary hypoplasia may be encountered in a child or an adult. The affected lung is small, and the mediastinum is displaced toward that side. The pulmonary vasculature may be deformed and stunted. The lateral chest film often shows a sharply marginated opacity behind and parallel to the

sternum. The appearance is similar to that seen in left upper lobe collapse or combined right upper and middle lobe collapse, but it is due to extrapleural areolar tissue occupying the space that should have been occupied by lung. Therefore there is no wedge or fan of tissue connected to the hilum. The presence of areolar tissue adjacent to the heart and mediastinum frequently results in lack of definition of these borders on the affected side (Figure 14-20).

PULMONARY SEQUESTRATION

Pulmonary sequestration is the presence of an abnormal mass of pulmonary tissue that does not communicate with the tracheobronchial tree through a normal bronchial connection and that receives its blood supply via an anomalous systemic artery. The arterial supply may arise from the descending thoracic aorta or from the abdominal aorta or one of its branches. Pulmonary sequestrations can be divided into the intralobar and the much less common extralobar types.[145] The differentiating features are best summarized in table form (Table 14-1).[34] However, the physician may encounter variants that do not fit neatly into these two categories.[13,44] For example, intralobar sequestrations may drain to the systemic venous system and extralobar sequestrations to the left atrium. Furthermore, a portion of normal lung may be supplied by an aberrant systemic artery or drained by a systemic vein.[79]

Intralobar sequestrations usually produce symptoms when they become infected, most commonly in adolescence or in early adult life. In very rare instances a considerable shunt through a sequestration may result in high-output cardiac failure.[89] This is most likely to occur with the extralobar variety and may compound associated

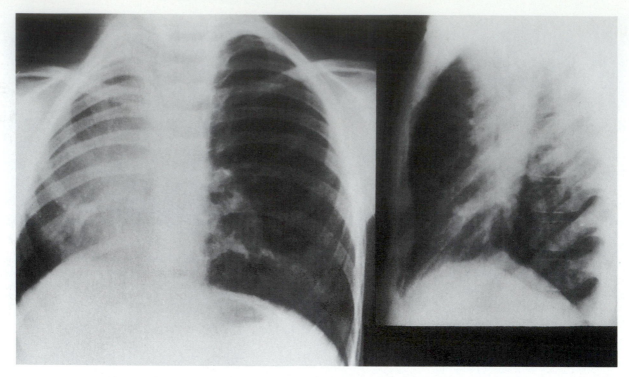

FIGURE 14-20
Frontal and lateral chest radiographs in an infant with hypoplasia of the right lung. Note the volume reduction and the retrosternal soft tissue density.

Table 14-1 Differentiation of extralobar and intralobular pulmonary sequestation

Parameter	Intralobar sequestration	Extralobar sequestration
Relation to normal lung	Within normal lung and its pleural cover	Separate with own pleural covering
Venous drainage	Pulmonary	Systemic
Side affected	Left 60%-70%	Left 90%
Associated congenital anomalies	Uncommon	Frequent
Age at diagnosis	50% 20 years	60% 1 year
Sex ratio	M = F	M/F = 4:1
Infection or communication with normal lung	Common	Rare

Modified from DeParades CG, Pierce WS, Johnson DG, et al: *Pediatr Surg* 5:136-147, 1970.

congenital cardiac problems. Extralobar sequestrations are usually asymptomatic and are often discovered incidentally on a chest radiograph, during angiocardiography, or during surgical repair of a congenital diaphragmatic hernia, with which they are frequently associated. Because extralobar sequestrations have a complete serosal covering and may have a narrow vascular pedicle, torsion may occur. The result may be a tension hydrothorax identified either by ultrasound in utero or on plain radiographs postnatally. An intrauterine tension hydrothorax may obstruct venous return to the heart, producing fetal hydrops.[63]

The appearances on plain chest radiography are typically those of an opacity at one or other base posteromedially (Figure 14-21). Sequestrations are found in the upper half of the thorax in only approximately 2% of cases.[66] There is a distinct affinity for the left side. In an uncomplicated lesion the mass is uniformly dense. With the extralobar variety the lateral margin is well defined because of the pleural envelope, while medially the lesion abuts the mediastinum so closely that it is usually confused with a mediastinal mass. Extralobar sequestrations may be found in a variety of other locations, including the pericardial space, mediastinum, and retroperitoneum. Communication with the esophagus or the stomach may be demonstrated by barium studies. These studies may be performed as a result of the feeding difficulties occasionally encountered.

Intralobar sequestrations are invariably supradiaphragmatic. They often have more ill-defined margins and resemble an area of pneumonia, although they may have rounded or lobulated contours and resemble an intrapul-

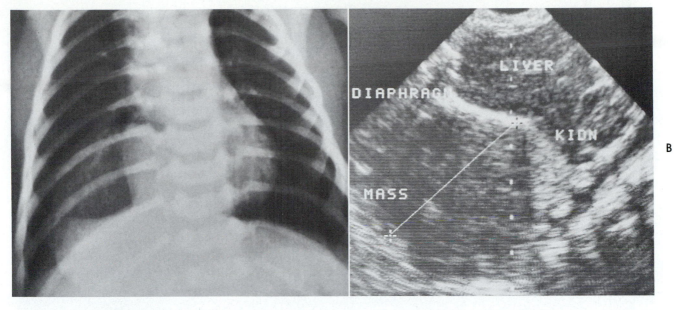

FIGURE 14-21
Extralobar sequestration in an infant. **A,** Well-circumscribed right posterior basal mass lesion is shown by, **B,** ultrasound to be a solid mass.

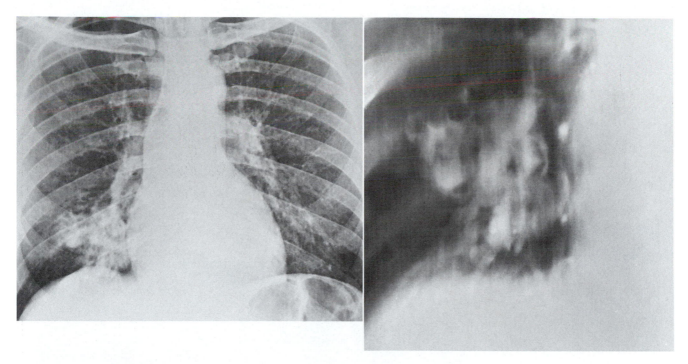

FIGURE 14-22
Intralobar sequestration in the right lower lobe. The lobulated mass contains some airspaces, indicating communication with bronchial tree.

monary mass (Figure 14-22). On occasion, one or more air-fluid levels are seen within sequestered segments. Such air-fluid levels are a consequence of infection with fistula formation to the adjacent bronchi. Although sequestrations may appear solid on plain radiographs, CT

usually shows an irregular cystic component to the lesion.[72] Ikezoe and associates[72] found a surprisingly high incidence of "emphysema" in the lung adjacent to both intralobar and extralobar sequestrations. Emphysema adjacent to intralobar sequestrations has been

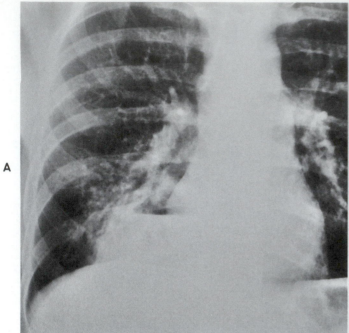

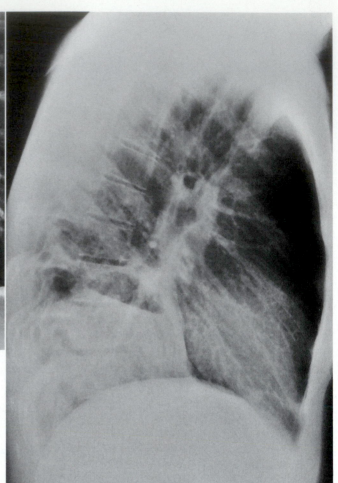

FIGURE 14-23
A, Posteroanterior and, B, lateral radiographs of a young man who had the sudden onset of fever and cough. (See Figure 14-24.)

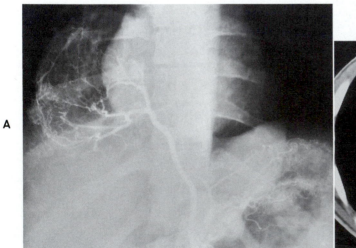

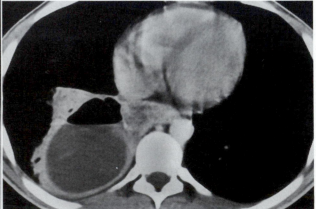

FIGURE 14-24
A, Same patient as in Figure 14-23. Large feeding vessel arising from the abdominal aorta supplies the intralobar sequestration. B, This vessel was not visualized on CT examination.

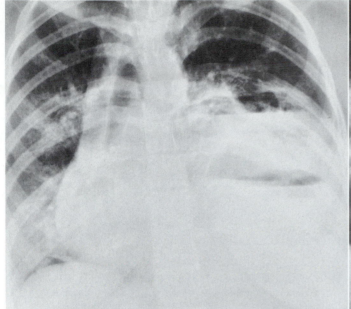

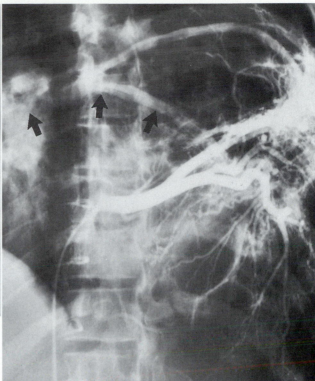

FIGURE 14-25
A, Infected intralobar sequestration in a young woman. B, Large feeding vessel arising from the descending thoracic aorta. Venous return is to the left atrium *(arrows)*.

explained on the basis of collateral air drift and air trapping caused by impaired ventilation.[141] Emphysema adjacent to extralobar sequestrations is more difficult to explain because the emphysematous portions of adjacent lung are distinctly separated from the actual sequestrations by the pleural envelope. Nevertheless, emphysema appeared to be a more constant finding in extralobar sequestration than in the intralobar variety. Occasionally, air trapping and bulla formation are the dominant features even on plain films. A cystic form of pulmonary sequestration may be encountered. This may be caused by infection of a previously solid mass with subsequent communication to the adjacent lung (Figures 14-23 and 14-24). However, a possible overlap between sequestrations and bronchogenic cysts has been proposed.[32]

The demonstration of a systemic artery supplying the lesion is the critical diagnostic feature. This can be readily shown by aortography and particularly by selective angiography, which also demonstrates the venous drainage (Figures 14-24 and 14-25). Arteriography is particularly important if surgical treatment is being considered because inadvertent damage to the artery during surgery can cause significant hemorrhage.[20] The systemic artery can also be demonstrated by CT using intravenous contrast enhancement[44,72,107] or occasionally by standard ultrasound.[77,153] However, the use of color flow Doppler ultrasound has allowed simple, reliable, noninvasive investigation of pulmonary sequestrations.[63,136,175] The systemic feeding artery is identified with certainty and its general morphology determined. Doppler ultrasound ap-

pears to permit a firm diagnosis of sequestration and to obviate further diagnostic studies. The systemic vascular perfusion of pulmonary sequestrations has also been demonstrated by comparison of the pulmonary and systemic phases at radionuclide angiography.[56,81] This method, however, is no longer of diagnostic importance, having been supplanted by CT, MRI, and particularly color flow Doppler ultrasound.

MRI is capable of clearly delineating the vascular supply of sequestrations.[108] Magnetic resonance angiography can provide an elegant demonstration of the vascular anatomy, almost on a par with conventional nonselective angiography (Figure 14-26).[38] However, these techniques are specialized, expensive, and not readily suited to infants. Surgeons vary in their demands for precision of information about the vascular anatomy, and the modality of investigation must cater to their individual requirements. The presence or absence of a systemic arterial supply is the critical feature in the differential diagnosis from bronchogenic cysts.

The infected pulmonary sequestration may contain fluid levels and have an ill-defined edge because of inflammatory changes in adjacent lung. The appearance therefore may exactly mimic a simple lung abscess, and only the position of the lesion and the clinical circumstances may lead to suspicion of an infected pulmonary sequestration. On the other hand, many cavitated sequestrations are sterile at the time of diagnosis or surgical removal. Communication with the bronchial tree may be demonstrated by bronchography, but bronchography has

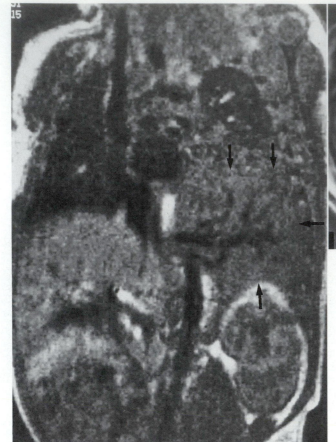

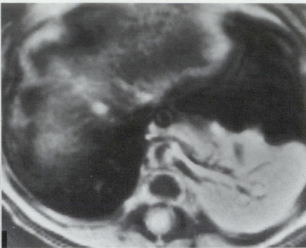

FIGURE 14-26

A, Coronal magnetic resonance (MR) image of an infant with intralobar sequestration *(arrows)*. **B,** Axial MR image showing a feeding vessel arising from the descending thoracic aorta.

no clinical value in evaluating bronchopulmonary sequestration. On rare occasion, calcifications occur in pulmonary sequestration and are readily detected by CT.[72,157] The differential diagnosis of lower paravertebral masses includes neurogenic tumors and lateral meningoceles. In these lesions pressure erosions of the vertebrae and the proximal ribs may be observed, a finding not seen with pulmonary sequestration. Other paravertebral masses such as extramedullary hematopoiesis or pleural tumors may be indistinguishable from pulmonary sequestration. In essence, the diagnosis of pulmonary sequestration depends as much on the position of the lesion and the clinical features as on the radiographic appearances alone.

Pulmonary sequestration has on several occasions been diagnosed by sonography in utero.[122,140] This might be only of academic interest except that the presence of a sequestration has sometimes caused an intrauterine tension hydrothorax and hydrops fetalis.[83,91,154] Such cases have been successfully treated by intrauterine tube drainage.[165]

PULMONARY ARTERIOVENOUS FISTULAS

Pulmonary arteriovenous fistulas may be single or multiple. Nearly 90% of cases are associated with Rendu-Osler-Weber disease (hereditary hemorrhagic telangiectasia), and especially in this disease the lesions are likely to

be multiple. Pulmonary arteriovenous fistulas may be associated with other congenital abnormalities, notably cardiac malformations. In infants and children the lesions may be large enough to cause a detectable bruit and enough right-to-left shunting to produce cyanosis (Figure 14-27). Even in adults the shunting often produces some hypoxia, particularly in the erect position, so-called orthodeoxia. The physiologic explanation for orthodeoxia is that the lesions have a predilection for the lower lung zones and shunting is increased in the upright position. The patient, however, is usually asymptomatic, having accommodated to the chronic hypoxia. On occasion the patient has systemic abscesses or infarction, notably of the brain, because the right-to-left shunting of blood bypasses the lung filter (Figure 14-28).[21,53,64] Fully one third of the patients in one large series had CT evidence of previous strokes.[168] Otherwise the lesions are detected by chance on chest radiographs or during screening of families with Rendu-Osler-Weber disease. A minority of patients have hemoptysis or hemothorax.[168]

On plain chest radiographs an arteriovenous malformation is seen as a well-circumscribed nodule, usually with a lobular outline. In peripheral lesions the vessels feeding and draining the lesion can usually be seen on the plain films, and this feature can be confirmed by conventional tomography or CT. More central lesions may be difficult to discern among the hilar vessels, and even if an abnormality is detected, the shorter feeding vessels may be difficult or impossible to identify. Multiple lesions may be confused with metastases if the enlarged feeding vessels are overlooked (Figure 14-29).[36] Contrast-en-

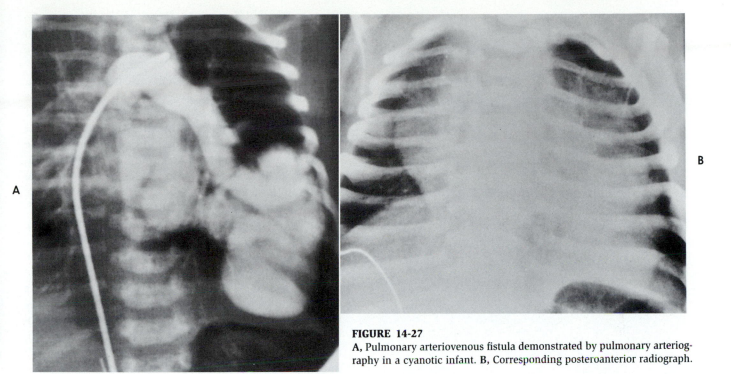

FIGURE 14-27
A, Pulmonary arteriovenous fistula demonstrated by pulmonary arteriography in a cyanotic infant. **B,** Corresponding posteroanterior radiograph.

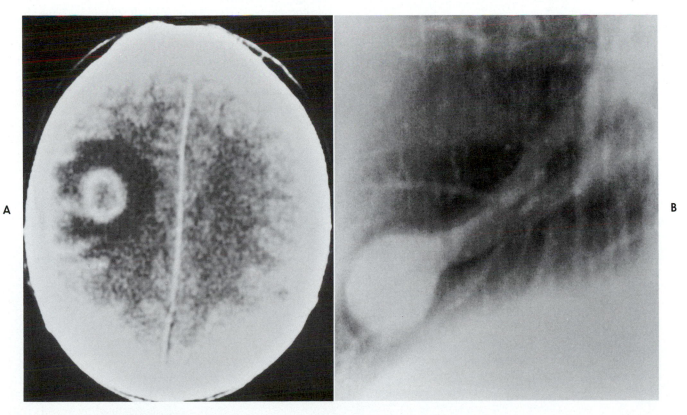

FIGURE 14-28
A, Brain abscess demonstrated by computed tomography scan in a previously healthy young male. **B,** Tomogram of the same patient shows a large arteriovenous malformation in the right lung. (Courtesy Dr. Bech-Olsen, Tonsberg, Norway.)

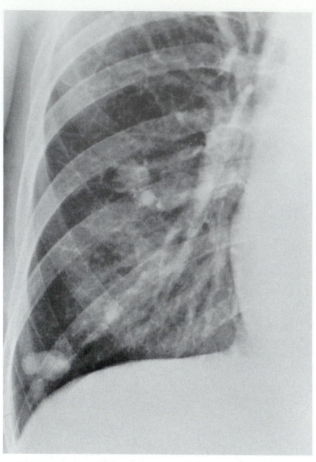

FIGURE 14-29
Multiple small arteriovenous malformations in a middle-aged woman with severe gastrointestinal bleeding. These lesions were initially suspected to be metastases from a neoplasm of the gastrointestinal tract.

hanced CT[87,121,124] or pulmonary angiography can be used not only to confirm the diagnosis, but also to search for additional lesions elsewhere in the lungs (Figure 14-30). Remy and co-workers[124] found somewhat surprisingly that CT was much more sensitive than pulmonary angiography in detecting pulmonary arteriovenous malformations. In their series 98% were detected by CT against 60% by pulmonary angiography. Admittedly the malformations found by CT and not by angiography were extremely small and thought to be clinically inconsequential. Such small malformations have not been observed to evolve into larger malformations. Furthermore, embolotherapy is usually restricted to malformations with feeding vessels 3 mm or greater in diameter.[168] Thus the finding of tiny malformations is not particularly critical.

Pulmonary angiography is vital for the planning of treatment. Some 80% of malformations have a single feeding vessel and are termed simple. The remainder have two or more feeding vessels and present a greater treatment challenge. Increasingly, pulmonary arteriovenous malformations are treated by embolotherapy with coils[58,126] or detachable balloons.[168] The purpose of such intervention is to reduce the risk of systemic embolization and the right-to-left shunting of blood in the lungs, thereby improving arterial oxygen saturation.[26] However, considerable experience is required for adequate interventional radiologic treatment, and this is best performed in specialist units.

Pulmonary arteriovenous malformations have been detected by MRI.[37] As yet MRI has no specific advantages over CT and may be inferior in terms of resolution. Thus small lesions may be overlooked, although this in itself is not critical. Shunting through arteriovenous malformations has been detected by echocardiography[6] and radio-

A

B

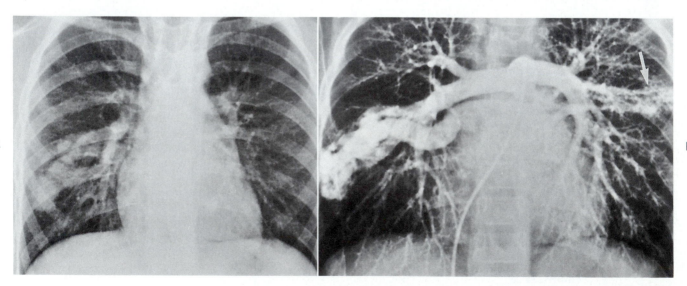

FIGURE 14-30
A, Large arteriovenous malformation in the right lung. No other lesion could be identified with certainty. **B,** Pulmonary arteriography reveals a second arteriovenous malformation in the left midzone *(arrow).*

scintigraphy,[25] but these methods have not evolved into techniques replacing oximetry.

CONGENITAL LYMPHANGIECTASIS

Generalized pulmonary lymphangiectasis may be seen in three distinct categories of patients[111]:

1. Primary lymphangiectasis. This condition is an extremely rare primary developmental abnormality of the lungs. At least half of afflicted individuals are stillborn, and the remainder die shortly after birth. The radiographs show a pattern of diffuse interstitial or alveolar edema. Echocardiography excludes a cardiac cause for the lung changes.

2. Secondary lymphangiectasis. These patients have severe pulmonary venous obstruction, most commonly obstructed total anomalous pulmonary venous return or the hypoplastic left heart syndrome. The condition is reversible if the cardiac condition can be surgically corrected; total anomalous pulmonary venous return, for example, is amenable to correction.

3. Lymphangiectasis as part of generalized lymphangiectasia. In these cases symptoms related to the lymphangiectasis are either delayed in onset or absent. A classic example of this type of lymphangiectasis occurs in Noonan's syndrome (Turner's syndrome phenotype with normal karyotype). These patients have clinical evidence of lymphangiectasis in the extremities and the cervical region; the webbed neck is thought to result from fibrosis in areas of cervical lymphedema. Radiographic evidence of diffuse or more focal interstitial infiltration may be seen, and there may be pleural effusions. Occasionally, localized pulmonary lymphangiectasis is seen, possibly representing a forme fruste of primary lymphangiectasis.[158]

CONGENITAL CYSTIC ADENOMATOID MALFORMATION OF THE LUNG

This rare, life-threatening condition usually manifests itself in the neonatal period, but approximately 10% of cases are manifested after the first year of life, usually with chronic respiratory infections.[118,159] The basic lesion is a hamartomatous mass of fibrous tissue and smooth muscle derived from the terminal respiratory tissues, usually containing numerous cystic spaces lined with bronchial or cuboidal epithelium.[131,144,145] Unlike the classic pulmonary hamartoma, cartilage is notably absent from the lesion.[73] The process usually involves just one lobe. Involvement of more than one lobe or bilateral lesions are exceedingly rare.[27,166] It is the expansile nature of the lesion that is life threatening, a feature frequently compounded by secondary hypoplasia of the uninvolved lung.

Radiographic study shows marked expansion of what appears to be an entire lung with consequent shift of the mediastinum and compression of the contralateral lung. The involved lung is composed of opaque tissue interspersed with cystic, air-containing spaces of varying size that may contain fluid levels (Figure 14-31). Occasionally

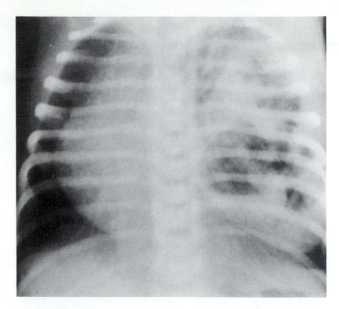

FIGURE 14-31
Radiograph of a neonate with a congenital cystic adenomatoid malformation of the left lung.

a single cyst predominates (Figure 14-32).[94] The lesion may initially appear solid if the radiograph is obtained before the fetal lung fluid has drained; it appears cystic only where air replaces the fluid. The similarity to a congenital diaphragmatic hernia can be striking.[60] In diaphragmatic hernia the abdomen tends to be scaphoid with a paucity of gas shadows in the abdomen. In congenital cystic adenomatoid malformation of the lung, both the abdominal gas pattern and the shape of the abdomen are normal. Immediate diagnosis is essential in both conditions, and the treatment for both is surgical. The extent of any associated pulmonary hypoplasia probably plays a significant role in determining the outcome. Congenital cystic adenomatoid malformation may be diagnosed antenatally by means of ultrasound.[30,74] The cardinal feature is the presence of a solid or cystic intrathoracic mass, often associated with polyhydramnios and nonimmune hydrops fetalis. Similar findings may be seen with pulmonary sequestration. Such findings would be academic were it not for the fact that seemingly successful antenatal interventions, either cyst drainage or even fetal lobectomies, have been performed on the basis of these studies.[84]

As previously indicated, in a small group of patients the disease is manifested after 1 year of age, usually with recurrent respiratory tract infections. Occasionally patients are found with an essentially asymptomatic solid or cystic mass in the chest. Pneumothorax has been described in rare cases.[105]

CYSTIC FIBROSIS OF THE PANCREAS (MUCOVISCIDOSIS)

This relatively common congenital disorder is variously termed cystic fibrosis of the pancreas, fibrocystic disease,

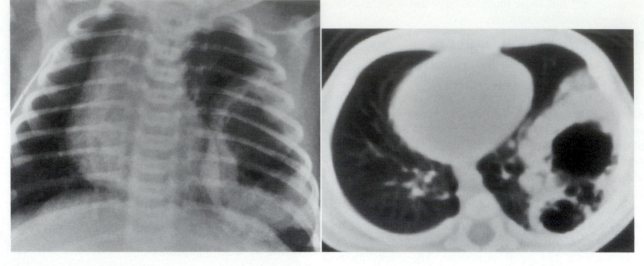

FIGURE 14-32
A, Radiograph of a neonate with a congenital cystic adenomatoid malformation of the left lung. B, Corresponding computed tomography scan showing a largely unilocular cavity.

EFFECTS OF MUCOVISCIDOSIS

INCIDENCE

1 in 1600 live births

INHERITANCE

Mendelian recessive

CARRIER STATE

1 in 20 are heterozygotes

RACE

High incidence in Caucasians

EFFECTS

Related to the viscid secretions

Pancreas
   Antenatal
      Meconium ileus
   Postnatal
      Pancreatitis
      Pancreatic insufficiency
      Diabetes mellitus
Liver
   Focal biliary cirrhosis
   Cirrhosis leading to portal hypertension, varices, hypersplenism
Gallbladder
   Thick walled with viscid secretions

Intestines
   Meconium ileus
   Atresia
   Constipation leading to rectal prolapse and inguinal hernias
Upper respiratory tract
   Abnormal salivary secretions
   Nasal polyps
   Sinusitis
Lower respiratory tract
   Bronchiectasis
   Bronchitis
   Bronchopneumonia
   Atelectasis
   Emphysema
   Hilar adenopathy
   Pulmonary hypertension
   Cor pulmonale
   Hemoptysis
   Respiratory failure
Female genital tract
   Reduced fertility
Exocrine gland abnormality
Salt depletion caused by increased salt content of sweat, heat stroke
Secondary aplasia in male genitalia (vas deferens, epididymis, seminal vesicles) leading to sterility

and mucoviscidosis. The term "mucoviscidosis" is used in this presentation because it underlines the primary feature of this condition, the presence of excessively viscid mucous secretions in a wide systemic distribution. Nevertheless, the term is not encompassing because it does not cover the associated abnormalities in the exocrine glands. A summary of mucoviscidosis and its diverse effects is given in the box on the facing page. The pulmonary manifestations are the most significant and cause the greatest morbidity and mortality.

The pulmonary manifestations of mucoviscidosis are progressive from birth but do not become radiologically apparent for months or years (Figure 14-33). The earliest changes are variable and may include focal atelectasis, recurrent pneumonias, diffuse peribronchial infiltration, emphysema, and hilar adenopathy. Clinical features, rather than chest radiographic findings alone, usually point to the diagnosis. The role of chest radiography is to follow the course of the pulmonary infections. Deteriora-

tion is inexorable despite treatment, but the rate of deterioration varies among patients. Patients with early manifestations of the disease tend to deteriorate the most rapidly. In the fully developed form of the disease the radiographic findings are remarkably uniform and include the following:

1. Emphysema. The widespread parenchymal changes may obscure the lung changes of emphysema, but the chest is usually barrel shaped with an increased sagittal diameter and low flat diaphragms.

2. Enlarged hilar shadows and diffuse increase in the perihilar shadows (Figure 14-34). The increase in size of the hila is probably caused by hilar adenopathy, dilatation of the pulmonary arteries with pulmonary hypertension, and inflammatory changes adjacent to the hila. The widespread peribronchial and bronchial infiltration causes the diffuse perihilar densities.

3. Bronchiectasis. Bronchiectasis may be either tubular or cystic. The cystic changes are perhaps a hallmark of the

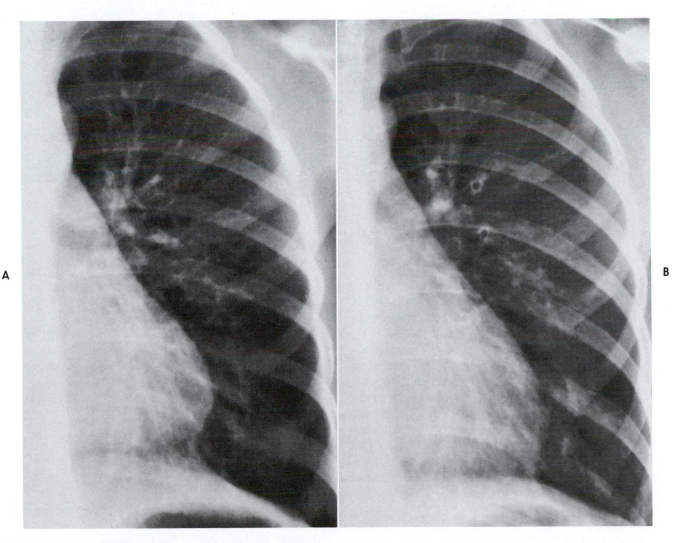

A   B

FIGURE 14-33
Series of radiographs over 13-year period in a patient with mucoviscidosis. A, Age 6 years. B, Age 10 years.   *Continued.*

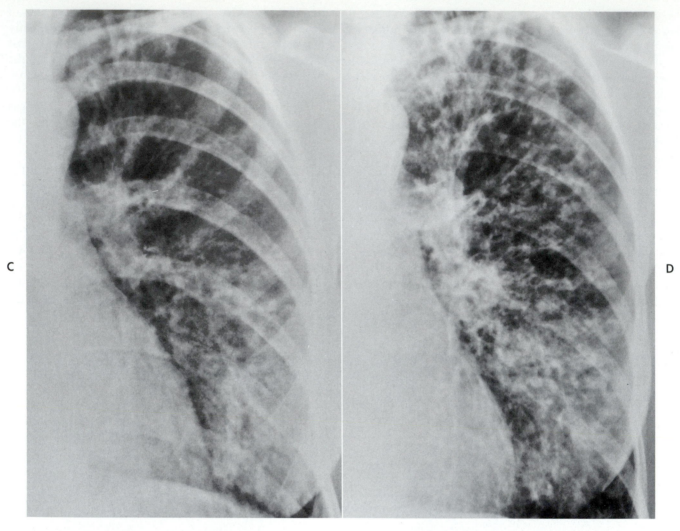

FIGURE 14-33, cont'd
C, Age 16 years. D, Age 19 years.

disease (Figure 14-35). The cysts may be as much as 2 cm in diameter and often have relatively thin walls. Walls may be thickened by associated infection, and the cysts may contain variable quantities of fluid.

4. Atelectasis and focal infiltration. Patchy focal parenchymal densities are common and may be observed to wax and wane in association with intercurrent infections.

Taken as a whole, the pulmonary shadows in mucoviscidosis are often predominant in the upper zones, a reverse of the usual situation with bronchiectasis. Pulmonary complications include pneumothorax caused by rupture of an emphysematous bleb and massive hemoptysis. Arteriography may be necessary to determine the site of bleeding. The hemoptysis can be abated by the interventional techniques of selective vascular occlusion. Lung abscess and empyema are surprisingly rare, probably because of a hyperimmune state resulting from prolonged chronic infection.

Chest radiographs over the years reflect the patient's deteriorating status, but short-term clinical fluctuations are not necessarily accompanied by any readily detectable radiographic changes. In part, this must be due to obscuration of minor changes by preexisting major chronic abnormalities. Eventually the patient dies, probably of respiratory failure, possibly precipitated by a major complication such as massive hemoptysis, or cor pulmonale, in which case increasing heart size may be apparent.

CONGENITAL DIAPHRAGMATIC ABNORMALITIES

Congenital diaphragmatic hernia

The exact embryologic basis for congenital diaphragmatic hernias is disputed. Some at least may be acquired through phrenic nerve trauma at birth. Wayne and co-workers[163] reviewed 60 cases of diaphragmatic eventration and found that 10 resulted from birth trauma.

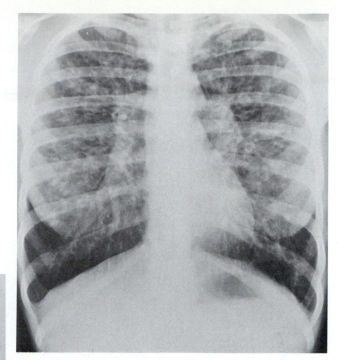

FIGURE 14-34
Mucoviscidosis. Enlarged hilar shadows and diffuse perihilar infiltration.

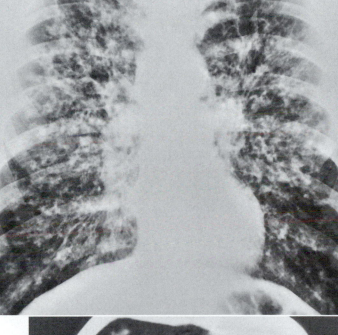

A

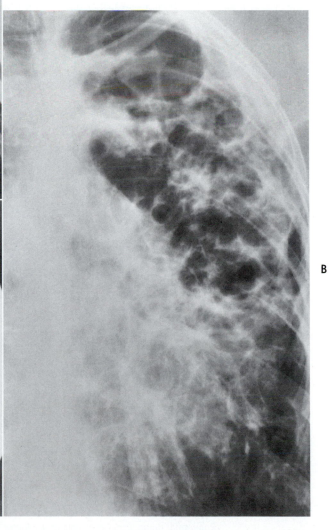

B

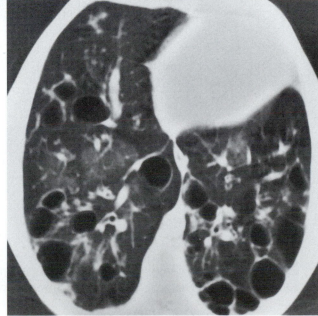

C

FIGURE 14-35
Mucoviscidosis. A, Widespread cystic changes in lungs with diffuse peribronchial infiltration. B, Advanced cystic changes in the lungs of a patient being assessed for lung transplantation. C, Computed tomography scan of the patient in B.

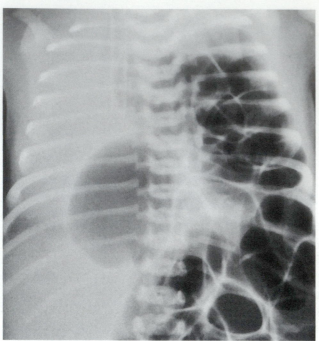

FIGURE 14-36
Congenital diaphragmatic hernia in a neonate with severe respiratory distress.

Nevertheless, 48 were truly congenital, and of these, 3 had coincident pulmonary hypoplasia. The most common congenital diaphragmatic hernia is a relatively central defect in one hemidiaphragm.

Classic congenital diaphragmatic hernias are first seen as an emergency in the neonatal period. A major portion of the abdominal viscera may be in one hemithorax with compressive effects on the lungs and mediastinum. Swallowed air enters the stomach and the bowel fairly quickly, and the diagnosis is not ordinarily difficult (Figure 14-36). The chest radiograph shows a mass of water or mixed water and gas density in one hemithorax, usually on the left. The diaphragmatic contour is lost, and it is usually evident that the lesion is centered in the lower chest because any air in the ipsilateral lung is seen in the upper chest. The mass effect may be considerable, with obvious shift of the mediastinum to the opposite side and evidence of compression of the contralateral lung. Gas in the lesion may be obviously in the stomach or collect as loculi of gas in small bowel. On the right side the contents of the hernia may be only liver and omentum, and the mass is then of uniform water density. If a nasogastric tube is inserted, this may either be impeded up in the region of the esophagogastric junction or turn up into the chest cavity (Figure 14-37). The abdomen is likely to be scaphoid instead of showing the protuberance normal in the infant. Aeration of the lungs may be severely restricted, and there may be underlying pulmonary hy-

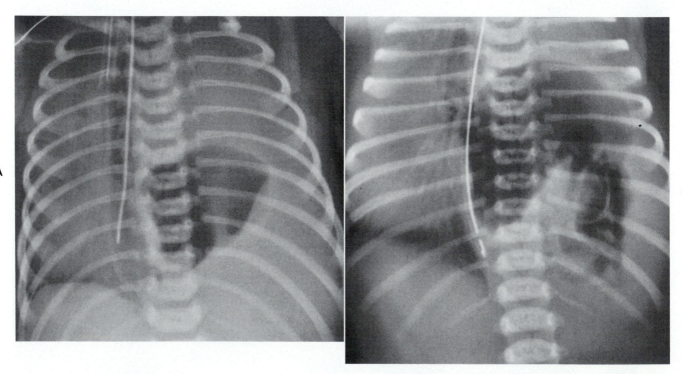

A   B

FIGURE 14-37
Congenital diaphragmatic hernia in a neonate with respiratory distress. Nasogastric tube could not be advanced into the stomach. **A,** Early image shows gas in stomach but not in the herniated small bowel. **B,** Later, gas appears in the small bowel.

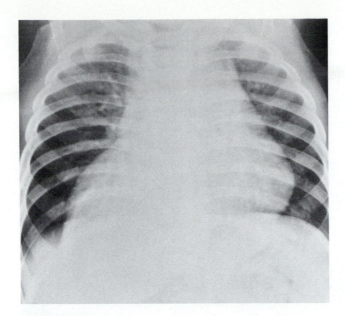

FIGURE 14-38
Morgagni hernia in the right cardiophrenic angle in a child. Hernia contained liver and omentum and was isodense with the heart.

poplasia, the extent of which cannot be determined with certainty on the initial radiographs. However, Saifuddin and Arthur[132] examined a series of preoperative radiographs and correlated the findings with the ultimate outcome. Absence of aeration of the contralateral lung or the preoperative presence of a contralateral pneumothorax was associated with mortality in all cases. On the other hand, all patients with visibly aerated ipsilateral lung survived. Other indicators of a poorer prognosis included right-sided defects and intrathoracic position of the stomach.

There are pitfalls in the diagnosis of diaphragmatic hernia, particularly in the right chest. The liver or omentum may plug the defect in the diaphragm, and herniation of abdominal contents into the chest may be delayed.[102] Indeed, in a number of cases the hernia is not manifested until later in childhood after chest radiographs had been normal.[12,95] Alternatively, the chest radiograph may be intermittently abnormal. Delayed appearance of right-sided hernias has been associated with group B streptococcal pneumonia in neonates.[101] Right-sided hernias have been noted to cause right pleural effusions, thought to be the result of obstructed hepatic venous outflow.[24] Such an effusion may not only obscure the hernia but also falsely raise the question of primary pulmonary disease such as pneumonia. Cystic adenomatoid malformation, particularly in the right side of the chest and before air has entered the lesion, may be difficult to differentiate from a hernia. Air in the cystic spaces of a congenital adenomatoid malformation may resemble bowel gas, but usually the air is seen to be within a circumscribed mass. Bowel gas may be identified

in a normally protuberant abdomen, and the course of a nasogastric tube is normal.

Ultrasound is useful in the diagnosis of congenital diaphragmatic hernia both prenatally and postnatally.[8,143] Peristalsis of bowel within the thorax may be observed, and the normal uninterrupted contours of the diaphragm are not seen. Ultrasound is of great use in differentiating other neonatal mass lesions such as pulmonary sequestration and congenital cystic adenomatoid malformations from hernias. The feeding artery of a pulmonary sequestration may be identified, particularly if Doppler ultrasound is used. Ultrasound examination of a cystic adenomatoid malformation should indicate the presence of an intact diaphragm and the cystic nature of the lesion.

Accessory diaphragm

Accessory diaphragm is a rare anomaly consisting of an accessory fibromuscular diaphragmatic sheet within the oblique fissure. The hemithorax is thereby separated into two compartments. In an uncomplicated case the only suggestion of the presence of an accessory diaphragm is the visualization of an unusually thick oblique fissure on that side. An accessory diaphragm may be associated with and be incidental to more significant pulmonary anomalies such as lobar hypoplasia or the scimitar syndrome.

Morgagni hernia

Morgagni hernias may be encountered at any age and represent herniation of abdominal contents through the diaphragm between its costal and sternal attachments. The hernia normally develops in the right cardiophrenic sulcus, presumably because the heart hinders herniation on the left. Morgagni hernias are normally small and often contain only liver or omentum, in which case they are of homogeneous density on plain radiographs. The margins are smooth and rounded, and the chief differential diagnoses include pericardial cysts, prominent cardiac fat pads, and focal pleural or pulmonary parenchymal masses (Figure 14-38). CT may be helpful in determining the high fat content of contained omentum or cardiac fat pads, in demonstrating liver in the hernia, or in confirming the presence of a pericardial cyst. MRI readily demonstrates a Morgagni hernia with the advantage that scanning may be performed in multiple planes (Figure 14-39).[31,173] Ultrasound and radionuclide imaging may also be useful in showing herniation of liver into the chest. Ultrasound can reasonably clearly distinguish fatty tissue from liver by their echo textures; fat is echodense and liver tissue is isoechoic with the rest of the liver. Loops of bowel can be identified by their peristaltic activity and the presence of gas. Radionuclide imaging is limited to determining that a cardiophrenic angle mass contains liver tissue. When the hernia contains bowel, usually transverse colon, the diagnosis is readily made based on plain radiographs. Morgagni hernias are more often a differential diagnostic problem on chest radiography than a clinical problem.

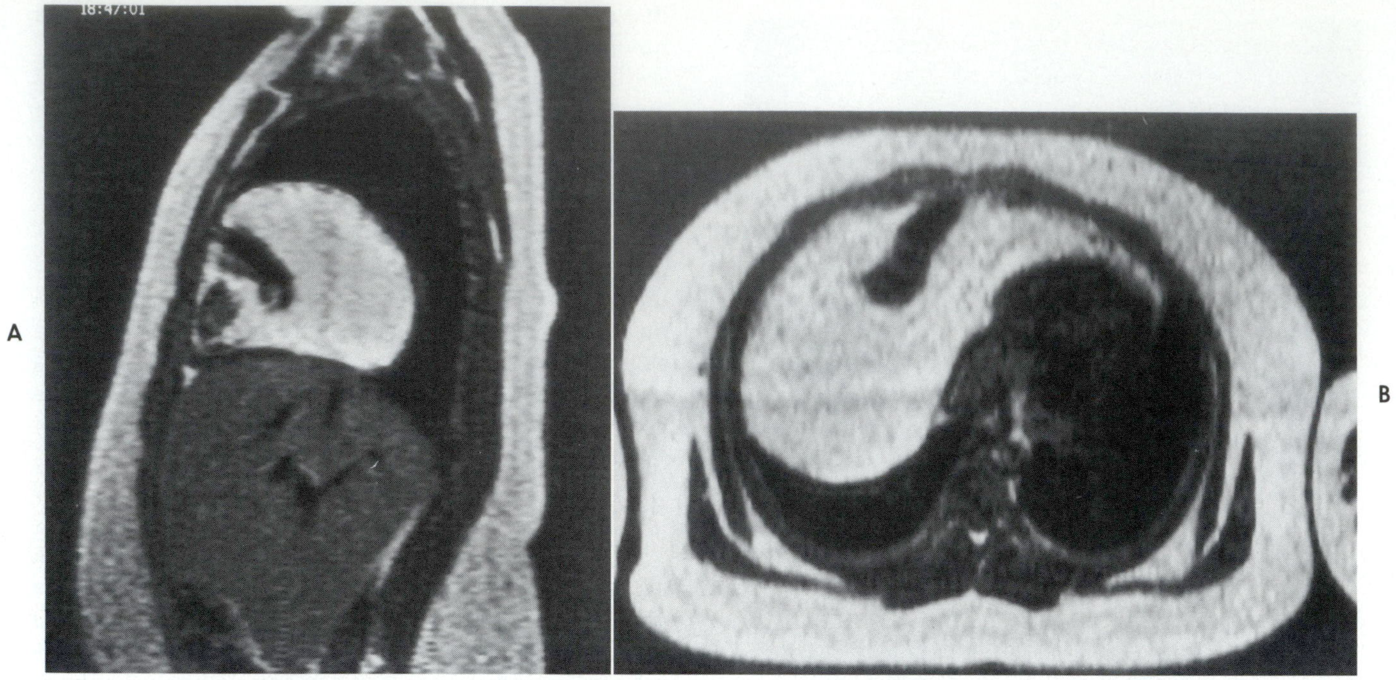

FIGURE 14-39
A, Sagittal magnetic resonance (MR) image of a child with a Morgagni hernia. Hernia contains omentum *(white)* and a loop of bowel *(black)*. B, Corresponding axial MR image.

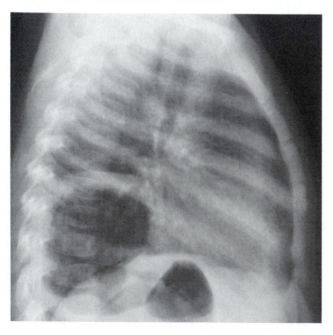

FIGURE 14-40
Bochdalek hernia containing herniated stomach in a child.

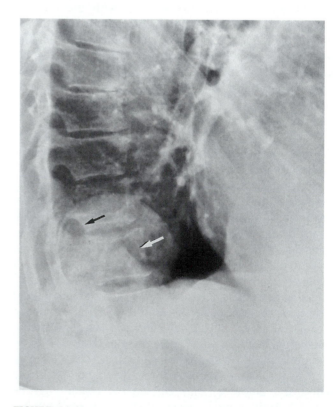

FIGURE 14-41
Bochdalek hernia containing a small knuckle of gas-filled bowel *(arrows)* in adult.

Bochdalek hernia

Bochdalek hernias represent herniations through a posterior diaphragmatic defect close to the crura. The defect is a relic of the pleuroperitoneal canal of the embryo. Bochdalek mistakenly believed that the herniation occurred under the lateral arcuate ligament of the diaphragm, but nevertheless his name is consistently applied to herniations through posterior diaphragmatic defects.[167] Bochdalek hernias usually become manifest in the neonatal period and are discussed previously under the heading "Congenital Diaphragmatic Hernia." The term "Bochdalek hernia" is not usually applied to such hernias but is customarily reserved for more localized herniations occurring later in life. Bochdalek hernias may be bilateral and symmetric. Minor degrees of herniation are fairly common and inconsequential, particularly in older individuals.[52] In these instances symmetric hemispherical bulges may be observed on the diaphragmatic contours posteriorly, slightly medial to the midlines of each lung. These small herniations contain only perinephric fat. Rarely, Bochdalek hernias are larger and contain portions of the kidney and even viscera such as the stomach and small bowel (Figures 14-40 and 14-41). Ordinarily the liver prevents visceral herniation on the right side.

REFERENCES

1. Allen RP, Taylor RL, Reiquam CW: Congenital lobar emphysema with dilated septal lymphatics, *Radiology* 86:929-931, 1966.
2. Atwell SW: Major anomalies of the tracheobronchial tree with a list of the minor anomalies, *Dis Chest* 52:611-615, 1967.
3. Bankoff MS, Daly BDT, Johnson HA, et al: Bronchogenic cyst causing superior vena cava obstruction: CT appearance, *J Comput Assist Tomogr* 9:951-952, 1985.
4. Barakos JA, Brown JJ, Bresain RJ, et al: High signal intensity lesions of the chest in MR imaging, *J Comput Assist Tomogr* 13:797-802, 1989.
5. Barnes JC, Smith WL: The VATER association, *Radiology* 126:445-449, 1978.
6. Barzilai B, Waggoner AD, Spessert C, et al: Two-dimensional echocardiography in the detection and follow-up of congenital pulmonary arteriovenous malformations, *Am J Cardiol* 68:1507-1510, 1991.
7. Bedard P, Girvan DP, Shandling B: Congenital H type tracheoesophageal fistula, *J Pediatr Surg* 9:663-668, 1974.
8. Benacerraf BR, Greene MF: Congenital diaphragmatic hernia: US diagnosis prior to 22 weeks gestation, *Radiology* 158:809-810, 1986.
9. Benisch BM, Wood WG, Kroeger GB, et al: Focal muscular hyperplasia of the trachea, *Arch Otolaryngol* 99:226-227, 1974.
10. Benson JE, Olsen MM, Fletcher BD: A spectrum of bronchopulmonary anomalies associated with tracheoesophageal malformations, *Pediatr Radiol* 15:377-380, 1985.
11. Bergstrom JF, Yost RV, Ford KT, et al: Unusual roentgen manifestations of bronchogenic cysts, *Radiology* 107:49-54, 1973.
12. Berman L, Stringer DA, Ein S, et al: Childhood diaphragmatic hernias presenting after the neonatal period, *Clin Radiol* 39:237-244, 1988.
13. Blesovsky A: Pulmonary sequestration: a report of an unusual case and a review of the literature, *Thorax* 22:351-357, 1967.
14. Boyd DP, Midell AI: Mediastinal cysts and tumors: an analysis of 96 cases, *Surg Clin North Am* 48:493-505, 1968.
15. Brasch RC, Gooding CA, Lallemond DP, et al: Magnetic resonance imaging of the thorax in childhood: work in progress, *Radiology* 150:463-467, 1984.
16. Brereton RJ, Rickwood AM: Esophageal atresia with pulmonary agenesis, *J Pediatr Surg* 18:618-620, 1983.
17. Bressler S, Wiener D: Bronchogenic cyst associated with an anomalous pulmonary artery arising from the thoracic aorta, *Surgery* 35:815-819, 1954.
18. Bruwer A, Clagett OT, McDonald JR: Anomalous arteries to the lung associated with congenital pulmonary abnormality, *J Thorac Surg* 19:957-972, 1950.
19. Cantrell JR, Guild HG: Congenital stenosis of the trachea, *Am J Surg* 108:297-305, 1964.
20. Carter R: Pulmonary sequestrations, *Ann Thorac Surg* 7:68-88, 1969.
21. Case records of the Massachusetts General Hospital (Case 16-1990), *N Engl J Med* 322:1139-1148, 1990.
22. Case records of the Massachusetts General Hospital (Case 32-1990), *N Engl J Med* 323:398-406, 1990.
23. Chang N, Hertzler JH, Gregg RH, et al: Congenital stenosis of the right main stem bronchus: a case report, *Pediatrics* 41:739-742, 1968.
24. Chilton HW, Chang JHT, Jones D, et al: Right-sided congenital diaphragmatic herniae presenting as pleural effusions in the newborn: dangers and pitfalls, *Arch Dis Child* 53:600-603, 1978.
25. Chilvers ER, Peters AM, George P, et al: Quantification of right to left shunt through pulmonary arteriovenous malformations using 99 Tcm albumin microspheres, *Clin Radiol* 39:611-614, 1988.
26. Chilvers ER, Whyte MKB, Jackson JE, et al: Effect of percutaneous transcatheter embolization on pulmonary function right-to-left shunt and arterial oxygenation in patients with pulmonary arteriovenous malformations, *Am Rev Respir Dis* 142:420-425, 1990.
27. Cloutier MM, Schaeffer DA, Hight D: Congenital cystic adenomatoid malformation, *Chest* 103:761-764, 1993.
28. Cumming WA: Esophageal atresia and tracheoesophageal fistula, *Radiol Clin North Am* 13:277-295, 1975.
29. Cunningham MD, Peter ER: Cervical hernia of the lung associated with cri du chat syndrome, *Am J Dis Child* 118:769-771, 1969.
30. Deacon CS, Smart PJ, Rimmers S: The antenatal diagnosis of congenital cystic adenomatoid malformation of the lung, *Br J Radiol* 63:968-970, 1990.
31. de Lange EE, Urbanski SR, Mugler JP, et al: Magnetization-prepared rapid gradient echo (MP-RAGE) magnetic resonance imaging of Morgagni's hernia, *Eur J Radiol* 11:196-199, 1990.
32. Demos TC, Budorick NE, Posniak HV: Benign mediastinal cysts: pointed appearance on CT, *J Comput Assist Tomogr* 13:132-133, 1989.
33. Demos NJ, Teresi A: Congenital lung malformations: a unified concept and case report, *J Thorac Cardiovasc Surg* 70:260-264, 1975.
34. De Parades CG, Pierce WS, Johnson DG, et al: Pulmonary sequestration in infants and children: a 20 year experience and review of the literature, *J Pediatr Surg* 5:136-147, 1970.
35. Di Lorenzo M, Collin PP, Vaillancourt R, et al: Bronchogenic cysts, *J Pediatr Surg* 24:988-991, 1989.
36. Dines DE, Seward JB, Bernatz PE: Pulmonary arteriovenous fistulas, *Mayo Clin Proc* 58:176-181, 1983.
37. Dinsmore BJ, Gefter WB, Hatabu H, et al: Pulmonary arteriovenous malformations: diagnosis by gradient-refocused MR imaging, *J Comput Assist Tomogr* 14:918-923, 1990.
38. Doyle AJ: Demonstration of blood supply to pulmonary sequestration by MR angiography, *AJR* 258:989-990, 1992.

39. Dupuis C, Charaf LAC, Breviere GM: The "adult" form of the scimitar syndrome, *Am J Cardiol* 70:502-507, 1992.
40. Eraklis AJ, Griscom NT, McGovern JB: Bronchogenic cysts of the mediastinum in infancy, *N Engl J Med* 281:1150-1155, 1969.
41. Ersöz A, Soncul H, Gökgöz L, et al: Horseshoe lung with left lung hypoplasia, *Thorax* 47:205-206, 1992.
42. Fagan CJ, Swischuk LE: The opaque lung in lobar emphysema, *AJR* 114:300-304, 1972.
43. Farnsworth AE, Ankeney JL: The spectrum of the scimitar syndrome, *J Thorac Cardiovasc Surg* 68:673-674, 1974.
44. Felker RE, Tonkin ILD: Imaging of pulmonary sequestration, *AJR* 154:241-249, 1990.
45. Felson B: Pulmonary agenesis and related anomalies, *Semin Roentgenol* 7:17-30, 1972.
46. Fitch SJ, Tonkin ILD, Tonkin AK: Imaging of foregut duplication cysts, *Radiographics* 6:189-201, 1986.
47. Fraga JR, Mirza AM, Reichelderfer TE: Association of pulmonary hypoplasia, renal anomalies and Potter's facies, *Clin Pediatr* 12:150-153, 1973.
48. France NE, Brown RJK: Congenital pulmonary lymphangectasis: report of 11 examples with special reference to cardiovascular findings, *Arch Dis Child* 46:528-532, 1971.
49. Frank JL, Poole CA, Rosas G: Horseshoe lung: clinical pathologic and radiologic features and a new plain film finding, *AJR* 146:217-226, 1986.
50. Freedom RM, Burrows PE, Moes CA: "Horseshoe" lung: report of five new cases, *AJR* 146:211-215, 1986.
51. Freedom RM, Culham JAG, Moes CAF: Anomalies of pulmonary arteries. In *Angiocardiography of congenital heart disease*, New York, 1984, Macmillan, pp 254-273.
52. Gale ME: Bochdalek hernias: prevalence and CT characteristics, *Radiology* 156:449-452, 1985.
53. Gibbons JR, McIlrath TE, Bailey IC: Pulmonary arteriovenous fistula in association with recurrent cerebral abscess, *Thorac Cardiovasc Surg* 33:319-321, 1985.
54. Godwin JD, Tarver RD: Scimitar syndrome: four new cases examined with CT, *Radiology* 159:15-20, 1986.
55. Gonzalez-Crussi F, Padilla LM, Miller JK, et al: "Bridging bronchus," a previously undescribed airway anomaly, *Am J Dis Child* 130:1015-1018, 1976.
56. Gooneratne N, Conway JJ: Radionuclide angiographic diagnosis of bronchopulmonary sequestration, *J Nucl Med* 17:1035-1037, 1976.
57. Harris KM, Lloyd DCF, Morrissey B, et al: The computed tomographic appearances in pulmonary artery atresia, *Clin Radiol* 45:382-386, 1992.
58. Hartnell GG, Allison DJ: Coil embolization in the treatment of pulmonary arteriovenous malformations, *J Thorac Imag* 4:81-85, 1989.
59. Hawass ND, Badawi MG, Al-Muzrakchi AM, et al: Horseshoe lung: differential diagnosis, *Pediatr Radiol* 20:580-584, 1990.
60. Heij HA, Ekkelkamp S, Vos A: Diagnosis of congenital cystic adenomatoid malformation of the lung in newborn infants and children, *Thorax* 45:122-125, 1990.
61. Heithoff KB, Sane SM, Williams MJ, et al: Bronchopulmonary foregut malformations: a unifying etiologic concept, *AJR* 126:46-55, 1976.
62. Hendren W, McKee DM: Lobar emphysema of infancy, *J Pediatr Surg* 1:24-39, 1966.
63. Hernanz-Schulman M, Stein SM, Neblett WW, et al: Pulmonary sequestration diagnosis with color Doppler sonography and a new theory of associated hydrothorax, *Radiology* 180:817-821, 1991.
64. Hewes RC, Auster M, White RI: Cerebral embolism—first manifestation of pulmonary arteriovenous malformation in patients with hereditary hemorrhagic telangiectasia, *Cardiovasc Intervent Radiol* 8:151-155, 1985.
65. Hislop A, Reid L: New pathological findings in emphysema of childhood. 1. Polyalveolar lobe with emphysema, *Thorax* 25:682-690, 1970.
66. Hoeffel JC, Bernard C: Pulmonary sequestration of the upper lobe in children, *Radiology* 160:513-514, 1986.
67. Holder TM, Cloud DT, Lewis JE, Pilling GP: Esophageal atresia and tracheoesophageal fistula, *Pediatrics* 34:542-549, 1964.
68. Hole BV, Wasserman K: Familial emphysema, *Ann Intern Med* 63:1009-1017, 1965.
69. Holinger PH, Johnstone KC, Schild JA: Congenital anomalies of the tracheobronchial tree and of the esophagus, *Pediatr Clin North Am* 9:1113-1124, 1962.
70. Hudson HL, McAlister WH: Obstructing tracheal hemangioma in infancy, *AJR* 93:428-431, 1965.
71. Hughes EW: Familial interstitial pulmonary fibrosis, *Thorax* 19:515-525, 1964.
72. Ikezoe J, Murayama S, Godwin JD, et al: Bronchopulmonary sequestration: CT assessment, *Radiology* 176:375-379, 1990.
73. Izzo C, Rickham PP: Neonatal pulmonary hamartoma, *J Pediatr Surg* 3:77-83, 1968.
74. Johnson JA, Rumack CM, Johnson ML, et al: Cystic adenomatoid malformations in antenatal demonstrations, *AJR* 142:483-484, 1984.
75. Johnston SRD, Adam A, Allison DJ, et al: Recurrent respiratory obstruction from a mediastinal bronchogenic cyst, *Thorax* 47:660-662, 1992.
76. Jones HE, Howells CHL: Pulmonary agenesis, *Br Med J* 2:1187-1189, 1961.
77. Kaude JV, Laurin S: Ultrasonographic demonstration of systemic artery feeding extrapulmonary sequestration, *Pediatr Radiol* 14:226-227, 1984.
78. Kennedy CD, Habili P, Matthew DJ, et al: Lobar emphysema: long-term imaging follow-up, *Radiology* 180:189-193, 1991.
79. Kirks DR, Kane PE, Free EA, et al: Systemic arterial supply to normal basilar segments of the left lower lobe, *AJR* 126:817-821, 1976.
80. Kirwan WO, Walbaum PR, McCormack RJM: Cystic intrathoracic derivatives of the foregut and their complications, *Thorax* 28:424-432, 1973.
81. Kobayashi Y, Abe T, Sato A, et al: Radionuclide angiography in pulmonary sequestration, *J Nucl Med* 26:1035-1038, 1985.
82. Koch B: Familial fibrocystic pulmonary dysplasia: observations in one family, *Am Med Assoc J* 92:801-808, 1965.
83. Kristoffersen SE, Ipsen I: Case report: ultrasonic real time diagnosis of hydrothorax before delivery in an infant with extralobar lung sequestration, *Acta Obstet Gynecol Scand* 63:721-723, 1984.
84. Kuller JA, Yankowitz J, Goldberg JD, et al: Outcome of antenatally diagnosed cystic adenomatoid malformations, *Am J Obstet Gynecol* 167:1038-1041, 1992.
85. Landing BH: Syndromes of congenital heart disease with tracheobronchial anomalies, *AJR* 123:679-686, 1975.
86. Landing BH, Wells TR: Tracheobronchial anomalies in children, *Perspect Pediatr Pathol* 1:1-32, 1973.
87. Langer R, Langer M: Value of computed tomography in the diagnosis of pulmonary arteriovenous shunts, *Cardiovasc Intervent Radiol* 7:277-279, 1984.
88. Leites V, Tannerbaum E: Familial spontaneous pneumothorax, *Am Rev Respir Dis* 82:240-241, 1960.
89. Levine MM, Nudel DB, Gootman N, et al: Pulmonary sequestration causing congestive heart failure in infancy: a report of two cases and review of the literature, *Ann Thorac Surg* 34:581-585, 1982.
90. Lincoln JCR, Deverall PB, Stark J, et al: Vascular anomalies compressing the esophagus and trachea, *Thorax* 24:295-306, 1969.
91. Lucaya J, Garcia-Conesa JA, Bernado L: Pulmonary sequestration associated with unilateral pulmonary hypoplasia and massive pleural effusion, *Pediatr Radiol* 14:228-229, 1984.

92. Lyon RD, Adams HP: Mediastinal bronchogenic cyst: demonstration of a fluid-fluid level at MR imaging, *Radiology* 186:427-428, 1993.

93. MacMahon HE, Ruggieri J: Congenital segmental bronchomalacia, *Am J Dis Child* 118:923-926, 1969.

94. Madewell JE, Stoacker JT, Korsower JM: Cystic adenomatoid malformation of the lung: morphologic analysis, *AJR* 124:436-448, 1975.

95. Malone PS, Brain AJ, Kiely EM, et al: Congenital diaphragmatic defects that present late, *Arch Dis Child* 64:1542-1544, 1989.

96. Maltz DL, Nadas AS: Agenesis of the lung: presentation of eight new cases and review of the literature, *Pediatrics* 42:175-188, 1968.

97. Mangiulea VG, Stingha RV: The accessory cardiac bronchus: bronchologic aspect and review of the literature, *Dis Chest* 54:433-436, 1968.

98. Marin ML, Romney BM, Grimes MM, et al: Bronchogenic cyst: a case report emphasizing the role of magnetic resonance imaging, *J Thorac Imag* 6:43-46, 1991.

99. Markowitz RI, Mercurio MR, Vahjen GA, et al: Congenital lobar emphysema: the roles of CT and V/Q scan, *Clin Pediatr* 28:19-23, 1989.

100. Matzinger MA, Matzinger FR, Sachs HJ: Intrapulmonary bronchogenic cyst: spontaneous pneumothorax as the presenting symptom, *AJR* 158:987-988, 1992.

101. McCarten KM, Rosenberg HK, Borden S, et al: Delayed appearance of right diaphragmatic hernia associated with group B streptococcal pneumonia in neonates, *Pediatr Radiol* 139:385-389, 1981.

102. McClead RE, Graham M, Fletcher BD: Postnatal appearance of diaphragmatic hernia, *Am J Dis Child* 132:1137-1138, 1978.

103. Mendelson DS, Rose JS, Efremedis SC, et al: Bronchogenic cysts with high CT numbers, *AJR* 140:463-465, 1983.

104. Meng RL, Jensik RJ, Faber LP, et al: Bronchial atresia, *Ann Thorac Surg* 25:184-192, 1978.

105. Merenstein GB: Congenital cystic adenomatoid malformation: report of a case and review of the literature, *Am J Dis Child* 118:772-776, 1979.

106. Miller DC, Walter JP, Guthaner DF, et al: Recurrent mediastinal bronchogenic cyst: cause of bronchial obstruction and compression of superior vena cava and pulmonary artery, *Chest* 74:218-220, 1978.

107. Miller PA, Williamson BRJ, Minor GR, Buschi AJ: Pulmonary sequestration: visualization of the feeding artery by CT, *J Comput Assist Tomogr* 6:828-830, 1982.

108. Naidich DP, Rumanak WM, Ettenger NA, et al: Congenital anomalies of the lungs in adults: MR diagnosis, *AJR* 151:13-19, 1988.

109. Nakata H, Nakayama C, Komoto T, et al: Computed tomography of mediastinal bronchogenic cysts, *J Comput Assist Tomogr* 6:733-738, 1982.

110. Neill CA, Ferencz C, Sabiston DC, et al: The familial occurrence of hypoplastic right lung with systemic arterial supply and venous drainage: scimitar syndrome, *Bull Johns Hopkins Hosp* 107:1-21, 1960.

111. Noonan JA, Walters LR, Reeves JT: Congenital pulmonary lymphangiectasis, *Am J Dis Child* 120:314-319, 1970.

112. Ochsner JL, Ochsner SC: Congenital cysts of the mediastinum: 20 year experience with 42 cases, *Ann Surg* 163:909-920, 1966.

113. Padilla L, Orzel JA, Kruns MK: Congenital lobar emphysema: segmental lobar involvement demonstrated on ventilation perfusion imaging, *J Nucl Med* 26:1343-1344, 1985.

114. Page DV, Stocker JT: Anomalies associated with pulmonary hypoplasia, *Am Rev Respir Dis* 125:216-221, 1982.

115. Palmer WE, Rivitz SM, Chew FS: Bilateral bronchogenic cysts, *AJR* 157:950, 1991.

116. Pardes JG, Auk YH, Blomquist K, et al: CT diagnosis of congenital lobar emphysema, *J Comput Assist Tomogr* 7:1095-1097, 1983.

117. Pena SDJ, Shokeir MJK: Syndrome of campotodactyly, multiple anklyoses, facial anomalies and pulmonary hypoplasia: a lethal condition, *J Pediatr* 85:373, 1974.

118. Pinson CW, Harrison MW, Thornburg KL, et al: Importance of fetal fluid imbalance in congenital cystic adenomatoid malformation of the lung, *Am J Surg* 163:510-514, 1992.

119. Potter EL: Bilateral renal agenesis, *J Pediatr* 29:68-76, 1946.

120. Ramenofsky ML, Leape Ll, McCauley RGK: Bronchogenic cyst, *J Pediatr Surg* 14:219-224, 1979.

121. Rankin S, Faling LJ, Pugatch RD: CT diagnosis of pulmonary arteriovenous malformations, *J Comput Assist Tomogr* 6:746-749, 1982.

122. Reece EA, Lockwood CJ, Rizzo N, et al: Intrinsic intrathoracic malformations of the fetus: sonographic detection and clinical presentation, *Obstet Gynecol* 70:627-632, 1987.

123. Reed JC, Sobonya RE: Morphologic analysis of foregut cysts in the thorax, *AJR* 120:851-860, 1974.

124. Remy J, Remy-Jardin M, Wattine L, et al: Pulmonary arteriovenous malformations: evaluation with CT of the chest before and after treatment, *Radiology* 182:809-816, 1992.

125. Remy J, Smith M, Marache P, et al: La bronche "trachéale" gauche pathogene: revue de la literature à propos de 4 observations, *Radiol Electrol Med Nucl* 58:621-630, 1977.

126. Remy-Jardin M, Wattine L, Remy J: Transcatheter occlusion of pulmonary arterial circulation and collateral supply: failures, incidents, and complications, *Radiology* 180:699-705, 1991.

127. Ries T, Currarino G, Nikaido H, et al: Real-time ultrasonography of subcarinal bronchogenic cysts, *Radiology* 145:121-122, 1982.

128. Rogers LF, Osmer JC: Bronchogenic cyst: a review of 46 cases, *AJR* 91:273-283, 1964.

129. Rogge JD, Mishkin ME, Genovese PD: The familial occurrence of primary pulmonary hypertension, *Ann Intern Med* 65:672-684, 1966.

130. Roghair GD: Non operative management of lobar emphysema: long-term follow-up, *Radiology* 102:125-127, 1972.

131. Rosado-de-Christenson M, Stocker JT: Congenital cystic adenomatoid malformation, *Radiographics* 11:865-886, 1991.

132. Saifuddin A, Arthur RJ: Congenital diaphragmatic hernia — a review of pre and postoperative chest radiology, *Clin Radiol* 47:104-110, 1993.

133. Sane SM, Sieber WK, Girdany BR: Congenital bronchobiliary fistula, *Surgery* 69:599-608, 1971.

134. Schwartz DB, Beals TF, Wimbish KJ, et al: Transbronchial fine needle aspiration of bronchogenic cysts, *Chest* 88:573-575, 1985.

135. Sener RN, Tugran C, Savas R, et al: CT findings in scimitar syndrome, *AJR* 60:1361, 1993.

136. Smart LM, Hendry GMA: Imaging of neonatal pulmonary sequestration including Doppler ultrasound, *Br J Radiol* 64:324-329, 1991.

137. Sotelo-Avila C, Shanklin DR: Congenital malformations in an autopsy series, *Arch Pathol* 84:272-279, 1967.

138. Starshak RJ, Sty JR, Woods G, et al: Bridging bronchus: a rare airway anomaly, *Radiology* 140:95-96, 1981.

139. Stephens RW, Lingeman RE, Lawson LJ: Congenital tracheoesophageal fistulas in adults, *Ann Otol Rhino Laryngol* 85:613-617, 1976.

140. Stern E, Brill PW, Winchester P, et al: Imaging of prenatally detected intraabdominal extralobar pulmonary sequestration, *Clin Imag* 14:152-156, 1990.

141. Stern EJ, Webb RW, Warnock ML, et al: Bronchopulmonary sequestration: dynamic ultrafast high-resolution CT evidence of air trapping, *AJR* 157:947-949, 1991.

142. St-Georges R, Deslauriers J, Duranceau A: Clinical spectrum of bronchogenic cysts of the mediastinum and lung in the adult, *Ann Thorac Surg* 52:6-13, 1991.

143. Stiller RJ, Roberts NS, Weiner S, et al: Congenital diaphragmatic hernia: antenatal diagnosis and obstetrical management, *J Clin Ultrasound* 13:212-215, 1985.

144. Stocker JT, Madewell JE, Drake RM: Congenital cystic adenomatoid malformation, *Hum Pathol* 8:155-171, 1977.

145. Stocker JT, Drake RM, Madewell JE: Cystic and congenital lung disease in the newborn. In Rosenberg H, Bolande R, eds: *Perspectives in pediatric pathology*, vol 4, Chicago, 1978, Year Book, pp 93-154.

146. Stovin PGI: Congenital lobar emphysema, *Thorax* 14:254-261, 1959.

147. Stringer DA, Ein SH: Recurrent tracheoesophageal fistula: a protocol for investigation, *Radiology* 151:637-641, 1984.

148. Suen HC, Mathisen DJ, Grills HC, et al: Surgical management and radiological characteristics of bronchogenic cysts, *Ann Thorac Surg* 55:476-481, 1993.

149. Swischuk LE, Richardson CJ, Nichols MM, et al: Bilateral pulmonary hypoplasia in the neonate, *AJR* 133:1057-1063, 1979.

150. Takeda K, Kato N, Nakagawa T, et al: Horseshoe lung without respiratory distress, *Pediatr Radiol* 20:604, 1990.

151. Tapper D, Schuster S, McBride J, et al: Polyalveolar lobe: anatomic and physiologic parameters and their relationship to congenital lobar emphysema, *J Pediatr Surg* 15:931-937, 1980.

152. Tederlinic PJ, Sicilian LS, Brigelman W, et al: Congenital bronchial atresia: a report of 4 cases and a review of the literature, *Medicine* 65:73-83, 1986.

153. Thind CR, Pilling DW: Case report: pulmonary sequestration; the value of ultrasound, *Clin Radiol* 36:437-439, 1985.

154. Thomas CS, Leopold GR, Hilton S, et al: Fetal hydrops associated with extralobar pulmonary sequestration, *J Ultrasound Med* 5:668-671, 1986.

155. Thomas PS, Chrispin AR: Congenital tracheo-esophageal fistula without esophageal atresia, *Clin Radiol* 20:371-374, 1969.

156. Toyama WM: Esophageal atresia and tracheoesophageal fistula in association with bronchial and pulmonary anomalies, *J Pediatr Surg* 7:302-307, 1972.

157. Van Dyke JA, Sagel SS: Calcified pulmonary sequestration: CT demonstrations, *J Comput Assist Tomogr* 9:372-374, 1985.

158. Wagenaar SS, Scvierenga J, Wagenvoort CA: Late presentation of primary pulmonary lymphangiectasis, *Thorax* 33:791-795, 1978.

159. Walker J, Andmore RE: Respiratory problems and cystic adenomatoid malformations of the lung, *Arch Dis Child* 65:649-650, 1990.

160. Warfel KA, Schulz DM: Agenesis of the trachea: report of a case and review of the literature, *Arch Pathol Lab Med* 100:357-359, 1976.

161. Waterston DJ, Carter REB, Aberdeen E: Oesophageal atresia, tracheooesophageal fistula: a study of survival in 218 infants, *Lancet* 1:819-822, 1961.

162. Watts WJ, Rotman HH, Patten GA: Pulmonary artery compression by a bronchogenic cyst simulating congenital pulmonary artery stenosis, *Am J Cardiol* 53:347-349, 1984.

163. Wayne ER, Campbell JB, Burrington JD, et al: Eventration of the diaphragm, *J Pediatr Surg* 9:643-651, 1974.

164. Weichert RF, Lindsey ES, Pearce CW, et al: Bronchogenic cyst with unilateral obstructive emphysema, *J Thorac Cardiovasc Surg* 59:287-291, 1970.

165. Weiner C, Varner M, Pringle K, et al: Case reports: antenatal diagnosis and palliative treatment of non-immune hydrops fetalis secondary to pulmonary extralobar sequestration, *Obstet Gynecol* 68:275-280, 1986.

166. Wexler HA, Dapena MV: Congenital cystic adenomatoid malformation: a report of three unusual cases, *Radiology* 126:737-741, 1978.

167. White JJ, Suzuki H: Hernia through the foramen of Bochdalek: a misnomer, *J Pediatr Surg* 7:60-61, 1972.

168. White RI, Lynch-Nyhan A, Terry P, et al: Pulmonary arteriovenous malformations: techniques and long-term outcome of embolotherapy, *Radiology* 169:663-669, 1988.

169. Whyte MKB, Dollery CT, Adam A, et al: Central bronchogenic cyst: treatment by extrapleural percutaneous aspiration, *Br Med J* 29:1457-1458, 1989.

170. Wittenborg MH, Gyepes MT, Crocker D: Tracheal dynamics in infants with respiratory distress, stridor and collapsing trachea, *Radiology* 88:653-662, 1967.

171. Woodring JH, Vandeviere HM, Dillon MJ: Air-filled, multilocular bronchiopulmonary foregut duplication cyst of the mediastinum: unusual computed tomography appearance, *Clin Imag* 13:44-47, 1989.

172. Worsnop CJ, Teichtahl H, Clarke CP: Bronchogenic cyst: a cause of pulmonary artery obstruction and breathlessness, *Ann Thorac Surg* 55:1254-1255, 1993.

173. Yeager BA, Guglielmi GE, Schiebler ML, et al: Magnetic resonance imaging of Morgagni hernia, *Gastrointest Radiol* 12:296-298, 1987.

174. Yernault JC, Kahn G, Dumortier P, et al: "Solid" mediastinal bronchogenic cyst: mineralogic analysis, *AJR* 146:73-74, 1986.

175. Yuan A, Yang PC, Chang DB, et al: Lung sequestration: diagnosis with ultrasound and triplex Doppler technique in an adult, *Chest* 102:1880-1881, 1992.

15 Pleura and Pleural Disorders

ALAN G. WILSON

PLEURAL ANATOMY

The pleural space is lined by a smooth serosal membrane of mesodermal origin and is lubricated by a small amount of fluid, which allows the lungs to change shape easily and provides low-friction mechanical coupling between the lungs and the chest wall. The visceral and parietal pleura is lined by a single layer of flat, and in part cuboidal, mesothelial cells. In the parietal pleura these mesothelial cells lie on loose, fat-containing, areolar connective tissue bounded externally by the endothoracic fascia.[133] In the visceral pleura five layers can be defined[240,349,680]: (1) a mesothelial layer; (2) a thin layer of connective tissue; (3) a strong layer of connective tissue — the chief layer; (4) a vascular layer; and (5) the limiting lung membrane, which is connected by collagen and elastic fibers to the chief layer.[349] The blood supply of

641

the parietal pleura is from systemic vessels, while the visceral pleura is supplied by both the pulmonary and bronchial circulation.[240,349] Both the parietal and the visceral pleura is supplied by lymphatics, but only parietal lymphatics communicate with the pleural space. Communication is by way of 2 to 12 μm stomata that lie over lacunae in the parietal lymphatics. Fluid, protein, and cells leave the pleural space by these stomata, which are confined to the low costal and mediastinal pleura and diaphragm.[240,559] Intercostal sensory nerves supply the pleura of the costal surface and peripheral diaphragm, and the phrenic nerve is sensory to the central diaphragm.[240] The visceral pleura lacks sensory nerves.

Pleural cavity and costal pleura

The parietal and visceral pleurae, which enclose the pleural cavity, are continuous with each other at the hilum of the lung and along the (inferior) pulmonary ligament. Inferiorly the parietal pleura is tucked into the costophrenic sulcus. The disposition of the sulcus helps to explain some of the radiologic findings in pleural disease and is important in upper abdominal interventional procedures. On the surface of the body the inferior edge of the sulcus crosses the xiphoid and eighth costochondral junction to reach the midaxillary line at the level of the tenth rib.[449,454] It then passes horizontally across the eleventh and twelfth ribs to reach the first lumbar vertebral body. The cephalad part of the sulcus is occupied to a variable extent by lung, whereas caudally the sulcus is empty and the diaphragm and chest wall are separated only by the two layers of the visceral pleura. The distance between the lowest part of the sulcus and the lung edge depends on the phase of respiration and the segment of sulcus being considered. The right intercostal midaxillary approach is often used for percutaneous introduction of needles into the upper abdomen, and because the pleural reflection reaches the tenth rib in this region, it would be usual for the pleura to be punctured, for example, during percutaneous transhepatic cholangiography or biliary drainage.[449,454] Somewhat surprisingly the complication rate of these procedures is low. In fine-needle transhepatic cholangiography, for example, only two pneumothoraces were recorded in 2005 procedures.[234] This low complication rate is undoubtedly because the lung rarely occupies the depth of the sulcus, except possibly in young patients taking a maximum inspiration. Bilious pleural effusion with liver biopsy is also rare.[489] The complications are more serious and frequent when drainage catheters pass through the pleural cavity because abdominal fluid collections and pus may then flow into the pleural space.[454]

The normal pleura cannot be imaged as such by computed tomography (CT) or high-resolution CT (HRCT) because it cannot be separated from adjacent structures at the lung–chest wall interface. The appearances of this interface on HRCT have been reported in detail by Im and co-workers,[271] and the following section

is based on their paper. Most of their findings can also be recognized on conventional (10 mm collimation) CT. In normal subjects examined by HRCT, at the lung–chest wall interface overlying an intercostal space there is a linear opacity of soft tissue density, 1 to 2 mm thick, connecting the inner aspects of the ribs (Figures 15-1 and 15-2). This opacity (the intercostal stripe) is produced by two layers of pleura, extrapleural fat, the endothoracic fascia, and the innermost intercostal muscle. It is marginated by air in the lung and by fat lying between the innermost and internal intercostal muscles. The intercostal stripe disappears on the inner aspect of ribs, since at this point it generally consists only of pleura, extrapleural fat, and endothoracic fascia, which are too thin to resolve. A linear soft tissue opacity on the inside of a rib is usually abnormal. However, in some circumstances such a finding may be normal:

1. Posteriorly, when ribs are parallel to the scan plane and sectioned toward their tapering edge. In this circumstance the intercostal stripe is projected on the inner aspect of the rib (Figure 15-2). The narrowness of the adjacent rib and the continuity of the stripe with that in adjacent intercostal spaces distinguish this finding from pathologic pleural thickening.

2. When there is significant fat between the parietal pleura and endothoracic fascia. This characteristically occurs laterally at the level of the fourth to eighth ribs and may not be appreciated on scans imaged on mediastinal settings, only becoming apparent with extended window widths (2000 HU). These findings are clarified and distinguished from pleural thickening by changing windowing parameters.

3. Low in the parasternal and paravertebral region. In these sites poorly developed muscle slips (anteriorly the sternocostal muscle and posteriorly the subcostal muscle) lie on the inside of the ribs, producing linear, soft tissue opacities 1 to 2 mm thick (Figure 15-1). The sternocostal muscle is commonly identified, but the subcostal muscle is seen less often — in 16% of examinations (Figure 15-3). These muscles are distinguished from pleural thickening by being smooth, uniform, and bilateral.

Paravertebrally, intercostal muscles are absent and the lung–soft tissue interface is formed by a very thin line produced by two layers of pleura and the endothoracic fascia (Figures 15-1 and 15-3). Linear soft tissue opacities 2 to 3 mm thick lying immediately underneath this interface are produced by intercostal veins, which can be positively identified when they join the azygos or hemiazygos vein.

Fissures and junctional lines

On a plain chest radiograph the pleura cannot be seen except where the visceral pleura invaginates into the lung to form the fissures and where the two lungs contact each other at junctional lines (see p. 40). Fissures are of two sorts: standard and accessory.

STANDARD FISSURES. Standard fissures consist of a

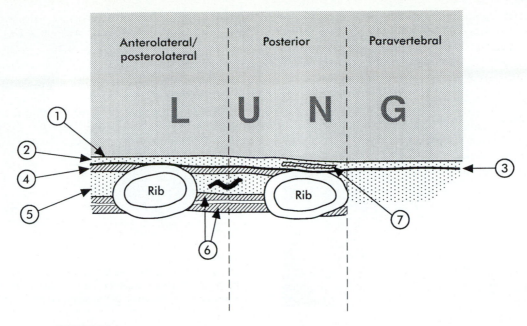

FIGURE 15-1
Diagramatic anatomy of lung–chest wall interface. Component layers vary in different segments. Anatomically identifiable layers (as illustrated) are not necessarily separately demonstrated on images and consist of (1) parietal and visceral pleura, which is too thin to image; (2) subpleural fat, which may be absent or if present is of variable thickness; (3) endothoracic fascia; (4) innermost intercostal muscle (3 and 4 appear as one structure on images); (5) intercostal fat and intercostal vessels; (6) internal and external intercostal muscles; and (7) subcostal muscle (anteriorly the transverse thoracic muscle).

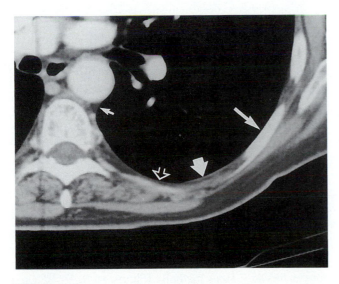

FIGURE 15-2
Lung–chest wall interface on computed tomography at 10 mm collimation. Joining inner rib margins is a soft tissue layer made up of pleura, endothoracic fascia, and innermost intercostal muscle *(broad arrow)*. It lies on intercostal fat, outside which are internal and external intercostal muscles. No soft tissue is seen inside ribs *(large arrow)* except where the thinner rib margin is sectioned *(open arrow)*. Paravertebral interface is marginated by a thin or invisible line *(small arrow)*, adjacent to which it is "thickened" by a posterior intercostal vein draining into hemiazygos vein.

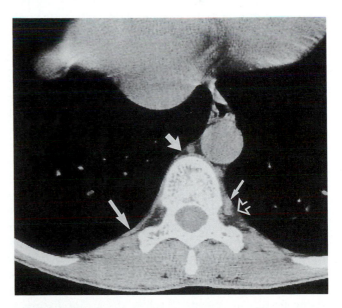

FIGURE 15-3
Lung–chest wall interface in paravertebral region on high-resolution computed tomography. Normal interface is marginated by layer that is undetectable *(open arrow)* or very thin *(broad arrow)*. Soft tissue density on left *(small arrow)* is a posterior intercostal vein. That on right *(large arrow)* is probably also venous but at this low level in the chest could be caused by subcostal muscle.

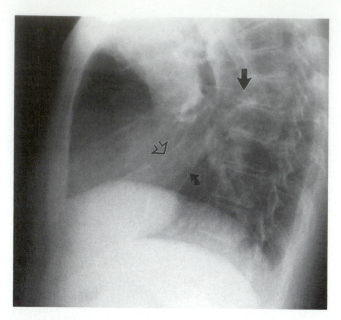

FIGURE 15-4
Major fissures. As is often the case, only lower halves of these major fissures are detectable. Right fissure *(open arrow)* is more oblique than left *(curved arrow)* and more anterior. Both fissures end up making contact with ipsilateral diaphragm 4 to 6 cm behind sternum. Posterior end of minor fissure *(straight arrow)* appears to cross general line of major fissures because the imaged structures are in different planes.

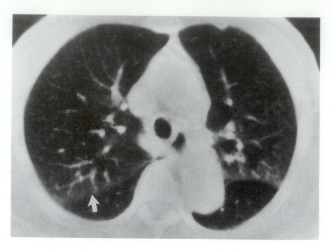

FIGURE 15-5
Upper part of major fissures shown as band opacities on computed tomography. That on right *(arrow)* is concave forward, the usual configuration at this level; left is atypical and convex forward.

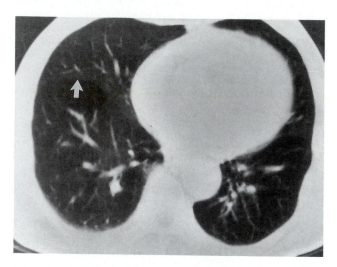

FIGURE 15-6
Inferior part of right oblique fissure. This is demonstrated on computed tomography as band opacity that is convex forward *(arrow)*.

double layer of infolded visceral pleura. They are normally very thin and are seen on plain radiographs only when they are tangential to the x-ray beam, appearing as a hairline of soft tissue density. Many fissures are incomplete and fail to extend all the way to the hilum. They are often partially hidden by ribs. As a result of these factors it is uncommon to see complete fissures on either frontal or lateral radiographs. There are two standard fissures: major and minor.

Major fissure. The major fissure, also called the oblique or greater fissure, separates the upper lobe from the lower lobe on the left and the upper and middle lobes from the lower lobe on the right. On plain chest radiographs the major fissures are most clearly seen on lateral projection (Figure 15-4). In Proto and Speckman's study of plain lateral radiographs, a part of a right fissure was seen in 22% of the images, a part of the left fissure was seen in 14%, and part of a major fissure of indeterminate side was seen in 62%; in only 2% of radiographs was a complete major fissure identified.[499] When the major fissure is incompletely seen, it is almost always the lower portion that is detected (Figure 15-4).

The right fissure is wider and shorter than the left and has a greater overall area.[505] Both fissures face forward and pass obliquely downward, parallel to the fifth rib, from about the body of the fifth thoracic vertebra, to meet the diaphragm several centimeters behind the sternum (Figure 15-4).[161] Neither fissure is flat; both are mildly

twisted in the middle, a configuration that has been likened to a propeller. The twist is such that the upper half, which is commonly concave forward (Figure 15-5), faces outward, while the lower half, which is usually convex forward, faces medially (Figure 15-6).[496,499] On a radiograph the fissure is detected where it becomes tangential to the x-ray beam. This means that generally on a lateral chest radiograph the caudad portion of the oblique fissure lies along the anterior edge of the lower lobe, whereas the cephalad portion is projected over the body of the lower lobe (Figure 15-7). Normal undulations in the oblique fissure can lead to the following misinterpretations on the *lateral* chest radiograph[499]:

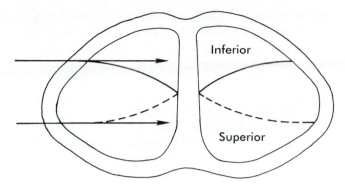

FIGURE 15-7
Major fissure. Diagram of computed tomography scan, oriented in conventional way, shows common configuration of major fissure in its upper half ("superior") and lower half ("inferior"). Upper segment is concave, facing forward and laterally, and lower is convex, facing forward and medially. Lateral x-ray beam *(long arrows)* is tangential to anterior aspect of lower part of fissure and to posterior aspect of upper part of fissure.

1. Because the lateral aspect of the minor fissure extends more posteriorly than the medial aspect of the right major fissure, the two can appear to cross in lateral view (Figure 15-4). This appearance can lead to problems in identifying the right major fissure and can also lead to mistaken identification of the posterior aspect of the minor fissure as a superior accessory fissure. Confusion between minor fissure and superior accessory fissure can be avoided if it is realized that the minor fissure usually ends before the vertebral bodies. Furthermore, the superior accessory fissure cannot appear to be continuous with the minor fissure because the fissures have to straddle the origins of the middle lobe and apical lower bronchi,[499] which arise at essentially the same level.

2. If because of undulations the medial aspect of the major fissure is visualized in the lower zone rather than the more usual lateral aspect, the apparent backward shift of the fissure may be erroneously interpreted as indicating volume loss in the lower lobe.

3. If lesions are close to but do not abut a major fissure, they cannot be localized with certainty to a particular lobe. CT, particularly HRCT, resolves this type of problem.

Fissures are commonly incomplete, failing to extend to the hilum or mediastinum,[237] and in these regions there is parenchymal fusion between lobes, often over quite a large area. The frequency of incomplete fissures in different series has ranged from 12.5% to 73% for the major fissure[505] and from 60% to 90% for the minor fissure.[237,294,405,725] An incomplete fissure allows pathologic processes such as pneumonia to spread easily from one lobe to another and also allows collateral air drift, so that even with complete large airway obstruction no atelectasis may occur.[255,573]

Distinguishing the left from the right major fissure on a lateral chest radiograph is sometimes useful (Figure

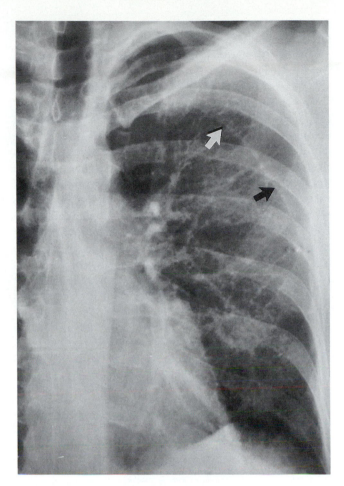

FIGURE 15-8
Superolateral major fissure. This curvilinear opacity *(arrows)* marks line along which major fissure contacts posterior chest wall.

15-4). The most helpful points are that the right fissure is more oblique, ends farther forward inferiorly, merges with the right hemidiaphragm, and joins with the minor fissure.

The major fissure is not usually seen on a frontal radiograph, but it may be detected under three circumstances. First, the upper edge where it contacts the posterior chest wall may become visible when extrapleural fat enters the lips of the fissure.[495] This generates the "superolateral major fissure" (Figure 15-8), a curved line or stripe that starts medially above the hilum and curves downward and laterally, concave to the mediastinum.[495] Second, the upper aspect of the major fissure can become tangential to the frontal x-ray beam, generating a hairline opacity that runs obliquely across the midzone (Figure 15-9). Medially this fissure line often crosses the hilum to end against the spine, allowing it to be distinguished from the minor fissure, which never crosses hilar vessels. This part of the major fissure becomes tangential to the frontal x-ray beam with lordotic projections and because of undulations in the fissure or volume loss of the lower lobe,[169] particularly the apical segment. Third, reorientation of the lateral aspect of the lower part of the oblique fissure probably accounts for the vertical fissure,[110,181,691] a vertical hairline seen particularly on the right, low and toward the chest wall. It is most often described in babies with lower lobe volume loss and cardiomegaly.[110]

The major fissure can be identified on standard CT sections in about 80% to 100% of patients.[201,496] The most common appearance, present in some 80% of cases, is a curvilinear avascular band (Figure 15-10) extending from the hilum to the chest wall, reflecting the lack of vessels in the subcortical zone of the lung.[184,212,383] In about 10% of cases the major fissure, particularly in the upper third, is seen as a curvilinear line or band density (Figures 15-5 and 15-6).[496] Low-level, narrow window settings promote this appearance. The upper part of the fissure is more easily detected with CT scanning, whereas the reverse is true of plain radiography. The left fissure is the longer; it is seen one or two sections higher than the right.[496] In about one fifth of patients supradiaphragmatic fat invaginates into the lower end of the major fissure and is detectable at CT scanning.[188]

On HRCT studies the major fissure appears as a dense line or much less commonly as a dense band (Figure 15-11). Imaging performed with a 25-degree cranial tilt of the scan section brings the imaging plane more nearly at right angles to the major fissure, increasing the probability that the fissure will be imaged as a line rather than as a band.[561] When fissures are imaged as lines, incomplete segments are commonly identified. In one study major fissures were incomplete on the left in 52% and on the right in 64%.[201] Incomplete segments of fissure were located medially and remote from the lung base.[201] Small

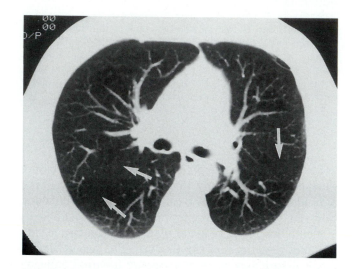

FIGURE 15-10
Oblique fissures on conventional computed tomography. Upper segments of both fissures are identified as broad avascular bands. Left lower lobe is longer than right and therefore the left fissure "leads" the right in upper part of chest.

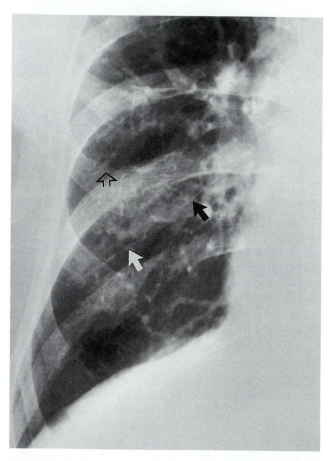

FIGURE 15-9
Major fissure on frontal radiograph. Reoriented major fissure *(closed arrows)* is visible on frontal radiograph as oblique line. It can be distinguished from minor fissure *(open arrow)* because it passes more medially, overlying right hilum and ending at spine.

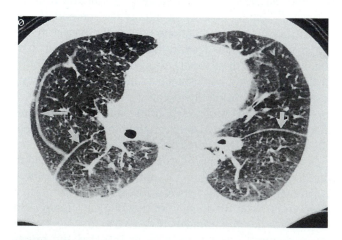

FIGURE 15-11
Fissures on high-resolution computed tomography (HRCT). On HRCT, fissures usually appear as dense lines or bands. Both major fissures *(broad arrows)* appear intact at this level. Lateral aspect of dome-shaped minor fissure *(long arrows)* has been sectioned, giving characteristic curvilinear opacity enclosing middle lobe with marginating tongue of upper lobe laterally. In this subject, most cephalad part of middle lobe is posteromedial, which is most common pattern.

bronchovascular structures, particularly veins, have been shown on HRCT to cross fissural defects.[476] Occasionally the major fissure on HRCT appears as two parallel lines because of motion artifact (Figure 15-12).[392] Movement is often cardiac in origin, and because of this, double fissures are commonly seen at the left base.

Minor fissure. The minor fissure separates the anterior segment of the right upper lobe from the right middle lobe, and because of its orientation it is seen on both frontal and lateral chest radiographs (Figures 15-4 and 15-13). It lies approximately horizontally on the right side

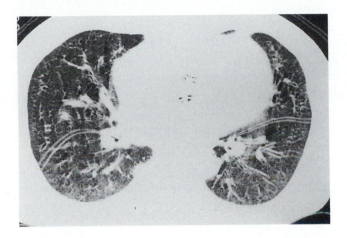

FIGURE 15-12
Major fissures — movement artifact. Major fissures (and also vessels) appear doubled in this high-resolution computed tomography scan because of lung movement during exposure. This example is so gross that misinterpretation of doubled structures is unlikely, but confusion between doubled vessels and bronchiectasis is possible when movement is less obvious.

at the level of the anterior fourth rib or interspace (Figure 15-13).[161] On frontal chest radiographs some or all of the fissure is seen in about 50% to 60% of patients.[161] The whole fissure is seen in only 7% of individuals, and when just a segment is seen, it is much more commonly the lateral portion than the medial. Felson[161] pointed out that on a frontal chest radiograph the fissure ends medially at the interlobar pulmonary artery within about 1 cm of the point at which the superior venous trunk crosses (Figure 15-13). This observation can be helpful in finding and identifying the fissure. Sometimes the upper lobe has a tonguelike projection on the inner aspect of the middle lobe, and in these circumstances part of the minor fissure becomes reoriented into a vertical and sagittal plane. This is visible on a frontal chest radiograph as a curvilinear hairline extending upward and outward from the region of the right cardiophrenic angle to join the horizontal part of the minor fissure.[223] On a lateral view (Figure 15-4) the minor fissure is seen in about half of the radiographs: in part in 44% and in toto in 6%.[499]

The upper surface of the middle lobe is either convex or, infrequently, flat, and the anterior and lateral aspects of the minor fissure commonly curve downward in a caudad direction. Because of undulations the minor fissure sometimes appears sigmoid or double.

Felson[161] has related the position of the minor fissure to the anterior ribs in order to assess pathologic displacement. He found that 67% of minor fissures were on a level with the fourth anterior interspace, with 15% above and 18% below. Two percent were above the anterior third rib, and 3% were below the anterior sixth rib. He thought that the variation was so great that, for diagnosis of pathologic shift, displacement had to be striking or the shape and direction of the fissure had to be altered.

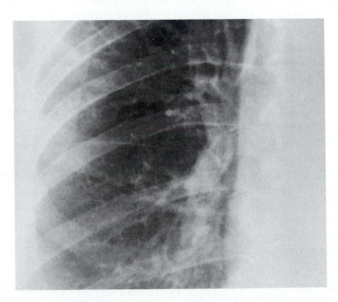

FIGURE 15-13
Minor fissure. Minor fissure stops medially at lateral margin of interlobar pulmonary artery at point about 1 cm beyond Y-point of hilum where artery and vein cross. This is a useful identifying feature of minor fissure.

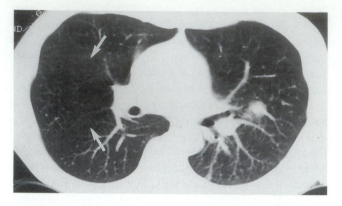

FIGURE 15-14
Minor fissure. On computed tomography, minor fissure gives rise to approximately triangular or oval avascular area *(arrows),* in front of major fissure and at level midway between right upper and middle lobar airways. Nodule in left midzone was carcinoma.

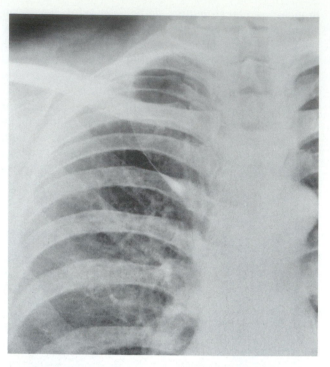

FIGURE 15-15
Azygos fissure. Plain radiograph of right upper zone, demonstrating hairline azygos fissure ending medially in teardrop of azygos vein.

On CT the minor fissure is manifest as an avascular zone extending from the major fissure to the chest wall (Figure 15-14). The avascular area is triangular or occasionally round or oval.[184,212,383] It is usually best seen on a single section midway between the origins of the upper and middle lobe bronchi. The overall detection rate in one series was 52%.[496]

With HRCT the typical upwardly convex configuration of the lesser fissure usually becomes apparent. In such studies the minor fissure is seen as a high-density curvilinear opacity usually forming a quarter or half circle (Figure 15-11).[39] The fissure is characteristically one to a few millimeters thick, but with decreasing slice thickness and reducing fissure angle with respect to the transaxial plane it becomes thicker (up to 15 mm)[39] and may form an oval opacity if the section passes through the apex of the dome-shaped fissure.[185] Berkmen and co-workers[39] distinguished four types of fissural configuration, characterized by the position of the highest portion of the fissure, which was predominantly posterior (81%) and medial (84%). Adjacent sections clarify the anatomy in atypical configurations, and the usefulness of the inferior tributary of the anterior segmental vein of the upper lobe (V^3b) in identifying the upper lobe has been stressed.[39] The relationship of subsegmental bronchi to their corresponding arteries can also be used to differentiate between the anterior segment of the upper lobe (airways lateral to artery) and the middle lobe (airways medial to artery).[475] In the series of Berkmen and co-workers[39] 30% of minor fissures were absent and 58% were incomplete as assessed by HRCT.

ACCESSORY FISSURES. Accessory fissures are clefts of varying depth in the outer surface of the lung that delineate accessory lobes. Six important accessory fissures are recognized, and one or more of these are commonly present. In a CT study of 50 patients, 22% had some form of accessory fissure.[207] Accessory fissures are important to recognize for the following reasons: to avoid their misinterpretation as pathologic structures such as bullae, scars, or pneumothorax[207]; to avoid incorrect localization of an intrapulmonary lesion; because they give consolidation a sharp margin so that the resulting opacity may be misinterpreted as atelectasis, consolidation of a whole lobe, or mediastinal mass[207]; and because of the atypical appearance of a pneumothorax in the presence of an azygos fissure.[697]

Azygos fissure. The azygos fissure is the best known accessory fissure, with a prevalence of 0.4% to 1% in various clinical and postmortem series.[613] Evidence suggests a male predominance,[170] and a familial occurrence has been described.[493] The azygos fissure produces a hairline curvilinear opacity, concave to the mediastinum, that extends obliquely across the right upper zone (Figure 15-15). It originates peripherally, where a small triangle of soft tissue density (trigonum parietale) may be present. The fissure ends medially in the teardrop of the displaced azygos vein above and to the right of the vein's normal location in the angle between trachea and right mainstem bronchus.

The segment of lung marginated by the fissure is the azygos lobe, which is not a true segment because it does not have a specific bronchial supply. Airways are derived from the apical or posterior segments of the right upper lobe.[50] The position of the trigonum in relation to the lung apex has been used to define three sizes of azygos

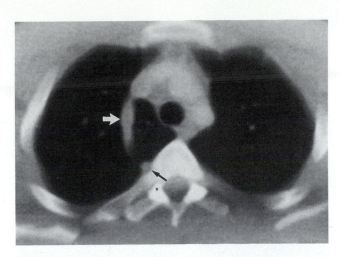

FIGURE 15-16
Azygos fissure. Computed tomography scan at level of lower trachea shows C-shaped band of displaced azygos venous arch *(white arrow)*. Note lateral displacement of ascending azygos vein *(black arrow)*, which must be distinguished from lung or pleural nodule.

lobe: type A (lateral to apex), type B (apical), and type C (medial to apex).[50] Occasionally the azygos lobe appears unduly opaque, and in one series this was found in 7 of 53 azygos lobes on plain chest radiography. In the majority (6 of 7) the increased opacity was due to overlap of tortuous supraaortic vessels.[69] Sometimes on the frontal chest radiograph a broad, somewhat vertical, bandlike apical opacity is seen passing down toward the azygos vein. This has been shown on CT to be the right brachiocephalic vein that has adopted an extramediastinal course, lying in the anterior part of the azygos fissure.[389] The main differential diagnoses of an azygos fissure are scars, bullae, a displaced minor fissure, and a supernumerary fissure such as may be associated with a tracheal bronchus.[388] On lateral view the azygos arch may be seen as a curvilinear band, situated higher than normal. In addition, the invagination of lung into the mediastinum, which is well demonstrated on CT (Figure 15-16), outlines the posterior wall of the superior vena cava.

The azygos fissure supports the azygos vein in a sling and is therefore sometimes called the mesoazygos. Unlike all other fissures it consists of four layers of pleura: two visceral and two parietal. These four layers are present because the precursor of the azygos vein, the right posterior cardinal vein, initially lies lateral to the lung and, instead of migrating over the lung apex, pushes through the upper lobe, taking both the visceral and the parietal pleura with it.[613] On CT (Figure 15-16) the azygos vein lies 2 to 4 cm higher than usual, forming a C-shaped band coursing through the lung.[613] The lung invaginates itself into the mediastinum, coming to lie behind the superior vena cava and sometimes the trachea (Figure 15-16). The azygos arch ends anteriorly at the junction of the right brachiocephalic vein and the supe-

rior vena cava. The cephalic part of the azygos vein as it runs upward in a paravertebral position courses more laterally than usual and can be mistaken for a lung nodule or subpleural mass on CT (Figure 15-16).[498] Below the carina the azygos vein returns to its usual prevertebral position.[613] Above the azygos arch the fissure is seen as a thin curvilinear line, its exact shape depending on the size of the lobe. On HRCT, caudal continuation of the fissure has been demonstrated below the azygos arch, the fissure becoming shorter and ending against the mediastinum in relation to the azygos vein.[389]

A left "azygos" fissure is rare[335,701] and most commonly involves the hemiazygos and left superior intercostal veins in an analogous way to the azygos vein on the right.[636] CT findings have been reported.[636]

Inferior accessory fissure. The inferior accessory fissure usually incompletely separates the medial basal segment from the rest of the lower lobe. Because this segment lies anteromedially in the lower lobe, the accessory fissure has components that are oriented both sagittally and coronally. As a result, parts of the fissure are tangential to frontal and lateral x-ray beams. Despite this the fissure is rarely seen on lateral radiographs. The frequency of occurrence is difficult to ascertain because the fissure varies greatly in depth and in its prominence from one examination to the next.[207] The reported prevalence also depends on the method of detection. The fissure is present in 30% to 50% of anatomic specimens,[161] in 16% of CT scans,[207] and in 5% to 10% of plain radiographs.[161,207,528]

On the frontal radiograph the fissure is a hairline that arises from the medial aspect of the hemidiaphragm and ascends obliquely toward the hilum (Figure 15-17). Sometimes there is a small triangular peak at its diaphragmatic end, and this, with a very short fissure line, may be all that is seen.[207] At the other extreme the fissure may be long, reaching all the way to the hilum.[161] Although the left lower lobe lacks a separate medial basal segment, the anteromedial basal bronchus divides early into two components analogous to the medial and anterior segmental bronchi on the right,[207] and an inferior accessory fissure is about as common on the left as the right. However, it is not detected with equal frequency on radiologic examination; in one series of 500 radiographs 80% of inferior accessory fissures were right sided, 12% left sided, and 7% bilateral.[528] On the lateral radiograph the inferior accessory fissure is occasionally seen as a vertical line, often associated with a diaphragmatic peak in the region of the esophagus.[207] The pulmonary ligament is close to the medial portion of the inferior accessory fissure, and some diaphragmatic peaks on the lateral radiograph in this region are really due to the inferior pulmonary ligament and its septum. On CT scans the fissure appears on sections near the diaphragm as an arc, concave to the mediastinum, extending from the major fissure back to the mediastinum near the esophagus. It is best demonstrated on HRCT.[207]

Should the inferior accessory fissure marginate a

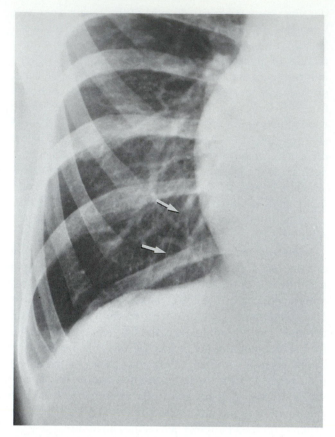

FIGURE 15-17
Inferior accessory fissure *(arrows).* This fissure separates medial basal segment from rest of lower lobe.

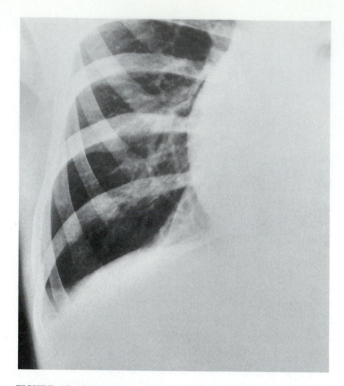

FIGURE 15-18
Inferior accessory fissure. Same patient as in Figure 15-17. Consolidation in medial basal segment of right lower lobe is sharply demarcated laterally by inferior accessory fissure. (Courtesy Dr. C.J. Dow, London.)

pneumonia in the medial basal segment, the triangular opacity has a sharp outer border (Figure 15-18),[652] which may mimic a collapsed lower lobe. Other lesions such as pleural effusion, mediastinal mass, hernia, or fat pad may be simulated.[207] Occasionally the appearance is reversed (Figure 15-19).

Superior accessory fissure. The superior accessory fissure separates the apical segment of a lower lobe from the basal segments and superficially resembles a minor fissure on a frontal radiograph. It was identified on 6% of lateral radiographs in one series,[499] a figure that seems high when judged by general experience. The minor fissure lies above the middle lobe bronchus, and the superior accessory fissure lies below the apical lower bronchus. Because both of these airways arise at approximately the same level, the superior accessory fissure is projected below the minor fissure on frontal radiographs (Figure 15-20). On the lateral view it differs from the minor fissure in that it extends backward across the vertebral bodies (Figure 15-21).[499] On CT, like the minor fissure, it appears as an avascular area, which should be distinguished from downward angulation of the upper end of the major fissure, a distinction that depends on identification of the apical lower bronchus.[207]

Left minor fissure. The left minor fissure is present in 8% to 18% of people but is only rarely detected on posteroanterior and lateral radiographs, with a reported frequency of 1.6%.[16] It separates the lingula from the rest of the left upper lobe and is analogous to the minor fissure. It is usually arched and located more cephalad than the minor fissure. It slopes medially and downward (Figure 15-22).

(INFERIOR) PULMONARY LIGAMENT. The pulmonary ligament is a double sheet of pleura that hangs down from the hilum like a curtain and joins the lung to the mediastinum and to the medial part of the diaphragm.[508] The two layers of pleura contact each other below the inferior pulmonary vein and end in a free border that usually lies over the inner third of the hemidiaphragm but is sometimes displaced toward the hilum. The right ligament is short and wide based and is related on its mediastinal aspect to the azygos vein. On the left the ligament is longer and attaches to the mediastinum close to the esophagus and anterior to the aorta (Figure 15-23).[508] The ligament overlies a septum within the lung that separates posterior and medial basal segments.[208] The bare area of the ligament contains connective tissue, bronchial veins, lymphatics, and nodes.[178]

The ligament is not visible on chest radiographs. On CT the "ligament" is visible in about 50% to 75% of patients (Figure 15-23).[97,208,545] It is best detected just above the

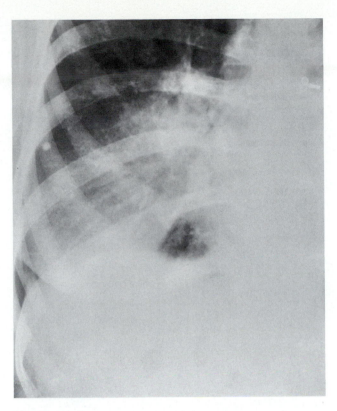

FIGURE 15-19
Inferior accessory fissure. The exudate of right lower lobe consolidation has been excluded from medial basal segment by inferior accessory fissure. (Courtesy Dr. C.J. Dow, London.)

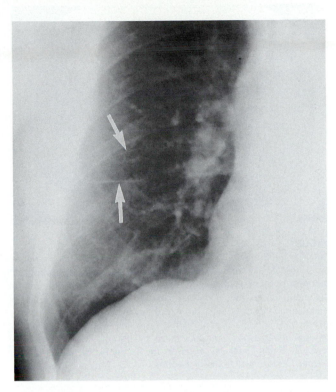

FIGURE 15-20
Superior accessory fissure. Superior accessory fissure *(lower arrow)* is projected below minor fissure *(upper arrow)* on posteroanterior chest radiograph. In this example, lateral aspect of minor fissure slopes downward, a normal finding when of this degree.

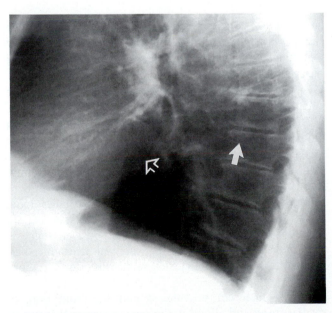

FIGURE 15-21
Superior accessory fissure (same patient as in Figure 15-20). On lateral view, superior accessory fissure *(closed arrows)* passes posteriorly from right major fissure *(open arrows)*, separating apical segment from rest of lower lobe.

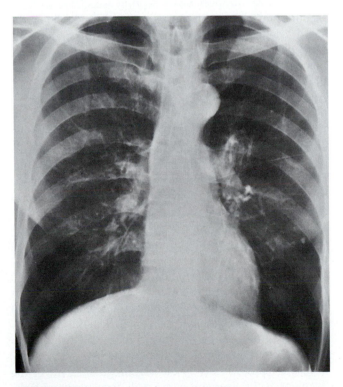

FIGURE 15-22
Left minor fissure. This separates lingula from rest of left upper lobe. It characteristically slopes downward and medially.

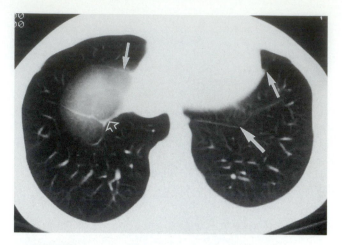

FIGURE 15-23
Inferior pulmonary ligament. Conventional computed tomography scan just above diaphragm shows septum associated with left inferior pulmonary ligament *(large arrow)*. Mediastinal end of ligament is marked by small triangular elevation at level of esophagus. On right side, branching linear structure *(open arrow)* arises from lateral aspect of inferior vena cava. It is too anterior to be pulmonary ligament and is caused by phrenic nerve or phrenic vessels. Small bilateral anterior mediastinal projections *(small arrows)* are related to major fissures.

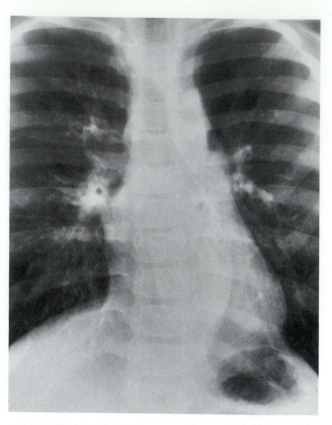

FIGURE 15-24
Convex paravertebral opacity is result of collapse of left lower lobe. This atypical appearance probably results from underdevelopment of pulmonary ligament, with resultant lack of tethering of lower lobe to diaphragm. Disposition of left mainstem bronchus and air bronchogram within opacity indicate correct diagnosis.

diaphragm[545] as a thin curvilinear line passing outward and slightly backward from the mediastinum at the level of the esophagus. There is strong evidence that this line represents an intrapulmonary septum associated with the ligament rather than the ligament itself.[41,208,660] Often a small, triangular elevation is present at the mediastinal base of the ligament. The linear opacity produced by the ligament should be distinguished from that produced by the phrenic nerve and pericardiophrenic vessels, which commonly branch and which arise more anteriorly, [639] at the level of the inferior vena cava on the right (Figure 15-23).[40] Some workers also using CT and cadaver-derived data consider that the latter structure is not the phrenic nerve or pericardiophrenic vessels but the inferior phrenic artery and vein.[660] The pulmonary ligament as identified by CT may appear thickened with asbestos exposure and with fat or fluid infiltration.[508]

The ligament and variations in its degree of development have been considered important for the following reasons:

1. The ligament determines the shape of a collapsed lower lobe[509] because the lobe, as it loses volume, folds backward, hinged along the line of the fixed mediastinal attachment of the ligament. In frontal view the characteristic triangular shape of lower lobe collapse occurs because the inferior part of the lobe is being held away from the mediastinum by the diaphragmatic part of the ligament. If the ligament is not well developed and lacks a diaphragmatic attachment, the whole lower lobe collapses against the mediastinum, resulting in an oval

paravertebral opacity (Figure 15-24).[508] This appearance can usually be distinguished from a mediastinal mass by identifying an air bronchogram or following the course of the left lower bronchus.

2. The ligament determines the ultimate shape of the collapsed lung in a pneumothorax.[509]

3. Pleural effusion collecting posterior to the ligament tends to produce a triangular opacity, not unlike a lower lobe collapse (see p. 90).[508]

4. The juxtaphrenic peak sign described with volume loss of an upper lobe[290] (see p. 84) may be due to reorientation and hyperexpansion of the lower lobe, which causes diaphragmatic traction by way of the ligament and septum. Some evidence, however, suggests that this is not the case and that the peak is produced by upward traction on the closely related inferior accessory fissure.[71,207]

5. The ligament provides a pathway from lung to mediastinum and allows pathologic processes to travel in either direction. It may contain lung tumors, esophageal varices, the vascular supply to sequestered segments, and lymph nodes.[545] Posttraumatic paramediastinal air cysts (Figure 15-25) (see p. 699) were at one time considered to

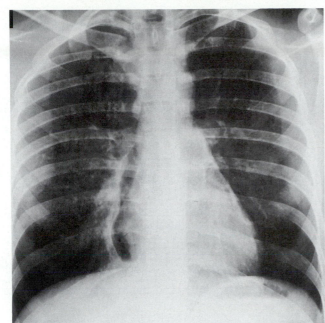

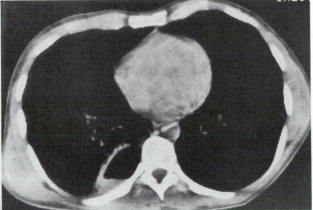

FIGURE 15-25
"Pulmonary ligament pneumatocele." **A,** Following closed chest trauma, triangular collection of air developed against lower right mediastinum, with its apex at hilum. **B,** Computed tomography of same patient shows that appearance in **A** is result of loculated posteromedial pneumothorax: it contains infected fluid, accounting for thick pleural wall. (Courtesy Dr. T. Bloomberg, Guildford, Surrey, U.K.)

be due to air collections within the inferior pulmonary ligament. More recent evidence shows that they represent loculated pneumothoraces or pneumomediastinum.[207]

PLEURAL PHYSIOLOGY

The outward pull of the chest wall and the inward recoil of the lung tend to separate the parietal and visceral pleurae. These membranes are permeable to both gases and liquid, and they are kept in apposition only because of mechanisms that keep the pleural space essentially free of gas and liquid.[7] Gas is removed by the venous blood because the total gas pressure in venous blood is about 70 cm H_2O subatmospheric, and this provides a steep absorption gradient.

The formation and absorption of pleural fluid are more complex. Until recently it was considered that both followed Starling's law, depending on the hydrostatic pressure of systemic (30 cm H_2O) and pulmonary capillaries (11 cm H_2O); the oncotic pressure of pleural fluid (5 cm H_2O) and blood (34 cm H_2O); and the pleural surface pressure (average value − 5 cm H_2O). The interplay of these various forces would be expected to cause a net flow of fluid across the pleural space from the parietal to the visceral pleura, and the flow per day has been estimated at 2.5 L.[349]

Work over the past decade[57] has radically altered the classic theory of pleural fluid kinetics.[57,240,559] It is now considered that pleural fluid forms principally as interstitial fluid in the parietal pleural (obeying Starling's law) and leaks through nontight mesothelial junctions into the pleural space, from which it is removed by bulk flow through the lymphatics via parietal pleural stomata. In this process the pleural space behaves essentially as

though it were part of the parietal pleural extracellular space. Under physiologic conditions the visceral pleura plays little part, generating only a small amount of fluid. The rate of fluid formation by the visceral pleura is low because the supplying arteries (bronchial) are relatively deep to the surface and have low pressure, since they drain into pulmonary veins. The entry rate of fluid into the pleural space is now thought to be low, for example, 7 ml per day in a 30 kg sheep.[705] Lymphatic drainage of the pleural space allows removal of proteins, particulates, and cells in addition to water and crystalloids. Protein removal is particularly important in pathologic states, but even under normal conditions some protein, possibly up to 4 g/day,[349] leaks into the pleural space. Were this not removed, the subsequent rise in oncotic pressure in the pleural fluid would lead to progressive pleural fluid accumulation. Although these mechanisms explain many aspects of pleural fluid dynamics, some findings are inexplicable. For example, the pleural space may be dry in cor pulmonale despite a right atrial pressure of 30 cm H_2O.[349] In addition, in pathologic states, critical factors affecting secretion and absorption may change (e.g., pleural thickening reduces permeability, and lymphatic stomata become blocked with cells and debris). Although the pleural space is gas free, it is normally lubricated by a small amount of pleural fluid. This liquid coupling provides instantaneous transmission of perpendicular forces between pleural surfaces and allows the pleural membranes to slide in response to shear forces.[6] The film of liquid is thin, only 10 to 30 μm.[8]

Normally the volume of pleural fluid is approximately 1 to 5 ml, but some persons have up to 15 ml, particularly in pregnancy or during exercise.[438,724] Using lateral decubitus chest radiographs to detect pleural fluid, a technique that has a threshold sensitivity of about 5 ml,[432] Hessen[243] found a 10% prevalence of definite or probable pleural fluid in healthy adults. This was sometimes unilateral and sometimes bilateral and varied in the same individual. Normal pleural fluid has a protein concentration of 1 to 2 g/dl, a cell count of 1500 to 4500/μl (60% to 70% monocytes), and less than half the serum concentration of large protein molecules such as lactic acid dehydrogenase (LDH).[680]

PLEURAL EFFUSION

Pleural effusions develop when the rate of entry and exit of pleural fluid is mismatched.[57] One or more of six mechanisms may be at work[559]: increased microvascular hydrostatic pressure, systemic venous pressure being the most important determinant; reduced vascular oncotic pressure, as occurs with hypoproteinemia; increased microvascular permeability, seen in inflammatory conditions; impaired lymphatic drainage from the pleural space, with the obstruction occurring at any point from stomata to mediastinal lymph nodes; reduced pleural space pressure, which may be important only with major atelectasis as seen with total lung collapse; and transdiaphragmatic passage of fluid from the peritoneum.

A variety of liquids may accumulate in the pleural space: transudate, exudate, blood, chyle, and occasionally more exotic liquids such as bile, cerebrospinal fluid, peritoneal dialysate, and intravenous infusions. By convention, and often in ignorance of the true contents of the pleural space, liquid in the pleural space is usually called pleural effusion. Alternative and more specific terms such as hemothorax, pyothorax, and chylothorax may be used as appropriate.

In clinical practice the majority of effusions are either transudates or exudates. This distinction is based on the specific gravity, protein, and LDH content of the fluid. Transudates classically have a specific gravity of 1.016 or less and a protein content of 3 g/dl or less. Recently more sophisticated and specific criteria have been introduced to define a transudate: a ratio of pleural fluid protein to serum protein of <0.5; an LDH ratio of <0.6; and an absolute pleural LDH level of <200 IU/L.[349] Some workers have suggested that the serum albumin/effusion albumin gradient is even more specific,[546] with a threshold level of 1.2 g/dl or less indicating an exudate.

Transudates develop because of a change in the physical factors that affect the rate of pleural fluid formation and resorption: microvascular pressure and plasma oncotic pressure. Because of the generalized nature of these changes, transudates are commonly bilateral. Once the altered factor or factors have been identified, attention can be directed away from the pleura, which is itself normal, to the underlying systemic abnormality. The important causes of transudative pleural effusions are listed in the box above right.

CAUSES OF PLEURAL TRANSUDATES

RAISED VENOUS PRESSURE

Heart failure
Constrictive pericarditis

REDUCED PLASMA ONCOTIC PRESSURE

Hepatic cirrhosis
Nephrotic syndrome
Hypoalbuminemia (other causes)

REDUCED PLEURAL SURFACE PRESSURE

Atelectasis

VARIOUS OTHER CAUSES

Nephrogenic effusion
Myxedema
Pulmonary embolism

An exudative effusion indicates that the pleural surface is pathologically altered, with an accompanying increase in permeability or a decrease in lymph flow. The list of possible causes for an exudative effusion is much longer than that for a transudate and is presented in the box below. The box on p. 655 gives a combined list of transudative and exudative effusions because a degree of overlap exists. This list is daunting, but in practice more than 90% of effusions result from heart failure, cirrhosis, ascites, pleuropulmonary infection, malignancy, or pulmonary embolism.[279] Very large effusions are seen especially in malignant disease as a result of metastases, notably from the lung and breast, but large effusions may also occur in heart failure, cirrhosis, tuberculosis, empyema, and hemothorax.[374] Bilateral effusions tend to be transudates, although there are notable exceptions, particularly with metastatic disease, lymphoma, pulmonary embolism, rheumatoid arthritis, and systemic lupus erythematosus.[507] The causes of asymptomatic and symptomatic effusions have recently been reviewed.[606] In both groups heart failure, malignancy, adjacent lung infection, and surgery accounted for more than 70% of cases.

Once the presence and location of a pleural effusion have been established by an imaging investigation, the next step is to establish its cause.[251] This depends on patient history, the examination, and a hierarchy of investigations that, depending on possible diagnoses, include blood and urine tests, thoracocentesis with an examination of the pleural fluid, and pleural biopsy. Exudates should be examined for microorganisms, malignant cells, autoantibodies, and in appropriate circumstances amylase and triglycerides.[240] Other investigations that may be used include thoracoscopy, bronchoscopy, and open biopsy. Imaging procedures play an early and important part in this workup and may disclose abnormalities both inside and outside the chest that can

CAUSES OF PLEURAL EFFUSION (EXCLUDING CHYLOTHORAX AND HEMOTHORAX)

PHYSIOLOGIC

Normal (exceptionally)
Postpartum

INFECTIOUS

Bacteria (including *Mycobacterium*)
Viruses, *Chlamydia*
Fungi
Protozoa, metazoa
Adjacent subphrenic abscess, hepatic abscess (including amebic)

NEOPLASTIC

Bronchial carcinoma, metastases (lung and pleura)
Lymphoma, leukemia, Castleman's disease,[17] macro-globulinemia
Pleural tumor (mesothelioma—diffuse, localized)
Chest wall neoplasm

CARDIOVASCULAR

Heart failure, constrictive pericarditis
Postcardiac injury syndrome
Superior vena cava obstruction
Pulmonary thromboembolism

HEPATIC

Cirrhosis
Hepatitis

PANCREATIC

Pancreatitis (acute, chronic)

RENAL

Uremic pleurisy
Nephrotic syndrome
Acute nephritic syndrome
Renal tract obstruction
Renal infection

SPLENIC

Abscess
Infarction
Hematoma

ASCITIC

Meigs' syndrome
Ascites (benign, malignant)
Peritoneal dialysis

TRAUMATIC

Open or closed chest trauma, including esophageal rupture, diaphragmatic hernia
Iatrogenic, including thoracic and abdominal surgery, esophageal sclerotherapy, radiation

INHALATIONAL

Asbestos

INFLAMMATORY

Rheumatoid disease
Systemic lupus erythematosus
Wegener's granulomatosis

DRUG INDUCED

Methotrexate and other drugs

MISCELLANEOUS

Sarcoidosis
Myxedema
Yellow nail syndrome
Familial Mediterranean fever
Atelectasis

---

establish or suggest a probable cause for the effusion. In addition, imaging techniques are used to direct biopsy or interventional therapy.

A subset of exudative pleural effusions are eosinophilic—ones in which eosinophils make up more than 10% of the total pleural fluid white blood cell count. In a literature review of 343 eosinophilic effusions the majority (63%) were either idiopathic (35%) or associated with air with or without blood in the pleural space (28%).[5] Other causes included infection (11%) with the majority parapneumonic (5%) or tuberculous (4%), malignancy (8%), pulmonary infarction (4%), benign asbestos-related effusion (4%), and rheumatologic disease (4%). Based largely on this study, an eosinophilic pleural effusion is generally considered benign and self-limiting and is commonly associated with air or blood in the pleural

space.[559] However, a recent report has emphasized the importance of disease prevalence in making judgments concerning the significance of an eosinophilic effusion. In this study, although only 4 of 84 effusions in patients with malignancy were eosinophilic, 48% of those with eosinophilic effusion were malignant.[313]

Several large series indicate that about one fifth of pleural effusions that are examined by thoracocentesis are of indeterminate cause despite extensive investigation.[251,337,606,626] Nearly half of such patients have a definite diagnosis, most commonly of a malignant disorder, made on follow-up.[224,557]

Imaging of pleural effusion

Conventional radiography, CT, and ultrasound are specific and sensitive ways of demonstrating pleural fluid.

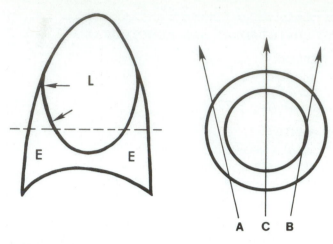

FIGURE 15-26
Left, Diagramatic vertical section through lung *(L)* and pleural effusion *(E)* to illustrate disposition of pleural fluid. Arrows mark lung–pleural fluid interface, which has meniscus-like shape. *Right,* Transaxial section at level indicated in diagram at left. Letters *A, B,* and *C* represent x-ray beams. See text for explanation. (From Wilson AG: *Br J Hosp Med* 37:526-534, 1987.)

The appearance of an effusion depends on the patient's position at the time of the examination and the mobility of the effusion, which may be free or constrained to a variable extent.

With a moderate-sized pleural effusion, fluid collects around and under the lung and takes on a characteristic configuration. This shape is determined by the interplay of the hydrostatic pressure in the effusion, the pleural liquid pressure, and the pleural surface pressure in the various zones from apex to base. In the erect subject, fluid collects mainly in the lower zone. Here the hydrostatic pressure is positive and the lung is compressed, so that it floats away from the chest wall and diaphragm.[6,8] Homeostatic mechanisms, particularly tissue interdependence, prevent the lower lung zones from collapsing as much as might be predicted from the local pleural liquid pressure.[197] In contrast, in the highest zone, normal conditions obtain and pleural liquid pressure is much lower than pleural surface pressure. In this zone the fluid is essentially normal in thickness and radiologically undetectable. In the middle zone the visceral-parietal pleural contact is lost and pleural liquid and surface pressures become identical. Descending in this zone pleural liquid pressure remains subatmospheric but becomes more positive because of the increasing head of effusion, and thus the recoil of the lung has to become less to allow the pleural surface pressure to rise (become less negative). This is achieved by a decrease in lung volume, since at smaller lung volumes recoil is less. Because lung volume decreases, the thickness of pleural fluid increases progressively. The result of the interactions between these forces is that the lung eventually sits in the pleural fluid rather like an egg in an egg cup and the upper surface of the effusion takes on a meniscus-like

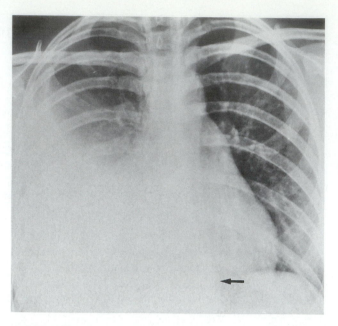

FIGURE 15-27
Pleural effusion. Right-sided opacity has classic features of free pleural effusion in erect patient. Opacity is homogeneous, occupies inferior part of chest, and has concave upper margin that extends higher laterally than medially. Medial to lateral limb of meniscus is characteristic haziness without clear upper border. At first glance, shadow low and to left *(arrow)* resembles displaced azygoesophageal recess, as sometimes occurs with pleural effusion. Its configuration is, however, not quite as expected, and it was found to result from tuberculous paravertebral abscess — cause of the effusion.

shape (Figure 15-26). The three-dimensional shape of effusions has been illustrated with casts.[111,173]

On plain radiographs the classic appearance of a moderate pleural effusion is a homogeneous lower zone opacity with a curvilinear upper border, quite sharply marginated and concave to the lung (Figure 15-27). A consideration of Figure 15-26 explains how this type of opacity is produced. The transaxial view shows that the x-ray beam is more attenuated laterally *(A)* than centrally *(C)* because the marginal beam passes through a greater thickness of fluid. A pleural effusion is therefore dense laterally, and because it presents a tangential fluid-air interface *(B)*, it has a sharp inner margin with the classic meniscus shape produced by the inner fluid envelope. More centrally the x-ray beam is less attenuated and the effusion produces only a general haziness, the upper edge of which cannot be seen because it has wedge-shaped geometry (Figure 15-27). The meniscus is often higher laterally than medially because lung attachments (hilum and pulmonary ligament) alter the distribution of forces (Figure 15-27).

Sometimes other types of shadow are seen with a moderate effusion. Most of these result from free pleural fluid within fissures, and the radiographic appearance depends on the shape and orientation of the fissure, the location of the fluid within it, and the direction of the

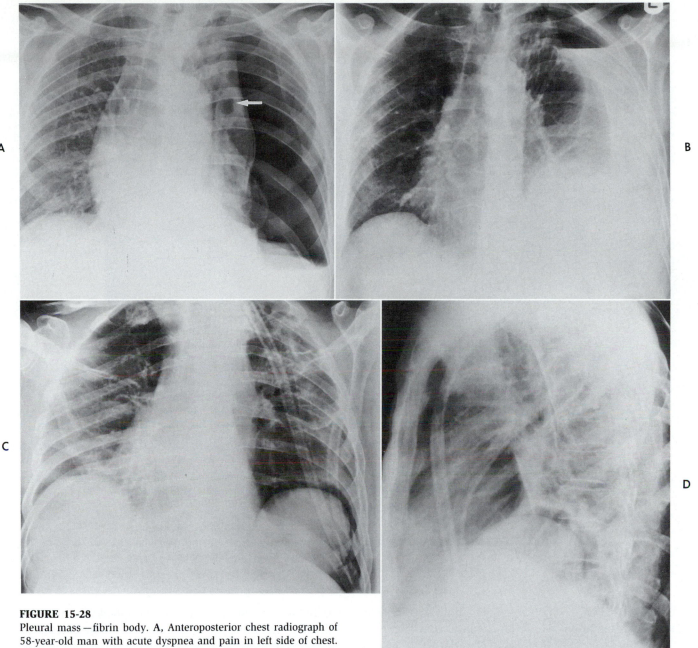

FIGURE 15-28

Pleural mass—fibrin body. **A**, Anteroposterior chest radiograph of 58-year-old man with acute dyspnea and pain in left side of chest. There was left pneumothorax with a little pleural fluid. Lung, which was prevented from collapsing completely by apical adhesion, contains cavity *(arrow)*. Appearances were caused by tuberculous bronchopleural fistula. **B**, Two months later there is persisting hydropneumothorax with great deal of protein-rich fluid despite repeated thoracocentesis. **C** and **D**, One month later drains have been inserted in left side of chest, draining fluid and revealing 10 cm rounded mobile mass lesion in pleural space. This is homogeneous and has smooth, sharp margin. There was no evidence of fungal infection of pleural space, and mass was assumed to be fibrin body despite its unusually large size.

x-ray beam.[506] A common appearance is a curvilinear interface on a frontal chest radiograph (Figure 15-28, *B*). Such an opacity may be faint; typically, it is relatively transradiant medially and more dense laterally and

superiorly.[506] The medial curvilinear interface marks the limit of fluid intrusion into the fissure, which may or may not be at the point of fissural fusion.[107] A similar shadow but higher and more peripheral may be produced by fluid accumulations between chest wall and the lips of contact of the major fissure (Figure 15-29, *C*).[237] Such tonguelike intrusions of fluid into the margins of fissures are common and may be seen quite early in the development of a pleural effusion, an observation that has been confirmed in studies with animals.[7] It gives rise to the

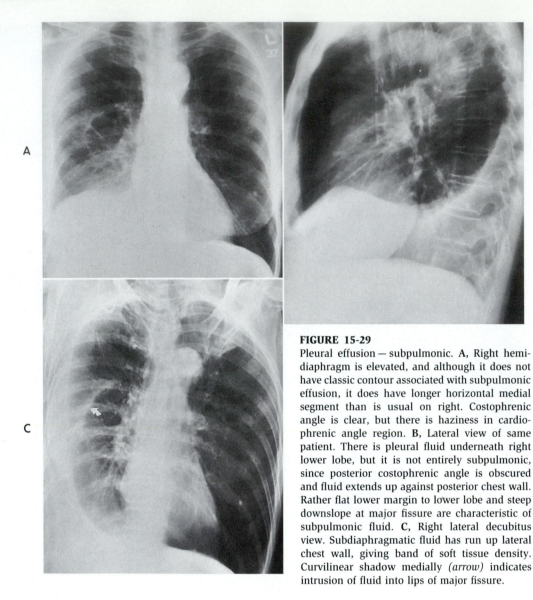

FIGURE 15-29
Pleural effusion — subpulmonic. **A,** Right hemidiaphragm is elevated, and although it does not have classic contour associated with subpulmonic effusion, it does have longer horizontal medial segment than is usual on right. Costophrenic angle is clear, but there is haziness in cardiophrenic angle region. **B,** Lateral view of same patient. There is pleural fluid underneath right lower lobe, but it is not entirely subpulmonic, since posterior costophrenic angle is obscured and fluid extends up against posterior chest wall. Rather flat lower margin to lower lobe and steep downslope at major fissure are characteristic of subpulmonic fluid. **C,** Right lateral decubitus view. Subdiaphragmatic fluid has run up lateral chest wall, giving band of soft tissue density. Curvilinear shadow medially *(arrow)* indicates intrusion of fluid into lips of major fissure.

thorn sign when a small amount of fluid accumulates laterally in the minor fissure on a frontal view.[466]

A more complex shadow also now attributed to fissural intrusion is the middle lobe step (Figure 15-30). It consists of a steplike accumulation of fluid laterally below the minor fissure. When originally described it was thought to indicate a diseased middle lobe with reduced compliance.[173] This explanation is no longer accepted, and it is now thought to result from overlapping fluid intrusion into incomplete major and minor fissures.[237,506]

Moderate or large right pleural effusions may displace the azygoesophageal interface to the left, producing a retrocardiac masslike lesion.[482] Fluid within the azygoesophageal recess may also simulate subcarinal adenopathy.[482]

Another unusual appearance with moderate-sized effusions is encapsulation of a lobe, particularly the lower lobe, simulating consolidation.[163,173,237] Sometimes fluid collects preferentially against the mediastinum, particu-

larly on the left, and gives a triangular retrocardiac density simulating lower lobe collapse, from which it can be differentiated by analysis of the position of the lower lobe bronchus. This distribution of fluid has been attributed to the modifying influence of the pulmonary ligament.[423,509]

Early in their development pleural effusions are small and collect between the lower lobes and the diaphragm (Figure 15-31).[8,243,527] After a variable amount of fluid has accumulated, it spills into the posterior and then into the lateral costophrenic angles[173] and may cause subtle changes in the contour of the inferior aspect of the lower lobe. The only study that has assessed the amount of pleural fluid needed to blunt the costophrenic angles on posteroanterior radiographs is a postmortem study in erect cadavers in which it was found that on average the required volume was 175 ml (range 25 to 525 ml).[93]

When effusions are too small to be detected on conventional posteroanterior and lateral chest radio-

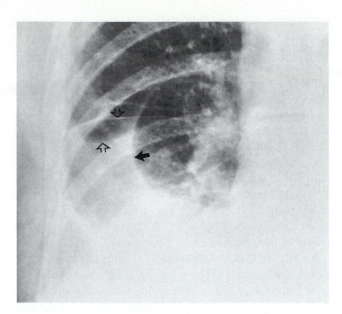

FIGURE 15-30
"Middle lobe step." There is steplike intrusion of pleural fluid into fissures below minor fissure. Features caused by minor fissure *(open arrows)* and major fissure *(closed arrow)* are indicated.

graphs, they may be demonstrated with special radiographic views or by ultrasound or CT. The most widely used special radiographic view is the lateral decubitus (Figure 15-29),[243,438,668] with which it may be possible to detect 3 to 10 ml of fluid.[432,438,668] A variant on this technique, the oblique semisupine view, can be performed in relatively immobile patients and by the bedside if necessary.[428] The sensitivity of ultrasound and CT has not been formally assessed, but it is probably similar to that of decubitus radiographs.

SUBPULMONIC EFFUSION. Occasionally, for reasons that are obscure, large quantities of pleural fluid accumulate in a subpulmonic location rather than escaping into the general pleural cavity. Attempts to attribute this distribution to an underlying abnormality in the lower lobe with subsequent distortion of pleural forces have not been convincing.[173,527] Pleural adhesions are not a factor either, since most subpulmonic effusions prove completely mobile with postural changes.[243] Also, for no clear reason, subpulmonic effusions are often transudates and associated with renal failure, liver cirrhosis, congestive heart failure, and nephrotic syndrome.[135,669] There are, however, many exceptions. Subpulmonic effusions may be unilateral or bilateral; when unilateral they are more commonly right sided,[486] and when bilateral they can easily be missed on the chest radiograph.[669]

The upper edge of the fluid mimics the contour of the diaphragm on the chest radiograph (Figure 15-32), so that the principal sign is an apparent elevation of the hemidiaphragm,[668] with the minor fissure appearing closer to the apparent diaphragm than usual. The "elevated hemidiaphragm" may have one or more of the

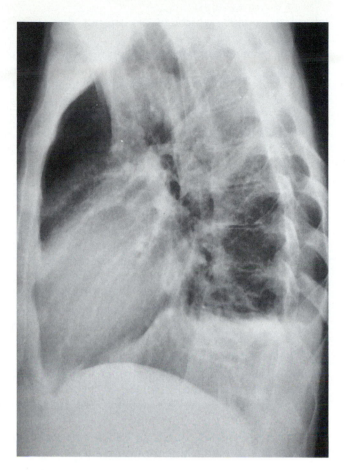

FIGURE 15-31
Pleural effusion — subpulmonic. Lateral radiograph with patient erect demonstrates characteristic horizontal upper border to effusion and abrupt angulation anteriorly against oblique fissure.

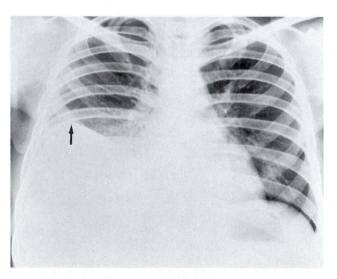

FIGURE 15-32
Pleural effusion — subpulmonic. Appearances on right superficially resemble those of elevated hemidiaphragm. Configuration is, however, unusual — with lateral peak that is characteristic of subpulmonic effusion.

following features, which should suggest the correct diagnosis:

1. The "hemidiaphragm" peaks more laterally than usual (Figure 15-32; see Figure 15-47, B), and the contour on either side of the peak is straighter. The medial slope tends to be gradual whereas the lateral one is steep.[61,173,486]

2. These appearances, particularly the lateral peaking, are accentuated on expiration,[61] a phenomenon that has been attributed to the presence of the pulmonary ligament.[552]

3. The costophrenic angle is usually ill defined, blunted (Figures 15-29 and 15-31), or shallow,[243,669] but exceptionally both the lateral and the posterior angles are clear.

4. In the lateral radiograph the posterior aspect of the "hemidiaphragm" tends to be flat beneath the lower lobe (Figure 15-31). At the major fissure the silhouette usually slopes steeply downward (Figures 15-29, B, and 15-31), and there may be a tail of fluid passing up into the fissure itself.[161,486,662] The perceived lack of fluid under the lung anteriorly may be more apparent than real.[506]

5. The rather flat upper surface of the fluid means that on frontal view there is not the usual wedge of lung passing down below the silhouette of the diaphragm. Thus on frontal view vessels are not seen below the superior surface of the diaphragm.[580]

6. On the left side the gastric air bubble and the upper surface of the "hemidiaphragm" are separated more than usual. Unfortunately, this distance is variable in healthy patients. Comparison with previous radiographs may help assessment. Some authors suggest that a distance of more than 2 cm is suggestive.[243]

7. The frontal radiograph occasionally shows a diaphragmatic spur associated with fluid entering the inferior accessory fissure[669] or a more substantial triangular retrocardiac shadow. This latter opacity, which effaces the medial "hemidiaphragmatic" contour and the left paravertebral interface, results from paramediastinal extension of the subpulmonic fluid.[135]

Subpulmonic pleural fluid is rarely loculated, and the diagnosis may therefore be confirmed by taking a decubitus radiograph (Figure 15-29, C).[243] Alternatively, its presence may be confirmed by ultrasound or CT.

LARGE PLEURAL EFFUSION. Large pleural effusions obscure the border of the heart and displace the mediastinum, airways, and diaphragm. Visualization of the pericardial fat as a curvilinear transradiancy sometimes allows assessment of heart size even when the heart border is completely obscured by pleural fluid.[186] Large pleural effusions should lead to contralateral displacement of the mediastinum (Figure 15-33), and right-sided ones may give a mediastinally based retrocardiac density convex to the left as a result of herniation of the fluid-filled azygoesophageal recess.[479] A central mediastinum in the presence of a large pleural effusion suggests that either the mediastinum is fixed (most commonly the

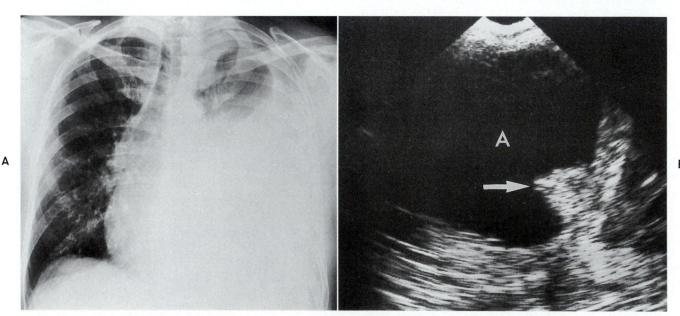

FIGURE 15-33
Pleural effusion — large. **A,** Mesothelioma is recognized cause for large pleural effusion unaccompanied by mediastinal shift. Exceptions to this finding are, however, not uncommon, as in this patient. **B,** Ultrasound examination demonstrates echo-free pleural fluid *(A)* and one of several areas of nodular pleural thickening *(arrow)*. Diagnosis was made by biopsy of local pleural mass under ultrasound control. (Courtesy Dr. A.E.A. Joseph, London.)

result of malignant infiltration by carcinoma or mesothelioma) or obstructive collapse has occurred, usually because of bronchial carcinoma of the underlying lung.[343,669] In contrast, relaxation collapse of the lung, which normally accompanies a large pleural effusion, is not usually so great that it makes up for the volume of the effusion. On lateral views posterior pleural collections cause anterior displacement of central airways, a helpful differentiating feature from collapse or consolidation.[497]

Inversion of the hemidiaphragm is an occasional but well-recognized finding.[161,439,632] It is seen with large or moderate effusions, more commonly on the left than on the right,[669] a difference ascribed to the lack of liver support on the left.[730] On plain chest radiography, diaphragmatic inversion is easier to recognize on the left, where displacement of gastric and colonic gas indicates the shape and position of the left hemidiaphragm (Figure 15-34). On the right side it is most easily diagnosed by ultrasound (Figures 15-35 and 15-36).[365,628,730] It has been brought to light by liver scintigraphy, which demonstrates deformity of the dome of the liver.[120,291] An inverted right hemidiaphragm on CT examination super-

ficially resembles a cystlike lesion of the liver (Figure 15-37).[242,291,341] Other lesions that may invert the hemidiaphragm include pneumothorax, lobar emphysema, diaphragmatic neoplasm, pericardial cyst, and myocardial aneurysm.[536] Diaphragm inversion generally produces few symptoms. However, the following effects have been described: (1) it may cause or simulate an upper abdominal mass[105,120]; (2) it leads to paradoxic diaphragmatic movement[628] that could cause dyspnea because of pendulum breathing (expired air from the ipsilateral lung being inspired contralaterally)[439]; and (3) should the inversion disappear following thoracocentesis, the apparent size of the pleural effusion on a chest radiograph may not change significantly.

LOCULATED PLEURAL EFFUSION. Pleural fluid may loculate (encyst) within the fissures, or between parietal and visceral pleura when the pleural layers are partly fused.

Loculations against the chest wall are the most frequent. They take on a variety of configurations, most commonly a dome-shaped projection into the lung (Figure 15-38). The appearance of this on plain radiographs

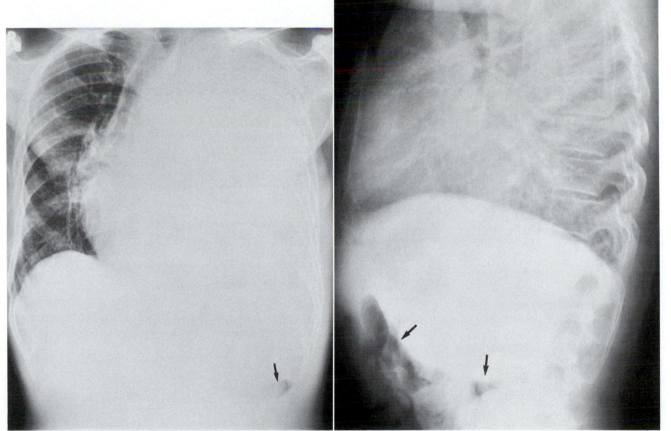

FIGURE 15-34
Pleural effusion — hemidiaphragm inversion. **A,** Posteroanterior chest radiograph shows large left pleural effusion displacing mediastinum to right and colonic gas inferiorly *(arrow)*. **B,** Lateral radiograph of same patient shows more clearly position of left hemidiaphragm, indicated by displaced bowel gas *(arrows)*.

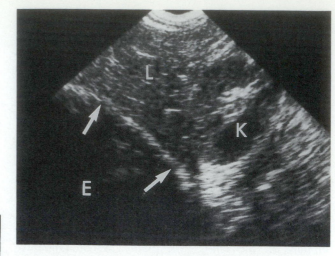

FIGURE 15-35
Pleural effusion — inverted hemidiaphragm. Ultrasound examination of right upper quadrant of abdomen. Liver *(L)* and kidney *(K)* to right are separated from essentially echo-free pleural effusion *(E)* by hemidiaphragm *(arrows)*, which is convex to liver. (Courtesy Dr. A.E.A. Joseph, London.)

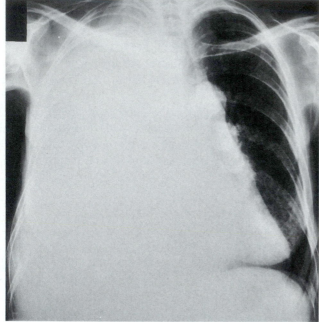

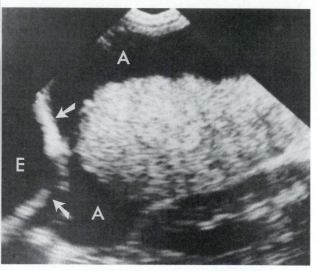

FIGURE 15-36
Pleural effusion — hepatic cirrhosis. **A,** Posteroanterior radiograph shows massive right pleural effusion with mediastinal displacement to left. Right-sided location of effusion is characteristic. **B,** Longitudinal ultrasound scan of right upper quadrant shows diaphragm *(arrows)* between pleural effusion *(E)* and ascites *(A)*. Diaphragm is convex to liver and inverted. Cirrhotic liver has nodular surface. (Courtesy Dr. A.E.A. Joseph, London.)

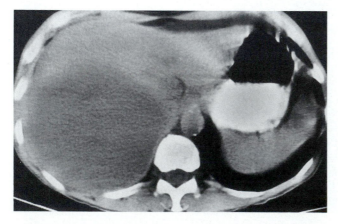

FIGURE 15-37
Pleural effusion — inverted hemidiaphragm. Computed tomographic examination of upper abdomen shows large, rounded, low-density area apparently lying posteriorly in liver and caused by right pleural effusion inverting right hemidiaphragm.

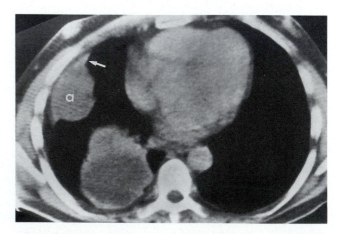

FIGURE 15-38
Pleural effusion — loculated. Opacities on right are loculated hematomas, in part clotted. Upper one is against chest wall, and lower is dome-shaped collection resting on hemidiaphragm. Opacity *a* has classic shape of loculated pleural collection; it is sharply marginated and convex to lung, and it lifts off tail of pleura *(arrow)*, giving its margin an obtuse angle with chest wall.

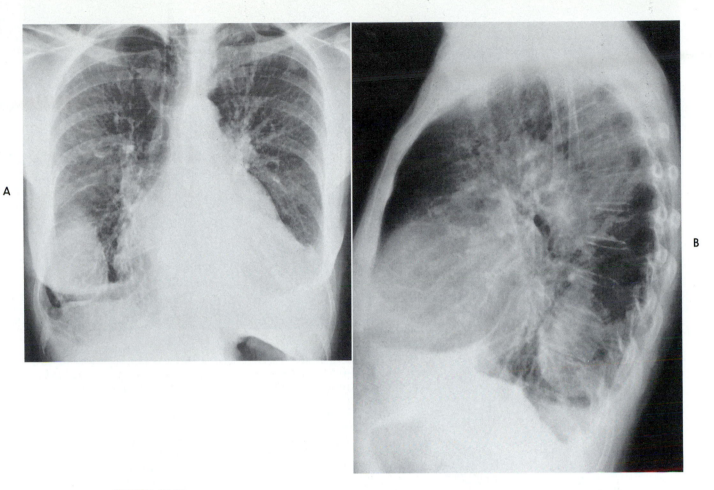

FIGURE 15-39

Pleural effusion — loculated. This 68-year-old woman was in heart failure because of mixed mitral valve disease. There is bilateral pleural fluid, which on right is loculated against chest wall. A, Posteroanterior radiograph shows oval right lower zone opacity with characteristics of chest wall or pleural lesion; it is homogeneous, margin in part sharp and in part ill defined. Much of sharp margin is on medial aspect of opacity, as is usually case with localized pleural/chest wall lesions. B, Lateral view of same patient confirms radiographic features of pleural loculation and shows blunting of posterior costophrenic angle and fluid entering major fissure on right.

depends on the projection. If the loculation is seen en face or obliquely, it produces a rounded opacity with part of the margin sharp and part ill defined. On a frontal radiograph the clear margin is usually medial and the hazy one lateral (Figure 15-39). This appearance is the same as that seen with a (sub)pleural lipoma (Figure 15-40). When viewed tangentially a loculation is classically convex to the lung and sharply demarcated on its pulmonary aspect because of its pleural covering, just as it appears on CT (Figure 15-38). These lesions tend to have greater length than height, and because of the weight of contained fluid the greatest height is not necessarily over the center of the lesion. The margins of the loculus make an obtuse angle with the chest wall, elevating a "tail" of pleura (Figure 15-38). Loculated pleural effusions share many radiologic features with chest wall or pleural masses,[162] and they are often

indistinguishable. Extrapleural chest wall lesions, however, tend to stand more proud, to be as high as they are long, to have their greatest depth opposite the center of attachment, and — most important — may show rib involvement.[162] A pleural lesion may well be accompanied by disease elsewhere in the pleural cavity.

Pleural fluid may also loculate within fissures, particularly in heart failure.[159,245,696] Because these collections tend to come and go, they have been called vanishing or phantom tumors and pseudotumors.[245] Such loculations are seen more commonly on the right[157] and in the minor rather than the major fissure despite the greater area of the latter (Figure 15-41).[245] In the minor fissure on a lateral radiograph, loculated fluid has a characteristic lenticular shape, often with a pathognomonic tail extending along the fissure for a short distance. In frontal view it usually appears rounded or oval and sharply demar-

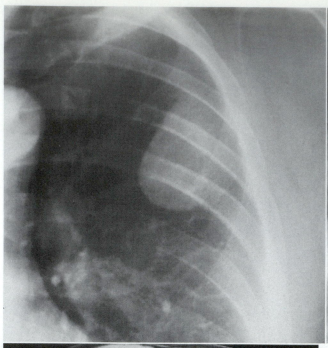

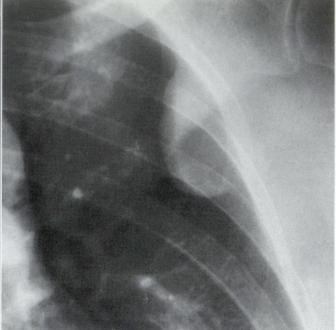

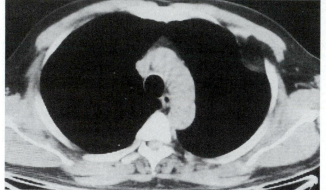

FIGURE 15-40

Pleural mass — lipoma. **A**, Localized view of left upper zone shows 3 × 5 cm homogeneous mass lesion. It is pleurally based and has sharp inner border, but its outer margin fades off into soft tissues of chest wall. Ribs are unaffected. Opacity could be pleural or extrapleural. **B**, Tangential view adds little information. Lesion makes obtuse angle where it contacts chest wall superiorly. Inferior angle cannot be analyzed. Inner margin of lesion is clear and sharp. **C**, Computed tomography shows low-density lesion that has attenuation of fat. Component of lesion lies in chest wall. Exact site of origin, although it could be pleural, is indeterminate.

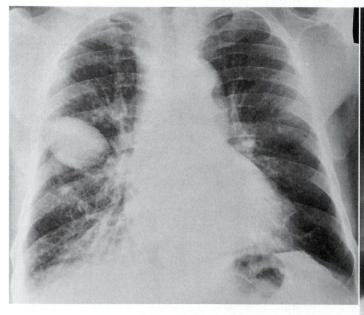

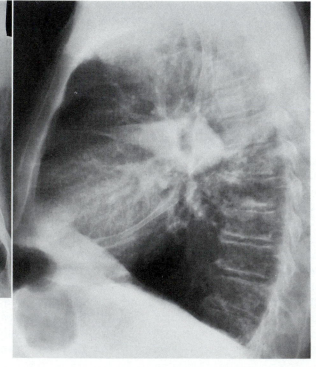

FIGURE 15-41

Pleural effusion — loculated. This 77-year-old man is in heart failure. **A**, Posteroanterior chest radiograph shows 7 × 4 cm well-demarcated oval opacity in right midzone projected in region of minor fissure. **B**, Lateral radiograph shows lenticular opacity occupying minor fissure, with characteristic tail anteriorly.

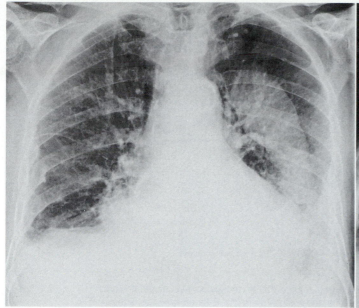

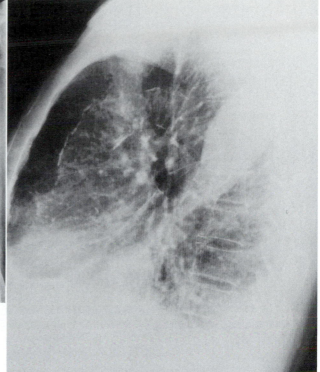

FIGURE 15-42
Pleural effusion — loculated. **A,** Anteroposterior (AP) and, **B,** lateral views of fluid encysted in major fissure. This effusion is unusual in that most of its margin is sharp in AP view. As with many loculated collections, there is also free fluid in pleural space.

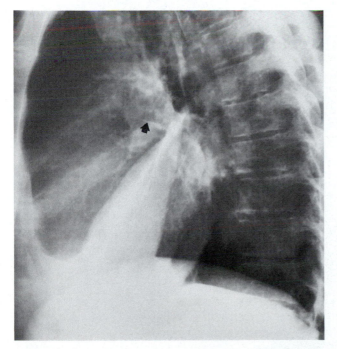

FIGURE 15-43
Pleural effusion — loculated. There is a homogeneous triangular opacity in this lateral view projected over lower end of major fissure. Features suggesting that it results from loculated fluid rather than middle lobe collapse are (1) contact with diaphragm rather than sternum anteriorly and (2) convex borders. Identification of separate minor fissure *(arrow)* confirms diagnosis.

cated. Usually the diagnosis is easily made if the distinctive shape and position of the lesion are considered, particularly in the presence of heart failure.

Loculated collections in the major fissure have the expected distinctive appearance in lateral views (Figure 15-42), but in frontal projection they commonly do not have the masslike features of those in the minor fissure. This is because the long axis of these lesions is tilted relative to the frontal x-ray beam and the shadow generated is either hazy and veil like or more discrete, with margins that are in part ill defined and in part distinct (Figure 15-42). Loculations in the caudad part of the major fissure (Figure 15-43) may resemble middle lobe collapse and consolidation (Figure 15-44). In this situation the following points favor loculated fluid rather than collapse (Figure 15-45): (1) identification of a separate minor fissure (Figure 15-43); (2) one or more convex margins in lateral projection (with collapse, usually at least one border is concave or straight); (3) right border of the heart not effaced on frontal view; and (4) both ends of the opacity tapering in lateral view (with collapse the anterior end is usually broad).[161] Two findings that favor collapse are (1) contact between the anterior end of the shadow and the chest wall and (2) an air bronchogram (Figure 15-45).[161]

Other peripheral fluid loculations (against diaphragm and mediastinum) are not so common as those against the chest wall, but they do occur and are being increas-

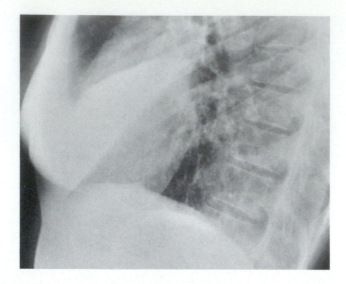

FIGURE 15-44
Right middle lobe collapse. In lateral view features that suggest this is collapsed and consolidated lobe rather than encysted fluid are (1) anterior contact of wedge-shaped opacity with sternum; (2) anterior end broader than posterior; (3) one straight border; and (4) absence of separate minor fissure. Convexity of upper border is atypical and more commonly a feature of encysted fluid.

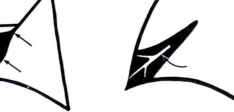

FIGURE 15-45
Diagram of collapse versus encysted fluid. Differential diagnosis of encysted fluid in oblique fissure *(left)* versus collapse and consolidation *(right)* of middle lobe are illustrated. For discussion see text.

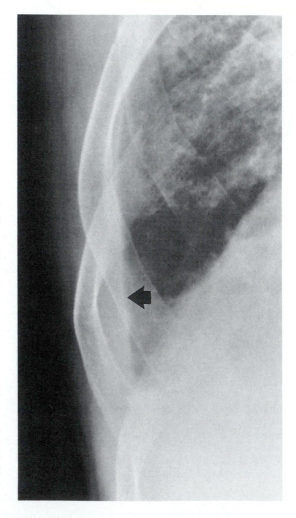

FIGURE 15-46
Effusion — laminar. Localized view of right costophrenic angle shows band of soft tissue density parallel to chest wall with edge enhancement caused by Mach effect *(arrow)*. This is not free pleural fluid but rather subvisceral pleural fluid, and it is seen when lung interstitium is waterlogged — as in this patient with heart failure. Note septal lines.

ingly recognized with CT. The plain radiographic features of these lesions are predictable.

So-called lamellar pleural effusions are, in fact, fluid collections in the loose connective tissue beneath the visceral pleura (Figure 15-46). They are seen with an edematous pulmonary interstitium, particularly in heart failure, and are discussed in Chapter 9.

On CT a loculated fluid collection usually produces a lenticular opacity with uniform, smooth inner walls. When the pleura of the envelope is thickened, a split pleura sign is produced, an appearance that can be mimicked by fluid accumulation in preexisting pulmonary airspaces.[735] In addition, loculated fluid produces a mass effect on adjacent lungs. CT of loculated fluid is discussed in more detail in relation to empyema, since it is in this condition that CT images play a critical role.

PLEURAL EFFUSION IN THE SUPINE PATIENT. When a patient is supine, free pleural fluid layers out posteriorly, and although a meniscus effect occurs at the lung-fluid interface, it is not appreciated on a frontal projection because it is oriented at right angles to the x-ray beam. The supine chest radiograph is not particularly sensitive or specific in the diagnosis of pleural effusion,[555] although in one study 90% of effusions between 200 and 500 ml were detected.[722] Sensitivity of detection falls when effusions are bilateral. The volume of pleural effusions is generally underestimated in supine patients.[555]

The signs produced by pleural effusions on supine radiographs are as follows:

1. Hazy, veil-like opacity of a hemithorax with preserved vascular shadows (Figure 15-47).[173,243] When effusions are small, this veiling may occupy only the lower chest, making the lower half of the hemithorax more opaque than the upper, which is the reverse of the normal situation.[722]
2. Loss of the sharp silhouette of the ipsilateral hemidiaphragm (Figure 15-47).[428,722]
3. Blunting of the costophrenic angle.[551] Although a common sign, it is often a false-positive finding.[555]
4. Capping of the lung apex with a pleural shadow (Figure 15-47).[506] Some regard this as a relatively early sign explicable because the chest apex has a small capacity and is the most dependent part of the pleural space tangential to a frontal x-ray beam in a supine patient.[506] Other workers, however, find that effusions have to be at least moderate (more than 500 ml) before they collect at the apex.[722] With the accumulation of more fluid a bandlike opacity develops and separates the lateral lung margin from the chest wall.
5. Thickening of the minor fissure.[506]
6. Widening of the paraspinal soft tissues.[650]
7. Apparent elevation of the hemidiaphragm and reduced visibility of lower lobe vessels behind the diaphragm.[551]

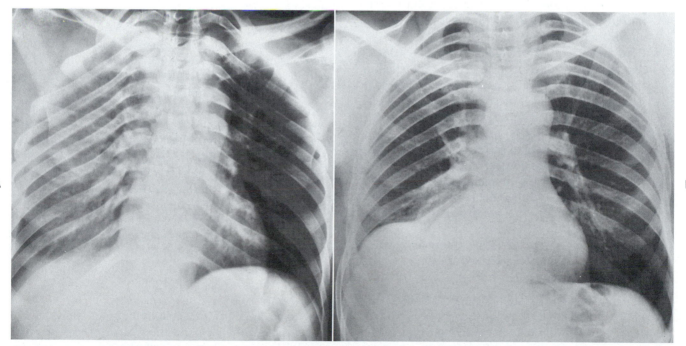

FIGURE 15-47
Effusion — supine. A, Supine view in patient with right-sided pleural effusion. There is hazy opacification of whole right hemithorax with preserved vascular markings. Diaphragm silhouette is hazy. Right costophrenic angle is, unfortunately, excluded from image, but with lateral band of fluid against chest wall it would almost certainly have been blunted. Lung is capped with apical fluid. B, Radiograph on same day with patient erect; effusion is largely in subpulmonic location.

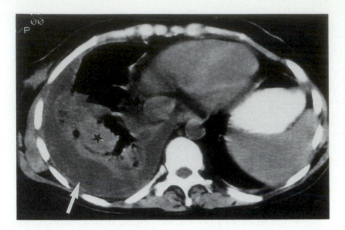

FIGURE 15-48
Pleural effusion on computed tomography (CT). Free pleural effusion of moderate size *(arrow)* lies in lower half of chest and has crescent shape. Effusions usually have obviously lower density than adjacent soft tissue. In this patient CT reveals underlying causal infective consolidation *(star)*.

The modifying effect of additional air in the pleural space on the signs of a supine effusion is discussed by Onik and co-workers.[473]

COMPUTED TOMOGRAPHY OF PLEURAL FLUID. In selected patients CT plays an important part in the assessment of pleural effusion:

1. It is a sensitive method, detecting and confirming the presence of early effusion.[400]
2. The configuration of the pleural opacity may allow a distinction between free and loculated fluid. When the effusion is loculated, CT can assess its extent and localization.
3. CT differentiates between pleural and parenchymal disease and is superior to the chest radiograph in this regard.[500] Such a distinction is greatly helped by a bolus injection of intravenous contrast material, which facilitates identification of lung parenchyma and pleura.[55]
4. CT allows assessment of pleural morphology. Some appearances (irregular thickening and focal masses) are highly suggestive of malignancy, and others (mild uniform thickening) of benignity.[371] A normal pleura or one that is thin yet irregular is indeterminate.[371]
5. CT allows underlying lung disease (tumor, pneumonia, abscess) to be characterized.
6. It facilitates percutaneous biopsy.

Although comparative studies have not been performed, CT is undoubtedly a more sensitive modality in the detection of pleural fluid than is an erect posteroanterior chest radiograph. Pleural effusion gives a homogeneous crescentic opacity in the most dependent part of the pleural cavity. The lower attenuation coefficient (CT number) of pleural fluid usually allows distinction from pleural thickening and masses (Figure 15-48),[371] but because of its variability the attenuation coefficient does

not allow a differentiation among exudate, transudate, and malignant effusion.[307,670] Many factors contribute to CT number variability, including scanner performance,[339] type of reconstruction algorithm,[734] beam hardening,[512] position of the lesion in the scanner field,[74,734] and motion artifact, particularly cardiac.[670] It may, however, be possible to identify a hemothorax with CT as a nonhomogeneous collection with an attenuation coefficient considerably higher than that of water.[713] The fat content of a chylothorax might be expected to produce low CT numbers, but the commonly high protein level usually militates against this, although occasionally modestly low numbers are recorded,[331] for example, −17 HU.[631] Small amounts of pleural fluid can be difficult to distinguish from pleural thickening, a situation that is clarified by repeat scanning in a changed position.[500]

Pleural fluid deep in the posterior and lateral costophrenic sulci may be confused with ascites, and a variety of signs have been described to differentiate pleural and ascitic fluid:

1. Displaced crus sign. Pleural fluid collects between the crus and the spine and displaces the crus anterolaterally (Figure 15-49), whereas ascitic fluid collects anterolateral to the crus and causes the opposite displacement.[136,444] The use of this sign is limited because it is commonly indeterminant, about one third of cases in one series.[231]

2. Interface sign. The interface between pleural fluid and liver or spleen is hazy (Figure 15-50),[642] probably because of a partial volume effect from the obliquely sectioned diaphragm. This sign must be assessed away from the dome of the diaphragm, and it becomes less discriminating with thin sections (1.5 to 5 mm).[642]

3. Diaphragm sign. If the diaphragm can be identified, fluid inside the dome must be ascites and fluid on the outside must be pleural, provided the diaphragm is not inverted.[11,444] The diaphragm is surprisingly difficult to identify because the diaphragm and liver have similar attenuation values; in a series of 38 patients with peridiaphragmatic fluid the diaphragm could not be identified in one fifth.[231] Sometimes the curvilinear opacity produced by atelectatic lung mimics the appearance of the diaphragm (Figure 15-51). In general, atelectatic lung is thicker than the diaphragm, tapers laterally, and may be interrupted.[158] In addition, contiguous cuts usually show continuity with air-containing lung (Figure 15-51) or lung that contains an air bronchogram.[158,598] Care must also be taken not to misidentify prominent parietal pleura as diaphragm.[598]

4. Bare area sign. Since the posterior portion of the diaphragm is difficult to identify in many individuals, a knowledge of the shape of the various spaces in which peridiaphragmatic fluid may collect is helpful in assessing whether fluid is pleural or ascitic on CT.[444] Pleural fluid is free to collect along the full width of the costophrenic recess behind the liver (Figure 15-50), whereas ascitic fluid is excluded from the large bare area over the posteromedial surface of the right lobe of the liver (Figure

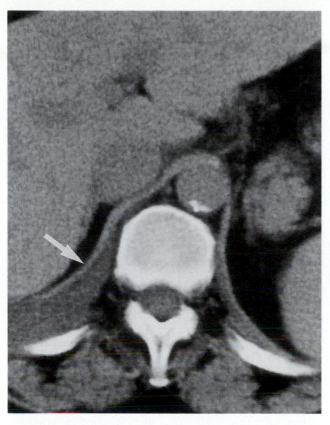

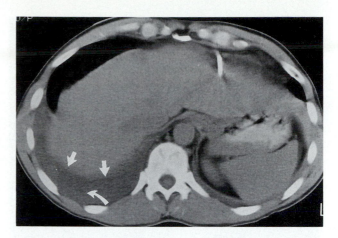

FIGURE 15-50
Pleural effusion versus ascites. Computed tomography at level of liver and posterior costophrenic sulcus. Homogeneous low-density opacity behind liver is caused by fluid. Hazy liver margin *(straight arrows)* and absence of bare area *(curved arrow)* indicate pleural effusion rather than ascites.

FIGURE 15-49
Pleural effusion versus ascites. Pleural effusion displaces diaphragmatic crus *(arrow)* away from adjacent vertebral body. Ascites has reverse effect.

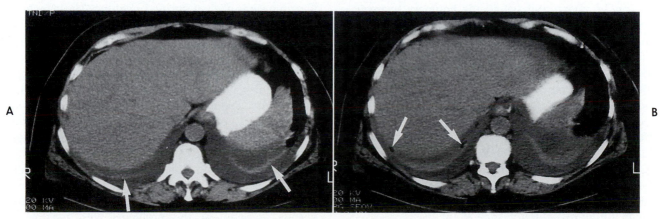

FIGURE 15-51
Pleural effusion versus ascites — diaphragm sign. **A,** There appears to be fluid on either side of diaphragm *(arrows)* at both bases, suggesting presence of both pleural effusion and ascites. However, section 10 mm above **(B)** shows apparent diaphragm to have nonuniform shape, to be too wide, and to contain gas *(arrows)*, proving it is collapsed lung surrounded by pleural fluid. No ascites is present.

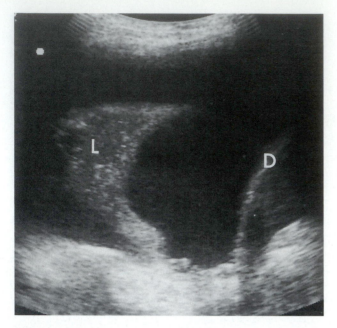

FIGURE 15-52
Free pleural effusion — ultrasound. Collapsed and partially consolidated lung (L) adopts characteristic beaklike configuration in
presence of pleural effusion between it and chest wall and diaphragm (D). Although effusion is overall echo poor, fine homogeneous echoes occurred in dependent half of effusion. Both these
echoes and collapsed lung showed evidence of movement, as would
be expected in presence of pleural fluid (metastatic hyperneph-
roma). (Courtesy of Dr. A.E.A. Joseph, London.)

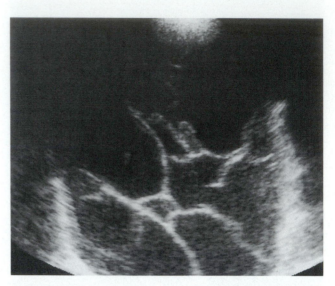

FIGURE 15-53
Ultrasound examination of empyema demonstrates multiple septa
and echo-rich spaces in between. Empyema fluid is commonly
echogenic because of its content of cells and debris.

15-50). This bare area, which lies between the upper and
lower layers of the coronary ligament, is extraperitoneal
and not accessible to ascitic fluid.[221] Therefore fluid
posteromedial to liver suggests a pleural location. Some
care in interpreting this sign is needed because ascitic
fluid can lie above and below the coronary ligament.
Therefore assessing multiple scan levels is important.[231]

In a study of 38 patients with peridiaphragmatic fluid
the interface and bare area signs proved the most accurate
(84% and 92%, respectively).[231] The diaphragm sign
(79%) and displaced crus sign (63%) were less accurate.
A notable feature of this study was significant intraobserver and interobserver variability.[231]

ULTRASOUND AND PLEURAL FLUID. Ultrasound can
be used to image pleural fluid provided there is no
intervening air-containing lung.[240,400,436] This situation
obtains for pleural fluid against the chest wall and for
fluid in other situations where there may be sonic access
through a lung-free window such as the liver.

Pleural fluid is commonly anechoic and delineated on
its lung aspect by a sharp, highly echogenic line (Figure
15-52).[400] This echogenic line is due not to posterior echo
enhancement but rather to high-impedance mismatch
resulting in high-amplitude reflections at the interface
between pleural fluid and air-filled lung. Anechoic or
hypoechoic effusions may be transudates or exudates.[252,726] Some fluid collections are echogenic, and the

pattern of echogenicity may be classified as complex,
nonseptated, complex septated, or homogeneously
echogenic. When pleural lesions are echogenic, a number
of signs indicate they are liquid and not solid: (1) change
in shape with breathing,[400] which may be relatively
subtle because pleural fluid collections often retain their
overall shape relatively unchanged despite maneuvers
designed to alter their position and outline; (2) presence
of septa (Figure 15-53)[385,539] or fibrinous strands; and (3)
dynamic signs elicited during breathing. These include a
flapping movement of septa, strands, and atelectatic lung
and a swirling motion of finely echogenic material
(debris).[361] Very occasionally fluid lesions are encountered that are diffusely and homogeneously echogenic
and that display no dynamic signs. These structures are
indistinguishable from solid pleural lesions. In one series
they made up 3 of 90 cases with pleural fluid collections;
one was an empyema and two were parapneumonic
exudates.[361]

Ultrasound examination is valuable in the evaluation
and management of pleural fluid for several reasons:

1. It is helpful in distinguishing solid from fluid pleural
lesions.[357] Some of the problems with making this
distinction are described previously in relation to fluid
collections that look solid. The reverse sometimes happens when hypoechoic solid lesions are interpreted as
fluid, as occurs occasionally with lymphoma and neurogenic tumors.[539]

2. Ultrasound also enables differentiation of peripheral
lung lesions from pleural fluid[127] and allows evaluation of
their relative extent. Findings that help in this assessment

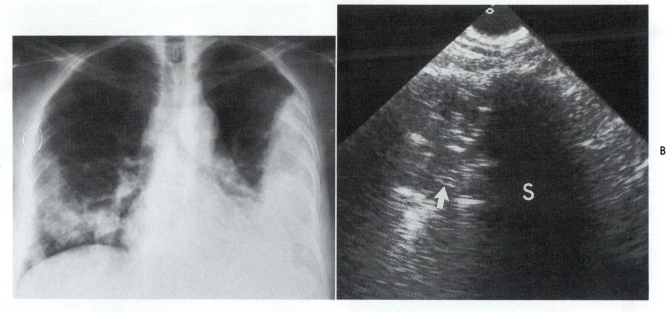

FIGURE 15-54
A, Posteroanterior chest radiograph of patient with pneumonia. It was questioned whether or not opacity against left chest wall was loculated pleural effusion. Its overall shape was suggestive, but irregular inner margin was atypical. **B,** Ultrasound examination shows acoustic shadowings because of rib. Lesion itself is echogenic and contains parallel linear reflections (*arrow*) that could be either airways or vessels. In either case this offers definite evidence that opacity is result of consolidated lung. Distinction between vessels and airways is academic but can be made by assessing pulsation. (Courtesy Dr. A.E.A. Joseph, London.)

include the angle between the lesion and the chest wall and in consolidation the presence of vessels on Doppler examination and of airways as evidenced by air or fluid bronchograms (Figure 15-54).[400] In general, peripheral lung lesions make an acute angle with the chest wall, whereas with pleural ones the angle is obtuse (Figures 15-55 and 15-56). Exceptions to this observation occur when peripheral lung lesions infiltrate the region of the adjacent visceral pleura. A specific example of the use of ultrasound in distinguishing between pleural and lung lesions is in the assessment of the opaque hemithorax. In this situation absence of air allows ultrasound to identify and quantitate possible consolidation, mass, collapse, and abscess in the underlying lung.

3. Ultrasound enables identification of pleural fluid in unusual sites such as in a subpulmonic location.

4. Ultrasound pinpoints localized fluid collections for aspiration, both diagnostic and therapeutic.[471]

5. Ultrasound may identify solid components of a large effusion, which enables directed biopsy.[400,726]

6. Ultrasound can suggest the nature of an effusion. Transudates are typically anechoic and unaccompanied by pleural thickening.[726] Exudates seen with empyema, malignancy, parapneumonic effusions, and hemothorax typically produce echoes that may be diffuse and homogeneous or structured and complex, for example, with septation and stranding.[248,252,726] Other features suggesting that an effusion may be an exudate are adjacent pleural thickening and an adjacent parenchymal lung lesion.[726] Effusions that are diffusely and homogeneously echogenic are commonly empyemas or caused by hemorrhage.[726]

7. Ultrasound is helpful in identifying the causes of some effusions, both inside the chest (e.g., pneumonia) and outside, such as those caused by subphrenic or hepatic abscesses.[451]

MAGNETIC RESONANCE IMAGING AND PLEURAL FLUID. Magnetic resonance imaging (MRI) does not have a significant role in the evaluation of pleural fluid. Pleural fluid has low signal intensity on T1-weighted images (Figure 15-57) and high signal intensity on T2-weighted images. It is often heterogeneous because motion within the effusion creates flow artifacts. Preliminary results of in vitro MRI analysis of pleural fluid analogues (saline with albumin or blood in various dilutions) have suggested that MRI signal intensity has the potential to differentiate among pleural effusions of different composition.[671] In vivo studies are limited. In one study performed on a 0.6 T system using an ungated, triple spin-echo multislice sequence, it was shown that both qualitative and quantitative assessment of signal from pleural effusions differentiated between exudates and transudates.[112] All effusions increased in signal as TE increased, but exudates produced higher signal than transudates, T2-weighted images being the most discriminatory.[112] Other studies have been unable to distinguish

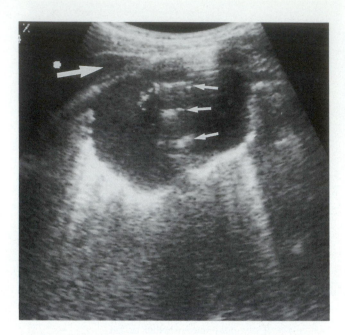

FIGURE 15-55
Lung versus pleural space opacity. Chest radiograph in this patient showed well-defined air containing ovoid opacity against chest wall. On ultrasound, opacity was shown to contain air *(small arrows)* and to be moderately echogenic. These small echoes displayed some mobility. Key finding is acute angle between lesion and chest wall *(large arrow)*, indicating intrapulmonary lesion (abscess). (Courtesy Dr. A.E.A. Joseph, London.)

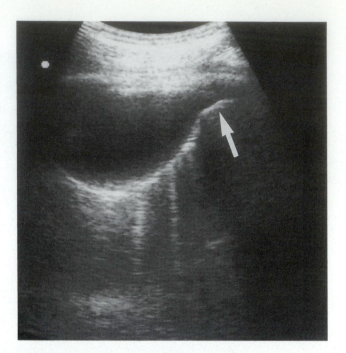

FIGURE 15-56
Lung versus pleural space opacity. Typically obtuse-angled, tapered margin *(arrow)* of pleural opacity, in this case loculated pleural fluid. (Courtesy Dr. A.E.A. Joseph, London.)

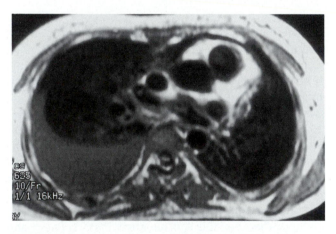

FIGURE 15-57
Transudative pleural effusion on magnetic resonance imaging. The pleural effusion is of low intermediate signal on the T1-weighted image. On T2-weighted image it was high signal.

between transudates and exudates.[654] These latter authors, however, have shown that subacute or chronic hemorrhage can be identified by the characteristically high signal on both T1- and T2-weighted images.[654] In such hematomas the central high signal may be surrounded by a low-signal rim caused by hemosiderin.[400]

In complex loculated effusions the multiplanar capability of MRI can be used to advantage.[112]

Specific pleural effusions

In this section, specific causes of pleural effusion are considered in detail. Effusions caused by pleuropulmonary infection, neoplasm, trauma, asbestos exposure, and collagen vascular diseases[287] are discussed elsewhere. The major causes of pleural effusion other than chylothorax and hemothorax are listed in the box on p. 655.

POSTPARTUM PLEURAL EFFUSION. Small pleural effusions are a normal finding on chest radiography within 24 to 48 hours of delivery. However, the true frequency is difficult to ascertain because selection criteria vary among reports and techniques have lacked specificity.[236] Prevalence rates in the two radiographic series following normal vaginal delivery have been 23%[243] and 67%.[262] Effusions are most commonly small and bilateral. An ultrasound series has failed to corroborate the preceding findings.[659] Other causes for pleural effusion associated with pregnancy have been reviewed.[236]

ADJACENT INFECTION. Infectious processes in the upper abdomen commonly cause pleural effusions, which are usually sterile transudates. This happens particularly with subphrenic (and hepatic) abscesses but also occurs with other forms of upper abdominal suppuration such as perinephric abscess.[560]

Subphrenic abscess. Subphrenic abscess most commonly follows upper abdominal surgery, particularly involving the stomach and spleen.[566] A significant pro-

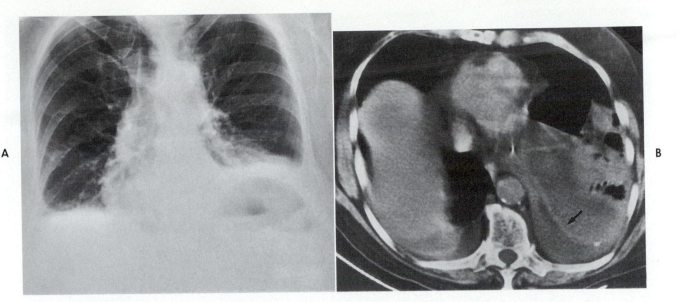

FIGURE 15-58
Pleural effusion — subphrenic abscess. **A,** Posteroanterior chest radiograph shows raised left hemidiaphragm, pleural fluid, two air-fluid levels underneath left hemidiaphragm, and collapse and consolidation of left lower lobe. **B,** Computed tomography of same patient shows slightly thickened diaphragm *(arrow)* between posterior pleural fluid and more anterior subdiaphragmatic fluid, which contains gas, at least some of which is in bowel.

portion of cases, between 10% and 20%,[115,566,592] are not directly related to surgery but follow perforation of a hollow viscus, pancreatitis, or trauma, and a small number are cryptogenic. A subphrenic abscess is commonly delayed to 1 to 3 weeks after surgery but may not develop until many months afterward.[349] With abscesses in contact with the diaphragm there are nearly always changes on the plain chest radiograph (Figure 15-58).[115] About 80% of patients have a pleural effusion,[115,419,566,702] which is usually small to moderate in size. Effusions are usually sterile, but occasionally they are empyematous.[22] Additional radiographic findings commonly include an elevated hemidiaphragm, basal collapse and consolidation, and an air-fluid level below the diaphragm (Figure 15-58). The diagnosis may be virtually established by ultrasound or CT scanning (Figure 15-58).[226]

Hepatic abscess. In a series of 53 patients with pyogenic liver abscesses the chest radiograph was abnormal in 53%.[549] The changes most commonly noted were basilar atelectasis and pneumonitis (44%), hemidiaphragm elevation (31%), and pleural effusion (20%). An air-fluid level was present below the hemidiaphragm in 7% of these patients. The possibility of a hepatic abscess (amebic or pyogenic) should be considered in all patients with an obscure right-sided exudative pleural effusion,[350] particularly if fever, anorexia, and abdominal pain are present. Investigation by ultrasound and CT plays a pivotal role in diagnosis and management, but their consideration is beyond the scope of this discussion.

CARDIOVASCULAR DISEASE

Heart failure. In clinical practice heart failure is probably the most common cause of a transudative pleural effusion; the volume ranges from barely detectable to considerable.[374] It is generally taught that pleural effusions in heart failure are more common and larger on the right, but a review of autopsy and clinical series shows that the excess of right effusions over the left side is not marked: 26% right sided, 16% left sided, 59% bilateral.* Some authors consider that isolated left pleural effusion in heart failure indicates an additional disease process such as pulmonary embolism.[360] This view receives some, but not strong, support from the autopsy series in which one fifth of those with right-sided and one third of those with left-sided effusions had pulmonary infarcts.[510,704] Left-sided pleural effusion following coronary artery bypass surgery has been ascribed to left ventricular failure combined with impaired drainage from the left pleural space following internal mammary artery dissection and pleurotomy.[306] Two unusually distributed forms of fluid collection occur particularly in heart failure: encysted effusion (see p. 661)[157,159] and lamellar "effusion" (see Chapter 9).

The mechanism responsible for the development of pleural effusion in heart failure is still under debate. Most authors have suggested that a mixture of left and right heart failure is necessary. A much quoted experiment

---

*References 29, 337, 403, 484, 510, 695, 704.

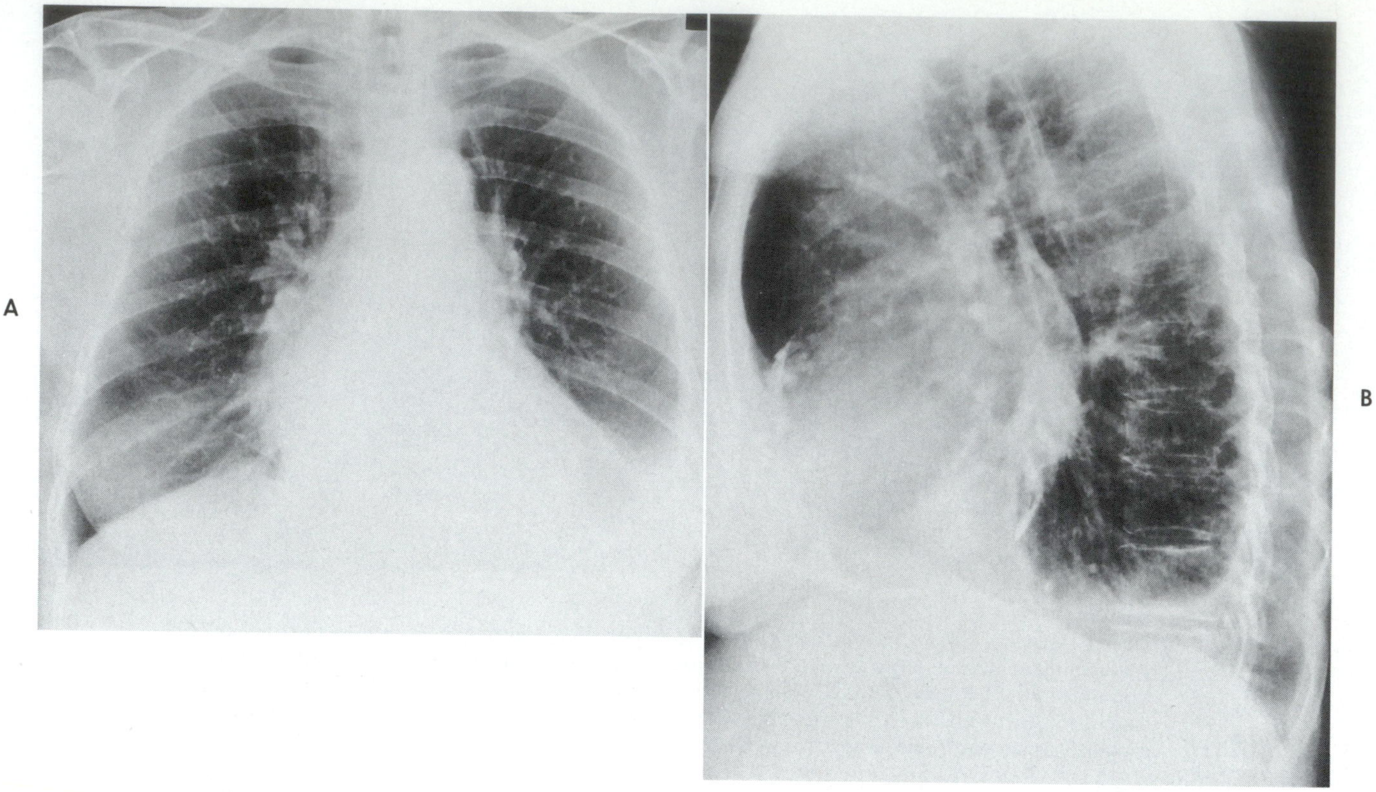

FIGURE 15-59
Pleural effusion — pericarditis. **A,** Posteroanterior chest radiograph in constrictive pericarditis. There is left-sided pleural effusion. **B,** Lateral chest radiograph of same patient shows that pleural fluid is confined to left side. There is heavy pericardial calcification.

conducted in dogs[410] showed that elevation of right-sided pressures caused a greater accumulation of pleural fluid than elevation of left-sided pressures, but that an increase of right- and left-sided pressures together was the most effective maneuver. On the other hand, a recent study of humans in heart failure following myocardial infarction showed that the presence of an effusion correlated much better with elevated left atrial pressure than it did with elevated right-sided pressures,[707] an observation that fits better with the low prevalence of pleural effusions in cor pulmonale.[706,707] On balance it seems likely that edema fluid in the lung interstitium moves across the nontight mesothelial barrier of the visceral pleura into the pleural space along an interstitial-pleural pressure gradient.[559] A number of studies have shown that long-standing effusions[559] or effusions following diuresis[82] may take on the biochemical characteristics of an exudate.

Pericardial disease. Pericardial disease, both inflammatory and noninflammatory, may be associated with pleural effusions. Weiss and Spodick[694] assessed a series of 35 patients with pleural effusions and a variety of pericardial diseases and found that effusions were solely left sided in 60% and predominantly left sided in 71% (9% were right predominant and 20% equal bilaterally) (Figure 15-59).

Post–cardiac injury syndrome. Post–cardiac injury syndrome follows a variety of myocardial and pericardial injuries and is most commonly seen after myocardial infarction (Dressler's syndrome)[130] or cardiac surgery (postpericardiotomy syndrome).[147] Other causes are described, including closed chest trauma.[559] The syndrome is characterized by fever, pleuritis, pneumonitis, and pericarditis days or weeks after the precipitating event and often runs an intermittent course. Study of the condition has been hampered by lack of a diagnostic test and by clinical similarities with pneumonia, extension of myocardial infarction, heart failure, and pulmonary embolism. The prevalence rate is probably a few percent following myocardial infarction[130,348] and somewhat higher after cardiac surgery.[558] Very high frequencies have been reported: 31% in 161 patients undergoing surgery for the Wolff-Parkinson-White syndrome.[288] In one series the syndrome developed on average 20 days after cardiac injury (range 2 to 86 days).[624] The most common symptoms and signs were pleuritic chest pain (91%), fever, pericardial rub, dyspnea, and pleural rub. Nearly all the patients had a high erythrocyte sedimentation rate, and 50% had leukocytosis. None had hemoptysis.

The post–cardiac injury syndrome is usually self-limiting. Should treatment be required, the usual drugs are aspirin, nonsteroidal antiinflammatory agents, or steroids. Relapse may follow drug withdrawal.[558]

The chest radiograph is abnormal in more than 90% of patients. The chief findings are pleural effusion, consolidation, and a large heart. Pleural effusions were present in 81% of patients in four combined series,[130,340,624,635] with unilateral and bilateral effusions approximately equally common. When unilateral, effusions are more common on the left than on the right.[624] About one half to three-fourths of the patients have consolidation, which is usually unilateral (left more than right), and about half have a large cardiac silhouette. In the appropriate clinical setting the diagnosis is suspected on radiologic grounds if pleural effusion(s) and consolidation develop with concomitant rapid enlargement of the cardiac silhouette without evidence of heart failure.[611] Echocardiography establishes the pericardial nature of the cardiac enlargement. The pleural fluid is a serosanguineous or bloody exudate.[624] The post–cardiac injury syndrome is important to identify if only to avoid iatrogenic complications from unnecessary therapy for incorrect diagnoses such as pulmonary embolism.[559]

Superior vena cava syndrome. Occlusion of the superior vena cava might be expected to predispose to the formation of pleural effusion[410] because it increases the parietal pleural hydrostatic pressure, thereby increasing fluid filtration from parietal pleural capillaries, and it reduces lymphatic flow from the thoracic duct and right bronchomediastinal trunk.[633] However, pleural effusion secondary to vena caval obstruction is uncommon. In a series of 35 patients with superior vena cava syndrome, eight had effusions but in only two did superior vena caval obstruction seem a reasonable explanation for its development.[266] In a larger series of 84 subjects with superior vena caval obstruction all four effusions were the result of malignancy.[483] Apart from these series there are isolated case reports of pleural effusion associated with obstruction of the innominate vein[278] and superior vena cava.[211] In the latter case the effusion followed iatrogenic thrombosis and was a transudate, but in other case reports effusions have been chylous.[122,582]

Pulmonary embolism. Pleural effusion is common in pulmonary embolism, occurring in one fourth to one half of the cases.* Effusions are more likely to occur with infarction but can be seen without it; in some series effusion without infarction was considered unusual.[68,104]

The characteristics of pleural effusions in pulmonary embolism have been well described in a prospective study of 155 patients with pulmonary embolism.[68] Effusion was the only chest radiographic sign in 18% of the patients; more commonly it was associated with other signs of pulmonary embolism. Effusions tended to be small, occupying 15% of a hemithorax on average, and none occupied more than one third of the hemithorax. The vast

majority (98%) were unilateral with no side predilection. This observation is somewhat at variance with other series, in which a higher prevalence of bilateral effusions was found.[104,172,638] The effusions were nearly always painful and tended to be maximal within the first 3 days of clinical illness. Only 3% enlarged after this time, an event that should suggest recurrent embolism, infection, or possibly anticoagulant-induced hemorrhage.[599] The effusions tended to disappear within about a week (72% disappearing by 7 days), but effusions accompanied by pulmonary consolidation usually took longer to clear.

CIRRHOSIS OF THE LIVER. Pleural effusion is a well-recognized finding in patients with hepatic cirrhosis. A prevalence varying between 0.4%[430] and 12%[273] is recorded in various series, a range that reflects the differing severity of the underlying liver disease. Effusions may be small to massive,[286,397] and they show a predilection for the right side (Figure 15-36). Thus, in 55 cases from six series, 60% were right sided, 22% left sided, and 18% bilateral.* In one series that looked at cirrhosis with isolated left pleural effusion, 18% of effusions were found to be tuberculous.[425] The authors concluded that isolated left-sided effusions in the context of cirrhosis should be fully investigated and not assumed to be the result of liver disease per se.[425]

Although raised lymphatic pressure, azygos vein hypertension, and hypoalbuminemia play a part in generating cirrhotic effusions,[43] evidence indicates that transdiaphragmatic passage of fluid is the most important mechanism.[347] Under these circumstances the development of pleural effusions depends on the presence of ascites, and this is an almost universal finding in cirrhotic pleural effusion (Figure 15-36),[273,286,397] with only a few exceptions having been reported.[79,179] The corollary, that all patients with cirrhotic ascites have pleural effusions, is by no means true. In one series of 330 patients with hepatic ascites only 5.5% had pleural effusions on plain chest radiography.[346] Transfer of fluid from the peritoneal cavity to the chest has been clearly demonstrated by studies in which blue dye, India ink, and labeled albumin have been introduced into ascitic fluid.[286,346] It is also well recognized that air in the peritoneal cavity can enter the pleural cavity, usually on the right.[51,346,347] Furthermore, defects have been identified in the diaphragm at postmortem examination,[144,346] at thoracotomy, and at thoracoscopy.[171,346,448] Fluid and air have been seen to pass through these defects.[346] The defects are usually found in the tendinous part of the diaphragm and are probably tears produced by the stretching that occurs in the presence of ascites.[347] Localized muscle thinning where vessels pass through the diaphragm may be another predisposing factor. The pathologic features of these lesions have been elegantly demonstrated by Lieberman and Peters.[347] Some of the defects were still closed by peritoneum and appeared as fluid-filled blebs

---

*References 68, 431, 594, 621, 638, 662.

*References 273, 286, 346, 347, 397, 711.

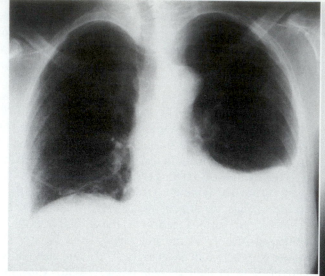

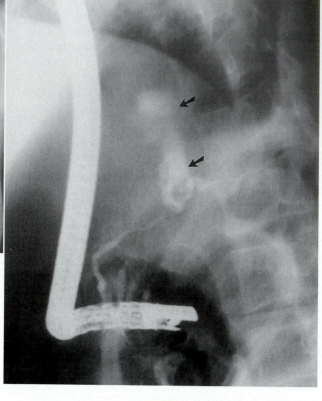

FIGURE 15-60
Pleural effusion—chronic pancreatitis. A 54-year-old woman with previous attacks of pancreatitis gave a short history of dyspnea, which was found to be due to moderate left pleural effusion. Possibility of pancreatic effusion was not considered at the time, but 3 months later serum and pleural amylase levels were found to be modestly raised and similar (1100 IU/L) and left effusion was settling (A). B, Endoscopic retrograde pancreatogram showed sinus track extending up into mediastinum *(arrows).* This was presumed to represent closed fistulous tract accounting for settling effusion and modestly raised pleural amylase level.

on the pleural side of the diaphragm, whereas in others the peritoneal membrane had ruptured, leaving a hole. The structure of the blebs, their possible sudden rupture, and their later occlusion by adhesions probably explains why many patients with ascites have no pleural effusion[346] and why effusions may develop or resolve suddenly.[346,347,711] The right-sided predilection of effusions in ascites may be related to the greater exposure of the tendinous diaphragm on the right, where it is not covered by the heart.

A number of papers have described pleural effusion occurring with hepatitis.[559]

PANCREATIC DISEASE. Pleural effusion occurs in both acute and chronic pancreatitis,[350] and several mechanisms may be pathogenetically important.[559]

The prevalence of pleural effusion in *acute pancreatitis* is about 10% to 20% but may range from 4%[167] to 38%.[442] The presence of an effusion suggests severe pancreatitis.[420] Because of the close relation of the pancreas, particularly the tail, to the left hemidiaphragm, effusions are usually left sided (70%) or bilateral (15%)[167,293,420,442] and are thought to be lymphatic or sympathetic in origin.[532] There may be additional elevation of the hemidiaphragm together with basal consolidation.[538] The clinical picture is usually dominated by abdominal symptoms, although occasionally the patient has dyspnea or pleuritic chest pain.[350]

The effusions are exudates and often hemorrhagic. The amylase levels of the pleural fluid are high and may exceed those in the serum. Pleural amylase values remain elevated even after serum levels have returned to normal values.[398] An elevated amylase level in pleural fluid is not, however, a specific indicator of pancreatitis and may be seen with esophageal perforation and occasionally with pleural malignancy.[350] The effusions usually resolve completely.

Effusions associated with *chronic pancreatitis* are often large and recurrent,[12,424,532,643] and in contrast to acute pancreatitis, chest symptoms usually dominate the clinical picture.[350] The pathogenesis of such effusions is thought to be posterior ductal rupture, allowing pancreatic fluid to move retroperitoneally into the chest via the aortic and esophageal hiatus (Figure 15-60).[72,298,364] Ninety-six cases are recorded in the English literature and have recently been comprehensively reviewed.[532] Patients were characteristically young to middle-aged men with a history of alcohol abuse (80%). At presentation 94% of patients had chest symptoms (67% without abdominal complaints) and only 52% gave a history of pancreatitis. Plain chest radiographs showed pleural effusions, often large with a left-sided predominance (left 67%, right 19%, bilateral 14%) (Figure 15-60). Since pleural fluid had drained directly from the pancreatic duct, pleural fluid amylase levels were dramatically high. Amylase diffuses into the bloodstream from the pleural effusion, usually causing a less striking elevation of *serum* amylase that was occasionally (3%) absent.

On CT nearly all patients had pancreatic pseudocysts (79%) and in 42% of patients the fistulous track was shown.[155,364] In the remaining patients the CT scan was normal or showed changes of pancreatitis. Endoscopic retrograde pancreatography (ERCP) showed the fistulous track[72,121] in 59% of patients (Figure 15-60), and when results from ERCP and CT were combined, the track was shown in 70% of patients and cysts and/or chronic pancreatitis in 25%. Excision of the pancreaticopleural fistula is the treatment of choice if a trial of 2 to 4 weeks of medical therapy fails.[532] Pleural effusions caused by chronic pancreatitis may cause gross pleural thickening requiring decortication.[350]

RENAL DISEASE. Nephrogenic effusions are associated with the following conditions and treatments.[204,560]

Uremic pleurisy and hemodialysis. A fibrinous pleuritis is common in uremia.[261] It may develop despite hemodialysis[37] and is often accompanied by pericarditis. Patients may be asymptomatic or have chest pain and fever.[37,455] The effusions are exudates[455] and are commonly bloody.[189] In one series 79% were unilateral.[37] The effusions may be small or large. In patients who continue to undergo hemodialysis they often subside over weeks. Sometimes, however, fibrous pleural thickening ensues and decortication is required.[196,533]

Urinothorax. Urinothorax is an unusual condition; only 22 cases were reported up to 1986.[563] It is usually an aftermath of obstruction and rupture of the urinary tract with urinoma formation.[26,27] It may also follow blunt[320] or penetrating trauma, particularly iatrogenic, such as renal biopsy,[563] nephrostomy,[519] or renal transplantation.[75] A few cases are described that are a result of hydronephrosis in which no urinoma is demonstrable.[99,319,464] It seems likely that a urinothorax develops when retroperitoneal urine dissects upward into the mediastinum, which then ruptures, allowing urine to escape into the pleural space.[563] The mediastinal widening that accompanies this process may be detectable radiographically.[27] The effusions are usually unilateral and on the same side as the obstructed or traumatized kidney.[560]

In the appropriate clinical setting a low-pH transudate with pleural fluid creatinine levels higher than in the serum establishes the diagnosis.[559] It is important that diagnostic thoracocentesis be performed early before equilibration between pleural and serum levels has had time to develop. The pleural collections subside following drainage of the urinomas and relief of the hydronephrosis.

Nephrotic syndrome. Transudative effusions develop in about 20% of patients with nephrotic syndrome because of the associated hypoalbuminemia.[559] The effusions tend to be bilateral and are commonly subpulmonic[135] and recurrent.[281] If the effusion is unilateral[559] or an exudate

or bloody, pulmonary embolism should be suspected.[359]

Acute glomerulonephritis. Effusions are also common in acute glomerulonephritis, occurring in some 50% of cases.[259,299] The effusions are often multifactorial in origin, with disturbed fluid balance playing an important role.

Peritoneal dialysis. Acute hydrothorax can develop during peritoneal dialysis.[139,553] The effusions most commonly develop within hours of the initiation of dialysis,[166] although effusions delayed a year or more are described.[649] Like ascites-related pleural effusions, those caused by dialysis are usually on the right,[560] although a few have been left sided.[447] Elevated levels of glucose confirm the presence of dialysate in the pleural effusion.[362] In some and possibly all of the cases the mechanism is believed to be direct transfer of fluid from the peritoneal cavity into the pleural space through diaphragmatic defects (see "Cirrhosis of the Liver"). There have, however, been several unsuccessful attempts to demonstrate such communications in patients with pleural effusions who are undergoing peritoneal dialysis.[312,362,447] Possibly therefore other mechanisms play a part in the development of dialysis-related effusions. Their appearance is a contraindication to peritoneal dialysis, since they usually recur when interrupted dialysis is restarted.[553]

Renal infection[491] and perinephric abscess.[560] Renal and perirenal infections are rare causes of ipsilateral sterile exudative pleural effusion.

SPLENIC DISEASE. Splenic disease is an uncommon cause of left-sided pleural effusion. Splenic abscess, most commonly caused by infective endocarditis, is associated with a left pleural effusion in 20% to 50% of patients and may be accompanied by basal collapse and consolidation and hemidiaphragm elevation.[87,284,569] Left pleural effusion is also described associated with splenic infarction[683] and splenic hematoma.[304]

ASCITIC EFFUSION. Ascitic fluid of any cause may be associated with a pleural effusion. The mechanism of pleural effusion formation in the majority of these patients seems to be transdiaphragmatic passage of fluid. The association of ascitic and pleural fluid is well recognized with hepatic cirrhosis, peritoneal dialysis, ovarian hyperstimulation syndrome,[394,575] intraperitoneal dextran,[418] and Meigs' syndrome. The first three conditions are considered elsewhere, and the pathogenesis of ascites-related effusion is discussed in some detail in the section on cirrhosis.

Meigs' syndrome. The earliest descriptions of Meigs' syndrome are those of Salmon in 1934 and Meigs and Cass in 1937.[408,564] The syndrome has four components: ascites, pleural effusion, ovarian fibroma, and resolution of ascites and hydrothorax with removal of the tumor. The definition was later extended[375,406] to include other ovarian tumors: theca cell, granulosa cell, and Brenner tumors. More recently there has been a tendency to include all female pelvic neoplasms, both ovarian and

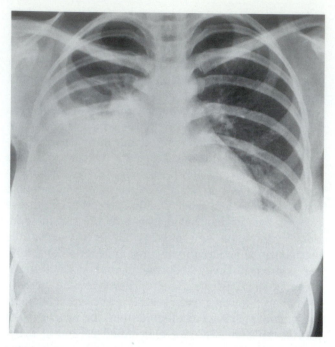

FIGURE 15-61
Pleural effusion—Meigs' syndrome. This 17-year-old had lower abdominal pain and irregular menstrual periods. There was large pleural effusion, which did not contain malignant cells, and also ascites with ovarian mass. Removal of mass (granulosa cell tumor) was followed by resolution of both ascites and pleural effusion. Three years later patient remained well.

uterine.[610] Some authors call this extended syndrome the atypical (pseudo) Meigs' syndrome.[233,467] Majzlin and Stevens[375] reviewed 128 cases of the more limited syndrome and found ovarian fibroma in 82%, theca cell tumor in 9.4%, granulosa cell tumor in 4.7%, and Brenner tumor in 1.6%. The fluid in the chest and abdomen was the same and usually clear, amber-colored transudates. However, various appearances of the effusions are described, including hemorrhagic.[407] Pleural effusions are more commonly right sided with a frequency of 65% on the right, 10% on the left, and 22% bilaterally (Figure 15-61).[375] Meigs' syndrome is uncommon; in one series, out of 283 patients with ovarian fibromas, 51 had ascites but only 2 had pleural effusions as well.[125] The source of the ascites is not clearly established, but evidence suggests that it is produced by transudation from the surface of the larger tumors, possibly resulting from vascular compromise.[125] Once formed, ascitic fluid almost certainly enters the chest through diaphragmatic defects (see earlier discussion in the section "Cirrhosis of the Liver" on p. 675).

The importance of Meigs' syndrome lies in the fact that neither ascites nor pleural effusion necessarily indicates that a pelvic mass is malignant and has metastasized. Furthermore, Meigs'-type syndromes have been described with malignant tumors.[427]

TRAUMATIC EFFUSION

Abdominal surgery. Half the patients in a series of 200 studied 2 to 3 days after abdominal surgery with bilateral decubitus chest radiographs had a pleural effusion.[352] Predisposing factors included upper rather than lower abdominal surgery and postoperative atelectasis. All but one of the effusions settled without complications. The benign nature of early effusions was confirmed in a prospective study of 128 patients having upper abdominal surgery, 70% of whom developed unilateral (37%) or bilateral (63%) effusion.[456]

Small early effusions should be distinguished from larger ones that develop later, since these are more commonly clinically significant, suggesting a complication such as subphrenic abscess (p. 672).[566]

The development of a unilateral effusion in patients with a chronic traumatic diaphragmatic hernia suggests strangulation and infarction of the contained bowel.[15]

Radiation. Pleural thickening[117] and effusion following radiation are recognized but unusual.[345,703] Two pathogenetic mechanisms may underlie pleural effusion: radiation pleuritis or lymphatic and venous obstruction caused by mediastinal fibrosis.[559] In one series of 11 patients with carcinoma of the breast, pleural effusions were mostly small, gradually decreasing and sometimes disappearing in an indolent fashion over many months or years.[21] Suggested criteria for the diagnosis of radiation pleuritis are effusion within 6 months of completing radiation therapy, coexisting radiation pneumonitis, and spontaneous resolution.[21] Reaccumulation or rapid increase in the pleural effusion suggests metastasis.

DRUGS AND THE PLEURA. A number of drugs may cause pleural effusions or pleural thickening. Relevant drugs are listed in the box at right, and all are considered in this section apart from those associated with systemic lupus erythematosus. Drug-induced pleural disease has recently been comprehensively reviewed.[418,559]

Cytotoxic drugs. Pleural changes are described with all types of methotrexate regimens: intermittent high dose,[661] intermittent low dose,[674] and maintenance.[152] Urban and colleagues[661] described a 9% prevalence of pleuritis with a high-dose regimen that produced thickening of fissures on the radiograph but no free fluid. In another series a 4% frequency of pleuritic pain and a 1% frequency of pleural effusion were described.[674] An intermittent low-dose regimen gave a 4% prevalence of pleuritis, but only about 1% had radiographic evidence of pleural effusion.[661] Maintenance therapy may be associated with pulmonary eosinophilia in which dominant parenchymal shadowing is occasionally accompanied by a small pleural effusion.[152] Procarbazine may cause an acute febrile syndrome within hours of its administration,[418] characterized by bilateral interstitial shadowing accompanied by blood eosinophilia and pleural effusions.[138] Pleural effusions have also been described with mitomycin,[474,559] busulfan,[604] and bleomycin.[258,480]

DRUGS CAUSING PLEURAL CHANGES

Drugs causing systemic lupus erythematosus
  Hydralazine
  Isoniazid
  Phenytoin
  Procainamide
  Others (rarely)
Cytotoxic drugs
  Bleomycin
  Busulfan
  Methotrexate
  Mitomycin
  Procarbazine
  Interleukin-2
Antibacterial drugs
  Nitrofurantoin
Antimigraine drugs
  Ergotamine
  Methysergide
Antiarrhythmic drugs
  Amiodarone
Antithyroid drugs
  Propylthiouracil
Skeletal muscle relaxants
  Dantrolene
Vasodilator antihypertensives
  Minoxidil
Dopaminergic receptor stimulants
  Bromocriptine
Beta-adrenergic blockers
  Acebutolol
  Practolol
  Propranolol
Gonadotropin

---

gide-induced pleuropulmonary disease have been reported in the literature since the first report in 1966.[216,418] The syndrome may appear between 1 month and 6 years after the beginning of therapy.[558] Radiography shows unilateral or bilateral pleural thickening and effusions.[215,250,305] Pleural effusions sometimes appear to be loculated.[193] Localized pleural and subpleural fibrosis can simulate a mass lesion.[215] Ergotamine has been implicated in causing unilateral pleural thickening with effusion,[418,634] and ergonovine may have the same effect.[193]

Antiarrhythmic drugs. Amiodarone may produce a variety of changes on the chest radiograph, most commonly parenchymal opacities with either acinar or interstitial characteristics.[98] Pleural thickening and effusions are occasionally present.[210,418,511,732] On average the onset is 6 months after the start of treatment, but the delay ranges from 1 month to several years and the changes are rarely seen if the dose is less than 400 mg/day. The prevalence varies between 1% and 6%.[98] All patients with pleural abnormality have had parenchymal involvement.[210]

Antithyroid drugs. Propylthiouracil has produced a unilateral, eosinophilic effusion.[415]

Skeletal muscle relaxants. Dantrolene may cause chronic symptomatic pleural effusion, which can be unilateral and rich in eosinophils.[487] Symptomatic improvement occurs within days after the drug is stopped, but radiologic clearing may take months.[418]

Vasodilator antihypertensives. There is one case report of minoxidil administration associated with bilateral pleural and pericardial exudative effusions.[688]

Dopaminergic receptor stimulants. Bromocriptine probably causes pleural changes in 2% to 5% of patients receiving the drug for long-term treatment of Parkinson's disease.[395] All patients have been male.[418] Symptoms consist of dyspnea, cough, and pleuritic pain, usually developing 1 to 2 years after the beginning of treatment. Radiologic findings are pleural thickening and effusion, either unilateral or bilateral.[395,418] Interstitial lung opacity may be present[342,529] but functionally appears to be a minor feature.[418] Symptoms resolve with bromocriptine withdrawal, but pleural thickening is usually a persistent feature.[395]

Beta-adrenergic blockers. Practolol, which was withdrawn from the market in 1976, caused a variety of side effects, including pleural thickening and effusion.[149,174,228,387] There is one case report of patchy visceral pleural thickening associated with lung fibrosis caused by acebutolol, which resembles practolol chemically. The radiologic changes were subtle and could be demonstrated only with CT.[720] Propranolol has been implicated in causing a pleural effusion in a patient with sclerosing peritonitis, but the effusion developed after surgery and a clear cause and effect was not established.[9] A single case report of pleural thickening thought to be

Interleukin-2, used for its cytotoxic activity in renal cell carcinoma and melanoma, can produce a capillary leak syndrome[418] characterized in the chest by pulmonary edema and pleural effusions.[381] Uncommonly, pleural effusions are isolated.[95]

Antibacterial drugs. Two syndromes are recognized with nitrofurantoin toxicity[418]: an acute syndrome that develops after hours or days and is probably immunologically based, because the patient usually has taken nitrofurantoin in the past and has eosinophilia, and a chronic syndrome, less commonly associated with eosinophilia, that appears months or years after therapy begins.[558] In one large series 35% of acute reactions were accompanied by interstitial lung opacities and pleural effusions, while isolated pleural effusions developed in a further 8%. In the chronic syndrome there was a 7% prevalence of effusions, which were never the sole manifestation.[257]

Antimigraine drugs. More than 30 cases of methyser-

due to the related drug oxprenolol was found later to be due to mesothelioma.[477]

Gonadotropin. Occasionally gonadotropins administered for infertility secondary to ovulation failure cause a syndrome characterized by abdominal pain and distension, cystic ovarian enlargement, and ascites with pleural effusion.[394,575] The syndrome is associated with high estrogen levels, and the ascites is caused by increased capillary permeability.[418] Pleural effusion is usually secondary to the ascites, but patients with isolated pleural effusion and no ascites are recorded.[283]

MISCELLANEOUS CAUSES OF PLEURAL EFFUSION

Myxedema. Pleural effusions are described in myxedema,[60] but whether they are more commonly transudates or exudates is not clear,[83,349] possibly because they have borderline characteristics.[214] In one series of patients with myxedema about half had a pleural effusion,[384] and these were usually accompanied by pericardial effusions although isolated pleural effusion is recorded.[578] In another series of 128 patients with hypothyroidism, 28 had a pleural effusion of which 79% were nonhypothyroid effusions, 4% were associated with pericarditis, and 18% were diagnosed as hypothyroid effusions by exclusion.[214] Effusions were as commonly bilateral as unilateral and occupied less than one third of the hemithorax. The presence and size of the effusion were not correlated with the degree of hypothyroidism.[214] Effusions disappear with treatment of the myxedema.[578]

Pleural effusion with yellow nails and primary lymphedema. The association between yellow nails and primary lymphedema was first described in 1964,[565] and in the same year the association between pleural effusion and primary lymphedema was recorded.[265] Two years after these accounts the triad of yellow nails, pleural effusion, and primary lymphedema was reported,[143] and by 1986 nearly 100 cases were on record.[459] The nails are not only yellow but also dystrophic[30] and subject to both onycholysis and infection. Lymphedema typically affects the lower legs and is mild.[729] The pleural effusions may be unilateral or bilateral, small or large,[30,246] and are characteristically chronic and persistent (Figure 15-62).[459] The exudates are rich in protein and lymphocytes, but since there is no reflux from the thoracic duct into the lungs, they are not chylous. Other respiratory manifestations are common and include recurrent bronchitis, pneumonia, pleurisy, bronchiectasis,[708] and sinusitis. Bronchiectasis was present in 25% of patients in two series totaling 32 cases.[30,246] Other, less common features are erysipelas and hypogammaglobulinemia.[459]

In a review of 97 patients the male/female ratio was 1:1.6 and the median age at presentation was 40 years.[459] However, the age at presentation and the severity of the manifestations vary widely. At presentation only about half of the patients have the classic triad. About one third of patients have respiratory symptoms at this time, often

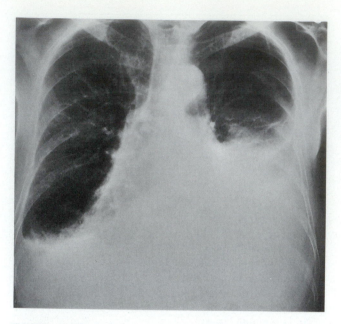

FIGURE 15-62
Pleural effusion — yellow nail syndrome. Bilateral pleural effusions in 74-year-old man. These had been present for several years, and this persistence is characteristic. Effusions are not chylous.

preceded by a long history of sinopulmonary infections.[559] All elements of the triad are thought to result from impaired lymphatic drainage.[559] In the visceral pleura are dilated lymphatics consistent with downstream obstruction,[609] and lymphatic drainage from the pleural space is reduced.[554] The exact mechanism of changes of the nails is, however, not clear.[729] Neither is the pathogenesis of recurrent sinusitis and bronchiectasis; in some they may be related to hypogammaglobulinemia.

The effusions may require pleurectomy or chemical pleurodesis.[265,459]

Familial Mediterranean fever. Familial Mediterranean fever is a rare, autosomal recessive disorder characterized by recurrent attacks of abdominal pain, arthralgia, and pleuritic pain accompanied by fever. It has several synonyms, including periodic disease, periodic fever, recurrent polyserositis, and familial paroxysmal polyserositis.[96] It occurs almost exclusively in non-Ashkenazic Jews, Armenians, Turks, and Arabs. The disease develops in the first decade in 50% of those affected and before the age of 20 years in 75% (range 1 to 40 years). Males outnumber females 2:1.[25] The most common presentation is with paroxysmal, recurrent peritonitis and fever lasting 1 to 4 days, which often lead to unnecessary laparotomy. The peritonitis is commonly accompanied by pleurisy, which is often overlooked. When first examined between 13% and 40% of patients have pleuritis.[25,238,462,597,608] Isolated pleurisy, however, is uncommon at presentation.[25,379,462] Febrile arthropathy, usually of large joints, is the second most common presentation. Colchicine prevents attacks and to some extent suppresses symptoms once an attack has begun.[96] The prognosis is good unless renal amyloidosis develops.

Radiologic manifestations in the chest are uncommon and include diaphragmatic elevation, small pleural effusions, diaphragmatic haziness, and discoid atelectasis.*

Atelectasis and trapped lung. If a portion of lung collapses or is reduced in volume and prevented from reexpanding by a postinflammatory pleural peel ("trapped lung"), the pleural pressure is reduced. This fall in pressure may disturb the balance of forces affecting pleural fluid formation and absorption, leading to the accumulation of pleural effusions. Although not well documented, such a mechanism may account for the presence of pleural effusions postoperatively and with neoplastic bronchial obstruction.[559]

CHYLOTHORAX

A chylothorax contains fluid that is largely chyle (lymph of intestinal origin). Because chyle usually contains suspended fat in the form of chylomicrons, chylothorax fluid is milky. A chylothorax should be distinguished from other milky effusions, particularly empyema and pseudochylothorax, which are discussed later. Before the causes of chylothorax are discussed, the anatomy of the thoracic duct and its tributaries and the physiology of chyle are briefly reviewed.

Anatomy of the thoracic duct and its tributaries†

The thoracic duct connects the cisterna chyli to the great veins in the root of the neck and transports all of the body lymph except that from most of the lungs and the right upper quadrant of the body (Figure 15-63).

The cisterna chyli is formed by the fusion of the two lumbar lymphatic trunks[542] and lies in front of D12 to L2 vertebral bodies. The thoracic duct arises from the cisterna chyli. It is 2 to 8 mm in diameter[463] and valved, particularly in its upper half,[292,463,542] which effectively prevents retrograde flow.[292] Although the thoracic duct is thought of as a single structure, it is commonly multiple in part of its course[664] and may consist of up to eight separate channels.[542] Indeed, in one study, entirely single ducts were less common than multiple ones and at the level of the diaphragms, where the duct is commonly ligated therapeutically, about one third were double.[292] The duct or ducts pass up from the cisterna behind the median arcuate ligament and ascend on the anterior aspect of the vertebral bodies and right intercostal arteries between the azygos vein and aorta. At the level of D6 the thoracic duct crosses to the left of the spine[404] and ascends along the lateral aspect of the esophagus behind the aorta and left subclavian artery. Having reached the

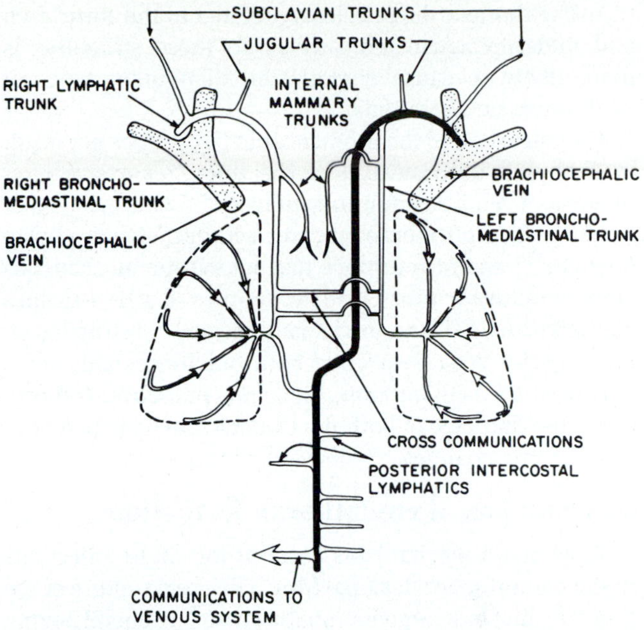

*References 25, 141, 142, 379, 414, 608.
†References 42, 103, 292, 542, 570, 579, 627.

FIGURE 15-63
Lymphatics of thorax. Thoracic duct is shown in black. Major feature is extensive lymphatic anastomoses between both lungs, right bronchomediastinal trunk, and thoracic duct. Another important feature is lymphatic-venous connections remote from brachiocephalic vein. Richness of these anastomoses and connections is such that simply obstructing thoracic duct does not produce chylothorax.

neck, it arches forward across the subclavian artery and inserts into a large central vein within 1 cm of the junction of the left internal jugular and subclavian veins. The number of channels and the site of insertion of the terminal thoracic duct vary.[367] Near its termination the thoracic duct receives the left bronchomediastinal trunk, which drains the left lung, the left jugular trunk, and the left subclavian trunk (Figure 15-63). Any or all of these vessels may end separately in the great veins.

On the right side is a right lymphatic duct that receives the right jugular, right subclavian, right internal mammary, and right bronchomediastinal trunk. The right bronchomediastinal trunk also receives communications from the left trunk (through which it commonly drains the caudad half of the left lung) and from the thoracic duct via the right posterior intercostal lymphatics (Figure 15-63).

The thoracic duct anatomy is clinically important for the following reasons:

1. Immediately after thoracic duct rupture, chyle commonly collects in the mediastinum and may cause a mediastinal swelling.[645] Eventually, however, it bursts through into the pleural space, after a delay that varies from days to months.

2. Because the thoracic duct crosses from right to left in the middorsal region, chylothorax tends to be right sided with low chest trauma and left sided with trauma high in the chest.

3. The thoracic duct is closely related to the aortic arch and midesophagus, and surgery to these structures is more likely to cause chylothorax than other types of cardiothoracic operations.

4. Obstruction to the thoracic duct per se does not result in a chylothorax because of the duct's extensive lymphatic and venous communications.[58,452] This means that it can be tied off therapeutically without adverse consequences[323] and also implies that neoplastic blockade, as with lymphoma, must lead to rupture if it is to cause chylothorax.[292,404] As might be expected, obstruction of the superior vena cava or of both brachiocephalic veins may produce a chylothorax, since this maneuver compromises the drainage of both the thoracic duct and potential anastomotic channels.[44,122,310,582,646]

Mechanisms of chylothorax formation

Three main mechanisms account for chyle collections in the pleural space: leakage from a discrete rupture of the thoracic duct or a large lymphatic vessel; a general oozing from pleural lymphatics; and passage of chylous ascites through the diaphragm.[458]

Direct leakage from the duct occurs with disruption because of trauma or neoplastic involvement. A phase of accumulation may occur within the mediastinum before the mediastinal pleura becomes breached and chyle spills over into the pleural cavity.

Blockage of the thoracic duct can cause extensive collateral formation in the parietal pleura, and these may rupture, allowing seepage of chyle from the parietal pleura (Figure 15-64). The degree and type of collateral formation with thoracic duct block vary depending on the richness of an individual's lymphatic-lymphatic and lymphatic-venous connections. Another factor that promotes pleural seepage is reflux of chyle into the lungs. With a few exceptions,[218] chyle does not gain access to the lungs or visceral pleura because both the intrapulmonary lymphatics and the thoracic duct are valved.[651] Valvular incompetence, however, allows chyle to reflux into the lungs and to ooze from the visceral pleura over the lung surface (Figure 15-64). The development of a "lymphangitic" radiologic pattern in the lungs and a chylothorax after obstruction of the thoracic duct and the right bronchomediastinal trunk has been described.[33,582] The "lymphangitic" pattern in these cases almost certainly represented dilated lung lymphatics distended by chylous reflux (Figure 15-64). Factors that promote reflux are lymphatic vessel dilation, increased thoracic duct and lymphatic vessel pressure, and maldevelopment of valves and lymphatic vessel walls.[693] Seepage of chyle from fragile lymphatic vessels and collaterals is possibly the mechanism for chylothorax formation associated with lymphangiomatous malformations.[131]

The third mechanism of chylous effusion formation is transdiaphragmatic passage of chylous ascites. This is a recognized but unusual occurrence.[458] The mechanism is the same as that involved with transdiaphragmatic passage of cirrhotic ascites (see "Cirrhosis of the Liver" earlier in this chapter).

Physiology of chyle[349,366,386,543,570]

Lymph flowing up the thoracic duct is derived principally from the gut (60%) and to a lesser extent from the liver (35%) and the peripheral lymphatics (5%). About 1.5 to 2.5 L/day is produced.[463,687] It flows upward because of contractions of the duct wall, adjacent arterial pulsations, gut contractions, the pressure gradient from the abdomen to the thorax, and vis a tergo.[42] Flow is increased by increased fluid intake and particularly by fat ingestion, an effect that may increase flow tenfold for several hours. Between 60% and 70% of the fat absorbed by the gut passes by way of the thoracic duct. Chyle contains about 0.5 to 6 g/dl fat, 3 g/dl of protein, and electrolytes as in serum. There are 2000 to 20,000 white cells, mostly T lymphocytes, per milliliter of chyle.[366] Loss of chyle from the body, as occurs with drainage of a chylothorax, has serious consequences, including inanition, lymphopenia, and immune compromise.

Most of the fat in chyle is carried as triglycerides in the form of chylomicrons, which gives chyle its characteristic milky appearance. Two other types of pleural fluid may appear milky and should be distinguished: (1) empyema, in which the milkiness is due to leukocytes that, unlike chylomicrons, settle out on standing or centrifugation, and (2) pseudochylous effusions, in which the milkiness is due to cholesterol or lecithin-globulin complexes. Pseudochylous effusions may be distinguished from true chylous effusions by their high cholesterol content and their occurrence in characteristic clinical settings in which there has been long-standing disease with pleural thickening. Not all chylous effusions are milky, and in one series 53% of 38 chylous effusions were initially not diagnosed because they were turbid or bloody.[618] Furthermore, during starvation, as may occur following surgery, flow is reduced and the characteristic milkiness may disappear.[49,543] The diagnosis of a chylous effusion is made by measuring the triglyceride levels of the effusion.[618] Levels above 110 mg/dl are taken as positive, levels below 50 mg/dl as negative. In patients with intermediate values, lipoprotein electrophoresis[584] should be performed. With bilateral effusions it should not be assumed that if one is chylous both are.[331] Chyle is bacteriostatic and does not irritate the pleura, so it does not cause pain, pleuritis, or fibrosis.

Causes of chylothorax

Chylothoraces can be conveniently classified (see box on p. 684) as neoplastic, traumatic, idiopathic, or of miscellaneous origins.[570] In most series, about 50% have been neoplastic,[49,370,663] 25% traumatic, and 15% idiopathic.[570]

NEOPLASTIC CAUSES. Lymphomas make up about 75% of the neoplastic lesions,[49,370,548,618] and chylotho-

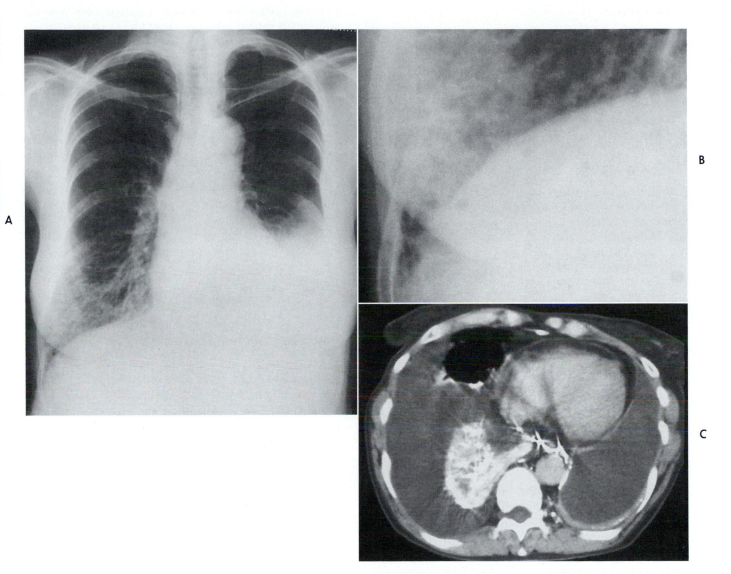

FIGURE 15-64
Chylothorax — cryptogenic. **A,** Posteroanterior chest radiograph of 64-year-old woman who presented with dyspnea and was found to have left chylothorax. At right lung base there are thick septal lines. Patient had had right chylothorax 7 years previously. **B,** Localized view of septal lines. **C,** Computed tomography (CT) following lymphangiogram shows multiple lymphatic channels in posterior mediastinum, lymphatic collaterals in left parietal pleura, as well as gross reflux of contrast medium into collapsed right lung. There are bilateral effusions (chylothoraces) at this stage with CT (Hounsfield) number of about 20. Lymphatic channels in mediastinum could not be traced above D3. Cause was obscure. Chylothorax presumably was formed by reflux into lung and seepage from visceral pleura. Contribution from parietal pleura seems likely as well.

CAUSES OF CHYLOTHORAX

NEOPLASTIC

Lymphoma
Metastatic carcinoma

TRAUMATIC

Operative
  Cardiac
  Esophageal
  Thoracic
  Cervical
Penetrating injuries
Closed injuries
  Major
  Minor

MISCELLANEOUS

Systemic venous hypertension
Obstruction of central systemic veins
Scarring processes
  Mediastinal
  Nodal (filariasis)
Developmental anomalies
  Thoracic duct atresia
  Lymphangioma
  Lymphangiectasia
  Lymphangioleiomyomatosis and tuberous sclerosis
Cryptogenic

---

rax can be the initial feature of lymphomas.[349] When chylothorax is associated with carcinoma, it suggests mediastinal metastasis.[543]

TRAUMA. The most common form of trauma is surgery, particularly cardiac surgery. The frequency of chylothorax with cardiothoracic surgery is between 0.2% and 0.56%,[49,81,377] and the condition is most commonly seen with surgery for Fallot's tetralogy, patent ductus arteriosus, and coarctation of the aorta. Chylothorax is also described with coronary artery surgery,[311,692] thoracoplasty and pneumonectomy (Figure 15-65), esophagoscopy and esophageal resection,[570] esophageal sclerotherapy,[465] thoracic sympathectomy, and block dissection of the neck.[570] Chylothorax may follow penetrating injuries such as stab and bullet wounds.

Closed chest trauma, ranging from major trauma with crush injuries and spinal fractures[134,366] to very minor injuries, is recognized as causing chylothorax. Minor injuries include childbirth,[73,236] vomiting and weight lifting,[570] coughing,[323] and the hyperextension and stretching that accompany yawning.[520] It has been suggested that for such trivial trauma to cause duct rupture, a duct must be distended by a high postprandial lymphatic flow.[42]

IDIOPATHIC CAUSES. A significant number of cases of chylothorax are cryptogenic (Figure 15-64), and in the

neonatal period this variety is the most common cause of a pleural effusion. Many of the adult cases arise following trauma that is so minor it is not recalled or recorded.

MISCELLANEOUS. The remaining 10% of chylothoraces have a great variety of causes, many of which fall into one of four subgroups:

1. Impaired venous drainage. This has been recorded with raised venous pressure caused by heart disease[54,370] and with central venous thrombosis that affects subclavian and brachiocephalic veins and the superior vena cava.* Despite a number of case reports chylothorax remains a rare complication of central venous thrombosis, and in one series of 25 cases no examples were encountered.[4]

2. Scarring. This is probably the common mechanism in chronic pancreatitis,[317] fibrosing mediastinitis, radiation exposure, tuberculosis,[665] and filariasis.[180,300]

3. Developmental anomalies. Under this broad heading can be included thoracic duct atresia[548]; tuberous sclerosis and lymphangioleiomyomatosis; pulmonary lymphangiectasia, either per se or as part of Noonan's syndrome[192,579]; and lymphangiomatous anomalies, which are often associated with massive osteolysis.[23,59,132,622]

4. Transdiaphragmatic passage of chylous ascites.[434,458]

Radiology of chylothorax

A chylous effusion on plain radiographs cannot be distinguished from other effusions. Chylothoraces vary from small to massive, can be unilateral or bilateral, and are slightly more frequent on the right side in large series.[366] Reference has already been made to the mass-like accumulation in the mediastinum that may precede the effusion[154,260,367,645] and the delay, which can vary from days to months, between trauma and the eventual development of chylothorax.[244,370,517,543,576] CT may demonstrate a causal mediastinal lymphoma that is covert on the chest radiograph. The CT attenuation density of chyle, despite the fat content, is usually indistinguishable from other effusions because it is protein rich (Figure 15-64), although in one report the CT density was significantly reduced.[331]

Lymphography has been commonly performed in assessments of chylothorax.[122,422,579,665] Lymphography can show leakage of contrast material into the pleural space[579] and may also demonstrate the exact site of thoracic duct rupture,[453] which may help in directing surgical repair. It also demonstrates lymphoma,[180] duct blockage with accompanying collaterals (Figure 15-64),[180,453,665] and lymphatic malformations, including lymphangiectasia.[23] The exact role of lymphography in the investigation of chylothorax is debatable, and with current surgical practice and the advent of CT it is not important. The thoracic duct can be opacified by the use

---

*References 122, 140, 249, 310, 582, 684.

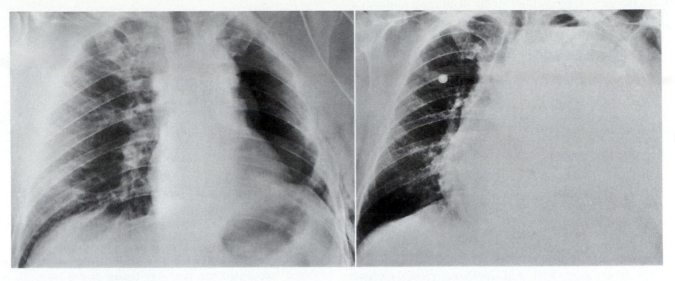

FIGURE 15-65
Chylothorax — traumatic. **A,** Anteroposterior chest radiograph immediately following left pneumonectomy for carcinoma of lung. **B,** Just over 1 week later, pleural effusion developed rapidly and proved
to be chylothorax. This complication of cardiothoracic surgery is seen especially following operations
for Fallot's tetralogy, patent ductus arteriosus, and coarctation of aorta.

of oral ethiodized oil before CT examination.[113] CT is
probably the best approach in screening for lymphoma.
Once neoplasia is excluded, details about the exact
mechanism and point of leakage often play little part in
treatment, because if medical management fails, the
usual approach is to tie the thoracic duct at the diaphragm[663] or perform a pleurodesis. Successful treatment
using a pleuroperitoneal shunt has recently been described.[300]

Pseudochylothorax

Pseudochylothorax is also a milky effusion, but the
milky appearance is the result of cholesterol or lecithin-
globulin complexes rather than chylomicrons. Several
reviews of the condition have been published.[90,247,349,570]
Pseudochylothorax characteristically occurs in pleural
disease of many years' duration, with chronic encysted
effusion, pleural thickening, and sometimes calcification.
It most commonly follows, or is associated with, tuberculosis[247] and rheumatoid disease.[90,164] Unusual causes,
including paragonimiasis,[285] are described.[570] The clinical context in which the effusion occurs is so characteristic that pseudochylothorax rarely causes diagnostic
confusion with a true chylothorax.

HEMOTHORAX

Hemothorax usually results from trauma,[222] but on
occasion it occurs in other conditions (see box above
right). The natural history of hemothorax depends in part
on the source of the bleeding. Low-pressure bleeding
from the lung tends to stop spontaneously because the
pleural fluid compresses and collapses the lung. High-

> ### CAUSES OF HEMOTHORAX
>
> Trauma
>   Open
>   Closed (with or without fracture)
>   Iatrogenic[421]
> Infection
>   Varicella[535]
> Coagulopathy
>   Hemophilia[513]
>   Anticoagulants[24,416,418]
> Vascular abnormality
>   Arteriovenous malformation[612]
>   Dissecting aortic aneurysm
>   Atherosclerotic aneurysm[118]
> Rib exostosis[80]
> Neurofibromatosis with pregnancy[236]
> Pulmonary neoplasm[118]
> Extramedullary hemopoiesis[315,630]
> Pneumothorax[70,714]
> Catamenial hemothorax (endometriosis)[591,727]
> Idiopathic[114,603,731]

pressure bleeding from systemic vessels is less susceptible
to the tamponade effect of pleural fluid,[524] and the
bleeding may be rapid and persistent with the formation
of a tension hemothorax.[24] In the context of trauma other
causes of rapidly accumulating pleural fluid should be
considered, including ruptured esophagus, ruptured thoracic duct, traumatic subarachnoid-pleural fistula,[504] and
iatrogenic causes, particularly those related to venous
lines.

In the acute state nothing on the plain chest radiograph distinguishes hemothorax from other collections of pleural fluid. However, on CT a hemothorax may show areas of hyperdensity.[719] With clotting of the blood, loculation tends to occur and fibrin bodies may form.[161,714] Hemothorax may eventually organize and cause massive pleural thickening (fibrothorax), necessitating decortication, a complication that can be avoided by early evacuation of the pleural space.

PLEURAL MASS

Pleural mass lesions are uncommon. Radiographically they may resemble pleural fluid collections loculated against the chest wall, chest wall masses, or pleurally based parenchymal lung masses. An important feature of these lesions on plain radiology is that they look entirely different when viewed en face and tangentially.

En face, chest wall and localized pleural lesions characteristically appear as homogeneous, often partly rounded opacities with a sharp medial edge and an ill-defined lateral margin (Figure 15-40). This typical appearance is produced because the medial border is usually aligned in a tangential fashion to the x-ray beam, generating a sharp marginal image. The lateral beam, on the other hand, is angled away from the tangent of the lung–soft tissue interface and passes through a wedge-shaped mass of soft tissue, which therefore has no clearly defined lateral margin (Figure 15-66). Tangentially both chest wall and localized pleural lesions are convex to the lung and sharply marginated, since they are both covered on the lung aspect by pleura. At their periphery these lesions often lift off a tail of pleura, creating an obtuse angle of contact with the chest wall (Figure 15-40). On plain radiographs localized lesions of the chest wall frequently cannot be distinguished from localized pleural lesions unless there is rib remodeling or destruction. These signs are characteristic of a chest wall lesion, and apart from the occasional neoplastic or infective lesion (actinomycosis, tuberculosis) they are rarely seen with pleural or lung processes. Rarely a chest wall lesion has a detectable layer of extrapleural fat on its inner aspect, allowing it to be unequivocally localized to the chest wall on a plain radiograph — the pleural coif sign.[521] The CT equivalent of this sign has also been described.[232]

Intrapulmonary lesions differ from pleural lesions in that they tend to have a less clearly defined lung interface (Figure 15-54) and may show characteristic inhomogeneities, such as an air bronchogram. Classically, they make an acute angle of contact with the visceral pleura, but with local infiltration, as may occur with a neoplasm, this can become obtuse.[713]

Ultrasound examination is helpful in establishing the solid nature of a pleural mass lesion.[357] Mass lesions are typically homogeneous and echogenic but may be hypoechoic.[321,501] Lymphoma and neurofibroma are recognized causes of solid hypoechoic lesions.[539] On the other hand, septation and dynamic signs elicited during breath-

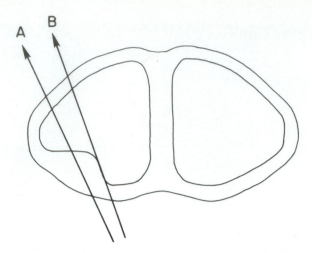

FIGURE 15-66
Diagramatic cross section of chest shows relationship between pleural mass lesion and two x-ray beams. Medial beam *(B)* is oriented tangentially to medial margin of mass, which will therefore have well-defined edge on radiograph. Lateral aspect of mass does not have tangential interaction with *A* and will not produce well-marginated image. Similar considerations will apply to chest wall lesions and loculated pleural collections. (From Wilson AG: *Br J Hosp Med* 37:526-534, 1987.)

ing are reliable indicators that a collection is fluid.[361,385,539] Disruption of the pleural line indicates chest wall invasion.[52]

CT provides a more sensitive way of detecting the signs that are assessed on plain radiographs and of placing a lesion in an anatomic compartment.[713] The presence of an obtuse angle between mass and chest wall, an important sign with all imaging modalities, indicating a pleural or extrapleural location, may be absent. Thus in a series of six benign fibrous pleural tumors not one made an obtuse angle with the chest wall.[116] However, the acute angles of such lesions were marginated by a tapered fringe. Pleural and extrapleural lesions displace the lung parenchyma, bowing adjacent airways and causing compression atelectasis.[400] CT is particularly helpful in detecting invasion of the chest wall with disruption of soft tissue planes and formation of masses (Figure 15-67).[501] In one study comparing plain radiography and CT in a variety of peripheral (lung, pleura, and chest wall) abnormalities, CT provided information that was not readily available on the plain radiograph in two thirds of patients.[500]

Conditions that produce local pleural masses are listed in the box on the facing page.

Lipoma

Lipomas are the most common benign soft tissue tumors of the chest wall.[470] Their exact origin is not always clear, but they can arise from subpleural adipose tissue and be present as a local pleural mass. They can extend into the chest wall (Figure 15-40), taking on an hourglass configuration[540] and remodeling adjacent

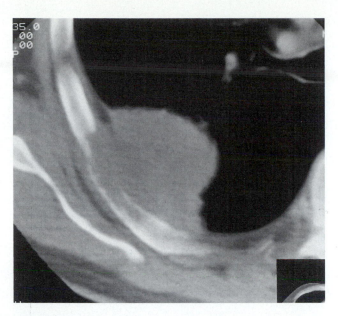

FIGURE 15-67
Pleural mass on computed tomography. Mass shows typical configuration with obtuse angle and tapered margin *(arrow)* under which there is local excess of extrapleural fat. There is also rib destruction. Such a lesion could be primarily pleural or chest wall. Asymmetry of mass and configuration of extrapleural fat suggest that its origin is pleural (metastatic adenocarcinoma).

CAUSES OF LOCALIZED PLEURAL MASSES

Metastasis extrathoracic, thymoma
Bronchial carcinoma (local spread)
Localized fibrous tumor (benign, malignant)[56,116,146,332]
Lymphoma[53,595]
Lipoma (rarely liposarcoma)[440]
Fibrin body
Thoracic splenosis
Others
    Endometriosis[269,727]
    Multiple benign fibromas[574]
    Amyloid[368]

---

ribs,[640] which may show hyperostosis.[66] Since they are soft lesions, they may change shape with respiration.[217] Although they are of soft tissue density on plain radiographs (Figure 15-40), they have a diagnostically low-fat density on CT (Figure 15-40)[148,501] and occasionally punctate calcification.[66] Lipomas on MRI are high signal on T1-weighted images and intermediate signal on T2-weighted images.[400]

Fibrin body

Fibrin bodies develop in the pleural cavity from fibrin-rich fluid,[63] particularly but not necessarily when both air and fluid are in the pleural space. They were common when therapeutic pneumothorax was used to treat tuberculosis and in one series were present in 21% of cases,[530] although the usual figure is about 1%.[150] Fibrin bodies are usually single, homogeneous, well-demarcated, spherical or ovoid mass lesions lying near the diaphragm (Figure 15-28).[63] They may be mobile or fixed[150] and are uncommonly more than 4 cm in diameter.[644] They may spontaneously and rapidly disappear or remain stable for many years.[63] Their only importance lies in possible confusion with a fungal or neoplastic mass.[191] They should always be considered in the differential diagnosis when a pleural mass or nodule develops after a pleural effusion or thoracotomy (Figure 15-28).[161]

Thoracic splenosis

Thoracic splenosis is a rare condition[106] in which tissue from a traumatized spleen crosses an injured diaphragm and proliferates within the left thorax.[572] The resulting pleural nodules are often multiple and usually less than 3 cm in diameter, but may be up to 7 cm.[572] The nodules are implanted on parietal or viscera pleura, including fissures.[429] On radiologic study they usually appear as pleural mass lesions of water density, but they may show intraparenchymal features both on conventional radiographs and with CT.[572] Probably the majority of these apparently intrapulmonary lesions have pleural contact, although possibly some have been implanted in a lung laceration rather than on the pleural surface. The presence of left-sided subpleural or pleural nodules in a patient with a history of splenic and diaphragmatic injury suggests thoracic splenosis.[572] Should the spleen have been removed at the time of trauma, the absence of Howell-Jolly bodies in a blood film would suggest persisting ectopic splenic activity.

The diagnosis may be confirmed with scintiscans using ^{99m}Tc sulfur colloid, ^{99m}Tc-labeled heat-damaged erythrocytes, or ^{111}In-labeled platelets, all of which are taken up by the ectopic splenic tissue.[109,572]

The importance of these lesions is that they may be misinterpreted as resulting from a neoplastic disorder.

PLEURAL THICKENING

Pleural thickening can be localized or generalized and usually represents the organized end stage of a variety of active processes, particularly infective and noninfective inflammation, hemothorax, and asbestos- and drug-related disease. It is virtually always present after thoracotomy and pleurodesis[401] and may follow irradiation. Particularly gross examples are seen following tuberculosis. Extensive unilateral pleural calcification, thickening, and evidence of previous parenchymal disease favor tuberculosis and (possibly to a lesser extent) empyema. A bilateral abnormality favors asbestos-related disease.[436] If pleural thickening is extensive, it is termed a fibrothorax. Fibrothorax may be associated with significant ipsilateral volume loss and ventilatory impairment.

The plain radiographic changes are more commonly unilateral than bilateral and consist of soft tissue shad-

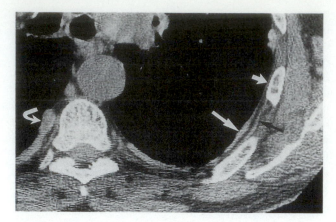

FIGURE 15-68
Pleural thickening—asbestos exposure. Thin soft tissue line on inside of rib *(broad arrow)* indicates pleural thickening. Nearby, pleural line *(large arrow)* becomes thicker and denser (calcified). Fatty layer below pleural thickening is subpleural and limited on outside by combined endothoracic fascia and innermost intercostal muscle layer *(black arrow)*. Widening of subpleural fatty layer commonly accompanies chronic pleural thickening. Paravertebral opacity *(curved arrow)* is local pleural thickening and not a vein, since it stands proud of pleural surface.

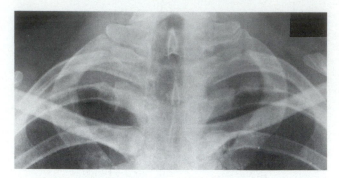

FIGURE 15-69
Apical pleural caps. Symmetric soft tissue opacities are projected under both second ribs. They are slightly atypical for pleural caps, being thicker (1 cm) than usual, with some irregularity of their lower margins. Appearance of pleural caps is quite variable.

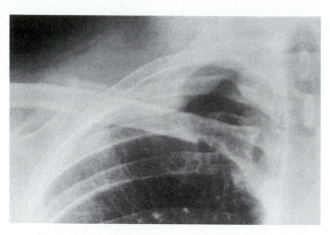

FIGURE 15-70
Pleural thickening—pseudoapical cap. Localized apical view in 27-year-old asymptomatic man shows lenticular soft tissue density projected under posterior aspect of second rib. Its maximum width is 2 cm, and it is sharply demarcated from lung. It has appearances of apical pleural cap, although some features are unusual: its particularly sharp demarcation from lung, its lateral offset from true apex, and its thickness. Ribs appear normal. Findings could indicate either pleural or extrapleural lesion, and final diagnosis was neurofibroma. There is rhomboid fossa in clavicle.

owing, characteristically in the more dependent lateral and posterior parts of the chest. Blunting of the costophrenic angle is common and is often angular, distinguishing it from the more smoothly curvilinear pleural fluid. Decubitus radiographs and ultrasound are particularly helpful in making this distinction. En face, extensive pleural thickening gives a veil-like opacity that has no clear margins and crosses known pulmonary boundaries. Tangentially, it appears as a soft tissue density immediately inside and parallel to the chest wall, sharply marginated on its inner aspect and fading into the soft tissues of the chest wall laterally. Such pleural thickening can extend into and thicken fissures.

On ultrasound, pleural thickening produces a homogeneously echo-dense layer subjacent to the chest wall, but it cannot be reliably detected unless it is about 1 cm or more thick.[400] There is no posterior echo enhancement, but this is often difficult to assess because the soft tissue–lung interface is normally so reflective (Figure 15-68).

On CT, pleural thickening is detected as a layer of soft tissue opacity lying at the chest wall–lung interface. It can be detected almost as well with conventional CT as with HRCT, although the latter is more sensitive in assessing asbestos-related plaques.[2] In addition, HRCT may sometimes clarify equivocal findings on CT.[338] On HRCT, pleural thickening is best assessed inside ribs where there should be no discernible soft tissue; exceptions to this "rule" are discussed on p. 642.[271] Paravertebrally any thickening of the normally insignificant pleural line is abnormal. HRCT is very sensitive and can detect thickening on the order of 1 to 2 mm. The

extrapleural fat layer, which is normally absent or relatively thin, thickens in chronic pleural disease, particularly with chronic empyema,[271,263,577,673] making appreciation of pleural thickening easier. When this fat has higher density than usual, it suggests that the pleural process is "active."[637] Both the distribution and morphology[371] of diffuse pleural thickening are helpful in identifying a cause. In one study the specificity of various CT signs in differentiating a malignant from a benign pleural process was measured. The four most useful signs of malignancy (with specificities) were circumferential thickening (100%), nodularity (94%), parietal thickening greater than 1 cm (94%), and mediastinal pleural involvement.[338]

A number of normal findings relating to the chest wall can closely resemble local or generalized pleural thickening:

1. Apical pleural cap. An idiopathic apical pleural cap is an irregular, usually homogeneous, soft tissue density that may be found at the extreme lung apex (Figure 15-69).[523] The lower border is usually sharply margined and may be smoothly curvilinear, tented, or undulating.[522] Caps are usually less than 5 mm thick, but the width is variable. In two series caps were about as common unilaterally (11% and 7%) as bilaterally (11% and 12%).[275,522] When bilateral the caps were usually asymmetric. The frequency of occurrence increased with age: 6.2% up to 45 years of age and 15.9% over 45 years of age.[523] The opacity is formed by an apical subpleural scar that is nonspecific and unrelated to tuberculosis.[65] The differential diagnosis of an idiopathic apical cap includes nongranulomatous and granulomatous (tuberculous, fungal) infection, radiation pleuritis, lymphoma, pleural and extrapleural neoplasms (Figure 15-70), extrapleural hematoma, prominent subclavian artery, mediastinal lipomatosis,[402] and apicolateral extrapleural fat.[494] It is particularly important that the cryptogenic variety be distinguished from a Pancoast tumor.[402] A recent HRCT study has shown somewhat surprisingly that the bulk of the apical "pleural" opacity associated with previous tuberculosis is caused by a greatly thickened (up to 25 mm) layer of fat between visceral pleura and the endothoracic fascia—innermost intercostal muscle stripe.[270]

2. Rib companion shadows. Rib companion shadows are bands of soft tissue density lying inside ribs. They have smooth margins and are almost parallel to the ribs.[523] Occasionally they appear as a line of soft tissue density separated from the rib by a less attenuating layer. This sandwich appearance could be due to subpleural fat but is more likely to be a Mach effect.[102,327] Companion shadows are the best developed posterolaterally inside the second and third ribs and are also present more caudad against the chest wall in relation to the sixth to ninth ribs.

3. Serratus anterior shadowing. Serratus anterior shadowing can produce a variety of soft tissue densities,[94,198] mostly low and laterally, overlying the anterolateral end of the ribs. Here the digitations of the serratus create repeating triangular shadows with sharp inner margins that fade laterally. The other common pattern is a convex, low-profile shadow that projects inward from the lateral chest wall and closely resembles asbestos-related pleural plaques. Muscle slips can usually be distinguished from plaques on plain radiographs.[568] CT allows unequivocal differentiation.

4. Extrapleural fat. Extrapleural fat may generate confusing shadows that can resemble generalized pleural thickening or plaques.[151,567,667] The distribution varies from patient to patient. Sometimes the fat is widely distributed in the form of a peel. More commonly it is

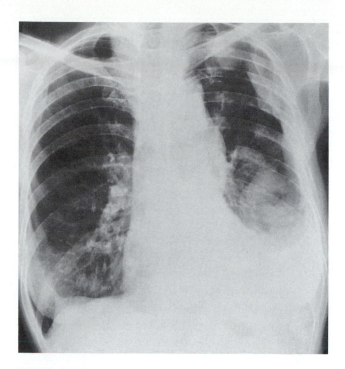

FIGURE 15-71
Pleural thickening—diffuse. In left hemithorax there is diffuse pleural thickening. It is irregular and coarsely nodular and is accompanied by pleural effusion. Pleural thickening also affects mediastinal pleura and distorts mediastinal silhouette. Combination of findings is very suggestive of malignant process, in this case metastatic adenocarcinoma. Mesothelioma could have identical appearance.

localized and develops particularly over the fourth to eighth ribs between the anterior axillary line and the rib angles.[567] Excess thoracic fat often occurs in obese patients, but there are exceptions. The more localized forms of fat deposition can be difficult to distinguish from plaques on plain radiographs, since both are of soft tissue density. Change over time on repeated radiographs may provide discriminative information, but if doubt remains, CT becomes the examination of choice because of its ability to identify fat.[567]

Pleural thickening, particularly when generalized, is often correctly dismissed as an inactive residuum. Care, however, must be taken to distinguish it from various active processes, some of which are neoplastic. Although a number of these conditions tend to give plaquelike, nodular or irregular shadowing (Figure 15-71), they occasionally closely resemble simple inactive pleural thickening. Disorders to consider include mycetoma-related pleural thickening, diffuse pleural mesothelioma, diffuse pleural metastases, leukemia, lymphoma, and Wegener's granulomatosis.

PLEURAL CALCIFICATION

Virtually any process that can cause pleural thickening can go on to calcify,[669] but in practice calcification is

CAUSES OF PLEURAL CALCIFICATION

Infection
   Tuberculous empyema
   Nontuberculous empyema
Hemothorax
Mineral inhalation
   Asbestos (including tremolite talc)
   Mica
   Zeolites
Miscellaneous
   Chronic pancreatitis[67]
   Chronic hemodialysis[685]
   Calcified metastasis
   Alveolar microlithiasis[308,478]

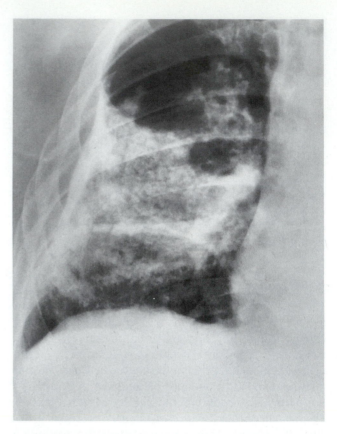

FIGURE 15-72
Pleural calcification. Localized view of right middle and lower zone shows sheetlike calcification. Laterally, where calcification is tangential to x-ray beam, it is dense and homogeneous, but medially—where it is seen en face—it is more broken up and nodular. On outside of axillary calcification is 1 cm soft tissue band as result of pleural thickening. Appearances occurring low down and unilaterally are characteristic of postempyema (tuberculous) pleural calcification. Calcification occurs in thickened pleura, both parietal and visceral.

usually due to infection, hemorrhage, or asbestos exposure. The recognized causes are listed in the box above.

Calcification in asbestos inhalation and related conditions is morphologically characteristic[568] and is considered elsewhere. Calcification following infection and hemorrhage generally cannot be distinguished from each other. Such calcification is usually unilateral and varies from barely detectable to massive (Figure 15-72). In the latter circumstance it becomes sheetlike and, reflecting the gravitationally determined distribution of the preceding pleural fluid, is often best developed posterolaterally.[669] En face it appears as a hazy veil-like opacity, but in profile it is dense and linear, often parallel to the inner chest wall. The calcification in old empyemas occurs in both visceral and parietal pleura.[577,586] Sometimes these calcified layers are separated, an observation that can be made on plain radiographs or more easily on CT (Figure 15-73).[577] In a series of 140 calcified fibrothoraces, 15.7% had a persistent effusion that was sandwiched between layers of thickened calcified pleura and was demonstrable on CT by virtue of its attenuation, location, homogeneity, and failure to enhance.[577] This can be suspected from the plain radiograph with pleural thickening of more than 2 cm and a double layer of calcification.[577] Active infection of these encysted collections is manifest by expansion of the pleural opacity and development of an air-fluid level signifying a bronchopleural fistula.[586]

Occasionally postempyema calcification in the pleural space is manifest as a milk of calcium collection. These are often lenticular in shape and surrounded by mildly thickened pleura. On CT they are high density (200 to 300 HU) and typically homogeneous.[268]

PNEUMOTHORAX

Traditionally, pneumothorax is divided into spontaneous and traumatic types. The most common causes in adults are listed in the box on the facing page. Only spontaneous pneumothorax is discussed in this chapter apart from a brief consideration of pneumothorax associated with mechanical ventilation.

Primary spontaneous pneumothorax

A pneumothorax occurring without an obvious precipitating traumatic event is spontaneous; if the individual is apparently healthy, it is also primary. Primary spontaneous pneumothorax is strongly associated with smoking.[277,351] The peak prevalence (two thirds of patients) is between 20 and 40 years of age.[295] The male/female ratio is approximately 5:1.[272,295,411] There is a slight predominance of right-sided over left-sided pneumothorax, which is thought simply to reflect the slightly larger volume of the right lung.[295] Bilateral pneumothoraces occur but are unusual[220] and are more likely to occur metachronously than simultaneously. Thus in one series of 242 cases 10% were bilateral but only 2.5% were simultaneous.[550] The incidence is about 10 per 100,000 population per year.[411]

Primary spontaneous pneumothorax is nearly always the result of rupture of an apical pleural bleb.[301] Blebs are said to be detectable on chest radiographs in 15% of cases in the presence of pneumothorax; they are seen in 54% of patients at thoracoscopy and in 92% at thoracotomy.[295]

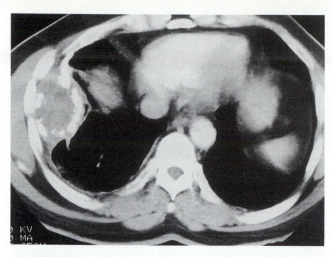

FIGURE 15-73
Pleural calcification — old tuberculous empyema. Lenticular pleural opacity is soft tissue density centrally and is marginated by heavy calcification both in visceral and parietal pleura.

They are rarely seen, however, on the interval chest radiograph. Interval CT is much more sensitive than chest radiography in detecting abnormal airspaces; in one study they were identified by CT in 85% of 20 patients (mean age 27 years) examined 2 months after spontaneous pneumothorax.[336] This is compared with a frequency of 30% in control subjects. The most common lesion was paraseptal emphysema (in 80%) with a subpleural and apical predilection, but centrilobular emphysema (in 60%) was almost as common.[336] In another CT study the size and number of apical "blebs" (cystic airspaces) was shown to correlate directly with likelihood of pneumothorax recurrence and need for surgical treatment.[682] The formation or rupture of blebs is probably encouraged by the greater mechanical stresses occurring at the lung apex,[700] where the pleural surface pressure is much more negative than at the base. The transpulmonary pressure, which is the force distending the lungs, is therefore greater at the apex than at the base, causing apical alveoli to be more distended.[203,256] These stresses are magnified in subjects with long lungs, possibly explaining why pneumothoraces are more common in tall, thin individuals.[175,717] Interestingly, if the prevalence of spontaneous pneumothorax is compared in male and female groups of the same height, any sex difference in prevalence disappears.[412] There is some difference of opinion regarding the importance of stressful activity in precipitating the actual event. Some authors suggest that this happens only occasionally,[200] but in other series about one fourth of patients were engaged in stressful activity, coughing, or sneezing.[295] Unusual atmospheric pressure swings may play a part in precipitating some pneumothoraces.[581]

On presentation patients may have chest pain (92%) and dyspnea (79%).[295] A few patients are asymptomatic. The pathophysiologic effect is usually mild, but there is a restrictive ventilatory defect[199] and sometimes transient

CAUSES AND VARIETIES OF PNEUMOTHORAX IN ADULTS

SPONTANEOUS

Primary
    Primary spontaneous pneumothorax*
    Familial pneumothorax*
Secondary
    Airflow obstruction*
        Asthma, COPD, cystic fibrosis*
    Infection
        Cavitary pneumonias
        Pneumatocele
        Tuberculous, fungal, hydatid disease
        AIDS[92,583]
    Infarction*
        Septic, aseptic
    Neoplasm*
        Primary, secondary, radiation*
    Diffuse lung disease
        Histiocytosis X, lymphangiomyomatosis, tuberous
          sclerosis, fibrosing alveolitis, sarcoidosis
    Catamenial pneumothorax*
    Heritable disorders of fibrous connective tissue*

TRAUMATIC

Iatrogenic
    Thoracotomy, thoracocentesis
    Percutaneous biopsy (lung, kidney, etc.)
    Tracheostomy
    Central venous punctures
    Artificial ventilation*
    Feeding tube perforation
Noniatrogenic
    Closed
        Ruptured esophagus
        Ruptured trachea
        Per se with or without rib fracture
    Penetrating

*Discussed in this section.

hypoxemia and widening of the $(A-a)O_2$ gradient.[460] The pneumothorax resorbs once the causal pleural break seals. Absorption is slow, occurring at a rate of about 1.25% of the hemithoracic volume per day.[297] Thus even a 15% pneumothorax takes 10 days to resolve. In one large series the average time for resorption was 25 days.[295] Breathing 100% oxygen increases the resorption rate.[461] Without definitive treatment the likelihood of having another pneumothorax is about 40%, and this is three times more likely on the ipsilateral than the contralateral side.[295] The chance of recurrence rises with each episode from about 25% with the first to about 50% after several episodes, at which point the risk flattens off.[295] More than 60% of recurrences occur within 2 years,[356] although they are reported up to 12 years after the initial pneumothorax.[295] Risk factors for recurrence include increasing age and height/weight ratio.[356]

Primary spontaneous pneumothorax may be treated conservatively, with chest tube drainage, or with chemical or surgical pleurodesis, the latter usually combined with bullectomy.[282,295] Management of pneumothorax during pregnancy has recently been reviewed.[236]

Familial pneumothorax has been occasionally reported since its first description in 1921.[587] The subject was reviewed in 1960[334] and again in 1979.[715] These last authors found reports of 61 pneumothoraces in 22 families. The male/female ratio was 1.8:1. The reported cases did not allow the mode of inheritance to be determined. Familial pneumothorax does not seem to be definitely related to stature, although in some reports patients have been marfanoid.[629] Other workers have raised the possibility of a relationship to human lymphocyte antigen haplotype (A2, B40) and alpha-1-antitrypsin phenotype.[587] Concurrent spontaneous pneumothoraces in 71-year-old identical twins were recently reported.[514] There is also a report of pneumothoraces associated with large bullae in sisters.[195]

Secondary spontaneous pneumothorax

A pneumothorax developing without a precipitating traumatic event in a patient with predisposing lung disease is said to be a spontaneous secondary pneumothorax. These are generally considered less common than primary spontaneous pneumothoraces. Important causes include the following.

AIRFLOW OBSTRUCTION. Chronic obstructive pulmonary disease is the most common cause of secondary spontaneous pneumothorax.[351,353] Patients are predominantly male (3:1 male/female preponderance in one series[666]) and older than patients with primary spontaneous pneumothorax (median age 59 years versus 32 years in the same series[666]). Pneumothorax is a serious complication that can lead to significant morbidity and possibly death.[123,194,666] The incidence in patients with chronic obstructive pulmonary disease has been estimated to be 0.4% per year, and the mortality is 3% or higher.[123,295]

Pneumothorax is a recognized complication of cystic fibrosis; it occurred in 8% of one large series of patients with cystic fibrosis.[614] It is a late complication (average age 19 years) and an ominous one, reflecting advanced disease.[614]

Pneumothorax is an unusual complication of asthma in adults. The frequency in patients with asthma severe enough to warrant hospitalization varies from 0.26%[518] to 2.5%.[64,333] The lower figure is probably the more reliable, since it is based on two very large series. The association is seen more often in children (p. 844), but even so is uncommon.[165]

PULMONARY INFARCTION. Pulmonary infarcts caused by aseptic emboli are occasionally associated with a pneumothorax; 25 cases were reported up to 1977.[229] At the time the pneumothorax develops, the infarct may be sterile[46,229,516] or it may have become secondarily in-

fected.[396] Such infarcts are usually large. Only about one third have had obvious cavities in the consolidation on the chest radiograph.[229] In half of the patients a large or persistent bronchopleural fistula develops. Septic pulmonary emboli may also cause pneumothorax.[274]

PRIMARY NEOPLASM. The association of primary bronchial neoplasm and pneumothorax has recently been reviewed.[329,623] The prevalence of this association is low; well under 1% of pneumothoraces are due to primary carcinoma of the lung.[124,623] Looked at the other way, pneumothorax is the initial manifestation in only 0.5% of lung carcinomas.[623] The suggested mechanisms include coincidental occurrence, possibly associated with chronic obstructive pulmonary disease[220,623]; tumor wall necrosis with direct pleural invasion and rupture (unexpectedly only a few of the carcinomas associated with pneumothorax have been cavitary[329]); rupture of lung that is overexpanded to compensate for adjacent carcinoma-induced collapse[623]; and endobronchial obstruction with a check valve effect.[19,623] The suspicion of an underlying bronchial carcinoma is usually raised by the finding of a mass or cavitary lesion in the reexpanded lung. Sometimes, however, the reexpanded lung appears radiographically normal.[88]

Pneumothorax is an unusual presenting feature of pleural mesothelioma; only 11 such cases are reported in the English literature.[589]

SECONDARY NEOPLASM. In a large series from the Mayo Clinic, about 0.5% of pneumothoraces were associated with lung metastases.[124] Of 45 cases in a literature review, 89% were caused by sarcoma (Figure 15-74) and only 11% by carcinoma.[723] Osteogenic sarcoma is by far the most common sarcoma.[276,615] Other tumors reported to cause pneumothorax include Wilms' tumor,[596] germ cell tumors,[600,601] and lymphoma.[490,728] Many of these patients have been on chemotherapy, and its role is not clear.[363] Pneumothoraces associated with metastases can occur before the deposits are radiologically detectable on the plain radiograph.[723]

RADIATION. The association of radiation and pneumothorax was first reported in 1974.[344] It is unusual, with only 11 cases found in the English literature in a 1985 review.[547] It was reported in 1% of patients receiving mantle irradiation for lymphoma.[547] Usually no malignancy is present in the chest at the time the pneumothorax develops. Typically pneumothoraces occur 4 to 16 weeks after the end of radiation therapy, and radiographically visible radiation pneumonitis is common. Patients without associated radiation changes in the lung have also been reported.[45] Pneumothoraces tend to be small or moderate in size and heal spontaneously, although some are recurrent and bilateral.[549,658]

Endometriosis and catamenial pneumothorax

Chest involvement in endometriosis is rare. The most common manifestation is catamenial pneumothorax. This disorder together with other aspects of endometriosis is

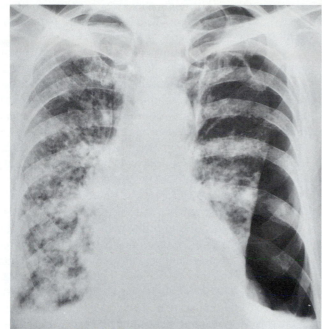

A

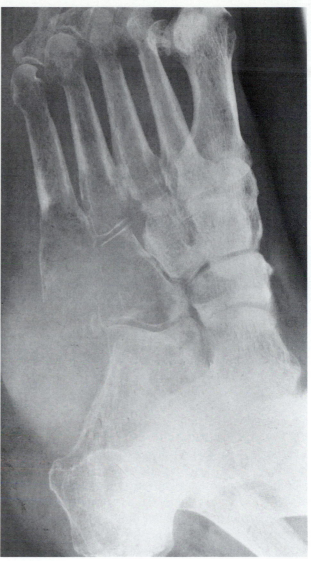

B

FIGURE 15-74
Secondary spontaneous pneumothorax. **A,** Left pneumothorax with multiple bilateral nodular shadows, more easily appreciated in right lung, caused by metastases from fibrosarcoma of foot (**B**).

discussed in this section. There are two distinct forms of chest endometriosis: pleurodiaphragmatic and bronchopulmonary.[727] Each has distinct demographic, pathogenetic, and clinical features.

PLEURODIAPHRAGMATIC ENDOMETRIOSIS. Pleurodiaphragmatic endometriosis is manifested clinically as catamenial pneumothorax or less commonly catamenial hemothorax.

Catamenial pneumothorax. Catamenial pneumothorax was first described by Maurer and co-workers in 1958.[390] It is uncommon; in females with spontaneous pneumothorax, catamenial pneumothorax has been recorded in 1% (6:664)[445] to 5.6% (11:196)[590] of patients. The second figure was recorded at a tertiary referral center and is higher than generally reported. Catamenial pneumothorax usually occurs in parous patients who are slightly older than patients with primary spontaneous pneumothorax.[78,544] Pneumothorax occurs only in relation to the menses, appearing 1 day before or up to 3 days after the periods. The pneumothorax is usually small and self-resolving.[602] It is nearly always right sided (87%) (Figure 15-75),[78,219] but left-sided (7%)[219,544] and bilateral instances (6%)[219,330,709] are recorded. Recurrence is a characteristic feature; indeed, without repeated episodes a clear relationship to the menses cannot be established. Ten or 20 recurrences are not uncommon, and some authors have reported 30 or more.[108,716] Another characteristic is that recurrence is prevented by pregnancy or drugs that suppress ovulation.[544]

Although 69 cases had been reported by 1987,[219] argument about the pathogenesis continues. No single concept can explain the occurrence of catamenial pneumothorax in all patients.[602] The most plausible theory is that air enters the peritoneal cavity by way of the genital tract during the menses, the only time the cervix is not occluded by a mucus plug.[437] Having entered the peritoneal cavity, the air passes into the pleural cavity through diaphragmatic holes, which may be either simple defects (see p. 675)* or defects associated with necrotic endometrial implants.[602,607,698] Some of these latter patients have pelvic endometriosis. In the review by Slasky and co-workers[602] one third of catamenial pneumothoraces were associated with simple diaphragmatic defects and one fifth with diaphragmatic endometrial implants. Further support for the genital-transdiaphragmatic theory is afforded when cure follows either hormonal suppression of ovulation[355,727] or tubal ligation.

*References 100, 129, 187, 390, 590, 602, 625.

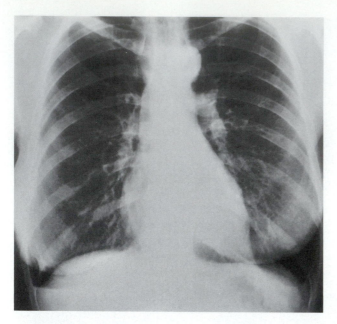

FIGURE 15-75
Catamenial pneumothorax in 34-year-old woman. This was third episode, and all had been right sided, as is usually the case. Air-fluid level in costophrenic angle draws attention to pneumothorax, which is otherwise easy to miss.

The preceding mechanisms cannot account for all cases.[219] In some patients pulmonary blebs seem to have been responsible just as in primary spontaneous pneumothorax.[219,355,393] In other cases endometriosis of the lung itself appears to have caused a direct air leak from the lung.[309,727] Another theory implicating prostaglandin-induced bronchiolar constriction in alveolar rupture has been proposed.[544] The role played by various mechanisms in catamenial pneumothorax has been critically reviewed.[219,602]

Catamenial hemothorax. A less common manifestation of pleurodiaphragmatic endometriosis in the chest is recurrent hemothorax occurring with the menses. Most patients are nulliparous with an average age of 32 years (range 24 to 42 years).[591] All patients have had right-sided hemothoraces, pleural endometriosis, and pelvic endometriosis with demonstrated diaphragmatic holes in some[727] and it seems likely in these patients that pleural implantation has followed transdiaphragmatic spread. Diaphragmatic defects and endometrial tissue in pleural and peritoneal cavities can be demonstrated by both CT and ultrasound.[269]

BRONCHOPULMONARY ENDOMETRIOSIS. Bronchopulmonary endometriosis is a disorder of parous women 30 to 50 years of age. There is often a clinical history of several spontaneous deliveries or uterine surgery, and the majority of patients do not have pelvic endometriosis.[176] Generally, postmenopausal patients have been symptomless while younger ones have had recurrent hemoptysis at the time of the menses (catamenial hemoptysis). There is usually a single focus of endometrial tissue in the lung parenchyma[280,309,328,426] and occasionally in an airway,[534] together with a variable amount of parenchymal hemorrhage.[534]

Radiologic study shows solitary, rounded nodules several centimeters in diameter[328,426] or thin-walled cavitary lesions with septation and focal mural irregularity.[280] Sometimes the dominant radiologic finding is the associated parenchymal bleeding, appearing as consolidation that comes and goes in phase with the menses and hemoptyses.[241,534] Two patients investigated by bronchial and pulmonary arteriography with a view to embolization had normal studies.[289] The chest radiograph can be normal in appearance.[541]

Catamenial hemoptysis has been successfully treated with the antigonadotropin danazol.[541] Probably pulmonary lesions are metastatic, since patients with bronchopulmonary involvement usually give a past medical history of pregnancy or obstetric or gynecologic surgery (cesarean section, dilatation and curettage, abortion, hysterectomy). Experimental evidence in rabbits suggests that this is a realistic possibility,[253] and the finding of decidua in the lungs at postmortem examination is well recognized.[280]

Heritable disorders of fibrous connective tissue

Four heritable disorders of fibrous connective tissue are associated with chest abnormalities. They may be classified as in Table 15-1.[502] These disorders are discussed here because pneumothorax is one of their more important respiratory manifestations.

MARFAN'S SYNDROME. Marfan's syndrome is an autosomal dominant disorder with a variable expression, involving particularly the eyes (myopia, ectopia lentis), aorta and heart (aortic aneurysm, aortic regurgitation, mitral valve disease), and musculoskeletal system (relatively long limbs in relationship to the trunk, arachnodactyly, pectus deformities, kyphoscoliosis, and joint laxity).[372] Recent studies have demonstrated abnormalities of fibrillin (a glycoprotein component of elastin-associated microfibrils) caused by mutations of the fibrillin gene on chromosome 15.[655] New mutations probably account for 15% of cases.[503] Life expectancy is greatly reduced, with most deaths caused by cardiovascular complications.[441]

The chief respiratory abnormalities in Marfan's syndrome are pneumothorax, bullae, cysts, and emphysema. These findings are present in some 5% to 10% of patients. Kyphoscoliosis may be gross and can lead to cor pulmonale and death.[679] Pneumothorax is 30 to several hundred times more likely to occur in patients with Marfan's syndrome than in unaffected individuals.[230,721] In such patients the frequency of pneumothorax ranges between 5% and 10%.[230,721] Pneumothoraces are commonly bilateral and recurrent. About two thirds of the affected patients have an underlying chest radiographic abnormality, either bullae or apical fibrosis.[126,230,721]

Table 15-1 Heritable disorders of connective tissue

Disorder	Major clinical features	Associated chest abnormality	
		Major	Minor
Marfan's syndrome	Myopia, ectopia lentis, aortic aneurysm, mitral valve disease, arachnodactyly, pectus deformity, lax joints	Emphysema, bullae, cysts, pneumothorax, skeletal deformity	Cor pulmonale, recurrent infection, bronchiectasis, mycetoma, pulmonary fibrosis, lobar hypoplasia
Ehlers-Danlos syndromes	Hyperextensible but elastic skin, lax joints, tissue fragility (bruising and bleeding)	Hemoptysis, bullae, pneumothorax, skeletal deformity	Recurrent infection, bronchiectasis, tracheobronchomegaly, pulmonary fibrosis
Cutis laxa	Loose inelastic skin, doleful facies	Emphysema, cor pulmonale	Recurrent infection, bronchiectasis, tracheobronchomegaly, laryngeal obstruction, tortuous and stenotic pulmonary artery, hernia, eventration of diaphragm
Pseudoxanthoma elasticum	Yellow skin papules	None	Small parenchymal nodules[378]

A particularly striking manifestation of Marfan's syndrome is bullae occurring in young patients.[126,721] The bullae may be apical in position[656] or widely distributed.[721] They can become occupied by an aspergilloma.[721] Other manifestations include emphysema, congenital pulmonary malformations, apical fibrosis, bronchiectasis, and an increased frequency of lower respiratory tract infections.[721] Emphysema has been recorded at all ages from neonates to adults.[47,126,137] It may cause cor pulmonale and death in the pediatric age group.[47,126] Upper zone fibrosis is rare; only six cases have been reported in the world literature.[358] Associated congenital pulmonary malformations consist mainly of "rudimentary" middle lobes, which do not contribute to mortality or morbidity.[137] Bronchiectasis has been reported in Marfan's syndrome,[177,641,721] but it is not clear if this is any more than a chance association.

The marfanoid hypermobility syndrome is classed as a separate entity that shares some of the features of both Marfan's and Ehlers-Danlos syndromes.[675] Chest abnormalities consist of cysts, pneumothorax, bronchomegaly, and hemoptysis.[435]

EHLERS-DANLOS SYNDROMES. The Ehlers-Danlos syndromes are a group of collagen disorders characterized by hyperextensible, doughy skin and joints and abnormal fragility of connective tissue that leads to bleeding, bruising, and atrophic scarring.[101,492] Ten clinical types are recognized.[492] The frequency of respiratory abnormality varies among types and is difficult to assess. Much of the literature has been confined to case reports, indicating a low prevalence, and in one series of 100 patients no respiratory disorder was detected.[32]

The common clinical respiratory findings are hemoptysis, pneumothorax, and bullae. In one series of 20 patients about 50% had respiratory symptoms or abnormal lungs on the chest radiograph[20] and 25% had hemoptysis, probably related to vascular fragility rather than a bleeding or clotting abnormality. Bullae can occur without pneumothorax[20] and in one patient were both transient and fluid filled.[28] Unlike in cutis laxa, emphysema is not a feature, although exceptional cases are reported.[101]

Pneumothorax is well described, particularly in type IV Ehlers-Danlos syndrome, but appears to be less common in Ehlers-Danlos syndromes than in Marfan's syndrome.[20] It may be encountered with[89,605] or without visible bullae on the plain chest radiograph.[20,472]

Other findings that have been noted include recurrent sinusitis and pneumonia[20] and rarely bronchiectasis,[531] tracheobronchomegaly,[1,20] and upper zone fibrosis.[20] Skeletal abnormalities are commonly seen on the chest radiograph. Of 20 cases in one series, 33% had pectus excavatum, 22% had scoliosis, 17% had straight back, and 17% had thin ribs.[20]

CUTIS LAXA (GENERALIZED ELASTOLYSIS). Cutis laxa may be acquired or congenital. Loose, inelastic skin is its characteristic feature. This results in a typical doleful facies with large earlobes, periorbital bagginess, and hook nose. Both forms demonstrate fragile, fragmented elastic tissue that shows normal collagen on histologic study. In the acquired form the abnormality is confined to the skin. Several congenital varieties are recognized. The autosomal recessive form is characterized by neonatal onset of respiratory disease with airflow obstruction, pneumonia, emphysema, and cor pulmonale, resulting in the patient's death in childhood.[86,209,227,391] The dominant form predominantly involves the skin, although other organ systems are sometimes involved.[31]

The most important respiratory abnormality accompanying this condition is emphysema, which usually develops shortly after birth[86,227] but may be delayed until adolescence[413,657] or adulthood.[235,322] Emphysema may be accompanied by bullae or pulmonary arterial hypertension.[657] It commonly leads to death from cor pulmonale or respiratory failure. Other features described in children include repeated pulmonary infections,[227,391] airflow obstruction caused by large floppy cords, tracheobronchomegaly,[678] and bronchiectasis.[31] The pulmonary arteries may become tortuous and stenotic,[409,413] causing abnormalities that appear on the plain chest radiograph. Hernias are a feature of cutis laxa and in the chest are manifest as hiatus hernias. In addition, the diaphragm may appear eventrated.[322,409]

Traumatic iatrogenic pneumothorax

Only one of the varieties of traumatic pneumothorax is discussed here.

MECHANICAL VENTILATION. Pneumothorax is common in patients undergoing ventilation. Because there are so many modifying factors, giving a prevalence rate is both difficult and meaningless. The likelihood of pneumothorax is increased by high airway pressures, long ventilation times, and abnormal lungs and is particularly associated with infection,[119] infarction, and chronic obstructive pulmonary disease.[220,537] Many factors cause high airway pressures: stiff lungs, volume cycling, unregulated manual inflation, large tidal volumes, endotracheal tube obstruction, right mainstem bronchus intubation, atelectasis, and positive end-expiratory pressure.[399,537] The development of a pneumothorax may be anticipated by the development of interstitial air, particularly in the form of "cysts."[10,537] These appear as rounded, thin-walled transradiancies, 2 to 9 cm in diameter; they occur anywhere in the lungs but particularly at the bases, medially, or along the diaphragm. These cysts almost invariably lead to a tension pneumothorax. Not only are pneumothoraces common with mechanical ventilation, but also they are more likely to be bilateral[220] and under tension (68% in one series).[537] Not surprisingly, pneumothorax occurring with mechanical ventilation may be rapidly fatal.[314] Immediate tube drainage is required.[620,738]

Radiographic signs of pneumothorax

As with other pleural processes, the radiologic appearance of a pneumothorax depends critically on the radiographic projection, the patient's position, and the presence or absence of loculation.

FREE PNEUMOTHORAX. In the erect patient, air rises in the pleural space and separates the lung from the chest wall, allowing the visceral pleural line to become visible as a thin curvilinear opacity between vessel-containing lung and the avascular pneumothorax space (Figure

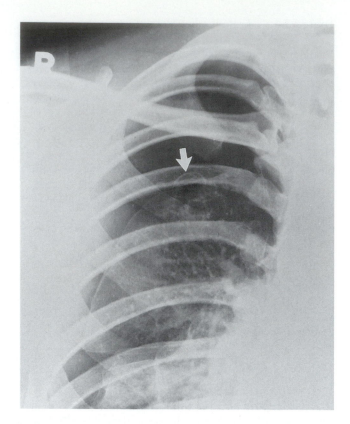

FIGURE 15-76
Primary spontaneous pneumothorax. Visceral pleural line is clearly demonstrated together with lateral avascular space. There is pleural bleb at apex of lung (*arrow*), a common finding. Such blebs are usually not detectable when lung reexpands.

15-76). The pleural line remains approximately parallel to the chest wall. It can be difficult to identify in shallow pneumothoraces, when it may be hidden by ribs and other bony structures. In this circumstance a radiograph taken in expiration may make the line easier to detect as it alters its orientation relative to ribs and also increases the volume of the pneumothorax space relative to the lung volume.[161] A lateral decubitus chest radiograph obtained with the suspect side uppermost may similarly be helpful.[369] In a study on cadavers with controlled pneumothoraces, lateral decubitus radiographs have been shown to be more sensitive than erect radiographs.[76] Somewhat surprisingly, this was not confirmed in an in vivo assessment comparing upright expiratory radiographs and lateral decubitus radiographs.[35] This study did, however, show that both views were equally good at excluding pneumothorax and that in 16% of cases the lateral decubitus view was critical in making the diagnosis of pneumothorax.[35] The difficulty in designing such studies has been discussed.[77]

Curvilinear shadows projected over the lung apex may mimic the visible visceral pleural line of a pneumothorax and cause difficulty in interpretation. Such opacities include those resulting from vascular lines, tubes, clothing, hair, scapulae, skinfolds, and the walls of bullae and cavities. Careful analysis of the structure and shape of these opacities — noting whether or not they extend beyond the inner margin of the chest wall — often allows correct identification. In practice, skinfolds and bullae are the most troublesome. Skinfold artifacts are seen on anteroposterior radiographs of very young or old, seriously ill patients and are produced when subjects with loose skin slump against a cassette. Sometimes it is clear that the skinfold shadow does not represent a pneumothorax, for instance, when vessels are seen beyond it, when it extends outside the margin of the chest cavity, or when it is located or oriented such that it could not possibly represent the edge of a slightly collapsed lung. A helpful feature is that a skinfold generates a broad bandlike opacity with a sharp outer edge that fades off medially and may have a transradiant lateral margin, whereas visceral pleura tends to produce a much thinner linear opacity.[168] The thin marginal transradiancy associated with a skinfold artifact is a Mach effect.[102,327] A somewhat similar shadow to that generated by a skinfold may be produced by the scapular companion shadow.[325]

Cysts, bullae, and cavities are probably the most troublesome mimics of pneumothorax because they produce both transradiancy and thin curvilinear opacities. These structures, however, have inner margins that are concave to the chest wall rather than convex.[220] They do not conform to the shape of the costophrenic angle when they are at the lung base,[36] and they may be demonstrably limited to a lobe.[161] Not only may a bulla mimic a pneumothorax, but the reverse sometimes occurs when synechiae cross the pleural space. Synechiae, however, are generally straight, allowing a distinction from the curved linear margins of a cyst or bulla.[220] CT may be used to differentiate bullae from pneumothorax.[48]

With a pneumothorax the transradiancy of the ipsilateral hemithorax is variable and is related to the degree of collapse, the presence or absence of disease in the lung itself, and the degree to which perfusion is reduced because of hypoventilation.[128] With a small pneumothorax, transradiancy is unchanged or occasionally slightly increased, but with progressive collapse the lobe's opacity increases until it eventually becomes a fistlike mass of soft tissue density at the hilum. An air bronchogram is often but not invariably present, and its absence does not necessarily mean obstruction of large airways as has been suggested.[450] As the lung loses volume, the small apical blebs that are almost invariably associated with primary spontaneous pneumothorax frequently become clearly visible (Figure 15-76). Searching the partially collapsed lung for other predisposing conditions (Figure 15-28) such as bullae, interstitial disease, or metastases is also worthwhile. Care should be taken not to misinterpret shadows that simply result from the collapse itself.[161]

On a lateral chest radiograph a pneumothorax is manifest most commonly as an anterior or posterior visceral pleural line (approximately 80% of patients).[202] In the same study 53% of patients had an air-fluid level

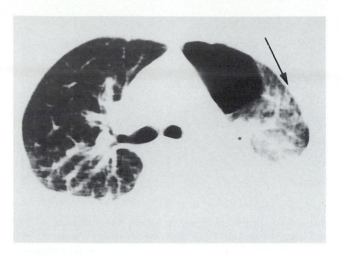

FIGURE 15-77

Pneumothorax in supine patient on computed tomography. There is left-sided pneumothorax. Lung falls away anteriorly from mediastinum but maintains chest wall contact almost to front of chest. Arrow represents lateral x-ray beam, tangential to chest wall as would be found when taking an anteroposterior supine chest radiograph. Resultant image would show lung and chest wall in contact laterally and fail to show visceral pleural line.

and in 9% this was the only sign of pneumothorax on the lateral view.[202]

Many patients, such as those who have sustained trauma and those in intensive care units, undergo radiography while supine. Chest radiographs of a supine patient are not sensitive in the detection of pneumothoraces; recent series suggest a sensitivity of 50% to 70%,[647,648,676] but clearly such figures depend critically on the size of the pneumothorax. Failure to diagnose pneumothorax under these circumstances may have serious consequences because, if untreated, many develop to tension.[537]

PNEUMOTHORAX IN THE SUPINE PATIENT. In the supine patient the highest part of the chest cavity lies anteriorly or anteromedially at the base and free pleural air rises to this region. If the pneumothorax is small to moderate in size, the lung is not separated from the chest wall laterally (Figure 15-77) or at the apex. In the absence of a displaced visceral pleural line in these regions the detection of pneumothorax depends on identification of one or more of the following signs:

1. Relative transradiancy in the hypochondrial region (Figure 15-78)[526,647,737] and even of the whole hemithorax.

2. Increased sharpness of the adjacent mediastinal margin (Figure 15-78) and diaphragm, which may become bordered by a band of relative transradiancy. This effect is particularly well seen in infants and neonates.[433]

3. A deep and sometimes rather tonguelike costophrenic sulcus (Figure 15-78).[213]

4. Visualization of the anterior costophrenic sulcus (Figure 15-78). This recess runs obliquely across the hypochondrium and is sigmoid shaped, with its most

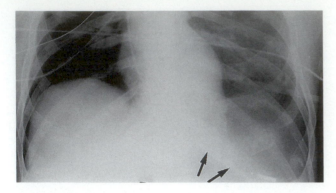

FIGURE 15-78
Bilateral pneumothorax in supine patient. Pneumothorax on right was large and obvious. Long, fingerlike costophrenic sulcus on right is characteristic of pneumothorax in supine patient. Pneumothorax was not obvious on left but was indicated by number of signs: sharp left cardiac border, hypochondrial transradiancy, and visible anterior costophrenic sulcus (arrows).

cephalad point medially.[303] It may be seen as an interface or, if the undersurface is bordered by gastric or colonic gas, as a line.[526,737] The term "double diaphragm sign" has been applied to the simultaneous visualization of the anterior sulcus and the dome of the true hemidiaphragm.[737]

5. Increased sharpness of the cardiac borders (Figure 15-78), particularly the apex and a lobulated, rounded, and often masslike appearance to the pericardial fat pads (Figure 15-79)[737] because they are no longer flattened against the heart.

6. Occasionally, anterior pleural air allows the middle lobe to retract medially away from the lateral chest wall while the lower and upper lobes still maintain chest wall contact. Under these circumstances the lateral border of the middle lobe becomes visible as a fine, linear opacity passing caudally from the lateral aspect of the minor fissure, parallel to the chest wall toward the diaphragm.[318]

7. Pleural air may also collect in the minor fissure, giving a characteristic transradiancy bounded by two visceral pleural lines.[200,616]

8. Visualization of the inferior edge of the collapsed lung[737] above the diaphragm. This must be distinguished from extrapleural extension of air above the diaphragm, described in pneumomediastinum.[468]

9. Depression of the ipsilateral hemidiaphragm.[737]

10. In infants the anterior junctional area is occupied by thymus and a junctional line is not normally seen on a frontal radiograph. Its identification on a frontal radiograph of a neonate signifies a bilateral pneumothorax.[382]

If a pneumothorax is suspected on a radiograph of a supine patient, it can be confirmed or excluded by other views, several of which were first described in infants and neonates. The cross-table lateral view[254] is probably the least satisfactory because of overlap of the other hemi-

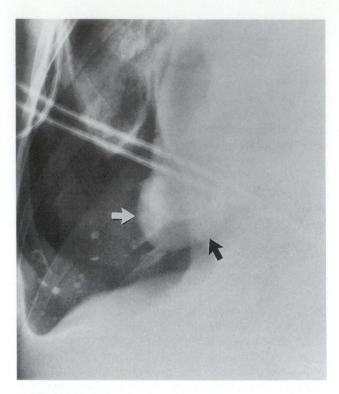

FIGURE 15-79
Pneumothorax in supine patient. Localized view of right lung base demonstrates fat pad in right cardiophrenic angle that has become rounded and masslike.

thorax. An alternative is to place a cassette 45 degrees dorsolaterally and angle the x-ray tube so that the central ray is perpendicular to the cassette. However, if the patient can be turned, the best image will result from a lateral decubitus view with the suspect side uppermost.[369] Clearly CT is more sensitive than conventional radiography in detecting pneumothorax in supine subjects.[647,648,677] Some authors recommend that a limited CT examination of the lung bases be performed in all patients with severe head trauma at the time of cranial CT[648] to exclude unsuspected pneumothorax. Surprisingly, the erect expiratory chest radiograph has been shown to be as sensitive as CT in detecting pneumothorax following percutaneous lung biopsy.[443]

Ultrasound is not recommended as a way of identifying a pneumothorax. Nevertheless, it may serendipitously demonstrate a pneumothorax by the loss of detectable visceral pleural movement and the absence of normal, intercostal, comet tail artifacts.[699]

LOCULATED AND LOCALIZED PNEUMOTHORAX. Sometimes a pneumothorax is truly loculated because of adhesions.[446] On other occasions a free pneumothorax shows an atypical distribution (Figure 15-80). Several patterns are recognized.

Subpulmonic pneumothorax. Several papers have described subpulmonic pneumothorax with the visceral pleural line visible just above the diaphragm. This unusual location has been ascribed to preferential collec-

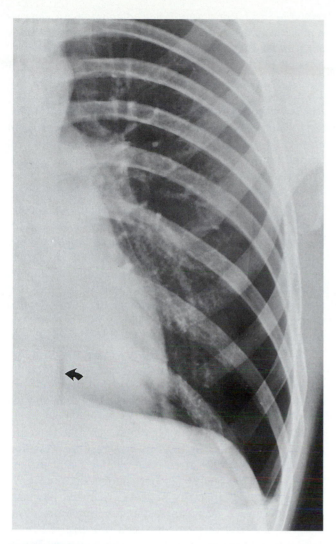

FIGURE 15-80
Left pneumothorax in erect patient. There is obvious pneumothorax. Pleural air is seen to collect in linear manner along left border of heart and behind heart *(arrow)* and must not be misinterpreted as pneumomediastinum.

tion around diseased basal lobes[316] or to scarring of the rest of the pleural space, for example, following tuberculosis.[85] In another series of patients with the adult respiratory distress syndrome (ARDS), subtle degrees of mediastinal shift and contour changes of the heart and hemidiaphragm suggested that these localized pneumothoraces were under tension.[205] Intrapleural air in this situation must be distinguished from extrapleural air that has dissected outward along the diaphragm from a pneumomediastinum[302,354,468] or from barotraumatic cysts.[10,537]

Encysted pneumothorax. This may occur in the oblique fissure, giving a cystic opacity in the right midzone[457,686] or an air-fluid collection with a hemopneumothorax.[14] It may also occur in the inferior accessory fissure.[380]

"Pulmonary ligament pneumatocele." Following trauma, particularly in children or young adults, a triangular collection of air sometimes develops against the mediastinum with its apex near the hilum (Figure 15-25). These air collections are more common on the left and may contain an air-fluid level.[153] An obvious ipsilateral pneumothorax may or may not be present, and the air collection generally clears in days or weeks.[206] In the past, these transradiancies have been ascribed to an air collection in the inferior pulmonary ligament.[160,267,515,672] Recent CT evaluation, which allows more accurate localization, indicates that such transradiancies are either localized posteromedial pneumothoraces (Figure 15-25) or air collections within the mediastinum.[182,206]

Pneumothorax adjacent to collapse. Pleural surface pressure would be expected to be more negative over collapsed lung and thus might favor the localization of pneumothorax to that region. Pneumothorax adjacent to collapsed lobes has been recognized in adults[326] and children.[34]

Complications of pneumothorax

About 20% to 50% of pnemothoraces are accompanied by *pleural fluid* (Figure 15-75), which is usually scant and inconsequential.[202,295] The fluid may be clear, serosanguineous, or sanguineous. On an erect frontal radiograph a small amount of fluid appears as a horizontal air-fluid level or as a C-shaped opacity in the costophrenic angle when its horizontal upper border is below the central ray and its anterior and posterior margins are projected separately. Sometimes the air-fluid level generated by a small effusion may be more eye catching than the visceral pleural line and induce the observer to scrutinize the lung apex (Figure 15-75). Rarely an air-fluid level is the only sign of a pneumothorax on an erect frontal radiograph, as occurred in 6 of 122 patients in one series.[202] If the pneumothorax is very small and pleural separation is present only at the apex, pleural fluid at the base will take on the classic meniscus form. In 3% or fewer of patients a hemothorax develops that is large enough to warrant treatment in its own right.[3,295,296] *Hemothorax* is much more frequent in primary than in secondary pneumothorax.[295] In keeping with this observation, 93% of patients with hemothorax in one review were men and 92% were under 39 years of age.[677] Torn adhesions between the parietal and visceral pleura are common sources of bleeding.[114] Blood can clot in the pleural space and produce a mass — a *fibrin body* or "pleural mouse" — that may mimic a pleural tumor.[714] Pleural thickening is common following hemopneumothorax; in one series 22% of patients needed subsequent decortication.[295]

Uncommonly, purulent fluid accompanies a pneumothorax, giving a *pyopneumothorax*. This is seen with esophageal perforation or necrotizing pneumonia caused most commonly by infection with *Staphylococcus aureus*, *Pseudomonas* spp., *Klebsiella* spp., or anaerobes.[282]

Tension pneumothorax is a life-threatening complication. It occurs when intrapleural pressure becomes posi-

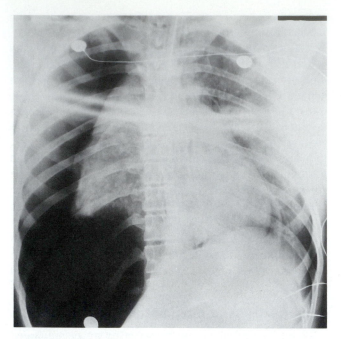

FIGURE 15-81

Right tension pneumothorax. There is marked depression of right hemidiaphragm and shift of mediastinum to left, indicated by position of heart and endotracheal tube. Patient was being mechanically ventilated, which may account for relative mildness of mediastinal shift compared with gross diaphragmatic depression. Complete collapse of right lung is prevented by consolidation. There is small left pneumothorax as well.

tive for a significant part of the respiratory cycle, compressing the normal lung and causing a restrictive ventilatory defect, an increase in the work of breathing, and a V/Q imbalance.[220] The cardiovascular effects probably result from respiratory failure rather than directly from the increased pleural pressure.[225,556] The condition must be treated by immediate decompression of the pleural space. It is usually diagnosed clinically by virtue of tachypnea, tachycardia, cyanosis, sweating, and hypotension. However, it sometimes is first detected on radiographic examination, and the most important signs are mediastinal shift and diaphragmatic depression (Figure 15-81). Contralateral mediastinal shift must be interpreted with caution because some movement toward the normal side is a frequent finding in a nontension pneumothorax, reflecting the fact that the pressure in the pneumothorax space is usually not as negative as on the normal side. If this shift is any more than mild or mild to moderate, true tension should be considered. Unfortunately, no way of quantitating such a shift has been worked out and it seems unlikely that it ever will because mediastinal compliance varies so much from person to person. The degree of depression of the ipsilateral hemidiaphragm is a more useful observation than the extent of mediastinal shift, and the hemidiaphragm is invariably depressed with significant tension. In patients receiving mechanical ventilation, diaphragmatic depression is the major sign. In such patients mediastinal shift is not a marked feature of tension because airway pressure remains positive.[220] It is important to remember that significant tension can occur with little lung collapse if the underlying lung is abnormal (e.g., consolidated).[220] Tension pneumothorax occurs when the leak is through a tear, which behaves like a valve. Tension is unusual in primary pneumothorax and is seen more commonly with trauma or mechanical ventilation,[537] particularly if positive end-expiratory pressure (PEEP) is employed.[620]

Following drainage of a pneumothorax, *acute pulmonary edema* may develop in the reexpanded lung (Figure 15-82). A similar sequence of events can follow drainage of a pleural effusion. Its mechanism is obscure; some authors suggest it is related to depletion of surfactant[417,481,585,653] and others that it is due to anoxic, mechanical, or mediator-induced capillary damage that leads to increased capillary permeability. Considerable evidence supports the latter view.[62,481,585,617,710] The edema usually develops within 2 hours of reexpansion and can progress for 1 or 2 days, resolving within 5 to 7 days. Reexpansion edema usually causes little morbidity, but patients can become hypotensive and hypoxic[239,282] and at least one death has been recorded.[571] Predisposing factors are generally considered to be complete pneumothoraces with gross lung collapse, chronicity of the pneumothorax, and high negative aspiration pressures. Most pneumothoraces have been complete and present for at least 3 days,[373,417,653] but shorter durations have been reported.[593] In many patients expansion has been rapid because negative aspiration pressure was used,[84,571,736] but this has not been universal.[264,653,681] The radiograph shows ipsilateral airspace opacity. Exceptional cases are reported with contralateral edema[239,619] and recurrent edema with recurrent pneumothorax.[588]

Pneumothoraces may be recurrent, and conditions that predispose to *recurrence* also predispose to bilateral pneumothoraces. *Bilateral pneumothoraces* may be synchronous or, much more commonly, metachronous. Conditions particularly associated with bilateral pneumothoraces have been reviewed.[91] They include primary spontaneous pneumothorax and a variety of secondary pneumothoraces, particularly those associated with malignant lung deposits, histiocytosis X, sarcoidosis, lymphangioleiomyomatosis, and exposure to radiation. Sometimes both pleural spaces are in communication following major cardiovascular surgery, so what would otherwise be a unilateral pneumothorax becomes bilateral[718] and behaves in an atypical shifting fashion.[145] Catamenial pneumothorax is almost invariably recurrent.

Pneumomediastinum is an unusual association of pneumothorax seen most commonly in neonates. In adults the combination may be seen in patients being mechanically ventilated and with rupture of the esophagus,[488] trachea, or bronchi. It is rare in primary spontaneous pneumothorax.

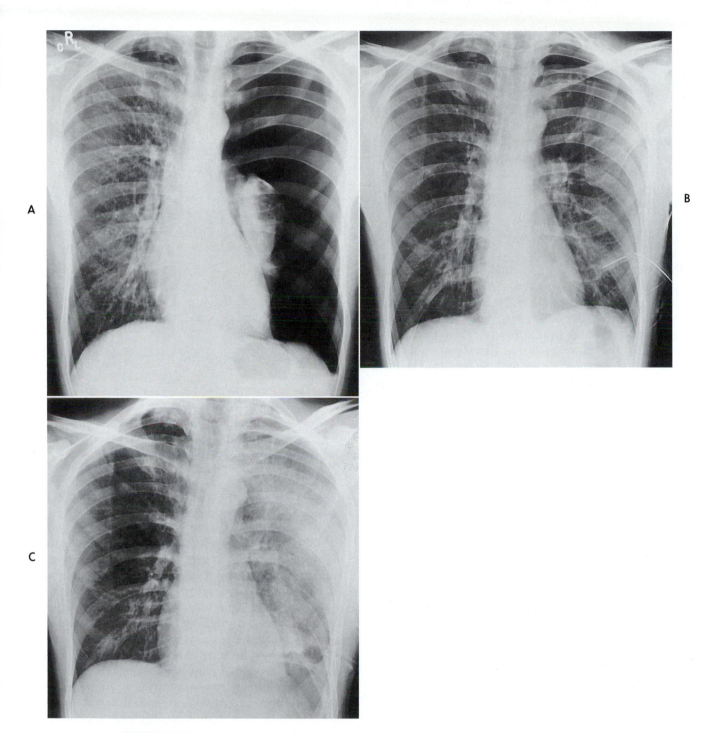

FIGURE 15-82
Reexpansion pulmonary edema. **A,** Complete collapse of left lung following primary spontaneous pneumothorax that had occurred 7 days previously. **B,** Diffuse consolidation of left lung 2 hours after insertion of left pleural drain attached to underwater seal drain. **C,** Twenty-four hours after radiograph in **B,** airspace shadowing has cleared.

Pneumoperitoneum is an extremely rare complication of pneumothorax. Diaphragmatic defects may allow pleural air to pass into the peritoneal cavity, resulting in a pneumoperitoneum.[156] Presumably because of the pressure gradient across the diaphragm, the development of pneumothorax after pneumoperitoneum is much more common.

Following progress and management

Changes in the size of a pneumothorax can be followed on serial radiographs by measuring the interpleural distance at the apex or along a specified rib. Numerical estimates of the size of a pneumothorax can be expressed as a percentage of hemithorax volume by making simple measurements.[18,525]

The causes to consider for failure of lung expansion include tube malplacement; large airway occlusion by blood, mucus, or foreign body; persistent air leak because of underlying lung disease, airway rupture, or pleural adhesions (Figure 15-28); visceral pleural thickening; and, possibly, acute depletion of surfactant.[190] A number of these conditions may be detected radiographically. Tube malposition may be obvious, but in some cases the radiographic signs are subtle. Malposition in the oblique fissure may be suspected on an anteroposterior radiograph if the chest tube follows a gently curved or straight course upward and medially from its entry point, rather than deviating soon after entry where it is deflected in front of or behind the lung.[690] The outer margin of pleural drainage tubes is seen by virtue of their contrast with surrounding air. Should such a tube become entirely displaced into the soft tissue of the chest wall, the outer margin of the tube will be no longer detectable.[689] Provided the degree of collapse is mild, it should be possible to detect any underlying lung diseases that may be responsible for persistent leakage, particularly diffuse interstitial fibrosis, cysts, bullae, or emphysema. Pleural adhesions that may hold open a visceral pleural tear will be seen as band shadows joining visceral to parietal pleura, distorting the lung envelope (Figure 15-28).

With failure of the lung to reexpand completely, the pneumothorax becomes chronic and persistent. This is an indication for surgery.

BRONCHOPLEURAL FISTULA

Bronchopleural fistula is an important cause of air in the pleural space (see top box at right). It is similar to a pneumothorax except that the pleural communication is with an airway rather than with distal gas exchange units. Although bronchopleural fistula has a number of causes, the bulk of cases are due to either surgical lung resection or necrotizing infections. Causes are listed in the second box at right.

Bronchopleural fistulas complicating infections (Figure 15-28) are considered in the discussion of empyema (see Chapter 6). Postsurgical fistulas are considered here. They occur with a frequency of about 2.5% to 3%[376,712]

CAUSES OF AIR IN THE PLEURAL SPACE

Pneumothorax
Iatrogenic causes
Infection with gas-forming organism (rare)
Fistulae
    Bronchopleural
    Esophagopleural
    Via diaphragm or chest wall

CAUSES OF BRONCHOPLEURAL FISTULA

TRAUMA

Thoracic surgery/lobectomy/pneumonectomy
Other iatrogenic causes (chest tubes, lung biopsy, thoracocentesis, nasogastric tube misplacement, oleothorax)

INFECTION

Necrotizing pneumonia/empyema (especially anaerobic, tuberculous, pyogenic)
Fungal infection

PULMONARY INFARCTION

Sterile/septic

MISCELLANEOUS

Neoplasms, radiation, rheumatoid nodules

Data from Friedman PJ, Hellekant CAG: *Radiology* 124:289-295, 1977; and Peters ME, Gould HR, McCarthy TM: *J Comput Tomogr* 7:267-270, 1983.

---

and usually develop within 2 weeks of surgery. They should be suspected with the postoperative development of fever, hemoptysis, cough (especially if productive of a large amount of brown sputum), and a persistent large air leak from the pleural drains.

With bronchopleural fistula following recent pneumonectomy the chest radiographic signs differ from those normally expected postoperatively because there are (1) an increased amount of air in the operated hemithorax, (2) a decreased amount of fluid, (3) loss of the normal mediastinal shift toward the operated side, and (4) sometimes an aspiration pneumonitis. Following lobectomy, or more than 6 months after a pneumonectomy, the pleural space is free of air, and the development of a bronchopleural fistula is then signaled by the appearance of air in the pleural space (Figure 15-83). Occasionally, unchanged persistence of an airspace following pneumonectomy indicates a fistula. This happens when the residual space is surrounded by pleural fibrosis and scarring so that it cannot change shape.[376] Extensive scarring may also prevent the mediastinal shift sign from being seen.[324] It is not uncommon for plain radiographic

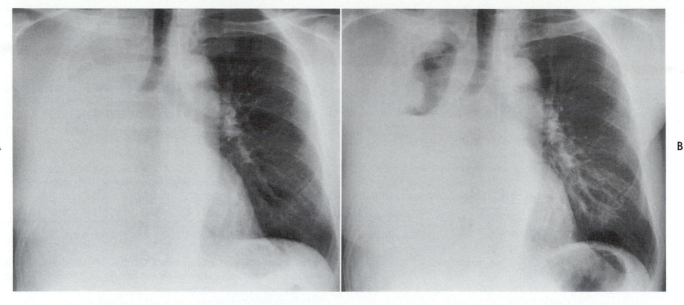

FIGURE 15-83
Bronchopleural fistula. A 62-year-old man had right pneumonectomy for squamous bronchial carcinoma. **A,** Appearance 2 years after surgery. **B,** Appearance 6 months later shows development of airspace with some fluid in upper right chest. Bronchoscopy showed bronchopleural fistula caused by tumor recurrence. There is no leftward mediastinal shift following development of fistula because, 2 to 3 years after surgery, mediastinum will be fixed by scar tissue.

signs (increasing pleural air) of bronchopleural fistula to appear in otherwise well patients who go on without complication or interference to successful obliteration of the pleural cavity.[469] This is ascribed to a flap valve type of fistula that is self-healing.

A fistula may be detected with scintigraphy and may for example be shown with xenon-133 lung scintigraphy in the washout phase.[733] Bronchography, sinography,[13] and even CT[485] can be used to demonstrate anatomic details.

REFERENCES

1. Aaby GV, Blake HA: Tracheobronchiomegaly, *Ann Thorac Surg* 2:64-70, 1966.
2. Aberle DR, Gamsu G, Ray CS: High-resolution CT of benign asbestos-related diseases: clinical and radiographic correlation, *AJR* 151:883-891, 1988.
3. Abyholm FE, Storen G: Spontaneous haemopneumothorax, *Thorax* 28:376-378, 1973.
4. Adams JT, McEvoy RK, DeWeese JA: Primary deep venous thrombosis of upper extremity, *Arch Surg* 91:29-42, 1965.
5. Adelman M, Abelda SM, Gottlieb J, et al: Diagnostic utility of pleural fluid eosinophilia, *Am J Med* 77:915-920, 1984.
6. Agostoni E: Mechanics of the pleural space, *Physiol Rev* 52:57-128, 1972.
7. Agostoni E: Mechanics of the pleural space. In Geiger SR, ed: *The handbook of physiology. Section 3. The respiratory system.* Vol III. *Mechanics of breathing, part 2,* Bethesda, Md, 1986. American Physiological Society.
8. Agostoni E, D'Angelo E: Thickness and pressure of the pleural liquid at various heights and with various hydrothoraces, *Respir Physiol* 6:330-342, 1969.
9. Ahmad S: Sclerosing peritonitis and propranolol, *Chest* 79:361-362, 1981.
10. Albelda SM, Gefter WB, Kelley MA, et al: Ventilator-induced subpleural air cysts: clinical, radiographic and pathologic significance, *Am Rev Respir Dis* 127:360-365, 1983.
11. Alexander ES, Proto AV, Clark RA: CT differentiation of subphrenic abscess and pleural effusion, *AJR* 140:47-51, 1983.
12. Anderson WJ, Skinner DB, Zuidema GD, et al: Chronic pancreatic pleural effusions, *Surg Gynecol Obstet* 137:827-830, 1973.
13. Andrews NC, VerMeulen VR, Christoforidis AJ: Injection of contrast media in postresection pleural spaces: diagnostic, prognostic and therapeutic value, *Dis Chest* 52:656-661, 1967.
14. Aronberg DJ, Brinkley AB, Levitt RG, et al: Traumatic fissural hemopneumothorax, *Radiology* 135:318, 1980.
15. Aronchick JM, Epstein DM, Gefter WB, et al: Chronic traumatic diaphragmatic hernia: the significance of pleural effusion, *Radiology* 168:675-678, 1988.
16. Austin JHM: The left minor fissure, *Radiology* 161:433-436, 1986.
17. Awotedu AA, Otulana BA, Ukoli CO: Giant lymph node hyperplasia of the lung (Castleman's disease) associated with recurrent pleural effusion, *Thorax* 45:775-776, 1990.
18. Axel L: A simple way to estimate the size of a pneumothorax, *Invest Radiol* 16:165-166, 1981.
19. Ayres JG, Pitcher DW, Rees PJ: Pneumothorax associated with primary bronchial carcinoma, *Br J Dis Chest* 74:180-182, 1980.
20. Ayres JG, Pope FM, Reidy JF, et al: Abnormalities of the lungs and thoracic cage in the Ehlers-Danlos syndrome, *Thorax* 40:300-305, 1985.
21. Bachman AL, Macken K: Pleural effusions following supervoltage radiation for breast carcinoma, *Radiology* 72:699-709, 1959.
22. Ballantyne KC, Sethia B, Reece IJ, et al: Empyema following intra-abdominal sepsis, *Br J Surg* 71:723-725, 1984.
23. Baltaxe HA, Lee JG, Ehlers KH, et al: Pulmonary lymphangiectasia demonstrated by lymphangiography in two patients with Noonan's syndrome, *Radiology* 115:149-153, 1975.

24. Banks J, Cassidy D, Campbell IA, et al: Unusual clinical signs complicating tension haemothorax, *Br J Dis Chest* 78:272-274, 1984.

25. Barakat MH, Karnik AM, Majeed HWA, et al: Familial Mediterranean fever (recurrent hereditary polyserositis) in Arabs — a study of 175 patients and review of the literature, *Q J Med* 60:837-847, 1986.

26. Barek LB, Cigtay OS: Urinothorax — an unusual pleural effusion, *Br J Radiol* 48:685-686, 1975.

27. Baron RL, Stark DD, McClennan BL, et al: Intrathoracic extension of retroperitoneal urine collections, *AJR* 137:37-41, 1981.

28. Baumer JH, Hankey S: Transient pulmonary cysts in an infant with the Ehler-Danlos syndrome, *Br J Radiol* 53:598-599, 1980.

29. Bedford DE, Lovibond JL: Hydrothorax in heart failure, *Br Heart J* 3:93-111, 1941.

30. Beer DJ, Pereira W, Snider GL: Pleural effusion associated with primary lymphedema: a perspective on the yellow nail syndrome, *Am Rev Respir Dis* 117:595-599, 1978.

31. Beighton P: Cutis laxa — a heterogeneous disorder, *Birth Defects* 10:126-131, 1974.

32. Beighton P, Thoma ML: The radiology of the Ehlers-Danlos syndrome, *Clin Radiol* 20:354-361, 1969.

33. Benninghoff D, Camiel M, Takashima T: Clinical and experimental studies of chylous reflux, *Prog Lymphol* 2:269-271, 1970.

34. Berdon WE, Dee GJ, Abramson SJ, et al: Localized pneumothorax adjacent to a collapsed lobe: a sign of bronchial obstruction, *Radiology* 150:691-694, 1984.

35. Beres RA, Goodman LR: Pneumothorax: detection with upright versus decubitus radiography, *Radiology* 186:19-22, 1993.

36. Berg RA: Giant congenital bronchogenic cyst, "pseudopneumothorax," *Postgrad Med* 48:121-126, 1970.

37. Berger HW, Rammohan G, Neff MS, et al: Uremic pleural effusion: a study in 14 patients on chronic dialysis, *Ann Intern Med* 82:362-364, 1975.

38. Berkmen YM: Uncomplicated torsion of the right upper lobe secondary to spontaneous pneumothorax, *Chest* 87:695-697, 1985.

39. Berkmen YM, Auh YH, Davis SD, et al: Anatomy of the minor fissure: evaluation with thin-section CT, *Radiology* 170:647-651, 1989.

40. Berkmen YM, Davis SD, Kazam E, et al: Right phrenic nerve: anatomy, CT appearance, and differentiation from the pulmonary ligament, *Radiology* 173:43-46, 1989.

41. Berkmen YM, Drossman SR, Marboe CC: Intersegmental (intersublobar) septum of the lower lobe in relation to the pulmonary ligament: anatomic, histologic, and CT correlations, *Radiology* 185:389-393, 1992.

42. Bessone LN, Ferguson TB, Burford TH: Chylothorax, *Ann Thorac Surg* 12:527-550, 1971.

43. Black LF: The pleural space and pleural fluid, *Mayo Clin Proc* 47:493-506, 1972.

44. Blalock A, Cunningham RS, Robinson CS: Experimental production of chylothorax by occlusion of the superior vena cava, *Ann Surg* 104:359-364, 1936.

45. Blane CE, Silberstein RJ, Sue JY: Radiation therapy and spontaneous pneumothorax, *J Can Assoc Radiol* 32:153-154, 1981.

46. Blundell JE: Pneumothorax complicating pulmonary infarction, *Br J Radiol* 40:226-227, 1967.

47. Bolande RP, Tucker AS: Pulmonary emphysema and other cardiorespiratory lesions as part of the Marfan abiotrophy, *Pediatrics* 33:356-366, 1964.

48. Bourgouin P, Cousineau G, Lemire P, et al: Computed tomography used to exclude pneumothorax in bullous lung disease, *J Can Assoc Radiol* 36:341-342, 1985.

49. Bower GC: Chylothorax: observations in 20 cases, *Dis Chest* 46:464-468, 1964.

50. Boyden EA: The distribution of bronchi in gross anomalies of the right upper lobe, particularly lobes subdivided by the azygos vein and those containing pre-arterial bronchi, *Radiology* 58:797-807, 1952.

51. Bradley JWP, Fielding LP: Hydropneumothorax complicating perforated peptic ulcer, *Br J Surg* 59:72-73, 1972.

52. Bradley MJ, Metrewelli C: Ultrasound in the diagnosis of the juxta-pleural lesion, *Br J Radiol* 64:330-333, 1991.

53. Bramson RT, Mikhael MA, Sagel SS, et al: Recurrent Hodgkin's disease manifesting roentgenographically as a pleural mass, *Chest* 66:89-91, 1974.

54. Brenner WI, Boal BH, Reed GE: Chylothorax as a manifestation of rheumatic mitral stenosis: its post operative management with a diet of medium-chain triglycerides, *Chest* 73:672-673, 1978.

55. Bressler EL, Francis IR, Glazer GM, et al: Bolus contrast medium enhancement for distinguishing pleural from parenchymal lung disease: CT features, *J Comput Assist Tomogr* 11:436-440, 1987.

56. Briselli M, Mark EJ, Dickerson GR: Solitary fibrous tumors of the pleura: eight new cases and review of 360 cases in the literature, *Cancer* 47:2678-2689, 1981.

57. Broaddus C, Staub NC: Pleural liquid and protein turnover in health and disease, *Semin Respir Med* 9:7-12, 1987.

58. Bron KM, Baum S, Abrams HL: Oil embolism in lymphangiography: incidence, manifestations, and mechanism, *Radiology* 80:194-202, 1963.

59. Brown LR, Reiman HM, Rosenow EC, et al: Intrathoracic lymphangioma, *Mayo Clin Proc* 61:882-892, 1986.

60. Brown SD, Brashear E, Schnute RB: Pleural effusion in a young woman with myxedema, *Arch Intern Med* 143:1458-1460, 1983.

61. Bryk D: Infrapulmonary effusion: effect of expiration on the pseudodiaphragmatic contour, *Radiology* 120:33-36, 1976.

62. Buczko GB, Grossman RF, Goldberg M: Re-expansion pulmonary edema: evidence for increased capillary permeability, *Can Med Assoc J* 125:460-461, 1981.

63. Bumgarner JR, Gahwyler M, Ward DE: Persistent fibrin bodies presenting as coin lesions, *Am Rev Tuberc* 72:659-662, 1955.

64. Burke GJ: Pneumothorax complicating acute asthma, *S Afr Med J* 55:508-510, 1979.

65. Butler C, Kleinerman J: The pulmonary apical cap, *Am J Pathol* 60:205-216, 1970.

66. Buxton RC, Tan CS, Khine NM, et al: Atypical transmural thoracic lipoma: CT diagnosis, *J Comput Assist Tomogr* 12:196-198, 1988.

67. Bydder GM, Kreel L: Pleural calcification in pancreatitis demonstrated by computed tomography, *J Comput Assist Tomogr* 5:161-163, 1981.

68. Bynum LJ, Wilson JE: Radiographic features of pleural effusions in pulmonary embolism, *Am Rev Respir Dis* 117:829-834, 1978.

69. Cáceres J, Mata JM, Alegret X, et al: Increased density of the azygos lobe on frontal chest radiographs simulating disease: CT findings in seven patients, *AJR* 160:245-248, 1993.

70. Calvert RJ, Smith E: An analytical review of spontaneous haemopneumothorax, *Thorax* 10:64-72, 1955.

71. Cameron DC: The juxtaphrenic peak (Katten's sign) is produced by rotation of an inferior accessory fissure, *Australas Radiol* 37:332-335, 1993.

72. Cameron JL: Chronic pancreatic ascites and pancreatic pleural effusions, *Gastroenterology* 74:134-140, 1978.

73. Cammarata SK, Brush RE, Hyzy RC: Chylothorax after childbirth, *Chest* 99:1539-1540, 1991.

74. Cann CE: Quantitative CT applications: comparison of current scanners, *Radiology* 162:257-261, 1987.

75. Carcillo J, Salcedo JR: Urinothorax as a manifestation of nondilated obstructive uropathy following renal transplantation, *Am J Kidney Dis* 5:211-213, 1985.

76. Carr JJ, Reed JC, Choplin RH, et al: Plain and computed radiography for detecting experimentally induced pneumothorax in cadavers: implications for detection in patients, *Radiology* 183:193-199, 1992.

77. Carr JJ, Reed JC, Choplin RH, et al: Pneumothorax detection: a problem in experimental design, *Radiology* 186:23-25, 1993.

78. Carter EJ, Ettensohn DB: Catamenial pneumothorax, *Chest* 98:713-716, 1990.

79. Case records of the Massachusetts General Hospital (Case 10, 1963), *N Engl J Med* 268:320-325, 1963.

80. Castells L, Comas P, Gonzalez A, et al: Case report: haemothorax in hereditary multiple exostosis, *Br J Radiol* 66:269-270, 1993.

81. Cevese PG, Vecchioni R, D'Amico DF, et al: Postoperative chylothorax, *J Thorac Cardiovasc Surg* 69:966-971, 1975.

82. Chakko S: Pleural effusion in congestive heart failure, *Chest* 98:521-522, 1990.

83. Chetty KG: Transudative pleural effusions, *Clin Chest Med* 6:49-54, 1985.

84. Childress ME, Moy G, Mottram M: Unilateral pulmonary edema resulting from treatment of spontaneous pneumothorax, *Am Rev Respir Dis* 104:119-121, 1971.

85. Christensen EE, Dietz GW: Subpulmonic pneumothorax in patients with chronic obstructive pulmonary disease, *Radiology* 121:33-37, 1976.

86. Christiaens L, Marchand-Alphant A, Favet A: Emphyseme congenital et cutix laxa, *Presse Med* 62:1799-1801, 1954.

87. Chun CH, Raff MJ, Contreras L, et al: Splenic abscess, *Medicine* 59:50-64, 1980.

88. Citron KM: Spontaneous pneumothorax complicating bronchial carcinoma, *Tubercle* 40:384-386, 1959.

89. Clark JG, Kuhn C, Uitto J: Lung collagen in type IV Ehlers-Danlos syndrome: ultrastructural and biochemical studies, *Am Rev Respir Dis* 122:971-978, 1980.

90. Coe JE, Aikawa JK: Cholesterol pleural effusion, *Arch Intern Med* 108:763-774, 1961.

91. Cohen HL, Cohen SW: Spontaneous bilateral pneumothorax in drug addicts, *Chest* 86:645-647, 1984.

92. Coker RJ, Moss F, Peters B, et al: Pneumothorax in patients with AIDS, *Respir Med* 87:43-47, 1993.

93. Collins JD, Burwell D, Furmanski S, et al: Minimal detectable pleural effusions: a roentgen pathology model, *Radiology* 105:51-53, 1972.

94. Collins JS, Pagani JJ: Extrathoracic musculature mimicking pleural lesions, *Radiology* 129:21-22, 1978.

95. Conant EF, Fox KR, Miller WT: Pulmonary edema as a complication of interleukin-2 therapy, *AJR* 152:749-752, 1989.

96. Cook GC: Periodic disease, recurrent polyserositis, familial Mediterranean fever, or simply "FMF," *Q J Med* 60:819-823, 1986.

97. Cooper C, Moss AA, Buy JN, et al: CT appearance of the normal inferior pulmonary ligament, *AJR* 141:237-240, 1983.

98. Cooper JAD, White DA, Matthay RA: Drug-induced pulmonary disease. 2. Noncytotoxic drugs, *Am Rev Respir Dis* 133:488-505, 1986.

99. Corriere JN, Miller WT, Murphy JJ: Hydronephrosis as a cause of pleural effusion, *Radiology* 90:79-84, 1968.

100. Crutcher RR, Waltuch TL, Blue ME: Recurring spontaneous pneumothorax associated with menstruation, *J Thorac Cardiovasc Surg* 54:599-602, 1967.

101. Cupo LN, Pyeritz RE, Olson JL, et al: Ehlers-Danlos syndrome with abnormal collagen fibrils, sinus of Valsalva aneurysms, myocardial infarction, panacinar emphysema and cerebral heterotopias, *Am J Med* 71:1051-1058, 1981.

102. Daffner RH: Visual illusions affecting perception of the roentgen image, *CRC Crit Rev Diagn Imag* 20:79-119, 1983-1984.

103. Dahlgren S: Anatomy of the thoracic duct from the standpoint of surgery for chylothorax, *Acta Chir Scand* 125:201-206, 1963.

104. Dalen JE, Haffajee CI, Alpert JS, et al: Pulmonary embolism, pulmonary hemorrhage and pulmonary infarction, *N Engl J Med* 296:1431-1435, 1977.

105. Dallemand S, Twersky J, Gordon DH: Pseudomass of the left upper quadrant from inversion of the left hemidiaphragm: CT diagnosis, *Gastrointest Radiol* 7:57-59, 1982.

106. Dalton ML, Strange WH, Downs EA: Intrathoracic splenosis: case report and review of the literature, *Am Rev Respir Dis* 103:827-830, 1971.

107. Dandy WE: Incomplete pulmonary interlobar fissure sign, *Radiology* 128:21-25, 1978.

108. Davies R: Recurring spontaneous pneumothorax concomitant with menstruation, *Thorax* 23:370-373, 1968.

109. Davis HH, Varki A, Heaton WA, et al: Detection of accessory spleens with indium 111–labeled autologous platelets, *Am J Hematol* 8:81-86, 1980.

110. Davis LA: The vertical fissure line, *AJR* 84:451-453, 1960.

111. Davis S, Gardner F, Qvist G: The shape of a pleural effusion, *Br Med J* 1:436-437, 1963.

112. Davis SD, Henschke CI, Yankelevitz DF, et al: MR imaging of pleural effusions, *J Comput Assist Tomogr* 14:192-198, 1990.

113. Day DL, Warwick WJ: Thoracic duct opacification for CT scanning, *AJR* 144:403-404, 1985.

114. Deaton WR, Johnston FR: Spontaneous hemopneumothorax, *J Thorac Cardiovasc Surg* 43:413-415, 1962.

115. DeCosse JJ, Poulin TL, Fox PS, et al: Subphrenic abscess, *Surg Gynecol Obstet* 138:841-846, 1974.

116. Dedrick CG, McLoud TC, Shepherd J-AO, et al: Computed tomography of localized pleural mesothelioma, *AJR* 144:275-280, 1985.

117. Deeley TJ: The effects of radiation on the lungs in the treatment of carcinoma of the bronchus, *Clin Radiol* 11:33-39, 1960.

118. DeFrance JH, Blewett JH, Ricci JA, et al: Massive hemothorax: two unusual cases, *Chest* 66:82-84, 1974.

119. de Lattore FJ, Tomasa A, Klamburg J, et al: Incidence of pneumothorax and pneumomediastinum in patients with aspiration pneumonia requiring ventilatory support, *Chest* 72:141-144, 1977.

120. Demos TC, Pieters C: Abdominal pseudotumor due to inverted hemidiaphragm, *Chest* 86:466-468, 1984.

121. Dewan NA, Kinney WW, O'Donohue WJ: Chronic massive pancreatic pleural effusion, *Chest* 85:497-501, 1984.

122. Diaconis JN, Weiner CI, White DW: Primary subclavian vein thrombosis and bilateral chylothorax documented by lymphography and venography, *Radiology* 119:557-558, 1976.

123. Dines DE, Clagett OT, Payne WS: Spontaneous pneumothorax in emphysema, *Mayo Clin Proc* 45:481-487, 1970.

124. Dines DE, Cortese DA, Brennan MD, et al: Malignant pulmonary neoplasms predisposing to spontaneous pneumothorax, *Mayo Clin Proc* 48:541-544, 1973.

125. Dockerty MB, Masson JC: Ovarian fibromas: a clinical and pathologic study of 283 cases, *Am J Obstet Gynecol* 47:741-752, 1944.

126. Dominguez R, Weisgrau RA, Santamaria M: Pulmonary hyperinflation and emphysema in infants with the Marfan syndrome, *Pediatr Radiol* 17:365-369, 1987.

127. Dorne HL: Differentiation of pulmonary parenchymal consolidation from pleural disease using the sonographic fluid bronchogram, *Radiology* 158:41-42, 1986.

128. Dornhorst AC, Pierce JW: Pulmonary collapse and consolidation: the role of collapse in the production of lung field shadows and the significance of segments in inflammatory lung disease, *J Fac Radiol* 5:276-281, 1954.

129. Downey DB, Towers MJ, Poon PY, et al: Pneumoperitoneum with catamenial pneumothorax, *AJR* 155:29-30, 1990.

130. Dressler W: The post-myocardial-infarction syndrome: a report on 44 cases, *Arch Intern Med* 103:28-42, 1959.

131. Ducharme J-C, Belanger R, Simard P, et al: Chylothorax, chylopericardium with multiple lymphangioma of bone, *J Pediatr Surg* 17:365-367, 1982.

132. Duckett JG, Lazarus A, White KM: Cutaneous masses, rib lesions, and chylous pleural effusion in a 20-year-old man, *Chest* 97:1227-1228, 1990.

133. Dugan DJ, Samson PC: Surgical significance of the endothoracic fascia: the anatomic basis for emphyemectomy and other extrapleural technics, *Am J Surg* 130:151-158, 1975.

134. Dulchavsky SA, Ledgerwood AM, Lucas CE: Management of chylothorax after blunt chest trauma, *J Trauma* 28:1400-1401, 1988.

135. Dunbar JS, Favreau M: Infrapulmonary pleural effusions with particular reference to its occurrence in nephrosis, *J Can Assoc Radiol* 10:24, 1959.

136. Dwyer A: The displaced crus: a sign for distinguishing between pleural fluid and ascites on computed tomography, *J Comput Assist Tomogr* 2:598-599, 1978.

137. Dwyer EM, Troncale F: Spontaneous pneumothorax and pulmonary disease in the Marfan syndrome, *Ann Intern Med* 62:1285-1292, 1965.

138. Ecker MD, Jay B, Keohane MF: Procarbazine lung, *AJR* 131:527-528, 1978.

139. Edwards SR, Unger AM: Acute hydrothorax — a new complication of peritoneal dialysis, *JAMA* 199:853-855, 1967.

140. Effmann EL, Ablow RC, Touloukian RJ, et al: Radiographic aspects of total parenteral nutrition during infancy, *Radiology* 127:195-201, 1978.

141. Ehrenfeld EN, Eliakim M, Rachmilewitz M: Recurrent polyserositis (familial Mediterranean fever, periodic disease): a report of fifty-five cases, *Am J Med* 31:107-123, 1961.

142. El-Kassimi FA: Roentgenogram of the month: acute pleuritic chest pain with pleural effusion and plate atelectasis, *Chest* 91:265-266, 1987.

143. Emerson PA: Yellow nails, lymphoedema, and pleural effusions, *Thorax* 21:247-253, 1966.

144. Emerson PA, Davies JH: Hydrothorax complicating ascites, *Lancet* 1:487-488, 1955.

145. Engeler CE, Olson PN, Engeler CM, et al: Shifting pneumothorax after heart-lung transplantation, *Radiology* 185:715-717, 1992.

146. England DM, Hochholzer L, McCarthy MJ: Localized benign and malignant fibrous tumors of the pleura: a clinicopathologic review of 223 cases, *Am J Surg Pathol* 13:640-658, 1989.

147. Engle MA, Ito T: The postpericardiotomy syndrome, *Am J Cardiol* 7:73-82, 1961.

148. Epler GR, McLoud TC, Munn CS, et al: Pleural lipoma: diagnosis by computed tomography, *Chest* 90:265-268, 1986.

149. Erwteman TM, Braat MCP, Van Aken WG: Interstitial pulmonary fibrosis: a new side effect of practolol, *Br Med J* 2:297-298, 1977.

150. Euphrat EJ, Beck E: Fibrin body following traumatic pneumothorax, *AJR* 74:86-89, 1955.

151. Evander LC: Pleural fat pads: a cause of thoracic shadows, *Am Rev Tuberc* 57:495-503, 1948.

152. Everts CS, Westcott JL, Bragg DG: Methotrexate therapy and pulmonary disease, *Radiology* 107:539-543, 1973.

153. Fagan CJ, Swischuk LE: Traumatic lung and paramediastinal pneumatoceles, *Radiology* 120:11-18, 1976.

154. Fairfax AJ, McNabb WR, Spiro SG: Chylothorax: a review of 18 cases, *Thorax* 41:880-885, 1986.

155. Faling LJ, Gerzof SG, Daly BDT, et al: Treatment of chronic pancreatitic pleural effusion by percutaneous catheter drainage of abdominal pseudocyst, *Am J Med* 76:329-333, 1984.

156. Fataar S, Morton P, Schulman A: Recurrent non-surgical pneumoperitoneum due to spontaneous pneumothorax, *Br J Radiol* 54:1100-1102, 1981.

157. Feder BH, Wilk SP: Localized interlobar effusion in heart failure: phantom lung tumor, *Dis Chest* 30:289-297, 1956.

158. Federle MP, Mark AS, Guillaumin ES: CT of subpulmonic pleural effusions and atelectasis: criteria for differentiation from subphrenic fluid, *AJR* 146:685-689, 1986.

159. Feldman DJ: Localized interlobar pleura effusion in heart failure, *JAMA* 146:1408-1409, 1951.

160. Felman AH, Rodgers BM, Talbert JL: Traumatic para-mediastinal air cyst: a case report, *Pediatr Radiol* 4:120-121, 1976.

161. Felson B: *Chest roentgenology*, Philadelphia, 1973, WB Saunders.

162. Felson B: The extrapleural space, *Semin Roentgenol* 12:327-333, 1977.

163. Felson B, Fleischner FG, McDonald JR, et al: Some basic principles in the diagnosis of chest diseases, *Radiology* 73:740-748, 1959.

164. Ferguson GC: Cholesterol pleural effusion in rheumatoid lung disease, *Thorax* 21:577-582, 1966.

165. Findley LJ, Sahn SA: The value of chest roentgenograms in acute asthma in adults, *Chest* 80:535-536, 1981.

166. Finn R, Jowett EW: Acute hydrothorax complicating peritoneal dialysis, *Br Med J* 2:94, 1970.

167. Fishbein R, Murphy GP, Wilder RJ: The pleuropulmonary manifestations of pancreatitis, *Dis Chest* 41:392-397, 1962.

168. Fisher JK: Skin fold versus pneumothorax, *AJR* 130:791-792, 1978.

169. Fisher MS: Significance of a visible major fissure on the frontal chest radiograph, *AJR* 137:577-580, 1981.

170. Fisher MS: Adam's lobe (letter), *Radiology* 154:547, 1985.

171. Fitzgerald TB, Johnstone MW: Diaphragmatic defects and laparoscopy, *Br Med J* 2:604, 1970.

172. Fleischner FG: Pulmonary embolism, *Clin Radiol* 13:169-182, 1962.

173. Fleischner FG: Atypical arrangement of free pleural effusion, *Radiol Clin North Am* 1:347-362, 1963.

174. Fleming HA, Hickling P: Pleural effusions after practolol, *Lancet* 2:1202, 1975.

175. Forgacs P: Stature in simple pneumothorax, *Guys Hosp Rep* 118:199-204, 1969.

176. Foster DC, Stern JL, Buscema J, et al: Pleural and parenchymal pulmonary endometriosis, *Obstet Gynecol* 58:552-556, 1981.

177. Foster ME, Foster DR: Bronchiectasis and Marfan's syndrome, *Postgrad Med J* 56:718-719, 1980.

178. Fraser RG, Pare JAP, Pare PD, et al: *Diagnosis of diseases of the chest*, vol 1, ed 3, Philadelphia, 1988, WB Saunders.

179. Frazer IH, Lichtenstein M, Andrews JT: Pleuroperitoneal effusion without ascites, *Med J Aust* 2:520-521, 1983.

180. Freundlich IM: The role of lymphangiography in chylothorax: a report of six nontraumatic cases, *AJR* 125:617-627, 1975.

181. Friedman E: Further observations on the vertical fissure line, *AJR* 97:171-173, 1966.

182. Friedman PJ: Adult pulmonary ligament pneumatocele: a loculated pneumothorax, *Radiology* 155:575-576, 1985.

183. Friedman PJ, Hellekant CAG: Radiological recognition of bronchopleural fistula, *Radiology* 124:289-295, 1977.

184. Frija J, Schmit P, Katz M, et al: Computed tomography of the pulmonary fissures: normal anatomy, *J Comput Assist Tomogr* 6:1069-1074, 1982.

185. Frija J, Yana C, Laval-Jeantet M, et al: Anatomy of the minor fissure: evaluation with thin-section CT, *Radiology* 173:571-572, 1989.

186. Frolich DJ, Clements JL, Weens HS: Epicardial fat line in left pleural effusion, *AJR* 124:394-396, 1975.

187. Furman WR, Wang KP, Summer WR, et al: Catamenial pneumothorax: evaluation by fiberoptic pleuroscopy, *Am Rev Respir Dis* 121:137-140, 1980.

188. Gale ME, Greif WL: Intrafissural fat: CT correlation with chest radiography, *Radiology* 160:333-336, 1986.

189. Galen MA, Steinberg SM, Lowrie EG, et al: Hemorrhagic pleural effusion in patients undergoing chronic hemodialysis, *Ann Intern Med* 82:359-361, 1975.

190. Galvis AG, Bowen AD, Oh KS: Nonexpandable lung after drainage of pneumothorax, *AJR* 136:1224-1226, 1981.

191. Gannon WE, Greenfield H: Fibrin body in an old abscess cavity, simulating a new growth, *Radiology* 66:564-566, 1956.

192. Gardner TW, Domm AC, Brock CE, et al: Congenital pulmonary lymphangiectasis: a case complicated by chylothorax, *Clin Pediatr* 22:75-78, 1983.

193. Gefter WB, Epstein DM, Bonavita JA, et al: Pleural thickening caused by Sansert and Ergotrate in the treatment of migraine, *AJR* 135:375-377, 1980.

194. George RB, Herbert SJ, Shames JM, et al: Pneumothorax complicating pulmonary emphysema, *JAMA* 234:389-393, 1975.

195. Gibson GJ: Familial pneumothoraces and bullae, *Thorax* 32:88-90, 1977.

196. Gilbert L, Ribot S, Frankel H, et al: Fibrinous uremic pleuritis: a surgical entity, *Chest* 67:53-56, 1975.

197. Gillett D, Ford GT, Anthonisen NR: Shape and regional volume in immersed lung lobes, *J Appl Physiol* 51:1457-1462, 1981.

198. Gilmartin D: The serratus anterior muscle on chest radiographs, *Radiology* 131:629-635, 1979.

199. Gilmartin JJ, Wright AJ, Gibson GJ: Effects of pneumothorax or pleural effusion on pulmonary function, *Thorax* 40:60-65, 1985.

200. Giuffre B: Supine pneumothoraces in adults, *Australas Radiol* 28:335-338, 1984.

201. Glazer HS, Anderson DJ, DiCroce JJ, et al: Anatomy of the major fissure: evaluation with standard and thin-section CT, *Radiology* 180:839-844, 1991.

202. Glazer HS, Anderson DJ, Wilson BS, et al: Pneumothorax: apparance on lateral chest radiographs, *Radiology* 173:707-711, 1989.

203. Glazier JB, Hughes JMB, Maloney JE, et al: Vertical gradient of alveolar size in lungs of dogs frozen intact, *J Appl Physiol* 23:694-705, 1967.

204. Glorioso LW, Lang EK: Pulmonary manifestations of renal disease, *Radiol Clin North Am* 22:647-658, 1984.

205. Gobien RP, Reines HD, Schabel SI: Localized tension pneumothorax: unrecognized form of barotrauma in adult respiratory distress syndrome, *Radiology* 142:15-19, 1982.

206. Godwin JD, Merten DF, Baker ME: Paramediastinal pneumatocele: alternative explanations to gas in the pulmonary ligament, *AJR* 145:525-530, 1985.

207. Godwin JD, Tarver RD: Accessory fissures of the lung, *AJR* 144:39-47, 1985.

208. Godwin JD, Vock P, Osborne DR: CT of the pulmonary ligament, *AJR* 141:231-236, 1983.

209. Goltz RW, Hult A-M, Goldfarb M, et al: Cutis laxa: a manifestation of generalized elastolysis, *Arch Dermatol* 92:373-387, 1965.

210. Gonzales-Rothi RJ, Hannan SE, Hood CI, et al: Amiodarone pulmonary toxicity presenting as bilateral exudative pleural effusions, *Chest* 92:179-182, 1987.

211. Good JT, Moore JB, Fowler AA, et al: Superior vena cava syndrome as a cause of pleural effusion, *Am Rev Respir Dis* 125:246-247, 1982.

212. Goodman LR, Golkow RS, Steiner RM, et al: The right mid-lung window, *Radiology* 143:135-138, 1982.

213. Gordon R: The deep sulcus sign, *Radiology* 136:25-27, 1980.

214. Gottehrer A, Roa J, Stanford GG, et al: Hypothyroidism and pleural effusions, *Chest* 98:1130-1132, 1990.

215. Graham JR: Cardiac and pulmonary fibrosis during methysergide therapy for headache, *Am J Med Sci* 254:1-12, 1967.

216. Graham JR, Suby HI, LeCompte PR, et al: Fibrotic disorders associated with methysergide therapy for headache, *N Engl J Med* 274:359-368, 1966.

217. Gramiak R, Koerner HJ: A roentgen diagnostic observation in subpleural lipoma, *AJR* 98:465-467, 1966.

218. Grant T, Levin B: Lymphangiographic visualization of pleural and pulmonary lymphatics in a patient without chylothorax, *Radiology* 113:49-50, 1974.

219. Gray R, Cormier M, Yedlicka J, et al: Catamenial pneumothorax: case report and literature review, *J Thorac Imag* 2:72-75, 1987.

220. Greene R, McLoud TC, Stark P: Pneumothorax, *Semin Roentgenol* 12:313-325, 1977.

221. Griffin DJ, Gross BH, McCracken S, et al: Observations on CT differentiation of pleural and peritoneal fluid, *J Comput Assist Tomogr* 8:24-28, 1984.

222. Groskin SA: Selected topics in chest trauma, *Radiology* 183:605-617, 1992.

223. Gross BH, Spizarny DL, Granke DS: Sagittal orientation of the anterior minor fissure: radiography and CT, *Radiology* 166:717-719, 1988.

224. Gunnels JJ: Perplexing pleural effusion, *Chest* 74:390-393, 1978.

225. Gustman P, Yerger L, Wanner A: Immediate cardiovascular effects of tension pneumothorax, *Am Rev Respir Dis* 127:171-174, 1983.

226. Haaga JR, Weinstein AJ: CT-guided percutaneous aspiration and drainage of abscesses, *AJR* 135:1187-1194, 1980.

227. Hajjar BA, Joyner EN: Congenital cutis laxa with advanced cardiopulmonary disease, *J Pediatr* 73:116-119, 1968.

228. Hall DR, Morrison JB, Edwards FR: Pleural fibrosis after practolol therapy, *Thorax* 33:822-824, 1978.

229. Hall FM, Salzman EW, Ellis BI, et al: Pneumothorax complicating aseptic cavitating pulmonary infarction, *Chest* 72:232-234, 1977.

230. Hall JR, Pyeritz RE, Dudgeon DL, et al: Pneumothorax in the Marfan syndrome: prevalence and therapy, *Ann Thorac Surg* 37:500-504, 1984.

231. Halvorsen RA, Fedyshin PJ, Korobkin M, et al: CT differentiation of pleural effusion from ascites: an evaluation of four signs using blinded analysis of 52 cases, *Invest Radiol* 21:391-395, 1986.

232. Hammerman AM, Susman N, Strzembosz A, et al: The extra pleural fat sign: CT characteristics, *J Comput Assist Tomogr* 14:345-347, 1990.

233. Handler CE, Fray RE, Snashall PD: Atypical Meigs' syndrome, *Thorax* 37:396-397, 1982.

234. Harbin WP, Mueller PR, Ferrucci JT: Transhepatic cholangiography: complications and use patterns of the fine-needle technique, *Radiology* 135:15-22, 1980.

235. Harris RB, Heaphy MR, Perry HO: Generalized elastolysis (cutis laxa), *Am J Med* 65:815-822, 1978.

236. Heffner JE, Sahn SA: Pleural disease in pregnancy, *Clin Chest Med* 13:667-678, 1992.

237. Heitzman ER: *The lung: radiologic-pathologic correlations*, ed 2, St Louis, 1984, Mosby.

238. Heller H, Sohar E, Sherf L: Familial Mediterranean fever, *Arch Intern Med* 102:50-71, 1958.

239. Henderson AF, Banham SW, Moran F: Re-expansion pulmonary oedema: a potentially serious complication of delayed diagnosis of pneumothorax, *Br Med J* 291:593-594, 1985.

240. Henschke CI, Davis SD, Romano PM, et al: The pathogenesis, radiologic evaluation, and therapy of pleural effusions, *Radiol Clin North Am* 27:1241-1255, 1989.

241. Hertzanu Y, Heimer D, Hirsch M: Computed tomography of pulmonary endometriosis, *Comput Radiol* 11:81-84, 1987.

242. Hertzanu Y, Solomon A: Inversion of the right diaphragm: a thoracoabdominal CT pitfall, *Gastrointest Radiol* 11:200-202, 1986.

243. Hessen I: Roentgen examination of pleural fluid: a study of the localization of free effusions, the potentialities of diagnosing minimal quantities of fluid and its existence under physiological conditions, *Acta Radiol (Stockh)* (suppl) 86:7-80, 1951.

244. Higgins CB, Mulder DG: Mediastinal chyloma: a roentgenographic sign of chylous fistula, *JAMA* 211:1188, 1970.

245. Higgins JA, Juergens JL, Bruwer AJ, et al: Loculated interlobar pleural effusion due to congestive heart failure, *Arch Intern Med* 96:180-187, 1955.

246. Hiller E, Rosenow EC, Olsen AM: Pulmonary manifestations of the yellow nail syndrome, *Chest* 61:452-458, 1972.

247. Hillerdal G: Chyliform (cholesterol) pleural effusion, *Chest* 88:426-428, 1985.

248. Himelman RB, Callen PW: The prognostic value of loculations in parapneumonic pleural effusions, *Chest* 90:852-856, 1986.

249. Hinckley ME: Thoracic-duct thrombosis with fatal chylothorax caused by a long venous catheter, *N Engl J Med* 280:95-96, 1969.

250. Hindle W, Posner E, Sweetnam MT, et al: Pleural effusion and fibrosis during treatment with methysergide, *Br Med J* 1:605-606, 1970.

251. Hirsch A, Ruffie P, Nebut M, et al: Pleural effusion: laboratory tests in 300 cases, *Thorax* 34:106-112, 1979.

252. Hirsch JH, Rogers JV, Mack LA: Real-time sonography of pleural opacities, *AJR* 136:297-301, 1981.

253. Hobbs JE, Bortnick AR: Endometriosis of the lungs: an experimental and clinical study, *Am J Obstet Gynecol* 40:832-843, 1940.

254. Hoffer FA, Ablow RC: The cross-table lateral view in neonatal pneumothorax, *AJR* 142:1283-1286, 1984.

255. Hogg JC, Macklem PT, Thurlbeck WM: The resistance of collateral channels in excised human lungs, *J Clin Invest* 48:421-431, 1969.

256. Hogg JC, Nepszy S: Regional lung volume and pleural pressure gradient estimated from the lung density in dogs, *J Appl Physiol* 27:198-203, 1969.

257. Holmberg L, Boman G: Pulmonary reactions to nitrofurantoin: 447 cases reported to the Swedish adverse drug reaction committee 1966-1976, *Eur J Respir Dis* 62:180-189, 1981.

258. Holoye PY, Luna MA, MacKay B, et al: Bleomycin hypersensitivity pneumonitis, *Ann Intern Med* 88:47-49, 1978.

259. Holzel A, Fawcitt J: Pulmonary changes in acute glomerulonephritis in childhood, *J Pediatr* 57:695-703, 1960.

260. Hom M, Jolles H: Traumatic mediastinal lymphocele mimicking other thoracic injuries: case report, *J Thorac Imag* 7:78-80, 1992.

261. Hopps HC, Wissler RW: Uremic pneumonitis, *Am J Pathol* 31:261-274, 1955.

262. Hughson WG, Friedman PJ, Feigin DS, et al: Postpartum pleural effusion: a common radiologic finding, *Ann Intern Med* 97:856-858, 1982.

263. Hulnick DH, Naidich DP, McCauley DI: Pleural tuberculosis evaluated by computed tomography, *Radiology* 149:759-765, 1983.

264. Humphreys RL, Berne AS: Rapid re-expansion of pneumothorax: a cause of unilateral pulmonary edema, *Radiology* 96:509-512, 1970.

265. Hurwitz PA, Pinals DJ: Pleural effusion in chronic hereditary lymphedema (Nonne, Milroy, Meige's disease), *Radiology* 82:246-248, 1964.

266. Hussey HH, Katz S, Yater WM: The superior vena caval syndrome: report of thirty-five cases, *Am Heart J* 31:1-26, 1946.

267. Hyde I: Traumatic para-mediastinal air cysts, *Br J Radiol* 44:380-383, 1971.

268. Im J-G, Chung JW, Han MC: Milk of calcium pleural collections: CT findings, *J Comput Assist Tomogr* 17:613-616, 1993.

269. Im J-G, Kang HS, Choi BI, et al: Pleural endometriosis: CT and sonographic findings, *AJR* 148:523-524, 1987.

270. Im J-G, Webb WR, Han MC, et al: Apical opacity associated with pulmonary tuberculosis: high-resolution CT findings, *Radiology* 178:727-731, 1991.

271. Im J-G, Webb WR, Rosen A, et al: Costal pleura: appearances at high-resolution CT, *Radiology* 171:125-131, 1989.

272. Inouye WY, Berggren RB, Johnson J: Spontaneous pneumothorax: treatment and mortality, *Dis Chest* 51:67-73, 1967.

273. Islam N, Ali S, Kabir H: Hepatic hydrothorax, *Br J Dis Chest* 59:222-227, 1965.

274. Jaffe RB, Koschmann FB: Septic pulmonary emboli, *Radiology* 96:527-532, 1970.

275. Jamison HW: Anatomic-roentgenographic study of pleural domes and pulmonary apices, with special reference to apical subpleural scars, *Radiology* 36:302-314, 1941.

276. Janetos GP, Ochsner SF: Bilateral pneumothorax in metastatic osteogenic sarcoma, *Am Rev Respir Dis* 88:73-76, 1963.

277. Jansveld CAF, Dijkman JH: Primary spontaneous pneumothorax and smoking, *Br Med J* 4:559-560, 1975.

278. Javaheri S, Hales CA: Sarcoidosis: a cause of innominate vein obstruction and massive pleural effusion, *Lung* 157:81-85, 1980.

279. Jay SJ: Diagnostic procedures for pleural disease, *Clin Chest Med* 6:33-48, 1985.

280. Jelihovsky T, Grant AF: Endometriosis of the lung: a case report and brief review of the literature, *Thorax* 23:434-437, 1986.

281. Jenkins PG, Shelp WD: Recurrent pleural transudate in the nephrotic syndrome: a new approach to treatment, *JAMA* 230:587-588, 1974.

282. Jenkinson SG: Pneumothorax, *Clin Chest Med* 6:153-161, 1985.

283. Jewelewicz R, Vandle Wiele RL: Acute hydrothorax as the only symptom of ovarian hyperstimulation syndrome, *Am J Obstet Gynecol* 121:1121, 1975.

284. Johnson JD, Raff MJ, Barnwell PA, et al: Splenic abscess complicating infectious endocarditis, *Arch Intern Med* 143:906-912, 1983.

285. Johnson JR, Falk A, Iber C, et al: Paragonimiasis in the United States: a report of nine cases in the Hmong immigrants, *Chest* 82:168-171, 1982.

286. Johnston RF, Loo RV: Hepatic hydrothorax: studies to determine the source of the fluid and report of thirteen cases, *Ann Intern Med* 61:385-401, 1964.

287. Joseph J, Sahn SA: Connective tissue diseases and the pleura, *Chest* 104:262-270, 1993.

288. Kaminsky ME, Rodan BA, Osborne DR: Postpericardiotomy syndrome, *AJR* 138:503-508, 1982.

289. Katoh O, Yamada H, Aoki Y, et al: Utility of angiograms in patients with catamenial hemoptysis, *Chest* 98:1296-1297, 1990.

290. Kattan KR, Eyler WR, Felson B: The juxtaphrenic peak in upper lobe collapse, *Semin Roentgenol* 15:187-193, 1980.

291. Katzen BT, Choi WS, Friedman MH, et al: Pseudomass of the liver due to pleural effusion and inversion of the diaphragm, *AJR* 131:1077-1078, 1978.

292. Kausel HW, Reeve TS, Stein AA, et al: Anatomic and pathologic studies of the thoracic duct, *J Thorac Surg* 34:631-642, 1957.

293. Kaye MD: Pleuropulmonary complications of pancreatitis, *Thorax* 23:297-306, 1968.

294. Kent EM, Blades B: Surgical anatomy of pulmonary lobes, *J Thorac Surg* 12:18-30, 1942.

295. Killen DA, Gobbel WG: *Spontaneous pneumothorax*, Boston, 1968, Little, Brown.

296. Kinmonth JB: *The lymphatics: diseases, lymphography and surgery*, London, 1972, Edward Arnold.

287. Kircher LT, Swartzel RL: Spontaneous pneumothorax and its treatment, *JAMA* 155:24-29, 1954.

298. Kirchner SG, Heller RM, Smith CW: Pancreatic pseudocyst of the mediastinum, *Radiology* 123:37-42, 1977.

299. Kirkpatrick JA, Fleisher DS: The roentgen appearance of the chest in acute glomerulonephritis in children, *J Pediatr* 64:492-498, 1964.

300. Kitchen ND, Hocken DB, Greenhalgh RM, et al: Use of the Denver pleuroperitoneal shunt in the treatment of chylothorax secondary to filariasis, *Thorax* 46:144-145, 1991.

301. Kjaergaard H: Spontaneous pneumothorax in the apparently healthy, *Acta Med Scand (suppl)* 43:1-159, 1932.

302. Kleinman PK, Brill PW, Whalen JP: Anterior pathway for transdiaphragmatic extension of pneumomediastinum, *AJR* 131:271-275, 1978.

303. Kleinman PK, Raptopoulos V: The anterior diaphragmatic attachments: an anatomic and radiologic study with clinical correlates, *Radiology* 155:289-293, 1985.

304. Koehler PR, Jones R: Association of left-sided pleural effusions and splenic hematomas, *AJR* 135:851-853, 1980.

305. Kok-Jensen A, Lindeneg O: Pleurisy and fibrosis of the pleura during methysergide treatment of hemicrania, *Scand J Respir Dis* 51:218-222, 1970.

306. Kollef MH: Chronic pleural effusion following coronary artery revascularization with the internal mammary artery, *Chest* 97:750-751, 1990.

307. Kollins SA: Computed tomography of the pulmonary parenchyma and chest wall, *Radiol Clin North Am* 15:297-308, 1977.

308. Korn MA, Schurawitzki H, Klepetko W, et al: Pulmonary alveolar microlithiasis: findings on high-resolution CT, *AJR* 158:981-982, 1992.

309. Kovarik JL, Toll GD: Thoracic endometriosis with recurrent spontaneous pneumothorax, *JAMA* 196:595-597, 1966.

310. Kramer SS, Taylor GA, Garfinkel DJ, et al: Lethal chylothoraces due to superior vena caval thrombosis in infants, *AJR* 137:559-563, 1981.

311. Kshettry VR, Rebello R: Chylothorax after coronary artery bypass grafting, *Thorax* 37:954, 1982.

312. Kuehnel E: Massive pleural effusion secondary to CAPD, *Kidney Int* 19:152, 1981.

313. Kuhn M, Fitting J-W, Leuenberger P: Probability of malignancy in pleural fluid eosinophilia, *Chest* 96:992-994, 1989.

314. Kumar A, Pontoppidan H, Falke KJ, et al: Pulmonary barotrauma during mechanical ventilation, *Crit Care Med* 1:181-186, 1973.

315. Kupferschmid JP, Shahian DM, Villanueva AG: Massive hemothorax associated with intrathoracic extramedullary hematopoiesis involving the pleura, *Chest* 103:974-975, 1993.

316. Kurlander GJ, Helmen CH: Subpulmonary pneumothorax, *AJR* 96:1019-1021, 1966.

317. Kutty CPK: Cause of chylous pleural effusion, *Chest* 78:357-358, 1980.

318. Lacombe P, Cornud F, Grenier P, et al: A new sign of right anterior pneumothorax in the supine adult: three case reports, *Ann Radiol* 25:231-236, 1982.

319. Laforet EG, Kornitzer GD: Nephrogenic pleural effusion, *J Urol* 117:118-119, 1977.

320. Lahiry SK, Alkhafaji AH, Brown AL: Urinothorax following blunt trauma to the kidney, *J Trauma* 18:608-610, 1978.

321. Laing FC, Filly RA: Problems in the application of ultrasonography for the evaluation of pleural opacities, *Radiology* 126:211-214, 1978.

322. Lally JF, Gohel VK, Dalinka MK, et al: The roentgenographic manifestations of cutis laxa (generalized elastolysis), *Radiology* 113:605-606, 1974.

323. Lampson RS: Traumatic chylothorax: a review of the literature and report of a case treated by mediastinal ligation of the thoracic duct, *J Thorac Surg* 17:778-791, 1948.

324. Lams P: Radiographic signs in post-pneumonectomy bronchopleural fistula, *J Can Assoc Radiol* 31:178-180, 1980.

325. Lams PM, Jolles H: The scapula companion shadow, *Radiology* 138:19-23, 1981.

326. Lams PM, Jolles H: The effect of lobar collapse on the distribution of free intrapleural air, *Radiology* 142:309-312, 1982.

327. Lane EJ, Proto AV, Phillips TW: Mach bands and density perception, *Radiology* 121:9-17, 1976.

328. Lattes R, Shepard F, Tovell H, et al: A clinical and pathologic study of endometriosis of the lung, *Surg Gynecol Obstet* 103:552-558, 1956.

329. Laurens RG, Pine JR, Honig EG: Spontaneous pneumothorax in primary cavitating lung carcinoma, *Radiology* 146:295-297, 1983.

330. Laws HL, Fox LS, Younger JB: Bilateral catamenial pneumothorax, *Arch Surg* 112:627-628, 1977.

331. Lawton F, Blackledge G, Johnson R: Co-existent chylous and serous pleural effusions associated with ovarian cancer: a case report of Contarinis syndrome, *Eur J Surg Oncol* 11:177-178, 1985.

332. Lee KS, Im J-G, Choe KO, et al: CT findings in benign fibrous mesothelioma of the pleura: pathologic correlation in nine patients, *AJR* 158:983-986, 1992.

333. Legge DA, Tiede JJ, Peters GA, et al: Death from tension pneumothorax and chlorpromazine cardiorespiratory collapse as separate complications of asthma, *Ann Allergy* 27:23-29, 1969.

334. Leites V, Tannenbaum E: Familial spontaneous pneumothorax, *Am Rev Respir Dis* 82:240-241, 1960.

335. Lesser MB: Left azygos lobe: report of a case, *Dis Chest* 46:95-96, 1964.

336. Lesur O, Delorme N, Fromaget JM, et al: Computed tomography in the etiologic assessment of idiopathic spontaneous pneumothorax, *Chest* 98:341-347, 1990.

337. Leuallen EC, Carr DT: Pleural effusion: a statistical study of 436 patients, *N Engl J Med* 252:79-83, 1955.

338. Leung AN, Müller NL, Miller RR: CT in differential diagnosis of diffuse pleural disease, *AJR* 154:487-492, 1990.

339. Levi C, Gray JE, McCullough EC, et al: The unreliability of CT numbers as absolute values, *AJR* 139:443-447, 1982.

340. Levin EJ, Bryk D: Dressler syndrome (postmyocardial infarction syndrome), *Radiology* 87:731-736, 1966.

341. Levitt RG, Sagel SS, Stanley RJ, et al: Accuracy of computed tomography of the liver and biliary tract, *Radiology* 124:123-128, 1977.

342. LeWitt PA, Calne DB: Pleuropulmonary changes during long term bromocriptine treatment for Parkinson's disease, *Lancet* 1:44-45, 1981.

343. Liberson M: Diagnostic significance of the mediastinal profile in massive unilateral pleural effusions, *Am Rev Respir Dis* 88:176-180, 1963.

344. Libshitz HI, Banner MP: Spontaneous pneumothorax as a complication of radiation therapy to the thorax, *Radiology* 112:199-201, 1974.

345. Libshitz HI, Southard ME: Complications of radiation therapy: the thorax, *Semin Roentgenol* 9:41-49, 1974.

346. Lieberman FL, Hidemura R, Peters RL, et al: Pathogenesis and treatment of hydrothorax complicating cirrhosis with ascites, *Ann Intern Med* 64:341-351, 1966.

347. Lieberman FL, Peters RL: Cirrhotic hydrothorax: further evidence that an acquired diaphragmatic defect is at fault, *Arch Intern Med* 125:114-117, 1970.

348. Liem K: Incidence and significance of heart muscle antibodies in patients with acute myocardial infarction and unstable angina, *Acta Med Scand* 206:473-475, 1979.

349. Light RW: *Pleural diseases,* Philadelphia, 1983, Lea & Febiger.

350. Light RW: Exudative pleural effusions secondary to gastrointestinal diseases, *Clin Chest Med* 6:103-111, 1985.

351. Light RW: Management of spontaneous pneumothorax, *Am Rev Respir Dis* 148:245-248, 1993.

352. Light RW, George RB: Incidence and significance of pleural effusion after abdominal surgery, *Chest* 69:621-625, 1976.

353. Light RW, O'Hara VS, Moritz TE, et al: Intrapleural tetracycline for the prevention of recurrent spontaneous pneumothorax, *JAMA* 264:2224-2230, 1990.

354. Lillard RL, Allen RP: The extrapleural air sign in pneumomediastinum, *Radiology* 85:1093-1098, 1965.

355. Lillington GA, Mitchell SP, Wood GA: Catamenial pneumothorax, *JAMA* 219:1328-1332, 1972.

356. Lippert HL, Lund O, Blegvad S, et al: Independent risk factors for cumulative recurrence rate after first spontaneous pneumothorax, *Eur Respir J* 4:324-331, 1991.

357. Lipscomb DJ, Flower CDR, Hadfield JW: Ultrasound of the pleura: an assessment of its clinical value, *Clin Radiol* 32:289-290, 1981.

358. Lipton RA, Greenwald RA, Seriff NS: Pneumothorax and bilateral honeycombed lung in Marfan syndrome: report of a case and review of the pulmonary abnormalities in this disorder, *Am Rev Respir Dis* 104:924-928, 1971.

359. Llach F, Arieff AI, Massry SG: Renal vein thrombosis and nephrotic syndrome: a prospective study of 36 adult patients, *Ann Intern Med* 83:8-14, 1975.

360. Logue RB, Rogers JV, Gay BB: Subtle roentgenographic signs of left heart failure, *Am Heart J* 65:464-473, 1963.

361. Lomas DJ, Padley SG, Flower CDR: The sonographic appearances of pleural fluid, *Br J Radiol* 66:619-624, 1993.

362. Lorentz WB: Acute hydrothorax during peritoneal dialysis, *J Pediatr* 94:417-419, 1979.

363. Lote K, Dahl O, Vigander T: Pneumothorax during combination chemotherapy, *Cancer* 47:1743-1745, 1981.

364. Louie S, McGahan JP, Frey C, et al: Pancreatic pleuropericardial effusions: fistulous tracts demonstrated by computed tomography, *Arch Intern Med* 145:1231-1234, 1985.

365. Lowe SH, Cosgrove DO, Joseph AEA: Inversion of the right hemidiaphragm shown on ultrasound examination, *Br J Radiol* 54:754-757, 1981.

366. Lowell JR: *Pleural effusions: a comprehensive review*, Baltimore, 1977, University Park Press.

367. Lowman RM, Hoogerhyde J, Waters LL, et al: Traumatic chylothorax: the roentgen aspects of this problem, *AJR* 65:529-546, 1951.

368. Lundin P, Simonsson B, Winberg T: Pneumonopleural amyloid tumour, *Acta Radiol* 55:139-144, 1961.

369. MacEwan DW, Dunbar JS, Smith RD, et al: Pneumothorax in young infants — recognition and evaluation, *J Can Assoc Radiol* 22:264-269, 1971.

370. MacFarlane JR, Holman CW: Chylothorax, *Am Rev Respir Dis* 105:287-291, 1972.

371. Maffessanti M, Tommasi M, Pellegrini P: Computed tomography of free pleural effusions, *Eur J Radiol* 7:87-90, 1987.

372. Magid D, Pyeritz RE, Fishman EK: Musculoskeletal manifestations of the Marfan syndrome: radiologic features, *AJR* 155:99-104, 1990.

373. Mahafan VK, Simon M, Huber GL: Re-expansion pulmonary edema, *Chest* 75:192-194, 1979.

374. Maher GG, Berger HW: Massive pleural effusion: malignant and nonmalignant causes in 46 patients, *Am Rev Respir Dis* 105:458-460, 1972.

375. Majzlin G, Stevens FL: Meigs' syndrome: case report and review of literature, *J Int Coll Surg* 42:625-630, 1964.

376. Malave G, Foster ED, Wilson JA, et al: Bronchopleural fistula — present-day study of an old problem, *Ann Thorac Surg* 11:1-10, 1971.

377. Maloney JV, Spencer FC: The nonoperative treatment of traumatic chylothorax, *Surgery* 40:121-128, 1956.

378. Mamtora H, Cope V: Pulmonary opacities in pseudoxanthoma elasticum: report of two cases, *Br J Radiol* 54:65-67, 1981.

379. Mancini JL: Familial paroxysmal polyserositis, phenotype I (familial Mediterranean fever), *Am Rev Respir Dis* 107:461-463, 1973.

380. Mandell GA, Pizzica AL: Air in the inferior accessory fissure of a neonate, *J Can Assoc Radiol* 32:249-250, 1981.

381. Mann H, Ward JH, Samlowski WE: Vascular leak syndrome associated with interleukin-2: chest radiographic manifestations, *Radiology* 176:191-194, 1990.

382. Markowitz RI: The anterior junction line: a radiographic sign of bilateral pneumothorax in neonates, *Radiology* 167:717-719, 1988.

383. Marks BW, Kuhns LR: Identification of the pleural fissures with computed tomography, *Radiology* 143:139-141, 1982.

384. Marks PA, Roof BS: Pericardial effusion associated with myxedema, *Ann Intern Med* 39:230-240, 1953.

385. Marks WM, Filly RA, Callen PW: Real-time evaluation of pleural lesions: new observations regarding the probability of obtaining free fluid, *Radiology* 142:163-164, 1982.

386. Marsac JH, Huchon GJ, Bismuth V: Pleural chylous effusion. In Chretien J, Bignon J, Hirsch A, eds: *The pleura in health and disease*, New York, 1985, Marcel Dekker.

387. Marshall AJ, Eltringham WK, Barritt DW, et al: Respiratory disease associated with practolol therapy, *Lancet* 2:1254-1257, 1977.

388. Mata JM, Cáceres J, Alegret X, et al: Imaging of the azygos lobe: normal anatomy and variations, *AJR* 156:931-937, 1991.

389. Mata J, Cáceres J, Llauger J, et al: CT demonstration of intrapulmonary right brachiocephalic vein associated with an azygos lobe, *J Comput Assist Tomogr* 14:305-306, 1990.

390. Maurer ER, Schaal JA, Mendez FL: Chronic recurring spontaneous pneumothorax due to endometriosis of the diaphragm, *JAMA* 168:2013-2014, 1958.

391. Maxwell E, Esterly NB: Cutis laxa, *Am J Dis Child* 117:479-482, 1969.

392. Mayo JR, Müller NL, Henkelman RM: The double-fissure sign: a motion artifact on thin section CT scans, *Radiology* 165:580-581, 1987.

393. Mayo P: Recurrent spontaneous pneumothorax concomitant with menstruation, *J Thorac Cardiovasc Surg* 46:415-416, 1963.

394. McArdle CR, Sacks BA: Ovarian hyperstimulation syndrome, *AJR* 135:835-836, 1980.

395. McElvaney NG, Wilcox PG, Churg A, et al: Pleuropulmonary disease during bromocriptine treatment of Parkinson's disease, *Arch Intern Med* 148:2231-2236, 1988.

396. McFadden ER, Luparello F: Bronchopleural fistula complicating massive pulmonary infarction, *Thorax* 24:500-505, 1969.

397. McKay DG, Sparling HJ, Robbins SL: Cirrhosis of the liver with massive hydrothorax, *Arch Intern Med* 79:501-509, 1947.

398. McKenna JM, Chandrasekhar AJ, Skorton D, et al: The pleuropulmonary complications of pancreatitis, *Chest* 71:197-204, 1977.

399. McLoud TC, Barash PG, Ravin CE: PEEP: radiographic features and associated complications, *AJR* 129:209-213, 1977.

400. McLoud TC, Flower CDR: Imaging the pleura: sonography, CT, and MR imaging, *AJR* 156:1145-1153, 1991.

401. McLoud TC, Isler R, Head J: The radiologic appearance of chemical pleurodesis, *Radiology* 135:313-317, 1980.

402. McLoud TC, Isler RJ, Novelline RA, et al: The apical cap, review, *AJR* 137:299-306, 1981.

403. McPeak EM, Levine SA: The preponderance of right hydrothorax in congestive heart failure, *Ann Intern Med* 25:916-927, 1946.

404. Meade RH, Head JR, Moen CW: The management of chylothorax, *J Thorac Surg* 19:709-723, 1950.

405. Medlar EM: Variations in interlobar fissures, *AJR* 57:723-725, 1947.

406. Meigs JV: Fibroma of the ovary with ascites and hydrothorax — Meigs' syndrome, *Am J Obstet Gynecol* 67:962-987, 1954.

407. Meigs JV: Pelvic tumours other than fibromas of the ovary with ascites and hydrothorax, *Obstet Gynecol* 3:471-485, 1954.

408. Meigs JV, Cass JW: Fibroma of the ovary with ascites and hydrothorax: with a report of seven cases, *Am J Obstet Gynecol* 33:249-267, 1937.

409. Meine F, Grossman H, Forman W, et al: The radiographic findings in congenital cutis laxa, *Radiology* 113:687-690, 1974.

410. Mellins RB, Levine OR, Fishman AP: Effect of systemic and pulmonary venous hypertension on pleural and pericardial fluid accumulation, *J Appl Physiol* 29:564-569, 1970.

411. Melton LJ, Hepper NGG, Offord KP: Incidence of spontaneous pneumothorax in Olmsted County, Minnesota: 1950-1974, *Am Rev Respir Dis* 120:1379-1382, 1979.

412. Melton LJ, Hepper NGG, Offord KP: Influence of height on the risk of spontaneous pneumothorax, *Mayo Clin Proc* 56:678-682, 1981.

413. Merten DF, Rooney R: Progressive pulmonary emphysema associated with congenital generalized elastolysis (cutis laxa), *Radiology* 113:691-692, 1974.

414. Meyerhoff J: Familial Mediterranean fever: report of a large family, review of the literature, and discussion of the frequency of amyloidosis, *Medicine* 59:66-77, 1980.

415. Middleton KL, Santella R, Couser JI: Eosinophilic pleuritis due to propylthiouracil, *Chest* 103:955-956, 1993.

416. Millard CE: Massive hemothorax complicating heparin therapy for pulmonary infarction, *Chest* 59:235-237, 1971.

417. Miller WC, Toon R, Palat H, et al: Experimental pulmonary edema following re-expansion of pneumothorax, *Am Rev Respir Dis* 108:664-666, 1973.

418. Miller WT: Drug-related pleural and mediastinal disorders, *J Thorac Imag* 6:36-51, 1991.

419. Miller WT, Talman EA: Subphrenic abscess, *AJR* 101:961-969, 1967.

420. Millward SF, Breatnach E, Simpkins KC, et al: Do plain films of the chest and abdomen have a role in the diagnosis of acute pancreatitis? *Clin Radiol* 34:133-137, 1983.

421. Milner LB, Ryan K, Gullo J: Fatal intrathoracic hemorrhage after percutaneous aspiration lung biopsy, *AJR* 132:280-281, 1979.

422. Mine H, Tamura K, Tanegashima K, et al: Non-traumatic chylothorax associated with diffuse lymphatic dysplasia, *Lymphology* 17:111-112, 1984.

423. Mintzer RA, Hendrix RW, Johnson CS, et al: The radiologic significance of the left pulmonary ligament, *Chest* 76:401-405, 1979.

424. Miridjanian A, Ambruoso VN, Derby BM, et al: Massive bilateral hemorrhagic pleural effusions in chronic relapsing pancreatitis, *Arch Surg* 98:62-66, 1969.

425. Mirouze D, Juttner H-U, Reynolds TB: Left pleural effusion in patients with chronic liver disease and ascites: prospective study of 22 cases, *Dig Dis Sci* 26:984-988, 1981.

426. Mobbs GA, Pfanner DW: Endometriosis of the lung, *Lancet* 1:472-474, 1963.

427. Mokrohisky JF: So-called "Meigs' syndrome" associated with benign and malignant ovarian tumors, *Radiology* 70:578-581, 1958.

428. Moller A: Pleural effusion: use of the semi-supine position for radiographic detection, *Radiology* 150:245-249, 1984.

429. Moncada R, Williams V, Fareed J, et al: Thoracic splenosis, *AJR* 144:705-706, 1985.

430. Morrow CS, Kantor M, Armen RN: Hepatic hydrothorax, *Ann Intern Med* 49:193-203, 1958.

431. Moses DC, Silver TM, Bookstein JJ: The complementary roles of chest radiography, lung scanning, and selective pulmonary angiography in the diagnosis of pulmonary embolism, *Circulation* 49:179-188, 1974.

432. Moskowitz H, Platt RT, Schachar R, et al: Roentgen visualization of minute pleural effusion: an experimental study to determine the minimum amount of pleural fluid visible on a radiograph, *Radiology* 109:33-35, 1973.

433. Moskowitz PS, Griscom NT: The medial pneumothorax, *Radiology* 120:143-147, 1976.

434. Moss R, Hinds S, Fedullo AJ: Chylothorax: a complication of the nephrotic syndrome, *Am Rev Respir Dis* 140:1436-1437, 1989.

435. Motoyoshi K, Momoi H, Mikomi R, et al: Pulmonary lesions seen in a family with marfanoid hypermobility syndrome, *Jpn J Thorac Dis* 11:138-143, 1973.

436. Muller NL: Imaging of the pleura, *Radiology* 186:297-309, 1993.

437. Muller NL, Nelems B: Postcoital catamenial pneumothorax, *Am Rev Respir Dis* 134:803-804, 1986.

438. Muller R, Lofstedt S: The reaction of the pleura in primary tuberculosis of the lungs, *Acta Med Scand* 122:105-133, 1945.

439. Mulvey RB: The effect of pleural fluid on the diaphragm, *AJR* 84:1080-1085, 1965.

440. Munk PL, Müller NL: Pleural liposarcoma: CT diagnosis, *J Comput Assist Tomogr* 12:709-710, 1988.

441. Murdoch JL, Walker BA, Halpern BL, et al: Life expectancy and causes of death in the Marfan syndrome, *N Engl J Med* 286:804-808, 1972.

442. Murphy D, Duncan JG, Imrie CW: The "negative chest radiograph" in acute pancreatitis, *Br J Radiol* 50:264-265, 1977.

443. Murphy FB, Small WC, Wichman RD, et al: CT and chest radiography are equally sensitive in the detection of pneumothorax after CT-guided pulmonary interventional procedures, *AJR* 154:45-46, 1990.

444. Naidich DP, Megibow AJ, Hilton S, et al: Computed tomography of the diaphragm: peridiaphragmatic fluid localization, *J Comput Assist Tomogr* 7:641-649, 1983.

445. Nakamura H, Konishiike J, Sugamura A, et al: Epidemiology of spontaneous pneumothorax in women, *Chest* 89:378-382, 1986.

446. Nashef SAM, Ferguson AD: Occult central pneumothorax, *Br J Radiol* 58:772-774, 1985.

447. Nassberger L: Left-sided pleural effusion secondary to continuous ambulatory peritoneal dialysis, *Acta Med Scand* 211:219-220, 1982.

448. Nayak IN, Lawrence D: Tension pneumothorax from a perforated gastric ulcer, *Br J Surg* 63:245-247, 1976.

449. Neff CC, Mueller PR, Ferrucci JT, et al: Serious complications following transgression of the pleural space in drainage procedures, *Radiology* 152:335-341, 1984.

450. Nelson SW: Large pneumothorax and associated massive collapse of the homolateral lung due to intrabronchial obstruction: a case report, *Radiology* 68:411-414, 1957.

451. Newlin N, Silver TM, Stuck KJ, et al: Ultrasonic features of pyogenic liver abscess, *Radiology* 139:155-159, 1981.

452. Neyazaki T, Kupic EA, Marshall WH, et al: Collateral lymphatico-venous communication after experimental obstruction of the thoracic duct, *Radiology* 85:423-432, 1965.

453. Ngan H, Fok M, Wong J: The role of lymphography in chylothorax following thoracic surgery, *Br J Radiol* 61:1032-1036, 1988.

454. Nichols DM, Cooperberg PL, Golding RH, et al: The safe intercostal approach? Pleural complications in abdominal interventional radiology, *AJR* 142:1013-1018, 1984.

455. Nidus BD, Matalon R, Cantacuzino D, et al: Uremic pleuritis—a clinicopathological entity, *N Engl J Med* 281:255-256, 1969.

456. Nielsen PH, Jepsen SB, Olsen AD: Postoperative pleural effusion following upper abdominal surgery, *Chest* 96:1133-1135, 1989.

457. Nightingale RC, Flower CDR: Encysted pneumothorax, a complication of asthma, *Br J Dis Chest* 78:98-100, 1984.

458. Nix JT, Albert M, Dugas JE, et al: Chylothorax and chylous ascites: a study of 302 selected cases, *Am J Gastroenterol* 28:40-53, 1957.

459. Nordkild P, Kromann-Andersen H, Struve-Christensen E: Yellow nail syndrome—the triad of yellow nails, lymphedema and pleural effusions, *Acta Med Scand* 219:221-227, 1986.

460. Norris RM, Jones JG, Bishop JM: Respiratory gas exchange in patients with spontaneous pneumothorax, *Thorax* 23:427-433, 1968.

461. Northfield TC: Oxygen therapy for spontaneous pneumothorax, *Br Med J* 4:86-88, 1971.

462. Nugent FW, Burns JR: Periodic disease, *Med Clin North Am* 50:371-378, 1966.

463. Nusbaum M, Baum S, Hedges RC, et al: Roentgenographic and direct visualization of thoracic duct, *Arch Surg* 88:105-113, 1964.

464. Nusser RA, Culhane RH: Roentgenogram of the month: recurrent transudative effusion with an abdominal mass, *Chest* 90:263-264, 1986.

465. Nygaard SD, Berger HA, Fick RB: Chylothorax as a complication of oesophageal sclerotherapy, *Thorax* 47:134-135, 1992.

466. Oestreich AE, Haley C: Pleural effusion: the thorn sign, *Chest* 79:365-366, 1981.

467. O'Flanagan SJ, Tighe BE, Egan TJ, et al: Meigs' syndrome and pseudo-Meigs' syndrome, *J R Soc Med* 80:252-253, 1987.

468. O'Gorman LD, Cottingham RA, Sargent EN, et al: Mediastinal emphysema in the new born: a review and description of the new extra pleural gas sign, *Dis Chest* 53:301-308, 1968.

469. O'Meara JB, Slade PR: Disappearance of fluid from the post-pneumonectomy space, *J Thorac Cardiovasc Surg* 67:621-628, 1974.

470. Omell GH, Anderson LS, Bramson RT: Chest wall tumors, *Radiol Clin North Am* 11:197-214, 1973.

471. O'Moore PV, Mueller PR, Simeone JF, et al: Sonographic guidance in diagnostic and therapeutic interventions in the pleural space, *AJR* 149:1-5, 1987.

472. O'Neill S, Sweeney J, Walker F, et al: Pneumothorax in the Ehlers-Danlos syndrome, *Ir J Med Sci* 150:43-44, 1981.

473. Onik G, Goodman PC, Webb WR, et al: Hydropneumothorax: detection on supine radiographs, *Radiology* 152:31-34, 1984.

474. Orwoll ES, Kiessling PJ, Patterson JR: Interstitial pneumonia from mitomycin, *Ann Intern Med* 89:352-355, 1978.

475. Otsuji H, Hatakeyama M, Kitamura I, et al: Right upper lobe versus right middle lobe: differentiation with thin-section, high-resolution CT, *Radiology* 172:653-656, 1989.

476. Otsuji H, Uchida H, Maeda M, et al: Incomplete interlobar fissures: bronchovascular analysis with CT, *Radiology* 187:541-546, 1993.

477. Page RL: Pleural thickening — oxprenolol exonerated, *Br J Dis Chest* 73:319, 1979.

478. Pant K, Shah A, Mathur RK, et al: Pulmonary alveolar microlithiasis with pleural calcification and nephrolithiasis, *Chest* 98:245-246, 1990.

479. Pantoja E, Kattan KR, Thomas HA: Some uncommon lower mediastinal densities: a pictorial essay, *Radiol Clin North Am* 22:633-646, 1984.

480. Pascual RS, Mosher MB, Sikand RS, et al: Effects of bleomycin on pulmonary function in man, *Am Rev Respir Dis* 108:211-217, 1973.

481. Pavlin J, Cheney FW: Unilateral pulmonary edema in rabbits after re-expansion of collapsed lung, *J Appl Physiol* 46:31-35, 1979.

482. Pecorari A, Weisbrod GL: Computed tomography of pseudotumoral pleural fluid collections in the azygoesophageal recess, *J Comput Assist Tomogr* 13:803-805, 1989.

483. Perez CA, Presant CA, Van Amburg AL: Management of superior vena cava syndrome, *Semin Oncol* 5:123-143, 1978.

484. Peterman TA, Brothers SK: Pleural effusions in congestive heart failure and in pericardial disease, *N Engl J Med* 309:313, 1983.

485. Peters ME, Gould HR, McCarthy TM: Identification of a bronchopleural fistula by computerized tomography — a case report, *J Comput Tomogr* 7:267-270, 1983.

486. Petersen JA: Recognition of infrapulmonary pleural effusion, *Radiology* 74:34-41, 1960.

487. Petusevsky ML, Faling LJ, Rocklin RE, et al: Pleuropericardial reaction to treatment with dantrolene, *JAMA* 242:2772-2774, 1979.

488. Phillips LG, Cunningham J: Esophageal perforation, *Radiol Clin North Am* 22:607-613, 1984.

489. Pisani RJ, Zeller FA: Bilious pleural effusion following liver biopsy, *Chest* 98:1535-1537, 1990.

490. Plowman PN, Stableforth DE, Citron KM: Spontaneous pneumothorax in Hodgkin's disease, *Br J Dis Chest* 74:411-414, 1980.

491. Polsky MS, Weber CH, Ball TP: Infected pyelocaliceal diverticulum and sympathetic pleural effusion, *J Urol* 114:301-303, 1975.

492. Pope FM: Ehlers-Danlos syndrome, *Ballière's Clin Rheumatol* 5:321-349, 1991.

493. Postmus PE, Kerstjens JM, Breed A, et al: A family with lobus venae azygos, *Chest* 90:298-299, 1986.

494. Proto AV: Conventional chest radiographs: anatomic understanding of newer observations, *Radiology* 183:593-603, 1992.

495. Proto AV, Ball JB: The superolateral major fissures, *AJR* 140:431-437, 1983.

496. Proto AV, Ball JB: Computed tomography of the major and minor fissures, *AJR* 140:439-448, 1983.

497. Proto AV, Merhar GL: Central bronchial displacement with large posterior pleural collections: findings on the lateral chest radiograph and CT scans, *J Can Assoc Radiol* 35:128-132, 1984.

498. Proto AV, Rost RC: CT of the thorax: pitfalls in interpretation, *Radiographics* 5:693-812, 1985.

499. Proto AV, Speckman JM: The left lateral radiograph of the chest, *Med Radiogr Photogr* 55:30-74, 1979.

500. Pugatch RD, Faling LJ, Robbins AH, et al: Differentiation of pleural and pulmonary lesions using computed tomography, *J Comput Assist Tomogr* 2:601-606, 1978.

501. Pugatch RD, Spirn PW: Radiology of the pleura, *Clin Chest Med* 6:17-32, 1985.

502. Pyeritz RE: Cardiovascular manifestations of heritable disorders of connective tissue. In Steinberg AG, Bearn AG, Motulsky AG, et al, eds: *Progress in medical genetics* (new series), vol 5, Philadelphia, 1983, WB Saunders.

503. Pyeritz RE, McKusick VA: The Marfan syndrome: diagnosis and management, *N Engl J Med* 300:772-777, 1979.

504. Qureshi MM, Roble DC, Gindin A, et al: Subarachnoid-pleural fistula, *J Thorac Cardiovasc Surg* 91:238-241, 1986.

505. Raasch BN, Carsky EW, Lane EJ, et al: Radiographic anatomy of the interlobar fissures, *AJR* 138:1043-1049, 1982.

506. Raasch BN, Carsky EW, Lane EJ, et al: Pictorial essay: pleural effusion; explanation of some typical appearances, *AJR* 139:899-904, 1982.

507. Rabin CB, Blackman NS: Bilateral pleural effusion: its significance in association with a heart of normal size, *Mount Sinai J Med* 24:45-53, 1957.

508. Rabinowitz JG, Cohen BA, Mendleson DS: The pulmonary ligament, *Radiol Clin North Am* 22:659-672, 1984.

509. Rabinowitz JG, Wolf BS: Roentgen significance of the pulmonary ligament, *Radiology* 87:1013-1020, 1966.

510. Race GA, Scheifley CH, Edwards JE: Hydrothorax in congestive heart failure, *Am J Med* 22:83-89, 1957.

511. Rakita L, Sobol SM, Mostow N, et al: Amiodarone pulmonary toxicity, *Am Heart J* 106:906-916, 1983.

512. Rao PS, Alfidi RJ: The environmental density artifact: a beam-hardening effect in computed tomography, *Radiology* 141:223-227, 1981.

513. Rasaretnam R, Chanmugam D, Sivathasan C: Spontaneous haemothorax in a mild haemophiliac, *Thorax* 31:601-604, 1976.

514. Rashid A, Sendi A, Al-Kadhimi A, et al: Concurrent spontaneous pneumothorax in identical twins, *Thorax* 41:971, 1986.

515. Ravin CE, Smith GW, Lester PD, et al: Post-traumatic pneumatocele in the inferior pulmonary ligament, *Radiology* 121:39-41, 1976.

516. Rawson AJ, Cocke JA: Infarction of an entire pulmonary lobe with subsequent aseptic softening causing sterile hemopneumothorax, *Am J Med Sci* 214:520-524, 1947.

517. Rea D: Traumatic chylothorax in a closed chest injury: report of a case, *Br J Dis Chest* 54:82-85, 1960.

518. Rebuck AS: Radiological aspects of severe asthma, *Australas Radiol* 14:264-268, 1970.

519. Redman JF, Arnold WC, Smith PL, et al: Hypertension and urino-thorax following an attempted percutaneous nephrostomy, *J Urol* 128:1307-1308, 1982.

520. Reilly KM, Tsou E: Bilateral chylothorax: a case report following episodes of stretching, *JAMA* 233:536-537, 1975.

521. Remy J, Mabille JP: La coiffe pleurale de le lesions parietales: un nouveau signe du syndrome extra-pleural, *Ann Radiol* 20:161-164, 1977.

522. Renner RR, Makarian B, Pernice NJ, et al: The apical cap, *Radiology* 110:569-573, 1974.

523. Renner RR, Pernice NJ: The apical cap, *Semin Roentgenol* 12:299-302, 1977.

524. Reynolds J, Davis JT: Injuries of the chest wall, pleura, pericardium, lungs, bronchi and esophagus, *Radiol Clin North Am* 4:383-401, 1966.

525. Rhea JT, DeLuca SA, Greene RE: Determining the size of pneumothorax in the upright patient, *Radiology* 144:733-736, 1982.

526. Rhea JT, vanSonnenberg E, McLoud TC: Basilar pneumothorax in the supine adult, *Radiology* 133:593-595, 1979.

527. Rigby M, Zylak CJ, Wood LDH: The effect of lobar atelectasis on pleural fluid distribution in dogs, *Radiology* 136:603-607, 1980.

528. Rigler LG, Ericksen LG: The inferior accessory lobe of the lung, *AJR* 29:384-392, 1933.

529. Rinne UK: Pleuropulmonary changes during longterm bromocriptine treatment for Parkinson's disease, *Lancet* 1:44, 1981.

530. Robins SA, Joress MH: Intrapleural fibrin bodies, *Am Rev Tuberc* 37:81-87, 1938.

531. Robitaille GA: Ehlers-Danlos syndrome and recurrent hemoptysis, *Ann Intern Med* 61:716-721, 1964.

532. Rockey DC, Cello JP: Pancreaticopleural fistula: report of 7 patients and review of the literature, *Medicine* 69:332-344, 1990.

533. Rodelas R, Rakowski TA, Argy WP, et al: Fibrosing uremic pleuritis during hemodialysis, *JAMA* 243:2424-2425, 1980.

534. Rodman MH, Jones CW: Catamenial hemoptysis due to bronchial endometriosis, *N Engl J Med* 266:805-808, 1962.

535. Rodriguez E, Martinez J, Javaloyas M, et al: Haemothorax in the course of chickenpox, *Thorax* 41:491, 1986.

536. Rogers CI, Meredith HC: Osler revisited: an unusual cause of inversion of the diaphragm, *Radiology* 125:596, 1977.

537. Rohlfing BM, Webb WR, Schlobohm RM: Ventilator-related extra-alveolar air in adults, *Radiology* 121:25-31, 1976.

538. Roseman DM, Kowlessar OD, Sleisenger MH: Pulmonary manifestations of pancreatitis, *N Engl J Med* 263:294-296, 1960.

539. Rosenberg ER: Ultrasound in the assessment of pleural densities, *Chest* 84:283-285, 1983.

540. Rosenberg RF, Rubinstein BM, Messinger NH: Intrathoracic lipomas, *Chest* 60:507-509, 1971.

541. Rosenberg SM, Riddick DH: Successful treatment of catamenial hemoptysis with danazol, *Obstet Gynecol* 57:130-131, 1981.

542. Rosenberger A, Abrams HL: Radiology of the thoracic duct, *AJR* 111:807-820, 1971.

543. Ross JK: A review of the surgery of the thoracic duct, *Thorax* 16:12-21, 1961.

544. Rossi NP, Goplerud CP: Recurrent catamenial pneumothorax, *Arch Surg* 109:173-176, 1974.

545. Rost RC, Proto AV: Inferior pulmonary ligament: computed tomographic appearance, *Radiology* 148:479-483, 1983.

546. Roth BJ, O'Meara TF, Cragun WH: The serum-effusion albumin gradient in the evaluation of pleural effusions, *Chest* 98:546-549, 1990.

547. Rowinsky EK, Abeloff MD, Wharam MD: Spontaneous pneumothorax following thoracic irradiation, *Chest* 88:703-708, 1985.

548. Roy PH, Carr DT, Payne WS: The problem of chylothorax, *Mayo Clin Proc* 42:457-467, 1967.

549. Rubin RH, Swartz MN, Malt R: Hepatic abscess: changes in clinical, bacteriologic and therapeutic aspects, *Am J Med* 57:601-610, 1974.

550. Ruckley CV, McCormack RJM: The management of spontaneous pneumothorax, *Thorax* 21:139-144, 1966.

551. Rudikoff JC: Early detection of pleural fluid, *Chest* 77:109-111, 1980.

552. Rudikoff JC: The pulmonary ligament and subpulmonic effusion, *Chest* 80:505-507, 1981.

553. Rudnick MR, Coyle JF, Beck LH, et al: Acute massive hydrothorax complicating peritoneal dialysis, report of two cases and a review of the literature, *Clin Nephrol* 12:38-44, 1979.

554. Runyon BA, Forker EL, Sopko JA: Pleural-fluid kinetics in a patient with primary lymphedema, pleural effusions, and yellow nails, *Am Rev Respir Dis* 119:821-825, 1979.

555. Ruskin JA, Gurney JW, Thorsen MK, et al: Detection of pleural effusions on supine chest radiographs, *AJR* 148:681-683, 1987.

556. Rutherford RB, Hurt HH, Brickman RD, et al: The pathophysiology of progressive tension pneumothorax, *J Trauma* 8:212-227, 1968.

557. Ryan CJ, Rodgers RF, Unni KK, et al: The outcome of patients with pleural effusion of indeterminate cause at thoracotomy, *Mayo Clin Proc* 56:145-149, 1981.

558. Sahn SA: Immunologic diseases of the pleura, *Clin Chest Med* 6:83-102, 1985.

559. Sahn SA: The pleura, *Am Rev Respir Dis* 138:184-234, 1988.

560. Sahn SA, Miller KS: Obscure pleural effusion: look to the kidney, *Chest* 90:631, 1986.

561. Sakai O, Takahashi K, Nakashima N, et al: CT visualization of the major pulmonary fissures: value of 25° cranially tilted axial scans, *AJR* 161:523-526, 1993.

562. Saks BJ, Kilby AE, Dietrich PA, et al: Pleural and mediastinal changes following endoscopic injection sclerotherapy of esophageal varices, *Radiology* 149:639-642, 1983.

563. Salcedo JR: Urinothorax: report of 4 cases and review of the literature, *J Urol* 135:805-808, 1986.

564. Salmon VJ: Benign pelvic tumours associated with ascites and pleural effusion, *J Mt Sinai Hosp* 1:169-172, 1934.

565. Samman PD, White WF: The "yellow nail" syndrome, *Br J Dermatol* 76:153-157, 1964.

566. Sanders RC: Post-operative pleural effusion and subphrenic abscess, *Clin Radiol* 21:308-312, 1970.

567. Sargent EN, Boswell WD, Ralls PW, et al: Subpleural fat pads in patients exposed to asbestos: distinction from non-calcified pleural plaques, *Radiology* 152:273-277, 1984.

568. Sargent EN, Jacobson G, Gordonson JS: Pleural plaques: a signpost of asbestos dust inhalation, *Semin Roentgenol* 12:287-297, 1977.

569. Sarr MG, Zuidema GD: Splenic abscess — presentation, diagnosis, and treatment, *Surgery* 92:480-485, 1982.

570. Sassoon CS, Light RW: Chylothorax and pseudochylothorax, *Clin Chest Med* 6:163-171, 1985.

571. Sautter RD, Dreber WH, MacIndoe JH, et al: Fatal pulmonary edema and pneumonitis after reexpansion of chronic pneumothorax, *Chest* 60:399-401, 1971.

572. Scales FE, Lee ME: Nonoperative diagnosis of intrathoracic splenosis, *AJR* 141:1273-1274, 1983.

573. Scanlon TS, Benumof JL: Demonstration of interlobar collateral ventilation, *J Appl Physiol* 46:658-661, 1979.

574. Scattini CM, Orsi A: Multiple bilateral fibromas of the pleura, *Thorax* 28:782-787, 1973.

575. Schenker JG, Weinstein D: Ovarian hyperstimulation syndrome: a current survey, *Fertil Steril* 30:255-268, 1978.

576. Schmidt A: Chylothorax: review of 5 years' cases in the literature and report of a case, *Acta Chir Scand* 118:5-12, 1959.

577. Schmitt WGH, Hubener KH, Rucker HC: Pleural calcification with persistent effusion, *Radiology* 149:633-638, 1983.

578. Schneierson SJ, Katz M: Solitary pleural effusion due to myxedema, *JAMA* 168:1003-1005, 1958.

579. Schulman A, Fataar S, Dalrymple R, et al: The lymphographic anatomy of chylothorax, *Br J Radiol* 51:420-427, 1978.

580. Schwarz MI, Marmorstein BL: A new radiologic sign of subpulmonic effusion, *Chest* 67:176-178, 1975.

581. Scott GC, Berger R, McKean HE: The role of atmospheric pressure variation in the development of spontaneous pneumothoraces, *Am Rev Respir Dis* 139:659-662, 1989.

582. Seibert JJ, Golladay ES, Keller C: Chylothorax secondary to superior vena caval obstruction, *Pediatr Radiol* 12:252-254, 1982.

583. Sepkowitz KA, Telzak EE, Gold JWM, et al: Pneumothorax in AIDS, *Ann Intern Med* 114:455-459, 1991.

584. Seriff NS, Cohen ML, Samuel P, et al: Chylothorax: diagnosis by lipoprotein electrophoresis of serum and pleural fluid, *Thorax* 32:98-100, 1977.

585. Sewell RW, Fewel JG, Grover FL, et al: Experimental evaluation of reexpansion pulmonary edema, *Ann Thorac Surg* 26:126-132, 1978.

586. Shapir J, Lisbona A, Palayew MJ: Chronic calcified empyema, *J Can Assoc Radiol* 31:24-27, 1981.

587. Sharpe IK, Ahmad M, Braun W: Familial spontaneous pneumothorax and HLA antigens, *Chest* 78:264-268, 1980.

588. Shaw TJ, Caterine JM: Recurrent re-expansion pulmonary edema, *Chest* 86:784-786, 1984.

589. Sheard JDH, Taylor W, Soorae A, et al: Pneumothorax and malignant mesothelioma in patients over the age of 40, *Thorax* 46:584-585, 1991.

590. Shearin RPN, Hepper NGG, Payne WS: Recurrent spontaneous pneumothorax concurrent with menses, *Mayo Clin Proc* 49:98-101, 1974.

591. Shepard MK, Mancini MC, Campbell GD, et al: Right-sided hemothorax and recurrent abdominal pain in a 34-year-old woman, *Chest* 103:1239-1240, 1993.

592. Sherman NJ, Davis JR, Jesseph JE: Subphrenic abscess: a continuing hazard, *Am J Surg* 117:117-123, 1969.

593. Sherman S, Ravikrishran KP: Unilateral pulmonary edema following reexpansion of pneumothorax of brief duration, *Chest* 77:714, 1980.

594. Short DS: A radiological study of pulmonary infarction, *Q J Med* 20:233-245, 1951.

595. Shuman LS, Libshitz HI: Solid pleural manifestations of lymphoma, *AJR* 142:269-273, 1984.

596. Siegel MJ, McAlister WH: Unusual intrathoracic complications in Wilms tumor, *AJR* 134:1231-1234, 1980.

597. Siegal S: Familial paroxysmal polyserositis: analysis of fifty cases, *Am J Med* 36:893-918, 1964.

598. Silverman PM, Baker ME, Mahony BS: Atelectasis and subpulmonic fluid: a CT pitfall in distinguishing pleural from peritoneal fluid, *J Comput Assist Tomogr* 9:763-766, 1985.

599. Simon HB, Daggett WM, DeSanctis RW: Hemothorax as a complication of anticoagulant therapy in the presence of pulmonary infarction, *JAMA* 208:1830-1834, 1969.

600. Singh A, Sethi RS, Singh G: Pneumothorax: an unusual complication of teratoma chest, *Chest* 63:1034-1036, 1973.

601. Slasky BS, Deutsch M: Germ cell tumors complicated by pneumothorax, *Urology* 22:39-42, 1983.

602. Slasky BS, Siewers RD, Lecky JW, et al: Catamenial pneumothorax: the roles of diaphragmatic defects and endometriosis, *AJR* 138:639-643, 1982.

603. Slind RO, Rodarte JR: Spontaneous hemothorax in an otherwise healthy young man, *Chest* 66:81, 1974.

604. Smalley RV, Wall RL: Two cases of busulfan toxicity, *Ann Intern Med* 64:154-164, 1966.

605. Smith J, Alberts C, Balk AG: Pneumothorax in the Ehlers-Danlos syndrome: consequences or coincidence? *Scand J Respir Dis* 59:239-242, 1978.

606. Smyrnios NA, Jederlinic PJ, Irwin RS: Pleural effusion in an asymptomatic patient: spectrum and frequency of causes and management considerations, *Chest* 97:192-196, 1990.

607. Soderberg CH, Dahlquist EH: Catamenial pneumothorax, *Surgery* 79:236-239, 1976.

608. Sohar E, Gafni J, Pras M, et al: Familial Mediterranean fever, *Am J Med* 43:227-253, 1967.

609. Solal-Celigny P, Cormier Y, Fournier M: The yellow nail syndrome, *Arch Pathol Lab Med* 107:183-185, 1983.

610. Solomon S, Farber SJ, Caruso LJ: Fibromyomata of the uterus with hemothorax — Meigs' syndrome? *Arch Intern Med* 127:307-309, 1971.

611. Soulen RL, Freeman E: Radiologic evaluation of myocardial infarction, *Radiol Clin North Am* 9:567-582, 1971.

612. Spear BS, Sully L, Lewis CT: Pulmonary arteriovenous fistula presenting as spontaneous haemothorax, *Thorax* 30:355-356, 1975.

613. Speckman JM, Gamsu G, Webb WR: Alterations in CT mediastinal anatomy produced by an azygos lobe, *AJR* 137:47-50, 1981.

614. Spector ML, Stern RC: Pneumothorax in cystic fibrosis: a 26-year experience, *Ann Thorac Surg* 47:204-207, 1989.

615. Spittle MF, Heal J, Harmer C, et al: The association of spontaneous pneumothorax with pulmonary metastases in bone tumours of children, *Clin Radiol* 19:400-403, 1968.

616. Spizarny DL, Goodman LR: Air in the minor fissure: a sign of right-sided pneumothorax, *Radiology* 160:329-331, 1986.

617. Sprung CL, Loewenherz JW, Baier H, et al: Evidence of increased permeability in reexpansion pulmonary edema, *Am J Med* 71:497-500, 1981.

618. Staats BA, Ellefson RD, Budahn LL, et al: Lipoprotein profile of chylous and nonchylous pleural effusions, *Mayo Clin Proc* 55:700-704, 1980.

619. Steckel RJ: Unilateral pulmonary edema after pneumothorax, *N Engl J Med* 289:621-622, 1973.

620. Steier M, Ching N, Roberts EB, et al: Pneumothorax complicating continuous ventilatory support, *J Thorac Cardiovasc Surg* 67:17-23, 1974.

621. Stein GN, Chen JT, Goldstein F, et al: The importance of chest roentgenography in the diagnosis of pulmonary embolism, *AJR* 81:255-263, 1959.

622. Steiner GM, Farman J, Lawson JP: Lymphangiomatosis of bone, *Radiology* 93:1093-1098, 1969.

623. Steinhauslin CA, Cuttat JF: Spontaneous pneumothorax: a complication of lung cancer, *Chest* 88:709-713, 1985.

624. Stelzner TJ, King TE, Antony VB, et al: The pleuropulmonary manifestations of the postcardiac injury syndrome, *Chest* 84:383-387, 1983.

625. Stern H, Toole AL, Merino M: Catamenial pneumothorax, *Chest* 78:480-482, 1980.

626. Storey DD, Dines DE, Coles DT: Pleural effusion: a diagnostic dilemma, *JAMA* 236:2183-2186, 1976.

627. Stranahan A, Alley RD, Kausel HW, et al: Operative thoracic ductography, *J Thorac Surg* 31:183-198, 1956.

628. Subramanyam BR, Raghavendra BN, Lefleur RS: Sonography of the inverted right hemidiaphragm, *AJR* 136:1004-1006, 1981.

629. Sugiyama Y, Maeda H, Yotsumoto H, et al: Short reports: familial spontaneous pneumothorax, *Thorax* 41:969-970, 1986.

630. Sulis E, Floris C: Haemothorax due to thoracic extramedullary erythropoiesis in thalassaemia intermedia, *Br Med J* 291:1094, 1985.

631. Sullivan KL, Steiner RM, Wechsler RJ: Lymphaticopleural fistula: diagnosis by computed tomography, *J Comput Assist Tomogr* 8:1005-1006, 1984.

632. Swingle JD, Logan R, Juhl JH: Inversion of the left hemidiaphragm, *JAMA* 208:863-864, 1969.

633. Szabo G, Magyar Z: Effect of increased systemic venous pressure on lymph pressure and flow, *Am J Physiol* 212:1469-1474, 1967.

634. Taal BG, Spierings ELH, Hilvering C: Pleuropulmonary fibrosis associated with chronic and excessive intake of ergotamine, *Thorax* 38:396-398, 1983.

635. Tabatznik B, Isaacs JP: Postpericardiotomy syndrome following traumatic hemopericardium, *Am J Cardiol* 7:83-96, 1961.

636. Takasugi JE, Godwin JD: Left azygos lobe, *Radiology* 171:133-134, 1989.

637. Takasugi JE, Godwin JD, Teefey SA: The extrapleural fat in empyema: CT appearance, *Br J Radiol* 64:580-583, 1991.

638. Talbot S, Worthington BS, Roebuck EJ: Radiographic signs of pulmonary embolism and pulmonary infarction, *Thorax* 28:198-203, 1973.

639. Taylor GA, Fishman EK, Kramer SS, et al: CT demonstration of the phrenic nerve, *J Comput Assist Tomogr* 7:411-414, 1983.

640. Ten Eyck EA: Subpleural lipoma, *Radiology* 74:295-297, 1960.

641. Teoh PC: Bronchiectasis and spontaneous pneumothorax in Marfan's syndrome, *Chest* 72:672-673, 1977.

642. Teplick JG, Teplick SK, Goodman L, et al: The interface sign: a computed tomographic sign for distinguishing pleural and intra-abdominal fluid, *Radiology* 144:359-362, 1982.

643. Tewari SC, Jayaswal R, Chauhan MS, et al: Bilateral recurrent haemorrhagic pleural effusion in asymptomatic chronic pancreatitis, *Thorax* 44:824-825, 1989.

644. Theros EG, Feigin DS: Pleural tumors and pulmonary tumors: differential diagnosis, *Semin Roentgenol* 12:239-247, 1977.

645. Thorne PS: Traumatic chylothorax, *Tubercle* 39:29-34, 1958.

646. Thurer RJ: Chylothorax: a complication of subclavian vein catheterization and parenteral hyperalimentation, *J Thorac Cardiovasc Surg* 71:465-468, 1976.

647. Tocino IM, Miller MH, Fairfax WR: Distribution of pneumothorax in the supine and semirecumbent critically ill adult, *AJR* 144:901-905, 1985.

648. Tocino IM, Miller MH, Frederick PR, et al: CT detection of occult pneumothorax in head trauma, *AJR* 143:987-990, 1984.

649. Townsend R, Fragola JA: Hydrothorax in a patient receiving continuous ambulatory peritoneal dialysis, *Arch Intern Med* 142:1571-1572, 1982.

650. Trackler RT, Brinker RA: Widening of the left paravertebral pleural line on supine chest roentgenograms in free pleural effusions, *AJR* 96:1027-1034, 1966.

651. Trapnell DH: The peripheral lymphatics of the lung, *Br J Radiol* 36:660-672, 1963.

652. Trapnell DH: The differential diagnosis of linear shadows in chest radiographs, *Radiol Clin North Am* 11:77-92, 1973.

653. Trapnell DH, Thurston JGB: Unilateral pulmonary oedema after pleural aspiration, *Lancet* 1:1367-1369, 1970.

654. Tscholakoff D, Sechtem U, de Geer G, et al: Evaluation of pleural and pericardial effusions by magnetic resonance imaging, *Eur J Radiol* 7:169-174, 1987.

655. Tsipouras P, Del Mastro R, Sarfarazi M, et al: Genetic linkage of the Marfan syndrome, ectopia lentis, and congenital contractural arachnodactyly to the fibrillin genes on chromosomes 15 and 5, *N Engl J Med* 326:905-909, 1992.

656. Turner JAMcM, Stanley NN: Fragile lung in the Marfan syndrome, *Thorax* 31:771-775, 1976.

657. Turner-Stokes L, Turton C, Pope FM, et al: Emphysema and cutis laxa, *Thorax* 38:790-792, 1983.

658. Twiford TW, Zornoza J, Libshitz HI: Recurrent spontaneous pneumothorax after radiation therapy to the thorax, *Chest* 73:387-388, 1978.

659. Udeshi UL, McHugo JM, Crawford JS: Postpartum pleural effusion, *Br J Obstet Gynaecol* 95:894-897, 1988.

660. Ujita M, Ojiri H, Ariizumi M, et al: Appearance of the inferior phrenic artery and vein on CT scans of the chest: a CT and cadaveric study, *AJR* 160:745-747, 1993.

661. Urban C, Nirenberg A, Caparros B, et al: Chemical pleuritis as the cause of acute chest pain following high-dose methotrexate treatment, *Cancer* 51:34-37, 1983.

662. Urokinase pulmonary embolism trial: a national cooperative study. Chapter B. Associated clinical and laboratory findings, *Circulation* 47(suppl II):II-81-II-85, 1973.

663. Valentine VG, Raffin TA: The management of chylothorax, *Chest* 102:586-591, 1992.

664. Van Pernis PA: Variations of thoracic duct, *Surgery* 26:806-809, 1949.

665. Vennera MC, Moreno R, Cot J, et al: Chylothorax and tuberculosis, *Thorax* 38:694-695, 1983.

666. Videm V, Pillgram-Larsen J, Ellingsen O, et al: Spontaneous pneumothorax in chronic obstructive pulmonary disease: complications, treatment and recurrences, *Eur J Respir Dis* 71:365-371, 1987.

667. Vix VA: Extrapleural costal fat, *Radiology* 112:563-565, 1974.

668. Vix VA: Roentgenographic recognition of pleural effusion, *JAMA* 229:695-698, 1974.

669. Vix VA: Roentgenographic manifestations of pleural disease, *Semin Roentgenol* 12:277-286, 1977.

670. Vock P, Effmann EL, Hedlund LW, et al: Analysis of the density of pleural fluid analogs by computed tomography, *Invest Radiol* 19:10-15, 1984.

671. Vock P, Hedlund LW, Herfkens RJ, et al: Work in progress: in vitro analysis of pleural fluid analogs by proton magnetic resonance; preliminary studies at I.S.T., *Invest Radiol* 22:382-387, 1987.

672. Volberg FM, Everett CJ, Brill PW: Radiologic features of inferior pulmonary ligament air collections in neonates with respiratory distress, *Radiology* 130:357-360, 1979.

673. Waite RJ, Carbonneau RJ, Balikian JP, et al: Parietal pleural changes in empyema: appearances at CT, *Radiology* 175:145-150, 1990.

674. Walden PAM, Mitchell-Heggs PF, Coppin C, et al: Pleurisy and methotrexate treatment, *Br Med J* 2:867, 1977.

675. Walker BA, Beighton PH, Murdoch JL: The marfanoid hypermobility syndrome, *Ann Intern Med* 71:349-352, 1969.

676. Wall SD, Federle MP, Jeffrey RB, et al: CT diagnosis of unsuspected pneumothorax after blunt abdominal trauma, *AJR* 141:919-921, 1983.

677. Walsh JJ: Spontaneous pneumohemothorax, *Dis Chest* 29:329-335, 1956.

678. Wanderer AA, Ellis EF, Goltz RW, et al: Tracheobronchiomegaly and acquired cutis laxa in a child: physiologic and immunologic studies, *Pediatrics* 44:709-715, 1969.

679. Wanderman KL, Goldstein MS, Faber J: Cor pulmonale secondary to severe kyphoscoliosis in Marfan's syndrome, *Chest* 67:250-251, 1975.

680. Wang N-S: Anatomy and physiology of the pleural space, *Clin Chest Med* 6:3-16, 1985.

681. Waqarrudin M, Bernstein A: Re-expansion pulmonary oedema, *Thorax* 30:54-60, 1975.

682. Warner BW, Bailey WW, Shipley RT: Value of computed tomography of the lung in the management of primary spontaneous pneumothorax, *Am J Surg* 162:39-42, 1991.

683. Warren MS, Gibbons RB: Left-sided pleural effusion secondary to splenic vein thrombosis: a previously unrecognized relationship, *Chest* 100:574-575, 1991.

684. Warren WH, Altman JS, Gregory SA: Chylothorax secondary to obstruction of the superior vena cava: a complication of the LeVeen shunt, *Thorax* 45:978-979, 1990.

685. Watanabe A, Kobayashi T: Pleural calcification: a type of "metastatic calcification" in chronic renal failure, *Br J Radiol* 56:93-98, 1983.

686. Watanabe A, Shimokata K, Nomura F, et al: Interlobar pneumothorax, *AJR* 155:1135-1136, 1990.

687. Watne AL, Hatiboglu I, Moore GE: A clinical and autopsy study of tumor cells in the thoracic duct lymph, *Surg Gynecol Obstet* 110:339-345, 1960.

688. Webb DB, Whale RJ: Pleuropericardial effusion associated with minoxidil administration, *Postgrad Med J* 58:319-320, 1982.

689. Webb WR, Godwin JD: The obscured outer edge: a sign of improperly placed pleural drainage tubes, *AJR* 134:1062-1064, 1980.

690. Webb WR, LaBerge JM: Radiographic recognition of chest tube malposition in the major fissure, *Chest* 85:81-83, 1984.

691. Webber MM, O'Loughlin BJ: Variations of the pleural vertical fissure line, *Radiology* 82:461-462, 1964.

692. Weber DO, Del Mastro P, Yarnoz MD: Chylothorax after myocardial revascularization with internal mammary graft, *Ann Thorac Surg* 32:499-502, 1981.

693. Weidner WA, Steiner RM: Roentgenographic demonstration of intrapulmonary and pleural lymphatics during lymphangiography, *Radiology* 100:533-539, 1971.

694. Weiss JM, Spodick DH: Association of left pleural effusion with pericardial disease, *N Engl J Med* 308:696-697, 1983.

695. Weiss JM, Spodick DH: Laterality of pleural effusions in chronic congestive heart failure, *Am J Cardiol* 53:951, 1984.

696. Weiss W, Boucot KR, Gefter WI: Localized interlobar effusion in congestive heart failure, *Ann Intern Med* 38:1177-1186, 1953.

697. Weissman JL: Pneumothorax and an azygos lobe (letter), *J Thorac Imag* 4:vi-ix, 1989.

698. Weldon CS, Tumulty PA: Topics in clinical medicine: recurrent pneumothorax associated with menstruation, *Johns Hopkins Med J* 123:259-263, 1968.

699. Wernecke K, Galanski M, Peters PE, et al: Pneumothorax: evaluation by ultrasound — preliminary results, *J Thorac Imag* 2:76-78, 1987.

700. West JB: Distribution of mechanical stress in the lung, a possible factor in the localisation of pulmonary disease, *Lancet* 1:839-841, 1971.

701. Weston WJ: Left-sided lobe of the azygos vein, *J Fac Radiol* 5:286-288, 1954.

702. Wetterfors J: Subphrenic abscess, a clinical study of 101 cases, *Acta Chir Scand* 117:388-408, 1959.

703. Whitcomb ME, Schwartz MI: Pleural effusion complicating intensive mediastinal radiation therapy, *Am Rev Respir Dis* 103:100-107, 1971.

704. White PD, August S, Michie CR: Hydrothorax in congestive heart failure, *Am J Med Sci* 214:243-247, 1947.

705. Wiener-Kronish JP, Albertine KH, Licko V, et al: Protein egress and entry rates in pleural fluid and plasma in sheep, *J Appl Physiol* 56:459-463, 1984.

706. Wiener-Kronish JP, Goldstein R, Matthay RA, et al: Lack of association of pleural effusion with chronic pulmonary arterial and right atrial hypertension, *Chest* 92:967-970, 1987.

707. Wiener-Kronish JP, Matthay MA, Callen PW, et al: Relationship of pleural effusions to pulmonary hemodynamics in patients with congestive heart failure, *Am Rev Respir Dis* 132:1253-1256, 1985.

708. Wiggins J, Strickland B, Chung KF: Detection of bronchiectasis by high-resolution computed tomography in the yellow nail syndrome, *Clin Radiol* 43:377-379, 1991.

709. Wilhelm JL, Scommegna A: Catamenial pneumothorax: bilateral occurrence while on suppressive therapy, *Obstet Gynaecol* 50:227-231, 1977.

710. Wilkinson PD, Keegan J, Davies SW, et al: Changes in pulmonary microvascular permeability accompanying re-expansion oedema: evidence from dual isotope scintigraphy, *Thorax* 45:456-459, 1990.

711. Williams MH: Pleural effusion produced by abdomino-pleural communication in a patient with Laennec's cirrhosis of the liver and ascites, *Ann Intern Med* 33:216-221, 1950.

712. Williams NS, Lewis CT: Bronchopleural fistula: a review of 86 cases, *Br J Surg* 63:520-522, 1976.

713. Williford ME, Hidalgo H, Putman CE, et al: Computed tomography of pleural disease, *AJR* 140:909-914, 1983.

714. Willson SA, Sawicka EH, Mitchell IC: Spontaneous pneumothorax: an unusual radiological appearance, *Br J Radiol* 58:173-175, 1985.

715. Wilson WG, Aylsworth AS: Familial spontaneous pneumothorax, *Pediatrics* 64:172-175, 1979.

716. Wingfield RC: Chronic recurring spontaneous pneumothoraces associated with menstruation, *Md State Med J* 10:344-345, 1961.

717. Withers JN, Fishback ME, Kiehl PV, et al: Spontaneous pneumothorax: suggested etiology and comparison of treatment methods, *Am J Surg* 108:772-776, 1964.

718. Wittich GR, Kusnick CA, Starnes VA, et al: Communication between the two pleural cavities after major cardiothoracic surgery: relevance to percutaneous intervention, *Radiology* 184:461-462, 1992.

719. Wolverson MK, Crepps LF, Sundaram M, et al: Hyperdensity of recurrent hemorrhage at body computed tomography: incidence and morphologic variation, *Radiology* 148:779-784, 1983.

720. Wood GM, Bolton RP, Muers MF, et al: Pleurisy and pulmonary granulomas after treatment with acebutolol, *Br Med J* 285:936, 1982.

721. Wood JR, Bellamy D, Child AH, et al: Pulmonary disease in patients with Marfan syndrome, *Thorax* 39:780-784, 1984.

722. Woodring JH: Recognition of pleural effusion on supine radiographs: how much fluid is required, *AJR* 142:59-64, 1984.

723. Wright FW: Spontaneous pneumothorax and pulmonary malignant disease — a syndrome sometimes associated with cavitating tumours, *Clin Radiol* 27:211-222, 1976.

724. Yamada S: Uber die serose Flussigkeit in der Pleurahohle der gesunden menschen, *Z Gesamte Exp Med* 90:342-348, 1933.

725. Yamashita H: *Roentgenologic anatomy of the lung*, Tokyo, 1978, Igaku-Shoin.

726. Yang P-C, Luh K-T, Chang D-B, et al: Value of sonography in determining the nature of pleural effusion: analysis of 320 cases, *AJR* 159:29-33, 1992.

727. Yeh TJ: Endometriosis within the thorax: metaplasia, implantation, or metastasis? *J Cardiovasc Surg* 53:201-205, 1967.

728. Yellin A, Benfield JR: Pneumothorax associated with lymphoma, *Am Rev Respir Dis* 134:590-592, 1986.

729. Yellow nails and oedema (editorial), *Br Med J* 4:130, 1972.

730. Yousef MMA: Case of the fall season, *Semin Roentgenol* 15:269-271, 1980.

731. Yung CM, Bessen SC, Hingorani V, et al: Idiopathic hemothorax, *Chest* 103:638-639, 1993.

732. Zaher C, Hamer A, Peter T, et al: Low-dose steroid therapy for prophylaxis of amiodarone-induced pulmonary infiltrates, *N Engl J Med* 308:779, 1983.

733. Zelefsky MN, Freeman LM, Stern H: A simple approach to the diagnosis of bronchopleural fistula, *Radiology* 124:843-844, 1977.

734. Zerhouni EA, Spivey JF, Morgan RH, et al: Factors influencing quantitative CT measurements of solitary pulmonary nodules, *J Comput Assist Tomogr* 6:1075-1087, 1982.

735. Zinn WL, Naidich DP, Whelan CA, et al: Fluid with preexisting pulmonary air-spaces: a potential pitfall in the CT differentiation of pleural from parenchymal disease, *J Comput Assist Tomogr* 11:441-448, 1987.

736. Ziskind MM, Weill H, George RA: Acute pulmonary edema following the treatement of spontaneous pneumothorax with negative intrapleural pressure, *Am Rev Respir Dis* 92:632-636, 1965.

737. Ziter FMH, Westcott JL: Supine subpulmonary pneumothorax, *AJR* 137:699-701, 1981.

738. Zwillich CW, Pierson DJ, Creagh CE, et al: Complications of assisted ventilation, *Am J Med* 57:161-170, 1974.

16 Mediastinal and Hilar Disorders

PETER ARMSTRONG

IMAGING TECHNIQUES

For plain films, high kilovoltage (greater than 120 KVp) has significant advantages over low kilovoltage (approximately 70 to 90 KVp) for demonstrating mediastinal interfaces; high kilovoltage also provides better penetration of the mediastinum. Several specially designed wedge filters have been constructed to achieve adequate penetration of the mediastinum without overexposing the lungs.[513,543] These filters are trough shaped so that they are thicker over the lungs and gradually taper over the mediastinum.

A standard computed tomography (CT) examination consists of images of the entire mediastinum from lung apices to costophrenic angles. Typically the section thickness is 8 to 10 mm, and sections are usually contiguous. Modern scanners are capable of 1-second scans with rapid acquisition of multiple sections, so that an entire examination can be performed in under 1 minute. With helical (spiral) scanners substantial portions of the mediastinum can be covered in a single breath hold. Such fast acquisition times permit excellent contrast enhancement following a single bolus. Ultrafast CT scanning with data acquisition in 100 msec or less per section is available in selected centers.

The use of intravenous contrast medium to opacify vessels in the mediastinum varies significantly from center to center. Since identifying vascular structures without additional opacification is usually possible, intravenous contrast medium often can be withheld. Dynamic contrast-enhanced scanning can then be performed at selected levels to clarify problems. In some centers intravenous contrast medium (usually 100 ml) is used routinely, except when specifically contraindicated. It is required for optimal evaluation of the hila. An appropriate technique for hilar CT is to obtain contiguous 5 mm sections, ensuring maximum contrast opacification with 50 ml of contrast medium, imaging as soon as half the bolus has been injected. The sections should be exposed as rapidly as possible from the level of the plane of the right upper lobe bronchus or from the level of the inferior pulmonary veins, depending on the direction of travel of the tabletop.[172] In those cases in which there is difficulty in deciding whether a density is a normal vessel, the specific level in question can be examined using contrast-enhanced dynamic scanning.

The major indications for magnetic resonance imaging (MRI) of the mediastinum are to demonstrate the status of the intrathoracic blood vessels and to clarify problems not solvable by CT. Unlike CT, MRI can provide images of the mediastinum in coronal, sagittal, and various angled planes with the same resolution as those obtained in the transaxial plane. These projections can be useful in evaluating the aortopulmonary window, imaging the aorta and its branches, defining the relationship of a mass to the spinal canal, and visualizing laterally placed hilar masses.[522,524] Regardless of projection, intraspinal extension of mediastinal masses is well evaluated with MRI because the subarachnoid space and spinal cord are so clearly visualized. Flowing blood alters signal on all MRI sequences. The difference in signal between flowing blood and stationary tissues can be used to demonstrate with relative ease invasion or narrowing of the large arteries and veins of the mediastinum.[326,397,443,527] With spin-echo techniques, fast-flowing blood produces no signal. As a result, hilar lymphadenopathy and other hilar masses can be easily identified against the signal void of flowing blood in hilar vessels.[15,86,522]

For standard spin-echo sequences, total time depends on the repetition time (TR), the number of signal averages, and the number of phase-encoding steps. Seven to 12 sections usually can be completed for each signal average, depending on the TR and echo time (TE) selected. For routine scans the section thickness is 7 to 10 mm. Electrocardiographic (ECG) gating improves the quality of the images, particularly those of the hila and lower mediastinum, and is often used routinely.[524,535] Respiratory gating is not currently in routine use. If an effective respiratory gate were to be manufactured, it would probably extend the imaging time. Reordered phase encoding (ROPE) can help reduce motion artifacts from breathing and should be used when available. Presaturation pulses to reduce phase wrap and flow artifacts are an advantage.[324]

With T1-weighted sequences, fat is of high intensity whereas tumors, except for fatty ones, are generally of appreciably lower intensity.[519] T2-weighted images show high signal in the fluid components of mediastinal cysts and in many inflammatory and neoplastic conditions, but the disadvantages are notably poor signal-to-noise ratio and poor fat to nonfat soft tissue contrast differences. Because their primary purpose is to characterize the signal in regions of abnormality, T2-weighted sequences can be omitted if the T1-weighted scans are normal. Fat suppression techniques or short tau inversion recovery (STIR) sequences can be used to increase the conspicuity of pathologic processes, since with these sequences fat has zero signal, whereas fluid, neoplasm, and active inflammatory tissues show high signal.

MRI may provide better tissue characterization than CT. Active inflammatory processes and neoplastic tissues tend to have long T1 and T2 relaxation values, whereas chronic inflammatory processes have intermediate T1 and T2 values.[443] Also, the long T1 and long T2 characteristics of fluid can be helpful in confirming that a mass is cystic,[397] thus limiting the differential diagnosis. This information is, however, only occasionally of diagnostic value, and initial hopes for improved tissue characterization based on signal differences have not yet been realized to any great extent.[524]

Magnetic resonance angiography, the technical details of which are beyond the scope of this book, can be used to demonstrate vascular disorders and stenosis, distortion, and displacement of vessels by mediastinal masses and other mediastinal processes.[257,305,306]

Ultrasound examination of the mediastinum is used for highly specific groups of patients. Transthoracic, that is, parasternal or suprasternal,[530] ultrasound examinations have been advocated for the following: follow-up of lymphadenopathy caused by lymphoma,[531] evaluating the thymus and mediastinal masses in adults[530,533] and children,[70,206,210,255] distinguishing cardiac from paracardiac masses in all ages,[206] and guiding mediastinal biopsy.[532,566] Juxtadiaphragmatic pathologic conditions can be demonstrated with a transabdominal approach. Transesophageal ultrasound has recently been introduced to demonstrate lymph nodes,[372] particularly the subcarinal nodes, and other masses adjacent to the esophagus and to demonstrate the descending aorta, notably for the diagnosis of aortic dissection and aortic aneurysms.

MEDIASTINAL MASSES

The relative incidence of various causes of mediastinal masses is difficult to ascertain because published surgical series are biased toward patients whose lesions undergo biopsy or resection. Some common mediastinal masses are not referred to a surgeon; therefore they are omitted from surgical reviews: notably thyroid masses, aortic aneurysms, and lymphadenopathy in patients with previously established diagnoses such as malignant lymphoma or sarcoidosis. The relative incidence of mediastinal masses in three large series is listed in Table 16-1; these masses were visible on plain chest radiographs and came to surgery.[34,85,556] In the Mayo Clinic series,[556] about 75% of mediastinal masses in both adults and children were benign and surgically resectable and 25% were malignant. Significant differences were seen between the masses encountered in children and those in adults. Neurogenic tumors, germ cell neoplasms, and foregut cysts accounted for almost 80% of the masses seen in children, whereas primary thymic neoplasms (only one case encountered), pericardial cysts, and thoracic goiters were rare in childhood.

The classification of mediastinal masses according to their location in the anterior, middle, or posterior mediastinal compartments is a matter of descriptive convenience because there are no anatomic boundaries to limit growth between these various compartments. Indeed, many radiologists do not even use these terms in the manner defined by anatomy textbooks. As Heitzman[217] has pointed out, apart from being useful for remembering that thymic, thyroid, and teratomatous masses are found in the anterior mediastinum and that most neurogenic tumors are posteriorly situated, this simple classification "tends to constrict thinking and minimizes more detailed anatomic analysis." What is needed is the most accurate assessment of the position of any mass, together with a description of its size, shape, and characteristics such as density and signal intensity. Cross-sectional imaging techniques, notably CT,[414] provide the best information with which to limit the number of possible diagnoses and on occasion permit a specific diagnosis to be made. The differential diagnosis of mediastinal masses is discussed on p. 802.

THYROID MASSES

An intrathoracic thyroid mass is usually a benign multinodular colloid goiter or an adenoma but occasionally may be a carcinoma. Intrathoracic thyroid masses are almost invariably a downward extension of a thyroid mass that originates in the neck and descends into the mediastinum, carrying with it a vascular pedicle.[556] Consequently the continuity between the mediastinal mass and the thyroid gland in the neck is an important diagnostic feature both on conventional films and at CT. An intrathoracic thyroid mass developing from heterotopic thyroid tissue without any connection to the thyroid in the neck is extremely rare.[136,205,433,487,556]

On plain films intrathoracic thyroid masses have a well-defined outline that may be spherical or lobular (Figures 16-1 and 16-2). Many masses displace and

Table 16-1 Incidence (percent) of mediastinal masses in two series

Masses	Wychulis et al.* (1064 cases)	Benjamin et al.† (214 cases)	Cohen et al.‡ (230 cases)
Neural tumors	19.9	22.9	16.9
Thymic tumors	19.4	20.6	24.3
Lymphoma	10.1	14.9	15.7
Teratoma/germ cell tumor	9.3	12.6	10.0
Benign cysts (foregut cysts)	18.4	7.0	20.0
Thyroid masses	5.3	11.2	1.7
Granuloma	6.3	§	0
Mesenchymal tumors	5.6	3.7	3.9
Primary carcinoma	2.3	§	§
Vascular tumor/malformation	§	7.5	1.7
Miscellaneous	3.4	§	5.7

*Data from Wychulis AR, Payne WS, Clagett OT, et al: *Thorac Cardiovasc Surg* 62:379-392, 1971.
†Data from Benjamin SP, McCormack LJ, Effler DB, et al: *Chest* 62:297-303, 1972.
‡Data from Cohen AJ, Thompson L, Edwards FH, et al: *Ann Thorac Surg* 51:378-386, 1991.
§Not listed as a separate category.

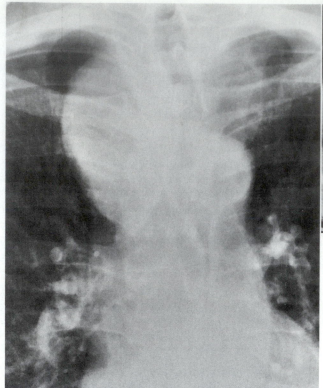

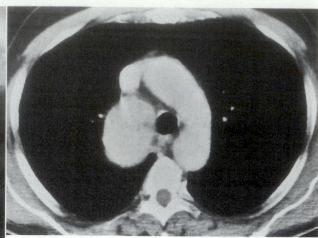

FIGURE 16-1
A, Plain film of benign intrathoracic goiter showing well-defined outline and tracheal deviation. **B,** CT scan shows the mass and contrast enhancement of thyroid tissue in the mass.

narrow the trachea; occasionally the narrowing is substantial and may result in cough or even stridor and shortness of breath. The pattern of tracheal displacement depends on the location of the mass, which is usually predominantly anterior or lateral to the trachea but may be posterior to it in as many as one fourth of cases. Posteriorly placed thyroid masses may separate the trachea and esophagus (Figure 16-2). This pattern may be encountered with bronchogenic cysts and anteriorly placed leiomyomas of the esophagus but almost never is seen with other mediastinal masses. Goiters very rarely pass posterior to the esophagus. Occasionally, intrathoracic goiters compress the brachiocephalic veins, a process that may result in superior vena cava (SVC) syndrome.[58] One case has been reported in which an intrathoracic goiter disappeared from the chest by moving into the neck.[482]

Calcification is common, mostly caused by benign disease (Figures 16-3 and 16-4). Its usual appearance is that of one or more dense, amorphous, well-defined calcifications, with a nodular, curvilinear or circular configuration. The longer the goiter is present, the more frequently calcifications are seen.[279] However, calcification may also be seen in carcinoma of the thyroid (Figure 16-3).[229,279,321,382,515] In general, malignant calcification is made up of fine dots grouped in a cloudlike formation corresponding to the psammoma bodies found pathologically in papillary and follicular carcinoma. The closest resemblance to benign calcifications occurs with medullary carcinoma, in which the conglomerate dots are very dense, can be remarkably well defined and even, on occasion, are arranged in a ring shape.

CT scanning[28,38,171,346] demonstrates the shape, size, and position of the mass (Figures 16-1 to 16-4). Diagnosing a thyroid origin is usually possible by noting a well-defined mass in the paratracheal or retrotracheal region cradled by brachiocephalic vessels. The mass is usually continuous with the thyroid gland in the neck (Figure 16-4). Occasionally the only connection is a narrow fibrous or vascular pedicle not visible at CT.[28] Another useful sign indicating a thyroid origin is the relatively high attenuation value of the thyroid tissue compared with the adjacent muscles on both precontrast and postcontrast CT images (Figure 16-4). The attenuation of normal thyroid tissue within a goiter is the same as thyroid tissue in the neck. At least some portion of the mass shows attenuation values at least 20 Hounsfield units (HU) above that seen in muscle both before and after administration of contrast medium.[171,346] Normal thyroid tissue enhances by more than 25 HU following intravenous contrast medium injection.[28]

Calcification is better seen at CT than on plain film; the pattern is similar to that described previously for plain films. It is a common finding that further aids differential diagnosis from other causes of mediastinal mass.[28] Rounded, focal, low-density areas are equally common (Figure 16-5). These low-density areas are more easily visible on the postcontrast films[28] because they do not enhance, whereas the surrounding normal thyroid gland shows substantial enhancement.

Distinguishing between benign and malignant masses at CT is not possible unless the tumor has clearly spread beyond the thyroid gland. If such spread is unequivocal, the mass should be considered malignant.

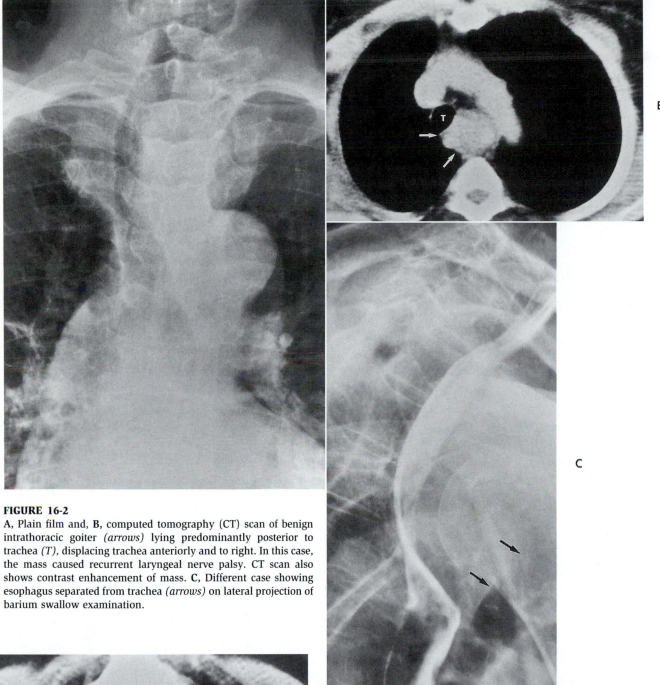

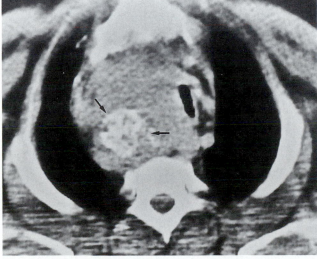

FIGURE 16-2
A, Plain film and, B, computed tomography (CT) scan of benign intrathoracic goiter *(arrows)* lying predominantly posterior to trachea *(T)*, displacing trachea anteriorly and to right. In this case, the mass caused recurrent laryngeal nerve palsy. CT scan also shows contrast enhancement of mass. C, Different case showing esophagus separated from trachea *(arrows)* on lateral projection of barium swallow examination.

FIGURE 16-3
Calcification *(arrows)* in a mucoepidermoid carcinoma of thyroid shown at contrast-enhanced computed tomography.

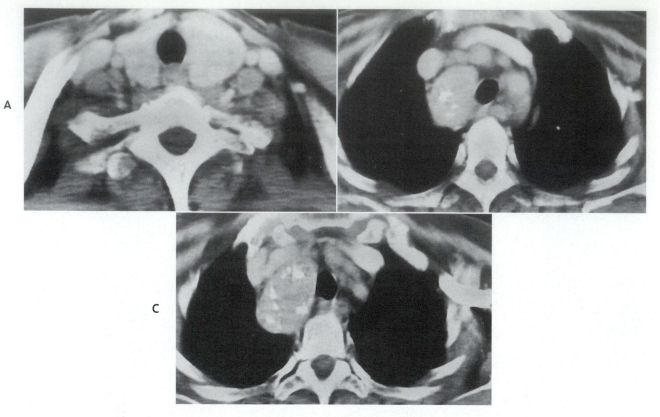

FIGURE 16-4
Benign intrathoracic goiter. Three levels (**A** to **C**) from contrast-enhanced computed tomography scan illustrate contiguity of the mass with thyroid in the neck. Note enhancement of both the mass and normal thyroid tissue. Also shown are multiple benign calcifications within mass.

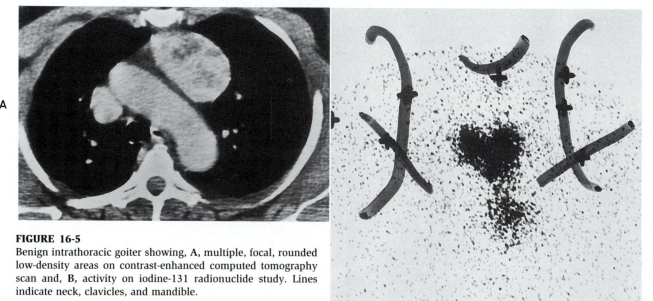

FIGURE 16-5
Benign intrathoracic goiter showing, **A**, multiple, focal, rounded low-density areas on contrast-enhanced computed tomography scan and, **B**, activity on iodine-131 radionuclide study. Lines indicate neck, clavicles, and mandible.

MRI, like CT, can identify cystic and solid components but does not demonstrate calcification.[221,222,443] T2-weighted images show heterogeneous increased intensity with very high signal in what are presumed to be the cystic portions of the goiter. Most reports of thyroid pathology refer to disease in the neck, rather than in the mediastinum. Here the T1-weighted images show intensity similar to muscle, but high-intensity regions can be seen in areas of hemorrhage or colloid cyst.[163,222,361] Adenomas cannot be distinguished from carcinomas based on signal intensities; both usually show increased signal on T2-weighted images.

Radionuclide imaging of the thyroid shows some functioning thyroid tissue in almost all intrathoracic goiters (Figure 16-5).[242] The appropriate agents are ^{131}I or ^{123}I, partly because they have a higher energy radiation that can penetrate the sternum, but more particularly because they can be seen on delayed images, thus avoiding appreciable background blood pool activity. Technetium-99m images are degraded by the background blood pool activity, and ^{125}I energy levels are too low to adequately penetrate the sternum.[242] Radionuclide imaging is a very sensitive and specific method of determining the thyroid nature of an intrathoracic mass. CT, however, is a more useful initial test to elucidate a possible intrathoracic thyroid mass because CT provides more information about the mass should it turn out to be something other than thyroid and is almost as specific for diagnosing a thyroid origin.

PARATHYROID MASSES

Hyperparathyroidism may be caused by parathyroid adenomas that arise in ectopic parathyroid glands in the mediastinum, usually in or near the thymus.[427] One case with multiple mediastinal hyperfunctional glands has been reported.[310] Mediastinal parathyroid adenomas vary greatly in size; they are often less than 2 cm in diameter (Figure 16-6). When larger than 2 cm they usually can be seen at CT; below 2 cm in diameter, the proportion detectable by CT drops considerably.[283]

Because smaller adenomas are the same size as normal mediastinal lymph nodes or normal thymic remnants, differential diagnosis at CT can be difficult. CT-directed needle aspiration of the suspected adenoma has proved helpful in making a distinction, since aspirates from adenomas contain significantly higher levels of parathormone than aspirates from lymph nodes or thymus.[113]

Mediastinal parathyroid glands also can be demonstrated using double tracer radionuclide imaging (thallium-201/^{99m}Tc-labeled MIBI or ^{99m}Tc-pertechnetate); arteriography; and MRI scanning, particularly using STIR sequences.[554]

THYMIC MASSES

The size of a normal thymus varies drastically with age. Differentiating between a large, normal thymus and a thymic mass can therefore be difficult in children[46] and some young adults. A normal thymus, in contradistinction to a thymic mass, conforms to the shape of the adjacent great vessels on CT and MRI. Also, a mass gives rise to focal swelling, usually centered away from the midline, whereas a normal gland is approximately symmetric, the left lobe usually being slightly larger than the right. Adjacent fat planes may be obliterated by invasive neoplasm or inflammation. The signal intensity at MRI can be useful because normal thymic tissue shows homogeneous signal similar to muscle on T1-weighted images, and similar or higher signal than fat on T2-weighted spin-echo sequences,[46,337,466] whereas thymic masses show altered, often inhomogeneous signal intensity.

Ultrasound can be used to establish the normality of a prominent thymus in infants. The suprasternal approach shows a homogeneous low-echo pattern without compression of the major vessels (Figure 16-7).[70,210,294] Tumors or lymph nodes, according to Carty,[70] show mixed echodensity or higher reflectivity than normal thymus.

Enlargement of the thymus is usually caused by a tumor. Occasionally it is caused by a cyst or, rarely, by hyperplasia or infection.[148] The most common thymic tumor in adults is thymoma. Other tumors of the thymus include thymolipoma; malignant lymphoma, notably Hodgkin's disease; thymic carcinoid, which may secrete adrenocorticotropic hormone (ACTH) and consequently may be responsible for Cushing's syndrome; germ cell tumors or teratomas; and thymic carcinoma.

Thymoma

Thymomas are tumors consisting of an admixture of cytologically bland thymic epithelial cells and reactive lymphocytes, with both circumscribed and invasive pat-

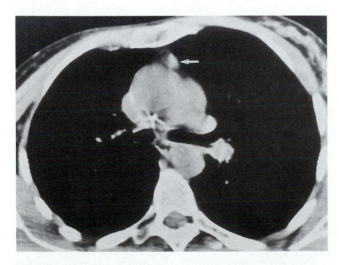

FIGURE 16-6
Functioning parathyroid adenoma *(arrow)* demonstrated by computed tomography. The patient had previously had parathyroidectomy for hyperparathyroidism.

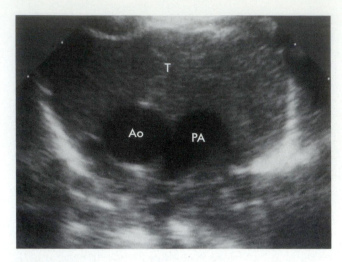

FIGURE 16-7
Transthoracic ultrasound scan in an infant showing normal thymus (T) anterior to the aorta (Ao) and pulmonary artery (PA). (Courtesy Dr. Helen Carty, Liverpool, U.K.)

terns of growth.[293] The proportion of lymphocytes to epithelial cells appears to comprise a continuous spectrum, but thymomas are sometimes divided into categories according to the relative proportion of these cells.[422] Providing thymic carcinoma is classified separately, it appears that the predominantly epithelial thymoma carries the poorest prognosis.[300] On pathologic study most thymomas show subdivisions into lobules by fibrous bands and have a lobular external contour.[225,300] Cystic change is common, and in some cases the majority of the tumor is cystic.[293,300] Foci of calcification, hemorrhage,[293] and necrosis may also be seen.[225] Thymomas, which vary in size from very small to larger than 20 cm in diameter, may be contained within or may penetrate capsule, eventually invading the mediastinum. The presence or absence of spread beyond the capsule rather than the histologic appearance within the thymus determines whether a tumor is labeled benign or malignant by the pathologist.[293] For this reason Zerhouni and others[300,571] use the term "invasive thymoma" to describe any tumor that has spread beyond the capsule. Some 15% to 40% of thymomas turn out to be invasive.[127,184,467]

There are several staging systems for invasive thymoma. The system advocated by Bergh and associates[35] classifies these tumors into the following stages: stage 1, in which the capsule is either intact, or the tumor has not spread beyond the capsule; stage 2, in which the tumor has spread into mediastinal fat; and stage 3, in which there is invasion of adjacent organs or pleural spread at a distance from the primary tumor. Newer staging systems subdivide these basic categories[509] or split off transpleural, pericardial, and distant metastases to form stage 4.[323] Surgery is undertaken in all three stages, with radiation therapy given for stage 2 and radiation therapy combined with chemotherapy given for stage 3.[546]

The average age at diagnosis is approximately 50,[293,300] or somewhat younger in those patients with myasthenia gravis. Thymomas are seen with virtually equal frequency in men and women[293,300] and are unusual below the age of 20.[251,293,300] They are exceptionally rare in patients less than 15 years old.

Most patients with noninvasive thymoma have no clinical symptoms from the tumor itself. When symptoms occur, they are caused by local compression.[300] Thymomas, however, are associated with a large variety of autoimmune diseases, most notably myasthenia gravis. Approximately 35% to 40% of patients with thymoma have myasthenia gravis.[300,474] The overall incidence of thymoma in patients with myasthenia gravis is 10% to 23%,[127,251,300] but is higher in the older patient groups.[251] The interrelationship between thymic disease and myasthenia gravis is not clearly understood. Thymectomy undoubtedly improves myasthenia in some patients, regardless of whether or not the thymus harbors a thymoma. Thymectomy therefore is used to treat the disease in selected patients when medical treatment fails. It is most likely to be successful in younger patients, particularly young females whose condition is not well controlled medically. For thymectomy to be effective, all thymic tissue must be removed. It rarely, however, improves myasthenia gravis in older patients, those with isolated ocular myasthenia gravis, or those without serum antibodies to acetylcholine receptors. Patients who have a thymoma are no more likely to show improvement in their myasthenia following surgery than those who are tumor free.[378] In fact, thymectomy for relieving myasthenia gravis is less effective in patients with thymoma than it is in patients without thymoma.[340] The decision to perform a thymectomy for alleviating myasthenia gravis should be based on clinical features. Thymic hyperplasia, even if it could be radiologically demonstrated, plays no part in this decision. The radiologist's role is to demonstrate a thymoma. When found, thymomas should be removed surgically, preferably while still confined to the thymus, in an attempt to stop the development of invasive thymoma.

Hematologic cytopenia,[474,509] notably pure red blood cell aplasia or aplastic anemia, is seen in 21% to 50% of patients,[425,474] and thymoma is associated with hypogammaglobulinemia in up to 10% of patients.[152,300,425,474,509] A number of other conditions have a definite association with thymoma, including[425,474] nonthymic cancers, such as thyroid carcinoma[293,474]; autoimmune disorders such as systemic lupus erythematosus,[300,509] polymyositis, Graves' disease,[293,300] or rheumatoid arthritis[300]; Crohn's disease[300] and ulcerative colitis[300]; pernicious anemia[300]; Sjögren's syndrome[509]; and alopecia areata.[300]

Most thymomas arise in the upper anterior mediastinum, but they may project into the adjacent middle or posterior mediastinum. They are usually found anterior to the ascending aorta above the right ventricular outflow

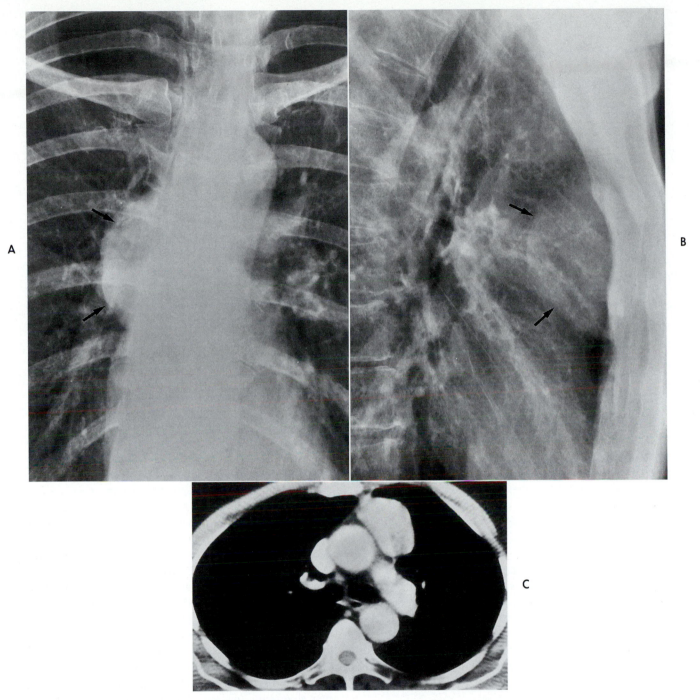

FIGURE 16-8
Thymoma. **A** and **B**, Plain films show mass *(arrows)* in anterior mediastinum lying anterior to ascending aorta above right ventricular outflow tract. The lesion was asymptomatic. **C**, Computed tomography scan in another patient showing asymptomatic benign thymoma. Note uniform contrast enhancement of thymoma.

tract and main pulmonary artery, and project into a hemithorax; less commonly they may extend to both sides of the midline (Figure 16-8).[422] A few are situated in the lower third of the mediastinum (Figure 16-9)[29] and occasionally as low as the cardiophrenic angles.[252] Large thymic masses may lie partly in the neck and partly in the

thorax.[193] A small percentage of thymomas are found exclusively in the neck, presumably in aberrant thymic tissue, and an occasional ectopic thymoma may project down from the neck and may mimic a thyroid mass.[335] A thymoma entirely in the middle or posterior mediastinum is rare but is reported.[94,493]

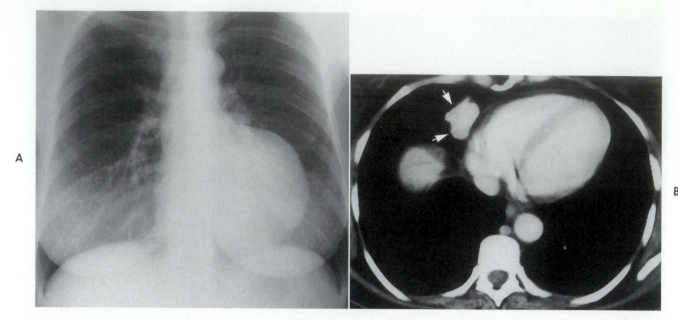

FIGURE 16-9
Low-lying thymomas. **A,** Plain chest film showing large benign thymoma lying against border of left side of heart. **B,** Computed tomography scan in different patient showing a small thymoma *(arrow)* at the right cardiophrenic angle. Note contrast enhancement of thymoma.

Thymomas are usually spherical or have lobulated borders. Only the larger tumors are visible on plain film. Sometimes the mass can be recognized only in one plain film projection, the opacity frequently being indefinite in the lateral view. Another problem on plain chest radiographs is overdiagnosis in obese patients in whom mediastinal fat can closely resemble a thymic swelling. CT is helpful in such cases because it readily distinguishes fat from tumor.

Punctate, curvilinear, or ringlike calcification is common in both benign and invasive thymomas.[128,212,345]

All plain film signs of thymic tumor are best seen with CT (Figures 16-8, *C,* 16-10, and 16-11),* and CT can provide information that significantly alters treatment decisions.[262] At CT, thymomas are usually of homogeneous density and show uniform enhancement, but they may on rare occasion appear cystic with discrete nodular components.[354]

CT is the most sensitive examination for the detection of thymoma in patients with myasthenia gravis. False-positive interpretations are unusual.[77] The diagnosis depends on identifying a focal swelling rather than applying a specific measurement. Recognizing focal swelling becomes easier as the thymus atrophies. Thymomas as small as 1.5 cm in diameter are readily identified over the age of 40. Before age 40, and particularly before 30, diagnosing a small thymoma can be difficult because the normal gland is variable in size and in myasthenia gravis the associated hyperplasia may lead to a bulky

gland. In these circumstances the fact that thymoma usually gives rise to an asymmetric focal swelling can be useful. Fortunately, thymoma is so infrequent in children that the potential difficulty of finding a thymoma rarely arises in a child with myasthenia gravis.

Invasive thymomas (Figures 16-10 and 16-11) invade the mediastinal fat and eventually spread to the pericardium and pleura; both mediastinal and pleural spread is best diagnosed with CT.[467,571] Blood-borne metastases are rare.[293] Until mediastinal invasion has occurred, distinguishing benign from invasive thymoma even with CT is not possible (Figure 16-11). Adjacent mediastinal fat planes are preserved when tumors are confined to the thymus, whereas they may be obliterated by invasive tumors. Complete obliteration of the adjacent fat planes at CT is highly suggestive of mediastinal invasion,[77] but partial obliteration is indeterminate. In one series invasive thymoma was present in only 8 of 15 patients showing this feature,[77] and the partial obliteration of fat planes was explained in some instances by adjacent inflammatory changes. Preservation of adjacent fat planes, of course, does not exclude capsular invasion, but when these fat planes are preserved, extensive invasive disease is unlikely.[77] Transpleural spread may occur as a sheet of neoplastic tissue extending outward from the primary thymic tumor, or it may manifest as a discrete "drop metastasis" at a distance from the primary lesion. Therefore, when potentially invasive thymoma is investigated, imaging the whole of both pleural cavities and the upper abdomen is important.[440] The pleural deposits may be so extensive that they mimic malignant pleural

---

*References 22, 52, 55, 127, 149, 259, 341, 342, 422, 467.

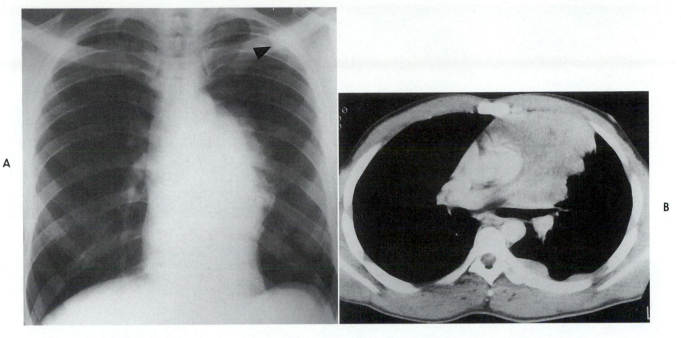

FIGURE 16-10

Invasive thymoma. **A,** Plain film shows a large mass projecting from the left side of the mediastinum and a small pleural deposit *(arrowhead)* at left apex. **B,** Contrast-enhanced computed tomography scan of same patient showing lobular-shaped, invading mediastinal mass plus two further "drop" pleural metastases lying posteriorly.

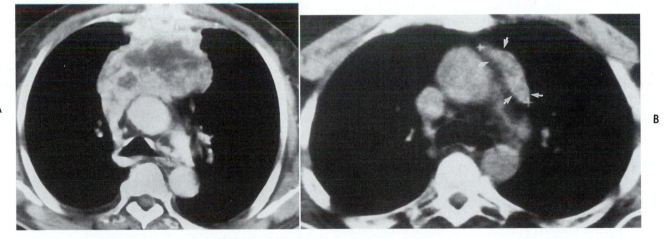

FIGURE 16-11

Invasive thymoma. **A,** Contrast-enhanced computed tomography (CT) scan shows a thymic mass of variable density invading the adjacent mediastinum and sternum. **B,** CT scan in another patient with an invasive thymoma *(arrows)* illustrates impossibility of distinguishing invasive from noninvasive thymoma before mediastinal or pleural invasion. Capsular invasion was present histologically, and the tumor recurred locally following thymectomy.

mesothelioma on imaging examination[190]; in some patients no visible mediastinal tumor is evident even at surgery.[343]

Early experience with MRI suggests that it provides little additional information compared with CT. Because there are no distinctive MR signal characteristics of thymoma, MRI can only document the presence of a mass and show its extent.[26,431] As always, MRI can more readily distinguish between mediastinal masses and the blood vessels traversing the mediastinum, a possible

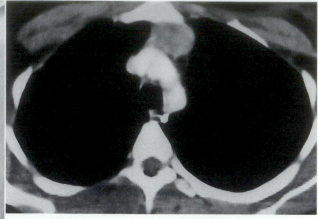

FIGURE 16-12
Hodgkin's disease of thymus. **A,** This asymptomatic mass in a 33-year-old man was discovered on routine chest radiography and was the only focus of disease. **B,** Contrast-enhanced computed tomographic scan of a similar case (11-year-old child).

advantage in selected cases when CT interpretation proves difficult. Thymomas have a signal intensity similar to muscle and normal thymic tissue on T1-weighted images.[239,337,431] On T2-weighted images the signal intensity, which may become inhomogeneous,[239,337] increases and approaches that of fat, so distinguishing thymic masses from surrounding mediastinal fat is more difficult. Low-intensity septations are seen with both benign and invasive thymomas, but inhomogeneous signal intensity with a visible lobular internal architecture is a particular feature of malignant thymoma.[239,431] Cysts and hemorrhagic areas also may be visible.[431]

Thymic carcinoma

Thymic carcinoma is sometimes classified as a subgroup of thymoma but may be classified separately; it is, however, a distinct entity that behaves more aggressively. It can be distinguished from thymoma by the presence of nucleolar prominence, vesicular chromatin, abundant mitotic activity, and markedly increased nucleus to cytoplasm ratio.[290,300,542] Thymic carcinoma cannot be distinguished from invasive thymoma by imaging examinations. CT shows local invasion along the pleura or mediastinum, often with necrosis and calcification.[290]

Thymic lymphoma and leukemia

Hodgkin's disease of the thymus is usually part of generalized disease. Its incidence is difficult to determine. Estimates have varied from 30% to 56%, with isolated involvement much rarer than combined thymic and mediastinal nodal disease.[219,264,534] The major imaging finding is thymic enlargement (Figure 16-12), either generalized thymic enlargement or single or multiple focal masses.[534] As with lymphoma in other sites, cystic degeneration may be present at initial presentation.[139] A major differential diagnostic problem in young patients without obvious focal masses is distinguishing between a large normal thymus and lymphomatous involvement.

Distinguishing rebound hyperplasia from recurrent lymphoma in children and young adults can be even more difficult. Unfortunately, neither CT density nor signal intensity at MRI is a reliable indicator of malignant infiltration because a normal gland, hyperplasia, and neoplastic infiltration may all show the same density or signal characteristics. Pronounced inhomogeneity of MR signal, which is a feature not seen in the normal or hyperplastic thymus, may be encountered with neoplastic involvement.[466]

Thymic carcinoid

Thymic carcinoid is histologically distinct from thymoma.[424] These tumors vary in their aggressiveness, and they may be frankly malignant,[122] particularly when responsible for Cushing's syndrome.[296] Thymic carcinoids may secrete ACTH and present with the so-called ectopic ACTH Cushing's syndrome.[45,114,249,511] In the review by Levine and Rosai,[296] 17 of 58 patients with thymic carcinoid had Cushing's syndrome. Thymic carcinoid may be part of the multiple endocrine adenoma syndrome, and thymic and pulmonary carcinoid may coexist.[296]

The plain film and CT features of thymic carcinoid

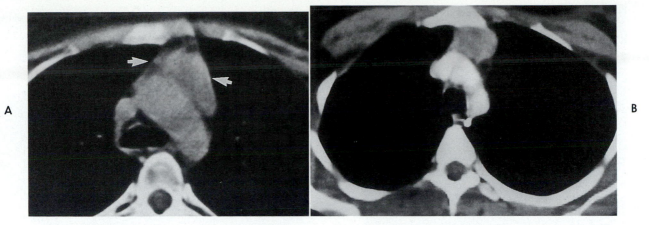

FIGURE 16-13
Thymic carcinoid. **A,** Contrast-enhanced computed tomographic (CT) scan shows thymic tumor *(arrows)* in a young woman with ectopic adrenocorticotropic hormone production by tumor. The tumor in this instance was invasive and recurred following surgery. **B,** Contrast-enhanced CT scan in another patient with a large carcinoid tumor of thymus who presented with chest pain. The mass shows areas of low density because of necrosis.

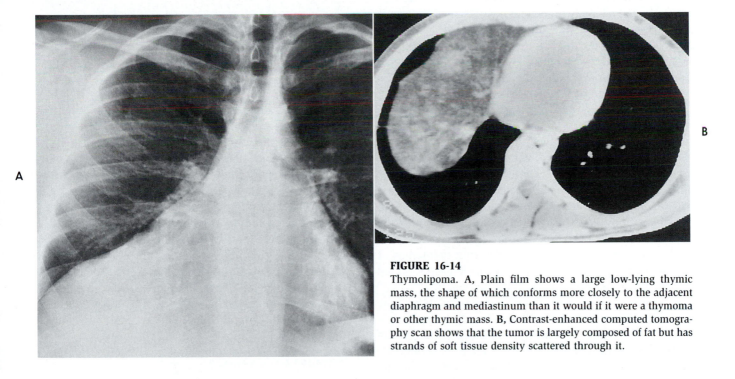

FIGURE 16-14
Thymolipoma. **A,** Plain film shows a large low-lying thymic mass, the shape of which conforms more closely to the adjacent diaphragm and mediastinum than it would if it were a thymoma or other thymic mass. **B,** Contrast-enhanced computed tomography scan shows that the tumor is largely composed of fat but has strands of soft tissue density scattered through it.

(Figure 16-13) are indistinguishable from thymoma[53] because both cause an anterior mediastinal mass resulting from thymic enlargement, which may contain calcification.

Thymolipoma

Thymolipomas (Figure 16-14) are rare tumors seen in both children and adults. The age range is 3 to 60 (mean 22 years).[73] The tumors are composed of a mixture of mature fat and normal looking or involuted thymic tissue. Individual cases have been reported in association with a variety of conditions, including myasthenia gravis,[368,373] aplastic anemia, Graves' disease, and hypogammaglobulinemia.[460] Thymolipomas can grow to be very large before discovery. They are soft and mold themselves to the adjacent mediastinum and diaphragm. They may

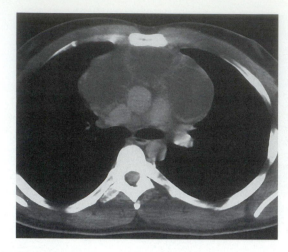

FIGURE 16-15
Thymic cyst that developed during chemotherapy treatment for Hodgkin's disease. (Courtesy Dr. J. Wong You Cheong, Manchester. From Radford JA, Wong You Cheong J: *Clinical radiology,* in press.)

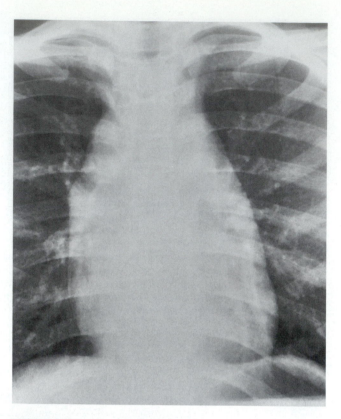

FIGURE 16-16
Substantial enlargement of thymus resulting from thymic hyperplasia in a 16-year-old girl with thyrotoxicosis.

mimic cardiomegaly or lobar collapse.[80,497] CT scanning shows the fatty density of the mass with islands of thymus and fibrous septa running through the lesion.[73,80,134,460,563] At MRI there is the expected high signal of fat on T1-weighted images and lower signal strands may course through the mass representing residual fibrous stroma or thymic tissue.[73,337,460]

Thymic cysts

Thymic cysts are usually simple cysts, some of which may be congenital in origin, within an otherwise normal or hyperplastic gland.[449] Simple thymic cysts may be unilocular or multilocular.[280] They are most frequently encountered in children.[25] They are usually asymptomatic[193] but may cause pain if bleeding occurs into the cyst.[74,347]

Thymic cysts also may be found within thymomas or thymic germ cell tumors.[119,193] They have been reported in Hodgkin's disease involving the thymus,[139,264,304,534] and in some cases the cysts develop after irradiation of the mediastinum or following chemotherapy (Figure 16-15).[23,407,508] Some are benign in nature. Others are caused by cystic change within a focus of Hodgkin's disease unrelated to therapy.[534] When radiation therapy eradicates the Hodgkin's disease, the size of the cysts may remain unchanged,[304] or they may disappear.[534] If a thymic mass develops in a patient with Hodgkin's disease following radiation therapy, the possibility of a benign cyst should be considered before giving further treatment for Hodgkin's disease.[268]

Suster and Rosai[488] believe that multilocular thymic cysts are the sequela of a variety of inflammatory processes, and Jaramillo, Perez-Atayde, and Griscom[248]

suggest that some thymic cysts may be associated with prior thoracotomy.

On plain film, simple thymic cysts are indistinguishable from other nonlobulated thymic masses, notably thymoma. Calcification of the wall of the cyst has been recorded.[193] CT may demonstrate water density of the cyst (Figure 16-15),[192] but some thymic cysts are of higher density and may be misdiagnosed as solid on CT.[55] On MRI the contents of a thymic cyst show the typical characteristics of fluid: low signal on T1-weighted images and uniform high signal on T2-weighted images. If spontaneous hemorrhage takes place, the mass shows high signal intensity in both the T1- and T2-weighted images.[337] Ultrasound can show the transsonic nature of the mass.[533]

Thymic hyperplasia

Thymic hyperplasia (lymphofollicular thymic hyperplasia, germinal centers in the medulla) is seen in over 50% of patients with myasthenia gravis.[296] Thymic hyperplasia is also found in other conditions, notably thyrotoxicosis (Figure 16-16),[22,154,296,553] as well as autoimmune diseases such as systemic lupus erythematosus, polyarteritis nodosa, Hashimoto's thyroiditis, Addison's disease, autoimmune hemolytic anemia, and Behçet's disease.[425]

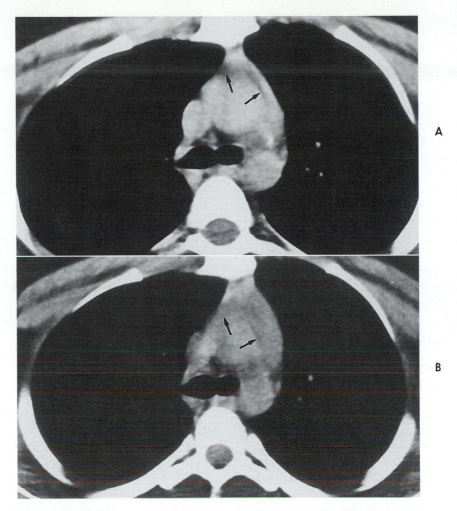

FIGURE 16-17
Rebound hyperplasia of thymus in a 13-year-old girl with osteosarcoma. **A,** Thymus *(arrows)* is normal in size before chemotherapy. **B,** Enlarged thymus *(arrows)* after completion of chemotherapy.

Thymic hyperplasia is rarely recognizable on plain film (Figure 16-16). On CT and MRI, patients with thymic hyperplasia may show enlargement of both lobes of an otherwise normally shaped gland with density or signal compatible with normal thymus,[337] but usually the size and shape of the thymus are within the normal range.[26,127] Thymic hyperplasia occasionally may cause a focal swelling that mimics a thymic mass.[22,55,149]

Rebound thymic hyperplasia

The thymus gland may atrophy rapidly in response to stress or to therapy with steroids and antineoplastic drugs. Such atrophy is seen in up to 90% of patients receiving chemotherapy for extrathoracic malignancies.[81,218] The gland will usually grow back to its original size on recovery or cessation of treatment. In the phenomenon known as rebound thymic hyperplasia,[4,81,218,271] the gland may grow back to a larger than normal size, and in patients younger than 35 years old, particularly children, the gland may exceed its original volume by more than 50% (Figure 16-17).[4,81] Histologically the gland shows hyperplasia of the cortex and medulla.[117] In a recent literature review the average interval between the termination of chemotherapy and the discovery of thymic rebound was 6 months for children and 9.3 months for adults.[547] The range appears to be 2 months to 5 years.[79,218,271,547] Rebound hyperplasia after steroid therapy can be more rapid and may be seen in children 2 or 3 weeks after cessation of therapy, and in adults after a slightly longer interval.[547]

Rebound thymic hyperplasia has been reported after treatment of Cushing's syndrome and after recovery from a wide variety of other stresses including burns, surgery, and tuberculosis.[63,115,165,417] When rebound thymic hyperplasia is seen in patients previously treated for a malignant neoplasm that might involve the thymus, distinguishing thymic involvement by neoplasm from thymic rebound may be difficult. The diagnosis depends on the absence of clinical or other features to indicate recurrence of tumor in a patient with a reason to have thymic rebound.[89] On CT (Figure 16-17) the appearance is a normally shaped although enlarged gland with a smooth nonlobular outline; the gland conforms to the shape of adjacent structures; and its enlargement is symmetric rather than asymmetric as is the case with most tumors (although leukemic involvement may be symmetric). The density of the hyperplastic gland is the same as that of the normal gland at CT, and the signal at MRI is also similar to normal thymic tissue,[466] although one case of transient calcification in a child has been reported.[151] A normal thymus shrinks with steroid therapy, and in those instances in which the diagnosis is uncertain a trial of steroids can be used to confirm thymic hyperplasia.[150] Lymphomas and leukemias, however, may also be responsive to steroid administration.[89]

TERATOMA AND GERM CELL TUMORS OF THE MEDIASTINUM

A teratoma is a neoplasm derived from more than one embryonic germ layer. Some authors use the term for the entire spectrum of mediastinal germinal tumors, both benign and malignant.[556] Others[97] divide such tumors into benign cystic teratoma (dermoid cyst) and a number of malignant forms, chiefly malignant germinal tumors normally found in the testes: seminoma, the most frequently encountered germ cell tumor; teratocarcinoma (teratoma with embryonal cell carcinoma), the next most frequent; and histologically restricted forms, namely embryonal carcinoma, endodermal sinus tumor (yolk sac tumor),[452] choriocarcinoma, and mixtures of these cell types. Malignant germ cell tumors secrete beta human chorionic gonadotropin (HCG), alpha-fetoprotein (AFP), and lactic dehydrogenase, which are used to diagnose and monitor the progress of the disease. Significant elevations in the concentrations of HCG or AFP imply a malignant component to the tumor and the presence of active tumor.

Most mediastinal teratomas are believed to develop in cell rests within, or in intimate contact with, the thymus.[296,359]

Benign cystic teratomas

Benign cystic teratomas are more common than the malignant forms.[314,423,556] They are found at all ages, but particularly in adolescents and young adults, with females slightly outnumbering males. They usually consist predominantly of ectodermal elements such as skin, sebaceous material, hair, and calcification — hence the expression ''dermoid cyst'' — along with smooth muscle and respiratory epithelium.[359] In most series half the cases are asymptomatic and diagnosed incidentally on chest radiography or CT. Symptoms are caused by local compression, rupture, or infection. The most common

symptoms are chest pain, a cough that is usually productive, dyspnea, and fever. An occasional patient initially has pneumonia, hemoptysis, or superior vena caval syndrome. Trichoptysis (expectoration of hair) has been reported.[359,556] Most of the lesions are single cysts containing a variety of tissues, notably fluid, hair, bone, cartilage, and fat. A few are made up of multiple cysts, some of which have intervening solid portions.[556] The cysts are frequently large and may be huge, occupying much of one hemithorax.

Benign cystic teratomas usually produce a well-defined, rounded or lobulated mass in the anterior mediastinum in front of the roots of the aorta and main pulmonary artery (Figures 16-18 and 16-19), but a few are found in the posterior mediastinum* or lung (see p. 317). Benign cysts grow slowly, but rapid increases in size may occur because of hemorrhage. Alternatively, they may rupture into the bronchial tree, in which case air may enter the cyst and be visible on imaging examinations. Rarely the cyst may rupture into the pericardium[362,451] or pleura, in which case a fat-fluid level may be visible in the pleural space.[564] Most teratomas project mainly to one side of the midline,[556] sometimes markedly so. Calcification, ossification, or even teeth[112] may be visible on a plain chest radiograph, and occasionally, sufficient fat is present to be detectable radiographically.

CT is more sensitive than plain films for detecting the various calcifications and particularly for showing fat.[423,525] The findings at CT (Figures 16-19 to 16-21) are variable.[54,239,489] Water density in the cystic component is common, and fat density (Figures 16-20 and 16-21) is seen in one fourth to one half of the patients. A fat-fluid level may be seen (Figure 16-20),[158,450] or fat and fluid may be more intimately mixed. A definite cyst wall, which may show curvilinear calcification, is often visible. The combination of a large anterior mediastinal mass, which is wholly or predominantly composed of a cyst, with a well-defined wall is highly suggestive of a benign cystic teratoma. With calcification in the wall of the cyst or small spherical or irregular calcifications (Figure 16-21) within the mass,[345] benign cystic teratoma is even more likely. Unequivocal fat within the mass, particularly a fat-fluid level, makes this diagnosis certain.

There are few reports of the use of MRI in mediastinal cystic teratoma.[239,429] The diagnostic information obtained is similar to that obtained from CT. Ultrasound examination may reveal useful information regarding the cystic components of the mass[238]; the lesions may appear cystic, solid, or complex.

Malignant germ cell tumors

Malignant germ cell tumors are usually encountered in young adults and are much more common in men than in women.[359] In Polansky and associates' review of 103

---

*References 112, 423, 429, 465, 525, 556.

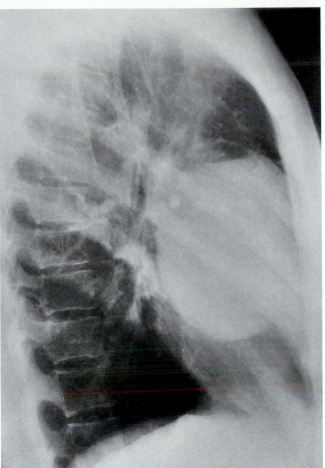

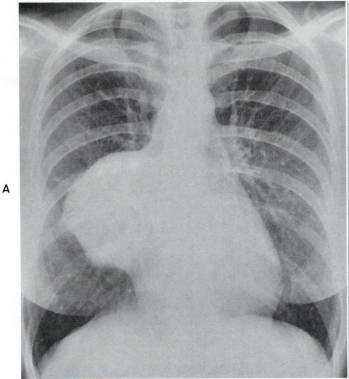

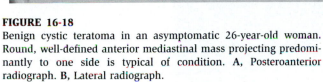

FIGURE 16-18
Benign cystic teratoma in an asymptomatic 26-year-old woman. Round, well-defined anterior mediastinal mass projecting predominantly to one side is typical of condition. **A,** Posteroanterior radiograph. **B,** Lateral radiograph.

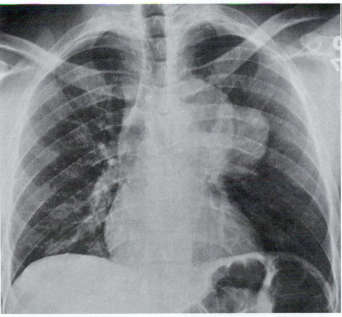

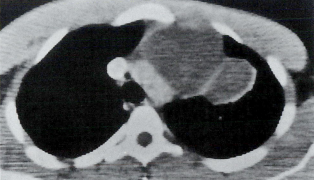

FIGURE 16-19
Benign cystic teratoma. **A,** Lobular anterior mediastinal mass projecting to left side discovered on routine chest radiographs in a 27-year-old man. **B,** Contrast-enhanced computed tomography scan shows fluid density and septations within the mass. (Courtesy Dr. Chuck Hubbard, Columbia, S.C.)

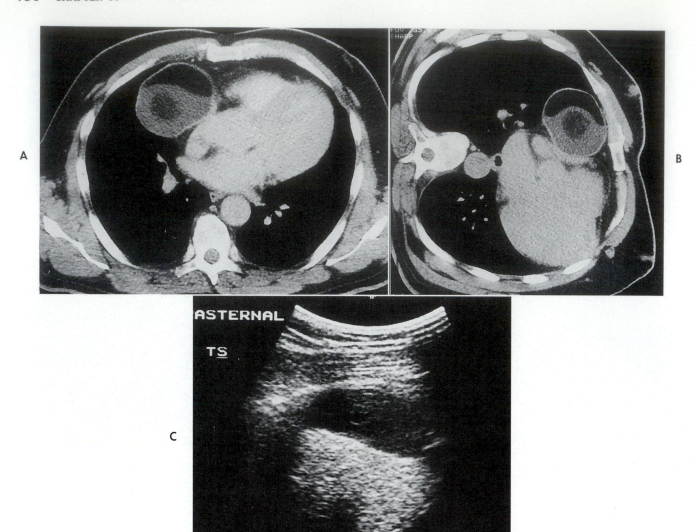

FIGURE 16-20
Cystic teratoma shows thin-walled cyst containing fluid and solid fat. **A,** Supine computed tomography (CT) scan. **B,** Lateral decubitus CT scan showing mobility of contents. **C,** Ultrasound scan. The fat *(top layer)* is echo free.

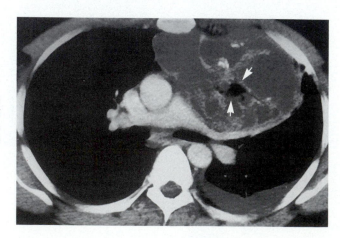

FIGURE 16-21
Cystic teratoma. Computed tomography scan shows an oval mass arising from anterior mediastinum. The mass contains areas of calcification, fat *(arrows),* and fluid density. This combination is diagnostic of cystic teratoma. The lesion was excised and shown to be benign.

cases of primary mediastinal seminoma only five were female.[394] Even mediastinal choriocarcinoma in adults is more common in men than in women. In children the male/female ratio is more even.[359]

Mediastinal malignant germ cell tumors give rise to symptoms similar to benign cystic teratoma, namely cough, dyspnea, and chest pain[394]; the great majority of patients are symptomatic.[359] Superior venal caval obstruction is not uncommon.[227] In a review of over 100 cases it was found in 10% of patients.[394] Weight loss also may be noted. About 10% to 30% of patients are asymptomatic, and the tumor is discovered as an anterior mediastinal mass on routine radiography.[359,394]

The plain film findings (Figure 16-22) are similar to benign teratoma except that the mass is often lobular in outline, fat density is not noted, and calcification is rare. Unlike benign teratoma, the malignant forms grow rapidly, and metastases may be seen in the lungs, bones, or pleura. CT shows an asymmetric mass,[44,291,423] which may have a lobular outline (Figures 16-22 and 16-23).[299,458] The adjacent mediastinal fat planes may be obliterated, and extensive local invasion may be identified.[452] The tumors are either of homogeneous soft tissue density or show multiple areas of contrast enhancement interspersed with rounded areas of decreased attenuation from necrosis and hemorrhage (Figure 16-23). Rarely, coarse tumor calcification may be evident.[299,345] A residual mass may be seen after successful treatment. This mass may be cystic, representing mature teratoma, and may grow with time despite being benign.[376] Although

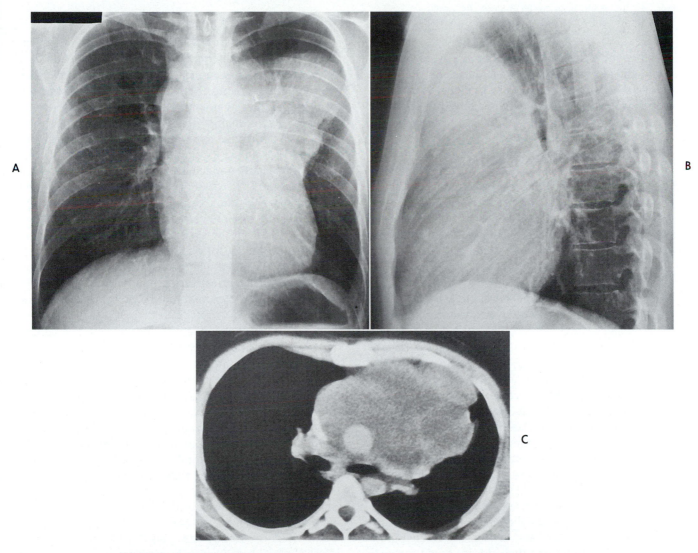

FIGURE 16-22
Malignant germ cell tumor (choriocarcinoma) of mediastinum. **A,** Posteroanterior and, **B,** lateral chest radiographs show a lobular asymmetric mediastinal mass and small metastases in both lungs. **C,** Contrast-enhanced computed tomography scan shows variable density in mass.

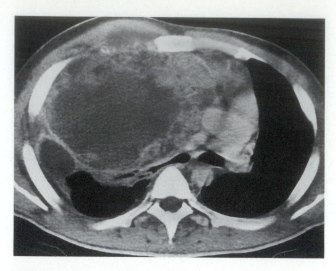

FIGURE 16-23
Malignant germ cell tumor. Contrast-enhanced computed tomography scan shows fluid density in widespread necrotic areas within the tumor. The tumor has invaded the anterior chest wall.

the benign or malignant nature of the residual mass cannot be stated with certainty on CT criteria, if the serum tumor markers are not elevated, the lesion may be benign. Surgical removal is currently recommended to detect the small number of cases with malignant transformation or residual malignancy.[376]

MRI shows the features of an invasive anterior mediastinal mass similar to CT.[239] CT and MRI cannot reliably distinguish malignant germ cell tumor from thymoma, and in the absence of calcification, the differential diagnosis includes lymphoma of the thymus, metastatic carcinoma, and other primary malignant tumors arising in the anterior mediastinum.

MEDIASTINAL CYSTS

Most mediastinal cysts are developmental in origin. Included in this category are bronchogenic (bronchial) cysts, esophageal duplication cysts, neurenteric cysts, and pericardial cysts. The distinction between these cysts is not always clear. For example, a cyst deep in the wall in the esophagus and unquestionably by all anatomic criteria an esophageal cyst may contain respiratory epithelium. Therefore bronchogenic, esophageal, and neurenteric cysts are frequently classified as foregut cysts to emphasize their origin from the embryologic foregut.[362,413] Mediastinal cysts containing cartilage are classified as definitely bronchogenic, and those with gastric epithelium are classified as definitely enteric. Those with seromucinous glands are considered as probably respiratory in origin. Most congenital mediastinal cysts are lined by respiratory epithelium and are usually labeled bronchogenic cysts even though their precise origin can only be conjectured.[413]

Bronchogenic cysts are discussed on p. 610.

Esophageal duplication cysts

Esophageal duplication cysts are uncommon. They may first present in adulthood or childhood. Initial presentation up to age 61 has been reported.[432] Many are clinically silent and discovered as an asymptomatic mass on an imaging examination of the chest, but they may cause dysphagia, pain, or other symptoms by compressing adjacent structures.[432] Ectopic gastric mucosa in the cyst may cause hemorrhage, infection, or perforation of the cyst.

The imaging features[284,432,529,538] are identical to those seen with bronchogenic cyst except that the wall of the lesion may be thicker and the mass may assume a more tubular shape with more intimate contact with the esophagus. Close contact with the esophagus means that barium swallow shows extrinsic or intramural compression.[432] Since the density at CT may be the same as that of soft tissue, the differential diagnosis includes any focal soft tissue mass appropriate to the location.

Pericardial cysts

Pericardial cysts are the result of anomalous outpouchings of the parietal pericardium, but only rarely do they have any visible communication with the pericardial sac. Pericardial diverticula are related anomalies of the visceral pericardium that communicate with the pericardial space.[371] Rapid change in size, particularly a decrease, suggests a pericardial diverticulum rather than a pericardial cyst.[273] The cysts contain clear yellow fluid. The interior is usually unilocular but is often trabeculated. In one series 20% of cases examined pathologically were multilocular,[141] although in another large series (72 patients) only one pericardial cyst was truly multilocular.[555] The wall of the cyst is composed of collagen and scattered elastic fibers lined by a single layer of mesothelial cells.[141] The great majority of these cysts are asymptomatic, but in surgical series symptoms such as chest pain, cough, and dyspnea may be present in up to one third of patients.[141,362,555]

A strong predilection exists for the anterior cardiophrenic angles, and the cysts typically contact the heart, diaphragm, and anterior chest wall. Cysts are more frequent on the right than the left. In the Mayo Clinic series[555] 37 of 72 pericardial cysts were in the right cardiophrenic angle and 17 were in the left cardiophrenic angle. The remaining 18 arose higher in the mediastinum, and 11 extended into the superior mediastinum. In a review of radiographs of 41 cases at the Armed Forces Institute of Pathology the right/left ratio was 4:3.[141]

On all imaging studies pericardial cysts are seen as smooth, round or oval, well-defined masses in contact with the heart (Figure 16-24). An oval shape coming to a point (Figure 16-25) has been observed in some cases.[57,108,141] Calcification is exceptional. On CT the cyst contents may be close to water density[403] or in the soft tissue range (Figure 16-25).[57] The cysts may be large;

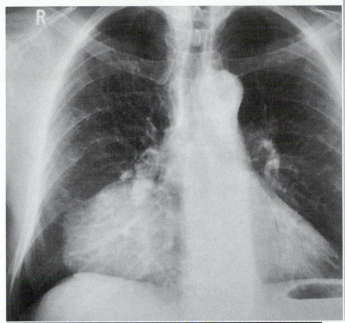

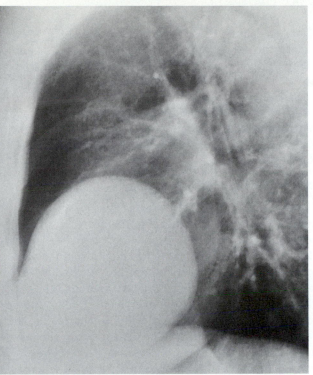

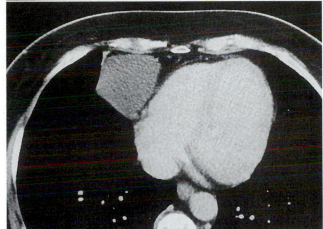

FIGURE 16-24
Pericardial cyst. **A,** Posteroanterior and, **B,** lateral radiographs show cyst in typical location in the right cardiophrenic angle. **C,** Contrast-enhanced computed tomography scan in another patient showing that the mass has uniform water density plus an imperceptible wall.

FIGURE 16-25
Pericardial cyst. **A,** Ultrasound scan shows echo-free, thin-walled cyst (*C,* cyst; *D,* diaphragm; *L,* liver). **B,** Pericardial cyst, in another patient, is oval and in contact with pericardium on contrast-enhanced computed tomography scan. Note oval shape coming to a point. In this case, the mass showed uniform soft tissue density, so the lesion was removed surgically.

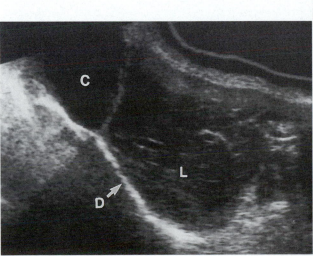

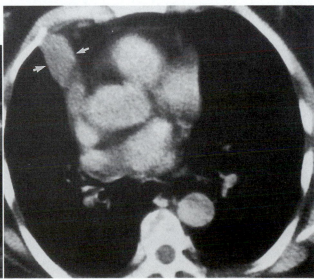

diameters up to 16 cm have been recorded.[141,555] Ultrasound can be used to demonstrate the cystic nature of these lesions (Figure 16-25). The role of MRI has yet to be ascertained, but clearly the fluid characteristics of the mass should be helpful in establishing the diagnosis. Cyst puncture with instillation of contrast medium to establish the diagnosis of a benign cyst has been performed with pericardial cysts just as it has with other benign mediastinal cysts.[275]

Neurenteric cysts

Neurenteric cysts are foregut cysts associated with anomalies of the vertebral column. In early embryogenesis the notochord lies against the embryonic foregut. Incomplete separation of the notochord from the alimentary tract may explain the various anomalies of the vertebrae seen in conjunction with neurenteric cysts.[362] The vertebral anomalies include hemivertebrae and sagittal clefts of the vertebral body (including butterfly vertebra and spina bifida). The vertebral anomaly may be located above the level of the cyst itself. Neurenteric cysts are relatively rare. They account for a small minority of mediastinal cysts; they were not encountered at all in three large surgical series.[47,362,556] On imaging (Figures 16-26 and 16-27),[317,548] neurenteric cysts are round, oval, or lobulated masses of water density in the posterior mediastinum or paravertebral region. Their transsonic nature can be demonstrated by ultrasound (Figure 16-27). The vertebral anomalies described above should be carefully sought because they may be difficult to see, but they are an important clue to the diagnosis. These cysts sometimes communicate with the subarachnoid space; this can be demonstrated by myelography.

Mediastinal pancreatic pseudocysts

On rare occasions a pancreatic pseudocyst extends into the mediastinum.[549,570] Most patients are adults and have clinical features of chronic pancreatitis, but only occasionally is an abdominal mass palpable. In children the usual cause of a pseudocyst is trauma.[269] On radiographic examination most patients have pleural effusion on the left or bilaterally. The mediastinal component of the pseudocyst is almost always in the posterior mediastinum, having gained access to the chest via the esophageal or aortic hiatus. In many instances the esophagus is deformed by the pseudocyst. CT is the optimum method of demonstrating the full extent of these pseudocysts.[370] It shows a thin-walled, fluid-containing cyst within the mediastinum in continuity with the pancreas and any peripancreatic fluid collections.

LYMPHANGIOMAS

Lymphangiomas (cystic hygromas) are tumorlike congenital malformations of the lymphatic system[37,456,568] consisting of lymph channels or cystic lymph spaces lined by endothelium, containing clear or straw-colored fluid. The walls are formed by fibrous tissue and smooth muscle. Lymphangiomas vary greatly in size and histologic characteristics. Some show a capillary or cavernous structure; others take the form of unilocular or multilocular cysts. They grow slowly and may envelop the adjacent structures but do not undergo malignant change.

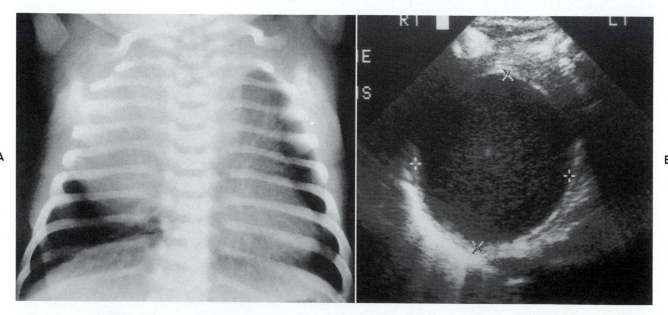

FIGURE 16-26
Neurenteric cyst. **A,** Plain chest radiograph shows large mass projecting from right mediastinum. **B,** Transthoracic ultrasound scan shows that the mass is a cyst.

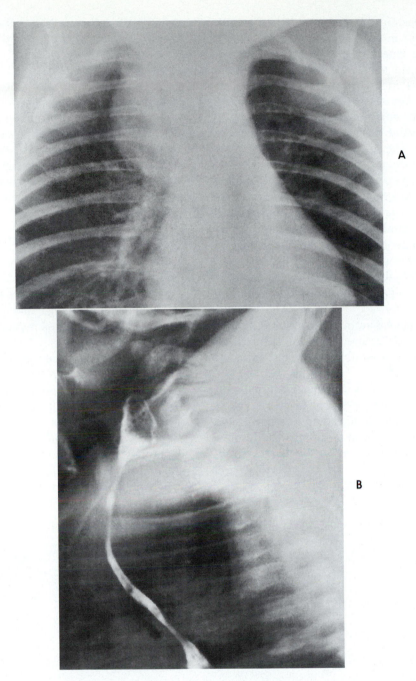

FIGURE 16-27
Neurenteric cyst. **A,** Plain film shows oval soft mass arising from mediastinum. Segmentation anomaly was present in lower cervical spine. **B,** Barium swallow study shows displacement of esophagus by mass, placing lesion between spine and esophagus. (Courtesy Dr. Helen Carty, Liverpool, U.K.)

Their invasive nature can make them difficult to resect, and recurrence rates are high. The most common location for lymphangiomas is the neck. Mediastinal lymphangiomas may be wholly confined to the mediastinum, or they may be an extension from the neck. The cervicomediastinal form, the usual form in infancy, is the more common. The form confined to the mediastinum is usually asymptomatic, is discovered on chest radiographs in older children or adults, and is rare.[56,144,386] Lymphangiomas may on rare occasions compress the surrounding structures such as the esophagus,[558] airway,[319] great veins,[103] or heart.[56]

On plain chest radiograph,[56,319] lymphangiomas form well-defined, round, lobular masses, usually in the anterior or superior mediastinum (Figures 16-28 and 16-29). Fewer than 10% occur in the posterior mediastinum.[456] Calcification does not appear to be a feature. Unilateral or bilateral pleural effusions may be present, and when present the effusion is often chylous.

CT shows a mass (Figures 16-28 and 16-29) that may mold to or envelop the adjacent mediastinal structures.* The CT attenuation value falls in the low soft tissue or water density range. The lesions may be recognizably unilocular or multilocular; septations are a frequent finding at CT. The septa may be thin or thick. Recognizing serpiginous, vessel-like structures in the lesion is sometimes possible, but regardless of shape, intravenous contrast administration enhances only the septa. Substantial dilatation of the superior vena cava was noted in more than one third of a series of 15 children with mediastinal cystic hygromas.[250] Whether this dilatation is caused by venous obstruction or is part of the congenital malformation is not clear.

The differential diagnosis from other cystic masses is based chiefly on location. Lymphangiomas are situated high in the superior mediastinum in contact with, or extending into, the neck.

Occasionally lymphangiomas visibly invade adjacent structures, notably pleura, pericardium, and chest wall.[66,392] Chest wall invasion may lead to recognizable rib thinning or destruction. A more widespread form of lymphangioma may relentlessly invade the thoracic struc-

*References 56, 66, 377, 392, 457, 495.

tures.[438] Chylothorax is a feature of this form of the disease.

Traumatic lymphoceles

Traumatic lymphoceles, also known as chylous pseudocysts, are rare lesions that may follow trauma,[230] particularly surgery. On radiographic examination they are enlarging mediastinal masses. CT demonstrates a low-density cystic mass with an imperceptible or very thin wall.[230,315,484] A single reported case examined by MRI showed low signal intensity on T1-weighted images.[230] Postoperative mediastinal seroma gives a similar appearance.[282]

BLOOD VESSEL TUMORS

Blood vessel tumors in the mediastinum are rare. Benign lesions are usually capillary or cavernous hemangiomas.[104] Mixed lymphatic and blood vessel lesions such as lymphangiohemangiomas,[10,504] hemangioendothelioma,[31,494] and hemangiosarcoma are also occasionally encountered.

Hemangiomas may be seen at any age but occur most often in the first decade. They are usually asymptomatic masses that arise in the anterior mediastinum (Figure 16-30). The next most common site is the posterior mediastinum.[84] Isolated involvement of the middle mediastinum was not found in an extensive review of the literature.[104] These lesions may extend into the neck and are almost always solitary.

Hemangiomas are recognized radiologically as masses

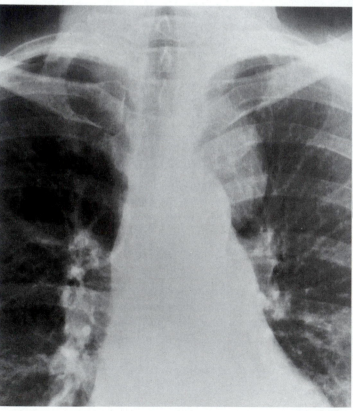

A

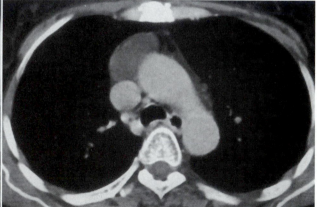

B

FIGURE 16-28
Lymphangioma (cystic hygroma) of superior mediastinum. **A,** Plain chest radiograph. Note contiguity of mass with anterior neck and lack of tracheal displacement. **B,** Contrast-enhanced computed tomography scan in another patient showing rounded, uniform water density mass with imperceptible wall in anterior mediastinum. The lymphangioma was an incidental finding in both patients.

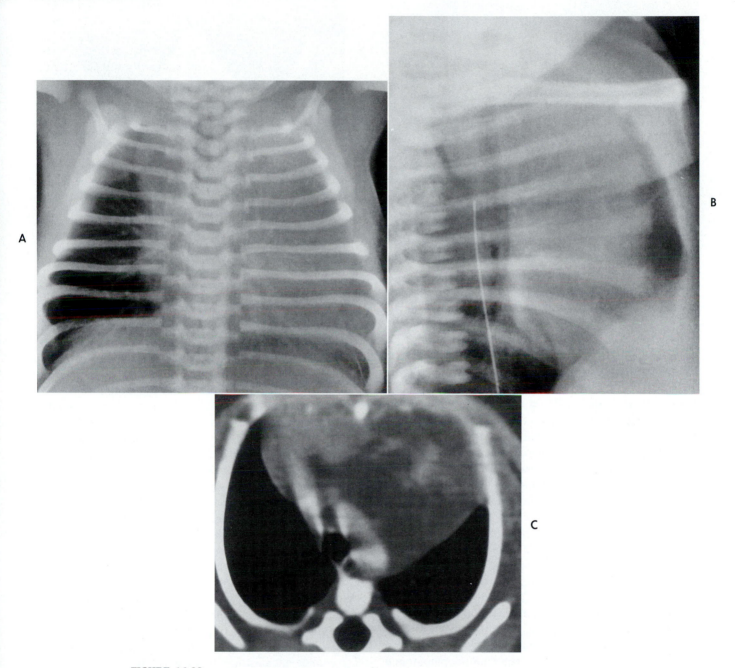

FIGURE 16-29
Lymphangioma (cystic hygroma) of mediastinum. This lesion is so large that, unusually, it displaces the great vessels and trachea backward. Computed tomography (CT) scan shows mixed density with large water-density areas. The patient, a newborn child, had respiratory distress. **A,** Posteroanterior radiograph. **B,** Lateral radiograph. **C,** Contrast-enhanced CT scan.

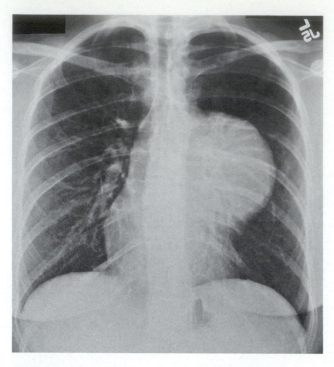

FIGURE 16-30
Hemangioma of anterior mediastinum in an asymptomatic 25-year-old woman. The mass has no specific radiologic features.

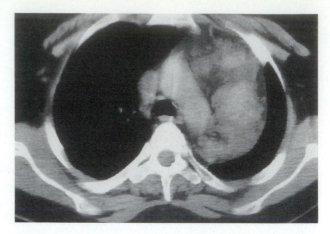

FIGURE 16-31
Extensive hemangioma in anterior mediastinum. Notice mixed attenuation: fat together with rounded and oval areas of contrast enhancement.

MEDIASTINAL LIPOMATOSIS

Excessive deposition of fat may give rise to mediastinal widening, a condition sometimes known as mediastinal lipomatosis.[217,231] When part of generalized obesity, the widening is fairly uniform and does not pose a diagnostic problem. However, in patients receiving steroid therapy and those with Cushing's disease, focal collections of histologically normal, unencapsulated fat occur in many sites in the body, including the mediastinum.[277,400,496] A similar phenomenon occasionally may be encountered as an incidental finding in patients with normal steroid hormone levels.[179,292] The usual appearance is a smooth widening of the upper anterior mediastinum, without tracheal deformity. If the fat deposition is symmetric, and particularly if it is widespread in the mediastinum, diagnosis is not difficult even on plain radiographic examinations. The observations that extrapleural fat is increased and that cardiophrenic fat pads are also often enlarged are helpful diagnostic features. In cases where the process is focal, CT is indicated to distinguish fat from neoplasm. This diagnostic problem arises most often in patients with lymphoma who are being treated with steroids. At CT the uniform low density of fat (−70 to −130 HU) is obvious (Figure 16-32).[33,179,481]

A rare condition called multiple symmetric lipomatosis resembles mediastinal lipomatosis but is linked to a specific biochemical abnormality in which multiple masses of benign fat may compress mediastinal structures, notably the trachea.[130]

FATTY TUMORS

True mediastinal tumors of fatty origin are uncommon, forming less than 1% of a series of 1064 surgically proven cases of mediastinal masses.[556] On plain film, regardless of whether they are benign or malignant, such tumors appear as well-defined, round or oval mediastinal

within the mediastinum. Phleboliths are an important diagnostic finding seen in 10% of cases. At CT (Figure 16-31),[84,444,448,494] the masses are usually complex in shape, similar to the clustered vessels that make up the lesion. The mass may clasp the adjacent mediastinal structures in a manner virtually specific to a vascular malformation. Before intravenous contrast administration the masses show soft tissue density of approximately 30 HU. Following contrast injection the mass may enhance brightly, but surprisingly, contrast enhancement can be minimal.[243,444,504] Only a few cases of MRI appearances have been reported.[243,444,448] The signal characteristics at MRI may be nonspecific but may show the more specific appearance of multiple high-signal foci of methemoglobin formation following hemorrhage in both T1- and T2-weighted images.

Mixed lymphangioma-hemangioendothelioma is a variant of these disorders. The condition may be widespread in the body. When encountered in the chest, the malformation may involve the mediastinum, pleura, and chest wall as a single continuous lesion causing widespread lobular soft tissue swelling, bone destruction, and chylous pleural effusion. This destructive form of the disease is known as Gorham's disease. Cystic angiomatosis is another, probably separate form of widespread lymphangiomatosis,[56] most frequently seen in children and young adults, in which lymphangiomas and hemangiomas may coexist. Many sites in the body may be involved, including the mediastinum, pericardium, and pleura, and multiple lytic lesions may be seen in bone.[207]

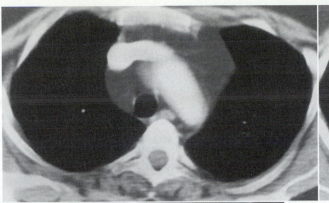

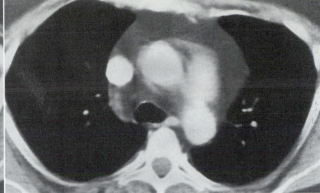

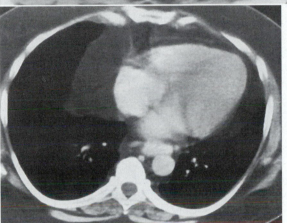

FIGURE 16-32
Mediastinal lipomatosis in a 47-year-old woman with Cushing's disease. Note masslike accumulations of fat on three representative contrast-enhanced computed tomography sections of the mediastinum in this typical example.

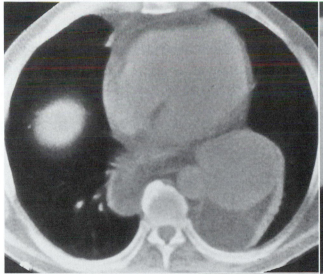

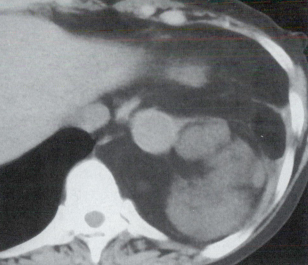

A

B

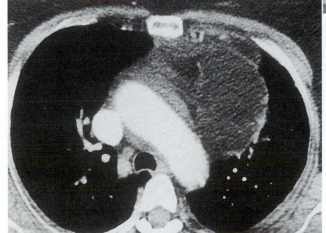

C

FIGURE 16-33
Liposarcoma of mediastinum. **A,** Fat density component indicates fatty origin of the tumor; soft tissue component within the tumor indicates its malignant nature. **B,** Another patient showing fatty mass that contains several rounded soft tissue density regions and has displaced aorta forward. **C,** Another patient, showing predominantly fat density with only a few soft tissue densities.

masses.[445] Benign lipomas are soft and therefore do not compress surrounding structures unless the tumors are very large. In one unusual case a lipoma extended into both the mediastinum and the spinal canal and produced pressure deformity of the adjacent bones.[405] The molding to the mediastinal contour can be so extreme that a large mediastinal lipoma may mimic cardiomegaly.[463] CT shows uniform fat density apart from a few strands of soft tissue.[330,405] Lipoblastoma, a benign tumor of childhood,[138] may show a few more soft tissue strands,[40,178,541] and in the occasional case the amount of fat density is relatively small.[447] Angiolipoma, a benign tumor, may show a combination of soft tissue density and fat that is indistinguishable from liposarcoma at CT.[276] Myelolipoma is another benign, fat-containing tumor that shows a combination of fat and soft tissue density. It is usually located in the adrenal but on very rare occasion may arise primarily in the mediastinum.[272]

In virtually every case liposarcomas show inhomogeneity of the fat on CT and often contain large areas of soft tissue density (Figure 16-33).

Other fat-containing mediastinal tumors are teratomas (see p. 732), thymolipomas (see p. 729), and extramedullary hemopoiesis (see p. 780).

HERNIATION OF ABDOMINAL FAT

Herniation of omental and perigastric fat is a common cause of localized fatty masses in the mediastinum. The fat may herniate through the esophageal hiatus, the foramen of Morgagni, or the foramen of Bochdalek. Such herniations are usually readily diagnosed on plain film because of their characteristic locations. A CT number in the fat range (-70 to -130 HU) eliminates confusion with other mediastinal masses[178,420]; the herniated omentum may contain streaky regions, presumably caused by omental vessels. Similarly, at MRI[562] high signal intensity on T1-weighted sequences and moderately high signal intensity on T2-weighted sequences — typical of fat — together with lower intensity linear regions representing omentum and omental blood vessels, enables a specific diagnosis to be made.

DESMOID TUMORS

Desmoid tumors, also known as aggressive fibromatosis, are locally invasive tumors of fibrous origin that primarily involve the soft tissues of the extremities, neck, and trunk.[8] They may arise in areas of previous trauma, notably previous surgery.[253] Distant metastasis is rare.[453] This tumor very rarely may be found in the mediastinum

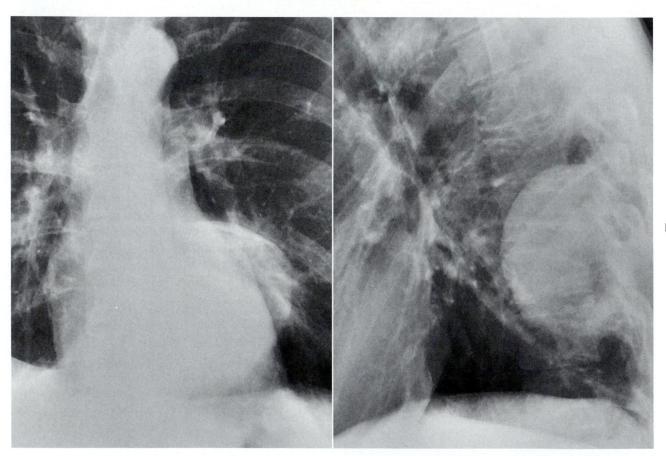

A

B

FIGURE 16-34
Desmoid tumor in a 34-year-old man. **A,** Posteroanterior radiograph. **B,** Lateral radiograph.

(Figure 16-34)[39,71] and chest wall.[253,384]

Plain radiographs show a soft tissue mass (Figure 16-34) and may show periosteal reaction or cortical erosion of adjacent bone. CT shows a mass that may be isodense with skeletal muscle on precontrast images and slightly hyperdense compared to muscle after intravenous contrast. The mass may show areas of cystic change.[384] At MRI, desmoids have low signal on T1-weighted images and variable signal on T2-weighted images compared with muscle.[485] They are very vascular at angiography.[235]

MEDIASTINAL SARCOMAS

Primary mediastinal sarcomas, other than neural tumors, are rare. Fibrosarcoma, osteosarcoma,[237,478] and liposarcoma (see p. 744) are occasionally encountered. Chest wall tumors, such as chondrosarcoma, may project so far into the mediastinum that a primary mediastinal origin may be mimicked.[391] The early symptoms depend on location. On radiographic study these lesions all appear as focal masses. In the case of osteosarcoma they characteristically show areas of dense calcification or ossification.[478] In the case of liposarcoma the fatty component is readily demonstrable by CT, in some cases together with foci of calcification.

HISTIOCYTOSIS X

Anterior mediastinal masses have been reported in a few infants with histiocytosis X (Langerhans' cell histiocytosis).[363] The mass can be quite large. Fine speckled calcification, visible at CT, and cavitation[6] have been documented.

MEDIASTINAL AND HILAR LYMPHADENOPATHY

Intrathoracic lymphadenopathy occurs frequently and has many causes. The two major imaging signs are change in density and enlargement of the nodes.

Intrathoracic lymph node calcification

Intrathoracic lymph node calcification is common following certain infections, notably tuberculous disease and fungal infections (particularly histoplasmosis) (Figure 16-35). It is also seen in other benign conditions such as sarcoidosis, silicosis, and coal worker's pneumoconiosis and more rarely in amyloidosis, Castleman's disease, and sclerodema.

Lymph node calcification is very rarely due to neoplastic disease. The tumors in which the primary neoplasm calcifies may also show calcification of lymph node metastases. These tumors include osteosarcoma, chon-

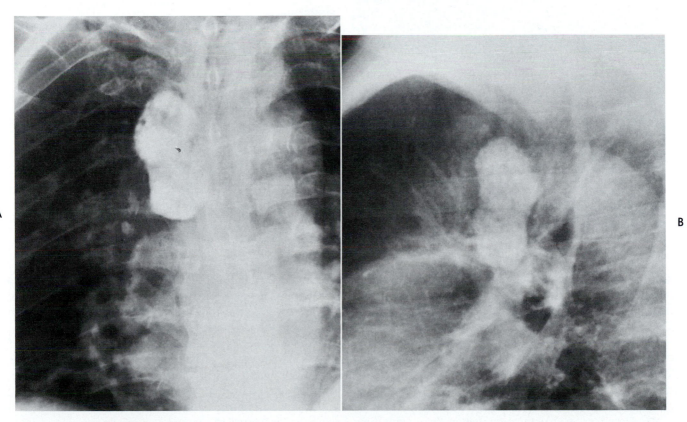

A   B

FIGURE 16-35
Lymph node calcification following histoplasmosis. The large size of the nodal mass illustrates how large infectious granulomatous lymph nodes can be. **A,** Posteroanterior radiograph. **B,** Lateral radiograph.

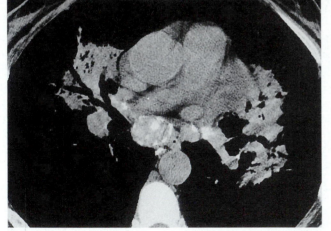

FIGURE 16-36
Eggshell calcification *(arrow)* in enlarged mediastinal lymph nodes.
A and **B**, In long-standing amyloidosis. **C**, In treated lymphoma
shown on computed tomography scan (no contrast enhancement).

drosarcoma, colorectal carcinoma, carcinoid tumors, and
lung carcinoma.[320] Single cases of nodal calcification in
untreated Hodgkin's disease have been reported.[289,375,557]
These examples are exceptions to a useful general rule:
lymph node calcification is not a feature of either primary
or secondary lymph node neoplasms before treatment.
Tumor-bearing nodes, however, may calcify following
radiation therapy. This phenomenon occurs most frequently in patients treated for lymphoma.

CT demonstrates calcification better than plain film
techniques. An important sign of benign lymph node
disease, namely calcification, is not usually visible at
MRI.[298]

Various patterns of calcification are seen. The two
common patterns are coarse, irregularly distributed
clumps within the node and homogeneous calcification of
the whole node. A strikingly foamy appearance is seen
with *Pneumocystis carinii* infection in AIDS patients[196,408]
and in some cases of metastatic carcinomatous involvement of lymph nodes. Sometimes a ring of calcification,
called eggshell calcification, appears at the periphery of
the node (Figure 16-36). Eggshell calcification is a
particular feature of prolonged dust exposure in coal and
metal mines and of sarcoidosis.[244,245] It is seen on plain
chest radiographs in 3% of those who have worked in the
coal industry for more than 30 years.[245] Eggshell calcifi-

cation is rare in other conditions but has been reported in amyloidosis, histoplasmosis, blastomycosis, and treated lymphoma (Figure 16-36).[197]

Low density on computed tomography

Areas of low CT density within enlarged nodes corresponding to necrosis may be seen in a variety of conditions, particularly infection, notably tuberculosis, fungal disease,[285] and infections in immunocompromised patients; metastatic neoplasm, notably from testicular tumors[439,565]; and malignant lymphoma. In one series of patients with Hodgkin's disease, 16 of 76 patients showed low-density nodes at diagnosis.[233] Nodes that are below water density are seen in fatty replacement of inflammatory nodes and also have been described in Whipple's disease.[436]

Contrast enhancement at computed tomography

Contrast enhancement in enlarged nodes, when moderate in degree, is nonspecific, being seen with inflammatory disorders, particularly tuberculosis,[240,396] fungal disease,[285] sarcoidosis, and neoplasm. When striking, it points particularly to the diagnosis of metastatic neoplasm from a primary tumor that itself is highly vascular, such as melanoma, renal and thyroid carcinoma, carcinoid tumor, leiomyoma, or sarcoma. A rare cause of striking uniform contrast enhancement is Castleman's disease (see p. 756).

A low-density center with rim enhancement can be a striking feature of tuberculous infection,[396] a feature of diagnostic value in young patients in whom tuberculosis is likely and metastatic carcinoma unlikely.[240]

Intrathoracic lymph node enlargement

CAUSES OF MEDIASTINAL AND HILAR NODE ENLARGEMENT. There are many causes of mediastinal and hilar lymph node enlargement, notably neoplasm, infection, sarcoidosis, and reactive hyperplasia. Neoplastic causes include malignant lymphoma, lymphoproliferative disorders, leukemia, and metastatic carcinoma; carcinomas of the bronchus, esophagus, breast, kidney, testis, and head and neck are the usual primary sites.[102,325]

Neoplastic lymph node enlargement is often markedly asymmetric in distribution. Paracardiac nodal enlargement has been shown to be caused by lymphoma approximately half of the time and by metastatic carcinoma in most other instances.[486,512] This is probably true for posterior mediastinal nodes as well.

Finding intrathoracic lymph node enlargement in patients being staged for a known lung carcinoma is an important topic discussed in Chapter 8 (see p. 286). A helpful feature when trying to distinguish between enlargement caused by a coincidental, clinically unimportant benign process (such as previous sarcoidosis, old granulomatous disease, or pneumoconiosis) and metastatic lymphadenopathy, is the distribution of the enlarged nodes. Enlarged nodes in the drainage areas of a primary tumor are more likely to be enlarged because of neoplastic involvement or reactive hyperplasia to the tumor than to be an incidental finding.

The most frequent infections that give rise to visibly enlarged intrathoracic lymph nodes are tuberculosis and fungal disease (particularly histoplasmosis), each of which may cause intrathoracic lymph node enlargement without visible pneumonia. Lymph node enlargement is now being encountered with increased frequency in AIDS patients, in whom it may have a variety of causes, notably AIDS-related lymphoma and granulomatous infections. Intrathoracic nodal enlargement may also be seen in tularemia, whooping cough, anthrax, plague, mycoplasmal and viral infections, and late stages of cystic fibrosis. Significantly enlarged hilar or mediastinal lymph nodes are rare in other infections, especially in the absence of visible consolidation in the lungs.

Sarcoidosis is a particularly frequent cause of intrathoracic lymph node enlargement in young adults. It is the most likely diagnosis when multiple node groups are involved and when the adenopathy is symmetrically distributed in the hila and mediastinum in young adults who either have no symptoms or have clinical features consistent with sarcoidosis. Lymphoma is an important differential diagnosis in such patients, but lymphoma is rarely symmetrically distributed with equal involvement of the hilar and mediastinal lymph node groups.

Reactive hyperplasia is a term that includes an acute or chronic, nonspecific, inflammatory response, in which both inflammation and hyperplasia are present. Lymph nodes undergo reactive changes whenever challenged by infection, cell debris, or foreign substances. Thus reactive hyperplasia is seen in nodes draining neoplasms or areas of pulmonary infection and in a variety of other inflammatory diseases. Generalized acute reactive inflammation is seen with virus infections and bacteremia.

Intrathoracic lymph node enlargement may occasionally result from a variety of other disorders, including silicosis; asbestos exposure[434]; Castleman's disease; angioimmunoblastic lymphadenopathy; amyloidosis; multiple myeloma[254]; chronic berylliosis; histiocytosis X[49]; Whipple's disease[436]; Wegener's granulomatosis[3]; mixed connective tissue disease[199]; chronic eosinophilic pneumonia[569]; severe raised pulmonary venous pressure[116]; and drug-induced lymphadenopathy, notably caused by methotrexate.[334]

PLAIN FILM SIGNS OF MEDIASTINAL LYMPH NODE ENLARGEMENT. Few studies have specifically addressed the relationship between the size of lymph nodes and their visibility on plain film. It would appear that most nodes with a short-axis diameter greater than 2 cm give rise to visible mediastinal widening if they lie in the right paratracheal area, the aortopulmonary window, the hilar regions, or the paravertebral areas. Pretracheal, left paratracheal, subcarinal, and paracardiac nodes may be

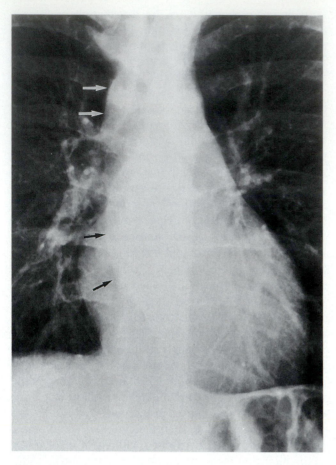

FIGURE 16-37
Right paratracheal lymph node enlargement *(white arrows)* resulting from Hodgkin's disease. The right paratracheal stripe is widened, and the right paratracheal area is as dense as the aortic knob. Note massive subcarinal lymph node enlargement *(black arrows).*

larger than 2 cm without being visible on plain chest radiographs.[350,486]

Enlargement of the right upper paratracheal nodes (Figure 16-37) (station 2R of the American Thoracic Society nomenclature[501]; see p. 38) causes uniform or lobular widening of the right tracheal stripe.[349] With substantial paratracheal nodal enlargement the border of the superior vena cava may be convex rather than flat or concave as in the normal subject. An additional or alternative feature is that the density of the superior vena cava increases and may equal the density of the aortic arch (normally the density of the superior vena cava in the right paratracheal area is significantly less than that of the aortic arch). When the right lower paratracheal (azygos) nodes (station 4R) enlarge, they push the azygos vein laterally so that the diameter of the combination shadow of the azygos node and vein enlarges (the normal diameter on an upright chest film should be 7 mm or less).[261]

The left upper paratracheal nodes (station 2L) must enlarge substantially if they are to cause recognizable mediastinal widening on plain chest radiograph because they have to project beyond the left carotid and left subclavian arteries to be visible. If the aortopulmonary nodes (station 5) are substantially enlarged, they project beyond the aortopulmonary window and cause a bulge in the angle between the aortic arch and the main pulmonary artery (Figure 16-38).[42] Nodes lateral to the aortic arch are visible as bulges even when relatively small (Figure 16-39).

Enlargement of the anterior mediastinal nodes, namely anterior to the aorta and innominate artery (station 6) and trachea (stations 2 and 4) must be substantial to be recognizable on plain chest radiographs (Figure 16-40). The resulting mediastinal widening is frequently bilateral and lobulated in outline. Sometimes the only sign of enlargement is increased opacity of the retrosternal area on the lateral view, a sign that is difficult to evaluate because it is also seen in normal people with abundant mediastinal fat. Enlargement of the anterior intercostal nodes is easiest to recognize on the lateral chest radiograph as extrapleural soft tissue swelling along the course of the internal mammary arteries.

The most useful plain film sign of subcarinal node (station 7) enlargement is a change in the contour of the superior portion of the azygoesophageal line (Figure 16-37) from its normal concave shape to a convex bulge. Alteration of the contour of the line, unfortunately, is a relatively insensitive sign of subcarinal adenopathy. It occurred in only 23% of the cases with subcarinal lymph node enlargement reported by Muller and associates.[350] Two other plain film signs of subcarinal node enlargement are increased opacity[209] and lack of visibility of the external surface of the medial wall of the right mainstem bronchus and bronchus intermedius.[350] Because the esophagus passes immediately behind the carina, subcarinal node enlargement causes posterior displacement of the esophagus. If the nodes are very large, the esophagus slips laterally. However, the hallmark of lymph node enlargement, namely lobulation, is not always evident, and the radiographic appearance may resemble left atrial enlargement.

Enlarged paraesophageal nodes and posterior mediastinal nodes (stations 8 and 9) produce displacement of the azygoesophageal and paraspinal lines (Figure 16-41).

COMPUTED TOMOGRAPHY OF MEDIASTINAL LYMPH NODE ENLARGEMENT. Lymph node enlargement is more readily demonstrated at CT than on plain film examination (Figures 16-38 to 16-40). The CT signs of lymph node enlargement (Figure 16-42) are an increase in size of individual nodes, focal bulges or lobulations of the interface between the mediastinum and lung, recognizable invasion of surrounding mediastinal fat, coalescence of adjacent and enlarged nodes to form larger masses, and diffuse soft tissue density throughout the mediastinum obliterating the mediastinal fat. Individually enlarged nodes are seen as round or oval soft tissue densities in the mediastinum. Distinguishing enlarged nodes from nor-

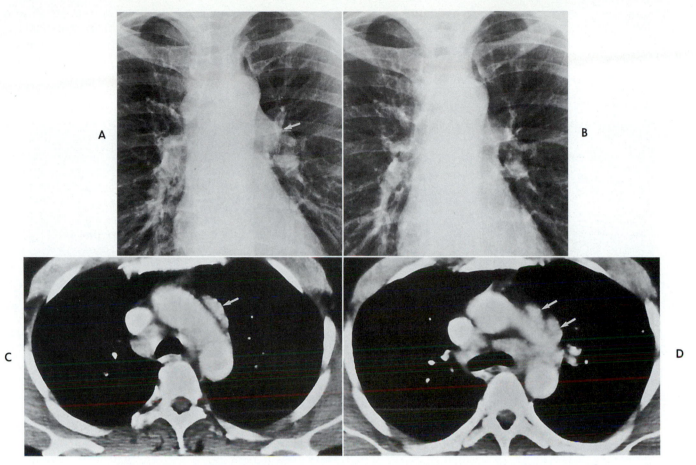

FIGURE 16-38
Aortopulmonary window lymph node enlargement in a patient with malignant lymphoma. (Note also the right paratracheal lymphadenopathy.) **A,** Plain radiograph shows bulge overlying main pulmonary artery *(arrow).* **B,** After treatment, the appearance has returned to nearly normal. **C** and **D,** Contrast-enhanced computed tomography scans through the aortopulmonary window and aortic arch show the many enlarged nodes *(arrows).* (Right paratracheal adenopathy is also demonstrated.)

mal vascular structures requires a secure knowledge of the normal arrangement of blood vessels and an understanding of the various anomalies and variations in the arrangement of the mediastinal vessels (see p. 793). In selected cases intravenous contrast enhancement is needed to help distinguish vessels from lymph nodes.

To date, four series have measured normal lymph node size at CT (see p. 39)[166,170,241,441] In summary, they showed that nodes less than 10 mm in short-axis diameter lie within the 95th percentile and should be considered normal. Nodes between 10 and 15 mm in short-axis diameter occur in certain sites, notably the subcarinal and tracheobronchial regions, in 5% to 7% of normal subjects. Short-axis diameter is the standard measurement because it shows the best correlation with lymph node volume at autopsy.[406]

Identifying and measuring right-sided mediastinal lymph nodes is easier than evaluating the left-sided nodes because mediastinal fat is more abundant and vascular anatomy is less complex on the right side.[406]

Subcarinal lymph node enlargement can be difficult to recognize even at CT (Figure 16-43). The signs to look for are (1) a soft tissue mass between the esophagus and either the left atrium or the intramediastinal portions of the right or left pulmonary arteries and (2) a soft tissue density bulging into the azygoesophageal recess posterior to the bronchus intermedius or left lower lobe bronchus.

MAGNETIC RESONANCE IMAGING OF MEDIASTINAL LYMPH NODE ENLARGEMENT. With current machines MRI and CT scans provide comparable information regarding enlargement of mediastinal nodes (Figure 16-44). MRI sometimes has the critical advantage of providing images in any desired plane.[393]

With spin-echo sequences the imaging times are long, and motion therefore degrades the image, which offsets the better contrast resolution of MRI. Measuring the

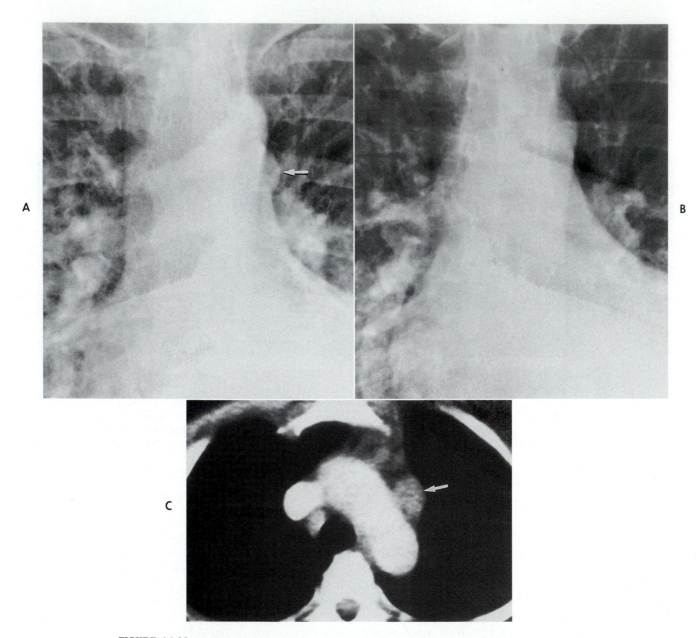

FIGURE 16-39
Aortopulmonary window lymph node enlargement caused by metastatic breast carcinoma. **A,** Plain radiograph demonstrates small bulge *(arrow)* just beneath the aortic knob. **B,** In contrast-enhanced computed tomography scan there is an enlarged node *(arrow)* projecting to the left of the aortic arch. **C,** Following treatment, the appearance of the aortopulmonary window region has returned to normal.

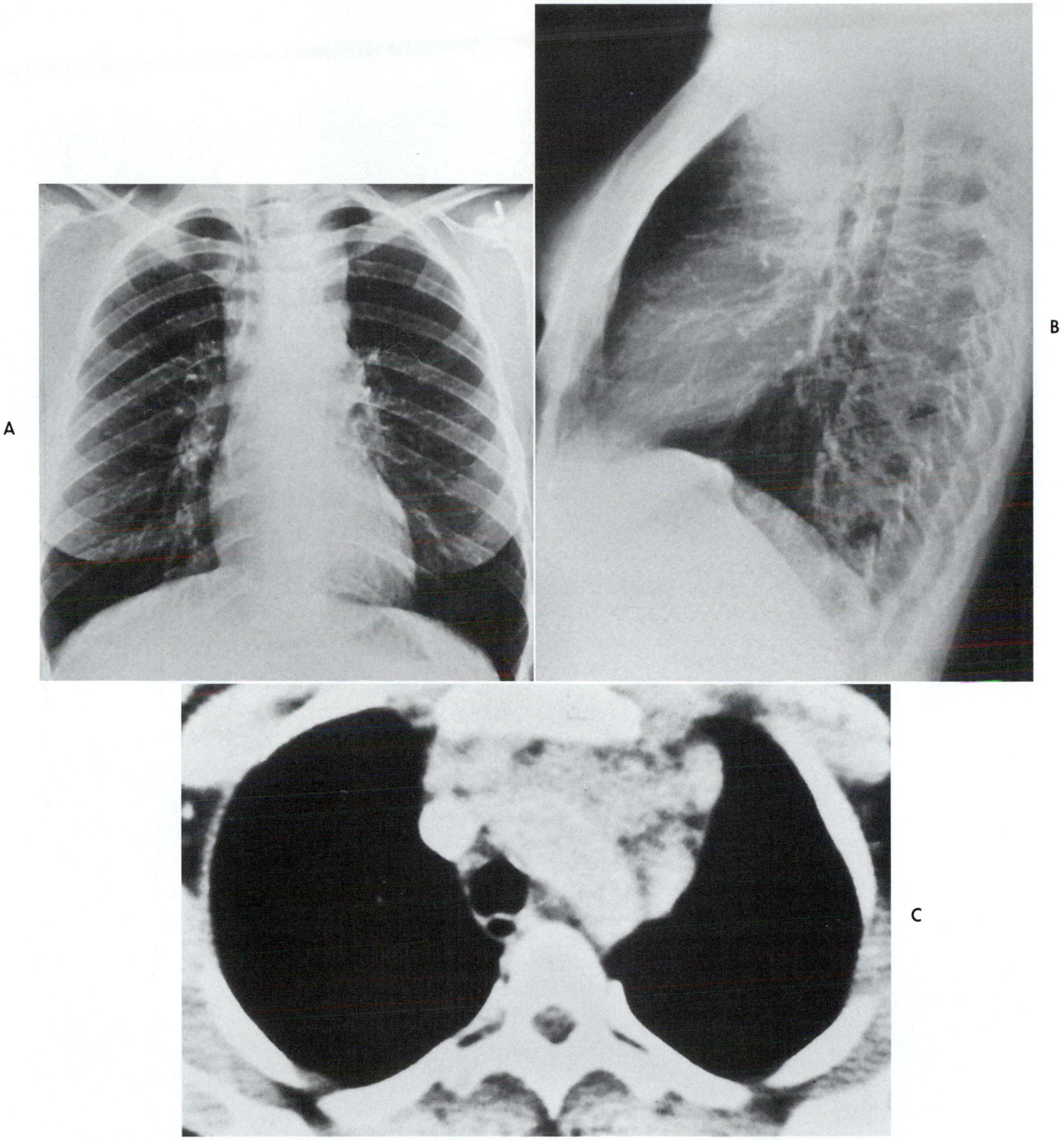

FIGURE 16-40
Anterior (prevascular) mediastinal lymph node enlargement caused by lymphoma. **A,** Posteroanterior radiograph shows lobular, left-sided widening of the upper mediastinum and aortopulmonary window. **B,** Lateral radiograph shows ill-defined increase in density in the anterior mediastinum. **C,** Contrast-enhanced computed tomography scan shows massive lymph node enlargement, predominantly anterior to and to the left of the aortic arch.

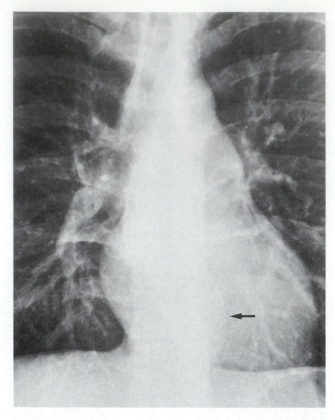

FIGURE 16-41
Enlarged paraesophageal and posterior mediastinal lymph nodes *(arrow)* in a patient with Hodgkin's disease.

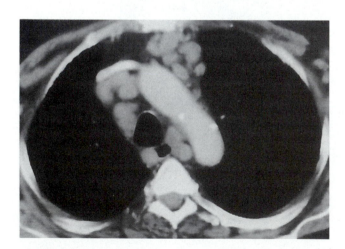

FIGURE 16-42
Mediastinal lymph node enlargement in Hodgkin's disease. In this contrast-enhanced computed tomography examination, the enlarged nodes are unusually discrete. (Courtesy Dr. Martin Wastie, Nottingham, U.K.)

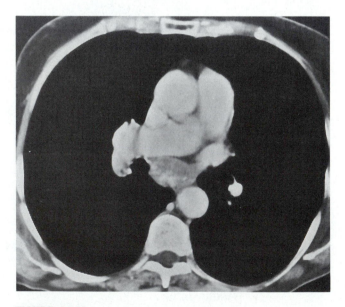

FIGURE 16-43
Subcarinal mediastinal adenopathy resulting from metastatic bronchial carcinoma. The mass of nodes interposes between the descending aorta and esophagus (not seen as a separate structure) posteriorly, and the right pulmonary artery anteriorly. Note also that the lymph node mass causes a convex bulge into the azygoesophageal recess of lung. Contrast-enhanced computed tomography scan.

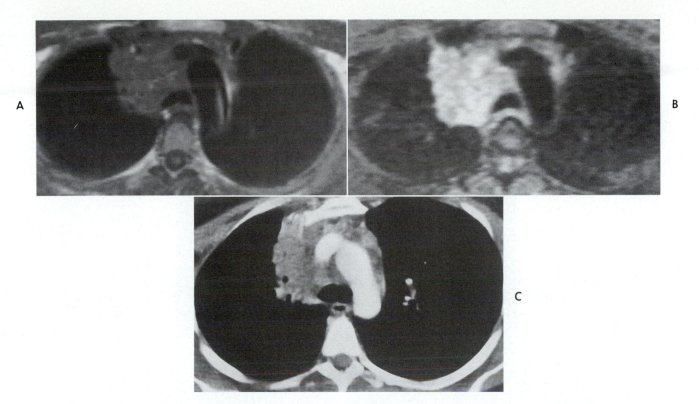

FIGURE 16-44
Comparison of magnetic resonance (MR) and computed tomography (CT) (contrast-enhanced) images of mediastinal lymph node enlargement in a patient with Hodgkin's disease. On these axial images, the information is comparable, but compression of the right and left brachiocephalic veins is shown well without intravenous contrast medium in MR images. All images are at same level. **A,** T1-weighted axial MR image. **B,** T2-weighted axial MR image. **C,** Contrast-enhanced CT scan. (Courtesy Dr. William C. Black, Washington, D.C.)

diameter of lymph nodes at MRI is frequently difficult, and distinguishing a cluster of small normal nodes from a single enlarged node may be impossible.[298] Fast-flowing blood in the larger arteries and veins can be recognized as signal void. This advantage is sometimes offset by averaging low signal from flowing blood and high signal from fat, both of which occupy part of the volume. Thus on the final image a normal vessel may be seen as a rounded area with a signal similar to soft tissue and resemble lymphadenopathy. This pitfall can be avoided by rescanning the patient with a long repetition time (for example, TR 2000 msec), so that signal intensity of a soft tissue mass increases, but the signal intensity of flowing blood remains low.[523] A problem with electrocardiographic gating of data acquisition is that some images of the blood vessels are obtained during periods of slow blood flow. Slow-flowing blood generates a signal that can be misinterpreted as a soft tissue mass.[535]

A clear disadvantage of MRI compared with CT is the inability of MRI to demonstrate most forms of calcification. Therefore enlarged, heavily calcified nodes, which on CT can be diagnosed as long-standing benign conditions such as old granulomatous infection, appear similar to neoplastic nodes on MRI.

Unfortunately, using magnetic resonance signal characteristics to distinguish between neoplastic and inflammatory causes for mediastinal lymphadenopathy has not proved possible.

PLAIN FILM SIGNS OF HILAR NODE ENLARGEMENT. The basic signs of hilar node enlargement are overall enlargement of the hilum, lobulation of outline, or the presence of a rounded mass of tissue in a portion of the hilum that does not contain major vascular trunks (Figure 16-45).[348] In portions of the hila that contain major blood vessels, such as the cross-over point of the right superior pulmonary vein and the descending limb of the right pulmonary artery, hilar node enlargement must be substantial to be recognized. Similarly, the inferior poles of both hila, where the inferior pulmonary veins intermingle with the segmental divisions of the lower lobe arteries, are a particularly difficult region to interpret. Enlarged nodes adjacent to the lower lobe arteries increase the diameter of the hilum (the transverse diameter of each lower lobe artery should be no greater than 16 mm) and create a lobular as opposed to a tubular configuration (Figure 16-46). Lymph node enlargement in the upper portions of the hila is often easy to recognize because the vessels in these regions are normally small and the nodes

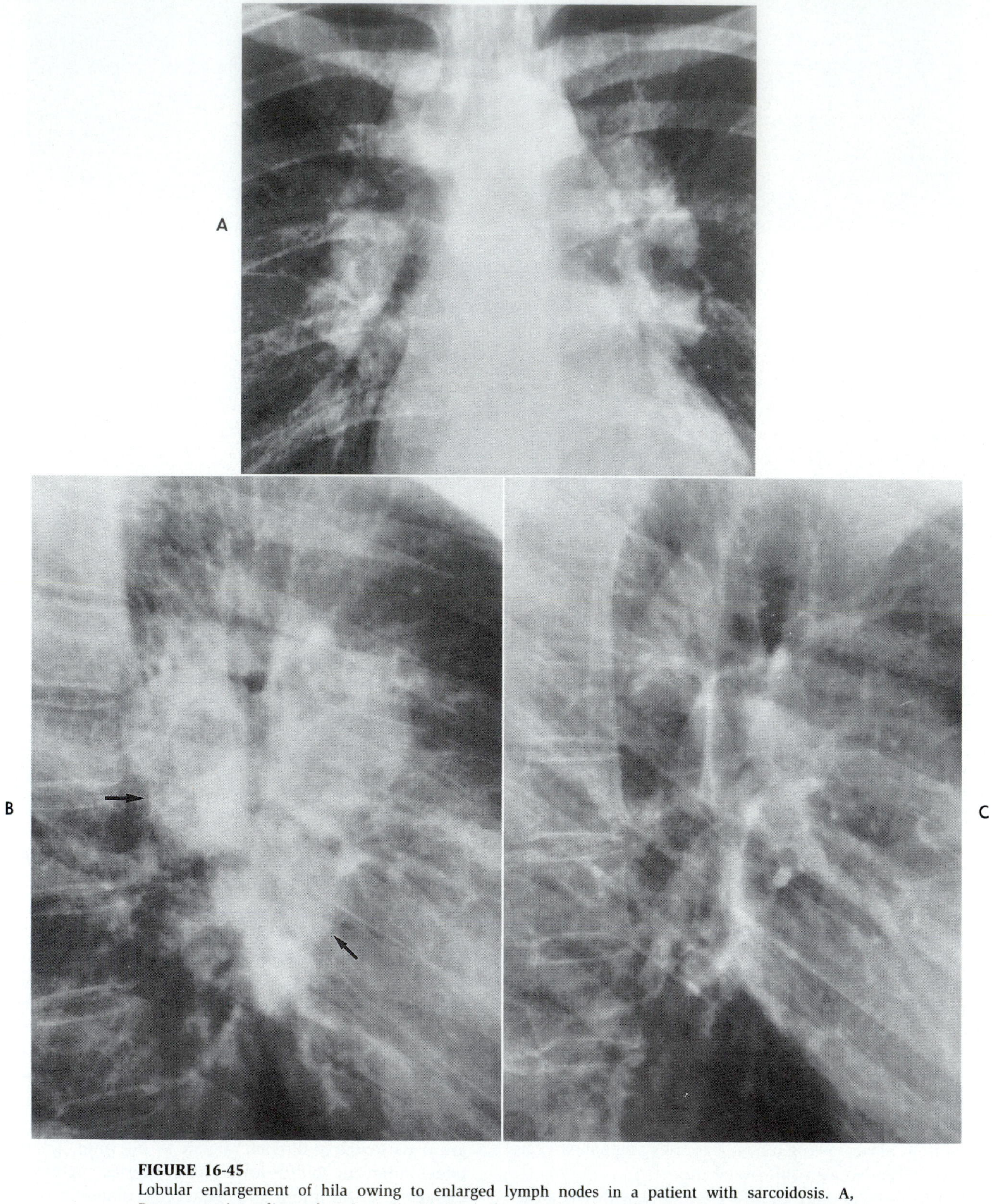

FIGURE 16-45
Lobular enlargement of hila owing to enlarged lymph nodes in a patient with sarcoidosis. **A,** Posteroanterior radiograph. **B,** Lateral radiograph. Recognizing adenopathy in this example is easy, but when in doubt the lateral projection should be examined for rounded densities in areas that are devoid of vessels. Arrows point to two such areas: posterior to the bronchus intermedius and anterior to the lower lobe bronchus below the level of middle lobe bronchus. **C,** Comparison lateral radiograph in another patient shows normal anatomy.

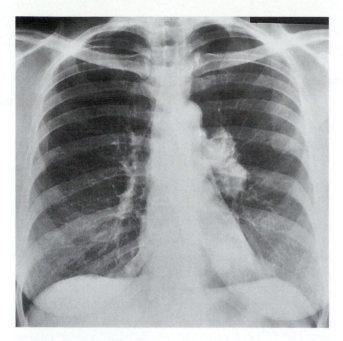

FIGURE 16-46
Left hilar lymph node enlargement caused by metastases from bronchial carcinoma in the left lower lobe; typical lobular enlargement of left hilum is seen.

stand out. Even mild nodal enlargement can be recognized when the enlarged nodes lie posterior to the right main bronchus and the bronchus intermedius (Figure 16-45) because in this region the lung normally contacts the posterior wall of the airway. Other sensitive sites in which to search for hilar node enlargement on lateral projection are the angles formed by the middle lobe or lingula bronchus and the lower lobe bronchi (Figure 16-45).

Distinguishing enlarged hilar lymph nodes from enlargement of the hilar arteries may at times be difficult (Figure 16-47). This analysis should concentrate on determining whether the enlargement is truly centered on the pulmonary arteries (any mass in a site that is normally devoid of vessels would clearly favor nodal enlargement) and on evaluating the degree of lobulation (central pulmonary arteries even when large should retain their basically tubular configuration).

COMPUTED TOMOGRAPHY OF HILAR NODE ENLARGEMENT. Recognition of hilar node enlargement at CT (Figure 16-48) is greatly facilitated by intravenous contrast opacification of the hilar vessels.[173] In general, lymph nodes do not enhance to the same degree as blood

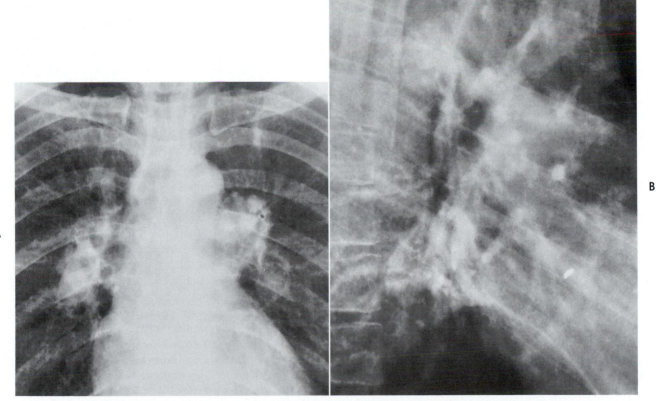

A

B

FIGURE 16-47
Enlarged hilar arteries in a patient with pulmonary hypertension caused by chronic pulmonary thromboembolism. Differentiation from hilar lymphadenopathy is best made by noting that hilar enlargement is not lobular and is centered on portions of the hila occupied by lobar divisions of the pulmonary arteries. A, Posteroanterior radiograph. B, Lateral radiograph.

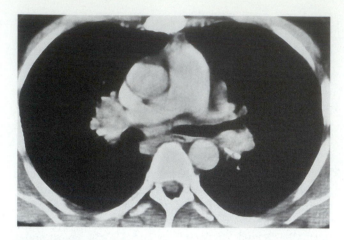

FIGURE 16-48
Bilateral hilar node enlargement caused by lymphoma. The right hilum shows lobular swelling that cannot be accounted for by normal vascular structures (right pulmonary artery and right superior pulmonary vein). Similarly, the bulk of tissue posterior to left bronchial tree is too great to be accounted for by the descending branch of the left pulmonary artery. (Note also subcarinal and aortopulmonary window adenopathy.) Contrast-enhanced computed tomography scan.

vessels. Any nonenhancing hilar tissue larger than 5 mm in short-axis diameter is considered abnormal.[174] If enhancement is uncertain or if the examination is performed without intravenous contrast medium, recognition of nodal enlargement depends on demonstrating rounded soft tissue densities that are too large to be blood vessels (Figure 16-48).[13,352,353,518] The required size varies according to location. Some portions of the hilum are normally devoid of vessels greater than 5 mm in diameter, and in other portions the vessel diameters may be 15 mm or even greater if there is increased pulmonary blood flow or pulmonary arterial hypertension. The most sensitive site to examine for lymph node enlargement is the region immediately behind the right mainstem bronchus and its divisions (the right upper lobe bronchus and the bronchus intermedius) because in these regions the lung contacts the posterior wall of the bronchial tree.[521] The equivalent area on the left is partially occupied by the descending aorta and descending left pulmonary artery, and therefore only a small tongue of lung can contact the posterior wall of the left main bronchus.[517] The most difficult and therefore the least sensitive area to evaluate is the central portion of the right hilum, where the right superior pulmonary vein passes directly anterior to the right pulmonary artery and its major divisions. Additionally, there are fat pads at the bifurcation of the right pulmonary artery that can resemble lymph node enlargement. Recognizing their fatty nature is not usually possible because of partial volume averaging with the adjacent central pulmonary arteries.

MAGNETIC RESONANCE IMAGING OF HILAR NODE ENLARGEMENT. Hilar node enlargement is easier to recognize at MRI than at CT[15,298,520] because the signal

from flowing blood is different compared with that returned from the stationary tissues, such as the walls of the blood vessels and bronchi, and the small amount of fat and connective tissue that surrounds the hilar structures. With spin-echo imaging no signal is generated by fast-flowing blood within the hilar blood vessels, nor is any signal generated from air within the bronchi. Hilar adenopathy therefore stands out as rounded or oval, relatively high-signal regions against a background of low signal (Figure 16-49).

Castleman's disease

Castleman's disease[72] (giant lymph node hyperplasia, angiofollicular lymph node hyperplasia, angiomatous lymphoid hamartoma) is a variety of lymph node hyperplasia of particular interest to chest radiologists because the usual hyaline vascular type is seen most frequently as an asymptomatic mass of mediastinal lymph nodes. (The lymph node mass, however, may press on mediastinal structures, causing pressure symptoms.) The less frequent plasma cell variety is associated with fever, fatigue, anemia, gamma globulin abnormalities, and elevated lactic dehydrogenase.[265]

Castleman's disease may occur at any age but frequently strikes young adults. Its etiology is uncertain, but it may be a chronic inflammatory response to as yet undefined antigens. It may be multifocal and can involve extrathoracic lymph nodes. Recently a multicentric form having a high association with Kaposi's sarcoma of the skin has been reported.[78,156] AIDS may be the underlying factor in these cases. On histologic study the hyaline form shows a follicular structure. The follicles consist predominantly of small lymphocytes with large numbers of blood vessels in the interfollicular areas. The plasma cell type shows sheets of interfollicular cells and fewer blood vessels.[265] Castleman's disease can be confused histologically with malignant lymphoma or with thymoma. Surgical excision is curative if the lesion is completely removed.[364] Vascular neoplasms have been reported to arise within lymph nodes affected by Castleman's disease.[167]

Radiologic examination[256,364] shows lobulated, well-defined, large or sometimes huge masses of lymph nodes in the mediastinum or proximal hilum (Figure 16-50). The enlarged lymph nodes may calcify[390]; this is a helpful feature in differential diagnosis. The lymph node masses may extend into the neck or retroperitoneum and are very vascular at angiography.[364,435,516]

CT* shows unilateral or bilateral masses of soft tissue density with striking uniform contrast enhancement. This feature helps in the differential diagnosis from cyst or lymphoma (Figure 16-50). CT also demonstrates any calcification to advantage (Figure 16-50).[76] MRI shows essentially the same features (Figures 16-50 and 16-51), including contrast enhancement.[234]

---

*References 2, 147, 168, 328, 367, 435.

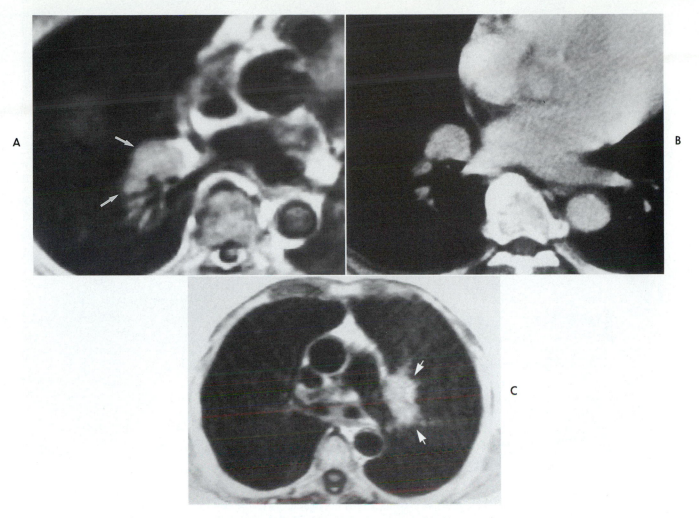

FIGURE 16-49
A, Magnetic resonance imaging (MRI) of hilar node enlargement. High signal from solid tissues *(arrows)* stands out clearly against the signal void of air in the bronchi and lungs, and signal void of flowing blood in the left atrium and hilar blood vessels. **B,** Contrast-enhanced computed tomography scan of same patient for comparison. **C,** MRI showing left hilar adenopathy *(arrows)* in another patient. (**C** courtesy Dr. Cynthia Janus, New York.)

Angioimmunoblastic lymphadenopathy

Angioimmunoblastic lymphadenopathy (immunoblastic lymphadenopathy) is another variety of lymph node hyperplasia that may be confused histologically with lymphoma.[303] It is a systemic disorder with a high mortality seen chiefly in individuals over 50 years of age and is characterized by fever, weight loss, and generalized lymph node enlargement, hepatosplenomegaly, a maculopapular rash, hypergammaglobulinemia, and a Coombs' positive hemolytic anemia.[402] It sometimes appears to be related to drug ingestion. Histologic examination reveals a combination of chronic inflammatory cellular infiltrate, hyperplasia of small blood vessels, and deposits of amorphous interstitial debris. The classification and nature of angioimmunoblastic lymphadenopathy are debated[402]; it may be caused by chronic antigenic stimulation inducing nonneoplastic proliferation of B lymphocytes. Immunoblastic sarcoma or immunoblastic lymphoma develops in approximately one third of cases.[303,357]

Paratracheal, anterior mediastinal, or hilar lymph node enlargement is the most common radiologic manifestation (Figure 16-52).[301,303] Widespread parenchymal infiltrates are infrequent, and a reticulonodular pattern with septal lines may be seen.[572] Pulmonary nodules are also encountered, and pleural effusions are not uncommon.

Pitfalls in the diagnosis of intrathoracic lymph node enlargement

A variety of anatomic structures can be confused with mediastinal lymph node enlargement.[59,175,401] Some of these are illustrated in Figures 16-53 through 16-58.

Text continued on p. 762.

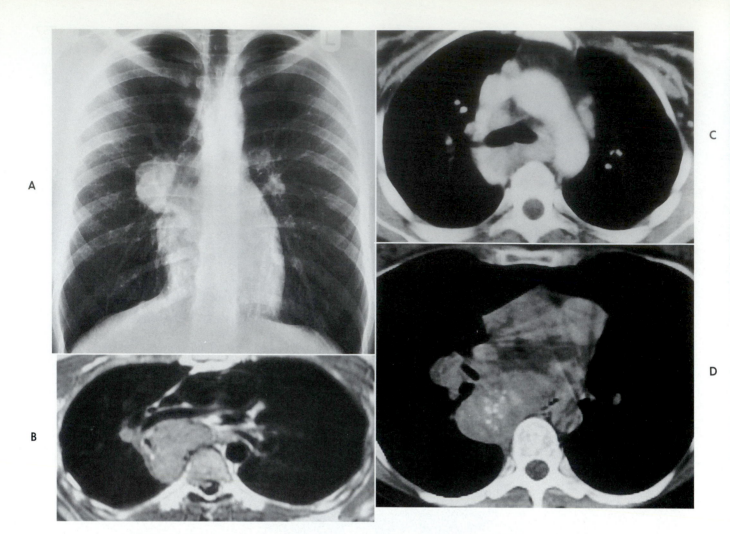

FIGURE 16-50
Castleman's disease. Four different patients. **A,** Massive right hilar enlargement visible on plain chest radiograph. **B,** Contrast enhancement of enlarged mediastinal nodes at computed tomography (CT). **C,** Flecks of calcification on precontrast CT scan. **D,** T1-weighted magnetic resonance image shows subcarinal lymph node enlargement. (**C** courtesy Dr. M.J. Charig, Oxford, U.K. From Charig MJ: *Clin Radiol* 42:440-442, 1990. **D** courtesy Dr. Frank Raila, Jackson, Miss.)

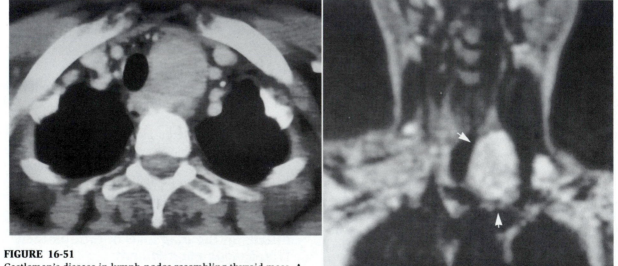

FIGURE 16-51
Castleman's disease in lymph nodes resembling thyroid mass. **A,** Computed tomography scan shows a mass that enhances with contrast medium and displaces the trachea and adjacent blood vessels similar to a thyroid mass. **B,** Magnetic resonance image shows high signal within the mass *(arrows)* on T2-weighted image.

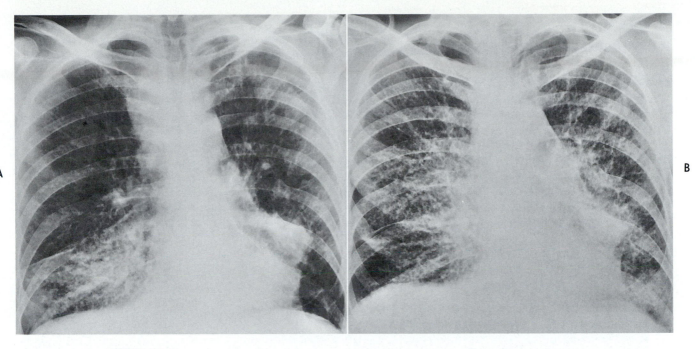

A B

FIGURE 16-52
Angioimmunoblastic lymphadenopathy in a 42-year-old man with generalized lymphadenopathy and hepatosplenomegaly. **A,** Obvious enlargement of right and left paratracheal lymph nodes as well as paracardiac nodes. Parenchymal reticulonodular shadowing is chiefly confined to the right base. **B,** Six months later, after an initial dramatic response to steroid therapy, the reticulonodular shadowing is seen in all lung zones. (Courtesy Dr. Keith Simpkins, Leeds, U.K.)

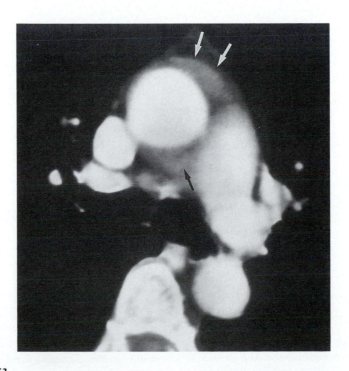

FIGURE 16-53
Superior pericardial recesses anterior *(white arrows)* and posterior *(black arrow)* to the proximal descending aorta mimicking lymphadenopathy. Contrast-enhanced computed tomography scan.

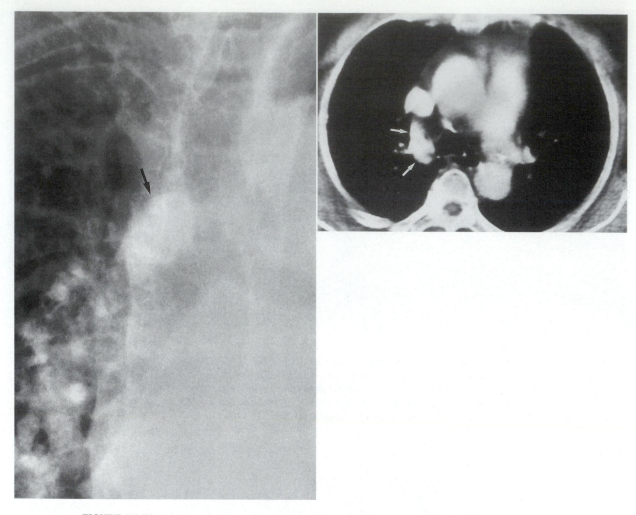

FIGURE 16-54
Azygos vein in right tracheobronchial angle *(arrow)* is difficult to distinguish from enlarged azygos node. Computed tomography proved that the opacity was a large azygos vein.

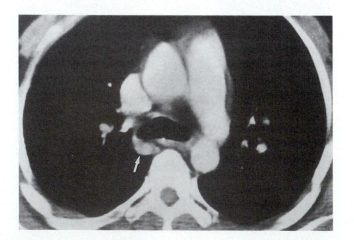

FIGURE 16-55
Azygos vein lying posterior to the right mainstem bronchus *(arrow)*, mimicking lymphadenopathy on computed tomography scan. Note that despite good contrast enhancement of aorta, pulmonary artery, and superior vena cava, the azygos vein is poorly opacified.

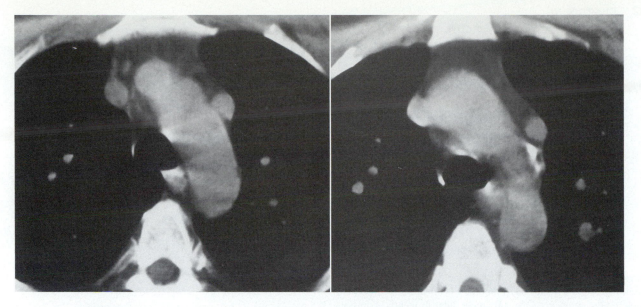

FIGURE 16-56
Persistent left superior vena cava mimicking anterior mediastinal and aortopulmonary lymph node enlargement. Confusion is avoided once the tubular nature of the density is appreciated. The vein could be traced from the left brachiocephalic vein to the upper posterior margin of the left atrium. Non-contrast-enhanced images are illustrated, since confusion with lymphadenopathy is greatest before administration of contrast material.

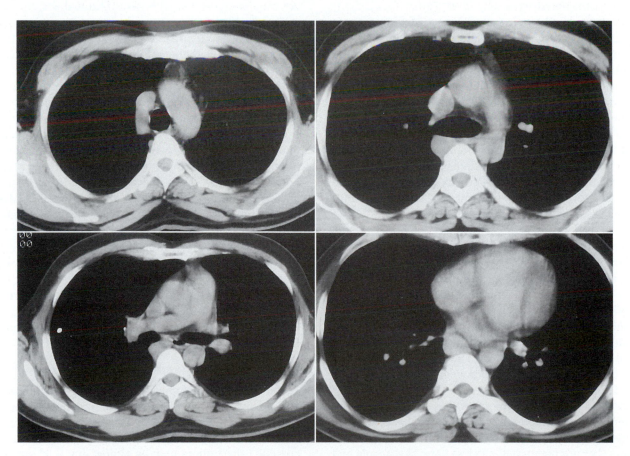

FIGURE 16-57
Azygos continuation of inferior vena cava (poorly contrast enhanced). The appearances on each image viewed separately could be confused with a mass or lymphadenopathy. Taken together, the tubular nature and conformity to the anatomy of the azygos vein establish the diagnosis.

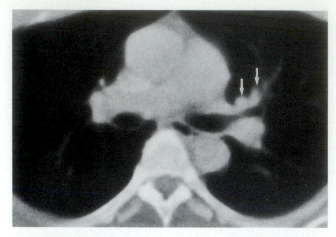

FIGURE 16-58
Tributaries of the left superior pulmonary vein *(arrows)* mimicking lymph nodes anterior to the left upper lobe bronchus. Contrast-enhanced computed tomography scan.

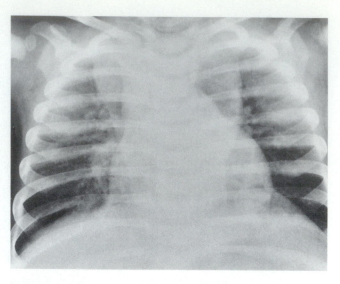

FIGURE 16-59
Plexiform neurofibroma in a young child with neurofibromatosis, producing extensive middle and posterior mediastinal widening.

NEURAL TUMORS

Neural tumors can be divided into nerve sheath tumors and ganglion cell tumors. (Tumors of the paraganglionic cells are considered separately on p. 768.)

The nerve sheath tumors comprise schwannomas (neurilemmoma), neurofibromas, and their malignant counterparts. The schwannoma is by far the most common intrathoracic nerve sheath tumor.[64,412] All of these tumors are more common in patients with neurofibromatosis. Although histologically distinct, both schwannomas and neurofibromas are derived from Schwann cells. In its classic form the schwannoma is eccentric and encapsulated and has no nerve fibers passing through it, whereas the neurofibroma is unencapsulated and has nerve fibers scattered through the tumor. Patients with neurofibromatosis may develop large plexiform masses of neurofibromatous tissue in the mediastinum (Figure 16-59).[64,75,191] Granular cell myoblastomas have been reported in the mediastinum; these tumors are believed to be of Schwann cell origin.[7]

Almost all intrathoracic nerve sheath tumors arise from either the intercostal or the sympathetic nerves, the rare exceptions being neurofibromas or schwannomas of the phrenic or vagus nerves.[358] Many arise close to the spine and may extend through the neural exit foramina into the spinal canal (dumbbell tumor). Though dumbbell tumors are a much talked about phenomenon, they occur in less than 5% of cases.[160,556]

Most nerve sheath tumors of the mediastinum are benign and asymptomatic and are usually discovered incidentally on chest imaging. In contrast to ganglion cell tumors they are rare in patients less than 20 years old and virtually nonexistent in patients less than 10 years old. The few cases encountered in children are likely to be associated with neurofibromatosis. Malignant nerve sheath tumors are infrequent. They may cause pain and are usually associated with neurofibromatosis.

The ganglion cell tumors form a spectrum: neuroblastomas are at the malignant end and ganglioneuromas at the benign end; ganglioneuroblastoma is an intermediate form. Neuroblastoma and ganglioneuroblastoma may occasionally mature into a more benign form.[9,120] The mediastinum is the second most common primary site for this spectrum of tumors, the adrenal gland being the most common. Approximately one third to one half of mediastinal neuroblastomas arise primarily in the mediastinum.[27,126] The remainder are secondary either to lymph node metastases or to thoracic spread from a tumor arising primarily in the adrenal gland. Primary mediastinal neuroblastomas appear to have a better prognosis than those that arise primarily in the abdomen.[126,145]

Neuroblastoma and ganglioneuroblastoma are essentially tumors of childhood[385]; less than 10% are seen in patients older than 20 years of age.[143,412] In children younger than 1 year of age a neural tumor is virtually certain to be one of these two types. Ganglioneuroma shows a wider and more even age distribution, ranging from 1 to 50 years.[412]

Imaging of neurogenic tumors

The cardinal imaging feature of neurogenic tumors is a well-defined mass with a smooth or lobulated outline (Figures 16-60 and 16-61).[24,143,412] When the tumors are localized, distinguishing benign from malignant is not possible. The tumors may be almost any size; some are very large, occupying most of a hemithorax. Except for vagal and phrenic nerve tumors and the occasional neuroblastoma, neural tumors are situated in the poste-

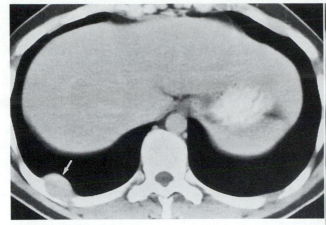

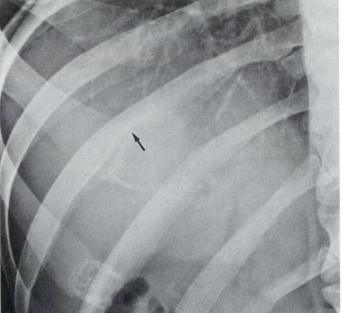

FIGURE 16-60
A, Contrast-enhanced computed tomography scan shows a schwannoma *(arrow)* arising from the intercostal nerve. B, Plain radiographs of ribs showing smooth, corticated pressure erosion of adjacent rib *(arrow)*.

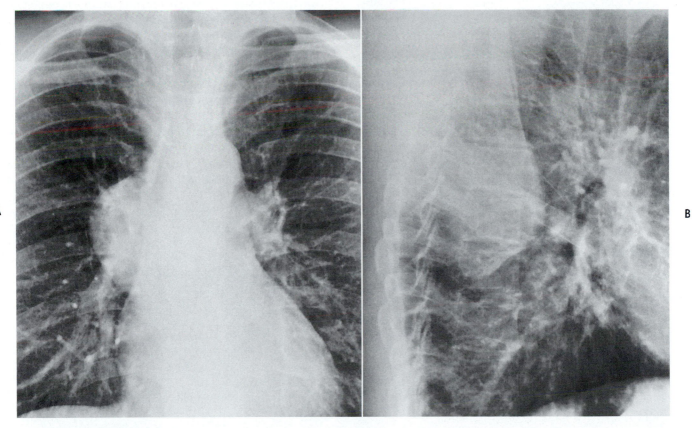

FIGURE 16-61
Schwannoma arising in posterior mediastinum of an asymptomatic young man. A, Posteroanterior radiograph. B, Lateral radiograph.

rior mediastinum. Those that arise adjacent to the upper thoracic spine and occupy the lung apex press down on the lung from above (Figure 16-62).

Most neurogenic tumors are approximately spherical,

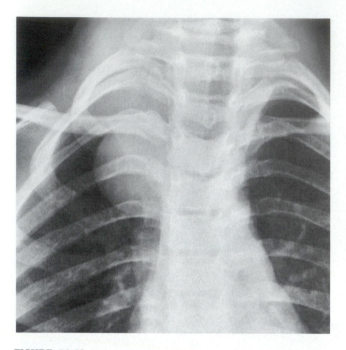

FIGURE 16-62
Ganglioneuroma arising from upper sympathetic chain in an older child. Note the smooth, lobulated outline and deformity of the adjacent ribs. The second interspace is widened, and the first interspace is correspondingly narrow. Adjacent ribs show pressure resorption but retain a corticated margin.

but some ganglion cell tumors are elongated, the axis following the vertical orientation of the sympathetic chain. It may be possible to distinguish between a ganglion cell tumor and a nerve sheath tumor by observing the shape and position of the tumor mass. Ganglion cell tumors may show a tapered interface with the adjacent chest wall or mediastinum, whereas nerve sheath tumors tend to show a sulcus at their margins. Ganglion cell tumors arise slightly more anteriorly with their epicenter against the vertebral body, whereas nerve sheath tumors are centered on the exit foramina or are plastered against the posterior chest wall.[498]

Calcification may be seen in all types of neural tumors (Figures 16-63 and 16-64). Approximately 10% of primary mediastinal neuroblastomas are visibly calcified on plain chest radiograph,[126,412] a figure considerably lower than that encountered with neuroblastoma arising in the adrenal gland. The incidence of calcification detectable at CT is substantially higher. In neuroblastoma the calcification is usually finely stippled. In ganglioneuroblastoma and ganglioneuroma it is denser and coarser, occurring most frequently in the larger, more benign lesions. Nerve sheath tumors calcify only occasionally. In one series of 65 cases examined by plain chest radiography,[412] only two cases with visible calcification were encountered; both were neurofibromas. In another series[64] calcification was seen seven times in 67 cases; all seven were schwannomas. In both series the calcification was curvilinear and lay in the walls of the larger masses, but it can be more widely distributed.[64]

Important diagnostic features of neurogenic tumors are pressure deformity and displacement of the adjacent ribs and vertebrae (Figures 16-60, 16-62, 16-65, and 16-66). The bone immediately adjacent to the tumor shows a scalloped edge; usually the bony cortex is preserved, and frequently it is thickened. The ribs may be thinned and

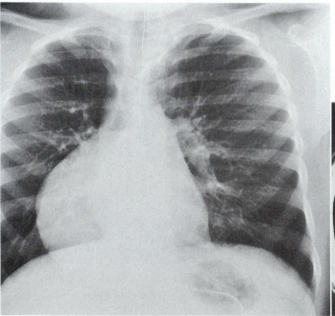

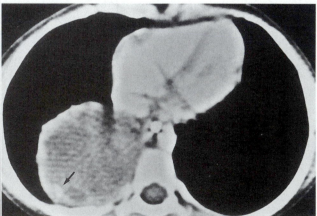

FIGURE 16-63
Ganglioneuroblastoma in a 7-year-old child. The mass is rounded and well defined. A small area of calcification *(arrow)* is noted on the computed tomography scan.

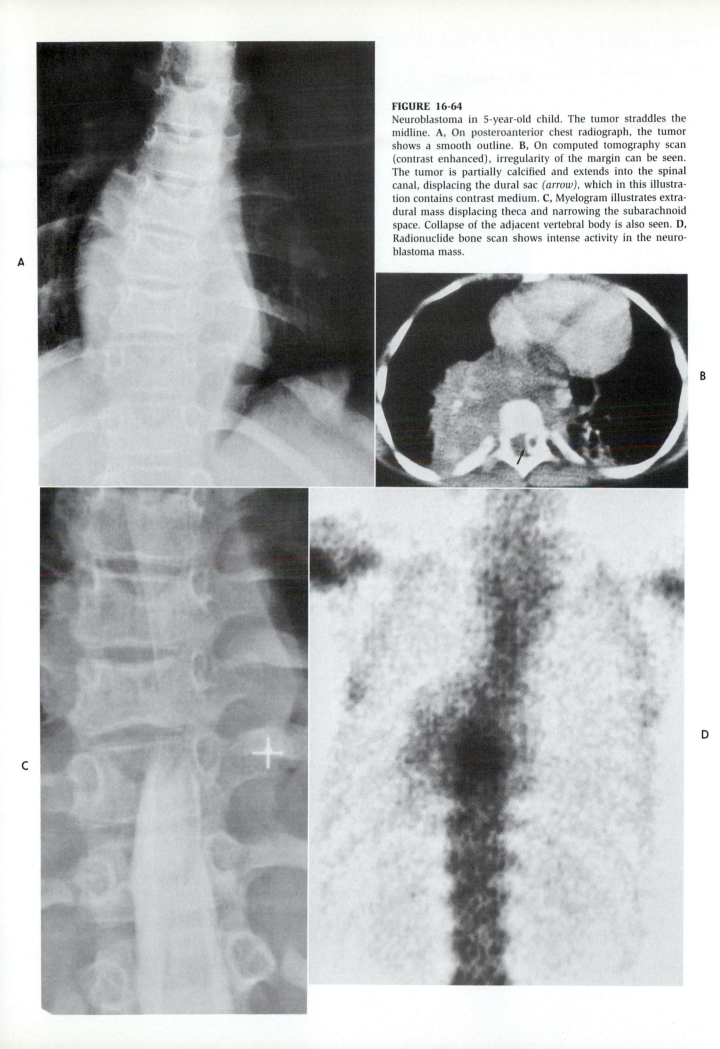

FIGURE 16-64
Neuroblastoma in 5-year-old child. The tumor straddles the midline. **A**, On posteroanterior chest radiograph, the tumor shows a smooth outline. **B**, On computed tomography scan (contrast enhanced), irregularity of the margin can be seen. The tumor is partially calcified and extends into the spinal canal, displacing the dural sac *(arrow)*, which in this illustration contains contrast medium. **C**, Myelogram illustrates extradural mass displacing theca and narrowing the subarachnoid space. Collapse of the adjacent vertebral body is also seen. **D**, Radionuclide bone scan shows intense activity in the neuroblastoma mass.

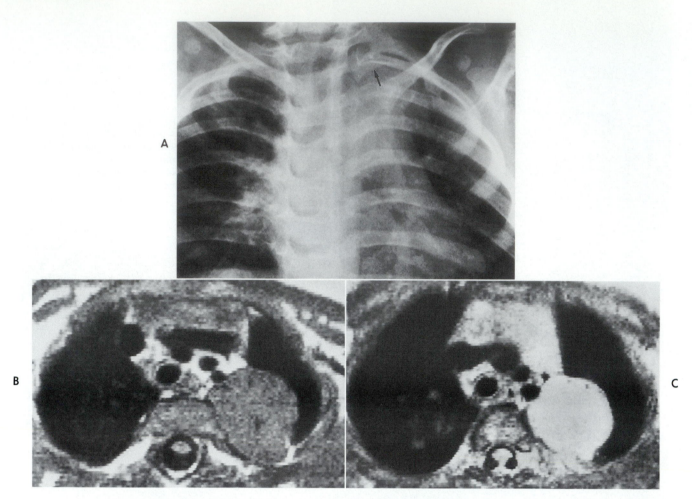

FIGURE 16-65
Neuroblastoma in a 2-year-old child. **A,** Posteroanterior radiograph shows the soft tissue mass plus splaying and deformity of the adjacent ribs *(arrow)*. **B,** T1-weighted and, **C,** T2-weighted magnetic resonance images show extent of mass between ribs but no evidence of extension into the spinal canal.

splayed apart, and the intervertebral foramina may appear widened. Bone changes are most frequently encountered with the neuroblastoma/ganglioneuroma range of tumors, perhaps because these particular tumors are frequently large when first diagnosed and the growing skeleton reacts relatively quickly. The large tumors may be associated with scoliosis.[64] Frank destruction of bone appears to be a sign of malignant invasion.[64,90,412]

At CT scanning many neural tumors have mixed density, including low-attenuation regions,[90,143] that are believed to represent hypocellularity and/or cystic degeneration (Figure 16-67).[88] Being vascular lesions they enhance on images taken after the administration of intravascular contrast medium (Figure 16-68).[561] One great advantage of CT is the superior demonstration of spinal and intraspinal involvement compared with plain films,[12,135,355] particularly if water-soluble contrast medium has previously been injected intrathecally. MRI

(Figures 16-65, 16-68, and 16-69) is even better than CT at demonstrating or excluding intraspinal involvement.[416] CT is superior to conventional radiography for detecting calcification,[12] whereas MRI is far inferior.

At MRI neurofibromas may show a so-called target pattern,[483] with a different signal in the central portion of the tumor compared with the peripheral zone.[60] On T1-weighted images the central portion is of higher signal. On T2-weighted spin-echo images the peripheral zone is of higher intensity than the center, corresponding to nerve tissue centrally and myxoid degeneration peripherally.[430] Schwannomas and ganglioneuromas apparently do not show this pattern on MRI; they show inhomogeneous high signal intensity throughout the lesion on T2-weighted images, and low to intermediate signal intensity on T1-weighted images. The high intensity on the T2-weighted images corresponds to cystic degeneration.[430] Ganglioneuromas may show a whorled appear-

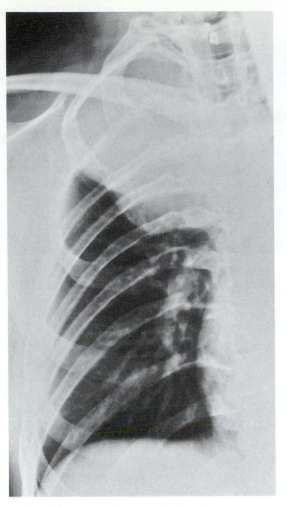

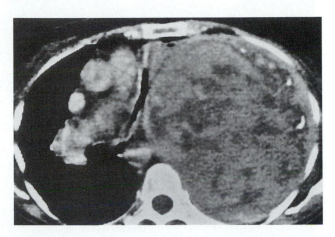

FIGURE 16-67
Malignant schwannoma. The huge mass shows both low-density areas corresponding to lipid elements in the tumor and high-density areas of calcification. Contrast-enhanced computed tomography scan.

FIGURE 16-66
Neurofibrosarcoma in young woman with neurofibromatosis. Note resemblance of the mass to a benign neurogenic tumor. The ribs are splayed and show corticated pressure erosion.

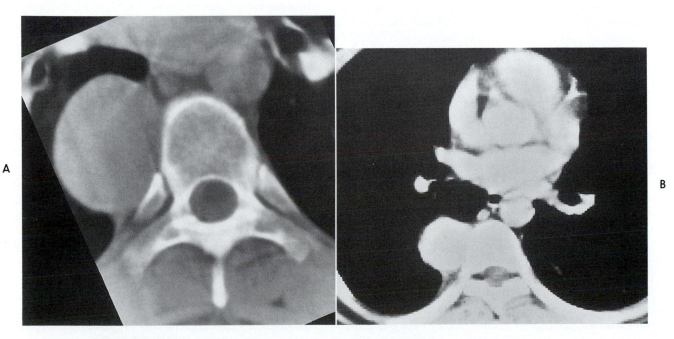

A

B

FIGURE 16-68
Benign schwannoma. A, Computed tomography (CT) scan before administration of contrast material. B, Following contrast material, CT scan shows intense enhancement of the tumor. Note that the schwannoma is as dense as the opacified left atrium.

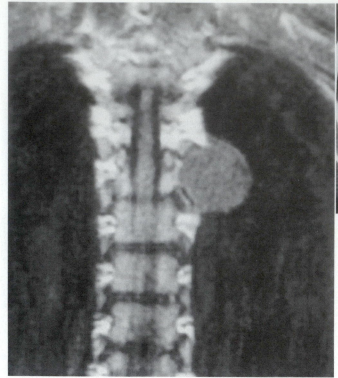

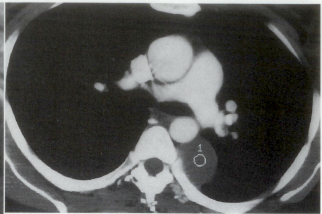

FIGURE 16-69

Schwannoma. A, Coronal T1-weighted magnetic resonance image excludes intraspinal extension. B, Contrast-enhanced computed tomography (CT) scan for comparison. CT density of the mass was between 30 and 40 HU.

ance, corresponding to whorls of collagenous fibrous tissue and neural tissue.

Mediastinal paragangliomas

Paragangliomas are tumors of the paraganglionic cells; they may be benign or malignant.[366,412,510] In the chest, paragangliomas may be chemodectomas or pheochromocytomas (functioning paragangliomas). Almost all the chemodectomas are aortic body tumors. Mediastinal paragangliomas are rare: they comprised only 2% of the large series of neural tumors of the thorax reported by Reed, Haller, and Feigin.[412] In a review of 51 cases of nonfunctioning paragangliomas, 39 were in the area of the aortic arch and therefore were classified as aortic body tumors; 12 were located near the sympathetic chain in the paravertebral area.[366] An aortic body tumor may be situated in one of four locations: lateral to the brachiocephalic artery, anterolateral to the aortic arch, at the angle of the ductus arteriosus, or above and to the right of the right pulmonary artery.[366] Multicentric cases are also reported.[203] In the review by Olson and Salyer,[366] 8 of 41 patients with aortic body tumors died either from metastasis or from local invasion.

Less than 2% of pheochromocytomas occur in the chest.[506] Most are found in the posterior mediastinum[327] in or adjacent to the heart and pericardium, particularly in the wall of the left atrium or the interatrial septum.[16,454,461] The left atrial lesions may indent the left atrium from the pericardial surface, rather than growing into the lumen of the heart.[454] Approximately one third of mediastinal pheochromocytomas are nonfunctioning and

asymptomatic; the remainder show symptoms, signs, and laboratory findings of overproduction of catecholamines.[327]

The various paragangliomas appear similar on plain chest radiography, CT, and angiography (Figure 16-70). They form rounded soft tissue masses that are usually extremely vascular and therefore enhance brightly at CT after administration of intravenous contrast material.[475] In one reported case of malignant paraganglioma the degree of contrast enhancement was minor.[41] Arteriography demonstrates enlarged feeding vessels, pathologic vessels within the tumor, and an intense tumor blush. Radioiodine metaiodobenzylguanidine (MIBG) and somatostatin receptor scintigraphy both show increased activity in paragangliomas and are good methods of identifying extraadrenal pheochromocytomas.[16,95,153,281,505]

At MRI (Figure 16-70), pheochromocytomas show signal intensity similar to muscle on T1-weighted images and very high signal intensity on T2-weighted images.[505] There are too few reports of MRI in other thoracic paragangliomas to be certain of the findings. In one reported case the signal intensity on T2-weighted images showed moderately high signal interspersed with low-intensity fibrous septa.[41] Paragangliomas in the head and neck[365] show numerous serpiginous vascular channels coursing through the stroma, which are isointense or slightly hyperintense compared with muscle on T2-weighted images and show substantially higher signal than muscle on T2-weighted images.

Lateral intrathoracic meningocele

Intrathoracic meningoceles are protrusions of the spinal meninges through the intervertebral foramina. They are usually detected in patients between 30 and 60 years of

FIGURE 16-70

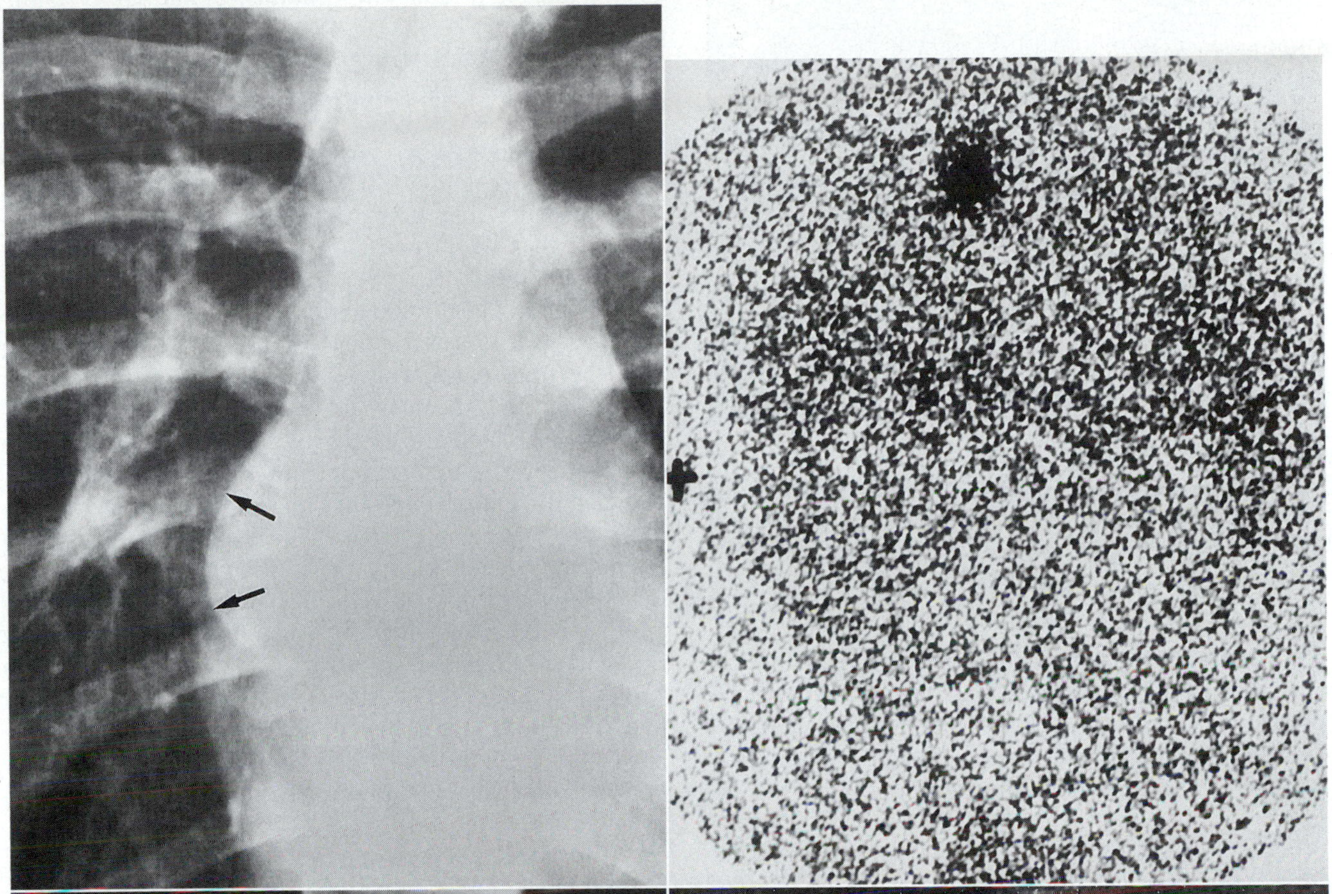

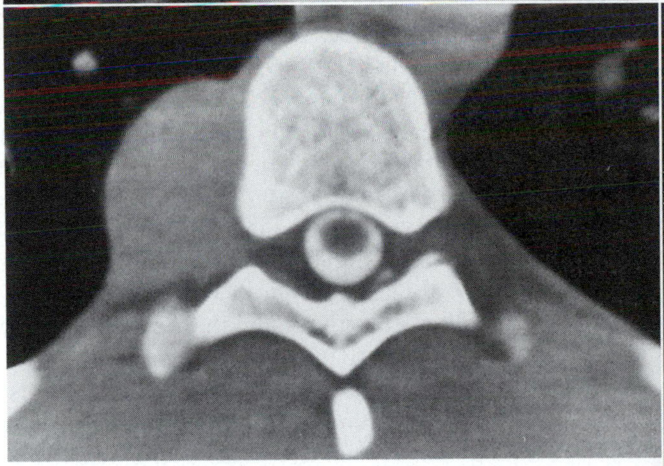

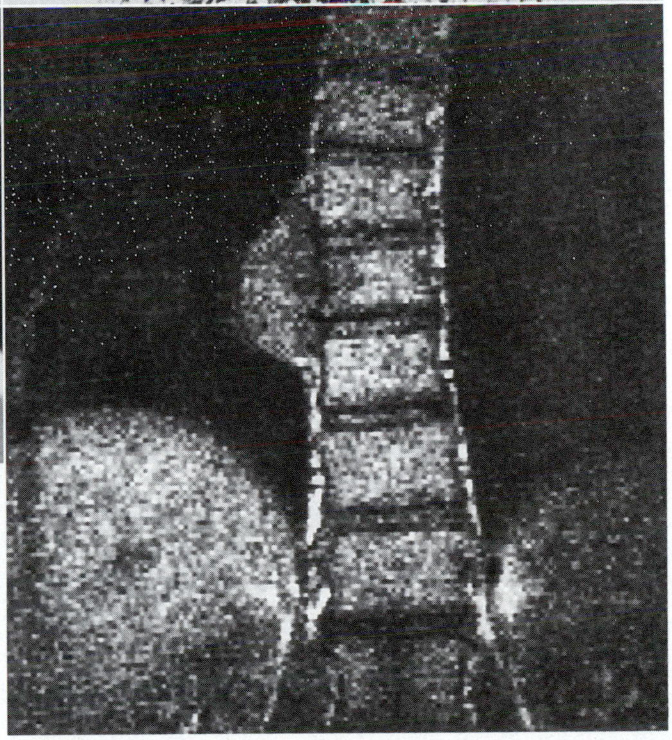

Mediastinal pheochromocytoma in an asymptomatic patient who was screened because of a strong family history of the condition and found to have high levels of urinary catecholamines. **A**, The mass *(arrows)*, which proved to be a solitary pheochromocytoma, was first discovered on plain film. **B**, MIBG scan shows increased activity in the mediastinal mass but no other site of tumor. **C**, Computed tomography scan (following myelography) shows posterior mediastinal mass centered on the sympathetic chain growing toward the adjacent neural exit foramen, but no displacement of the dural sac. **D**, T1-weighted magnetic resonance image shows an oval mass with a flat base against the thoracic spine and signal intensity similar to muscle.

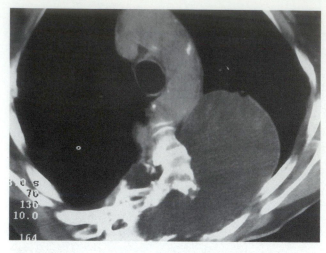

FIGURE 16-71
Lateral thoracic meningocele. Computed tomography scan showing a smoothly marginated mass of fluid density with a very thin wall arising from the spinal canal and widening the neural exit foramina.

age.[332] Most are asymptomatic, but occasionally they are associated with pain or neurologic abnormality.[332] Approximately two thirds of cases occur in association with neurofibromatosis.[332] On rare occasions, multiple or bilateral intrathoracic meningoceles are encountered.[43,123,464]

On plain chest radiograph[123] a well-defined paravertebral mass is seen, usually with scalloping and deformity of the adjacent ribs, pedicle, or vertebral body. Enlargement of the adjacent intervertebral foramen is an important diagnostic feature. Kyphoscoliosis is often present. These signs are identical to those seen with dumbbell nerve sheath tumors — a diagnostic problem complicated by the fact that both conditions are frequently associated with neurofibromatosis.

CT scanning[356,526] documents the features listed previously and also shows the expected low attenuation value of the mass because much of its bulk consists of cerebrospinal fluid (CSF) (Figure 16-71). If the examination is performed with intrathecal contrast medium, the contrast medium enters the meningocele, confirming the diagnosis. Similarly, uniform CSF signal is seen throughout the lesion on MRI.[356] Ultrasound can show the fluid content of appropriately situated lateral thoracic meningoceles. Before CT or MRI was available, the diagnosis was established by using conventional myelography.

MEDIASTINAL HEMORRHAGE

Trauma (penetrating or blunt) to the aorta or one of its major branches is a frequent cause of mediastinal hemorrhage. The usual spontaneous causes are dissecting hematoma, rupture of an aneurysm, and bleeding disorders or anticoagulant therapy. Other causes of spontaneous mediastinal hemorrhage are extremely unusual. They include chronic hemodialysis,[129] bleeding into preexist-

ing mediastinal tumors such as thymic masses and thyroid goiter,[1] radiation vasculitis,[2,36] and severe vomiting.[389,480]

Mediastinal hemorrhage can be asymptomatic or give rise to varying degrees of substernal chest pain, which often radiates to the back. Its investigation depends on the probable cause. When further tests are indicated, aortography, rather than CT or MRI, is frequently undertaken; although CT and MRI can confirm or exclude hemorrhage, they might not show the underlying cause with sufficient detail.

On plain chest radiography, mediastinal hemorrhage causes widening of the mediastinal shadow and widening of the right paratracheal stripe (Figure 16-72).[552] The widening may be focal or general, depending on how freely the blood tracks through the mediastinum. The blood may also track extrapleurally over the lung apices, giving rise to the important sign of apical capping (Figure 16-72).[468] When the hemorrhage is severe, it may rupture into the pleural cavity or track into the lung along perivascular and peribronchial sheaths, giving rise to pulmonary shadowing that may resemble pulmonary edema.[374] Generalized widening is often difficult to diagnose unless comparison can be made with previous examinations; focal hematoma around a bleeding site causes a homogeneous mass that is far easier to recognize. Rapid widening on serial films is a useful clue to the diagnosis.

The appearance of mediastinal hemorrhage on CT scanning may be fairly characteristic (Figure 16-73). Streaky soft tissue densities are often seen interspersed through the mediastinal fat. On occasion, high density associated with fresh thrombus can be seen; precontrast CT images are needed to recognize this high density. A focal hematoma, however, may be difficult to distinguish from a solid mediastinal mass on CT findings alone (Figure 16-73), but usually the clinical situation is sufficiently different to prevent confusion.

The appearance of hemorrhage on MRI varies primarily with the age of the hemorrhage and the degree of T1 and T2 weighting. Relatively specific patterns have been described for hematomas in the brain[186] and soft tissues[490]; whether the patterns for mediastinal hematoma and infiltrating hemorrhage will be as specific remains to be seen. The hyperacute phase shows low signal on T1-weighted and high signal on T2-weighted images. Over the ensuing days the signal on the T1-weighted images rises, and during the subacute phase, high signal may be seen on both T1- and T2-weighted images. Thereafter complex signal patterns are seen in which the signal depends on the amount of water in the area of hemorrhage and the degree of conversion from methemoglobin to ferritin and hemosiderin.[48]

PNEUMOMEDIASTINUM

The presence of a pneumomediastinum indicates perforation of some portion of either the respiratory or

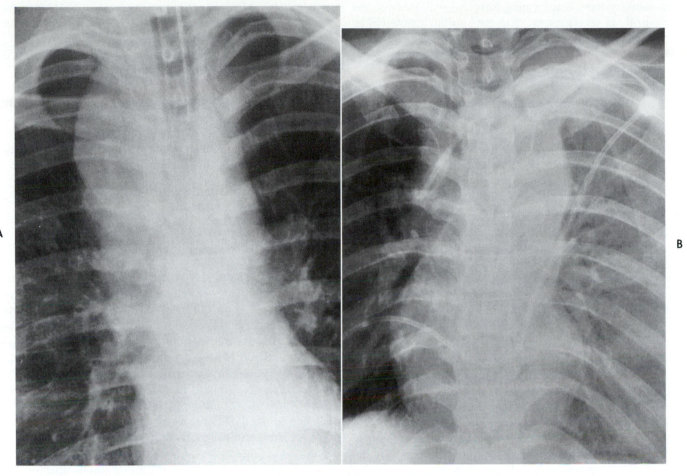

FIGURE 16-72
Two examples of mediastinal hemorrhage following inadvertent arterial puncture during placement of an intravenous line. **A,** Right paratracheal hemorrhage. **B,** Left superior mediastinal hemorrhage tracking extrapleurally over left lung apex.

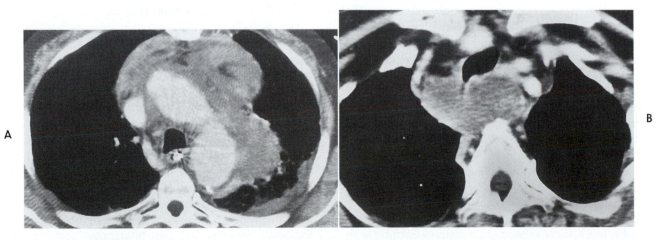

FIGURE 16-73
Mediastinal hemorrhage on computed tomography (CT). **A,** In a case of aortic dissection, showing blood with islands of mediastinal fat. **B,** Following spinal fracture. Note that from this image alone it would not be possible to distinguish a hematoma from a solid mediastinal mass. Contrast-enhanced CT scan.

alimentary tract. Gas-forming infection may increase the quantity of gas present. The perforation need not be within the mediastinum; indeed, it often lies beyond the confines of the mediastinum itself. The causes[195] are categorized as follows:

1. Alveolar rupture
   a. Spontaneous
   b. In patients receiving mechanical ventilation
   c. Following compressive trauma to thorax
   d. Following rupture of lung by rib fracture with tracking of air into mediastinum by way of chest wall and neck.
2. Traumatic laceration of trachea or central bronchus
3. Perforation of esophagus
   a. Spontaneous
   b. Following instrumentation
4. Perforation of pharynx,[437,502] duodenum,[476] colon, or rectum,[32] with tracking of air into mediastinum

Alveolar rupture

In spontaneous alveolar rupture the patients are usually healthy young men or women with a history of an attack of asthma or a bout of severe coughing, vomiting, or some other cause of sudden rise of intrathoracic pressure.[351] Other reported associations[100,195,351] include strenuous exercise, marijuana smoking, nitrous oxide inhalation,[307] pneumonia, diabetic ketoacidosis,[169,428] diffuse interstitial pulmonary fibrosis,[157] and childbirth. The air leak from alveolar rupture tracks through the interstitial tissues of the lung to accumulate in the mediastinum,[316] but the interstitial air is visible only if the adjacent lung is opaque, as in hyaline membrane disease or adult respiratory distress syndrome. Associated rupture of air into the pleural space to produce pneumothorax may occur.

The patient may complain of chest pain aggravated by deep breathing and dyspnea. Fever and leukocytosis without apparent infection are frequently encountered[351] and may cause confusion with acute mediastinitis. If the air has tracked into the neck, crepitus may be palpable in the supraclavicular areas. The equivalent of crepitus may be heard as a crackling sound through a stethoscope. Hammond's sign, a crunching sound synchronous with the heartbeat that may be heard in half of the patients, was at one time thought to be diagnostic of pneumomediastinum, but a similar clicking sound is heard with small pneumothoraces.[195] Spontaneous pneumomediastinum resulting from alveolar rupture, although it may cause symptoms and signs, does not in itself affect patient outcome and therefore is not treated.[169,195]

Alveolar rupture is common in patients who are receiving mechanical ventilation, particularly those with small airway obstruction or noncompliant lungs.[421] This combination is frequent in patients in intensive care units, particularly neonates. Hyaline membrane disease, meconium aspiration, and neonatal pneumonia are among the many neonatal pulmonary disorders that require mechanical ventilation and produce stiff lungs. In adults the pneumomediastinum itself rarely affects the outcome of the disease and does not require treatment, although reduction of ventilatory pressure to the minimum needed is advisable.

Air in the chest wall following rib fracture or placement of a chest tube may track into the mediastinum, usually by way of the neck. This is a particularly common occurrence in patients receiving mechanical ventilation. Usually chest wall emphysema is severe and the cause of the pneumomediastinum is obvious.

Radiographic findings in pneumomediastinum

Air in the mediastinum is seen on plain chest radiograph as streaks, bubbles, or larger collections of air outlining the mediastinal blood vessels, major airways, or esophagus (Figure 16-74).[100,419] The dissection of air along tissue planes may be more obvious in the lateral projection than on the frontal view. The air may dissect under the parietal layer of the mediastinal pleura so that a line shadow representing the combined parietal and visceral pleura is seen separate from the heart and great vessels. The amount of air is usually greatest anteriorly. When air is limited in quantity, the only sign of pneumomediastinum on plain chest radiography may be a line or band of transradiancy in the retrosternal area.

An important plain film sign of pneumomediastinum is air dissecting under and medial to the thymus. The outlining of the thymus by air is quite specific for pneumomediastinum and may be the most striking sign of the condition (Figure 16-74). Air may also track extrapleurally along the upper surface of the diaphragm. Air between the heart and diaphragm gives rise to the continuous diaphragm sign,[295] so-called because air beneath the heart may form a visible line of transradiancy that permits the diaphragm to be seen even within the confines of the mediastinum (Fig. 16-75).

Occasionally, distinguishing pneumomediastinum from pneumothorax or pneumopericardium on plain chest radiograph may be difficult (Figure 16-75). The distinction depends on the anatomic extent of the air.[100] Pneumothorax is rarely confined to the mediastinal border but can usually be traced out over the lung apex to the lateral portion of the thoracic cavity. A lateral decubitus view confirms the pleural location, although it is rarely needed. Pneumopericardium may extend from the diaphragm to just below the aortic knob but does not extend around the aortic knob or into the superior mediastinum. Pneumopericardium can mimic the continuous diaphragm sign and can lift the thymus away from the great vessels, but the bilaterality and anatomic conformity to the pericardium are usually evident.

A thin line of apparent radiolucency is frequently seen against the heart borders and aortic knob in healthy individuals because of the Mach band phenomenon. The Mach band may have the same degree of radiolucency as

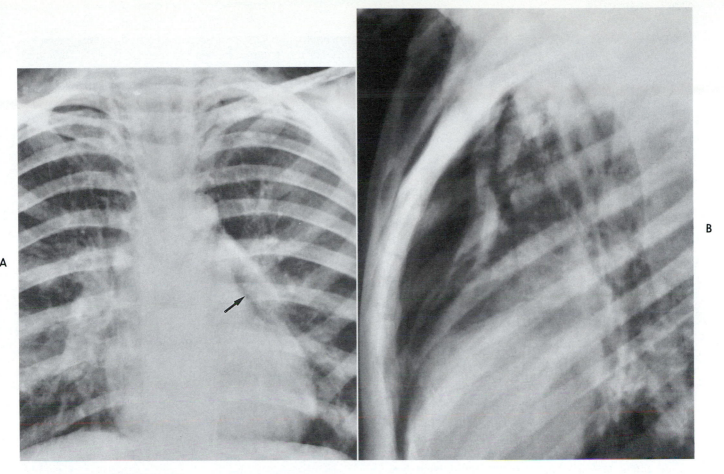

FIGURE 16-74
Pneumomediastinum in an asthmatic child showing air in mediastinal tissue planes. Note air deep to the thymus *(arrow)*. A, Posteroanterior radiograph. B, Lateral radiograph.

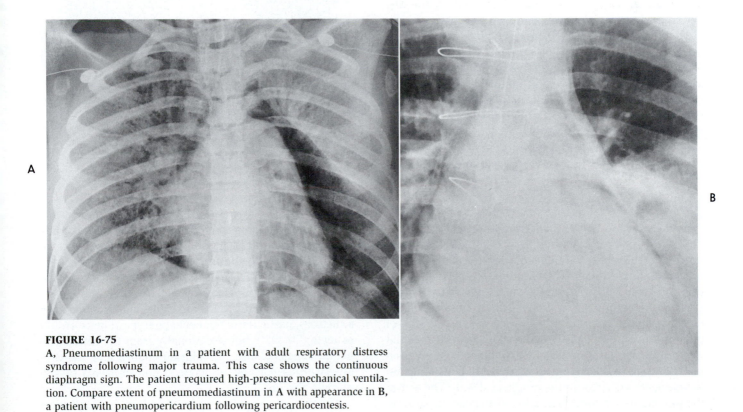

FIGURE 16-75
A, Pneumomediastinum in a patient with adult respiratory distress syndrome following major trauma. This case shows the continuous diaphragm sign. The patient required high-pressure mechanical ventilation. Compare extent of pneumomediastinum in A with appearance in B, a patient with pneumopericardium following pericardiocentesis.

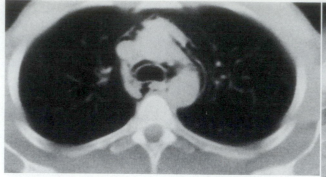

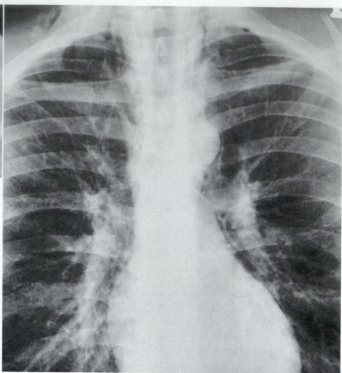

FIGURE 16-76
A, Computed tomography scan of pneumomediastinum in a young man following bout of marijuana inhalation with subsequent retching and coughing. B, Plain chest radiograph at same time for comparison.

a small pneumomediastinum. The distinction from pneumomediastinum[155] depends on analyzing both the anatomic extent and the border of the radiolucent line. A Mach band is adjacent to a normally visualized contour, and its lateral boundary is either unrecognizable or formed by a pulmonary blood vessel. The outer margin of a pneumomediastinum, on the other hand, is the displaced mediastinal pleura.

The diagnosis of mediastinal emphysema is made easily at CT (Figure 16-76) because the anatomic location of the air is self-evident on cross-sectional display. CT scanning is more sensitive and more specific than plain chest radiography and can be used to make the diagnosis in clinically suspected cases when the plain chest radiograph is normal or equivocal. Usually this is necessary only in patients with suspected rupture of the trachea or central bronchi or in cases of suspected esophageal perforation.

ACUTE MEDIASTINITIS

Acute infection of the mediastinum is relatively rare. The most common causes are esophageal perforation[61,383] or postoperative infection, for example, following median sternotomy.[247] Esophageal perforation is usually a result of penetrating trauma, particularly from surgery, endoscopy, or swallowing sharp objects such as chicken bones. In young children the possibility of pharyngeal or esophageal perforation as part of child abuse must be borne in mind.[5] Spontaneous perforation may occur, as in Boerhaave's syndrome, in which forceful vomiting causes a tear in the esophageal wall. The tear in the esophagus is almost invariably just above the gastroesophageal junction and may be of any depth. Usually it is

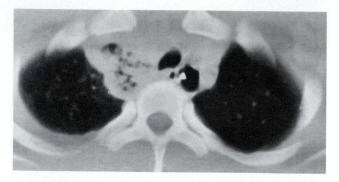

FIGURE 16-77
Acute mediastinitis from a peritonsillar abscess that had tracked into the mediastinum. The mediastinal infection required surgical drainage. CT scan shows mediastinal widening caused by fluid containing numerous air bubbles.

confined to the mucosa, in which case bleeding may occur, but there is no immediate danger of mediastinitis. If the tear is complete, air, alimentary juices, and food will leak into the mediastinum.

Other causes of acute mediastinal infection are leakage from the esophagus into the mediastinum through necrotic neoplasm and extension of infection from adjacent structures, particularly the neck, pharynx (Figure 16-77), or teeth,[297,339,472] but occasionally from the retroperitoneum, lungs, pleura, or adjacent bones and joints.[395] Mediastinitis may be associated with empyema or subphrenic abscess.

The patients are often very ill with chills, high fever, tachycardia, and chest pain. Circulatory shock is com-

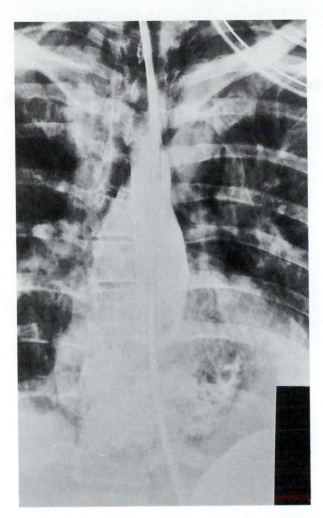

FIGURE 16-78
Acute mediastinitis resulting from spontaneous perforation of the esophagus during severe vomiting (Boerhaave's syndrome). This image, taken during esophagography, shows the pneumomediastinum and contrast material leaking into the mediastinum through a perforation of the left lower wall of esophagus.

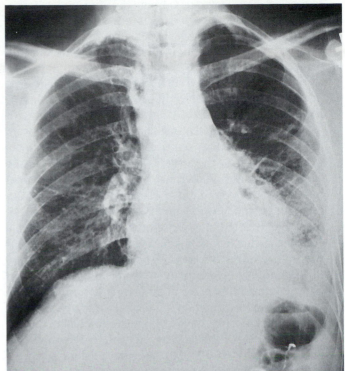

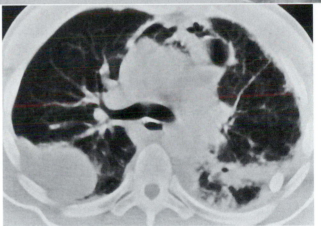

FIGURE 16-79
Acute mediastinitis following perforation of pharynx by a chicken bone. The patient, a 30-year-old man, had swallowed a chicken bone 3 weeks earlier. **A,** Plain chest radiograph shows features typical of pneumomediastinum: left lower lobe consolidation and left pleural effusion. **B,** Computed tomography scan following placement of a tube in the left side of the chest shows extensive air-fluid collection in the mediastinum and a right pleural empyema.

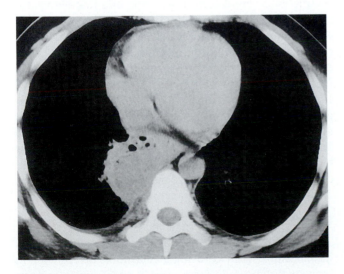

FIGURE 16-80
Acute mediastinitis with mediastinal abscess formation, following ingestion of a kebab skewer, shown by computed tomography scan.

mon.[247] Dysphagia may occur if the mediastinitis is caused by perforation of the esophagus.[383] Diffuse mediastinitis has a particularly high mortality.

The major radiologic features of acute mediastinitis are mediastinal widening, pneumomediastinum, obliteration of fat planes, localized fluid collections, and abscess formation (Figures 16-78 to 16-80). Accompanying pleural effusions in one or both pleural cavities are common.

In cases of Boerhaave's syndrome the effusion is particularly striking on the left and is often accompanied by consolidation of the left lower lobe.[419] All of these features are better demonstrated on CT scans than on plain radiographs.[50,67] CT may also show important associated abnormalities such as jugular vein thrombosis, pericardial effusion, or rupture of the hypopharynx or esophagus.

The widening of the mediastinum is the result of inflammatory swelling or abscess formation; therefore the size and shape of the widening are determined by the cause of the infection. Because so many acute mediastinal infections are secondary to esophageal perforation, an important clue to the diagnosis is air within the mediastinum, a feature that may be difficult to see on plain films. The air may be bubbly or streaky and may be localized or widespread in distribution. As with all types of pneumomediastinum, the air may extend into the neck or retroperitoneum. In cases of diffuse mediastinitis without discrete abscess formation, CT shows widespread infiltration of the mediastinum with obliteration of the normal fat planes. Gas bubbles may be scattered through the mediastinum (Figure 16-79). Where walled-off abscesses occur, the gas may be seen in more discrete rounded collections, together with air-fluid levels. Abscesses may be single but are frequently multiple. Discrete fluid collections within the mediastinum on CT may serve as an invaluable guide should percutaneous drainage be indicated.[50,180] MRI shows the expected signal intensity of fluid: low to intermediate intensity on T1-weighted images and high signal intensity on proton density and T2-weighted images, with a recognizable abscess wall in patients with discrete abscess.[202]

Barium swallow examination can be critical in determining the presence and precise location of esophageal perforation or underlying tumor.[419]

The radiologic evaluation of possible complications of median sternotomy is a separate subject.[50,187,258] When acute mediastinitis is suspected clinically following sternotomy, CT shows the extent of inflammation and any drainable mediastinal or pericardial fluid collections.[50,258] With chronically draining wounds the role of CT is uncertain. Distinguishing retrosternal hematomas from reactive granulation tissues or cellulitis is difficult, as is distinguishing osteomyelitis from the direct effects of the surgical incision. Minor degrees of sternal separation and step-off are common in asymptomatic uncomplicated operations.[187,258] Substernal fluid collections and dots of air are normal in the first 20 days following sternotomy, and therefore the anterior mediastinum may not appear normal until 2 months have passed. Similarly, air trapped in the presternal or retrosternal soft tissues, although it usually dissipates within a few weeks, may be visible for up to 50 days on plain chest radiographs. Therefore, before gas-forming infections can be diagnosed, the air collections must appear de novo or must progressively increase without other explanation.[68]

SUPERIOR VENA CAVAL OBSTRUCTION

The most common cause of superior vena caval obstruction is compression and invasion by bronchogenic carcinoma either because of primary tumor invasion into the mediastinum or because of lymph node metastases.[381] Other causes include mediastinal malignant neoplasms, notably metastatic breast and testicular neoplasm, and lymphoma; mediastinal fibrosis (see later discussion); and thrombosis, usually around a transvenous catheter.[381] In one large review 78% of cases were the result of malignant neoplasm (two thirds of which were lung carcinoma) and 22% were the result of benign causes.[381]

Clinically, the features of obstruction are edema and visible distension of the veins of the face, neck, arms, and anterior chest wall. Dyspnea, choking, dysphagia, and a feeling of congestion are common symptoms. Cerebral edema may occur. The severity of the symptoms and signs depends on the degree of venous collateral formation.[318] No symptoms may be seen at all even with total obstruction, particularly if the obstruction is slow in developing.

A variety of imaging techniques have been used to document superior vena caval syndrome. On occasion the dilated collaterals, particularly enlargement of the azygos vein or enlargement of the superior intercostal vein (aortic nipple) draining the hemiazygos system, are visible on plain film.[69] In cases of superior vena caval thrombosis around an indwelling catheter the superior mediastinum may be visibly widened on plain chest radiography.[51] The explanation for this widening is not clear, but the observation may allow the diagnosis of superior vena caval thrombosis before it is clinically suspected.[51] Venography shows the obstruction and demonstrates collateral pathways and intraluminal thrombus. In general, however, venography provides relatively little information about the cause of the obstruction. Radionuclide venography is a simple technique that can readily confirm or exclude superior vena caval obstruction,[91] but it contributes little information regarding the cause. CT with intravenous contrast material enhancement is an excellent all-purpose test that shows caval narrowing or filling defects in the superior vena cava and demonstrates the responsible pathologic process (Figures 16-81 and 16-82).[18,30,338] MRI (Figure 16-82) can show the same features[326,527] and has the advantages of sagittal and coronal imaging as well as the ability to distinguish rapidly flowing blood from both slowly flowing blood and thrombus.[326] A disadvantage of MRI is that it does not demonstrate calcification, which is an important feature in the diagnosis of granulomatous mediastinal fibrosis.

FIBROSING MEDIASTINITIS

The most common cause of fibrosing mediastinitis is histoplasmosis, but fibrosing mediastinitis is rare, even in individuals who come from areas in which histoplasmosis is endemic. Other causes of mediastinal fibrosis include

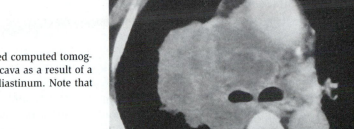

FIGURE 16-81
Superior vena cava syndrome. Contrast-enhanced computed tomography scan shows obstruction of superior vena cava as a result of a small cell carcinoma of lung involving the mediastinum. Note that the superior vena cava has been obliterated.

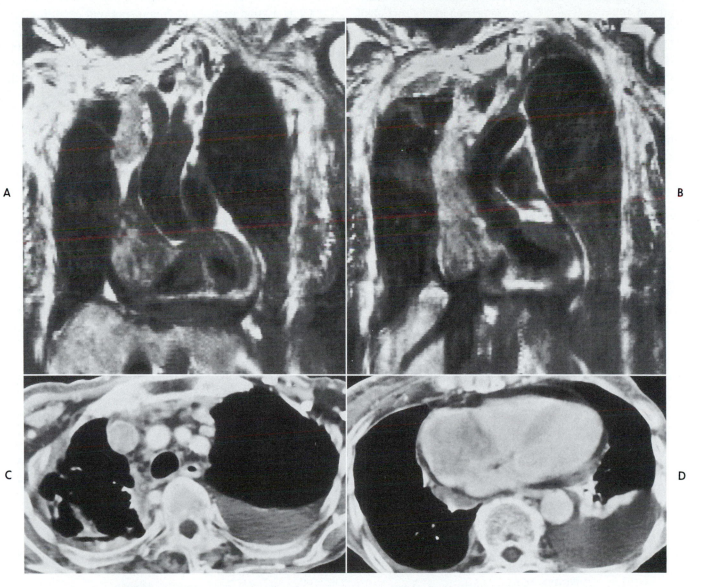

FIGURE 16-82
Superior vena cava syndrome. **A** and **B**, Magnetic resonance images of an intraluminal thyroid carcinoma growing in the superior vena cava and right atrium. **C** and **D**, Contrast-enhanced computed tomography scans at level of the right brachiocephalic vein and right atrium showing an intraluminal filling defect.

tuberculosis, syphilis,[226] and drug or radiation therapy. An idiopathic variety, which may be autoimmune in origin and is sometimes combined with retroperitoneal fibrosis, has also been described.[274,302]

When caused by histoplasmosis, dense fibrosis progressively encases and may eventually obliterate the lumen of the mediastinal vessels and airways. This fibrotic response may be a response to a focus of granulomatous adenitis or the result of an idiosyncratic tendency to develop excessive fibrosis in response to a fungal antigen escaping from adjacent lymph nodes.[189,308] The condition may be similar to the layers of fibrosis that form within an enlarging histoplasmoma of the lung.[188,189] The fact that histoplasma organisms are rarely identifiable is believed to be related to the inactivity of the infection at the time of nodal biopsy.

The signs and symptoms develop most often between 20 and 40 years of age[308] and are related to obstruction of the structures that traverse the mediastinum, most notably the superior vena cava. They include swelling of the face, distention of the veins in the neck, cough, pulmonary infection, wheezing, hemoptysis, dyspnea, and hoarse voice.*

The radiologic features† vary according to the site and bulk of the adenopathy and the severity of the obstructive phenomena. Plain films of the chest may be normal, but cases related to histoplasmosis almost always demonstrate enlargement or calcification of at least some of the mediastinal or hilar lymph nodes (Figure 16-83). The

adenopathy may be unilateral or bilateral. It is most often asymmetric and is usually maximal in the superior mediastinum. Narrowing of the lower trachea or major bronchi may be detectable, and if a pulmonary artery is severely obstructed, the resulting pulmonary oligemia may be identified, even on plain films. Pulmonary consolidation or atelectasis resulting from bronchial, venous, or lymphatic obstruction or pleuropulmonary scarring may be seen. Mediastinal venography (Figure 16-84) and pulmonary arteriography show smooth, tapered narrowing of the superior vena cava and brachiocephalic veins together with numerous dilated collateral veins, and may also show narrowing of the central pulmonary arteries (Figure 16-85).[308,545] Barium swallow examination may show narrowing of the esophagus and in rare instances may show varices, the so-called downhill varices, resulting from esophageal venous collaterals.

CT is a good method of diagnosing and assessing the site and severity of mediastinal fibrosis (Figures 16-83, 16-84, and 16-86).* CT shows the enlarged calcified nodes to advantage. Lymph node calcification is present in many of the patients in whom the process is the result of histoplasmosis. CT scanning also demonstrates airway narrowing, pulmonary or systemic vein compression, collateral venous pathways, arterial compression, and pulmonary shadows resulting from the central obstructive processes. The noncalcified fibrotic tissue may be difficult to identify; with the obliteration of fat planes, identifying normal vascular landmarks is difficult.

---

*References 111, 188, 189, 270, 308, 410, 442.
†References 82, 92, 111, 140, 270, 278, 544, 545.

*References 20, 278, 308, 415, 459, 528.

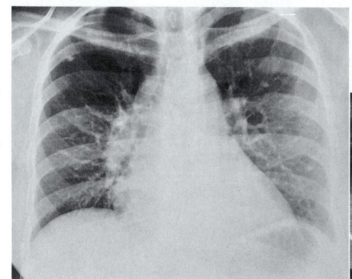

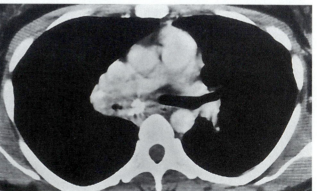

FIGURE 16-83
Mediastinal fibrosis resulting from histoplasmosis. **A,** Plain chest radiograph shows enlarged right hilar and paratracheal nodes as well as subcarinal lymph node enlargement. Note small calcified granulomas in the lungs. **B,** Contrast-enhanced computed tomography scan through the subcarinal region shows enlarged, partially calcified nodes and severe narrowing of the bronchus intermedius.

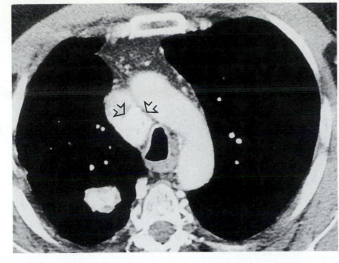

A

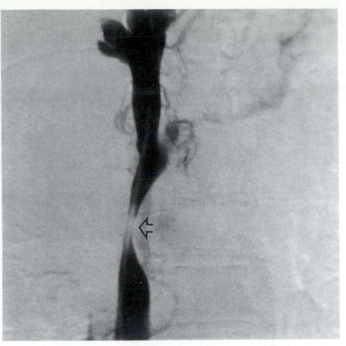

B

FIGURE 16-84
Superior vena cava *(SVC)* obstruction resulting from mediastinal fibrosis associated with calcified tuberculous adenopathy. **A,** Computed tomography scan showing enlarged calcified nodes *(arrows)* adjacent to the superior vena cava, which is not visible at this level. A calcified granuloma is seen lying posteriorly in right lung. **B,** Venogram showing narrowed superior vena cava at same level *(arrow)*.

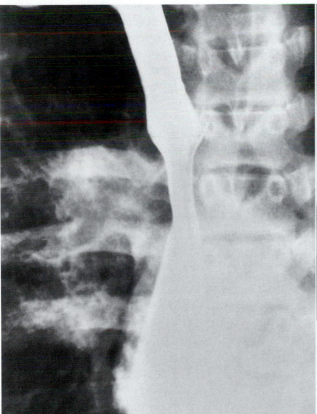

A

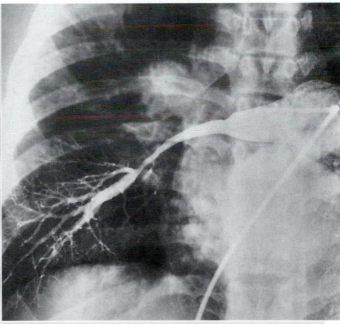

B

C

FIGURE 16-85
Mediastinal fibrosis resulting from histoplasmosis. **A,** Superior vena cavogram shows smooth focal narrowing. **B,** Pulmonary arteriogram shows long, smooth stricture through the right lower lobe artery and occlusion of the truncus anterior. **C,** ^{99m}Tc pulmonary perfusion radionuclide scan indicates substantial reduction in blood flow to the right lung.

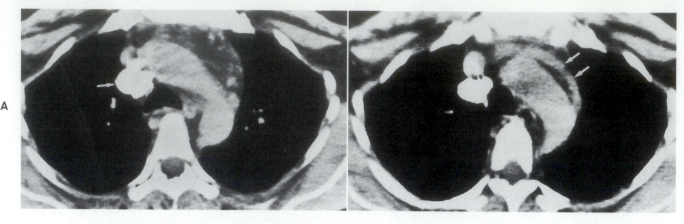

FIGURE 16-86
Mediastinal fibrosis resulting from histoplasmosis. **A,** Contrast-enhanced computed tomography scan shows enlarged calcified nodes *(arrow)* adjacent to the narrowed right brachiocephalic vein. **B,** Adjacent level shows collateral venous channels *(arrows)*. Note that the noncalcified fibrous tissue in the mediastinum is not visualized in these or other sections.

MRI[137,270,415,527] can demonstrate narrowing of the major vessels and bronchi as well as, if not better than, CT scanning and has an additional advantage of not requiring contrast media. A major disadvantage of MRI is that it cannot reliably show calcification. Consequently an important diagnostic sign of histoplasmosis or tuberculosis is not available. On T2-weighted spin-echo sequences, however, the adenopathy seen in fibrosing mediastinitis may be lower in signal intensity than is generally seen with malignancy, probably because of the presence of calcification.[415]

Radionuclide ventilation-perfusion scanning can be used to demonstrate the pulmonary arterial flow and to show which areas are underventilated.[344]

EXTRAMEDULLARY HEMOPOIESIS

Extramedullary hemopoiesis in potential blood-forming organs such as the liver, spleen, and lymph nodes is a common condition in various anemias, but only rarely does it cause masslike collections within the chest. Usually the anemia in question is one of the congenital hemolytic anemias, notably thalassemia and sickle cell disease, although the condition may be seen in other anemias and even in patients without anemia.[426] The masses themselves are usually asymptomatic, although paraplegia from cord compression may occur.[309,379]

On plain film[200,224,379,426] and CT,[200,322] focal masses are found in the paravertebral regions, usually in the lower chest (Figure 16-87). Further foci of extramedullary hemopoiesis may be seen as subpleural masses adjacent to ribs. These subpleural masses may be continuous or discontinuous with the paravertebral masses. The hemopoietic masses may be unilateral but are usually bilateral. They are smoothly marginated because they are covered by pleura, and are of homogeneous soft tissue or

slightly higher density. On CT the mass may have a large fatty component.[559] Calcification does not appear to be a feature. Sometimes the masses occur at multiple levels and involve the entire paravertebral area,[200] in which case the symmetric lobular arrangement conforming to the segmental divisions of the body produces a striking and characteristic appearance.[379] The intervening or adjacent bone may be normal or show marrow expansion. CT is particularly useful in demonstrating the lacelike marrow expansion in the adjacent bones (Figure 16-87).[200] A radionuclide bone marrow scan may demonstrate activity in the mass[200,479] but may be negative.[200,211]

The condition should be considered in the differential diagnosis of a paravertebral mass in a patient with severe chronic anemia, particularly if the mass is multifocal. Unlike neurogenic tumors, the major differential diagnosis, extramedullary hemopoiesis does not appear to cause pressure erosion of the adjacent spine or ribs.[426]

AORTIC ANEURYSMS
Atherosclerotic aortic aneurysms

Atherosclerotic aneurysms and generalized ectasia are extremely common aging or degenerative phenomena. Systemic hypertension is a clearly identified risk-factor for atherosclerotic aortic aneurysms. Degenerative aneurysms are often discovered on imaging studies when still asymptomatic. Chest pain and compression effects are the most common symptoms. A hoarse voice may occur because of pressure on the recurrent laryngeal nerve as it passes around and under the aortic arch. Compression of the left main or lower lobe bronchus may lead to atelectasis of the left lung (Figure 16-88), and compression of the esophagus may cause dysphagia with extrinsic deformity that is seen on barium swallow. Compression of the right and left pulmonary arteries has also been

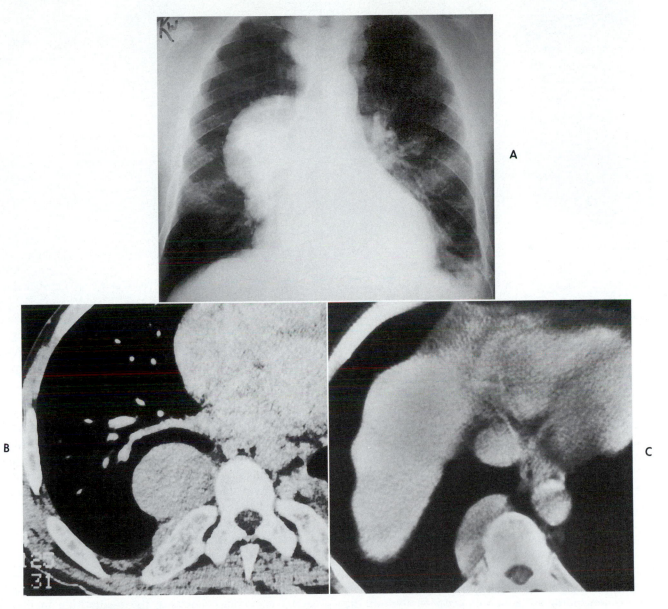

FIGURE 16-87
Extramedullary hemopoiesis. **A,** Chest radiograph in a patient with thalassemia. Note bilateral paravertebral masses. **B,** Computed tomography (CT) scan in the same patient shows mediastinal mass and bone changes of hemolytic anemia. **C,** Contrast-enhanced CT scan in another patient showing nonspecific paravertebral mass that proved to be extramedullary hemopoiesis. (**A** and **B** courtesy Dr. Philip Gishen, London.)

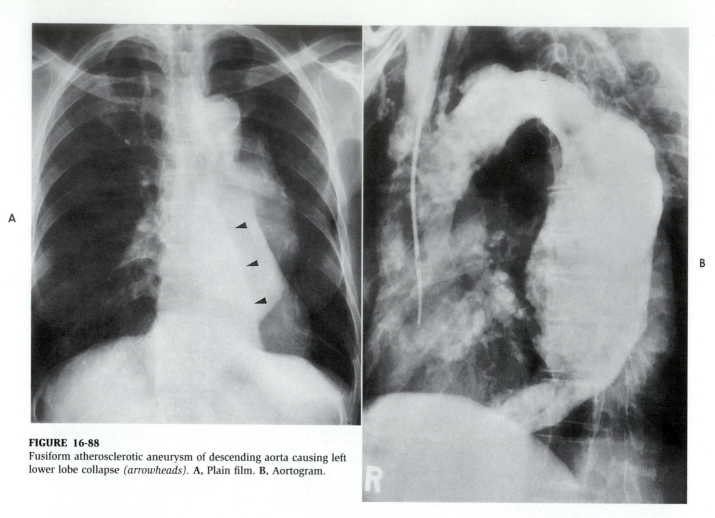

FIGURE 16-88
Fusiform atherosclerotic aneurysm of descending aorta causing left lower lobe collapse *(arrowheads)*. **A**, Plain film. **B**, Aortogram.

reported.[98,118] Rupture is the most feared complication. An aortic arch or descending aortic aneurysm with a diameter exceeding 6 cm is at significant risk of rupture, and many surgeons consider surgical intervention for such large aneurysms. Saccular aneurysms are at particular risk of rupture without warning.

Most atherosclerotic aneurysms are fusiform in shape; a few are saccular. Fusiform aneurysms usually arise in the aortic arch or descending aorta. They do not pose a diagnostic problem because their anatomic conformity to the aorta is obvious. Saccular aneurysms usually arise from the descending aorta, or very occasionally from the aortic arch, but are extremely unusual in the ascending aorta. Occasionally they are misdiagnosed on plain films as a neoplastic mediastinal mass.[471] They are usually differentiated from the majority of neoplastic or cystic masses by their conformity to the aorta and by the presence of curvilinear calcification in the wall of the aneurysm (Figure 16-89). Such calcification is usually present, although it may be difficult to see on plain chest radiographs. Peripheral calcification of the aneurysm wall is well demonstrated at CT,[398] particularly before contrast enhancement. Most degenerative aneurysms show significant amounts of lining thrombus, which may have flecks of calcification on the inner margin of the thrombus (Figure 16-89).[215] The thrombus is usually shaped like a crescent wedged against the outer wall of the aorta, and some luminal dilatation at the level of the aneurysm is almost invariable (Figure 16-90). Only a few cases have been reported in which the lumen of the aneurysm is totally occupied by thrombus.[471]

The ease of multiplanar imaging and the ability to differentiate between the wall, lumen, and lining thrombus without contrast media makes MRI an excellent method for assessing the size and shape of stable thoracic aortic aneurysms, showing the relationship to branch vessels, and demonstrating compressive effects.[305,306,539] MRI can also be of value in showing mediastinal hematoma if an aneurysm is leaking.

Traumatic aneurysms

Traumatic laceration of the aorta is discussed in Chapter 18. In patients who do not receive surgery soon after the trauma, a chronic false aneurysm may develop in characteristic sites.[201,220] With few exceptions[223] they arise from the anteromedial wall of the distal arch or upper descending aorta close to the ligamentum arteriosum (Figure 16-91). It has been suggested that hemato-

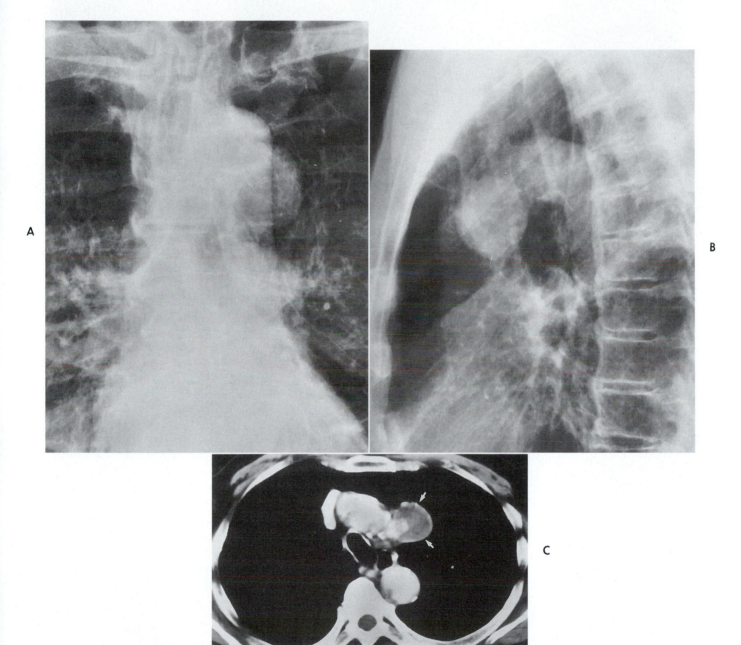

FIGURE 16-89
Saccular aneurysm of aortic arch resembling a mediastinal mass in a patient with recurrent laryngeal nerve paralysis. **A** and **B,** Plain chest radiographs showing a round mass in contact with the upper ascending aorta. Curvilinear calcification is visible in the wall of the aneurysm but is seen only with difficulty. **C,** Computed tomography scan showing contiguity of the mass *(arrows)* with the ascending aorta, crescentic lining thrombus, opacified central lumen, and calcification of wall.

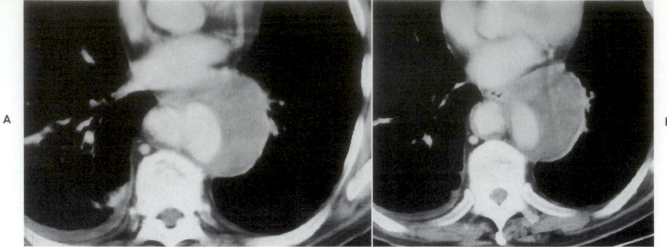

FIGURE 16-90
Saccular atherosclerotic aneurysm of descending aorta. **A** and **B**, Adjacent, contrast-enhanced computed tomography sections. The aneurysm is partially lined by thrombus. In this case, unusually, no calcification in the wall of the aneurysm is apparent.

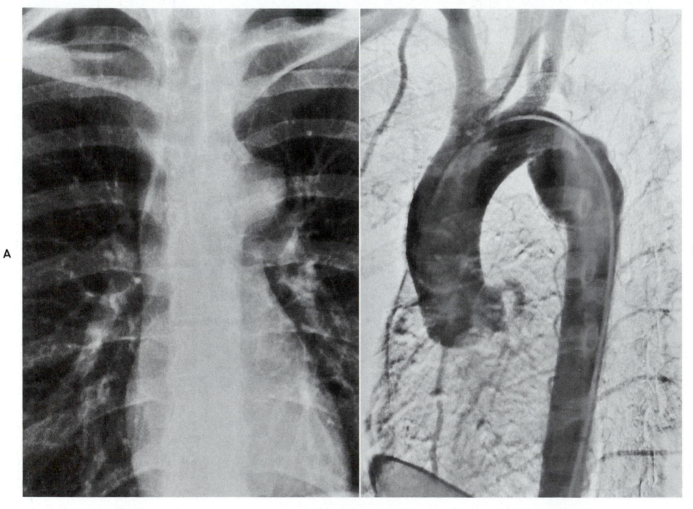

FIGURE 16-91
Traumatic aortic aneurysm in a typical location in the distal aortic arch close to the level of the ligamentum arteriosum. Trauma had taken place 3 years previously. **A**, Plain film. **B**, Aortogram.

mas at this site may be contained by the surrounding structures, whereas more posterior lacerations tend to bleed extensively and do not develop false aneurysms.[201] A hoarse voice may develop because of pressure on the recurrent laryngeal nerve, and dysphagia may be present if the aneurysm presses on the esophagus. Other symptoms include chest pain, dyspnea, and shortness of breath. When small, these aneurysms often project into the aortopulmonary window and therefore may be invisible on plain chest radiograph. As they enlarge, they form a bulge projecting from the aortopulmonary window (Figure 16-91). Chronic posttraumatic false aneurysms are saccular in shape and in time develop calcification in the wall or lining thrombus.[201,220] At this stage they are identical in appearance to degenerative saccular aneurysms on both plain chest radiographs and CT, except that the patient is often younger with no other evidence of atherosclerotic disease in the remainder of the aorta.

Mycotic aneurysms

Mycotic aneurysms of the aorta are confined to patients with predisposing causes: intravenous drug abusers, patients with valvular disease or congenital disorders of the heart or aorta, patients who have undergone previous cardiac or aortic surgery, those with adjacent pyogenic infection,[411] and subjects who are immunocompromised. A recent review of 20 mycotic aneurysms of the aortic root serves to emphasize that all patients had aortic valve disease or had an infected aortic valve prosthesis.[142] Mycotic aneurysms may occur in any site, depending on the predisposing factors. Unlike other aneurysms, mycotic aneurysms usually have fever and leukocytosis as early symptoms. Because the process is basically a form of abscess, it may be discovered first on a radionuclide scan such as an indium-111 leukocyte scintigram.[446] Mycotic aneurysms are usually saccular in shape. The major radiologic differences between mycotic aneurysms and other saccular aneurysms of the aorta are rapid enlargement and absence of calcification of the wall. These aneurysms are rapidly fatal unless treated.

Cystic medial necrosis and aortic dissection

Cystic medial necrosis is characterized by deposition of acellular basophilic material within the media that, when significant in amount, is associated with disruption of the aortic wall.[124] Severe cystic medial necrosis is seen in Marfan's syndrome and in an idiopathic form known as primary dilatation of the aorta. Focal aneurysms caused by cystic medial necrosis usually involve the ascending aorta and are an important cause of aortic regurgitation.[263] Lesser degrees of the condition are common in older individuals, probably in response to hemodynamic stresses such as hypertension and aortic stenosis.[124] Carlson, Lillehei, and Edwards[65] examined the ascending aorta in 250 autopsies. Having excluded cases of Marfan's syndrome, idiopathic dilatation of the aorta, and aortic dissection, they found that the incidence of cystic medial

necrosis increased progressively with age, from 10% in the first two decades to 60% and 64% in the seventh and eighth decades, respectively. Also the incidence of cystic medial necrosis was consistently higher in hypertensive patients than in normotensive subjects of comparable ages. Because much of the ascending aorta is not border-forming on plain chest radiography, even very large aneurysms when confined to the proximal half of the ascending aorta may be invisible on plain chest films.[263,491] However, identifying displaced mediastinal fat planes may be possible even if no visible widening of the mediastinal contour is evident.[491] This sign is difficult to evaluate, and in general the diagnosis is suspected only when the ascending aorta is clearly dilated. Confusion with mediastinal masses is rare because the lesion in question is so clearly the result of dilatation of the ascending aorta.

Aortic dissections, sometimes called dissecting aneurysms, are collections of blood within the media of the aortic wall that communicate with the true aortic lumen through one or more tears in the intima. It is assumed that most dissections begin within an intimal tear,[124] and bleeding then splits the aortic media. Degenerative changes in the media, cystic medial necrosis, and hypertension are important predisposing factors.[14,288]

Aortic dissections are divided into acute (first 14 days) and chronic.[99] Three fourths of deaths occur within the acute phase. Patients who survive 2 weeks are more stable and have a better prognosis.[99] The dissection channel usually spirals so that the false lumen lies anterior and to the right in the ascending aorta, and posterior and to the left in the descending aorta. The classic deBakey classification divides aortic dissection into types I to III.[105] Type I refers to dissections that commence in the ascending aorta and extend into the descending aorta, type II to dissections confined to the ascending aorta, and type III to dissections that commence just beyond the right subclavian artery and are confined to the descending aorta. The more recent classifications divide dissecting hematomas into two types depending on whether they involve the ascending aorta (type A) or are confined to the descending aorta (type B), irrespective of the site of the primary intimal tear.[11,101,333] The rationale for this division is that the survival of patients with acute ascending aortic dissections is significantly better when they are treated surgically than when they are treated medically.[11,99,101,336,536] Patients with acute descending aortic dissections (type B) fare equally well with medical or surgical therapy, and therefore such patients are usually treated initially with medical therapy, reserving surgery for patients with persistent symptoms, progression of dissection, or life-threatening ischemic complications.[11,99,536] Medical treatment is based on hypotensive therapy designed to prevent propagation of the hematoma.[537] Surgical treatment entails the obliteration of the false lumen close to the entry site and, when necessary, aortic valve replacement.

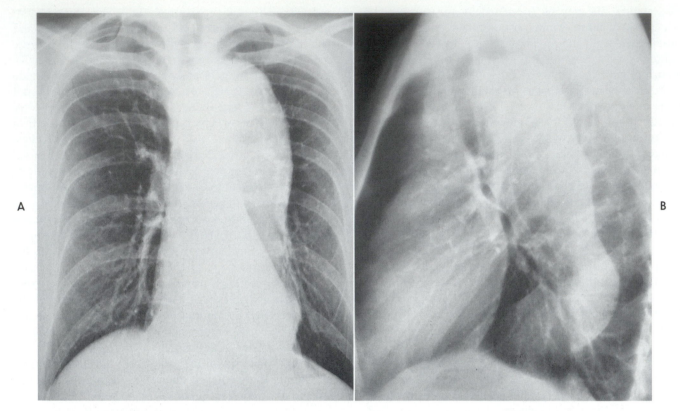

FIGURE 16-92
Acute aortic dissection. Plain chest radiographs show undulating widening of the arch and descending aorta. **A,** Posteroanterior radiograph. **B,** Lateral radiograph.

Patients usually have high blood pressure or other clinical evidence of hypertension, severe chest pain, often with midscapular radiation, circulatory shock, pulse deficits, and ischemic problems resulting from compression of the origins of the arteries arising from the affected portions of the aorta. Ascending aortic dissections may show the signs and symptoms of left ventricular failure resulting from aortic regurgitation. Pericardial tamponade is a life-threatening complication.

The main role of the plain chest film is to exclude other conditions. Plain films cannot be relied on either to confirm or to deny the diagnosis; an entirely normal plain chest radiograph is unusual but occasionally encountered in aortic dissection.[121] Occasionally it provides the first clue to the diagnosis of aortic dissection.[21] A major problem in many cases is that films are obtained with portable equipment in critically ill patients who cannot take a deep breath and who cannot stand or sit up. All these factors make the mediastinum appear wide even in a patient with no intrathoracic disorder.

Dissecting hematomas confined to the aortic root are often hidden on plain films, whereas the arch and descending aorta are border-forming structures. Therefore dissections involving these portions of the aorta usually produce recognizable signs (Figure 16-92). The widening of the aorta in dissecting hematoma tends to involve long segments, although short segment involvement is occasionally seen. Sometimes the widening is distinctly undulating in appearance, and occasionally the dissection may be manifest as a focal aneurysm of the aorta.[107] The distinction from degenerative widening and unfolding may not be possible on plain films.[246] Progressive widening over a few hours or days is an almost specific sign and is therefore an important observation.

The position of calcification in the aortic wall on plain film examination may help establish that a dissecting hematoma is present.[133] In the correct clinical circumstances, atheromatous calcification more than 1 cm inside the aortic contour can be regarded as suggestive evidence of aortic dissection. Displacement of this degree is not a common finding; in one large series, it was seen in only 4% of cases.[121] The sign, however, must be used with caution. Calcification must be unequivocally profiled against the outer aortic contour and is of no use in the aortic arch because the aortic knob in the frontal projection represents a foreshortened view of an obliquely curving tube. It is not a specific sign because the wall of the aorta may be substantially thickened in atherosclerosis or in aortitis, and clearly it is not applicable when the soft tissue outside the aorta is tumor or mediastinal fat. The sign cannot be used in reverse; calcification along the outermost aspect of the wall of the aneurysm on plain film and CT, while a feature of atherosclerotic aneurysms, is also seen in a small proportion of aortic dissections.[204]

Bleeding from aortic dissection may cause recognizable mediastinal widening on plain chest radiograph. This widening may be well or ill defined, and perihilar pulmonary consolidation caused by bleeding into the lung may be seen. Pleural effusions from seepage of blood from the mediastinum are a common accompaniment of aortic dissection. They are usually left sided or, if bilateral, are often worse on the left than on the right. Rupture into the pericardium is an extremely serious, often fatal, complication. The presence of pericardial fluid rarely can be diagnosed using plain films.

CT provides a highly sensitive and specific technique with which to diagnose or exclude the presence of a dissecting hematoma of the aorta.* Demos, Posniak, and Marsan,[110] in their review of the literature, found the average accuracy of CT to be 95%. The CT technique varies from center to center. With modern spiral (helical)[96] or ultrafast scanners[208,477,499] the images can be obtained so rapidly that timing the postcontrast images is no longer a problem and all desired levels in the thorax can be imaged. If spiral or ultrafast scanning is not available, a suggested protocol[110,540] uses precontrast scans at 2 cm intervals through the aorta or at selected levels. These may be at the level of the arch, the midascending aorta, and the distal descending aorta (through mid–left atrium or left ventricular apex). Dynamic scans at these levels are then carried out as follows: during each of three dynamic series, a 35 to 40 ml bolus injection of intravenous contrast material is rapidly administered at each level, and if necessary, further boluses or a slow infusion of contrast material is given while contiguous 1 cm sections are obtained from just above the aortic arch to the level of the diaphragm (or below, if necessary).

The diagnostic feature on contrast-enhanced CT scans[181] is similar to that seen at aortography (Figure 16-93), namely, two lumina separated by an intimal flap (Figure 16-94). The intimal flap is seen as a curvilinear lucency within the opacified aorta. Sometimes, particularly in the aortic arch, the intimal flap may assume a serpiginous course. Plaques of calcification are sometimes seen within the displaced intima (Figure 16-95). A false lumen usually fills and empties in a delayed fashion compared with a true lumen, a finding that is best interpreted on dynamic scans at a single level. Differential opacification can be a useful sign in cases where the intimal flap is invisible or uncertain. The false lumen may be partially or on occasion totally filled by thrombus (Figure 16-96). The true lumen is usually compressed by the false lumen, sometimes to a substantial degree.

*References 125, 183, 198, 214, 369, 387, 469, 500, 507, 540.

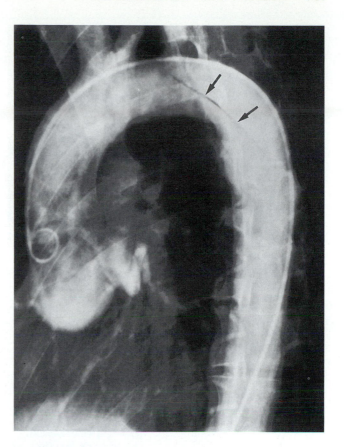

FIGURE 16-93
Angiogram of type B dissection in a patient with Marfan's syndrome showing little or no widening of the aorta but an obvious intimal flap (*arrows*) separating two lumina.

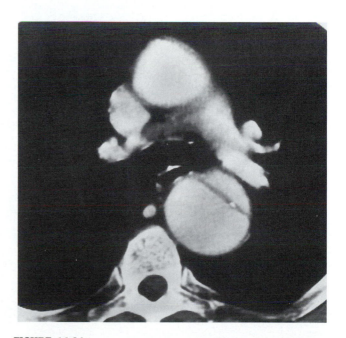

FIGURE 16-94
Contrast-enhanced computed tomography scan showing type B dissection with an intimal flap, containing focal calcification, separating two lumina. Notice pronounced dilatation of the affected descending aorta.

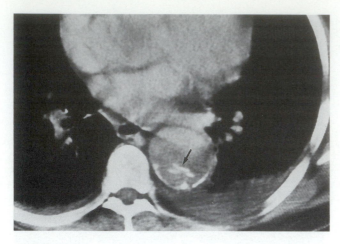

FIGURE 16-95
Displaced calcification in an intimal flap *(arrow)* on precontrast computed tomography scan in a patient with aortic dissection.

The appearance of two lumina separated by an intimal flap is specific for aortic dissection, but care must be taken not to misdiagnose an extraaortic structure as a false lumen.[182] The left innominate vein, superior vena cava, left superior intercostal vein, left superior pulmonary vein, and superior pericardial recesses can all mimic a false channel, as can adjacent pleural or pericardial thickening and adjacent atelectasis of the lung (Figure 16-97). Another potential mimic of a false lumen is apparent asymmetric thickening of the wall of the aorta caused by motion artifact.[62,399] Partial volume averaging of densities in the section above or below may also closely resemble a false lumen and can give the impression of displaced intimal calcification.[181] Streak artifacts can mimic an intimal flap (Figure 16-98).[162,182] Intimal flaps are gently curved structures of uniform thickness conforming to the configuration of the aorta. Streak artifacts are straight and vary in thickness; their orientation may change markedly from one CT section to the next, and

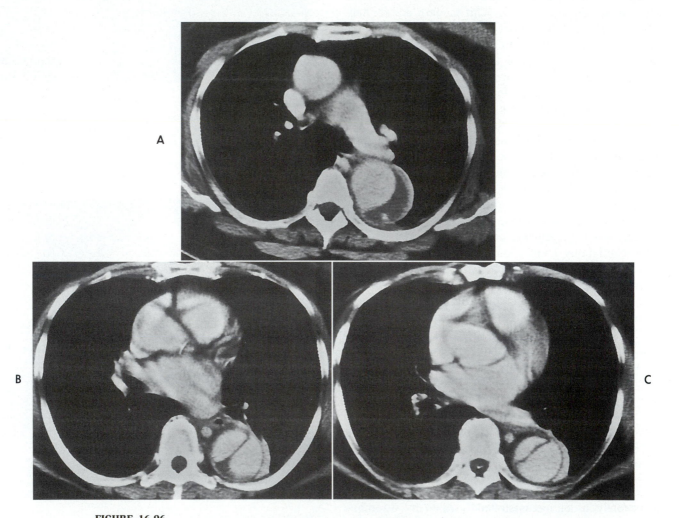

FIGURE 16-96
Partial thrombosis of false lumen in aortic dissection. Three levels from a contrast-enhanced computed tomography scan in a patient with type B dissection 15 days after onset of symptoms. **A,** The almost completely thrombosed false lumen. **B,** Thrombus-free false lumen. **C,** Partially thrombosed false lumen.

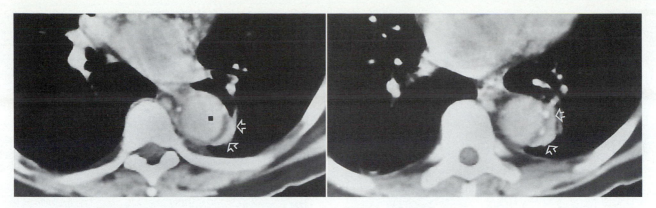

FIGURE 16-97
Adjacent contrast-enhanced computed tomography sections showing atheromatous disease of the descending aorta in a patient with atelectasis of lung adjacent to the aorta (arrows) closely mimicking an aortic dissection.

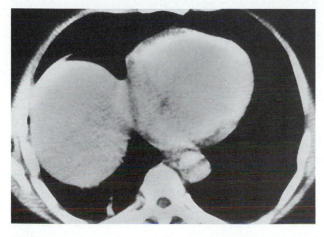

FIGURE 16-98
Streak artifacts across descending aorta mimicking aortic dissection on a contrast-enhanced computed tomography scan.

they often extend outside the aorta.

Another common but subtle CT sign of acute aortic dissection is a moderate increase in density of the false lumen owing to recently clotted blood.[215] This sign can be appreciated only on precontrast scans by comparing the density of the nonopacified true and false lumina. The sign can be mimicked by asymmetric disease of the aortic wall in patients who do not have aortic dissection.[286]

The shape of the opacified lumen may help in diagnosis. In atherosclerotic aneurysm the lumen is almost always round, whereas in aortic dissection the lumen is flattened in over half the cases.[215]

Displacement of calcified atheromatous plaques by the dissection can be demonstrated on precontrast scans (Figure 16-95) and is a useful CT sign in cases where contrast enhancement of the two lumina cannot be achieved as, for example, when the false lumen is thrombosed. The sign is seen only in a minority of patients.[507] Occasionally the intimal flap can be seen even without contrast material,[507] particularly in patients who are anemic.[109] This sign clearly should not be relied on but could be useful if for some reason only precontrast CT images are available for review.

The affected portions of the aorta are often enlarged. In some reports[198,287] dilatation is always present, but in the largest series reported to date, almost 60% of patients with dissection show no aortic dilatation.[507] Enlarged portions of the aorta should be carefully examined, using dynamic scanning if necessary, for the more specific signs of dissection.[507]

Distinguishing between an aortic dissection with a completely thrombosed false lumen and an atheromatous aneurysm with thrombus lining the wall of the aorta can be difficult. The thrombosis of the false lumen means that neither the double channel nor the intimal flap can be demonstrated. In these circumstances the displacement of intimal calcification becomes a useful sign of dissection, but calcification on occasion may be seen lining the inner surface of the thrombus in an atherosclerotic aneurysm.[182,215]

MRI is being used with increasing frequency to demonstrate aortic dissection. The ability to recognize flowing blood without contrast media together with the multiplanar imaging capability is a significant advantage, and the sensitivity and specificity of MRI are at least as good as with CT.[19,164,266,360] However, the difficulties associated with monitoring sick patients within the very high magnetic fields and enclosed environment of a magnetic resonance imager limit the use of MRI.

A variety of techniques can be used.[306,539] Electrocardiography-gated spin-echo images show fast-flowing blood as a signal void. When the blood flow is above a critical rate, the intimal flap and the aortic wall are readily demonstrated as separately definable curvilinear structures. For the most part, blood in the true lumen of the aorta flows above this threshold.[539] Slow-flowing blood in

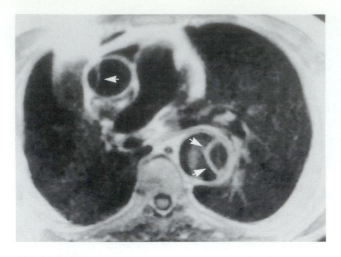

FIGURE 16-99
Magnetic resonance image of aortic dissection. T1-weighted spin-echo sequence. The intimal flap *(arrows)* in ascending and descending aorta is well seen against background of fast-flowing blood in the true and false lumens. (Courtesy Cynthia Janus, New York.)

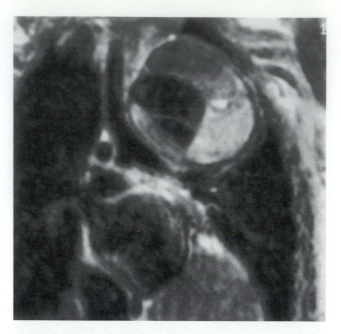

FIGURE 16-100
Magnetic resonance image of aortic dissection. Coronal section through aortic arch showing differential flow in false lumen (high signal resulting from slow flow) and true lumen (signal void resulting from fast flow).

the false lumen produces a variety of signal patterns that can be difficult to distinguish from thrombus, but gradient echo and magnetic resonance angiographic sequences can usually help resolve this problem.[305,306]

The basic sign of aortic dissection at MRI (Figures 16-99 and 16-100) is the same as that described for CT: an intimal flap separating true and false lumina. On occasion eccentric or concentric aortic wall thickening may be the only MR finding.[550]

The multiplanar imaging capability of MRI is a particular advantage[232] compared with CT; oblique sagittal and coronal imaging planes may be optimal for demonstrating the extent of dissection and the relationship of the dissection to the major aortic branches, particularly those arising from the aortic arch.

As with CT, MRI has a number of diagnostic pitfalls.[311,473] At MRI, adjacent structures, such as the left brachiocephalic vein, left superior intercostal vein, left superior pulmonary vein, or azygos vein, may mimic a false lumen. The superior pericardial recesses and the origins of the arteries arising from the aortic arch can also be misleading. Apparent thickening of the aortic wall from motion artifact, atherosclerotic plaques, or fibrosing mediastinitis also may be confused with a thrombosed false lumen.[473]

Echocardiography is proving increasingly useful for aortic dissection. Standard transthoracic cardiac echocardiography can be used to show the proximal aorta, aortic valve, and any hemopericardium that may have occurred. Doppler ultrasound can be used to diagnose and grade aortic regurgitation. Cardiac ultrasound can also show the proximal ascending aorta in enough detail to show a false lumen and intimal flap in the great majority of type A

dissections.[194,503] Doppler techniques can be used to assess flow in the true and false lumens.

Transthoracic ultrasound cannot see reliably beyond the proximal ascending aorta. Transesophageal ultrasound, which allows examination of the aorta at multiple levels,[462] has an extensive view of the aorta. Some early reports suggest close to 100% sensitivity and specificity for combined transthoracic and transesophageal ultrasound.[132,213] The poor visibility of ascending aortic dissections by transesophageal ultrasound alone must be borne in mind.[360] The basic sign of dissection is the same as that described for CT, MRI, and aortography, namely, a double lumen separated by an intimal flap. If the false lumen is thrombosed, the observer should look for central displacement of intimal calcification or separation of intimal layers. The entry tear can be identified at ultrasound as an interruption in the continuity of the intimal flap with associated fluttering of the edges.[131,132] A potentially major advantage of transthoracic and transesophageal ultrasound is that they can be performed at the patient's bedside.[462,492]

Choosing a test for patients with possible aortic dissection is not always easy.[83] Aortography[387] has a sensitivity and specificity above 88%,[132] usually closer to 97%,[121] but false-negative results can occur when the flow through the true and false lumens is such that the true and false channels opacify equally and the intimal flap is not tangential to the x-ray beam. Also dissection can be overlooked if the false lumen is thrombosed. Conversely, aortic wall thickening may mimic dissection. Also, aortography is invasive, and complications can be catastrophic. The main advantages of aortography over CT are that aortography can demonstrate aortic regurgitation and can best demonstrate the degree of involvement of major aortic branches, which may be useful preoperative information. It can also show which arteries are perfused from which lumen and often can demonstrate with greater precision the entry point of the dissection. However, CT is safer and at least as accurate as aortography for demonstrating the extent of the dissection.[369] This is true even for thrombosed portions of the false lumen. CT also allows recognition of pericardial fluid, pleural fluid, mediastinal bleeding, and any spread of hemorrhage into the lung parenchyma. CT does not allow evaluation of aortic regurgitation, nor does it show adequately the origins of the major aortic branches. MRI, which can provide images of similar or greater diagnostic value than CT, is limited in that only hemodynamically stable patients can be examined.[387] As magnetic resonance–compatible monitoring and life support systems become available, the use of MRI as the primary imaging modality for acute aortic dissections is likely to increase. By then, the main alternative may well be combined transthoracic and transesophageal ultrasound. The final choice will depend on the patient's clinical state, the preferences of the thoracic surgeon, and the questions being asked.[83,106] A growing number of surgeons now operate on selected patients after a cross-sectional imaging examination without prior angiography.[110]

Where a treatment decision can be based on the findings at CT, MRI, or ultrasound, angiography should be held in reserve. For example, a patient with severe chest pain would be a good candidate for CT or MRI, if the likelihood of dissection is low but clinical examination or plain chest films show features that require a diagnosis of dissection be excluded. This is also true for a patient thought likely to have dissection in whom medical therapy is the treatment of choice; here the prime purpose is to confirm the diagnosis and to provide a baseline for follow-up. CT, MRI, and ultrasound are clearly also the diagnostic tests of choice for follow-up of a previously treated dissection and for chronic dissections. If aortography is likely to be needed before surgery, great care must be taken not to delay the aortogram or to compromise the examination by large doses of contrast medium for a CT scan.

Penetrating atherosclerotic ulcer

A newly described entity, "penetrating atherosclerotic ulcer of the thoracic aorta,"[93,236,260] has many clinical features that are similar to aortic dissection, in particular the searing chest and back pain and the propensity for systemic hypertension. Cases of this entity appear to have been included in previously published series of aortic dissection.[260] The atherosclerotic ulcer penetrates the internal elastic lamina with resultant hematoma formation within the aortic wall. The hematoma may rupture

through the aortic wall to become a false aneurysm or may produce widespread, life-threatening mediastinal hemorrhage. Whether these patients should be treated conservatively, similarly to type B aortic dissections, or with early surgical intervention is debated.[260]

The ulcer, a major feature on imaging studies such as aortography, CT, and MRI, is typically seen in the middle or distal third of the descending thoracic aorta in association with adjacent intramural hematoma, but without an intimal flap.[260,567] Displaced intimal calcification similar to that seen with classic aortic dissection is a common finding on CT. One practical point of CT technique is that the diagnosis depends largely on demonstrating a focal ulcer, which could be overlooked unless contiguous CT scans of the whole of the thoracic aorta are performed.[260]

Congenital aneurysms

Congenital aneurysms of the aorta are rare. Almost all of those encountered in clinical practice are sinus of Valsalva aneurysms. Normally, the media of the wall of the proximal aorta is firmly attached to the fibrous annulus of the aortic valve. In congenital sinus of Valsalva aneurysm, the media avulses from its attachment to the annulus, and an aneurysm results.[124] These aneurysms most commonly arise from the posterior or right aortic sinus. An aneurysm of the posterior aortic sinus bulges into the right atrium, and if it ruptures, an aortic to right atrial shunt results. An aneurysm of the right aortic sinus bulges into the right ventricle, and rupture therefore causes an aortic to right ventricular shunt. The aortic valve lies deep within the mediastinal shadow on plain chest radiograph, and congenital aortic sinus aneurysms must therefore reach substantial size to be recognizable on plain film. Occasionally they do reach such a size. Calcification may be visible in the wall of the aneurysm. The signs of left-to-right shunt may be visible if rupture has occurred. CT and MRI show the aneurysm to advantage.[185]

Very occasionally, aneurysms are associated with coarctation of the aorta (Figure 16-101) or other aortic anomalies, such as right-sided aortic arch.[228] Whether the aneurysms in patients with coarctation are truly congenital or acquired secondary to prolonged hypertension is debatable.

Aneurysms resulting from aortitis

Aneurysms from aortitis are rare now that syphilis[226] is so uncommon. Takayasu's disease is the best known arteritis; although it is more often a stenosing disease, it may on occasion cause saccular or fusiform aortic aneurysms (Figure 16-102).[312,388,455,560] It is a chronic inflammatory condition of unknown origin that affects the aorta, its main branches, and the pulmonary arteries. It occurs most commonly in the Orient but has a worldwide distribution. Aneurysms in this condition may be single or multiple and may be seen anywhere in the

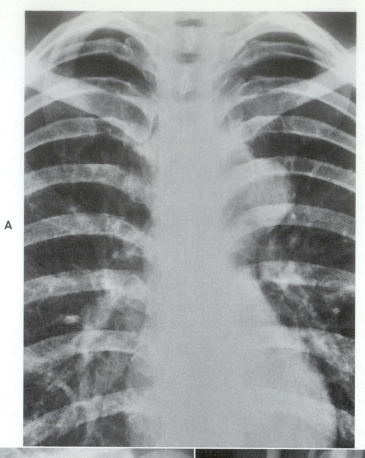

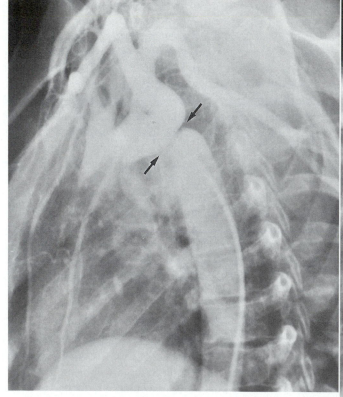

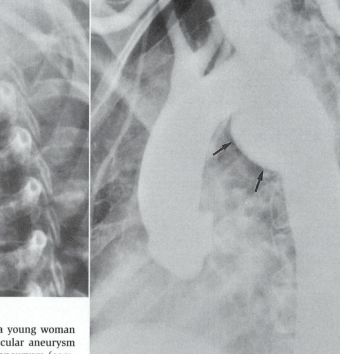

FIGURE 16-101
Slowly enlarging congenital aneurysm of aorta in a young woman with coarctation of aorta. **A,** Plain film shows saccular aneurysm indistinguishable from atherosclerotic or traumatic aneurysm (compare with Figure 16-91). **B,** Early phase of aortogram showing the coarctation *(arrows).* **C,** Later phase of aortogram showing contrast opacification of aneurysm *(arrows).*

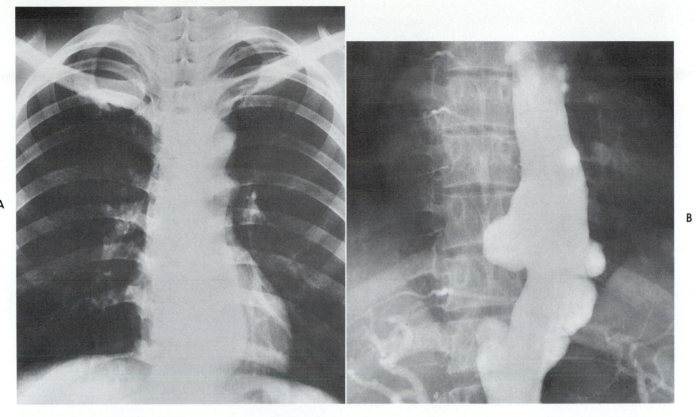

FIGURE 16-102
Arteritis causing aortic aneurysms in a young Nepalese man. A, Posteroanterior radiograph. B, Aortogram.

aorta. Calcification of the wall of the aorta and of the aneurysms may be present, and aortic dissection may be a complication.

AORTIC ANOMALIES THAT MAY SIMULATE A MEDIASTINAL MASS

Three congenital variations of the aorta can simulate a mediastinal mass on plain chest radiographs or unenhanced CT scans: right aortic arch, double aortic arch, and pseudocoarctation of the aorta.

Right aortic arch

Right aortic arch is a common finding in a number of congenital heart disorders. This discussion is confined to right aortic arch in patients without cardiac malformation. A right aortic arch passes to the right of the trachea and usually descends in the right posterior mediastinum; only rarely is the descending aorta on the left. In the usual branching pattern the left carotid artery arises first, followed by the right carotid and right subclavian arteries. The left subclavian artery, which arises as the fourth and most distal branch of the aortic arch, is known as an aberrant subclavian artery to distinguish it from the so-called mirror image arrangement, which is seen when right aortic arch accompanies complex congenital heart

disease. (In mirror image branching the left subclavian artery is a branch of the first vessel to arise from the aortic arch, namely the left brachiocephalic artery.) The aberrant left subclavian artery passes behind the esophagus to reach the root of the neck on the left side. The left subclavian artery may take origin from a diverticulum in the proximal descending aorta, which embryologically represents a remnant of the left arch.

The radiographic appearances (Figures 16-103 and 16-104) consist of a visible right aortic arch and a density posterior to the esophagus that varies in size from small to large. This density is caused by the diverticulum or by medial displacement of the proximal descending aorta. The posterior impression on the esophagus at barium swallow and on the trachea at plain film and CT is often striking (Figure 16-105). Although no left aortic arch is visible, great caution is needed here because either the diverticulum or the leftward displacement of the aortic arch may resemble a small left aortic knob.

The combination of these features makes it possible to diagnose almost every right aortic arch with aberrant left subclavian artery on plain chest radiograph (or barium swallow study). CT scanning (Figure 16-105) shows the same features and also shows contrast enhancement of the aorta and its branches.

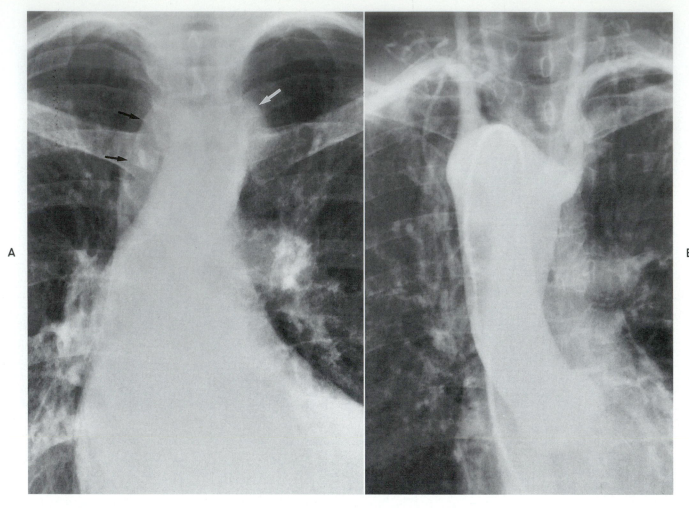

FIGURE 16-103
Right aortic arch with aberrant left subclavian artery mimicking lymphadenopathy. **A,** Posteroanterior radiograph shows aortic arch *(black arrows)* to the right of the trachea. Density to the left of the trachea *(white arrow)* is a diverticulum from which the left subclavian artery originates. **B,** Aortogram of right aortic arch with aberrant left subclavian artery. Note midline position of distal arch and diverticulum from which the left subclavian artery originates. These two phenomena together give rise to the posterior impression on the esophagus shown in Figure 16-104, *B.*

Double aortic arch

In most cases double aortic arch is diagnosed early in life because of tracheal obstruction and swallowing difficulties. Occasionally the anomaly remains undetected until later childhood or adult life. The two aortic arches pass to either side of the trachea and join posteriorly, at which point they often displace the trachea and esophagus forward and may be confused with a mass. The descending aorta is usually in the midline. The following are the diagnostic features:

1. The right arch is almost always larger and higher than the left arch (Figure 16-106). This observation is particularly important at barium swallow, when the arches are seen to indent the esophagus from both sides.

2. At CT scanning the branching pattern of the vessels to the head and neck is distinctive. Each arch gives rise to

two vessels: a carotid and a subclavian artery. Each artery of the pair lies one in front of the other (Figure 16-106).

3. The arches fuse posterior to the esophagus and trachea and may create a masslike density in the posterior mediastinum.

Pseudocoarctation of the aorta

Pseudocoarctation of the aorta is a congenital anomaly that many authorities believe is part of the spectrum of true coarctation, but without a gradient-producing narrowing of the aorta. The aorta is kinked at the level of the ligamentum arteriosum, the same position as the usual site of coarctation (Figure 16-107). The aortic arch therefore rises higher than usual, the ascending aorta being more vertical and the curve of the arch tighter. The high aortic arch, or the kinking, may simulate a mass

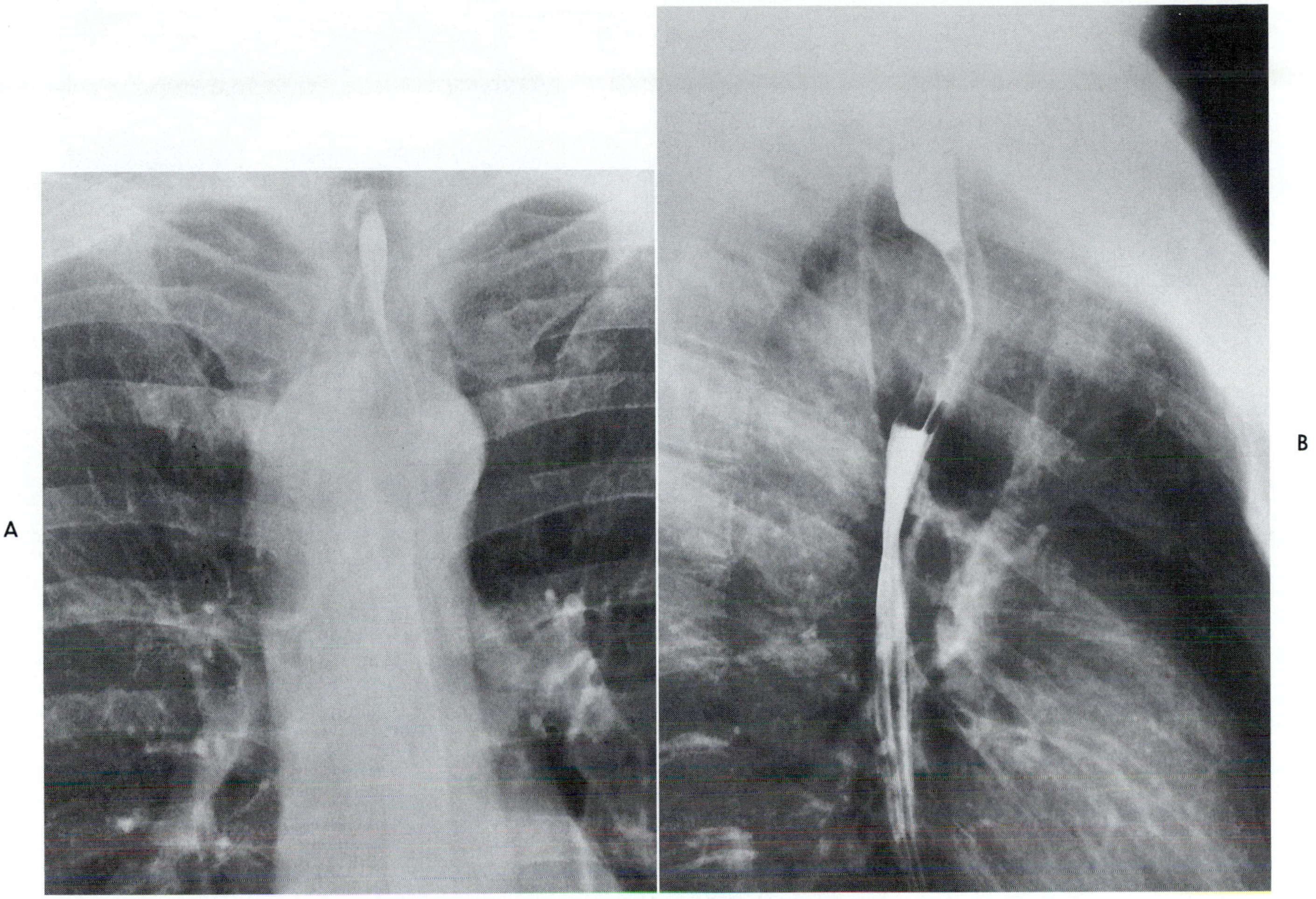

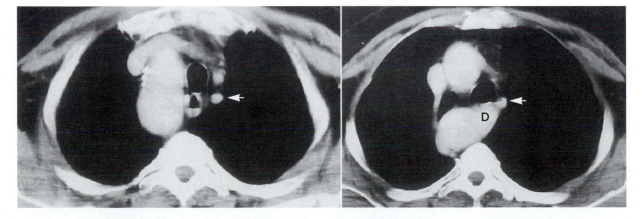

FIGURE 16-104
Right aortic arch. **A,** Posteroanterior and, **B,** lateral radiographs taken during passage of a bolus of barium. Confusion with lymphadenopathy is particularly great in this case because, unusually, the descending aorta is on the left. Note characteristic forward displacement of the esophagus and trachea on the lateral view.

FIGURE 16-105
Right aortic arch. Contrast-enhanced computed tomography scans 2 cm apart. Right-sided aortic arch and aberrant left subclavian *(arrow)* arising from the aortic diverticulum *(D)* posterior to the esophagus are well seen.

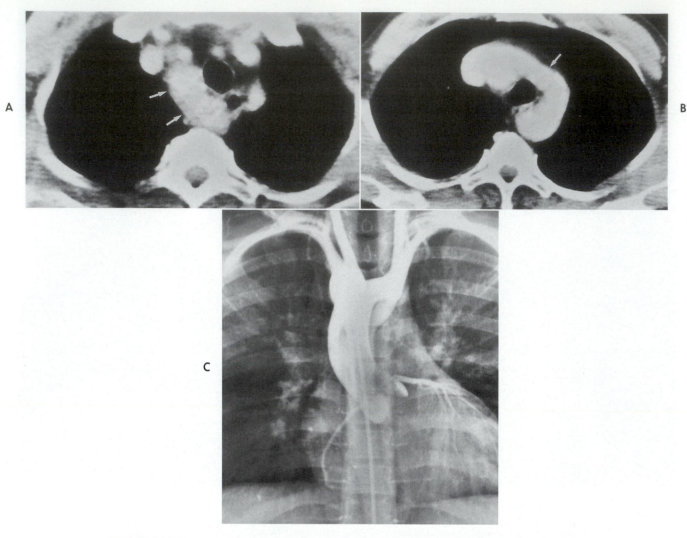

FIGURE 16-106
Double aortic arch. **A,** Computed tomography (CT) section at the level of the left brachiocephalic vein illustrates a high right-sided aortic arch *(arrows)* mimicking right paratracheal adenopathy. **B,** CT section 3 cm lower illustrates the left-sided aortic arch *(arrow)*. Contrast-enhanced scans. **C,** Aortogram in a child, showing anatomic features. Note that the right arch is larger and higher, and that two main branches arise from each arch.

(Figures 16-108 and 16-109). Pseudocoarctation, like true coarctation, is associated with an increased tendency for aneurysm formation and aortic dissection, in which case the aorta above or below the kink may be significantly enlarged and may be confused with a mass (Figure 16-110).[267]

ESOPHAGEAL TUMORS PRESENTING AS MEDIASTINAL MASSES

Carcinoma of the esophagus, the most common neoplasm to affect the esophagus, only occasionally gives rise to recognizable plain film findings. Presentation as a mediastinal mass is almost never seen. The most frequent sign is visible dilatation of the esophagus, which may be accompanied by recognizable thickening of the esophageal wall. Esophageal dilatation is usually easiest to

recognize posterior to the trachea on the lateral view. The fluid-filled, dilated esophagus displaces the trachea and carina forward.[409] Normally the lung invaginates posterior to the right half of the trachea, so that the posterior tracheal band can be seen (see Chapter 2). With esophageal dilatation the esophagus displaces the lung, and recognizing a thick band of tissue between air in the trachea and air in the lumen of the esophagus may be possible. This thickened band represents the combined thickness of the walls of the trachea and esophagus. In addition, in carcinoma of the esophagus, periesophageal lymphatic involvement contributes to the thickening of the posterior tracheal band.[404] As an isolated sign, increased thickness of the posterior tracheal band has little value because the collapsed normal esophagus can interpose between the lung and the trachea and cause

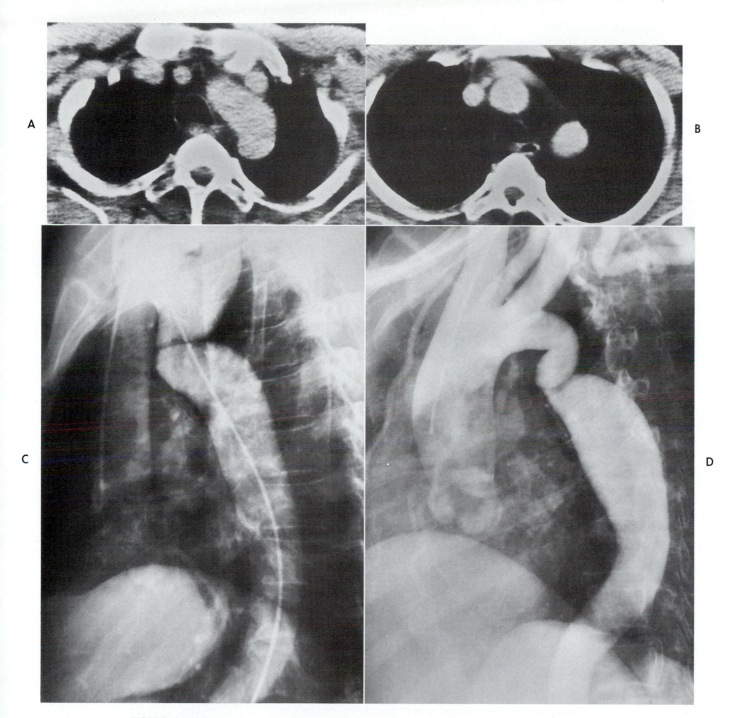

FIGURE 16-107
Pseudocoarctation of aorta simulating a mass. **A,** The arch is seen in an unexpectedly high position on contrast-enhanced computed tomography scan. **B,** Section 2 cm lower at expected level of the top of the arch shows ascending and descending aorta. **C,** Aortogram of same patient. (Plain chest radiograph in this patient is shown in Figure 16-108.) **D,** True aortic coarctation for comparison. Features are similar except that there are large collaterals and a pressure gradient was present.

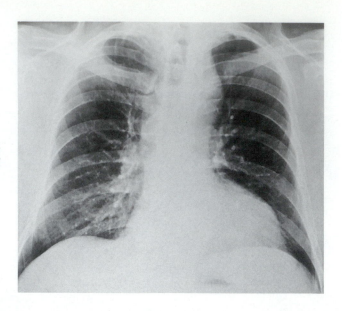

FIGURE 16-108
Pseudocoarctation of the aorta mimicking a left-sided superior mediastinal mass. Angiogram and computed tomography scan of this patient are shown in Figure 16-107.

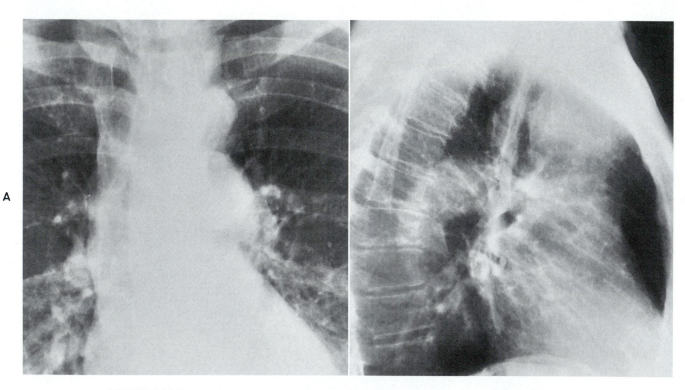

A
B

FIGURE 16-109
Pseudocoarctation of aorta. Kinked aorta is aligned such that the portion distal to the kink simulates either an enlarged pulmonary artery or a mediastinal mass. **A,** Posteroanterior radiograph. **B,** Lateral radiograph.

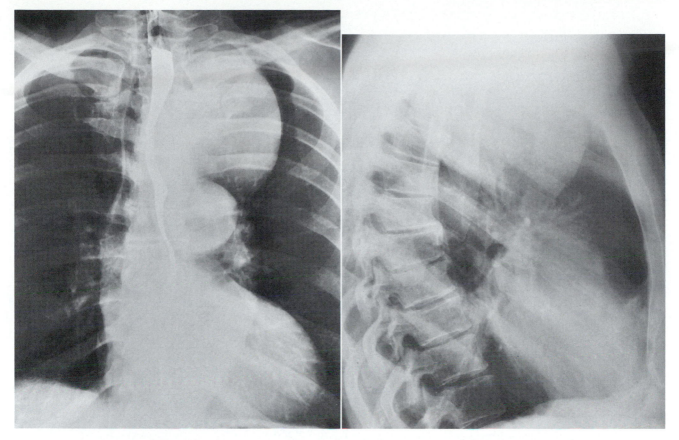

FIGURE 16-110
Aneurysm formation of aortic arch proximal to a pseudocoarctation. **A,** Posteroanterior radiograph with barium in the esophagus. **B,** Lateral radiograph.

marked thickening of the band. However, if the sign is accompanied by forward bowing of the trachea and anterior displacement of the carina, esophageal dilatation can be confidently diagnosed (Figure 16-111).

Smooth muscle tumors (leiomyomas and leiomyosarcomas) may grow to a substantial size without causing dysphagia and therefore may first appear as an asymptomatic mediastinal mass.[87] When barium swallow was the automatic next test for posterior mediastinal masses, the diagnosis was readily made by observing the characteristic signs of an intramural extramucosal mass. Now CT often is performed without preliminary barium swallow. CT shows a smooth, round, well-defined, enhancing mass in the posterior mediastinum inseparable from the esophagus (Figure 16-112). The esophagus is usually not dilated above the level of the tumor. This lack of dilatation can be an important differential diagnostic point in reducing the likelihood of carcinoma of the esophagus.

HIATUS HERNIA

Hiatus hernias are frequent incidental findings on chest radiographs and CT examinations. They may produce pain as a result of gastroesophageal reflux and may be responsible for anemia or upper gastrointestinal bleeding.

On plain chest radiograph they produce a smooth, focal widening of the posterior junction anatomy extending down to the diaphragm. Varying amounts of fat surround the hernia itself, and in most instances some air is seen within the hernia on plain film; often there is a visible air-fluid level. At CT the esophagus can be traced down into the hernia, and air (and contrast material) within the lumen usually enables the diagnosis to be made without difficulty. The fat surrounding the hernia may be a striking feature. Hiatus hernias can be huge and may contain a major portion of the stomach. With large paraesophageal hernias the stomach frequently undergoes organoaxial rotation and therefore may contain two air-fluid levels.

HERNIA THROUGH THE FORAMEN OF BOCHDALEK

The pleuroperitoneal hiatus in each hemidiaphragm closes early in fetal life. The major component of the developing diaphragm is the septum transversum. During the seventh week of development the pleuroperitoneal folds fuse with the mesentery of the esophagus and migrate anteriorly to join the septum transversum, closing two large posterolateral openings. Failure of closure

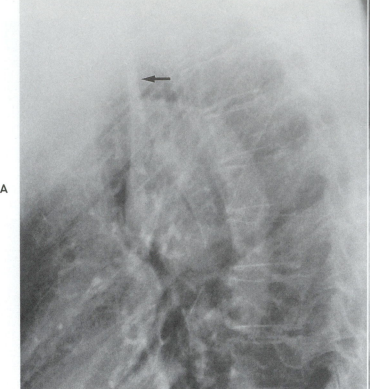

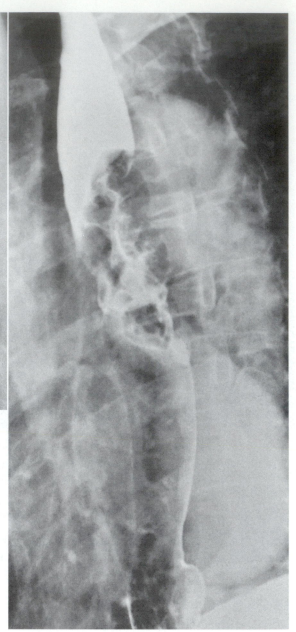

FIGURE 16-111
Esophageal dilatation resulting from carcinoma of esophagus. **A,** Lateral radiograph shows forward bowing of the trachea and a thick posterior tracheal band *(arrow)*. **B,** Corresponding features at barium swallow examination.

results in congenital diaphragmatic hernia. Small defects of closure are common and usually are not discovered until late in adult life when they appear as rounded "humps" on one or both hemidiaphragms (Figure 16-113). They are particularly common in patients over 70 years of age. Gale found a prevalence of 6% when he reviewed the chest and abdominal CT scans of 940 patients[161]; left-sided hernias were approximately twice as common as those on the right, and bilateral hernias were present in just over 15% of patients with hernias. These humps are seen posteriorly, usually close to the spine; they represent collections of herniated retroperitoneal fat and sometimes kidney or a portion of spleen. They are typically found about 4 to 5 cm from the posterior attachment of the diaphragm. The herniation of the kidney may be so striking that the term "intrathoracic kidney" has been used.[313] The radiographic appearance of the chest in elderly individuals is sufficiently characteristic that further investigation is not warranted. When alternative causes for a diaphragmatic or paraspinal swelling are being entertained, CT scanning[161] can demonstrate the fatty nature of the hernial content and can often show the accompanying muscle defect in the diaphragm (Figure 16-114). Identifying the muscle defect may be difficult in patients who have little retroperitoneal fat, but most patients have relatively abundant subdiaphragmatic fat on the left. On the right the liver may obscure the details of the superior portion of the right hemidiaphragm and make it difficult to recognize a high Bochdalek defect. Typically, however, the defects are lower and lie against retroperitoneal fat.[161] CT scanning also may reveal an ipsilateral kidney in a high position. Extrapleural lipomas in contact with the diaphragm may appear similar, but they are not accompanied by a diaphragmatic defect or displacement of abdominal viscera.

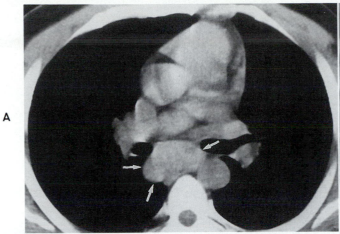

FIGURE 16-112
Leiomyoma of esophagus presenting as a mediastinal mass. **A,** Contrast-enhanced computed tomography scan shows smooth homogeneous mass centered on the esophagus *(arrows).* **B,** Barium swallow study shows an intraluminal extramucosal mass.

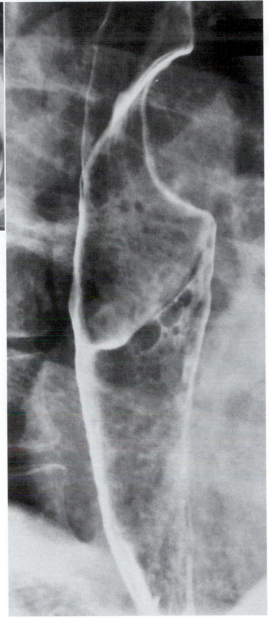

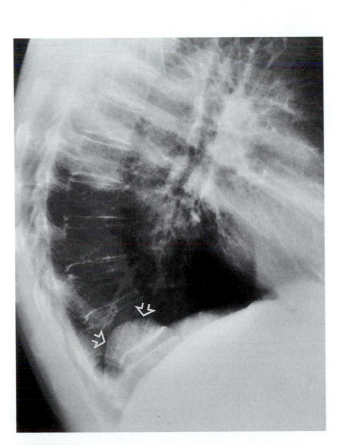

FIGURE 16-113
Bochdalek hernia in typical location on the posterior surface of dome of the hemidiaphragm *(arrows).*

HERNIA THROUGH THE FORAMEN OF MORGAGNI

The foramina of Morgagni (space of Larrey) are V-shaped developmental diaphragm defects between the muscle origins from the sternum and adjacent ribs.[380] Morgagni hernias are often confined to the right side, presumably because herniation is prevented on the left side by the pericardium beneath the heart. Herniation into the pericardial sac, however, has been reported in both children and adults.[470,514] In adults these hernias are mostly asymptomatic, although lower sternal discomfort, cough, dyspnea, and nonspecific gastrointestinal symptoms may occur.[380]

On plain chest radiographs,[380,418] hernias through the foramen of Morgagni produce opacities in the right

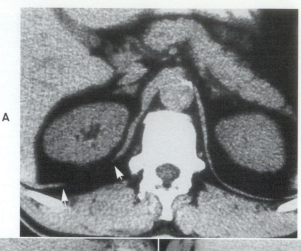

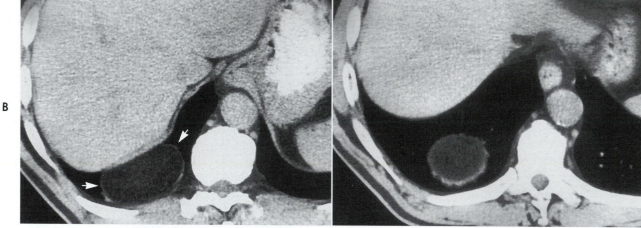

FIGURE 16-114
Bochdalek hernia. Typical computed tomography appearances. **A,** Section at the level of the defect in the right hemidiaphragm. (Arrows point to edges of the defect.) Note that the kidney is higher on the right than on the left. **B,** Higher section showing fat-containing hernia *(arrows).* **C,** Even higher section showing Bochdalek hernia mimicking an intrapulmonary abnormality.

cardiophrenic angle. The shadow may be well defined and resemble a mass, or it may be ill defined and resemble pneumonia. The contents are mostly fat, and therefore on plain chest radiograph the density resembles soft tissue. Air-containing loops of bowel are only occasionally seen. Examination of the bowel with contrast material may show contrast medium in the hernia or may show a loop of small or large bowel hooked up toward the hernial sac. Radionuclide liver scans may show liver herniating into the chest.

DIFFERENTIAL DIAGNOSIS OF MEDIASTINAL MASSES

The differential diagnosis of mediastinal masses is a common problem. The first step is to be sure that the mass arises within the mediastinum rather than from contiguous lung, pleura, spine, or sternum. Clearly, masses that lie deep to mediastinal vessels are mediastinal in origin, and masses arising from the sternum or

spine should be obvious at CT. The interface with the adjacent lung is a useful sign, particularly at CT. With few exceptions a mass with a spiculated, nodular, or irregular edge arises in the lung, and a mass with a broad base on the mediastinum and a smooth edge arises in the mediastinum or mediastinal pleura.[551] Masses arising from the mediastinal pleura project into the lung and usually show obtuse rather than acute angles at their margins. Using these criteria, Woodring and Johnson[551] were able to correctly localize 99% of masses to the lung, pleura, or mediastinum.

Because the choice of likely diagnoses depends on the age of the patient; the position, shape, size, density, and intensity of any mass; and the number of masses, the radiologist must construct a mental grid incorporating all these items.

Traditionally mediastinal masses have been divided by their location and then subdivided according to their other radiographic features. These divisions are used in the following discussion, but some general points about age, density and signal intensity, and multiplicity are relevant whatever the site of the mass:

1. Malignant lymphoma, benign thymic enlargement, germ cell tumors and teratomas, foregut cysts, and the ganglion cell range of neurogenic tumors make up 80% of mediastinal masses in children.[331] In adults, lymphoma, metastatic carcinoma to lymph nodes, intrathoracic thyroid, thymoma, neurofibroma, aortic aneurysms, germ cell tumors, and foregut cysts are the prime considerations.

2. On CT, higher attenuation of a mass than of muscle before contrast enhancement may be caused by calcium deposition, high iodine content (indicating thyroid tissue or previous lymphography), or areas of acute hemorrhage within the mass.[176]

Irregular, granular, or eggshell calcification within multiple small mediastinal masses limits the differential diagnosis for practical purposes to lymphadenopathy caused by such benign conditions as granulomatous infections (tuberculosis and histoplasmosis are the most common and *Pneumocystis carinii* infection in patients with AIDS is an increasingly common cause), coal worker's pneumoconiosis, silicosis, and old sarcoidosis. Amyloidosis, treated lymphoma, metastasis, and Castleman's disease may be occasional causes. Calcification in a solitary mass has a wider differential diagnosis. Neural tumors may calcify, as may thymoma and germ cell tumors, and solitary nodules in the thyroid frequently show calcification. Curvilinear calcification is also seen in the walls of congenital cystic lesions, notably cystic teratoma, and in bronchogenic, pericardial, and foregut duplication cysts. The important practical point here is that untreated lymphoma or untreated metastatic neoplasm in lymph nodes almost never results in calcification.

Aneurysms of the aorta or its major branches frequently show curvilinear calcification in their walls or in thrombus lining the aneurysm. This calcification allows a confident distinction to be made between aneurysms and other causes of mediastinal mass, when taken with the observations that aneurysms always arise from and are in intimate contact with the aorta or one of its branches, and that they almost always have blood swirling within them.

3. Uniform water density in a mass with a thin wall of uniform thickness at CT suggests the presence of a congenital cyst, superior pericardial recess, meningocele, or cystic hygroma. A precise diagnosis depends on the size and location of the mass. Variable density within a mass, even including some regions of less than 10 HU, may be seen in necrotic malignant neoplasms and abscesses and in benign masses that undergo cyst formation, such as thyroid and thymic masses. Therefore the low density of a mass can be used to diagnose a true cyst only if all the preceding criteria are met. Thickness or irregularity of the wall and variability in the density of the remainder of the mass mean that more sinister lesions must be included in the differential diagnosis.[177]

Attenuation, lower than that of muscle but higher than that of water, is seen in some neural tumors.

4. Fat density within a mass limits the diagnostic possibilities to collections of normal fat, such as epicardial fat pads, lipomatosis, and herniated abdominal fat; lipomas, lipoblastomas, and liposarcomas; extramedullary hematopoiesis; fat in cystic teratomas or thymolipoma; and fatty replacement within lymph nodes.[178] A fat-fluid level within a cystic mass is pathognomonic of benign cystic teratoma. Benign lipomas and thymolipomas are composed entirely of fat, containing a few thin strands of soft tissue stroma. Liposarcoma usually shows fat intermingled with masses of soft tissue density.

5. Intravenous contrast enhancement may show opacification of a portion of the mass at CT, particularly opacification of the lumen of an aneurysm or enhancement of the soft tissue component of the mass. Minor degrees of enhancement of the soft tissue component of the mass are nonspecific, but marked enhancement[475] suggests thyroid tissue; a paraganglioma, including pheochromocytoma; a neurogenic tumor; vascular malformations; or the rare conditions Castleman's disease and aggressive fibromatosis. Thyroid tissue shows higher attenuation than the other soft tissues even before contrast administration and enhances brightly after contrast is given.

6. Multiple small masses within the mediastinum are almost specific for lymphadenopathy, particularly if they are concentrated in the node-bearing areas. The nodes may be physically isolated from one another or form conglomerate masses; in the latter, they usually have lobular outlines. Lobulation of a single mass, although frequently seen with lymphadenopathy, is not specific for any one type of mediastinal mass.

7. At MRI, most mediastinal masses show low signal on T1-weighted images and high signal on T2-weighted images. Fat and subacute hemorrhage show substantially higher signal than muscle on T1-weighted images,[17] but the differential diagnosis of masses with high signal areas on T1-weighted images is wide because a large variety of primary and secondary tumors occasionally show such high signal even if they do not contain fat or recent hemorrhage. Barakos and co-workers[17] reported 20 patients with mediastinal masses containing areas of high signal intensity on T1-weighted images (greater than 70% of signal seen in fat). These diagnoses included neurogenic tumor, lipoma, teratoma, bronchogenic cyst, lymphangioma, pheochromocytoma, carcinoid tumor, and a variety of primary and secondary carcinomas. In some the high signal is explained by fat or recent hemorrhage, in others by myxoid degeneration or collections of cells with high cytoplasmic to nuclear ratios, but the reason for the shortened T1 is not always clear. MRI signal intensity can be helpful but must be used with great care when limiting the differential diagnosis of a mediastinal mass.

Masses anterior to the ascending aorta and the arteries arising from the aortic arch

Almost all masses anterior to the ascending aorta and the arteries arising from the aortic arch are thyroid masses, thymic masses, germ cell tumors or cysts, or lymphadenopathy. Thyroid masses usually can be specifically diagnosed or excluded based on their contiguity with the thyroid gland in the neck and their high CT density on both contrast-enhanced and non-contrast-enhanced scans. In addition, many show cystic areas close to water density, as well as one or more areas of discrete calcification. Any mass located superiorly in the anterior mediastinum that causes focal deviation of the trachea is likely to be of thyroid origin. Exceptions to this rule are relatively rare although they are well recognized. Thymic masses and germ cell tumors can be grouped together because most germ cell tumors arise within the thymus. Clinical and laboratory features may help distinguish between the two. For example, myasthenia gravis, red blood cell aplasia, and hypogammaglobulinemia are associated with thymoma, whereas high alpha fetoprotein or high HCG levels may be seen with malignant germ cell tumors. If a pleural mass is associated, transpleural spread of thymoma becomes a strong possibility. If fat, cartilage calcification, or teeth are present in the mass, teratoma is the diagnosis.

Rarer causes of masses anterior to the aorta and the branches of the aortic arch are parathyroid adenoma, lymphangioma (cystic hygroma), pericardial cyst, aortic body paraganglioma, lipoma and liposarcoma or other mesenchymal tumors, and aneurysms. (Aneurysms are extremely rare in this location and are likely to be congenital or mycotic in origin.) Many of these masses have features that permit a specific diagnosis to be made. Parathyroid adenomas are usually associated with hyperparathyroidism and are discovered during a search for an ectopic parathyroid. Lymphangiomas almost always have broad contact with the root of the neck, and because they are composed largely of lymph-filled spaces, show numerous areas of nonenhancing, water or near water density on CT scanning. Cystic hygroma should be a serious consideration for an anteriorly located mass in contact with the neck in a child. Lipomas may be indistinguishable from normal fat collections but are readily distinguished from more significant mediastinal masses. Liposarcomas show a unique mixture of fat interspersed with irregular strands or masses of soft tissue density. Aneurysms show contrast opacification of their lumens. Pericardial cysts are generally of uniform water density with a thin, uniform thickness wall, and they need be considered only when the mass in question is in contact with the pericardium. It should be remembered, however, that the pericardium extends to the level of the junction point between the proximal and middle thirds of the ascending aorta. Mesenchymal tumors such as fibrosarcomas or blood vessel tumors have no distinguishing features.

Paracardiac masses

The likely diagnoses for paracardiac masses in contact with the diaphragm are pericardial cyst, diaphragmatic hernia, fat pad, or lymphadenopathy. If the mass is separated from the diaphragm, the likely differential diagnoses widen to include germ cell, mesenchymal and pericardial tumors, and thymic masses. Approximately 20% of thymomas are found in a paracardiac location, although contact with the diaphragm is unusual. Lack of connection with the diaphragm eliminates the possibility of a diaphragmatic hernia.

Most paracardiac masses are in the cardiophrenic angles; the right cardiophrenic angle is more often the site of a mass than the left because pericardial cysts are more often right-sided than left-sided and because foramen of Morgagni hernias can occur on the right but are usually prevented on the left by the presence of the heart. CT has proved extremely helpful in the diagnosis of paracardiac masses. Most pericardial cysts can be diagnosed by their uniform low density and their thin walls. Morgagni hernias are recognized by the omental fat within the hernia and sometimes by opacified bowel either within the mass or leading to it. Thus diagnostic difficulty is confined to distinguishing thymic tumor, germ cell tumor, localized lymphadenopathy, or mesenchymal tumor. Biopsy is appropriate for all these lesions.

Paratracheal, subcarinal, and paraesophageal masses

Paratracheal, subcarinal, and paraesophageal sites are considered together because the trachea, central bronchi, and esophagus are contained within a common fascial sheath. This compartment continues into the neck around the airway, esophagus, and pharynx. The prime considerations for nonvascular masses in these locations are lymphadenopathy, intrathoracic thyroid mass, developmental foregut cysts, esophageal tumors, hiatus hernia, and paraspinal masses encroaching on the middle mediastinum. Lymphadenopathy has by far the greatest incidence. Masses beneath the azygos vein in either the right paratracheal area or the pretracheal or precarinal space are almost invariably lymphadenopathy. For masses arising in the aortopulmonary window the only alternative is aortic aneurysm, which can be readily confirmed or excluded with contrast-enhanced CT. As mentioned earlier, lymphadenopathy is frequently multifocal, and in the case of metastatic carcinoma the primary tumor usually is already known. Bronchogenic cyst can be diagnosed with confidence if the criteria for a simple cyst are met. Many bronchogenic cysts, however, do not show the diagnostic features of uniform low density and these therefore are included in the differential diagnosis of a single mass of lymph nodes.[329] The presence of curvilinear calcification in the wall of the cyst, although a rare sign, makes the distinction between bronchogenic cyst and untreated malignant lymphadenopathy possible. Thyroid masses that pass laterally to or posteriorly to the trachea are distinctive, partly because of the signs already described but also because thyroid masses show far greater contact, displacement, and compression of the trachea than do lymph nodes. Splitting of the trachea from the esophagus is a characteristic shared only by thyroid masses, bronchogenic cysts, esophageal tumors, and an aberrant origin of the left pulmonary artery. Aortic arch anomalies, although they deform the trachea and esophagus in various ways, do not pass between these two structures.

Esophageal tumors very rarely occur as an asymptomatic mediastinal mass. Patients with esophageal carcinoma, the most common esophageal tumor, nearly always experience dysphagia when the tumor mass is relatively small. Although the tumor can sometimes be seen as a mass on plain chest radiographs and can nearly always be recognized at CT, the diagnosis of esophageal carcinoma is made at barium swallow examination and is not part of the differential diagnosis of a mediastinal mass. Leiomyoma or other mesenchymal tumors of the muscle layer may grow to a considerable size without causing dysphagia and may occasionally be seen as a mediastinal mass at plain chest radiography or CT scanning. The intimate relationship to the esophagus leads to a barium swallow examination, at which time the typical features of an intramural-extramucosal esophageal mass limit the diagnosis to leiomyoma, leiomyosarcoma, or rarely some other tumor or cyst of the esophageal wall.

Hiatus hernia is a common cause of enlargement of the mediastinum in the region of the lower esophagus. The plain film diagnosis is so easy and reliable that barium swallow is rarely required for diagnosis.

As discussed on p. 793, a number of vascular anomalies may mimic a mediastinal mass on plain chest radiographs and sometimes even on CT scans.

Paravertebral masses

Masses on either side of the vertebral column are outside the mediastinum because according to anatomists' definitions, the mediastinum lies anterior to the spine. However, standard practice among radiologists and thoracic surgeons labels all masses against the spine as posterior mediastinal masses.

Neurogenic lesions and neoplastic lymphadenopathy dominate the differential diagnosis for paraspinal masses. Neurogenic lesions consist of nerve sheath tumors (schwannoma, neurofibroma, and their malignant counterparts); ganglion cell tumors (ganglioneuroma, ganglioneuroblastoma, and neuroblastoma); paragangliomas, including pheochromocytoma; lateral thoracic meningoceles; and neuroenteric cysts. Lymphadenopathy is rarely confined to the paraspinal areas; usually it is accompanied by enlarged lymph nodes in adjacent mediastinal or retroperitoneal areas. The most common causes of posterior mediastinal lymph node enlargement are lymphoma and metastatic carcinoma from genitourinary primary tumors. Other, less common causes of paraspinal masses

include metastases from other sites; extramedullary hemopoiesis; pancreatic pseudocyst; mesenchymal tumors such as lipoma, fibroma, and hemangioma; and lesions arising from the esophagus, pharynx, spine, or aorta. The esophageal or pharyngeal lesions that may project posteriorly include leiomyoma, foregut cyst, and congenital or acquired diverticula of the esophagus. The spinal origin of lesions such as paraspinal abscess, tumors of the vertebral body that have spread into the adjacent paravertebral or mediastinal space, or hematoma from trauma to the spine is usually readily recognized by observing corresponding changes in the spine. Aneurysms of the descending aorta truly mimicking a mediastinal mass are uncommon. Most large aneurysms in this location are obvious dilatations of the descending aorta. Saccular aneurysms that could be confused with a mass show a broad base on the aorta and almost always have curvilinear calcification in their walls. The diagnosis is easily made at CT when opacification of the lumen can be demonstrated. Most contain thrombus within the aneurysm, but not enough to obliterate the lumen totally.

REFERENCES

1. Aalbers R, Piers B, Eygelaar A, et al: Sudden superior mediastinal enlargement, *Chest* 99:209-210, 1991.
2. Aalbers R, van dam Jagt E, Poppema S, et al: Left paravertebral mass, *Chest* 91:889-890, 1987.
3. Aberle DR, Gamsu G, Lynch D: Thoracic manifestations of Wegener's granulomatosis: diagnosis and course, *Radiology* 174:703-709, 1990.
4. Abildgaard A, Lien HH, Fossa SD, et al: Enlargement of the thymus following chemotherapy for non-seminomatous testicular cancer, *Acta Radiol* 30:259-262, 1989.
5. Ablin DS, Reinhart MA: Esophageal perforation with mediastinal abscess in child abuse, *Pediatr Radiol* 20:524-525, 1990.
6. Abramson SJ, Berdon WER, Reilly BJ, et al: Cavitation of anterior mediastinal masses in children with histiocytosis X: report of four cases with radiographic pathologic and clinical follow-up, *Pediatr Radiol* 17:10-14, 1987.
7. Aisner SC, Chakravarthy AK, Joslyn JN, et al: Bilateral granular cell tumors of the posterior mediastinum, *Ann Thorac Surg* 46:688-689, 1988.
8. Allen PW: The fibromatoses: a clinicopathologic classification based on 140 cases, Part I, *Am J Surg Pathol* 1:255-270, 1977.
9. Alterman K, Shueller EF: Maturation of neuroblastoma to ganglioneuroma, *Am J Dis Child* 120:217-222, 1970.
10. Angtuaco EJC, Jimenez JF, Burrows P, et al: Lymphatic-venous malformation (lymphangiohemangioma) of mediastinum: case report, *J Comput Assist Tomogr* 7:895-897, 1983.
11. Appelbaum A, Karp RB, Kirklin JW: Ascending vs descending aortic dissection, *Ann Surg* 183:296-300, 1976.
12. Armstrong EA, Harwood-Nash DCF, Ritz CR, et al: CT of neuroblastomas and ganglioneuromas in children, *AJR* 139:571-576, 1982.
13. Armstrong P: Tomographic evaluation of the questionably enlarged pulmonary hilum. In Armstrong P, ed: *Critical problems in diagnostic radiology*, Philadelphia, 1983, JB Lippincott.
14. Asfoura JY, Vidt DG: Acute aortic dissection, *Chest* 99:724-729, 1991.
15. Baker HL, Berquist TH, Kispert DB, et al: Magnetic resonance imaging in a routine clinical setting, *Mayo Clin Proc* 60:75-90, 1985.

16. Banzo J, Prats E, Velilla J, et al: Functioning intrapericardial paraganglioma diagnosed by I-123 MIBG imaging, *Clin Nucl Med* 16:860-861, 1991.

17. Barakos JA, Brown JJ, Brescia RJ, et al: High signal intensity lesions of the chest in MR imaging, *J Comput Assist Tomogr* 13:797-802, 1989.

18. Barek L, Lautin R, Ledor S, et al: Role of CT in the assessment of superior vena caval obstruction: CT, *J Comput Tomogr* 6:121-126, 1982.

19. Barentz JO, Rujis JHJ, Heystarten JMJ, et al: Magnetic resonance imaging of the dissected thoracic aorta, *Br J Radiol* 60:499-502, 1987.

20. Barnett SM: CT findings in tuberculous mediastinitis, *J Comput Assist Tomogr* 10:165-166, 1986.

21. Baron MG: Dissecting aneurysm of the aorta, *Circulation* 63:933-943, 1971.

22. Baron RL, Lee JKT, Sagel SS, et al: Computed tomography of the abnormal thymus, *Radiology* 142:127-134, 1982.

23. Baron RL, Sagel SS, Baglan RJ: Thymic cysts following radiation therapy for Hodgkin's disease, *Radiology* 141:593-597, 1981.

24. Barrett AF, Toye DKM: Sympathicoblastoma: radiological findings in forty-three cases, *Clin Radiol* 14:33-42, 1963.

25. Barrick B, O'Kell RT: Thymic cysts and remnant cervical thymus, *J Pediatr Surg* 4:355-358, 1969.

26. Bartra P, Herrmann C, Mulder D: Mediastinal imaging in myasthemia gravis: correlations of chest radiography, CT, MR, and surgical findings, *AJR* 148:515-519, 1987.

27. Bar-Ziv J, Nogrady MB: Mediastinal neuroblastoma and ganglioneuroma, *AJR* 125:380-390, 1975.

28. Bashist B, Ellis K, Gold RP: Computed tomography of intrathoracic goiter, *AJR* 140:455-460, 1983.

29. Batata MA, Martini N, Huvos AG, et al: Thymomas: clinicopathologic features, therapy and prognosis, *Cancer* 34:389-396, 1974.

30. Bechtold RE, Wolfman NT, Karstaedt N, et al: Superior vena caval obstruction: detection using CT, *Radiology* 157:485-487, 1985.

31. Bedros AA, Munson J, Toomey FE: Hemangioendothelioma presenting as posterior mediastinal mass in a child, *Cancer* 46:801-803, 1980.

32. Beerman PJ, Gelfand DW, Ott DJ: Pneumomediastinum after double-contrast barium enema examination: a sign of colonic perforation, *AJR* 136:197-198, 1981.

33. Bein ME, Mancuso AA, Mink JH, et al: Computed tomography in the evaluation of mediastinal lipomatosis, *J Comput Assist Tomogr* 2:379-383, 1978.

34. Benjamin SP, McCormack LJ, Effler DB, et al: Primary tumors of the mediastinum, *Chest* 62:297-303, 1972.

35. Bergh NP, Gatzinsky P, Larsson S, et al: Tumors of the thymic region. 1. Clinicopathological studies on thymomas, *Ann Thorac Surg* 25:91-98, 1978.

36. Bethancourt B, Pond GD, Jones SE, et al: Mediastinal hematoma simulating recurrent Hodgkin disease during systemic chemotherapy, *AJR* 142:1119-1120, 1984.

37. Bill AH, Sumner DS: A unified concept of lymphangioma and cystic hygroma, *Surg Gynecol Obstet* 120:79-86, 1965.

38. Binder RE, Pugatch RD, Faling J, et al: Diagnosis of posterior mediastinal goiter by computer tomography, *J Comput Assist Tomogr* 4:550-552, 1980.

39. Black WC, Armstrong P, Daniel TM, et al: Computed tomography of aggressive fibromatosis in the posterior mediastinum, *J Comput Assist Tomogr* 11:153-155, 1987.

40. Black WC, Burke JW, Feldman PS, et al: CT appearance of cervical lipoblastoma, *J Comput Assist Tomogr* 10:696-698, 1986.

41. Blandino A, Salvi L, Faranda C, et al: Unusual malignant paraganglioma of the anterior mediastinum: CT and MR findings, *Eur J Radiol* 15:1-3, 1992.

42. Blank N, Castellino RA: Patterns of pleural reflections of the left superior mediastinum: normal anatomy and distributions produced by lymphadenopathy, *Radiology* 102:585-589, 1972.

43. Blewett JH, Szypulski JT: Double unilateral intrathoracic meningocele: report of a case, *J Thorac Cardiovasc Surg* 67:481-483, 1974.

44. Blomlie V, Lien HH, Fossa SD: Computed tomography in primary non-seminomatous germ cell tumors of the mediastinum, *Acta Radiol* 29:289-292, 1988.

45. Blunt SB, Sandler LM, Burrin JM, et al: An evaluation of the distinction of ectopic and pituitary ACTH dependent Cushing's syndrome by clinical features, biochemical tests and radiological findings, *Q J Med* 77:1113-1133, 1990.

46. Boothroyd AE, Hall-Craggs MA, Dicks-Mireaux C, et al: The magnetic resonance appearances of the normal thymus in children, *Clin Radiol* 45:378-381, 1992.

47. Boyd DP, Midell AI: Mediastinal cysts and tumors: an analysis of 96 cases, *Surg Clin North Am* 48:493-505, 1968.

48. Bradley WG: MR appearance of hemorrhage in the brain, *Radiology* 189:15-26, 1993.

49. Brambilla E, Fontaine E, Pison CM, et al: Pulmonary histiocytosis X with mediastinal lymph node involvement, *Am Rev Respir Dis* 142:1216-1218, 1990.

50. Breatnach E, Nath PH, Delany DJ: The role of computed tomography in acute and subacute mediastinitis, *Clin Radiol* 37:139-145, 1986.

51. Brown G, Husband JE: Mediastinal widening—a valuable radiographic sign of superior vena caval thrombosis, *Clin Radiol* 47:415-420, 1993.

52. Brown LR, Aughenbaugh GL: Masses of the anterior mediastinum: CT and MR imaging, *AJR* 157:1171-1180, 1991.

53. Brown LR, Aughenbaugh GL, Wick MR, et al: Roentgenologic diagnosis of primary corticotropin-producing carcinoid tumors of the mediastinum, *Radiology* 142:143-148, 1982.

54. Brown LR, Muhm JR, Aughenbaugh GL, et al: Computed tomography of benign mature teratomas of the mediastinum, *J Thorac Imag* 2(2):66-71, 1987.

55. Brown LR, Muhm JR, Sheedy PF, et al: The value of computed tomography in myasthenia gravis, *AJR* 140:31-35, 1983.

56. Brown LR, Reiman HM, Rosenow EC, et al: Intrathoracic lymphangioma, *Mayo Clin Proc* 61:882-892, 1986.

57. Brunner DR, Whitley NO: A pericardial cyst with high CT numbers, *AJR* 142:279-280, 1984.

58. Bryk D: Venous compression and obstruction by intrathoracic goiter, *J Can Assoc Radiol* 25:300-302, 1974.

59. Buirski G, Jordan SC, Joffe HS, et al: Superior vena caval abnormalities: their occurrence rate, associated cardiac abnormalities and angiographic classification in a paediatric population with congenital heart disease, *Clin Radiol* 37:131-138, 1986.

60. Burk DL, Brunberg JA, Kanal E, et al: Spinal and paraspinal neurofibromatosis: surface coil MR imaging at 1.5 T, *Radiology* 162:797-801, 1987.

61. Burnett CM, Rosemurgy AS, Pfeiffer EA: Life-threatening acute posterior mediastinitis due to esophageal perforation, *Ann Thorac Surg* 49:979-983, 1990.

62. Burns MA, Molina PL, Gutierrez FR, et al: Motion artifact simulating aortic dissection on CT, *AJR* 157:465-467, 1991.

63. Caffey J, Silbey R: Regrowth and overgrowth of the thymus after atrophy induced by the oral administration of adrenocorticosteroids to human infants, *Pediatrics* 26:762-770, 1960.

64. Carey LS, Ellis FH, Good CA, et al: Neurogenic tumors of the mediastinum: a clinicopathologic study, *AJR* 84:189-205, 1960.

65. Carlson RG, Lillehei CW, Edwards JE: Cystic medial necrosis of the ascending aorta in relation to age and hypertension, *Am J Cardiol* 25:411-415, 1970.

66. Caro PA, Mahboubi S, Faerber EN: Computed tomography in the diagnosis of lymphangiomas in infants and children, *Clin Imag* 15:41-46, 1991.

67. Carrol CL, Jeffrey RB, Federle MP, et al: CT evaluation of mediastinal infections, *J Comput Assist Tomogr* 11:449-454, 1989.

68. Carter AR, Sostman HD, Curtis AM, et al: Thoracic alterations after cardiac surgery, *AJR* 140:475-481, 1983.

69. Carter MM, Tarr RW, Mazer MJ, et al: The "aortic nipple" as a sign of impending superior vena caval syndrome, *Chest* 87:775-777, 1985.

70. Carty H: Ultrasound of the normal thymus in the infant: a simple method of resolving a clinical dilemma, *Br J Radiol* 63:737-738, 1990.

71. Casillas J, Sais GJ, Greve JL, et al: Imaging of intra- and extraabdominal desmoid tumours, *Radiographics* 11:959-968, 1991.

72. Castleman B, Iverson L, Menendez VP: Localized mediastinal lymph node hyperplasia resembling thymoma, *Cancer* 9:822-830, 1956.

73. Casullo J, Palayew MJ, Lisbona A: General case of the day, *Radiographics* 12:1250-1254, 1992.

74. Chalaoui J, Samson L, Rubillard P, et al: General case of the day, *Radiographics* 10:957-958, 1990.

75. Chalmers AH, Armstrong P: Plexiform mediastinal neurofibromas: a report of two cases, *Br J Radiol* 50:215-217, 1977.

76. Charig MJ: Case report: mediastinal Castleman's disease; a missed pre-operative diagnosis? *Clin Radiol* 42:440-442, 1990.

77. Chen J, Weisbroad GL, Herman SJ: Computed tomography and pathologic correlations of thymic lesions, *J Thorac Imag* 3(1):61-65, 1988.

78. Chen KTK: Multicentric Castleman's disease and Kaposi's sarcoma, *Am J Surg Pathol* 8:287-293, 1984.

79. Chertoff J, Barth RA, Dickerman JD: Rebound thymic hyperplasia five years after chemotherapy for Wilms' tumor, *Pediatr Radiol* 21:596-597, 1991.

80. Chew FS, Weissleder R: Mediastinal thymolipoma, *AJR* 157:468, 1991.

81. Choyke PL, Zeman RK, Gootenberg JE, et al: Thymic atrophy and regrowth in response to chemotherapy: CT evaluation, *AJR* 149:269-272, 1987.

82. Christoforidis AJ: Radiologic manifestations of histoplasmosis, *AJR* 109:478-490, 1970.

83. Cigarroa JE, Isselbacher EM, De Sanctis RW, et al: Medical progress: diagnostic imaging in the evaluation of suspected aortic dissection: old standards and new directions, *AJR* 161:485-493, 1993.

84. Cohen AJ, Sbaschnig RJ, Hochholzer L, et al: Mediastinal hemangiomas, *Ann Thorac Surg* 43:656-659, 1987.

85. Cohen AJ, Thompson LN, Edwards FH, et al: Primary cysts and tumors of the mediastinum, *Ann Thorac Surg* 51:378-386, 1991.

86. Cohen AM, Creviston S, Lipuma JP, et al: NMR evaluation of hilar and mediastinal lymphadenopathy, *Radiology* 148:739-742, 1983.

87. Cohen AM, Cunat JS: Giant esophageal leiomyoma as a mediastinal mass, *J Can Assoc Radiol* 32:129-130, 1981.

88. Cohen LM, Schwartz AM, Rockoff SD: Benign schwannomas: pathologic basis for CT inhomogeneities, *AJR* 147:141-143, 1986.

89. Cohen M, Hill CA, Cangir A, et al: Thymic rebound after treatment of childhood tumors, *AJR* 135:151-156, 1980.

90. Coleman BG, Arger PH, Dalinka MK, et al: CT of sarcomatous degeneration in neurofibromatosis, *AJR* 140:383-387, 1983.

91. Coltart RS, Wraught EP: The value of radionuclide venography in superior vena caval obstruction, *Clin Radiol* 36:415-418, 1985.

92. Connell JV, Muhm JR: Radiographic manifestations of histoplasmosis: a 10 year review, *Radiology* 121:281-285, 1976.

93. Cooke JP, Kazmier FJ, Orszulak TA: The penetrating aortic ulcer: pathologic manifestations, diagnosis, and management, *Mayo Clin Proc* 63:718-725, 1988.

94. Cooper GN, Narodick BG: Posterior mediastinal thymoma, *J Thorac Cardiovasc Surg* 63:561-563, 1972.

95. Cornford EJ, Wastie ML, Morgan DAL: Malignant paraganglioma of the mediastinum: a further diagnostic and therapeutic use of radiolabelled mIBG, *Br J Radiol* 65:75-78, 1992.

96. Costello P, Ecker CP, Tello R, et al: Assessment of the thoracic aorta by spiral CT, *AJR* 158:1127-1130, 1992.

97. Cox JD: Primary malignant germ cell tumors of the mediastinum, *Cancer* 36:1162-1168, 1975.

98. Cramer M, Foley WD, Palmer TE, et al: Compression of the right pulmonary artery by aortic aneurysms: CT demonstration, *J Comput Assist Tomogr* 9:310-314, 1985.

99. Crawford ES: The diagnosis and management of aortic dissection, *JAMA* 264:2537-2541, 1990.

100. Crylak D, Milne ENC, Imray TJ: Pneumomediastinum: a diagnostic problem, *Crit Rev Diagn Imag* 23:75-117, 1984.

101. Daily PO, Trueblood HW, Stinson EB, et al: Management of acute aortic dissections, *Ann Thorac Surg* 10:237-247, 1970.

102. Daly BD, Leung SF, Cheung H, et al: Thoracic metastases from carcinoma of the nasopharynx: high frequency of hilar and mediastinal lymphadenopathy, *AJR* 160:241-244, 1993.

103. Daniel TM, Staub EW, Clark DE: Symptomatic venous compression from a mediastinal cystic lymphangioma, *Chest* 63:834-835, 1973.

104. Davis J, Mark G, Green R: Benign blood vascular tumors of the mediastinum: report of four cases and review of the literature, *Radiology* 126:581-587, 1987.

105. DeBakey ME, Henly WS, Cooley DA, et al: Surgical management of dissecting aneurysms of the aorta, *J Thorac Cardiovasc Surg* 49:130-149, 1965.

106. Dee P, Granato JE, Gibson RS: The CT and ultrasound diagnosis of aortic dissection, *Semin Ultrasound CT MR* 6:146-155, 1985.

107. Dee P, Martin R, Oudkerk M, et al: The diagnosis of aortic dissection, *Curr Probl Diagn Radiol* 12:8-55, 1983.

108. Demos TC, Budorick NE, Posniak HV: Benign mediastinal cysts: pointed appearance on CT, *J Comput Assist Tomogr* 13:132-133, 1989.

109. Demos TC, Posniak HV, Churchill RJ: Detection of intimal flap of aortic dissection on unenhanced CT images, *AJR* 146:601-603, 1986.

110. Demos TC, Posniak HV, Marsan RE: CT of aortic dissection, *Semin Roentgenol* 24:22-37, 1989.

111. Dines DE, Payne WS, Bernatz PE, et al: Mediastinal granuloma and fibrosing mediastinitis, *Chest* 75:320-324, 1979.

112. Dobranowski J, Martin LFW, Bennett WF: CT evaluation of posterior mediastinal teratoma, *J Comput Assist Tomogr* 11:156-157, 1987.

113. Doppman JL, Krudy AG, Masx SJ, et al: Aspiration of enlarged parathyroid glands for parathyroid hormone assay, *Radiology* 148:31-35, 1983.

114. Doppman JL, Nieman L, Miller DL, et al: Ectopic adrenocorticotropic hormone syndrome: localization studies in 28 patients, *Radiology* 172:115-124, 1989.

115. Doppman JL, Oldfield EH, Chrousos CP, et al: Rebound thymic hyperplasia after treatment for Cushing's syndrome, *AJR* 147:1145-1147, 1986.

116. Drent M, Gelissen J-P, Ascoop CAPL, et al: Mediastinal lymph node enlargement as a result of mitral valve stenosis, *Chest* 102:1269-1271, 1992.

117. Due W, Dieckmann KP, Stein H: Thymic hyperplasia following chemotherapy of a testicular germ cell tumor: immunohistological evidence for a simple rebound phenomenon, *Cancer* 63:446-449, 1989.

118. Duke RA, Barrett MR, Payne SD, et al: Compression of left main bronchus and left pulmonary artery by thoracic aortic aneurysm, *AJR* 149:261-263, 1987.

119. Dyer NH: Cystic thymomas and thymic cysts: a review, *Thorax* 22:408-421, 1967.

120. Dyke PC, Mulkey DA: Maturation of ganglioneuroblastoma to ganglioneuroma, *Cancer* 20:1343-1349, 1967.

121. Earnest F, Muhm JR, Sheedy PF: Roentgenographic findings in thoracic aortic dissection, *Mayo Clin Proc* 54:43-50, 1979.

122. Economopoulos GC, Lewis JW, Lee MW, et al: Carcinoid tumors of the thymus, *Ann Thorac Surg* 50:58-61, 1990.

123. Edeiken J, Lee KF, Libshitz H: Intrathoracic meningocele, *AJR* 106:381-384, 1969.

124. Edwards JE: Manifestations of acquired and congenital diseases of the aorta, *Curr Probl Cardiol* 3:7-62, 1979.

125. Egan TJ, Neiman HL, Herman RJ, et al: Computed tomography in the diagnosis of aortic aneurysm dissection or traumatic injury, *Radiology* 136:141-146, 1980.

126. Eklof O, Gooding CA: Intrathoracic neuroblastoma, *AJR* 100:202-207, 1967.

127. Ellis K, Austin JHM, Jaretzki A: Radiologic detection of thymoma in patients with myasthenia gravis, *AJR* 151:873-881, 1988.

128. Ellis K, Gregg HE: Thymomas: Roentgen considerations, *AJR* 91:105-119, 1964.

129. Ellison RT, Corrao WM, Fox MJ, et al: Spontaneous mediastinal hemorrhage in patients on chronic hemodialysis, *Ann Intern Med* 95:704-706, 1981.

130. Enzi G, Biondetti PR, Fiore D, et al: Computed tomography of deep fat masses in multiple symmetrical lipomatosis, *Radiology* 144:121-124, 1982.

131. Erbel R, Borner N, Steller D, et al: Detection of aortic dissection by transesophageal echocardiography, *Br Heart J* 58:45-51, 1987.

132. Erbel R, Engberding R, Daniel W, et al: Echocardiography in diagnosis of aortic dissection, *Lancet* 4:457-460, 1989.

133. Eyler WR, Clark MD: Dissecting aneurysms of the aorta: Roentgen manifestations including a comparison with other types of aneurysms, *Radiology* 85:1047-1057, 1965.

134. Faerber EN, Balsara RK, Schidlow DV, et al: Thymolipoma: computed tomographic appearances, *Pediatr Radiol* 20:196-197, 1990.

135. Faerber EN, Carter BL, Sarno RC, et al: Computed tomography of neuroblastic tumors in children, *Clin Pediatr* 23:17-21, 1984.

136. Falor WH, Kelly TR, Krabill WS: Intrathoracic goiter, *Ann Surg* 142:238-247, 1955.

137. Farmer DW, Moore E, Amparo E, et al: Calcific fibrosing mediastinitis: demonstration of pulmonary vascular obstruction by magnetic resonance imaging, *AJR* 143:1189-1191, 1984.

138. Federici S, Cuoghi D, Sciutti R: Benign mediastinal lipoblastoma in a 14-month-old infant, *Pediatr Radiol* 22:150-151, 1992.

139. Federle MP, Callen PW: Cystic Hodgkin's lymphoma of the thymus: computed tomographic appearance, *J Comput Assist Tomogr* 3:542-544, 1979.

140. Feigin DS; Eggleston JC, Siegelman SS: The multiple roentgen manifestations of sclerosing mediastinitis, *Johns Hopkins Med J* 144:8, 1979.

141. Feigin DS, Fenoglio JJ, McAllister HA, et al: Pericardial cysts: a radiologic-pathologic correlation and review, *Radiology* 125:15-20, 1977.

142. Feigl D, Feigl A, Edwards JE: Mycotic aneurysms of the aortic root: a pathologic study of 20 cases, *Chest* 90:553-557, 1986.

143. Feinstein RS, Gatewood OMB, Fishman EK, et al: Computed tomography of adult neuroblastoma, *J Comput Assist Tomogr* 8:720-726, 1984.

144. Feutz EP, Yune HY, Mandelbaum I, et al: Intrathoracic cystic hygroma, *Radiology* 108:61-66, 1973.

145. Filler RM, Traggis DG, Jaffe N, et al: Favorable outlook for children with mediastinal neuroblastoma, *J Pediatr Surg* 7:136-143, 1972.

146. Findling JW, Tyrrell JB: Occult ectopic secretion of corticotropin, *Arch Intern Med* 146:929-933, 1986.

147. Fiore D, Biondetti PR, Calabro F, et al: CT demonstration of bilateral Castleman tumors in the mediastinum, *J Comput Assist Tomogr* 7:719-720, 1983.

148. FitzGerald JM, Mayo JR, Miller RR, et al: Tuberculosis of the thymus, *Chest* 102:1604-1605, 1992.

149. Fon GT, Bein ME, Mancuso AA, et al: Computed tomography of the anterior mediastinum in myasthenia gravis, *Radiology* 142:135-141, 1982.

150. Ford EG, Lockhart SK, Sullivan MP: Mediastinal mass following chemotherapeutic treatment of Hodgkin's disease: recurrent tumor or thymic hyperplasia? *J Pediatr Surg* 22:1155-1159, 1987.

151. Foulner D: Transient thymic calcification: association with rebound enlargement, *Clin Radiol* 44:428-429, 1991.

152. Fox MA, Lynch DA, Make BJ: Thymoma with hypogammaglobulinemia (Good's syndrome): an unusual case of bronchiectasis, *AJR* 158:1229-1230, 1992.

153. Francis IR, Glazer GM, Shapiro B, et al: Complementary roles of CT and ^{131}I-MIBG scintigraphy in diagnosing pheochromocytoma, *AJR* 141:719-725, 1983.

154. Franken EA: Radiologic evidence of thymic enlargement in Graves' disease, *Radiology* 91:20-22, 1969.

155. Friedman AC, Lautin E, Rothenberg L: Mach bands and pneumomediastinum, *J Can Assoc Radiol* 32:232-235, 1981.

156. Frizzera G, Banks PM, Massarelli G, et al: A systemic lymphoproliferative disorder with morphologic features of Castleman's disease, *Am J Surg Pathol* 7:211-231, 1983.

157. Fujiwara T: Pneumomediastinum in pulmonary fibrosis: detection by computed tomography, *Chest* 104:44-46, 1993.

158. Fulcher AS, Proto AV, Jolles H: Cystic teratoma of the mediastinum: demonstration of fat/fluid level, *AJR* 154:259-260, 1990.

159. Furman WL, Buckley PJ, Green AA, et al: Thymoma and myasthenia gravis in a 4-year-old child: case report and review of the literature, *Cancer* 56:2703-2706, 1985.

160. Gale AW, Jelihovsky T, Grant AF, et al: Neurogenic tumors of the mediastinum, *Ann Thorac Surg* 17:434-443, 1974.

161. Gale ME: Bochdalek hernia: Prevalence and CT characteristics, *Radiology* 156:449-452, 1985.

162. Gallagher S, Dixon AK: Streak artifacts of the thoracic aorta: pseudodissection, *J Comput Assist Tomogr* 8:688-693, 1984.

163. Gefter WB, Spritzer CE, Eisenberg B, et al: Thyroid imaging with high-field-strength surface-coil, *MR Radiol* 164:483-490, 1987.

164. Geisinger MA, Risius B, O'Donnell JA, et al: Thoracic aortic dissections: magnetic resonance imaging, *Radiology* 155:407-412, 1985.

165. Gelfand DW, Goldman AS, Law EJ: Thymic hyperplasia in children recovering from thermal burns, *J Trauma* 12:813-817, 1972.

166. Genereux GP, Howie JL: Normal mediastinal lymph node size and number: CT and anatomic study, *AJR* 142:1095-1100, 1984.

167. Gerald W, Kostianovsky M, Rosai J: Development of vascular neoplasia in Castleman's disease: report of seven cases, *Am J Pathol* 14:603-614, 1990.

168. Gibbons JA, Rosencrantz H, Posey DJ, et al: Angiofollicular lymphoid hyperplasia (Castleman's tumor) resembling a pericardial cyst: differentiation by computerized tomography, *Ann Thorac Surg* 32:193-196, 1981.

169. Girard DE, Carlson V, Natelson EA, et al: Pneumomediastinum in diabetic ketoacidosis: comments on mechanism, incidence, and management, *Chest* 60:455-459, 1971.

170. Glazer BH, Gross BH, Quint LE, et al: Normal mediastinal lymph nodes: number and size according to American Thoracic Society mapping, *AJR* 144:261-265, 1985.

171. Glazer GM, Axel L, Moss AA: CT diagnosis of mediastinal thyroid, *AJR* 138:495-498, 1982.

172. Glazer GM, Francis IR, Gebarski K, et al: Dynamic incremental computed tomography in the evaluation of the pulmonary hili, *J Comput Assist Tomogr* 7:59-64, 1983.

173. Glazer GM, Francis IR, Shirazi KK, et al: Evaluation of the pulmonary hilum: comparison of conventional radiography, 55° oblique tomography and dynamic computed tomography, *J Comput Assist Tomogr* 7:983-989, 1983.

174. Glazer GM, Gross BH, Francis IR, et al: Evaluation of the pulmonary hili. In Siegelman SS, ed: *Computed tomography of the chest*, New York, 1984, Churchill Livingstone.

175. Glazer HS, Aronberg DJ, Sagel SS: Pitfalls in CT recognition of mediastinal lymphadenopathy, *AJR* 144:267-274, 1985.

176. Glazer HS, Molina PL, Siegel MJ, et al: High-attenuation mediastinal masses on unenhanced CT, *AJR* 156:45-50, 1991.

177. Glazer HS, Siegel MJ, Sagel SS: Low-attenuation mediastinal masses on CT, *AJR* 152:1173-1177, 1989.

178. Glazer HS, Wick MR, Anderson DJ: CT of fatty thoracic masses, *AJR* 159:1181-1187, 1992.

179. Glickstein MF, Miller WT, Dalinka MK, et al: Paraspinal lipomatosis: a benign mass, *Radiology* 163:79-80, 1987.

180. Gobien RP, Stanley JH, Gobien BS, et al: Percutaneous catheter aspiration and drainage of suspected mediastinal abscesses, *Radiology* 151:69-71, 1984.

181. Godwin JD: Conventional CT of the aorta, *J Thorac Imag* 5(4):18-31, 1990.

182. Godwin JD, Breiman RS, Speckman JM: Problems and pitfalls in the evaluation of thoracic aortic dissection by computed tomography, *J Comput Assist Tomogr* 6:750-756, 1982.

183. Godwin JD, Herfkens RL, Skioldebrand CG, et al: Evaluation of dissections and aneurysms of the thoracic aorta by conventional and dynamic CT scanning, *Radiology* 136:125-133, 1980.

184. Goldman AJ, Herrmann C, Keesey JC, et al: Myasthenia gravis and invasive thymoma: a 20 year experience, *Neurology* 25:1021-1025, 1975.

185. Gomes AS, Lois JF, George B, et al: Congenital abnormalities of the aortic arch: MR imaging, *Radiology* 165:691-695, 1987.

186. Gomori JM, Grossman RI, Goldberg HI, et al: Intracranial hematomas: imaging by high field MR, *Radiology* 157:87-93, 1985.

187. Goodman LR, Kay HR, Teplick SK, et al: Complications of median sternotomy: computed tomographic evaluation, *AJR* 141:225-230, 1983.

188. Goodwin RA, Loyd JE, Des Prez RM: Histoplasmosis in normal hosts, *Medicine* 60:231-266, 1981.

189. Goodwin RA, Nickell JA, Des Prez RM: Mediastinal fibrosis complicating healed primary histoplasmosis and tuberculosis, *Medicine* 51:227-246, 1972.

190. Gorich J, Beyer-Enke SA, Schmitterckert H, et al: Pleural metastasis of malignant thymoma, a pitfall in the CT-diagnosis of pleural mesothelioma, *Comput Med Imag Graph* 13:169-170, 1989.

191. Gossios KJ, Guy RL: Case report: Imaging of widespread plexiform neurofibromatosis, *Clin Radiol* 47:211-213, 1993.

192. Gouliamos A, Striggaris K, Lolas C, et al: Thymic cyst, *J Comput Assist Tomogr* 6:172-174, 1982.

193. Graeber GM, Thompson LD, Ronnigen DL, et al: Cystic lesion of the thymus, *J Thorac Cardiovasc Surg* 87:295-300, 1984.

194. Granato JE, Dee P, Gibson RS: Utility of two-dimensional echocardiography in suspected ascending aortic dissection, *Am J Cardiol* 56:123-129, 1985.

195. Gray JM, Hanson GC: Mediastinal emphysema: aetiology, diagnosis, and treatment, *Thorax* 21:325-332, 1966.

196. Groskin SA, Massi AF, Randall PA: Calcified hilar and mediastinal lymph nodes in an AIDS patient with *Pneumocystis carinii* infection, *Radiology* 175:345-346, 1990.

197. Gross BH, Schneider HJ, Proto AV: Eggshell calcification of lymph nodes, *AJR* 135:1265-1268, 1980.

198. Gross SC, Barr I, Eyler WR, et al: Computed tomography in dissection of the thoracic aorta, *Radiology* 136:135-139, 1980.

199. Guit GL, Shaw PC, Ehrlich J, et al: Mediastinal lymphadenopathy and pulmonary arterial hypertension in mixed connective tissue disease, *Radiology* 154:305-306, 1985.

200. Gumbs RV, Higginbotham-Ford EA, Teal JS, et al: Thoracic extramedullary hematopoiesis in sickle-cell disease, *AJR* 149:889-893, 1987.

201. Gundry SR, Burney RE, Mackenzie JR, et al: Traumatic pseudoaneurysms of the thoracic aorta: anatomic and radiologic correlations, *Arch Surg* 119:1055-1060, 1984.

202. Gupta RK, Sharma BK, Jena A, et al: Primary mediastinal tuberculous abscess: demonstration with MR, *Pediatr Radiol* 19:330-332, 1989.

203. Haber S: Retroperitoneal and mediastinal chemodectoma: report of a case and review of the literature, *AJR* 92:1029-1041, 1964.

204. Hachiya J, Nitatori T, Yoshino A, et al: CT of calcified chronic aortic dissection simulating atherosclerotic aneurysm, *J Comput Assist Tomogr* 17:374-378, 1993.

205. Hall TS, Caslowitz P, Popper C, et al: Substernal goiter versus intrathoracic aberrant thyroid: a critical difference, *Ann Thorac Surg* 46:684-685, 1988.

206. Haller JO, Schneider M, Kassner EG, et al: Sonographic evaluation of the chest in infants and children, *AJR* 134:1019-1027, 1980.

207. Halliday DR, Dahlin DC, Pugh DG, et al: Massive osteolysis and angiomatosis, *Radiology* 82:637-643, 1964.

208. Hamada S, Takamiya M, Kimura K, et al: Type A aortic dissection: evaluation with ultrafast CT, *Radiology* 183:155-158, 1992.

209. Hammersley JR, Grum CM, Green RA: The correlation of subcarinal density visualized on plain chest roentgenograms with computed tomographic scans, *Chest* 97:869-872, 1990.

210. Han BK, Babcock DS, Oestreich AE: Normal thymus infancy: sonographic characteristics, *Radiology* 170:471-474, 1989.

211. Harnsberger HR, Datz FL, Knockel JQ, et al: Failure to detect extramedullary hematopoiesis during bone-marrow imaging with indium-111 or technetium-99m sulfur colloid, *J Nucl Med* 23:589-591, 1982.

212. Harper RAK, Guyer PB: The radiological features of thymic tumours: a review of sixty-five cases, *Clin Radiol* 16:97-100, 1965.

213. Hashimoto S, Kumada T, Osakada G, et al: Assessment of transesophageal Doppler echography in dissecting aortic aneurysm, *J Am Coll Cardiol* 14:1253-1262, 1989.

214. Heiberg E, Wolverson MK, Sundaram M, et al: CT findings in thoracic aortic dissection, *AJR* 136:13-17, 1981.

215. Heiberg E, Wolverson MK, Sundaram M, et al: CT characteristics of aortic atherosclerotic aneurysm versus aortic dissection, *J Comput Assist Tomogr* 9:78-83, 1985.

216. Heitzman ER: Radiological diagnosis of mediastinal lymph node enlargement, *J Can Assoc Radiol* 29:151-157, 1987.

217. Heitzman ER: *The mediastinum: radiologic correlations with anatomy and pathology*, ed 2, Berlin, 1988, Springer-Verlag.

218. Hendrickx P, Döhring W: Thymic atrophy and rebound enlargement following chemotherapy for testicular cancer, *Acta Radiol* 30:263-267, 1989.

219. Heron CW, Husband JE, Williams MP: Hodgkin disease: CT of the thymus, *Radiology* 167:647-651, 1988.

220. Heystraten FM, Rosenbusch G, Kingma LM, et al: Chronic posttraumatic aneurysm of the thoracic aorta: surgically correctable occult threat, *AJR* 146:303-308, 1986.

221. Higgins CB, Auffermann W: MR imaging of thyroid and parathyroid glands: a review of current status, *AJR* 151:1095-1106, 1988.

222. Higgins CB, McNamara MT, Fisher MR, et al: MR imaging of the thyroid, *AJR* 147:1255-1261, 1986.

223. Hirsch JH, Carter SJ, Chikos PM: Traumatic pseudoaneurysms of the thoracic aorta: two unusual cases, *AJR* 130:157-160, 1978.

224. Hockholzer L, Theros EG, Rosen EH: Some unusual lesions of the mediastinum: roentgenologic and pathologic features, *Semin Roentgenol* 4:74-90, 1979.

225. Hoffmann WJ, Otto HF: Epithelial tumors of the thymus. In Walter E, Willich E, Webb WR, eds: *The thymus: diagnostic imaging, functions and pathologic anatomy*, Berlin, 1992, Springer-Verlag.

226. Hofmann-Wellenhof R, Domej W, Schmid C, et al: Mediastinal mass caused by syphilitic aortitis, *Thorax* 48:568-569, 1993.

227. Holbert BL, Libshitz HI: Superior vena caval syndrome in primary germ cell tumors, *J Can Assoc Radiol* 37:182-183, 1986.

228. Holland P, Fitzpatrick JD: Case report: magnetic resonance imaging of a right-sided cervical aortic arch with a congenital aneurysm, *Clin Radiol* 43:352-355, 1991.

229. Holtz S, Powers WE: Calcification in papillary carcinoma of the thyroid, *AJR* 80:997-1000, 1958.

230. Hom M, Jolles H: Traumatic mediastinal lymphocele mimicking other thoracic injuries: case report, *J Thorac Imag* 7(3):78-80, 1992.

231. Homer MJ, Wechsler RJ, Carter BL: Mediastinal lipomatosis: CT confirmation of a normal variant, *Radiology* 128:657-661, 1978.

232. Honda T, Yano K, Hamada M, et al: Usefulness of multiangle MRI in aortic arch dissection, *J Comput Assist Tomogr* 16:646-648, 1992.

233. Hopper KD, Diehl LF, Cole BA, et al: The significance of necrotic mediastinal nodes on CT in patients with newly diagnosed Hodgkin disease, *AJR* 155:267-270, 1990.

234. Hsieh ML, Quint LE, Faust JM, et al: Enhancing mediastinal mass at MR: Castleman disease, *Magnet Res Imag* 11:599-601, 1993.

235. Hudson TM, Vandergriend RA, Springfield DS, et al: Aggressive fibromatosis: evaluation by computed tomography and angiography, *Radiology* 150:495-501, 1984.

236. Hussain S, Glover JL, Bree R, et al: Penetrating atherosclerotic ulcers of the thoracic aorta, *J Vasc Surg* 9:710-717, 1989.

237. Ikeda T, Ishihara T, Yoshimatsu H, et al: Primary osteogenic sarcoma of the mediastinum, *Thorax* 29:582-588, 1974.

238. Ikezoe J, Morimoto S, Arizawa J, et al: Ultrasonography of mediastinal teratoma, *J Clin Ultrasound* 14:513-520, 1986.

239. Ikezoe J, Takeuchi N, Johkoh T, et al: MRI of anterior mediastinal tumors, *Radiat Med* 10:176-183, 1992.

240. Im JG, Song KS, Kang HS, et al: Mediastinal tuberculous lymphadenitis: CT manifestations, *Radiology* 164:115-119, 1987.

241. Ingram CE, Belli AM, Lewars MD, et al: Normal lymph node size in the mediastinum: a retrospective study in two patient groups, *Clin Radiol* 40:35-39, 1989.

242. Irwin RS, Braman SS, Arvanitidis AN, et al: [131]I thyroid scanning in preoperative diagnosis of mediastinal goiter, *Ann Intern Med* 89:73-74, 1978.

243. Ishii K, Maeda K, Hashihira M, et al: MRI of mediastinal cavernous hemangioma, *Pediatr Radiol* 20:556-557, 1990.

244. Israel HL, Lenchner G, Steiner GM: Late development of mediastinal calcifications in sarcoidosis, *Am Rev Respir Dis* 124:302-305, 1981.

245. Jacobson G, Felson B, Prendergrass EP, et al: Eggshell calcifications in coal and metal miners, *Semin Roentgenol* 2:276-282, 1967.

246. Jagannath AR, Sos TA, Lockhart SH, et al: Aortic dissection: a statistical analysis of the usefulness of plain chest radiographic findings, *AJR* 147:1123-1126, 1986.

247. Jamplis RW: Infections of the mediastinum and the superior vena caval syndrome. In Shields TW, ed: *General thoracic surgery*, ed 2, Philadelphia, 1983, Lea & Febiger.

248. Jaramillo D, Perez-Atayde A, Griscom NT: Apparent association between thymic cysts and prior thoracotomy, *Radiology* 172:207-209, 1989.

249. Jex RK, van Heerden JA, Carpenter PC, et al: Ectopic ACTH syndrome: diagnostic and therapeutic aspects, *Am J Surg* 149:276-282, 1985.

250. Joseph AE, Donaldson JS, Reynolds M: Neck and thorax venous aneurysm: association with cystic hygroma, *Radiology* 170:109-112, 1989.

251. Juliani G: Radiological diagnosis of thymoma in myasthenia gravis (MG): review of a series of 523 surgically controlled patients, *Clin Imag* 14:48-54, 1990.

252. Kaplan IL, Swayne LC, Widmann W, et al: CT demonstration of "ectopic" thymoma, *J Comput Assist Tomogr* 12:1037-1038, 1988.

253. Kaplan J, Davidson T: Intrathoracic desmoids: report of two cases, *Thorax* 41:894-895, 1986.

254. Kaplan JO, Morillo G, Weinfeld A, et al: Mediastinal adenopathy in myeloma, *J Can Assoc Radiol* 31:48-49, 1980.

255. Kapoor R, Saha MM: Sonographic evaluation of chest masses in children, *Australas Radiol* 35:233-236, 1991.

256. Katz I, Dziadiw R: Localised mediastinal lymph node hyperplasia, *AJR* 84:206-212, 1960.

257. Kauczor H-U, Layer G, Schad LR, et al: Clinical applications of MR angiography in intrathoracic masses, *J Comput Assist Tomogr* 15:409-417, 1991.

258. Kay HR, Goodman LR, Teplick SK, et al: Uses of computed tomography to assess mediastinal complications after median sternotomy, *Ann Thorac Surg* 36:706-714, 1983.

259. Kaye AD, Janssen R, Arger PH, et al: Mediastinal computed tomography in myasthenia gravis, *J Comput Tomogr* 7:273-279, 1983.

260. Kazerooni EA, Bree RL, Williams DM: Penetrating atherosclerotic ulcers of the descending thoracic aorta: evaluation with CT and distinction from aortic dissection, *Radiology* 183:759-765, 1992.

261. Keats TE, Lipscomb GE, Betts CS: Mensuration of the arch of the azygos vein and its application to the study of cardiopulmonary disease, *Radiology* 90:990-994, 1968.

262. Keen SJ, Libshitz HI: Thymic lesions: experience with computed tomography in 24 patients, *Cancer* 59:1520-1523, 1987.

263. Keene RJ, Steiner RE, Olsen EJG, et al: Aortic root aneurysm — radiographic and pathologic features, *Clin Radiol* 22:330-340, 1971.

264. Keller AR, Castleman B: Hodgkin's disease of the thymus gland, *Cancer* 33:1615-1623, 1974.

265. Keller AR, Hochholzer L, Castleman B: Hyaline-vascular and plasma cell types of giant lymph node hyperplasia of the mediastinum and other locations, *Cancer* 29:670-683, 1972.

266. Kersting-Sommerhoff BA, Higgins CB, White RD, et al: Aortic dissection: sensitivity and specificity of MR imaging, *Radiology* 166:651-655, 1988.

267. Kessler RM, Miller KB, Pett S, et al: Pseudocoarctation of the aorta presenting as a mediastinal mass with dysphagia, *Ann Thorac Surg* 55:1003-1005, 1993.

268. Kim HC, Nosher J, Haas A, et al: Cystic degeneration of thymic Hodgkin's disease following radiation therapy, *Cancer* 55:354-356, 1985.

269. Kirchner SG, Heller RM, Smith CW: Pancreatic pseudocyst of the mediastinum, *Radiology* 123:37-42, 1977.

270. Kirchner SG, Hernanz-Schulman M, Stein SM, et al: Imaging of pediatric mediastinal histoplasmosis, *Radiographics* 11:365-381, 1991.

271. Kissin CM, Husband JE, Nicholas D, et al: Benign thymic enlargement in adults after chemotherapy: CT demonstration, *Radiology* 163:67-70, 1987.

272. Kitai K, Koo BC, Davis TD, et al: Primary myelolipoma of mediastinum, *CT: Comput Tomogr* 8:119-123, 1984.

273. Kittredge RD, Finby N: Pericardial cysts and diverticula, *AJR* 99:668-673, 1967.

274. Kittredge RD, Nash AD: The many facets of sclerosing fibrosis, *AJR* 122:288-298, 1974.

275. Klatte EC, Yune JY: Diagnosis and treatment of pericardial cysts, *Radiology* 104:541-544, 1972.

276. Kline ME, Patel BU, Agosti SJ: Non-infiltrating angiolipoma of the mediastinum, *Radiology* 175:737-738, 1990.

277. Koerner HJ, Sun DIC: Mediastinal lipomatosis secondary to steroid therapy, *AJR* 98:461-464, 1966.

278. Kountz PD, Molina PL, Sagel SS: Fibrosing mediastinitis in the posterior thorax, *AJR* 153:489-490, 1989.

279. Kowolafe F: Radiological patterns and significance of thyroid calcification, *Clin Radiol* 32:571-575, 1981.

280. Krech WG, Storey CF, Umiker WC, et al: Thymic cysts: a review of the literature and report of two cases, *J Thorac Surg* 27:477-493, 1954.

281. Krenning EP, Kwekkeboom DJ, Bakker WH, et al: Somatostatin receptor scintigraphy with [^{111}In-DTPA-D-Phe^1]- and [^{123}I-Tyr^3]-octreotide: the Rotterdam experience with more than 1000 patients, *Eur J Nucl Med* 20:716-731, 1993.

282. Kronthal AJ, Heitmiller RF, Fishman EK: Mediastinal seroma after esophagogastrectomy, *AJR* 156:715-716, 1991.

283. Krudy AG, Doppman JL, Brennan MF, et al: The detection of mediastinal parathyroid glands by computed tomography, selective arteriography, and venous sampling: an analysis of 17 cases, *Radiology* 140:739-744, 1981.

284. Kuhlman JE, Fishman EK, Wang KP, et al: Esophageal duplication cyst: CT and transesophageal needle aspiration, *AJR* 145:531-532, 1985.

285. Landay MJ, Rollins NK: Mediastinal histoplasmosis granuloma: evaluation with CT, *Radiology* 172:657-659, 1989.

286. Landay MJ, Virolainen H: "Hyperdense" aortic wall: potential pitfall in CT screening for aortic dissection, *J Comput Assist Tomogr* 15:561-564, 1991.

287. Larde D, Belloir C, Vasile N, et al: Computed tomography of aortic dissection, *Radiology* 136:147-151, 1980.

288. Larson EW, Edwards WD: Risk factors for aortic dissection: a necropsy study of 161 cases, *Am J Cardiol* 53:849-855, 1984.

289. Lautin EM, Rosenblatt M, Friedman AC, et al: Calcification in non-Hodgkin lymphoma occurring before therapy: identification on plain films and CT, *AJR* 155:739-740, 1990.

290. Lee JD, Choe KO, Kim SJ, et al: CT findings in primary thymic carcinoma, *J Comput Assist Tomogr* 15:429-433, 1991.

291. Lee KS, Im JG, Han CH, et al: Malignant primary germ cell tumors of the mediastinum: CT features, *AJR* 153:947-951, 1989.

292. Lee WJ, Fattal G: Mediastinal lipomatosis in simple obesity, *Chest* 70:308-309, 1976.

293. Le Golvan DP, Abell MR: Thymomas, *Cancer* 39:2142-2157, 1977.

294. Lemaitre L, Marconi V, Avni F, et al: The sonographic evaluation of normal thymus in infants and children, *Eur J Radiol* 7:130-136, 1987.

295. Levin B: The continuous diaphragm sign: a newly recognized sign of pneumomediastinum, *Clin Radiol* 24:337-338, 1973.

296. Levine GD, Rosai J: Thymic hyperplasia and neoplasia: a review of current concepts, *Hum Pathol* 9:495-515, 1978.

297. Levine TM, Wurster CF, Krespi YP: Mediastinitis occurring as a complication of odontogenic infections, *Laryngoscope* 96:747-750, 1986.

298. Levitt RG, Glazer HS, Roper CL, et al: Magnetic resonance imaging of mediastinal and hilar masses: comparison with CT, *AJR* 145:9-14, 1985.

299. Levitt RG, Husband JE, Glazer HS: CT of primary germ-cell tumors of the mediastinum, *AJR* 142:73-78, 1984.

300. Lewis JE, Wick MR, Scheithauer BW, et al: Thymoma: a clinicopathological review, *Cancer* 60:2727-2743, 1987.

301. Libshitz HI, Clouser M, Zornoza J, et al: Radiographic findings of immunoblastic lymphadenopathy and related immunoblastic proliferations, *AJR* 129:875-878, 1977.

302. Light AM: Idiopathic fibrosis of mediastinum: a discussion of three cases and review of the literature, *J Clin Pathol* 31:78-88, 1978.

303. Limpert J, MacMahon H, Variakajis D: Angioimmunoblastic lymphadenopathy: clinical and radiological features, *Radiology* 152:27-30, 1984.

304. Lindfors KK, Meyer JE, Dedrick CG, et al: Thymic cysts in mediastinal Hodgkins disease, *Radiology* 156:37-41, 1985.

305. Link KM, Lesko NM: The role of MR imaging in the evaluation of acquired diseases of the thoracic aorta, *AJR* 158:1115-1125, 1992.

306. Link KM, Loehr SP, Baker DM, et al: Magnetic resonance imaging of the thoracic aorta, *Semin Ultrasound CT MRI* 14:91-105, 1993.

307. LiPuma JP, Wellman J, Stern HP: Nitrous oxide abuse: a new cause of pneumomediastinum, *Radiology* 145:602, 1982.

308. Lloyd JE, Tillman BF, Atkinson JB, et al: Mediastinal fibrosis complicating histoplasmosis, *Medicine* 67:295-309, 1988.

309. Long JA, Doppman JL, Nienhius AW: Computed tomographic studies of thoracic extramedullary hematopoiesis, *J Comput Assist Tomogr* 4:67-70, 1980.

310. Lossef SV, Ziessman HA, Alijani MR, et al: Multiple hyperfunctioning mediastinal parathyroid glands in a patient with tertiary hyperparathyroidism, *AJR* 161:285-286, 1993.

311. Lotan CS, Cranney GB, Doyle M, et al: Fat-shift artifact simulating aortic dissection on MR images, *AJR* 152:385-386, 1989.

312. Lui YQ: Radiology of aortoarteritis, *Radiol Clin North Am* 23:671-688, 1985.

313. Lundius B: Intrathoracic kidney, *AJR* 125:678-681, 1975.

314. Lyons HA, Calvy GL, Sammons BP: The diagnosis and classification of mediastinal masses. 1. A study of 782 cases, *Ann Intern Med* 51:897-932, 1959.

315. Mack JW, Heyden WH, Pauling FW, et al: Postoperative chylous pseudocyst, *J Thorac Cardiovasc Surg* 77:773-776, 1979.

316. Macklin MT, Macklin CC: Malignant interstitial emphysema of the lungs and mediastinum as an important occult complication in many respiratory diseases and other conditions, *Medicine* 23:281-358, 1944.

317. Madewell JE, Sobonya RE, Reed JC: Neurenteric cyst: RPC from the AFIP, *Radiology* 109:707-712, 1973.

318. Mahajan V, Strimlan V, van Ordstrand HS, et al: Benign superior vena cava syndrome, *Chest* 68:32-35, 1975.

319. Maier HC: Lymphatic cysts of the mediastinum, *AJR* 73:15-18, 1955.

320. Mallens WMC, Nijhius-Heddes JMA, Bakker W: Calcified lymph node metastases in bronchioloalveolar carcinoma, *Radiology* 161:103-104, 1986.

321. Margolin FR, Winfield J, Steinbach HL: Patterns of thyroid calcification: roentgenologic-histologic study of excised specimens, *Invest Radiol* 2:208-212, 1967.

322. Martin J, Palacio A, Petit J, et al: Fatty transformation of thoracic extramedullary hematopoiesis following splenectomy: CT features, *J Comput Assist Tomogr* 14:477-478, 1990.

323. Masaoka A, Monden Y, Nakahara K, et al: Follow-up study of thymomas with special reference to their clinical stages, *Cancer* 48:2485-2492, 1981.

324. Mayo JR, Culham JAC, MacKay AL: Blood MR signal suppression by preexcitation with inverting pulse, *Radiology* 173:269-271, 1989.

325. McLoud TC, Kalisher L, Stark P, et al: Intrathoracic lymph node metastases from extrathoracic neoplasms, *AJR* 131:403-407, 1978.

326. McMurdo KK, de Geer C, Webb WR, et al: Normal and occluded mediastinal veins: MRI imaging, *Radiology* 159:33-38, 1986.

327. McNeill AD, Groden BM, Neville AM: Intrathoracic phaeochromocytoma, *Br J Surg* 57:457-462, 1970.

328. Meisel S, Rozenman J, Yellin A, et al: Castleman's disease: an uncommon computed tomographic feature, *Chest* 93:1306-1307, 1988.

329. Mendelson DS, Rose JS, Efremidis SC, et al: Bronchogenic cysts with high CT numbers, *AJR* 140:463-465, 1983.

330. Mendez G, Isikoff MB, Isikoff SK, et al: Fatty tumors of the thorax demonstrated by CT, *AJR* 133:207-212, 1979.

331. Merten DF: Diagnostic imaging of mediastinal masses in children, *AJR* 158:825-832, 1992.

332. Miles J, Pennybacker J, Sheldon P: Intrathoracic meningocele: its development and association with neurofibromatosis, *J Neurol Neurosurg Psychiatry* 32:99-110, 1969.

333. Miller DC, Stinson EB, Oyer PE, et al: Operative treatment of aortic dissection: experience with 125 patients over a sixteen-year period, *J Thorac Cardiovasc Surg* 78:365-382, 1979.

334. Miller WT: Drug-related pleural and mediastinal disorder, *J Thorac Imag* 6(1):36-49, 1991.

335. Miller WT, Gefter WB, Miller WT: Thymoma mimicking a thyroid mass, *Radiology* 184:75-76, 1992.

336. Mills SE, Teja K, Crosby IK, et al: Aortic dissection: surgical and nonsurgical treatments compared: an analysis of seventy-four cases at the University of Virginia, *Am J Surg* 137:240-243, 1979.

337. Molina PL, Siegel MJ, Glazer HS: Thymic masses on MR imaging: a pictorial essay, *AJR* 155:495-500, 1990.

338. Moncada R, Cardella R, Demos T, et al: Evaluation of superior vena cava syndrome by axial CT and CT phlebography, *AJR* 143:731-736, 1984.

339. Moncada R, Warpeha R, Pickleman J, et al: Mediastinitis from odontogenic and deep cervical infection, *Chest* 73:497-500, 1978.

340. Monden Y, Nakahara K, Kagotina K, et al: Myasthenia gravis with thymoma: analysis of and postoperative prognosis for 65 patients with thymomatous myasthenia gravis, *Ann Thorac Surg* 38:46-52, 1984.

341. Moore AV, Korobkin M, Powers B, et al: Thymoma detection by mediastinal CT: patients with myasthenia gravis, *AJR* 138:217-222, 1982.

342. Moore AV, Silverman PM, Putman CE: Current concepts in computerized tomography of the mediastinum, *CRC Crit Rev Diagn Imag* 24:1-38, 1985.

343. Moran CA, Travis WD, Rosado-de-Christenson M, et al: Thymomas presenting as pleural tumors, *Am J Surg Pathol* 16:138-144, 1992.

344. Morens AJ, Weismann I, Billingsley JL, et al: Angiographic and scintigraphic findings in fibrosing mediastinitis, *Clin Nucl Med* 8:167-169, 1983.

345. Mori K, Moriyama E, Miyazawa N: Computed tomography of anterior mediastinal tumors: differentiation between thymoma and germ cell tumor, *Acta Radiol* 28:395-398, 1987.

346. Morris UL, Colletti PM, Ralls PW, et al: CT demonstration of intrathoracic thyroid tissue, *J Comput Assist Tomogr* 6:821-824, 1982.

347. Moskowitz PS, Noon MA, McAlister WH, et al: Thymic cyst hemorrhage: a cause of acute, symptomatic widening in a child with aplastic anemia, *AJR* 134:832-836, 1980.

348. Müller NL, Webb WR: Imaging of the pulmonary hila, *Invest Radiol* 20:661-671, 1985.

349. Müller NL, Webb WR, Gamsu G: Paratracheal lymphadenopathy: radiographic findings and correlation with CT, *Radiology* 156:761-765, 1985.

350. Müller NL, Webb WR, Gamsu G: Subcarinal lymph node enlargement: radiographic findings and CT correlation, *AJR* 145:15-19, 1985.

351. Munsell WP: Pneumomediastinum: a report of 28 cases and review of the literature, *JAMA* 202:129-133, 1967.

352. Naidich DP, Khouri NF, Scott WW, et al: Computed tomography of the pulmonary hila. 1. Normal anatomy, *J Comput Assist Tomogr* 5:459-467, 1981.

353. Naidich DP, Khouri NF, Stitik FP, et al: Computed tomography of the pulmonary hila. 2. Abnormal anatomy, *J Comput Assist Tomogr* 5:468-475, 1981.

354. Naidich DP, Zerhouni EA, Siegelman SS: *Computed tomography and magnetic resonance of the thorax*, ed 2, New York, 1991, Raven Press.

355. Nakagawa H, Huang YP, Malis LI, et al: Computed tomography of intraspinal and paraspinal neoplasms, *J Comput Assist Tomogr* 1:377-390, 1977.

356. Nakasu Y, Minouchi K, Hatsuda N, et al: Thoracic meningocele in neurofibromatosis: CT and MR findings, *J Comput Assist Tomogr* 15:1062-1064, 1991.

357. Nathwani BN, Rappaport H, Moran EM, et al: Malignant lymphoma arising in angioimmunoblastic lymphadenopathy, *Cancer* 41:578-606, 1978.

358. Newman A, So SK: Bilateral neurofibroma of the intrathoracic vagus nerve associated with von Recklinghausen's disease, *AJR* 112:389-392, 1971.

359. Nichols CR: Mediastinal germ cell tumors: clinical features and biologic correlates, *Chest* 99:472-479, 1991.

360. Nienaber CA, Spielmann RP, von Kodalitsch Y, et al: Diagnosis of thoracic aortic dissection: magnetic resonance imaging versus transesophageal echocardiography, *Circulation* 85:434-447, 1992.

361. Noma S, Nishimura K, Togashi K, et al: Thyroid gland: MR imaging, *Radiology* 164:495-499, 1987.

362. Ochsner JL, Ochsner SC: Congenital cysts of the mediastinum: 20 year experience with 42 cases, *Ann Surg* 163:909-920, 1966.

363. Odagiri K, Nishihara K, Hatekeyama S, et al: Anterior mediastinal masses with calcifications in children with histiocytosis X (Langerhans' cell histiocytosis), *Pediatr Radiol* 21:550-551, 1990.

364. Olscamp G, Weisbrod G, Sanders D, et al: Castleman disease: unusual manifestations of an unusual disorder, *Radiology* 135:43-48, 1980.

365. Olsen WL, Dillon WP, Kelly WM, et al: MR imaging of paragangliomas, *AJR* 148:201-204, 1987.

366. Olson JL, Salyer WR: Mediastinal paragangliomas (aortic body tumor): a report of four cases and a review of the literature, *Cancer* 41:2405-2412, 1978.

367. Onik G, Goodman PC: CT of Castleman's disease, *AJR* 140:691-692, 1983.

368. Otto HF, Loning I, Lachenmayer L, et al: Thymolipoma in association with myasthenia gravis, *Cancer* 50:1623-1628, 1982.

369. Oudkerk M, Overbosch E, Dee P: CT recognition of acute aortic dissection, *AJR* 141:671-676, 1983.

370. Owens GR, Arger PH, Mulhern CB, et al: CT evaluation of mediastinal pseudocyst, *J Comput Assist Tomogr* 4:256-259, 1980.

371. Pader E, Kirschner PA: Pericardial diverticulum, *Dis Chest* 55:344-346, 1969.

372. Page JE, Wilson AG, de Belder MA: The value of transoesophageal ultrasonography in the management of a mediastinal foregut cyst, *Br J Radiol* 62:986-988, 1989.

373. Pan CH, Chiang CY, Chen SS: Thymolipoma in patients with myasthenia gravis: report of two cases and review, *Acta Neurol Scand* 78:16-21, 1988.

374. Panicek DM, Ewing DK, Markarian B, et al: Interstitial pulmonary hemorrhage from mediastinal hematoma secondary to aortic rupture, *Radiology* 162:165-166, 1987.

375. Panicek DM, Harty MP, Scicutella CJ, et al: Calcification in untreated mediastinal lymphoma, *Radiology* 166:735-736, 1988.

376. Panicek DM, Toner GC, Heelan RT, et al: Nonseminomatous germ cell tumors: enlarging masses despite chemotherapy, *Radiology* 175:499-502, 1990.

377. Pannell TL, Jolles H: Adult cystic mediastinal lymphangioma simulating a thymic cyst, *J Thorac Imag* 7(1):86-89, 1991.

378. Papatestas AE, Alpert LI, Osserman K, et al: Studies in myasthenia gravis: effects of thymectomy; results on 185 patients with nonthymomatous and thymomatous myasthenia gravis, 1941-1969, *Am J Med* 50:465-474, 1971.

379. Papavasiliou C, Gouliamos A, Andreou J: The marrow heterotopia in thalassemia, *Eur J Radiol* 6:92-96, 1986.

380. Paris F, Tarazona V, Casillas M, et al: Hernia of Morgagni, *Thorax* 28:631-636, 1973.

381. Parish JM, Marschke RF, Dines DE, et al: Etiologic considerations in superior vena cava syndrome, *Mayo Clin Proc* 56:407-413, 1981.

382. Park CH, Rothermel FJ, Judge DM: Unusual calcification in mixed papillary and follicular carcinoma of the thyroid gland, *Radiology* 119:554, 1976.

383. Payne WS, Larson RH: Acute mediastinitis, *Surg Clin North Am* 49:999-1009, 1969.

384. Peled N, Babyn PS, Manson D, et al: Aggressive fibromatosis simulating congenital lung malformation, *Can Assoc Radiol J* 44:221-223, 1993.

385. Perez CA, Vietti T, Ackerman LV, et al: Tumors of the sympathetic nervous system in children, *Radiology* 88:750-760, 1967.

386. Perkes EA, Haller JO, Kassner EG, et al: Mediastinal cystic hygroma in infants, *Clin Pediatr* 18:168-170, 1979.

387. Petasnick JP: Radiologic evaluation of aortic dissection, *Radiology* 180:297-305, 1991.

388. Peterson IM, Futhaner DF: Aortic pseudoaneurysm complicating Takayasu disease: CT appearance, *J Comput Assist Tomogr* 10:676-678, 1986.

389. Pezzulli FA, Aronson DA, Goldberg N: Computed tomography of mediastinal hematoma secondary to unusual esophageal laceration: a Boerhaave variant, *J Comput Assist Tomogr* 13:129-131, 1989.

390. Phelan MS: Castleman's giant lymph node hyperplasia, *Br J Radiol* 55:158-160, 1982.

391. Phillips GWL, Choong M: Chondrosarcoma presenting as an anterior mediastinal mass, *Clin Radiol* 43:63-64, 1991.

392. Pilla TJ, Wolverson MK, Sundaram M, et al: CT evaluation of cystic lymphangiomas of the mediastinum, *Radiology* 144:841-842, 1982.

393. Platt JF, Glazer GM, Orringer MB, et al: Radiologic evaluation of the subcarinal lymph node: a comparative study, *AJR* 151:279-282, 1988.

394. Polansky SM, Barwick KW, Ravin CE: Primary mediastinal seminoma, *AJR* 132:17-21, 1979.

395. Pollack MS: Staphylococcal mediastinitis due to sternoclavicular pyarthrosis: CT appearance, *J Comput Assist Tomogr* 14:924-927, 1990.

396. Pombo F, Rodriguez E, Mato J, et al: Patterns of contrast enhancement of tuberculous lymph nodes demonstrated by computed tomography, *Clin Radiol* 46:13-17, 1992.

397. Poon PY, Bronskill MJ, Henkelman M, et al: Magnetic resonance imaging of the mediastinum, *J Can Assoc Radiol* 37:173-181, 1986.

398. Posniak HV, Olson MC, Demos TC, et al: CT of thoracic aortic aneurysms, *Radiographics* 10:839-855, 1990.

399. Posniak HV, Olson MC, Demos TC: Aortic motion artifact simulating dissection on CT scans: elimination with reconstructive segmented images, *AJR* 161:557-558, 1993.

400. Price JE, Rigler LG: Widening of the mediastinum resulting from fat accumulation, *Radiology* 96:497-500, 1970.

401. Proto AV, Rost RC: CT of the thorax: pitfalls in interpretation, *Radiographics* 5:693-812, 1985.

402. Pruzanski W: Lymphadenopathy associated with dysgammaglobulinaemia, *Semin Hematol* 17:44-62, 1980.

403. Pugatch RD, Braver JH, Robbins AH, et al: CT diagnosis of pericardial cysts, *AJR* 131:515-516, 1978.

404. Putman CE, Curtis AM, Westfried M, et al: Thickening of the posterior tracheal stripe: a sign of squamous cell carcinoma of the esophagus, *Radiology* 121:533-536, 1976.

405. Quinn SF, Monson M, Paling M: Spinal lipoma presenting as a mediastinal mass: diagnosis by CT, *J Comput Assist Tomogr* 7:1087-1089, 1983.

406. Quint LE, Glazer GM, Orringer MB, et al: Mediastinal lymph node detection and sizing at CT and autopsy, *Radiology* 147:469-472, 1986.

407. Radford JA, Wong You Cheong J: Enlargement of a mediastinal mass during treatment for Hodgkin's disease may be due to accumulation of fluid within thymic cysts, *Clin Radiol*, in press.

408. Radin DR, Baker EL, Klatt EC, et al: Visceral and nodal calcification in patients with AIDS-related *Pneumocystis carinii* infection, *AJR* 154:27-31, 1990.

409. Raider L, Landry BA, Brogdon BG: The retrotracheal triangle, *Radiographics* 10:1055-1079, 1990.

410. Ramakantan R, Shah P: Dysphagia due to mediastinal fibrosis in advanced pulmonary tuberculosis, *AJR* 154:61-63, 1990.

411. Reed DH: Case report: mycotic pseudoaneurysm of the descending thoracic aorta associated with vertebral osteomyelitis, *Clin Radiol* 41:427-429, 1990.

412. Reed JC, Haller KK, Feigin DS: Neural tumours of the thorax: subject review from the AFIP, *Radiology* 126:9-17, 1978.

413. Reed JC, Sobonya RE: Morphologic analysis of foregut cysts in the thorax, *AJR* 120:851-860, 1974.

414. Rendina EA, Venuta F, Ceroni L, et al: Computed tomographic staging of anterior mediastinal neoplasms, *Thorax* 43:441-445, 1988.

415. Rholl KS, Levitt RE, Glazer HS: Magnetic resonance imaging of fibrosing mediastinitis, *AJR* 145:255-259, 1985.

416. Ricci C, Rendina EA, Venuta F, et al: Diagnostic imaging and surgical treatment of dumbbell tumors of the mediastinum, *Ann Thorac Surg* 50:586-589, 1990.

417. Rizk G, Cuteo L, Amplatz K: Rebound enlargement of the thymus after successful corrective surgery for transposition of the great vessels, *AJR* 116:528-530, 1972.

418. Robinson AE, Gooneratne NS, Blackburn WR, et al: Bilateral anteromediastinal defect of the diaphragm in children, *AJR* 135:301-306, 1980.

419. Rogers LF, Puig AW, Dooley BN, et al: Diagnostic considerations in mediastinal emphysema: a pathophysiologic-roentgenologic approach to Boerhaave's syndrome and spontaneous pneumomediastinum, *AJR* 115:495-511, 1972.

420. Rohlfing BM, Korobkin M, Hall AD: Computed tomography of intrathoracic omental herniation and other mediastinal fatty masses, *J Comput Assist Tomogr* 1:181-183, 1977.

421. Rohlfing BM, Webb WR, Schlobohm RM: Ventilator-related extra-alveolar air in adults, *Radiology* 121:25-31, 1976.

422. Rosado-de-Christenson ML, Galabardes J, Moran CA: Thymoma: radiologic-pathologic correlation, *Radiographics* 12:1013-1030, 1992.

423. Rosado-de-Christenson ML, Templeton PA, Moran CA: Mediastinal germ-cell tumours: radiologic and pathologic correlation, *Radiographics* 12:1013-1030, 1992.

424. Rosai T, Higa E: Mediastinal endocrine neoplasm of probably thymic origin, related to carcinoid tumor: clinicopathologic study of 8 cases, *Cancer* 29:1061-1074, 1992.

425. Rosenow EC, Hurley BT: Disorders of the thymus, *Arch Intern Med* 144:763-770, 1984.

426. Ross P, Logan W: Roentgen findings in extramedullary hematopoiesis, *AJR* 106:604-613, 1969.

427. Russel CF, Edis AJ, Scholz DA, et al: Mediastinal parathyroid tumors: experience with 38 tumors requiring mediastinotomy for removal, *Ann Surg* 193:805-809, 1981.

428. Ruttley M, Mills RA: Subcutaneous emphysema and pneumomediastinum in diabetic keto-acidosis, *Br J Radiol* 44:672-674, 1971.

429. Ruzal-Shapiro C, Abramson SJ, Berdon WE: Posterior mediastinal cystic teratoma surrounded by fat in a 13 month old boy: value of magnetic resonance imaging, *Pediatr Radiol* 20:107-109, 1989.

430. Sakai F, Sone S, Kiyono K, et al: Intrathoracic neurogenic tumors: MR-pathologic correlation, *AJR* 159:279-283, 1992.

431. Sakai F, Sone S, Kiyono K, et al: MR imaging of thymoma: radiologic-pathologic correlation, *AJR* 158:751-756, 1992.

432. Salo JA, Ala-Kulju K: Congenital esophageal cysts in adults, *Ann Thorac Surg* 44:135-138, 1987.

433. Salvatore M, Gallo A: Accessory thyroid in the anterior mediastinum: case report, *J Nucl Med* 16:1135-1136, 1975.

434. Sampson C, Hansell DM: Prevalence of enlarged mediastinal lymph nodes in asbestos-exposed individuals: a CT study, *Clin Radiol* 45:340-342, 1992.

435. Samuels TH, Hamilton PA, Ngan B: Castleman's disease: demonstration with computed tomography and angiography, *J Can Assoc Radiol* 41:380-383, 1990.

436. Samuels T, Hamilton P, Shaw P: Whipple disease of the mediastinum, *AJR* 154:1187-1188, 1990.

437. Sandler CM, Libshitz HI, Marks G: Pneumoperitoneum, pneumomediastinum and pneumopericardium following dental extraction, *Radiology* 115:539-540, 1975.

438. Scalzetti EM, Heitzman ER, Groskin SA, et al: Developmental lymphatic disorders of the thorax, *Radiographics* 11:1069-1085, 1991.

439. Scatarige JC, Fishman EK, Kuhajda FP, et al: Low attenuation nodal metastases in testicular carcinoma, *J Comput Assist Tomogr* 7:682-687, 1983.

440. Scatarige JC, Fishman EK, Zerhouni EA, et al: Transdiaphragmatic extension of invasive thymoma, *AJR* 144:31-35, 1985.

441. Schnyder PA, Gamsu G: CT of the pretracheal retrocaval space, *AJR* 136:303-308, 1981.

442. Schowengerdt CG, Suyemoto R, Main FB: Granulomatous and fibrous mediastinitis: a review and analysis of 180 cases, *J Thorac Cardiovasc Surg* 57:365-379, 1969.

443. Schulthess GK, McMurdo K, Tscholakoff D, et al: Mediastinal masses: MR imaging, *Radiology* 158:289-296, 1986.

444. Schurawitzki H, Stiglbauer R, Klepetko W, et al: CT and MRI in benign mediastinal haemangioma, *Clin Radiol* 43:91-94, 1991.

445. Schweitzer DL, Aguam AS: Primary liposarcoma of the mediastinum: report of a case and review of the literature, *J Thorac Cardiovasc Surg* 74:83-97, 1977.

446. Seabold JE, Binet EF, Schaefer RF: Mycotic aortic aneurysm diagnosed by In-111 leukocyte scintigraphy and computed tomography, *Clin Nucl Med* 8:486-487, 1983.

447. Seidel FG, Magill HL, Burton EM: Case of the day (lipoblastoma), *Radiographics* 10:728-731, 1990.

448. Seline TH, Gross BH, Francis IR: CT and MR imaging of mediastinal hemangioma, *J Comput Assist Tomogr* 14:766-768, 1990.

449. Seltzer RA, Mills DS, Baddock SS, et al: Mediastinal thymic cyst, *Dis Chest* 53:186-196, 1968.

450. Seltzer SE, Herman PG, Sagel SS: Differential diagnosis of mediastinal fluid levels visualized on computed tomography, *J Comput Assist Tomogr* 8:244-246, 1984.

451. Serlo WS, Heikkinen E: Cardiac tamponade caused by a mediastinal teratoma, *Scand J Thorac Cardiovasc Surg* 17:323-325, 1983.

452. Sham JST, Chan FL, Lau WH, et al: Primary mediastinal endodermal sinus tumors: CT evaluation, *Clin Imag* 13:299-304, 1989.

453. Shankwiler RA, Athey PA, Lamki N: Aggressive infantile fibromatosis: pulmonary metastases documented by plain film and computed tomography, *Clin Imag* 13:127-129, 1989.

454. Shapiro B, Sisson J, Kalff V, et al: The location of middle mediastinal pheochromocytomas, *J Thorac Cardiovasc Surg* 87:814-820, 1984.

455. Sharma S, Rajani M, Kamalakar T, et al: Association between aneurysm formation and systemic hypertension in Takayasu's arteritis, *Clin Radiol* 42:182-187, 1990.

456. Shenoy SS, Barua NR, Patel AR, et al: Mediastinal lymphangioma, *J Surg Oncol* 10:523-528, 1978.

457. Shin MS, Berland LL, Ho KJ: Mediastinal cystic hygromas: CT characteristics and pathogenetic consideration, *J Comput Assist Tomogr* 9:297-301, 1985.

458. Shin MS, Ho KJ: Computed tomography of primary mediastinal seminoma, *J Comput Assist Tomogr* 7:990-994, 1983.

459. Shin MS, Ho KJ: Computed tomography evaluation of bilateral bronchostenosis caused by sclerosing granulomatous mediastinitis: a complication of histoplasmosis, *J Comput Tomogr* 8:345-350, 1984.

460. Shirkhoda A, Chasen MH, Eftekhari F, et al: MR imaging of mediastinal thymolipoma, *J Comput Assist Tomogr* 11:364-365, 1987.

461. Shirkhoda A, Wallace S: Computed tomography of juxtacardiac phaeochromocytoma, *J Comput Tomogr* 8:207-209, 1984.

462. Shively BK: Transesophageal echocardiography in the diagnosis of aortic disease, *Semin Ultrasound CT MRI* 14:106-116, 1993.

463. Shub C, Parkin TW, Lie T: An unusual mediastinal lipoma simulating cardiomegaly, *Mayo Clin Proc* 54:60-62, 1979.

464. Sickles EA, Winestock D: Bilateral intrathoracic meningoceles, *J Can Assoc Radiol* 28:79-81, 1977.

465. Sidani AH, Oberson R, Deleze G, et al: Infected teratoma of a lower posterior mediastinum in a six-year-old boy, *Pediatr Radiol* 21:438-439, 1991.

466. Siegel MJ, Glazer HS, Wiener JI, et al: Normal and abnormal thymus in childhood, *Radiology* 172:367-371, 1989.

467. Siegelman SS, Scott WW, Baker RR, et al: CT of the thymus. In Siegelman SS: *Computed tomography of the chest*, New York, 1984, Churchill Livingstone.

468. Simeone JF, Minagi H, Putman CE: Traumatic disruption of the thoracic aorta: significance of the left apical extrapleural cap, *Radiology* 117:265-268, 1975.

469. Singh H, Fitzgerald E, Ruttley MST: Computed tomography: the investigation of choice for aortic dissection, *Br Heart J* 56:171-175, 1986.

470. Smith L, Lippert KM: Peritoneo-pericardial diaphragmatic hernia, *Ann Surg* 148:798-804, 1958.

471. Smith TR, Khoury PT: Aneurysm of the proximal thoracic aorta simulating neoplasm: the role of CT and angiography, *AJR* 144:909-910, 1985.

472. Snow N, Lucas AE, Grau M, et al: Purulent mediastinal abscess secondary to Ludwig's angina, *Arch Otolaryngol* 109:53-55, 1983.

473. Solomon SL, Brown JJ, Glazer HS, et al: Thoracic aortic dissection: pitfalls and artifacts in MR imaging, *Radiology* 177:223-228, 1990.

474. Souadjian JV, Enriquez P, Silverstein MN, et al: The spectrum of diseases associated with thymoma: coincidence or a syndrome? *Arch Intern Med* 134:374-379, 1974.

475. Spizarny DL, Rebner M, Gross BH: CT evaluation of enhancing mediastinal masses, *J Comput Assist Tomogr* 11:990-993, 1987.

476. Stahl JD, Goldman SM, Minkin SD, et al: Perforated duodenal ulcer and pneumomediastinum, *Radiology* 124:23-25, 1977.

477. Stanford W, Rooholamini SA, Galvin JR: Ultrafast computed tomography in the diagnosis of aortic aneurysms and dissections, *J Thorac Imag* 5(4):32-39, 1990.

478. Stark P, Smith DC, Watkins GE, et al: Primary intrathoracic extraosseus osteogenic sarcoma: report of three cases, *Radiology* 174:725-726, 1990.

479. Stebner FC, Bishop CR: Bone marrow scan and radioiron uptake of an intrathoracic mass, *Clin Nucl Med* 7:86-87, 1982.

480. Stilwell ME, Weisbrod GL, Ilves R: Spontaneous mediastinal hematoma, *J Can Assoc Radiol* 32:60-61, 1981.

481. Streiter ML, Schneider HJ, Proto AV: Steroid-induced thoracic lipomatosis: paraspinal involvement, *AJR* 139:679-681, 1982.

482. Strickland NH, Lavender JP: Case report: spontaneous radiographic "resolution" of retrosternal goitre, *Clin Radiol* 44:430-431, 1991.

483. Suh JS, Abenoza P, Galloway HR, et al: Peripheral (extracranial) nerve tumors: correlation of MR imaging and histologic findings, *Radiology* 183:341-346, 1992.

484. Sullivan KL, Wechsler RJ: CT diagnosis of lymphocele, *J Comput Assist Tomogr* 9:1110-1111, 1985.

485. Sundaram M, McGuire MH, Schajowicz F: Soft-tissue masses: histologic basis for decreased signal (short T_2) on T_2-weighted images, *AJR* 148:1247-1250, 1987.

486. Sussman SK, Halvorsen RA, Silverman PM, et al: Paracardiac adenopathy: CT evaluation, *AJR* 149:29-34, 1987.

487. Sussman SK, Silverman PM, Donnal JP: CT demonstration of isolated mediastinal goiter, *J Comp Assist Tomogr* 10:863-864, 1986.

488. Suster S, Rosai J: Multilocular thymic cyst: an acquired reactive process: study of 18 cases, *Am J Surg Pathol* 15:388-398, 1991.

489. Suzuki M, Takashima T, Itoh H, et al: Computed tomography of mediastinal teratomas, *J Comput Assist Tomogr* 7:74-76, 1983.

490. Swenson SJ, Keller PL, Berquist TH, et al: Magnetic resonance imaging of hemorrhage, *AJR* 145:921-927, 1985.

491. Szamosi A: Radiological detection of aneurysms involving the aortic root, *Radiology* 138:551-555, 1981.

492. Taams MA, Gussenhoven WJ, Schippers LA, et al: The value of transesophageal echocardiography for diagnosis of thoracic aorta pathology, *Eur Heart J* 9:1308-1316, 1988.

493. Tan A, Holdener GP, Hecht A, et al: Malignant thymoma in an ectopic thymus: CT appearance, *J Comput Assist Tomogr* 15:842-844, 1991.

494. Tarr RW, Page DL, Glick RG, et al: Benign hemangioendothelioma involving posterior mediastinum: CT findings, *J Comput Assist Tomogr* 10:865-867, 1986.

495. Tatu WF, Pope TL Jr, Daniel TM, et al: Computed tomography of mediastinal cystic hygroma in an adult, *J Comput Tomogr* 9:233-236, 1985.

496. Teates CD: Steroid induced mediastinal lipomatosis, *Radiology* 96:501-502, 1970.

497. Teplick JG, Nedwich A, Haskin ME: Roentgenographic features of thymolipoma, *AJR* 117:873-877, 1973.

498. Theros EG: RPC of the month from the AFIP, *Radiology* 93:677-681, 1969.

499. Thompson BH, Stanford W: Utility of ultrafast computed tomography in the detection of thoracic aortic aneurysms and dissections, *Semin Ultrasound CT MRI* 14:117-128, 1993.

500. Thorsen MK, San Dretto MA, Lawson TL, et al: Dissecting aortic aneurysms: accuracy of computed tomographic diagnosis, *Radiology* 148:773-777, 1983.

501. Tisi GM, Friedman PJ, Peters RM, et al: Clinical staging of primary lung cancer: official ATS statement, *Am Rev Respir Dis* 127:659-664, 1983.

502. Tomsick TA: Dental surgical subcutaneous and mediastinal emphysema: a case report, *J Can Assoc Radiol* 25:49-51, 1974.

503. Tottle AJ, Wilde P, Hartnell GG, et al: Diagnosis of acute thoracic aortic dissection using combined echocardiography and computed tomography, *Clin Radiol* 45:104-108, 1992.

504. Toye R, Armstrong P, Dacie JE: Lymphangio-haemangioma of the mediastinum, *Br J Radiol* 64:62-64, 1991.

505. van Gils APG, Falke THM, van Erkel AR, et al: MR imaging and MIBG scintigraphy of pheochromocytomas and extraadrenal functioning paragangliomas, *Radiographics* 11:37-57, 1991.

506. van Heerden JA, Sheps SG, Hamberger B, et al: Pheochromocytoma: current status and changing trends, *Surgery* 91:367-373, 1982.

507. Vasile N, Mathieu D, Keita K, et al: Computed tomography of thoracic aortic dissection: accuracy and pitfalls, *J Comput Assist Tomogr* 10:211-215, 1986.

508. Veeze-Kuijpers B, Van Andel JG, Stiegelis WF, et al: Benign thymic cyst following mantle radiotherapy for Hodgkin's disease, *Clin Radiol* 38:289-290, 1987.

509. Verley J, Hollman KH: Thymoma: a comparative study of clinical stages, histologic features, and survival in 200 cases, *Cancer* 55:1074-1086, 1985.

510. Victor S, Anand KV, Andappan P, et al: Malignant mediastinal chemodectoma, *Chest* 68:583-584, 1975.

511. Vincent JM, Trainer PJ, Reznek RH, et al: The radiological investigation of occult ectopic ACTH-dependent Cushing's syndrome, *Clin Radiol* 48:11-17, 1993.

512. Vock P, Hodler J: Cardiophrenic angle adenopathy: update of causes and significance, *Radiology* 159:395-399, 1986.

513. Vyborny C, MacMahon H: Foil filters for equalized chest radiography, *Radiology* 151:524, 1984.

514. Wallace DB: Intrapericardial diaphragmatic hernia, *Radiology* 122:596, 1977.

515. Wallace S, Hill CS, Paulus DD, et al: The radiologic aspects of medullary (solid) thyroid carcinoma, *Radiol Clin North Am* 8:463-474, 1970.

516. Walter JF, Rottenberg RW, Cannon WB, et al: Giant mediastinal lymph node hyperplasia (Castleman's disease): angiographic and clinical features, *AJR* 130:447-450, 1978.

517. Webb WR, Gamsu G: Computed tomography of the left retrobronchial stripe, *J Comput Assist Tomogr* 7:65-69, 1983.

518. Webb WR, Gamsu G, Glazer GM: Computed tomography of the abnormal pulmonary hilum, *J Comput Assist Tomogr* 5:485-490, 1981.

519. Webb WR, Gamsu G, Stark DD, et al: Evaluation of magnetic resonance sequences in imaging mediastinal tumors, *AJR* 143:723-727, 1984.

520. Webb WR, Gamsu G, Stark DD, et al: Magnetic resonance imaging of the normal and abnormal pulmonary hila, *Radiology* 152:89-94, 1984.

521. Webb WR, Hirji M, Gamsu G: Posterior wall of the bronchus intermedius: radiographic-CT correlation, *AJR* 142:907-911, 1984.

522. Webb WR, Jensen BG, Gamsu G, et al: Coronal magnetic resonance imaging of the chest: normal and abnormal, *Radiology* 153:729-735, 1984.

523. Webb WR, Moore EH: Differentiation of volume averaging and mass on magnetic resonance images of the mediastinum, *Radiology* 155:413-416, 1985.

524. Webb WR, Sostman HD: MR imaging of thoracic disease: clinical uses, *Radiology* 182:621-630, 1992.

525. Weinberg B, Rose JS, Efremidis SC, et al: Posterior mediastinal-teratoma (cystic dermoid): diagnosis by computerized tomography, *Chest* 77:694-695, 1980.

526. Weinreb JC, Arger PH, Grossman R, et al: CT metrizamide myelography in multiple bilateral intrathoracic meningoceles, *J Comput Assist Tomogr* 8:324-326, 1984.

527. Weinreb JC, Mootz A, Cohen JM: MRI evaluation of mediastinal and thoracic inlet venous obstruction, *AJR* 146:679-684, 1986.

528. Weinstein JB, Aronberg DJ, Sagel SS: CT of fibrosing mediastinitis: findings and their utility, *AJR* 141:247-251, 1983.

529. Weiss LM, Fagelman D, Warhit JM: CT demonstration of an esophageal duplication cyst, *J Comput Assist Tomogr* 7:716-718, 1983.

530. Wernecke K, Peters PE, Galanski M: Mediastinal tumors: evaluation with suprasternal sonography, *Radiology* 159:405-409, 1986.

531. Wernecke K, Vassallo P, Hoffmann G, et al: Value of sonography in monitoring the therapeutic response of mediastinal lymphoma: comparison with chest radiography and CT, *AJR* 156:265-272, 1991.

532. Wernecke K, Vassallo P, Peters PE, et al: Mediastinal tumors: biopsy under US guidance, *Radiology* 172:473-476, 1989.

533. Wernecke K, Vassallo P, Potter R, et al: Mediastinal tumours: sensitivity of detection with sonography compared with CT and radiography, *Radiology* 175:137-143, 1990.

534. Wernecke K, Vassallo P, Rutsch F, et al: Thymic involvement in Hodgkin's disease: CT and sonographic findings, *Radiology* 181:375-383, 1991.

535. Westcott JL, Henschke CI, Berkmen Y: MR imaging of the hilum and mediastinum: effects of cardiac gating, *J Comput Assist Tomogr* 9:1073-1078, 1985.

536. Wheat MW: Acute dissection of the aorta, *Cardiovasc Clin* 17:241-262, 1987.

537. Wheat MW, Palmer RF, Bartley TD, et al: Treatment of dissecting aneurysms of the aorta without surgery, *J Thorac Cardiovasc Surg* 50:364-373, 1965.

538. Whitaker JA, Defenbaugh LD, Cooke AR: Esophageal duplication cyst: case report, *Am J Gastroenterol* 73:329-332, 1980.

539. White RD, Higgins CB: Magnetic resonance imaging of thoracic vascular disease, *J Thorac Imag* 4(2):34-50, 1989.

540. White RD, Lipton MJ, Higgins CB, et al: Noninvasive evaluation of suspected thoracic aortic disease by contrast-enhanced computed tomography, *Am J Cardiol* 57:282-290, 1986.

541. Whyte AM, Powell N: Case report: mediastinal lipoblastoma of infancy, *Clin Radiol* 42:205-206, 1990.

542. Wick MR, Scheithauer BW, Weiland LH, et al: Primary thymic carcinomas, *Am J Surg Pathol* 6:613-630, 1982.

543. Wieder S, Adams PL: Improved routine chest radiography with a trough filter, *AJR* 137:695-698, 1981.

544. Wieder S, Rabinowitz JC: Fibrous mediastinitis: a late manifestation of mediastinal histoplasmosis, *Radiology* 125:305-312, 1977.

545. Wieder S, White TJ, Salazar J, et al: Pulmonary artery occlusion due to histoplasmosis, *AJR* 138:243-251, 1982.

546. Wilkins EW, Grillo HC, Scannel G, et al: Role of staging in prognosis and management of thymoma, *Ann Thorac Surg* 51:888-892, 1991.

547. Willich E: Clinical features of thymic hyperplasia. In Walter E, Willich E, Webb WR, eds: *The thymus: diagnostic imaging, functions and pathologic anatomy*, Berlin, 1992, Springer-Verlag.

548. Wilson ES: Neurenteric cyst of the mediastinum, *AJR* 107:641-646, 1969.

549. Wittich GR, Karnel F, Schurawitzki H, et al: Percutaneous drainage of mediastinal pseudocysts, *Radiology* 167:51-53, 1988.

550. Wolff KA, Herold CJ, Tempany CM, et al: Aortic dissection: atypical patterns seen at MR imaging, *Radiology* 181:489-495, 1991.

551. Woodring JH, Johnson PJ: Computed tomography distinction of central thoracic masses, *J Thorac Imag* 6(2):32-39, 1991.

552. Woodring JH, Loh FK, Kryscio RJ: Mediastinal hemorrhage: an evaluation of radiographic manifestations, *Radiology* 151:15-21, 1984.

553. Wortsman J, McConnachie P, Baker JR, et al: Immunoglobulins that cause thymocyte proliferation from a patient with Graves' disease and an enlarged thymus, *Am J Med* 85:117-121, 1988.

554. Wright AR, Goddard PR, Nicholson S, et al: Fat-suppression magnetic resonance imaging in the preoperative localization of parathyroid adenomas, *Clin Radiol* 46:324-328, 1992.

555. Wychulis AR, Connolly DC, McGoon DC: Pericardial cysts, tumors, and fat necrosis, *J Thorac Cardiovasc Surg* 62:294-300, 1971.

556. Wychulis AR, Payne WS, Clagett OT, et al: Surgical treatment of mediastinal tumors: a 40 year experience, *J Thorac Cardiovasc Surg* 62:379-392, 1971.

557. Wycoco D, Raval B: An unusual presentation of mediastinal Hodgkin's lymphoma on computed tomography, *J Comput Tomogr* 7:187-188, 1983.

558. Yacoub MH, Lise M: Intrathoracic cystic hygromas, *Br J Dis Chest* 63:107-111, 1969.

559. Yamato M, Fuhrman CR: Computed tomography of fatty replacement in extramedullary hematopoiesis, *J Comput Assist Tomogr* 11:541-542, 1987.

560. Yamato M, Lecky JW, Hiramatsu K, et al: Takayasu arteritis: radiographic and angiographic findings in 59 patients, *Radiology* 161:329-334, 1986.

561. Yang WC, Zapulla R, Malis L: Neurilemmoma in lumbar intervertebral foramen, *J Comput Assist Tomogr* 5:904-906, 1981.

562. Yeager BA, Guglielmi GE, Schiebler ML, et al: Magnetic resonance imaging of Morgagni hernia, *Gastrointest Radiol* 12:296-298, 1987.

563. Yeh HC, Gordon A, Kirschner PA, et al: Computed tomography and sonography of thymolipoma, *AJR* 140:1131-1133, 1983.

564. Yeoman LJ, Dalton HR, Adam EJ: Fat-fluid level in pleural effusion as a complication of mediastinal dermoid: CT characteristics, *J Comput Assist Tomogr* 14:307-309, 1990.

565. Youssem DM, Scatarige JC, Fishman EK, et al: Low-attenuation thoracic metastases in testicular malignancy, *AJR* 146:291-293, 1986.

566. Yu CJ, Yang PC, Chang DB: Evaluation of ultrasonically guided biopsies of mediastinal masses, *Chest* 100:399-405, 1991.

567. Yucel EK, Steinberg FL, Egglin TK, et al: Penetrating aortic ulcers: diagnosis with MR imaging, *Radiology* 177:779-781, 1990.

568. Zadvinskis DP, Benson MT, Kerr HH, et al: Congenital malformations of the cervicothoracic lymphatic system: embryology and pathogenesis, *Radiographics* 12:1175-1189, 1992.

569. Zaki I, Wears R, Parnell A, et al: Case report: mediastinal lymphadenopathy in eosinophilic pneumonia, *Clin Radiol* 48:61-62, 1993.

570. Zeilender S, Turner MA, Glauser FL: Mediastinal pseudocyst associated with chronic pleural effusions, *Chest* 97:1014-1016, 1990.

571. Zerhouni EA, Scott WW, Baker RR, et al: Invasive thymomas: diagnosis and evaluation by computed tomography, *J Comput Assist Tomogr* 6:92-100, 1982.

572. Zylak CJ, Banerjee R, Galbraith PA, et al: Lung involvement in angioimmunoblastic lymphadenopathy (AIL), *Radiology* 121:513-519, 1976.

17 Diseases of the Airways

ALAN G. WILSON

TRACHEA
Anatomy

The trachea extends from the lower border of the cricoid cartilage to the main carina at approximately the level of D5. The cervical portion is midline, but the intrathoracic part usually deviates slightly to the right to accommodate the left-sided aortic arch. With increasing age and aortic unfolding, this tracheal deviation becomes more pronounced. The wall of the trachea contains 16 to 20 incomplete rings of hyaline cartilage. Rings are C, U, or horseshoe shaped and are closed posteriorly by a fibromuscular membrane. During childhood and adolescence the trachea is rounded.[182] The normal dimensions in this age group have been studied on plain radiographs and computed tomography (CT).[113,178,182] In adults, particularly men, the trachea tends to be slightly flattened from side to side, with sagittal diameters exceeding coronal by about 1 mm.[59] Most cross-sectional tracheal growth occurs in the first two decades of life, but a further modest increase in dimensions often occurs in the third and fourth decades.[59] Normal values for tracheal dimensions in adults have been assessed by plain radiographs[59,168,249] and CT.[508] The most comprehensive plain radiographic study was of 808 subjects (53% male) in whom the internal diameter of the trachea was measured 2 cm above the aortic arch. Measurements were magnified by 8%. Mean values with standard deviation (SD) for men were 19.3 ± 2.2 mm (coronal) and 20.2 ± 2.3 mm (sagittal) and for women were 16.3 ± 1.9 mm (coronal) and 16.6 ± 2.1 mm (sagittal). On CT the mean inspiratory sagittal and coronal diameters of the adult trachea (measured at the thoracic inlet, just above the carina, and halfway between) were 15.2 mm (SD 1.4 mm) in women and 18.2 mm (SD 1.2 mm) in men.[508] In the same study the mean area at the same levels was found to be 194 mm^2 (SD 35 mm^2) in women and 272 mm^2 (SD 33 mm^2) in men.[508] The technical aspects of measuring true tracheal dimensions have been discussed.[179]

The pressure gradient across the intrathoracic tracheal wall varies with lung volume, and extramural pressure is generally assumed to be the same as pleural space pressure. Thus with an open glottis the static transmural gradient is about 0 mm H_2O on maximal expiration and approximately 25 mm H_2O on maximal inspiration. These gradients are exaggerated by forced respiratory maneuvers. Stern and co-workers[475] have studied cross-sectional tracheal dimensions and contour during forced inspiratory and expiratory maneuvers using fast dynamic CT (100 msec exposures every 600 msec). Ten adult volunteers had a 35% ± 18% (SD) reduction in cross-sectional area from inspiration to expiration. The round or oval tracheal configuration became horseshoe shaped at end expiration with a variable degree of invagination of the posterior membrane.

Cartilage rings calcify as part of the aging process. In one series about 50% were calcified on CT in subjects in their seventh and eighth decades.[291] Tracheal ring calcification is also described in a number of rare conditions in childhood[190,339] and with warfarin therapy in both adults[339] and children.[419,491]

At approximately the level of D5 the trachea divides at the main carina into the right and left mainstem bronchi, the right deviating from the general direction of the trachea less than the left. The subcarinal angle is variable and has been measured on the erect posteroanterior chest radiograph.[195] The mean angle was approximately 60 degrees with an SD of about 10 degrees. There was a weak correlation between subcarinal angle and chest shape, with the angle becoming more acute as the chest became longer and narrower.[195]

Tracheal disorders[40,80,487]

Tracheal lesions that are part of a generalized pulmonary or systemic disorder, together with congenital, traumatic, and neoplastic processes, are discussed in the relevant chapters. With a few exceptions, detailed consideration in this section is given only to conditions in adults that are essentially confined to the trachea. CT has become the examination of choice for investigating tracheal disorders.[148,149,268,269]

The trachea may be affected by extrinsic or intrinsic processes. Extrinsic processes, particularly masses, displace and distort the trachea, while intrinsic ones cause narrowing, widening, or a mass effect.

Tracheal narrowing

Tracheal narrowing may affect a long or short segment, and since the distinction is not always clear, both types are considered together. The important causes are listed in the box at right.

TUBERCULOSIS. Although common in the past,[453] tracheal tuberculosis is now rare. It is almost always associated with cavitary lung disease and grossly infected sputum.[80] Pathologic study shows mucosal thickening and ulceration and subsequent healing by fibrosis with stricture formation.[80] Very occasionally the trachea is involved by direct spread from adjacent nodes and fistula formation subsequent to this is described.[3]

SCLEROMA. Scleroma is a chronic progressive granu-

CAUSES OF TRACHEAL NARROWING

EXTRINSIC

Mass lesions
  Thyroid
  Nodes
  Vessels[289]
  Mediastinal mass
Invading lesions
  Thyroid or esophageal carcinoma
Mediastinal fibrosis
  Tuberculosis
  Histoplasmosis[530]

INTRINSIC

Congenital[36,75,273]
  Tracheal narrowing[71,218]
Infective
  Croup, laryngotracheobronchitis[191]
  Papillomatosis[170]
  Tuberculosis[453]
  Scleroma
  Fungal[85]
    Histoplasmosis
    Coccidioidomycosis[151]
    Mucormycosis
    Candidiasis[80]
    Necrotizing tracheobronchial aspergillosis[112,204]
Granulomatous
  Necrotizing cytomegalovirus tracheitis[225]
  Wegener's granulomatosis
  Sarcoidosis[57]
Neoplastic
  Benign or malignant neoplasm[131]
  Lymphoma[392]
  Sinus histiocytosis[374]
Traumatic
  Tracheostomy or endotracheal intubation
  Right pneumonectomy syndrome[445]
  Blunt or penetrating trauma[537]
Postinflammatory[212]
  Epidermolysis bullosa[494]
Deposition or dysplastic
  Mucopolysaccharidoses[386]
  Chondrodysplasia punctata[251]
Immunologic
  Amyloidosis[88]
  Relapsing polychondritis
Cryptogenic
  Tracheopathia osteoplastica
  Saber-sheath trachea
  Idiopathic

Modified from Berkmen YM: *Radiol Clin North Am* 22:539-562, 1984.

lomatous infection that affects primarily the nose but may also involve the nasopharynx, larynx, trachea, and bronchi. It is caused by the gram-negative bacterium *Klebsiella rhinoscleromatis.* Scleroma is uncommon in the West, occurring mainly in Asia, North Africa, Central and South America, and Eastern Europe. It affects principally rural people from low socioeconomic groups.[80] The disease passes through three phases: catarrhal, granulomatous and proliferative, and scarring.[33] Patients usually present with symptoms related to the nose and paranasal sinuses, and the majority have radiographic signs of sinusitis.[33] Occasionally there is a soft tissue mass or bone destruction suggesting a nasal carcinoma. Laryngeal involvement is usually manifest as transglottic narrowing and vocal cord thickening. About 5% of patients have tracheal involvement, which is nearly always accompanied by laryngeal disease and often, although not necessarily, by paranasal sinus disease.[80]

All or more commonly part of the trachea is involved, typically the proximal rather than the distal segment.[211] Stenoses are usually concentric and may be nodular or smooth.[130] Less commonly there is diffuse uniform narrowing or multiple masses.[149] Bronchial involvement is described.[330]

TRACHEO(BRONCHO)PATHIA OSTEO(CHONDRO) PLASTICA. Tracheopathia osteoplastica was first described more than 100 years ago,[533] yet it remains a curiosity of obscure etiology. Although rare, it is more common than airway amyloidosis, a closely allied condition that some workers consider identical.[15] In 1974 it was possible to collect 245 cases of tracheopathia from the world literature.[315]

Pathologic characteristics include the development of cartilaginous and bony submucosal nodules[80] in the trachea and proximal airways. The nodules are typically found in the lower two thirds of the trachea and in the main, lobar, and segmental bronchi.[295] The disorder, however, sometimes starts more proximally and affects the first tracheal ring region.[550] The osteochondral nodules develop adjacent to the airway cartilages and therefore usually occur anterolaterally in the trachea,[295] only occasionally involving the membranous part.[511] The nodules give rise to sessile and polypoidal elevations of the mucosa, which produce airway narrowing.[550] The overlying mucosa usually remains intact, but sometimes it ulcerates, causing hemoptysis.[15] The cause of the condition is obscure, with two theories currently commanding the most support. One theory considers the nodules to be a form of ecchondrosis of the airway cartilage because of their distribution in the airways and because they have bony, cartilaginous, and fibrous connections to the cartilage rings themselves.[550] The other theory is that the disorder is due to amyloidosis, a condition in which cartilage and bone formation is known to occur. Several workers have in fact found evidence of amyloid in pathologic specimens from patients with tracheopathia.[15,432,451]

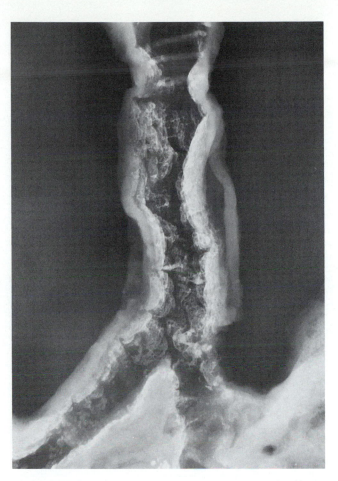

FIGURE 17-1

Tracheopathia osteoplastica. Radiograph of autopsy specimen of trachea and mainstem bronchi opened from back, showing extensive nodular thickening of tracheal wall. Nodules are calcified and extend down into mainstem bronchi. Subglottic trachea is relatively spared.

Seventy-five percent of patients are male, and the disease usually develops in middle age (sixth decade), although the age range is wide, from 11 to 78 years.[80] The common early symptoms are dyspnea, hoarseness, cough that is often productive, hemoptysis, and recurrent pulmonary infections.[295] The disease progresses very slowly. In one report of nine patients, seven had had symptoms for more than 10 years and one had had symptoms for about 20 years.[295]

The chest radiograph may be normal[295] or may demonstrate evidence of collapse or infective consolidation. Airway calcification has diagnostic value but can be surprisingly difficult to detect.[80] Tracheal calcification (Figure 17-1) is manifest as irregular or scalloped opacities lying inside the cartilage rings.[550] Although this calcification may be seen on a well-penetrated posteroanterior chest radiograph, it is better appreciated on a lateral view.[550] When the calcification extends more distally, the chest radiograph may show linear opacities radiating out from the hila, representing thickened and calcified airway walls.[15] If the tracheal air column is

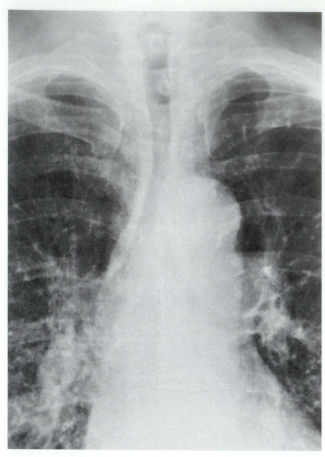

FIGURE 17-2
Saber-sheath trachea. Posteroanterior radiograph in which coronal diameter of trachea in cervical region is 19 mm, decreasing to 9 mm in intrathoracic portion. Transitional zone is at level of thoracic inlet, and narrowing affects whole of intrathoracic trachea. Patient was male and had chronic bronchitis.

clearly seen, the irregular nodularity of the tracheal wall and the encroachment of these nodules on the lumen can be appreciated. Conventional tomography[222,526] and particularly CT[184,375] show all these features to better advantage. The definitive diagnosis is made with bronchoscopy, during which the passage of the instrument may generate a grating sensation. However, the diagnosis may be missed even on bronchoscopy, and some patients have needed several examinations before the diagnosis was eventually made.[295]

SABER-SHEATH TRACHEA. The saber-sheath deformity is limited to the intrathoracic part of the trachea, which is flattened from side to side so that the coronal diameter is two thirds or less of the sagittal diameter at the same level. The condition is virtually confined to men, who are usually more than 50 years of age; the youngest recorded patient was 37 years of age.[168] Saber-sheath trachea is strongly associated with the presence of chronic obstructive pulmonary disease (COPD), and in one series COPD was present in 93% of patients with the deformity compared with 18% of control subjects.[168] The pathogen-

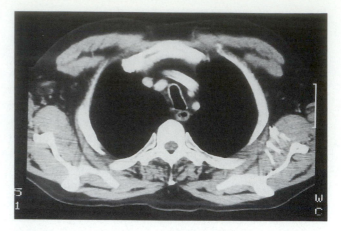

FIGURE 17-3
Saber-sheath trachea. Computed tomographic scan showing coronal diameter of trachea at level of left brachiocephalic vein to be 1 cm whereas sagittal diameter is 2.6 cm. This represents about 50% coronal reduction and 15% sagittal increase from normal dimensions.

esis of the lesion is obscure, but probably it is an acquired deformity related to the abnormal pattern and magnitude of intrathoracic pressure changes in COPD.

Saber-sheath trachea can be detected on the plain chest radiograph (Figure 17-2) but is better demonstrated on CT (Figure 17-3). The narrowing usually affects the whole of the intrathoracic trachea, with an abrupt return to normal caliber at the thoracic inlet.[169] In Greene's series of 60 patients with saber-sheath trachea and 60 control subjects, the mean coronal diameter of the deformed trachea was reduced to 61% and the sagittal diameter increased to 115%, giving a mean tracheal area of 75% compared with control subjects.[168] Cartilage rings are commonly calcified or ossified both pathologically and radiologically.[148,169] The inner wall of the trachea is usually smooth (Figure 17-3), but examples with nodular irregularity have been described.[429] Patients with both saber-sheath trachea and mediastinal lipomatosis are described in whom the appearance on the plain radiograph strongly resembles a mediastinal mass.[219] The original studies described the trachea as displaying the usual changes in configuration in relation to respiration and considered the trachea to be normally compliant (Figure 17-4).[168] Other workers, however, have described an abnormal degree of narrowing on forced expiration[148] and have noted that the cross-sectional area was reduced mainly by apposition of the lateral walls with slight invagination of the posterior membrane.[149]

CRYPTOGENIC STENOSIS. Intrinsic, fibrotic, tracheal stenoses of obscure origin have been described.[232] These may occur at any site and be multiple.[80] In a recently described series of 15 cases of idiopathic laryngotracheal stenoses, patients were predominantly female (94%) and middle aged (30 to 60 years).[44] One third of the stenoses were tracheal, and these were hourglass or eccentric in

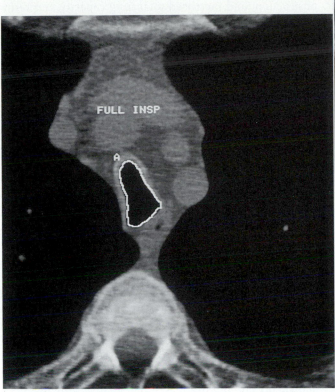
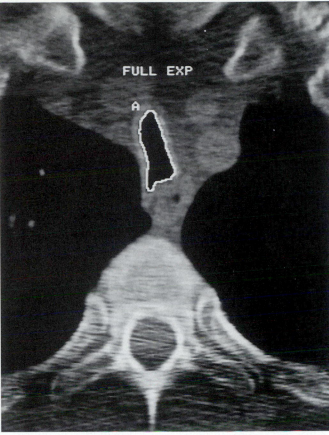
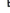

A

B

FIGURE 17-4
Saber-sheath trachea. Ultrafast computed tomography images at beginning and end of rapid expiratory maneuver. **A,** At maximum inspiration. **B,** At maximum expiration. Cross-sectional area of trachea is essentially the same in **A** and **B,** but its configuration has changed with development of coronal narrowing and sagittal widening on expiration. Trachea is not hypercompliant.

configuration with smooth or less commonly irregular lobulated margins. Stenoses were 2 to 4 cm long and 3 to 5 mm wide. The histologic changes were nonspecific, consisting of scarring of the adventitia and lamina propria.

Some patients with cryptogenic stenoses have positive titers of antineutrophil cytoplasmic antibodies.[150] In these patients stenoses have been recurrent and the histologic features either granulomatous or nonspecific. It seems highly likely that these cases are part of the Wegener's granulomatosis spectrum.

Tracheal widening

A number of studies[59,168,234,249,508] have assessed the normal tracheal dimensions in adults using plain radiographs, bronchography, and CT. The most useful study using plain chest radiographs is that of Breatnach, Abbott, and Fraser,[59] who studied 808 subjects. Measurements were made 2 cm above the aortic arch and were subject to 8% magnification. Tracheal diameter increased slightly with age, and taking the largest measurements (between 60 and 80 years of age) the coronal diameter in males (mean ± SD) was 19.7 ± 2.2 mm and in females 16.8 ± 2.0 mm. In light of these data a coronal diameter on a

---

CAUSES OF LOCAL AND GENERALIZED TRACHEAL WIDENING

Tracheobronchomegaly (Mounier-Kuhn syndrome)
Heritable connective tissue disorders
    Ehlers-Danlos complex[1]
    Cutis laxa[509]
Immune deficiency states and recurrent childhood infections
    Ataxia telangiectasia[271]
    Immunoglobulin deficiency[271]
    Cystic fibrosis[180]
Endotracheal cuff damage
Relapsing polychondritis[129]
Tracheocele[183]
Diffuse pulmonary fibrosis[541]

---

chest radiograph of 26 mm in males and 23 mm in females is considered abnormal. The CT coronal diameter is smaller, since it is not subject to magnification; values are 3 to 4 mm less.

A limited number of disorders cause tracheal widening, and these are listed in the box above. In some of the conditions the widening is generalized, and in others it is local, as with a tracheocele or following endotracheal tube cuff damage. In some forms of diffuse disease, widening is mild and confined to one diameter. Thus in cystic fibrosis the sagittal diameter is mildly (about 3 to 5 mm) increased while the coronal dimension remains normal.[180] In day to day clinical practice the most common cause of mild enlargement of the trachea is upper zone or diffuse lung fibrosis as seen in sarcoidosis, fibrosing alveolitis, and histoplasmosis.[541]

TRACHEOBRONCHOMEGALY (MOUNIER-KUHN SYNDROME). The most striking diffuse increase in tracheal diameter is seen in tracheobronchomegaly (Mounier-Kuhn syndrome). This is a rare abnormality of the trachea and large airways that is associated with recurrent respiratory tract infection and was first described in 1932.[349] Atrophy affects the elastic and muscular elements of both the cartilaginous and membranous parts of the trachea.[14,152,249,542] In the past the condition was considered to be acquired and to be caused by recurrent infections weakening the airway walls. However, evidence strongly suggests that this is a primary process.[542] Thus in some patients the condition is familial with an autosomal recessive pattern of transmission.[237] There is a recognized association with anatomic variants of the lungs, ribs, and bronchial tree (including a double tracheal lumen, tracheal trifurcation, and a short left main bronchus).[31,542] Many patients have a history of disease dating back to childhood; presentation as early as 18 months of age is recorded.[223] Furthermore, pathologic findings of tracheobronchomegaly without inflammation of the tracheal wall are described.[249] The probable chance association of tracheobronchomegaly and ankylosing spondylitis is recorded.[379]

No reliable data on prevalence are available, but in 1800 bronchograms the frequency was about 1%.[152] However, it seems likely that the condition is underdiagnosed, since some patients are asymptomatic or have only minor symptoms.[542] It is markedly male predominant (only about 5% of patients are female) and has a possible racial predisposition for blacks.[31] In a recent review of 27 patients 52% were black,[542] indicating a significant excess of blacks if, as seems likely, most of the populations from which cases were derived were predominantly white. The condition most commonly presents in the third or fourth decade and in more than three fourths of the patients have presented by the age of 40 years.[31] Symptoms, however, often date back a decade or even into childhood.[152,249] Ineffective cough, because of widened central airways, and diverticula predispose the patient to pulmonary infections. The typical history is of chronic cough that is characteristically loud and productive. Other clinical features include recurrent chest infections and occasionally hoarseness, hemoptysis, and dyspnea. Symptoms therefore closely resemble those of chronic bronchitis or bronchiectasis. A minority of patients have no or very mild symptoms.[1,108,237,542] Respiratory func-

tion tests usually show increased dead space, airflow obstruction, and increased total lung capacity and residual volume,[31,152,237] but occasionally findings are normal.[542] Airway compliance is increased, and dynamic airway collapse on expiration and cough can be demonstrated.* The prognosis is variable; some patients have recurrent infections leading to progressive lung damage, bronchiectasis, scarring, and eventual respiratory failure, whereas others survive into old age with relatively mild, nonprogressive disease.[542]

The diagnosis is based on radiologic findings. The immediately subglottic trachea has a normal diameter, but it expands as it passes to the carina (Figures 17-5 and 17-6) and this dilatation often continues into the major bronchi.[31,152,400] A coronal diameter of more than 26 mm for the trachea in men and 23 mm in women on a postero-anterior radiograph is required for the diagnosis. These values represent the normal mean diameter plus 3 SD. The dilatation may vary from segment to segment but overall tends to be relatively even. Atrophic mucosa prolapses between cartilage rings and gives the trachea a characteristically corrugated outline that on a plain radiograph is best appreciated in the lateral view.[1,237,480] Corrugations may become exaggerated to form sacculations or diverticula.[31,105,124] Tracheal changes are well shown on CT (Figure 17-7)[105,108,149,450] and magnetic resonance imaging.[420] Large vessels may indent the compliant trachea.[105]

The dilated proximal airways in the lung show changes of bronchiectasis (Figures 17-7 and 17-8),[31,152,450] and this affects particularly first- to fourth-order branches.[237] Characteristically there is an abrupt transition from large central airways to normal peripheral ones (Figure 17-8).[105,152] Small branches that arise from bronchiectatic segments tend to remain patent (Figure 17-8); this is atypical of bronchiectasis in general, in which they are usually occluded by a bronchiolitis obliterans. This characteristic feature[152] is shared only by allergic bronchopulmonary aspergillosis.[439] Dynamic collapse of the trachea and central airways on expiration and cough can be demonstrated by a variety of imaging techniques, including cine fluoroscopy and CT.[14,70,152,249]

Dilatation of the trachea is generalized in tracheobronchomegaly. Occasionally in other conditions the trachea is locally dilated. This may be seen with a tracheocele, a localized ballooning of the membranous posterior tracheal wall of obscure etiology.[183] Tracheoceles tend to arise from the right posterior tracheal wall, and their size varies with transmural tracheal pressure.[480] They may affect the cervical[183] or thoracic trachea and in the latter instance may be seen as a paratracheal, thin-walled ring opacity with or without an air-fluid level. Smaller, frequently multiple outpouchings (diverticula) may arise from the trachea and mainstem airways.[26] They are a

---

*References 14, 70, 152, 223, 249, 542.

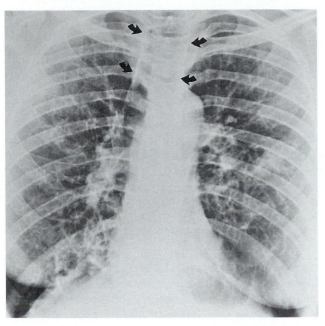

FIGURE 17-5
Tracheobronchomegaly on posteroanterior radiograph. Trachea *(arrows)* is just over 3 cm wide. There is evidence of airflow obstruction with low, flat right hemidiaphragm. Throughout lungs, but particularly in left middle and lower zones, are line and ring opacities consistent with bronchiectasis.

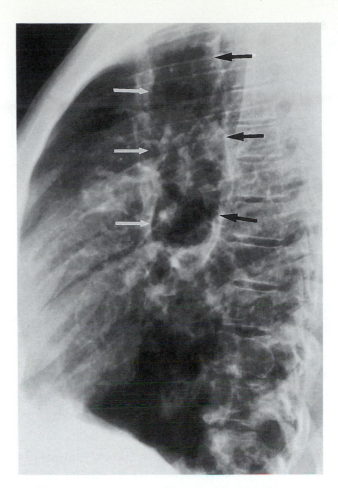

FIGURE 17-6
Tracheobronchomegaly. Lateral view of trachea of same patient as in Figure 17-5 showing grossly dilated trachea *(arrows)*.

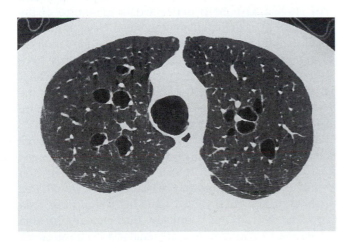

FIGURE 17-7
Tracheobronchomegaly. High-resolution computed tomogram taken through midthoracic trachea of 39-year-old black man with slowly resolving pneumonia. He had had previous episode of pneumonia but was otherwise well and symptom free despite being physical training instructor. Tracheal diameter is considerably widened at 30 mm. Fourth- and fifth-order airways show marked varicose bronchiectasis.

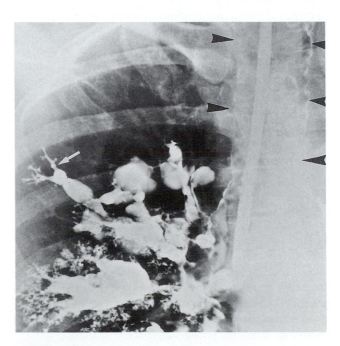

FIGURE 17-8
Tracheobronchomegaly in 53-year-old woman with recurrent lower respiratory tract infections. Bronchogram with contrast medium outlining dilated trachea (3.3 cm coronal diameter; *black arrowheads*). There is varicose and cystic bronchiectasis with characteristic filling of distal bronchi *(white arrow)*, a feature otherwise seen only in allergic aspergillosis.

CAUSES OF TRACHEOMALACIA

CONGENITAL[75]

Cartilage deficiency[534]
Generalized tracheomalacia[484]
Tracheoesophageal fistula[75]

ACQUIRED

Associated with endotracheal tubes and tracheo-
stomy[404,514]
After closed chest trauma[129]
After lung resection[129,445]
After radical neck dissection[116]
After radiation therapy[116]
Chronic obstructive pulmonary disease[236]
Relapsing polychondritis[116]
Lunate trachea[70,286,292]

feature of tracheobronchomegaly[124] but are also described as occurring with cystic dilatation of mucous gland ducts.[480]

Tracheomalacia

Tracheomalacia is present when tracheal compliance is increased. It is usually a localized rather than a generalized process and may be congenital or acquired. Important causes are listed in the box above. The increase in compliance is due to the loss of integrity of the wall's structural components and is particularly associated with damaged or destroyed cartilage.

Tracheomalacia is diagnosed when changes in the transmural pressure gradient produce undue tracheal wall movements. The pressure outside the intrathoracic trachea approximates to pleural pressure and outside the cervical trachea is atmospheric. When the glottis is open, the luminal pressure is atmospheric. Thus imaging the intrathoracic trachea at full inspiration and expiration permits observation of the effect of a modest change in transmural pressure (circa 25 cm H_2O). Static maneuvers such as the Valsalva or Müller can produce bigger pressure gradients across the cervical trachea. Cervical tracheal compliance has been measured by use of this method with CT imaging.[181] For a 40 cm H_2O change in transmural pressure the cross-sectional area of the cervical trachea changed by about one third.[181] During dynamic maneuvers such as cough, forced expiration, and forced inspiration the luminal pressure of the intrathoracic trachea is modestly increased or decreased. At the same time large excursions in pleural pressure are generated, and with suitable imaging intrathoracic tracheal compliance can be assessed under more stressful conditions than are produced by static maneuvers.

Until recently the most common cause of tracheomalacia in adults was damage following placement of tracheostomy and endotracheal tubes. However, since the introduction of wide, low-pressure cuffs the problem has largely disappeared. Tracheostomy-related compliant segments may develop at the site of the stoma, at the level of the cuff, or in between; in the last instance the pathogenesis is thought to be damage caused by infection associated with stagnant secretions.[514] A compliant tracheal segment may or may not be accompanied by a stenosis.[145] An endotracheal tube cuff lying in a hyper-compliant segment appears overinflated, and this may provide an early clue to the presence of tracheomalacia.[404]

Normally the intrathoracic trachea is slightly oval with coronal diameters less than sagittal. Occasionally, however, coronal diameters become significantly larger than sagittal ones, producing a lunate configuration to the trachea. A lunate trachea is easily deformed in a sagittal direction, giving rise to a form of tracheomalacia. In a number of patients a lunate trachea has been associated with COPD,[70] but in others it has been cryptogenic[286] and in one case radiation therapy may have been contributory.[292] Collapse of the affected segment has been observed bronchoscopically.[70]

A suspected diagnosis of tracheomalacia can be confirmed with a flow-volume loop,[145] but tracheomalacic segments are best identified and characterized by use of fluoroscopy with video or cine recording.[129] Contrast enhancement is not necessary for these studies, but it usually improves the image.[129] The trachea is studied in anteroposterior, lateral, and oblique views during forced inspiration and expiration and during cough. Under these conditions a normal trachea shows narrowing both coronally and sagittally, the latter caused by invagination of the membranous posterior wall. Reliable data on the degree of narrowing to be expected are not available, and most studies have been performed in ignorance of the transmural pressure gradient generated. Several authors consider that caliber changes of more than 50% indicate increased wall compliance.[70,236] In patients who have COPD with high downstream resistance, particularly high dynamic pressure gradients can be generated across the tracheal wall, and it is likely that caliber changes of more than 50% can occur with normal tracheal compliance.[210]

With the advent of ultrafast CT it has become possible to image the trachea during quiet breathing[243] and forced dynamic maneuvers.[475] During forced inspiration and expiration the intrathoracic tracheal cross-sectional area varies by 35% ± 18% (SD),[475] and in view of these data Stern and co-workers[475] suggest that changes in area greater than 70% indicate tracheomalacia.[475] Ultrafast CT has been used to identify tracheomalacic segments.[243,475]

Tracheal filling defects

In adults tracheal filling defects are most commonly produced by neoplasms (see Chapter 8), but there are a number of other causes (see box at left on p. 825).

ECTOPIC THYROID. Ectopic thyroid is a rare cause of an intratracheal filling defect,[104,403] with about 150 cases in the literature,[515] mostly from endemic goitrous ar-

TRACHEAL FILLING DEFECTS

NEOPLASM[515]

Benign (epithelial and mesenchymal)
Malignant
    Carcinoma (squamous, adenoid cystic, adenocarcinoma)
    Sarcoma
    Plasmacytoma[32]
    Lymphoma
Malignant invasion from without

INFECTION OR GRANULOMA

Viral papilloma[159]
Membranous croup
Fungal infection
Tuberculosis
Rhinoscleroma
Wegener's granulomatosis

TRAUMA

Hematoma

MISCELLANEOUS

Ectopic thyroid and thymus
Amyloidosis
Tracheopathia osteoplastica
Foreign body
Mucoid pseudotumor[244]
Cyst or mucocele

Modified from Rost RC: *Semin Roentgenol* 18:4, 1983.

CAUSES OF TRACHEOESOPHAGEAL FISTULA IN ADULTS

Congenital[47,474]
Neoplasm[317]
    Carcinoma of esophagus[290] or trachea
    Lymphoma[41,317]
Trauma
    Closed chest[189,471]
    Penetrating[547]
    Postendoscopy or postoperative
    Endotracheal intubation[177]
    Corrosive esophagitis[16,461]
    Esophageal foreign body[318]
    Postirradiation
Infection
    Histoplasmosis[240]
    Actinomycosis[547]
    Tuberculosis
    Other bacteria

congenital fistulas are first manifested in adults.[47,474] Recognized causes of TEF are listed in the box above. Malignant neoplasia, particularly esophageal, is the most common cause in adults. Infection and trauma are the most frequent nonmalignant causes.[547] The etiology of bronchoesophageal fistulas is similar to that of TEF.

BRONCHI
Anatomy

The division of the trachea gives rise to the left and right mainstem bronchi. In adults the right mainstem bronchus is more vertical than the left and wider by about 2 mm (approximately 15 versus 13 mm). It is also half the length of the left (approximately 25 versus 50 mm). The end of the right mainstem bronchus is marked by the lateral origin of the right upper lobar airway, and the mainstem continues as the intermediate-stem bronchus. This terminates at the point where the middle lobar airway originates anterolaterally and the superior (apical) segmental airway to the right lower lobe originates posteriorly. The main airway continues as the lower lobar bronchus. This eventually divides into four basal segmental branches, which in a frontal view are arranged from laterally to medially in the order anterior, lateral, posterior, and medial (Figure 17-9). On the left side is a short left upper lobar bronchus, which usually bifurcates into the lingular bronchus (caudad) and a short trunk (cephalad) that almost immediately divides into anterior and common apicoposterior segmental airways. Having given rise posteriorly to the superior (apical) segmental bronchus the lower lobar airway continues inferiorly dividing into three or four basal segmental bronchi. In Figure 17-9, which is taken from Boyden,[55] four basal segmental airways are shown with a separate medial branch. In

eas.[131] Females outnumber males by about 3:1.[104] The ectopic thyroid may be histologically normal, although it is usually goitrous. Occasionally it is malignant.[104,131] Three fourths of intratracheal thyroid nodules are associated with extratracheal goiter. Sometimes they declare themselves years after the removal of an extratracheal goiter because of compensatory hypertrophy. Tumors may occur anywhere between the subglottis and main carina,[515] but typically they are a few centimeters below the vocal cords, arising as smooth, sessile nodules from the posterolateral wall of the trachea.[104]

Ectopic thymus has also been described as causing a submucosal intratracheal mass.[316]

TRACHEAL PAPILLOMA. Squamous papillomas of the trachea in children are usually multiple and a manifestation of laryngeal papillomatosis with tracheobronchial dissemination (see p. 318).[69,131,170,425,460] Similar cases are rarely reported in adults.[159,170] Solitary squamous cell papillomas of the trachea are also recognized in adults and may undergo malignant transformation.[98,131]

Tracheoesophageal fistula

In the pediatric age group tracheoesophageal fistula (TEF) is commonly congenital.[273] Occasionally such

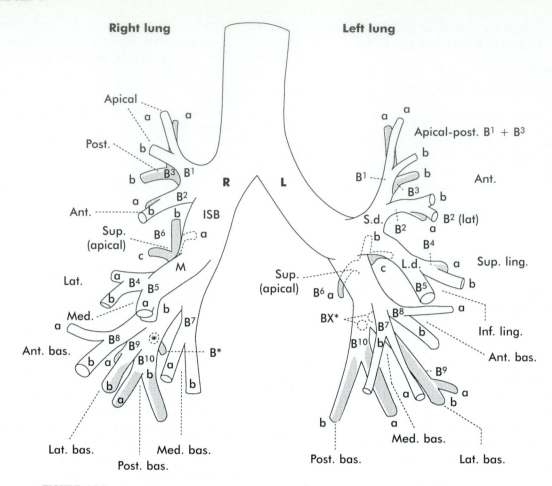

FIGURE 17-9
Anterior view of bronchial tree illustrating branches to segmental level and their alphanumeric designation. *ISB,* Intermediate stem bronchus; *S.d.,* superior division of left upper lobar bronchus; *L.d.,* lingular division of left upper lobar bronchus. (Modified from Boyden EA: *Segmental anatomy of the lungs,* New York, 1955, McGraw-Hill.)

other classifications,[227] it is shown as arising from a common anterobasal segmental airway.

Various alphanumeric systems of identifying segmental and subsegmental airways have been described.[55,227,548] The one illustrated here (Figure 17-9, Table 17-1) is taken from Boyden.[55]

Central airways to subsegmental level are well shown on CT if thin (3 to 5 mm) contiguous sections are taken. Some authors recommend 20-degree oblique CT in selected patients because it allows more adequate evaluation of segmental and subsegmental airways.[415] The CT anatomy of central airways has been discussed,[149,363,376,513] and CT images of central airways are illustrated in the section on hilar anatomy (pp. 23 and 24). The reader is referred to a number of detailed articles concerning the CT appearance of the segmental and subsegmental airways: upper lobes,[279,378] lower lobes,[230,364] and lingular segments.[280]

Bronchial anomalies

Variations in bronchial anatomy[22,56] particularly affecting segmental and subsegmental airways are com-

mon and are not often clinically significant. The two kinds of anomalous airways are the displaced, in which a standard airway arises from an unusual site, and the supernumerary, an additional airway. Displaced airways are much more common than supernumerary ones. The following are a few of the more important variations:

1. Tracheal bronchus.[75] This arises from the lateral wall of the trachea,[347] usually within a few centimeters of the main stem takeoff, and is much more common on the right side than on the left. The anomalous airway is usually a displaced apical segmental bronchus, but it may be a supernumerary apical segmental bronchus, a displaced upper lobar airway, or even a supernumerary upper lobar airway.[326] This anomaly is usually clinically inapparent, but occasionally the orifice is narrow[326,421] or the airway bronchiectatic,[326,421] which may lead to recurrent distal pneumonia and abscess formation. Apical cyst formation in the lung supplied by the anomalous bronchus is also described.[452] When the tracheal bronchus is a displaced upper lobar airway, the more distal trachea is narrowed.[218]

Table 17-1 Bronchial anatomy nomenclature

Jackson-Huber (Thoracic Society of Great Britain) nomenclature		Boyden nomenclature	
Lobar	Segmental	Lobar	Subsegmental
Right lung			
Right upper lobe	Apical	B^1	B^1a apical
			B^1b anterior
	Anterior	B^2	B^2a posterior
			B^2b anterior
	Posterior	B^3	B^3a apical
			B^3b posterior (axillary)
Middle lobe	Lateral	B^4	B^4a posterior
			B^4b anterior
	Medial	B^5	B^5a superior
			B^5b inferior
Right lower lobe	Superior (apical)	B^6	B^6a medial
			B^6b superior
			B^6c lateral
	Subsuperior	B^*	
	Medial basal	B^7	B^7a anterior
			B^7b medial
	Anterior basal	B^8	B^8a lateral
			B^8b basal
	Lateral basal	B^9	B^9a lateral
			B^9b basal
	Posterior basal	B^{10}	$BX^*(10)$ accessory subsuperior
			$B^{10}a$ laterobasal
			$B^{10}b$ mediobasal
Left lung			
Left upper lobe — upper division	Apicoposterior	$B^{1\ \&\ 3}$	B^1 apical
			B^3 posterior
	Anterior	B^2	B^2a posterior
			$B^2(lat)$ lateral
			B^2b anterior
Left upper lobe — lower (lingular) division	Superior	B^4	B^4a posterior
			B^4b anterior
	Inferior	B^5	
Left lower lobe	Superior (apical)	B^6	B^6a medial
			B^6b superior
			B^6c lateral
	Subsuperior	B^*	
	Medial basal	B^7	B^7a anterolateral
			B^7b anteromedial
	Anterior basal	B^8	B^8a lateral
			B^8b basal
	Lateral basal	B^9	$BX^*(9)$ accessory subsuperior
			B^9 basal
	Posterior basal	B^{10}	$BX^*(10)$ accessory subsuperior
			$B^{10}a$ laterobasal
			$B^{10}b$ mediobasal

2. Common origin of the right upper and middle lobar airways.[310]

3. Accessory cardiac bronchus. This is a supernumerary bronchus arising from the medial aspect of the intermediate-stem bronchus proximal to the origin of the superior (apical) segmental airway to the lower lobe. The cardiac bronchus passes downward and medially toward the heart. It is either blind ending, in which case it may have a nodule of unaerated lung tissue at its tip, or supplies a small ventilated "lobule."[309,324] The CT appearances have been described.[324] An accessory cardiac bronchus may be associated with local infection or hemoptysis. The simultaneous occurrence of an accessory cardiac and tracheal bronchus has been reported.[228]

4. Bridging bronchus. This is a displaced right lower lobar bronchus that arises from the left mainstem bronchus, crossing the mediastinum to reach the right lower lobe.[472]

5. Lateral inversion of right- and left-sided airways. This occurs in situs inversus. With situs ambiguus the airway has either a bilateral right-sided or left-sided configuration. Such anomalies are strongly associated with serious congenital heart disease.[272,274] The central airway abnormality associated with situs ambiguus may be detected on the chest radiograph.[469]

Bronchiectasis

Bronchiectasis is a chronic condition characterized by local, irreversible dilatation of bronchi, usually associated with inflammation.[200] The qualification "irreversible" is included in the definition to exclude the transient airway dilatation that has been observed in pneumonia and atelectasis.* Dilatation of the airway in these circumstances is probably partly related to inflammatory changes in the wall, altering compliance, and to exaggerated lung stresses after collapse. Bronchiectasis may be regional or widespread. The generalized mild bronchial dilatation seen in chronic bronchitis is not considered a form of bronchiectasis.

On pathologic study, bronchiectasis may be divided into obstructive and nonobstructive forms. The latter shows a basilar predilection and is commonly bilateral.[84] When unilateral it shows a preference for the left side.[528] The lingula and the middle lobe are also commonly affected. On gross examination, bronchiectatic lungs are small in volume, gray-blue, and rubbery. On macroscopic study, the airways are dilated in a variety of patterns that may be classified into two[200] or three subtypes.[413] The three-part Reid classification is widely used and is equally applicable to gross pathologic, bronchographic, and CT appearances. It uses the following divisions:

1. Cylindrical bronchiectasis. This is the least severe form. Dilatation is mild, and the bronchi retain their regular and relatively straight outline (Figure 17-10). The bronchiectatic airways terminate abruptly with squared-

*References 24, 49, 134, 366, 390, 463.

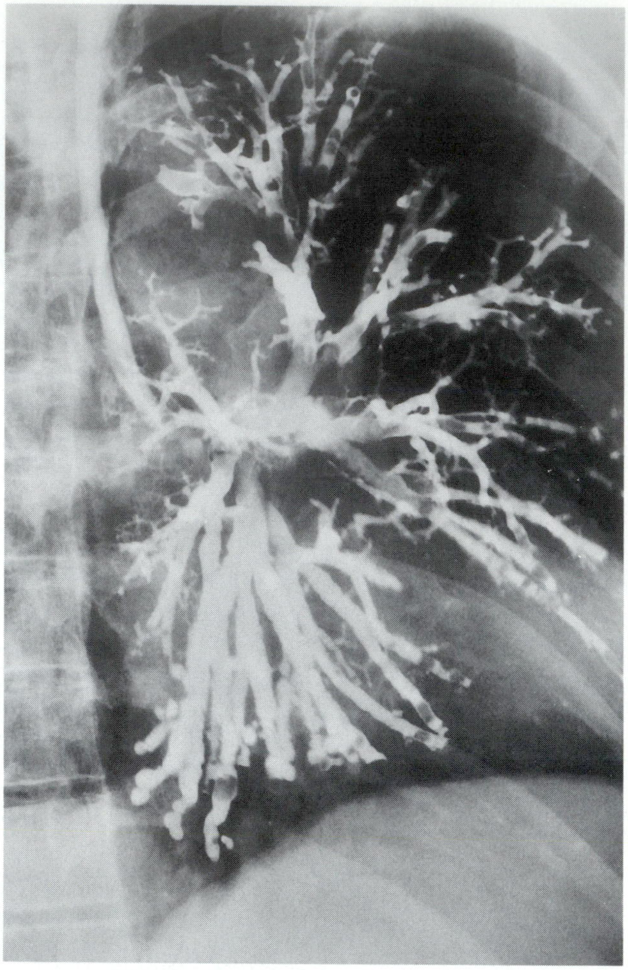

FIGURE 17-10
Cylindrical bronchiectasis. Left posterior oblique projection of left bronchogram showing cylindrical bronchiectasis affecting whole of lower lobe except for superior segment. Few side branches fill. Basal airways are crowded together, indicating volume loss of lower lobe, a common finding in bronchiectasis.

off ends, and smaller bronchi and bronchioles are plugged with secretions. The number of bronchial subdivisions from the hilum to the periphery is normal.

2. Varicose bronchiectasis. In this form, bronchial dilatation is greater and is accompanied by local constrictions that give the airway an irregular outline with a typically bulbous termination (Figure 17-11). Obstruction of small airways is more pronounced, and some are irreversibly obliterated by scarring. The number of generations of patent airways from hilum to periphery, which is normally in the order of 17 to 20, is reduced to six or seven.

3. Cystic (saccular) bronchiectasis. This is the most severe form of bronchiectasis (Figure 17-12). The airway takes on a ballooned appearance and dilates progressively as it passes distally. The number of bronchial divisions is greatly reduced, and although the terminal sacs are subpleural, they represent only fourth- or fifth-generation

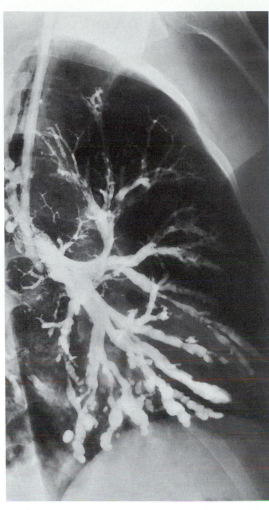

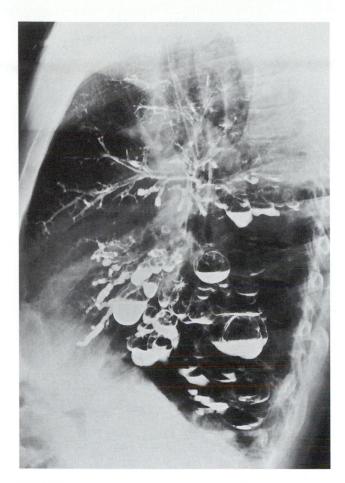

FIGURE 17-12
Cystic bronchiectasis. Right lateral bronchogram showing cystic bronchiectasis affecting mainly lower lobe and posterior segment of upper lobe.

FIGURE 17-11
Varicose bronchiectasis. Left posterior oblique projection of left bronchogram in patient with ciliary dyskinesia syndrome. All basal bronchi are affected by varicose bronchiectasis.

airways, indicating that considerable parenchymal loss has occurred. Small airway branches are occluded and obliterated by a bronchiolitis obliterans.

Histologic study shows the airway walls to be thickened and chronically inflamed with chronic granulation tissue and the bronchial arteries to be hypertrophied.[27,250] Ciliated epithelium is largely replaced by squamous epithelium or areas of squamous metaplasia. The mucosa is sometimes ulcerated or thrown into transverse ridges by circular muscle hypertrophy. Airways are surrounded by fibrosis with acute and organizing pneumonia in the adjacent parenchyma,[250] leading to volume loss and distortion.

The pathogenesis of bronchiectasis is complex, as shown by the large number of recognized causes.[27] The most important and commonly implicated pathogenic factors are bronchial wall weakness, often brought about by infective inflammatory damage, and an increased transmural distending pressure. Recognized etiologic

conditions[27] are listed in the box on p. 830.

Gross bronchiectasis is characterized by persistent cough, with copious purulent sputum and recurrent pulmonary infections. Symptoms frequently date from childhood, when a precipitating pneumonic event may have occurred. With widespread disease there may be dyspnea and, ultimately, cor pulmonale. Such gross bronchiectasis is becoming unusual and is largely limited to patients with impaired defense mechanisms. A recognized presentation of mild bronchiectasis is recurrent hemoptysis,[361] but mild bronchiectasis is often asymptomatic. This is particularly true of some forms such as that following granulomatous disease of the upper zones.

The classic description of the plain radiologic changes in bronchiectasis is that of Gudbjerg.[185] In this old series only 7% of radiographs were normal, although this is a low figure judged by current clinical experience.[89,94] Some varieties of bronchiectasis such as occur in cystic fibrosis and the ciliary dyskinesia syndrome[360] almost invariably show plain radiographic changes:

1. The bronchial walls are visible either as single thin lines or as parallel line opacities (Figure 17-13). With the

---

CAUSES OF BRONCHIECTASIS

CONGENITAL

Cartilage deficiency[242,336,510,512,534]
Cystic bronchiectasis[13]

POSTINFECTION

Childhood pneumonia, measles, pertussis, *Mycoplasma* pneumonia,[529] tuberculosis[367]
Swyer-James syndrome[498]

OBSTRUCTION

Neoplasm
Nodes (including "middle lobe syndrome")[43]
Broncholith
Foreign body[266]
Bronchostenosis

INHALATION AND ASPIRATION

Ammonia[207,247]
Riley-Day syndrome
Gastric aspiration[536]
Heroin overdose[25]

IMPAIRED HOST DEFENSE AND IMMUNOLOGIC

Primary ciliary dyskinesia
Cystic fibrosis[193]
Primary impaired humoral or cell immunity[535]
  Infantile X-linked agammaglobulinemia (Bruton's disease)
  Variable immunodeficiency[97,106]
  Selective immunoglobulin deficiency
  Good's syndrome[139]
  Wiskott-Aldrich syndrome
  Ataxia telangiectasia (Louis-Bar syndrome)
  Chédiak-Higashi syndrome
HIV associated[213,323]
Lung transplant[462]
Inflammatory bowel disease[68,155,338]

ALLERGY

Allergic bronchopulmonary aspergillosis

PULMONARY FIBROSIS

End-stage lung[523]
Radiation[90,285]

MISCELLANEOUS

Tracheobronchomegaly (Mounier-Kuhn syndrome)
Alpha$_1$-antitrypsin deficiency[238,241,293]
Obstructive azoospermia (Young's syndrome)[192,368]
Anhidrotic ectodermal dysplasia[406]
Rheumatoid disease, Sjögren's syndrome[125]
Ehlers-Danlos syndromes
Marfan's syndrome
Yellow nail syndrome[531]
Cryptogenic

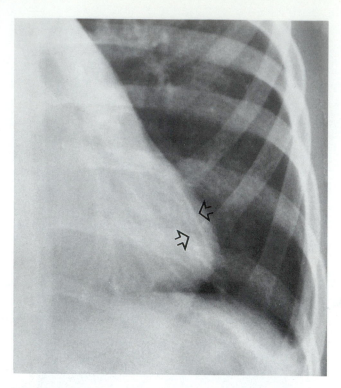

FIGURE 17-13
Bronchiectasis. Posteroanterior radiograph on which thickened bronchial walls are seen as line opacities through heart. Some lines appear paired *(arrows)* and probably represent opposite walls of a single airway. Separation of these lines is such that airway must be dilated.

latter finding the lines representing bronchial walls are more widely separated than would be expected with airways of normal diameter.

2. Ring and curvilinear opacities are generated by thickened airway walls seen end on (Figure 17-14). Ring opacities range in size from 5 to 20 mm and have thin (hairline) walls. They may contain air-fluid levels (Figure 17-15).

3. Dilated airways filled with secretions give rise to band shadows about 5 to 10 mm wide and several centimeters long (Figures 17-16 and 17-17). Band shadows may branch, giving V, Y, or more complex shaped opacities. They point toward the hilum. Seen end on, such dilated fluid-filled airways generate rounded or oval nodular opacities.

4. Vascular opacities are increased in size and show loss of definition because of adjacent peribronchial fibrosis.

5. Volume changes vary. In generalized forms, such as that associated with cystic fibrosis and the ciliary dyskinesia syndrome, there is often generalized overinflation (Figures 17-14 and 17-15).[360] Localized forms, however, are frequently accompanied by atelectasis (Figure 17-18), which may be mild and detected only because of vascular crowding or fissural displacement. Volume loss may, on the other hand, be marked with a grossly collapsed airless lobe (Figure 17-19). Occasionally, collateral air drift

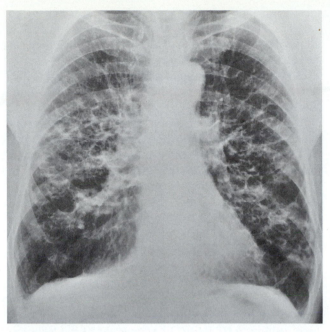

FIGURE 17-14
Gross cystic bronchiectasis. Posteroanterior chest radiograph showing overinflated lungs. There is diffuse lung shadowing with nodular and linear elements. In addition, there are multiple ring opacities ranging from 3 to 15 mm.

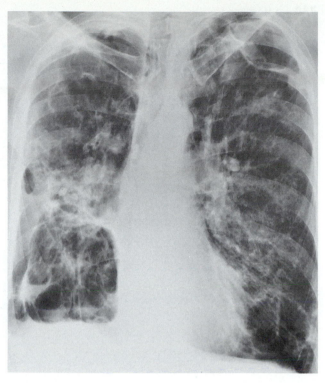

FIGURE 17-15
Bronchiectasis in patient with ciliary dyskinesia syndrome. Overall lung volume is increased. At left base are multiple linear opacities caused by bronchial wall thickening. On right is small hydropneumothorax. Multiple ring shadows at right base are due to bronchiectatic airways, which contain air-fluid levels.

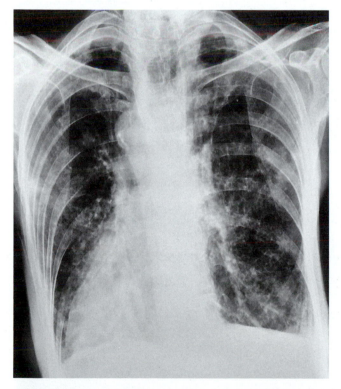

FIGURE 17-16
Ciliary dyskinesia syndrome–Kartagener's syndrome. This 62-year-old woman gave 40-year history consistent with bronchiectasis. Aortic arch, descending aorta, heart, and gastric air bubble are all on right. Diffuse complex pulmonary shadowing with many ring opacities is visible. Broad-branching band shadow can just be seen through heart and represents dilated fluid-filled airways.

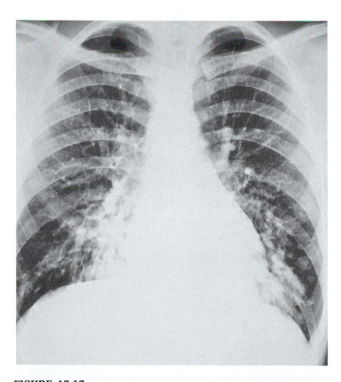

FIGURE 17-17
Ciliary dyskinesia syndrome. Patient, a 20-year-old man, had had recurrent pneumonia, otitis, and sinusitis. In paracardiac region are bilateral broad linear shadows caused by dilated, fluid-filled bronchi. Like 50% of patients with ciliary dyskinesia, this patient does not have dextrocardia.

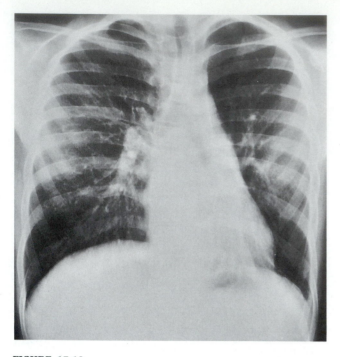

FIGURE 17-18
Left lower lobe bronchiectasis. Marked volume loss of left lower lobe is indicated by depressed hilum, vertical left mainstem bronchus, mediastinal shift, and left-sided transradiancy. Just visible through heart are parallel line opacities ("tubular shadows").

allows continued aeration of the distal lung, in which case there may be a localized increase in volume.

6. Other radiologic signs include infective consolidation, evidence of scarring, bulla formation, and pleural thickening.

In the past the definitive diagnosis of bronchiectasis has been made by bronchography, despite difficulties with interpretation of this examination.[94] The types of change observed are those mentioned previously in the discussion of pathologic manifestations. However, over the last 5 to 10 years this invasive and relatively unpleasant procedure has been largely replaced by CT. A number of reports have correlated bronchographic and CT findings. Several studies, particularly the earlier ones, used standard CT techniques and employed thick (10 mm) sections.[89,342,352,362,454] Although they had high specificity, sensitivity was generally only about 50% to 80% when compared with bronchography. More recently, high-resolution CT (HRCT) has emerged as the technique of choice, using thin sections (1.5 to 3 mm) and a high–spatial frequency ("bone") reconstruction algorithm. Reports of studies using HRCT are not easy to

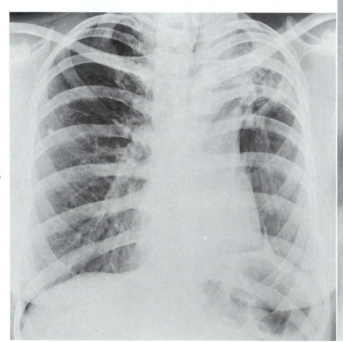

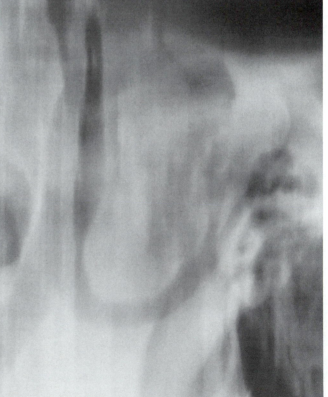

A

B

FIGURE 17-19
Left upper lobe bronchiectasis. **A,** Posteroanterior chest radiograph showing grossly collapsed left upper lobe caused by previous tuberculosis. **B,** Midlung tomogram of left upper lobe shows bronchiectatic airways as air bronchograms in collapsed lobe. Such airways drain well and are rarely associated with infective complications.

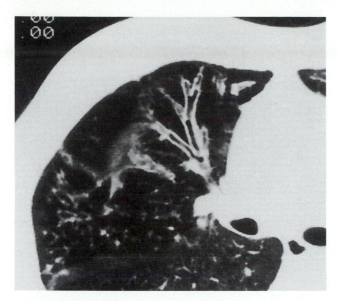

FIGURE 17-20
Cylindrical bronchiectasis. On high-resolution computed tomogram, airways parallel to plane of section in anterior segment of right upper lobe show changes of cylindrical bronchiectasis; bronchi are wider than normal and fail to taper. Airway walls are thickened, so that airways are seen more peripherally than normal.

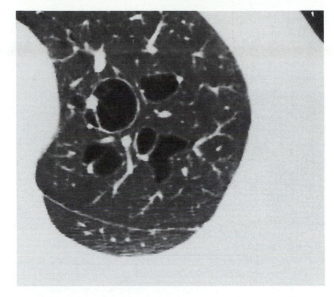

FIGURE 17-21
Bronchiectasis in segmental and subsegmental airways of left upper lobe. On high-resolution computed tomogram, dilated airways are perpendicular to plane of section and, along with their accompanying arteries, resemble signet rings. Note that bronchiectatic airway walls need not be thickened.

compare because of variation in section thickness, section spacing, severity of disease, and type of assessment; some correlate the presence or absence of whole lung disease and others correlate segmental disease. Three of these HRCT studies[176,235,549] give sensitivities and specificities in excess of 95% when compared with bronchography. Joharjy, Bashi, and Abdullah[235] used 4 mm sections every 5 mm, whereas the other two studies generally employed 1.5 mm sections every 10 mm.[176,549] A fourth study, using 3 mm sections every 10 mm, found lower sensitivities and specificities, just over 80%.[354] Probably these lower values are largely related to the type and severity of disease in the study population, with most patients having relatively mild, predominantly cylindrical bronchiectasis. Ten millimeter collimation is now considered inferior to thin sections (1.5 to 3 mm).[175] The protocol used has to be a compromise among absorbed dose, examination time, and the risk of missing lesions when sections are not contiguous.[175] The best compromise seems to be 1.5 mm thick sections every 10 mm from lung apex to base, decreasing intersection separation to 5 mm in questionable areas. The matrix should be 512 × 512, the reconstruction algorithm should have a high spatial frequency ("bone" algorithm), and times must be short (about 2 seconds) to minimize motion artifacts. Artifacts are particularly troublesome adjacent to the left heart border in the left lower zone, where they appear as doubled vascular structures simulating a "tubular" opacity, and as lucencies simulating airways in the elbow of U-shaped vascular artifacts.[490] HRCT performed as sug-

gested has a resolution of about 300 μm, and airway walls thinner than this are not resolvable. This means that the smallest detectable normal airways, which are fifth- to tenth-order branches, have an overall diameter of about 2 mm.[175] Such airways are not seen closer than 3 cm to the visceral pleura.

The signs of bronchiectasis on HRCT depend on the morphologic type of bronchiectasis (cylindrical, varicose, or cystic) and the orientation of the airway in question to the scan plane. Findings in cylindrical bronchiectasis have been reported. Airway dilatation (Figure 17-20) is easy to access when the airway is in the plane of section. When the airway is not parallel to the plane of section, it appears as an oval or circle and its size can be judged by comparison with the adjacent artery. Normally these two structures have approximately the same diameter. In making this comparison it is important to avoid bifurcations and to use the smallest airway diameter, making sure also that vessels are not pathologically large and not small as might occur in an oligemic area.[175,362] When the airway is moderately or markedly dilated, the combination of airway and artery produces a signet ring appearance (Figure 17-21).[362] Airways fail to taper as they extend peripherally, an assessment that can be made easily when they are parallel to the plane of section (Figure 17-20) but with difficulty when they cross obliquely from section to section. Airway walls are thickened (Figure 17-20). Bronchiectatic airways often have thickened walls, particularly in some conditions such as hypogammaglobulinemia.[97] However, walls are

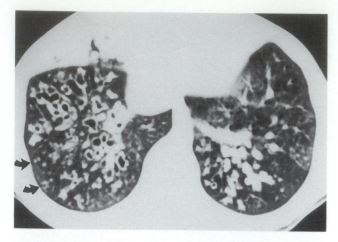

FIGURE 17-22
Extensive cylindrical and varicose bronchiectasis in ciliary dyskinesia, seen on conventional computed tomogram through lung bases. Many of bronchiectatic airways are filled with secretions (bronchoceles) and, depending on how they are sectioned, appear as rounded, oval, bandlike, or branching structures. Bronchiolar impaction can be seen as prominent centrilobular structures (arrows).

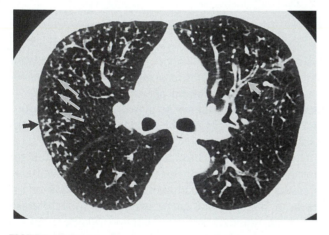

FIGURE 17-23
Diffuse panbronchiolitis on high-resolution computed tomogram. Characteristic findings include centrilobular nodules, 1 to 2 mm diameter (large arrows); branching linear opacities contacting centrilobular nodules (short black arrow); and bronchial wall thickening (short white arrow). Histologic study shows that nodules are caused by bronchial and peribronchial cellular infiltration, and branching linear structures by bronchiolectastis and bronchiolar impaction.

not necessarily thickened, and furthermore bronchial wall thickening may be seen in the absence of bronchiectasis. Airways with thickened walls may be seen closer to the periphery than normal (Figure 17-20). Secretion-filled airways (bronchoceles) appear as linear bandlike opacities that characteristically branch, giving rise to Y- or V-shaped structures (Figure 17-22). In cross section such airways produce rounded or oval opacities (Figure 17-22). Following such lesions from section to

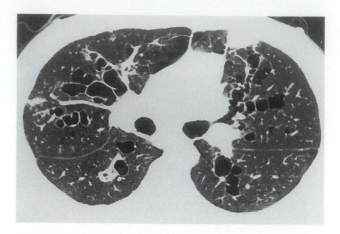

FIGURE 17-24
Varicose bronchiectasis in tracheobronchomegaly on high-resolution computed tomogram.

section usually allows their correct identification. The contents of these bronchoceles have a variable density that may even be calcific if long standing.[325] When contrast medium is administered, the contents fail to opacify.[325] Sometimes there is distal small airway impaction in bronchiectasis, reflecting the bronchiolitis obliterans of bronchioles arising from a more central, bronchiectatic parent airway. Distal impaction is manifest as centrilobular small nodules and branching structures, some of which may be just a few millimeters from the pleura (Figures 17-22 and 17-23). Geographic areas of reduced density and reduced vessel size (oligemia) are additional features of bronchiolitis obliterans.

Varicose bronchiectasis when imaged in cross section is easily misinterpreted as cystic or cylindrical bronchiectasis, but when airways are parallel to the plane of section, the corrugation of bronchial walls produced by sacculations in series is characteristic (Figure 17-24).[175,176]

Cystic bronchiectasis produces cystlike lesions that may or may not contain air-fluid levels. Sometimes they produce a characteristic linear array ("string of cysts"), which can be followed (possibly on adjacent sections) from the hilar region to the lung periphery. Other common patterns include a cluster of cysts (Figure 17-25) and cysts arranged in a segmental fashion. Differentiation from other cystic lesions can be difficult. The characteristic combination of cyst and accompanying artery (Figure 17-21) is sometimes helpful, but it is not pathognomonic of bronchiectasis, since such a combination can occur by chance in other cystic conditions such as bullous disease, histiocytosis X, or lymphangioleiomyomatosis. A sign that helps in this situation is the variation in size of bronchiectatic cysts with inspiration and expiration, a feature that is usually absent with other types of cystic lesions.[313] In general a careful analysis, attempting to follow cystlike lesions from one section to another and also noting their relation to central airways, allows

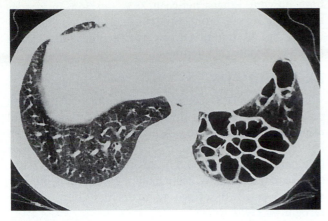

FIGURE 17-25
Cystic bronchiectasis of unknown etiology. High-resolution computed tomogram shows aggregated ring opacities in basal segments of left lower lobe.

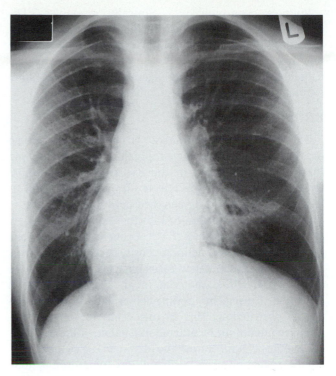

FIGURE 17-26
Ciliary dyskinesia syndrome–Kartagener's syndrome in 14-year-old boy with recurrent pneumonic episodes. Dextrocardia and situs inversus are present. Border of left side of heart is obscured by confluent nodular and linear opacities caused by bronchiectatic and shrunken left middle lobe.

the observer to make a diagnosis of cystic bronchiectasis with a reasonably high degree of certainty. CT also detects the secondary effects of bronchiectasis: parenchymal consolidation and scarring, atelectasis, and pleural thickening.

Scintiscan abnormalities have been described in bronchiectasis, but scintigraphy has never achieved much popularity as a diagnostic tool. On ventilation-perfusion (V/Q) scintiscans perfusion and ventilation are both impaired, with ventilation more affected.[162] Several workers using either xenon-133 or krypton-91m have concluded that a normal V/Q scintiscan coupled with a normal chest radiograph virtually excludes bronchiectasis.[162,481,506] Aerosol ventilation scintigraphy, as might be expected, is less sensitive (56%) than gas ventilation scintigraphy.[21] Indium 111–labeled autologous neutrophils migrate to bronchiectatic areas of the lung, but this has not been adopted as a useful clinical technique.[95,96]

Ciliary dyskinesia syndrome (immotile cilia syndrome)

The ciliary dyskinesia syndrome (CDS) is one of the specific causes of bronchiectasis, and with changing patterns of etiology it is becoming relatively more important. In this condition, first identified in 1976,[4] a variety of genetically determined defects in ciliary structure and function[430] interfere with mucociliary clearance. This impaired clearance is associated with recurrent upper and lower respiratory tract infections.[5,115] Another factor contributing to recurrent infection is defective neutrophil chemotaxis, a common association.[430] CDS shares many features with cystic fibrosis but is less disabling and carries a better prognosis.[360] Kartagener's syndrome (Figures 17-16 and 17-26)[246]—situs inversus, paranasal sinusitis, and bronchiectasis—is a subset of CDS, and about 50% of patients with CDS have Kartagener's syndrome.[5,172,360] About one fifth of subjects with dextrocardia have Kartagener's syndrome.[331] CDS has auto-

somal recessive transmission[427] with an equal sex incidence. In Europe and the United States CDS has a prevalence of about 1:20,000 people.[430] Ciliary function is abnormal throughout the body, and sperm are immotile. Thus males are infertile. Fertility in females is generally unaffected, although there are exceptions.[172] Respiratory symptoms may be delayed in onset but can generally be traced back to childhood, and CDS is even described as causing neonatal respiratory distress.[527] Symptoms are those of bronchitis, rhinitis, and sinusitis, which are universal, and otitis, which is less common. Bronchiectasis develops in childhood and adolescence (Figure 17-17)[360] and is associated with recurrent pneumonia. Prognosis is generally good,[5] and the diagnosis is compatible with a full life span.[331] The diagnosis is regarded as established in the following circumstances: (1) complete Kartagener's syndrome, (2) men with normal situs but a classic history and immotile sperm, (3) women and children with normal situs but typical history and an affected sibling, and (4) subjects with normal situs but with a classic history and ultrastructural defects of nasal or bronchial cilia on biopsy.[5] Patients with Kartagener's syndrome and morphologically normal cilia have been described.[173,430] Findings on the chest radiograph (Figures 17-16 and 17-17) and CT are of bronchiectasis with a predilection for involvement of the anatomic middle lobe (Figure 17-26).[360]

Young's syndrome[192,368] clinically resembles CDS. However, in Young's syndrome ciliary function is normal and infertility is due to obstructive azoospermia. Obstruction occurs at the level of the epididymis, which is palpably enlarged. The pathogenesis of increased sinopulmonary infection in these patients is obscure.

BRONCHOLITHIASIS

The term "broncholithiasis" is generally interpreted more widely than meaning simply the condition resulting from calcified material in the airway.[507] Most authors include, in addition, the effects of airway distortion or inflammation caused by calcified peribronchial nodes.[20] Nearly all cases are due to infective nodes, particularly following histoplasmosis.[101,516] Other causal infections include tuberculosis, actinomycosis, coccidioidomycosis, and cryptococcosis. A few cases have been reported with silicosis.[72] Calcified material in an airway or luminal distortion caused by peribronchial disease results in airway obstruction. This in turn leads to collapse, obstructive pneumonitis, mucoid impaction, or bronchiectasis. Fistulas can form from the airway to the esophagus,[99] pleural space, or aorta.[101] Symptoms commonly include cough, hemoptysis, and recurrent episodes of fever and purulent sputum.[87,101] The classic symptom of lithoptysis is uncommon, with a frequency of just 16% in one series[101] and 13% in another.[87]

In a review of the plain radiographic findings three major types of change were distinguished[507]: (1) disappearance of a previously identified calcified nidus; (2) change in position of a calcified nidus; and (3) evidence of airway obstruction including segmental or lobar atelectasis, mucoid impaction, obstructive pneumonitis, and obstructive overinflation with air trapping. There may be signs of bronchiectasis.[101] Calcified hilar or mediastinal nodes are a key feature of the radiograph, and it is important to inspect all calcifications, assessing their position and looking for evidence of movement on serial films. Movement can be difficult to detect and may just be a relatively subtle rotation.[507] Broncholithiasis is more common on the right,[101] and obstructive changes particularly affect the right middle lobe.

Once the diagnosis is suspected on plain radiographs, confirmation may be sought by CT and fiberoptic bronchoscopy. These examinations often complement each other, neither on its own being necessarily diagnostic. Principal findings on CT[87,263,449] are a calcified lymph node within an airway or immediately adjacent to a distorted airway, distal changes secondary to bronchial obstruction, and absence of an associated soft tissue mass. CT is not always correct in accurately localizing calcification because of partial volume effects, and in one series 40% of truly endobronchial lesions were interpreted on CT as extrabronchial.[87] Thin section CT should avoid this problem. The CT appearance of broncholithiasis can be mimicked by calcifying endobronchial hamartomas or carcinoid tumors.[448] The sensitivity of fiberoptic

bronchoscopy ranges between 28% and 56% in various series.[87] In some patients bronchoscopy is used therapeutically, but in others technical difficulties and excess bleeding obviate this approach.

BRONCHIOLITIS

Bronchiolitis is a spectrum of inflammatory disorders predominantly affecting small airways (membranous and respiratory bronchioles). These disorders show great heterogeneity as regards cause, clinical features, and histopathologic changes. A number of attempts to classify these conditions have been made,[86,119,358] and the one used here is that described by Myers and Colby.[358] They recognized eight types:

1. Constrictive bronchiolitis (obliterative bronchiolitis, bronchiolitis obliterans)
2. Cryptogenic organizing pneumonia (bronchiolitis obliterans organizing pneumonia [BOOP], proliferative bronchiolitis)
3. Acute bronchiolitis (infectious bronchiolitis)[382]
4. Small airways disease (adult bronchiolitis)
5. Respiratory bronchiolitis (smoker's bronchiolitis, respiratory bronchiolitis–associated interstitial lung disease)
6. Mineral dust airways disease (early pneumoconiosis)[546]
7. Follicular bronchiolitis
8. Diffuse panbronchiolitis

A number of these conditions are discussed elsewhere, and only five are considered in detail here.

Constrictive bronchiolitis

Constrictive bronchiolitis (CB) is a syndrome of airflow limitation caused by bronchiolar and peribronchiolar inflammation and fibrosis.[358] It has a number of synonyms, including bronchiolitis obliterans and obliterative bronchiolitis. In addition, adult bronchiolitis and small airways disease are included under this heading by some authors. CB is an unusual disorder that in most cases is associated with a recognized predisposing condition but occasionally is cryptogenic. Recognized associations are listed in the box on the facing page.

Histologic changes in CB are patchy and can easily be missed unless techniques are meticulous and samples adequate. A variety of abnormalities may be demonstrated, ranging from a cellular bronchiolitis to scarring and complete occlusion of small airways.[86] The early change is a cellular inflammation that is intraluminal, mural, and peribronchial, affecting membranous and respiratory bronchioles. Inflammatory cells are a mixture of neutrophils, lymphocytes, and plasma cells. The mature lesion is a peribronchiolar fibrosis, encroaching on the lumen and narrowing and eventually occluding the airway.[358] Other features include smooth muscle hyperplasia and bronchiolectasis with mucoid impaction.[86]

Clinical findings vary according to cause but have

Data from Myers JL, Colby TV: *Clin Chest Med* 14:611-622, 1993; and Wright JL, Cagle P, Churg A, et al: *Am Rev Respir Dis* 146:240-262, 1992.

common features. Symptoms consist of progressive dyspnea and nonproductive cough unaccompanied by significant wheezing. On auscultation of the chest, crackles and inspiratory squeaks are heard. Respiratory function tests show airflow obstruction with a normal gas transfer adjusted for alveolar volume (KCO).[505] There is evidence of gas trapping with a low forced vital capacity (FVC) and a high residual volume (RV). Airflow limitation is volume dependent and may be demonstrated by use of flow volume loops that allow calculation of maximum midexpiratory flow rates (MMEFR). However, a reduced MMEFR is not specific for small airways disease.[522]

Constrictive bronchiolitis is well recognized following the inhalation of toxic fumes and gases. It has been most frequently described following nitrogen dioxide inhalation (silo-filler's disease),[34,294,334,348] when it follows 2 to 6 weeks after acute symptoms caused by diffuse alveolar damage.[91,239,402] The prevalence of CB in exposed individuals is low,[118] and the condition responds to steroid administration. Viruses, particularly respiratory syncytial virus and adenovirus,[35,296,335] are the most commonly implicated infectious agents in CB.[6,23,538] Nonviral agents are much less common, with some specific reports, such as *Legionella pneumophila*,[438] *Mycoplasma pneumoniae*,[194,391] and others.[384] Postinfectious CB is largely

confined to children and has been recently reviewed.[384] Among the connective tissue disorders[120] the association is strongest with rheumatoid arthritis[153,202,299,522] and has been described rarely in systemic lupus erythematosus[256] and eosinophilic fasciitis.[120] Constrictive bronchiolitis associated with rheumatoid arthritis is usually manifest as rapidly advancing, refractory airflow obstruction and is associated with a poor prognosis; death from respiratory failure occurred in the majority of patients in one series 5 to 18 months after presentation.[153] About 50% of patients with rheumatoid arthritis and CB have been taking penicillamine,[153,505] and a cause and effect relationship has been proposed.[120,357] This is supported by a study of 602 patients with rheumatoid arthritis in which there was a 3% prevalence of CB in patients receiving penicillamine but there were no cases of CB in those not taking the drug.[539] Furthermore, a close temporal relationship often exists between starting penicillamine medication and the onset of symptoms.[522] A granulomatous bronchiolitis has been described in a patient with rheumatoid arthritis during gold treatment.[270]

In the last few years a clear association between lung transplantation and CB has emerged,[117,383,493] and it is a major determinant of long-term mortality and morbidity.[383] Posttransplant CB is caused by immunologically mediated damage to pulmonary or airway epithelium. It has a prevalence of between 25% and 50% and usually manifests itself between 9 and 15 months (range 60 days to 5.6 years) after transplantation.[383] It is seen particularly in patients who have had frequent and severe episodes of acute rejection and in patients who have had cytomegalovirus pneumonitis. Treatment is with augmented immunosuppression, which usually leads to improvement or a halt in progression. Although such remissions are common and are sometimes permanent, relapses are common.[383] Constrictive bronchiolitis is also recognized as a delayed complication of bone marrow transplantation.[117,377,423] The disorder develops usually within 500 days of transplantation [92] and has a prevalence of about 10%.[77,83] The main risk factors for the development of CB are old age, chronic graft versus host disease, and methotrexate immunosuppression.[92] It is associated with morbidity and an increased mortality — a 65% 3-year mortality compared with 44% in a group with chronic graft versus host disease alone.[82] Treatment is with augmented immunosuppression.

Rarely CB is cryptogenic.* It seems likely that patients described by these authors as cryptogenic do not constitute a homogeneous group, and indeed some cases were associated with bronchiectasis and others would probably now be classified as respiratory bronchiolitis–interstitial lung disease.[359]

A limited number of changes are described on the chest radiograph in CB, with some variation depending on the

---

*References 153, 163, 186, 253, 302, 476, 505.

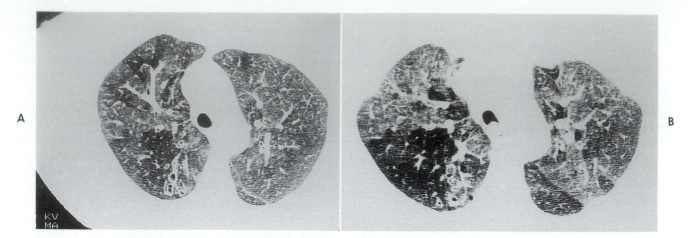

FIGURE 17-27
Constrictive bronchiolitis after infection on high-resolution computed tomogram. **A,** On full inspiration there are areas of low density, particularly in right lung, distributed in geographic fashion with intervening lung of normal density. **B,** On full expiration low-density areas persist and are accentuated.

cause of the disease:

1. The chest radiograph is sometimes normal; this is described with inhalation, transplantation, or rheumatoid disease; following infection; and in cryptogenic CB.

2. Hyperinflation is described following toxic fume inhalation,[327,540] in rheumatoid disease,[153] following marrow transplantation,[377] and in cryptogenic disease.[60]

3. Hypovascularity is described in cryptogenic CB,[60,483] with rheumatoid disease,[483] and with lung transplantation.[346] It is characterized by a reduction in size and number of vessels, particularly peripheral ones. In the report by Turton and co-workers,[505] oligemia was accompanied by matched V/Q defects on scintiscans.

4. Reticulonodular patterns. CB associated with nitrogen dioxide inhalation (silo-filler's disease) is characterized by small nodules (1 to 5 mm) distributed diffusely or with an upper zone predominance[91] that may become confluent.[217,294,334] Nodules following inhalation may resolve completely or incompletely with time.[296] Nodular and reticulonodular opacity has also been described in cryptogenic CB,[196,302] in CB following infection,[163] and in CB associated with heart-lung transplantation[462] and rheumatoid disease.[202]

5. Bronchiectatic changes. In some disorders the agent or condition causing CB also causes damage to larger airways. This situation is seen with lung transplantation,[283,346,462] viral infections,[194] and toxic inhalation.[466] In such disorders linear and ring opacities characteristic of bronchiectasis may be seen — changes that may be useful markers of significant small airway obstruction in the appropriate clinical context.[296]

6. Consolidation. Patchy airspace opacity is not a feature of CB but is recorded in lung transplants, possibly on the basis of infection.[346,462] Areas of persisting consolidation and collapse are also seen in postinfection CB.[296,438]

A number of studies have looked at changes on CT and HRCT. The majority of patients in these series have had lung or heart-lung transplants.[283,346,380,462] Other types of CB studied include cryptogenic CB[483] and CB related to rheumatoid disease, infection, and penicillamine.[380] The principal findings in these series follow:

1. Peripheral vessels are attenuated.

2. Patchy areas of low and high parenchymal density give an overall mosaic that is accentuated on expiration (Figure 17-27).[483] Sweatman and co-workers[483] considered that low-density areas were caused by air trapping with diversion of blood elsewhere and that high-density areas were the result of impaired alveolar ventilation. The sharp lobular[110] and segmental distribution of low-attenuation areas (Figure 17-27) in CB usually allows a distinction from the low-density areas of emphysema.[296,297]

3. Although not a manifestation of CB, bronchiectatic change is a common association in posttransplant CB[283,346,380] and postinfection CB.[297] Bronchiectasis is manifest as bronchial dilatation at segmental and subsegmental level and may be unaccompanied by bronchial wall thickening.[380]

4. Centrilobular branching structures, which almost certainly represent "mucoid" impaction at a bronchiolar level, were seen in 28% of cases of CB of mixed etiology in one series (Figure 17-23).[380]

Respiratory bronchiolitis–associated interstitial lung disease

Respiratory bronchiolitis–associated interstitial lung disease (RB-ILD) is a recently recognized clinicopathologic syndrome that is usually seen in current heavy cigarette smokers.[254,359,553] Pathologic findings are nonspecific, consisting of an excess of pigmented macrophages in respiratory bronchioles and adjacent alveolar ducts and alveoli, a membranous and respiratory mononuclear bronchiolitis, fibrous scarring extending outward from airways into alveolar walls, and an abnormal airway epithelium.[553] Patients have cough and dyspnea, and on examination there are bibasal end-inspiratory crepitations.[254]

The chest radiograph is usually abnormal in RB-ILD, and in two series with a total of 24 patients 70% had reticulonodular opacities,[359,553] typically fine and diffuse or basally predominant.[553] A few patients have had bibasal atelectasis.[214,359,553] Before the recognition of RB-ILD a number of studies have noted the presence of low-profusion, small, irregular opacities on the chest radiographs of smokers.[74,100,519,520] It seems highly likely that these abnormalities were due to RB-ILD. In a major study comparing HRCT of 98 current smokers with 175 nonsmoking control subjects,[416] parenchymal micronodules (upper zone predominant, ill-defined, 2 to 3 mm nodules) were found in 27% of smokers but in no control subjects. Comparable values were noted for areas of ground-glass attenuation (20% of smokers, and none of the control group).[416] Histologic examination in a number of these patients showed RB-ILD changes.[417] In a second study HRCT findings were described in five patients with biopsy-proven RB-ILD.[214] The most common finding was areas of ground-glass opacity. One patient had interlobular and intralobular thickening. No patient had nodular opacities.[214]

Follicular bronchiolitis

Follicular bronchiolitis has characteristic pathologic changes consisting of lymphoid follicular hyperplasia and lymphocytic infiltration of bronchiolar walls.[522,551] The hyperplastic lymphoid follicles narrow airways by external compression. The condition has been most commonly described in patients with rheumatoid arthritis and Sjögren's syndrome,[136,551] but other associations are recognized, including a familial form with immunodeficiency.[551] Patients have a restrictive respiratory defect, and the disorder has a variable natural history. CT changes are not described, but the plain chest radiograph shows diffuse, small nodular or reticulonodular opacities.[136,552]

Diffuse panbronchiolitis

Diffuse panbronchiolitis (DPB) is a disorder characterized by chronic sinusitis and bronchial inflammation[479] and found almost exclusively in Japanese, Chinese, and Koreans. Initial symptoms usually occur between 20 and 50 years of age, and there is no sex predilection. Some cases are familial, and an association with B54 human leukocyte antigen has been shown. Patients have cough, sputum, and signs and symptoms of progressive obstruc-

tive airways disease. Later the disorder is punctuated by episodic bacterial infections (especially caused by *Pseudomonas*) until the picture becomes one of marked bronchiectasis with terminal chronic respiratory failure. Respiratory function tests show gross airflow obstruction with or without mild restriction, hypoxemia, and increased residual volume. Treatment is with long-term, low-dose erythromycin. This leads to subjective and objective improvement, but its effect on prognosis remains to be evaluated. Without treatment the prognosis is poor, with a 42% 5-year survival and a 25% 10-year survival.[479]

The histologic findings[358] center on respiratory bronchioles, where there is a dense peribronchial and intraluminal infiltrate of acute and chronic inflammatory cells, particularly mononuclear cells, with striking hyperplasia of lymphoid follicles.[437] These bronchiolocentric lesions are visible macroscopically as yellow nodules. Accumulations of foamy macrophages in alveolar ducts and septa are also characteristic. Other findings include dilatation of membranous airways, which may be plugged with mucus and inflammatory cells, and in some cases bronchiectasis.

The principal finding on the plain chest radiograph is multiple small (1 to 5 mm), ill-defined nodules.[8,215,296,372] These are symmetrically distributed and initially most prominent basally. Later they spread to involve all zones, at which time small ring and tramline opacities appear particularly at the bases, to be joined later by large thin-walled ring opacities.

A number of studies have described the HRCT changes,[7,8] and one study gives a detailed pathologic correlation.[372] Findings include the following:

1. Small (1 to 3 mm), ill-defined, rounded nodules distributed in a centrilobular fashion (Figure 17-23). The nodules are 2 to 3 mm inside the lobular envelope, at the point where respiratory bronchioles might be expected. These opacities are produced by the bronchiolocentric inflammatory lesions described previously.

2. Thin, branching, linear opacities that contact the nodules (Figure 17-23). Histologic study has shown these to be widened bronchioles with thickened, inflamed walls containing intraluminal secretions. When these small airways lose their contents, they become visible as small ring-shaped or oval structures joining nodules to the centrilobular bronchovascular bundles. With progression the whole of the intralobular airway becomes visible, since it is dilated and has thicker than normal walls.[8]

3. Beyond the margin of peripheral lobules bronchi and bronchioles have thickened walls and widened lumina.

4. The peripheral rim of lung is less dense than normal because of air trapping.[355] The reduced ventilation of this region has been demonstrated by positron emission tomography using ^{13}N.[355]

Swyer-James (MacLeod's) syndrome

The Swyer-James or MacLeod's syndrome is a form of bronchiolitis obliterans that has special features: it occurs following an insult to the developing lung; small bronchi are affected in addition to bronchioles; the lung served by abnormal airways remains inflated by collateral air drift; and by definition the airway disease as assessed by the chest radiograph is predominantly unilateral, giving rise to the key finding of unilateral transradiancy.

The condition was first described in the early 1950s, and a variety of noneponymous terms have been used to identify it, particularly unilateral or lobar emphysema. However, these terms may lead to confusion with, for example, congenital lobar emphysema, and the current practice of using eponymous titles seems likely to continue and is probably to be recommended. On several grounds Swyer-James syndrome seems to be the most acceptable.

The first accounts were of a 6-year-old boy who had the abnormal lung removed and studied pathologically[485] and in the following year of nine healthy adults aged 18 to 41 years.[304] The condition is characterized by bronchitis, bronchiolitis, bronchiolitis obliterans, and emphysema. Typically the condition is unilateral and a whole lung is affected, but changes may be confined to a lobe or segment.[412] Other recognized patterns are of segmental sparing with the rest of the lung involved[412] and of bilateral lobar or segmental disease. The patchy nature of lung involvement in some patients is particularly well demonstrated on CT examination.[341] Bronchi and bronchioles from the fourth generation to terminal bronchioles have submucosal fibrosis, causing luminal irregularity and occlusion.[412,485] Pulmonary tissue is hypoplastic, including the pulmonary artery and its branches, which are reduced in both size and number. Lung distal to diseased airways is hyperinflated and supplied by collateral air drift. Sometimes panacinar emphysematous changes are present.[496]

The Swyer-James syndrome is caused by injury of the immature lung. Injury most commonly follows an acute viral infection occurring during the first 8 years of life, before the lung has completed its development.[221] Viruses implicated include adenovirus[306,387] and measles virus.[311] Nonviral causes include infections such as *Mycoplasma* pneumonia,[477] tuberculosis,[401,412] and pertussis[311] and noninfectious causes such as aspirated foreign bodies,[311,517] irradiation,[37] and hydrocarbon ingestion.[261]

Patients are typically asymptomatic and commonly present as adults with an abnormal radiograph. Less commonly patients have exertional dyspnea,[311] which may be progressive and, exceptionally, quite marked,[304] or repeated respiratory infections.[311,485] When coincidental acute lung disorders occur in the presence of the Swyer-James syndrome, the chest radiograph may show a unilateral distribution of acute abnormality, as is recorded with pulmonary edema[433] and pulmonary hemorrhage.[340] Respiratory function tests show a reduced vital capacity, some airflow obstruction, and a reduced steady-state diffusing capacity. Lung scintigraphy shows a decrease or absence of perfusion in the affected lung[525] and impaired ventilation with delayed xenon washout.[373] Although a matched perfusion-ventilation defect might raise the possibility of embolic pulmonary artery obstruction, this is rarely a diagnostic problem in the clinical setting. Furthermore, delayed xenon washout indicating air trapping is not a feature of pulmonary embolism.

Findings on the plain chest radiograph are characteristic. Unilateral transradiancy is caused by reduced lung perfusion (Figure 17-28). If the condition is confined to a lobe, the transradiancy is lobar. Lesser degrees of involvement are not detectable on the plain radiograph. On the affected side the size and number of midlung and peripheral vessels are reduced (Figure 17-28). Blood flow in the contralateral lung is increased, and frequently this lung looks plethoric, an abnormality that may be more striking than the unilateral transradiance. The hilum of the involved lung is small (Figure 17-28), but lung volumes are normal or only slightly decreased. The mediastinum may show some shift to the affected side at total lung capacity.[304] The fact that the ipsilateral lung volume does not increase is helpful in distinguishing Swyer-James syndrome from emphysema per se.[304] Ipsilateral air trapping is a key finding and a sine qua non of the condition. It can be demonstrated with a pair of chest radiographs — one taken on inspiration and one on expiration (Figure 17-28). The expiratory radiograph should be exposed during a forced expiratory maneuver because the short expiratory time maximizes volume differences between the obstructed and nonobstructed lung.[171] Air trapping can also be demonstrated by xenon ventilation scintigraphy[373] or inspiratory-expiratory CT.[341]

Pulmonary angiography and bronchography have been performed in the past, and at the time they contributed significantly to an understanding of the pathophysiology of the Swyer-James syndrome. However, their use is no longer justified. Pulmonary angiography shows small hilar and peripheral lung vessels (Figure 17-28).[221,485] Typically on bronchography, segmental airways are irregular in outline and end abruptly at the fifth or sixth generation in square or tapered ends,[311,401,412,485] with no filling of peripheral airways despite maneuvers designed to correct this (Figure 17-29).

CT findings (Figure 17-30) have been described.[314,341] CT shows changes that are often more complex than suspected from the chest radiograph, and while it may confirm that transradiancy is unilateral, it more commonly shows bilateral transradiancy. Transradiant regions are often inhomogeneous, containing a patchwork of local low-density and hypovascular areas interspersed with lung of normal density.[341] Such small low-density areas may be poorly or sharply marginated, possibly representing areas of emphysema and air trapping, respectively.[341] Air trapping can be confirmed with

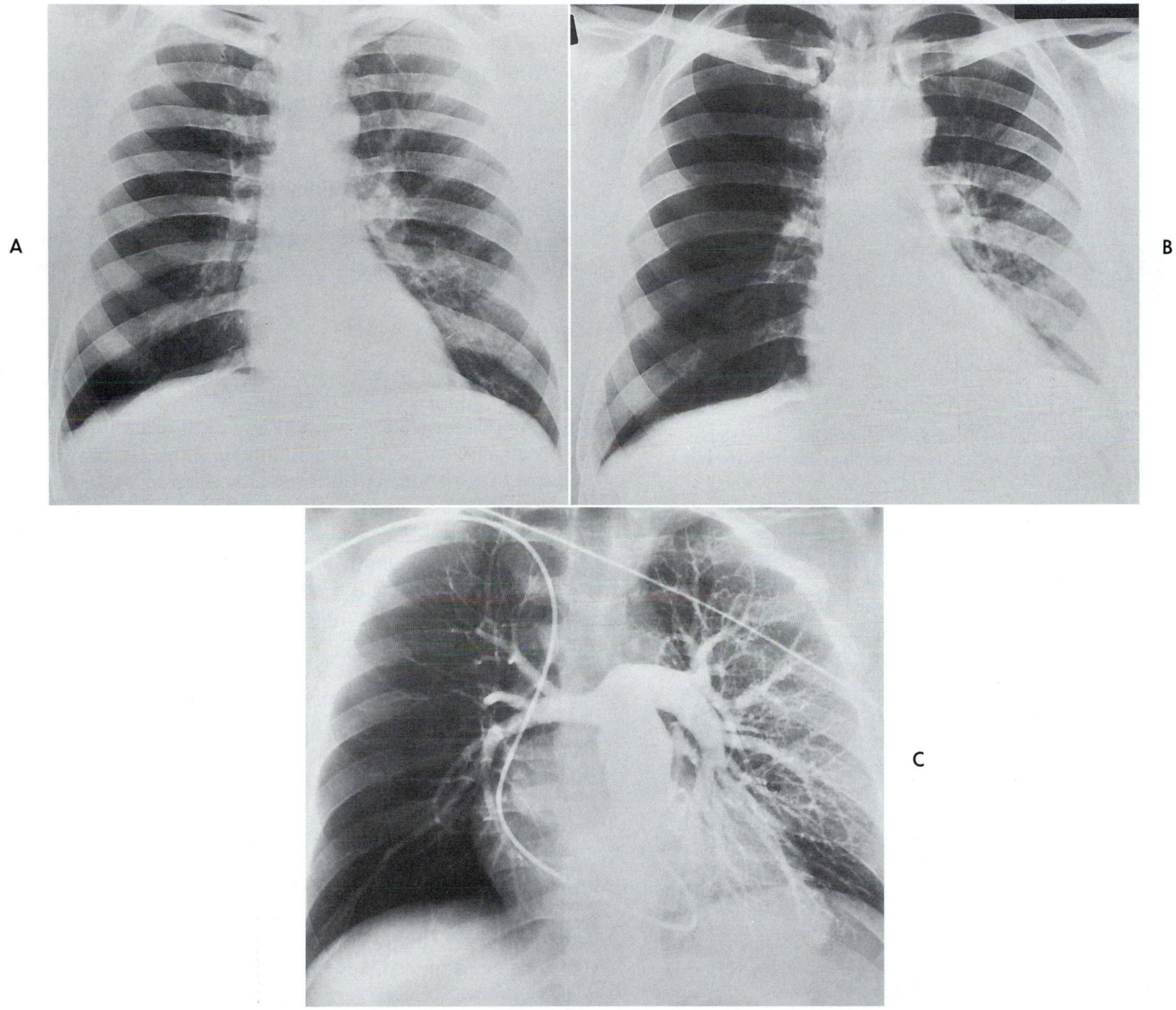

FIGURE 17-28
Swyer-James (Macleod's) syndrome. **A,** Posteroanterior chest radiograph on inspiration shows transradiant right lung with reduced number and size of vessels and small right hilum. Lung volume on right is probably slightly increased, and there is blunt costophrenic angle. **B,** Same patient. Expiratory radiograph demonstrates air trapping with relative elevation of left hemidiaphragm, vascular crowding on left, and mild mediastinal shift. **C,** Same patient. Pulmonary angiogram shows reduction in size and number of vessels to right lung. Compare size of right and left pulmonary arteries.

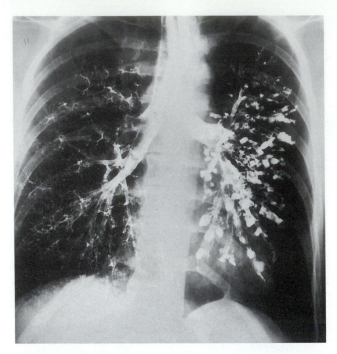

FIGURE 17-29
Swyer-James (Macleod's) syndrome. Bronchography shows diffuse left-sided bronchiectatic changes more marked in lower zones.

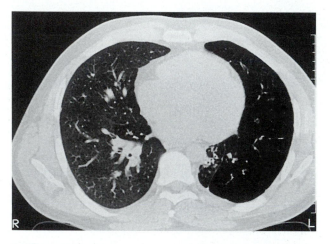

FIGURE 17-30
Swyer-James syndrome on high-resolution computed tomogram. Left lung shows lower density than right, and vessels are reduced in size and number. Left lung volume is slightly reduced.

expiratory CT scans. Other changes on CT include bronchiectasis,[314] which is not a universal finding,[341] and areas of collapse and scarring.

The described combination of radiographic findings usually allows exclusion of other conditions that may resemble the Swyer-James syndrome. These conditions include congenital hypoplastic lung, pulmonary artery hypoplasia, and proximal interruption of the pulmonary artery. The greatest worry is that signs are being produced by a central, large airway obstruction causing lung

hypoventilation and a compensatory ipsilateral reduction in perfusion. This is a problem that may be resolved only by bronchoscopy or a tailored CT examination of central airways.

CHRONIC OBSTRUCTIVE PULMONARY DISEASE

COPD (chronic airflow obstruction, chronic obstructive airway disease) encompasses a group of disorders characterized by chronic or recurrent obstruction to airflow. Four principal disorders fall under this heading: asthma, chronic bronchitis, emphysema, and bronchiectasis.[135,495] Although some purists object to the use of all-embracing, generic terms such as chronic obstructive airway disease or COPD, they are necessary in clinical practice because the various forms are sometimes difficult to identify and often coexist to a variable extent in the same patient.

Asthma

Asthma is a recurrent disorder that is defined functionally as a "disease characterized by wide variations over short periods of time in resistance to air flow in intrapulmonary airways."[440] This definition does not specify the degree of variation, but it is usually taken to be 15% to 20%.

Radiologic findings in uncomplicated asthma are due to both pathologic and pathophysiologic changes. Pathologic changes have been studied largely,[73,109] but not exclusively,[160] by postmortem examination of lungs in patients who died of asthma. Such findings represent the severe end of a spectrum of change. On gross examination the lungs are overinflated and fail to deflate because of tenacious mucus plugs in medium-sized airways. Bronchial mucosa is damaged or shed, and there are submucosal edema and inflammatory cell infiltrates of eosinophils, sometimes with lymphocytes and plasma cells, causing bronchial wall thickening. Other changes contributing to a general thickening of the bronchial walls include mucous gland hypertrophy, basement membrane thickening, and smooth muscle hyperplasia.[220] The lung parenchyma, in addition to being generally hyperinflated, may show patchy collapse and consolidation.

Routine respiratory function tests demonstrate pathophysiologic changes in attacks but are often normal in remission. Even in remission, however, results of sophisticated tests, particularly of small airway function, may be abnormal.[203,321] In acute asthma the findings are increased airway resistance, increased total lung capacity (TLC), and increased residual volume and functional residual capacity (FRC) with decreased vital capacity (VC), indicating air trapping.[328,543] Changes in TLC and FRC may be at least 20% in an acute attack.[544] With recovery, falls in the TLC and FRC may anticipate increases in the forced expiratory volume in 1 second (FEV$_1$). Changes in lung volumes assessed by planimetric measurement of the chest radiograph in acute asthma are documented[48] and have been used to follow the course of the disease.[312] Nonuniform ventilation and perfusion lead to mismatch and hypoxemia in attacks. Steady-state diffusing capacity for carbon monoxide is normal.

Radiographic findings in simple asthma are due to pathologic and functional changes, and in complicated asthma they are also due to the complications. The main radiographic findings in simple asthma, in decreasing order of frequency, are hyperinflation, bronchial wall thickening, and hilar prominence.

Hyperinflation may be seen in asthma in both relapse and remission. The prevalence of hyperinflation depends on many factors and is generally higher in children and in patients needing hospital admission. It is also more frequent in patients with an onset of asthma in the first or second decade than in those with a later onset.[206,258] These latter findings may be related to remodeling of the lungs and thoracic cage induced by airway obstruction during the growing phase.[48] With overinflation, diaphragms become depressed. Although less curved, they rarely become flat or inverted in asthma per se. The frequency of hyperinflation in adults with acute asthma has varied between approximately 20% and 70% in various series, reflecting different patient populations and hyperinflation criteria.* In one series of 117 patients with a mean age of 41 years (range 13 to 75) admitted to the hospital with acute asthma and in whom strict criteria for hyperinflation were applied, the prevalence was 39%.[388] While hyperinflation is often short lived, lasting perhaps just 24 hours,[405] it may be a permanent change; in the study of 117 patients mentioned previously, 19% showed hyperinflation when in remission.[388] Hyperinflation in such patients is due to a change in lung compliance and is not caused by generalized emphysema, which can be shown to be absent by use of CT.[258] However, if the patient is a smoker, emphysema may be a factor.[262]

In asthmatic patients the walls of end-on segmental airways become thickened (more than 1 mm) and the normally invisible airways parallel to the radiograph appear as parallel- or single-line opacities (Figure 17-31). The most comprehensive study of bronchial wall thickening in asthma was that of Hodson and Trickey[205] in 1960, in which they assessed the finding on plain radiographs in 190 asthmatic patients ranging in age from 3 to 74 years. Bronchial wall thickening was found to be more common in children, and in the small number of children analyzed it was a universal finding. Its frequency in adults was less but still surprisingly high, for example, 50% in the third and fourth decades. Other studies in adults also find that radiographic bronchial wall thickening is common: 71% in 48 asthmatic patients, nearly half of whom were smokers.[298] Bronchial wall thickening was 10 times more common in patients with an infective element to their asthma (asthma-bronchitis) than in those whose asthma was thought to be purely allergic. Its

*References 132, 298, 388, 405, 524, 554.

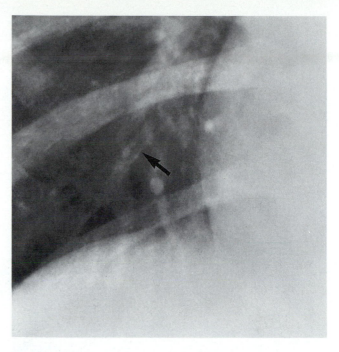

FIGURE 17-31
Asthma. Localized view of right lower zone shows bronchial wall thickening *(arrow).*

frequency correlated also with severity of asthma. In adults bronchial wall thickening, once developed, became a permanent feature. The nontransient nature of bronchial wall thickening has also been noted on CT.[381]

About 10% of asthmatic patients show slight prominence of hilar shadows. This is ascribed variously to nodal enlargement[428] and vascular enlargement.[50,154,388] Peripheral lung vessels are generally considered normal, but some authors describe diffuse narrowing or subpleural oligemia.[154]

A number of complications and associations of asthma may be detected on the chest radiograph, including consolidation, atelectasis and mucoid impaction, pneumothorax, pneumomediastinum, and allergic bronchopulmonary aspergillosis. Allergic aspergillosis apart, such complications are more common in children than in adults. In one series of 479 hospital patients with a median age of nearly 4 years, 22% had radiographic abnormalities, excluding signs of bronchial wall thickening and hyperinflation.[114] Other pediatric series bear these figures out.[62,157] In adults the prevalence of similar abnormalities is generally less than 10% even in admissions for acute asthma and is only about 1% to 2% in series drawn from emergency room patients.[50,132,388,428,554] However, higher figures are reported: in one series of patients with acute asthma, admitted after 12 hours of bronchodilator therapy in the emergency room, one third of chest radiographs were abnormal.[524]

Consolidation in asthma is most commonly infective (Figure 17-32),[50] but in some cases it is due to eosino-

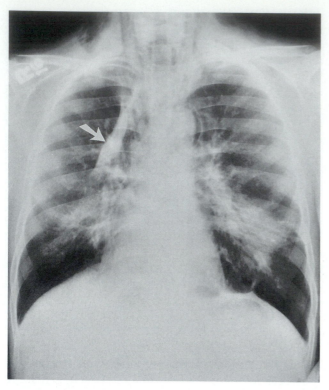

FIGURE 17-32
Acute asthma. Radiograph of 10-year-old boy shows three complications of acute asthma. In right upper zone, oblique band shadow is due to segmental collapse *(arrow),* and in left lower zone there is infective consolidation. Third complication is pneumomediastinum with air tracking into neck.

philic consolidation, probably associated with allergic aspergillosis. Collapse (Figure 17-32) ranges from subsegmental to lobar but occasionally involves a whole lung.[58] Such episodes of collapse are not necessarily associated with an acute illness, a respiratory tract infection, or a worsening of the asthma.[216,428] When segmental or lobar collapse occurs, the middle lobe is commonly affected both in children[114] and in adults.[428] Collapse is due to mucoid impaction in large airways or, more commonly, mucus plugging in many small airways. The frequency of occurrence of collapse per se is difficult to determine because in many series consolidation and collapse are considered together.[388] In adults it is probably only a few percent.[132,428]

Pneumothorax is, unexpectedly, an unusual complication of acute asthma in adults, and in combined series consisting largely of adults with acute disease* only three pneumothoraces in 566 patients were recorded. In a retrospective survey based on a region of the United Kingdom with over 6 million inhabitants, a frequency of pneumothorax in asthma of between 1:300 and 1:1,100 was recorded,[64] which was almost identical to figures from a large retrospective study at the Mayo Clinic (Rochester, Minnesota).[281] In the series reported by

Burke[64] it was noted that pneumothorax did not lead to death or morbidity and was usually not suspected clinically. Other workers agree that pneumothorax is not an important factor in mortality except when patients are being treated by positive-pressure ventilation.[50,245] A condition that may simulate tension pneumothorax in asthmatic patients receiving mechanical ventilation is described. This is due to a ball valve mucus plug causing localized or unilateral obstructive hyperinflation.[370]

Pneumomediastinum in adults is as uncommon as pneumothorax, and in the combined series of 566 patients discussed previously, only two had a pneumomediastinum. Pneumomediastinum is considerably more common in children (Figure 17-32), with a prevalence of 5.4% in 515 acute asthma admissions.[114] In children it is much more common than pneumothorax, by a factor of 10:1 in one series.[46] Spinal epidural emphysema is a complication of mediastinal emphysema in asthma.[502] Pneumopericardium has been reported rarely.[501]

A clear picture of CT and HRCT findings to be expected in asthma has not emerged from the few studies so far performed.[298,365,381] In the two main studies HRCT was abnormal in over 90%[298] and 68%[381] of patients. Principal abnormalities involved the airways. Both series showed bronchial wall thickening—in 16%[381] and 92%[298]—a discrepancy that may be related to the high proportion of smokers (nearly 50%) in the latter series. In a pathologic and HRCT study of 41 smokers 39% were found to have bronchial wall thickening.[417] Comparing bronchial dilatation in the series of Paganin and co-workers[381] with that of Lynch and co-workers[298] is difficult because patients with bronchiectasis (clinically and on CT tapering criteria) were excluded from the latter study.[298] If cylindrical bronchiectasis and airway dilatation are taken as equivalent terms, the findings are similar: cylindrical bronchiectasis in 56% of one series[381] and bronchial dilatation in 77% of the other.[298] However, the significance of the latter finding is not clear because airway dilatation was found in 59% of the control series. Other HRCT changes noted in these two studies included mucoid impaction, collapse, acinar opacities, emphysema, and hyperlucent areas ascribed to air trapping with secondarily reduced perfusion.

The indications for a chest radiograph in adults with asthma are not clearly established. Most authors would recommend chest radiography in all patients who are ill enough to justify admission to a hospital.[132,388,446,524,554] In the series described by Petheram, Kerr, and Collins,[388] of 117 patients admitted to the hospital with acute asthma, 9% of chest radiographs showed abnormalities that altered management.[388] White and co-workers[524] recorded an even higher figure, 22%, in 58 patients who were admitted after 12 hours of bronchodilator therapy in the emergency ward. Most would consider radiography essential before mechanical ventilation is initiated,[111,405] and failure to respond to therapy is also considered an indication by some.[50,132,554]

*References 132, 154, 206, 388, 405, 554.

Chronic bronchitis

Chronic bronchitis is defined, using clinical criteria, as a chronic or recurrent increase in the volume of mucoid bronchial secretions sufficient to cause expectoration and occurring on most days for 3 months in 2 or more successive years, other causes for expectoration having been excluded.[81,135,200]

At one time chronic bronchitis was thought to be an important cause of chronic airflow obstruction, but this idea is no longer accepted.[135,371,389] Evidence for this view comes from clinical studies showing that chronic expectoration and airflow obstruction behave largely as independent variables.[135,229] This is perhaps not surprising because bronchial gland hypertrophy, the major pathologic change in chronic bronchitis, occurs in large airways,[409] whereas the dominant site of irreversible airflow obstruction is in peripheral airways less than 3 mm in diameter.[209,455]

Chronic bronchitis is a common disease, affecting up to 20% of the adult population in some studies.[350] It is much more common in males than females,[350] but when smoking habits are taken into account the difference is only 2:1.[495] Most studies show an increasing prevalence with age. Cigarette smoking is the most important factor associated with the development of chronic bronchitis. In eight combined series in England there was a sixfold rise in prevalence of chronic bronchitis, from 6.3% in nonsmokers to 40% in heavy smokers.[495] In epidemiologic studies a linear relationship exists between the amount smoked and the frequency of chronic bronchitis.[486] The quantitative contribution made by other factors to the development of chronic bronchitis is small by comparison. Such factors include occupation, environment, age, and gender. Some of these factors appear to have a stronger association with acute infective exacerbations than with chronic bronchitis itself. The epidemiology of COPD has been recently reviewed.[447]

The major pathologic changes are in the mucous glands, which show hypertrophy and hyperplasia and develop enlarged ducts. The enlargement of mucous glands can be quantified histologically using either the proportional mucous gland area or the Reid index, which is the ratio of gland thickness to bronchial wall thickness measured from epithelial basement membrane to perichondrium.[409] These indexes unfortunately do not clearly distinguish normal subjects from those with chronic bronchitis, since there is considerable overlap.[197,497] A correlation has been demonstrated in chronic bronchitis between gland mass and sputum production.[229] Study of these indexes has shown that mucous glands also enlarge with age and in cigarette smokers.[337,371] There is in addition a positive association between increased mucous gland mass and emphysema,[337] probably reflecting the common etiology of smoking.

Other pathologic changes in chronic bronchitis include goblet cell hyperplasia, squamous metaplasia of the epithelium, and a variable and often mild[409] chronic inflammatory cell infiltrate.[200] Mucus plugs occur in the smaller airways, which themselves may be stenotic.[123,319,495] Cartilage atrophy probably occurs, but the evidence is conflicting,[166,418,488] and atrophy seems to be more a feature of emphysema than of chronic bronchitis.[141] Muscle hypertrophy is seen in patients with chronic bronchitis who have episodes of wheezing.

Chronic bronchitis typically occurs as a persistent productive cough following an acute chest infection. Such symptoms may persist for years with normal respiratory function tests and chest radiographs. Indeed the majority of such patients do not develop chronic airway obstruction, although they are at risk for recurrent episodes of purulent bronchitis. Such infections cause short-term illnesses requiring time off work, but they have no significant long-term effect on the rate of deterioration, disability, or prognosis.[29] In addition, in these patients the annual decrease in FEV_1 is within the normal range.[29,61] In some patients with chronic bronchitis, however, particularly those who smoke heavily, there is detectable airflow obstruction with a greater than predicted annual fall in FEV_1. These patients become dyspneic, with copious sputum, and tend to become hypoxemic.[66] In such patients pulmonary arterial hypertension and cor pulmonale may develop and an acute infective exacerbation may lead to respiratory failure.

Radiologic signs in pure chronic bronchitis are poorly documented. Nearly all the available information is derived from three series of patients in whom coexistent emphysema was not excluded.[30,456,458] Overinflation of the lung described in these reports is in conflict with the normal total lung capacity (TLC) usually found in chronic bronchitis.[300] Overinflation and oligemia described in these studies are now generally ascribed to coexistent emphysema.

The majority of patients with chronic bronchitis have a normal chest radiograph.[147] Radiographic signs that are ascribed to chronic bronchitis include bronchial wall thickening and "increased lung markings." Bronchial wall thickening might be expected in chronic bronchitis because of the known pathologic changes in the airways: mucous gland hypertrophy, cellular infiltration, and muscle hypertrophy. However, some histologic studies suggest that the magnitude of these changes is small; in one report the absolute increase in gland thickness was only 0.1 mm.[497] Admittedly in Reid's report[409] the mean increase in gland thickness was 0.47 mm, but this has to be set against probable cartilage atrophy.[141] Bates and co-workers[30] described parallel line shadows on radiographs representing large airways seen side on (tramline opacities) in 42% of patients with chronic bronchitis. However, this sign was not described by Simon and Galbraith,[456,458] who did not consider radiologic bronchial wall thickening a part of chronic bronchitis. Airways may also be seen end on as small ring opacities in the perihilar region. Ring shadows vary between 4 and 7 mm in diameter and most commonly represent the end-on

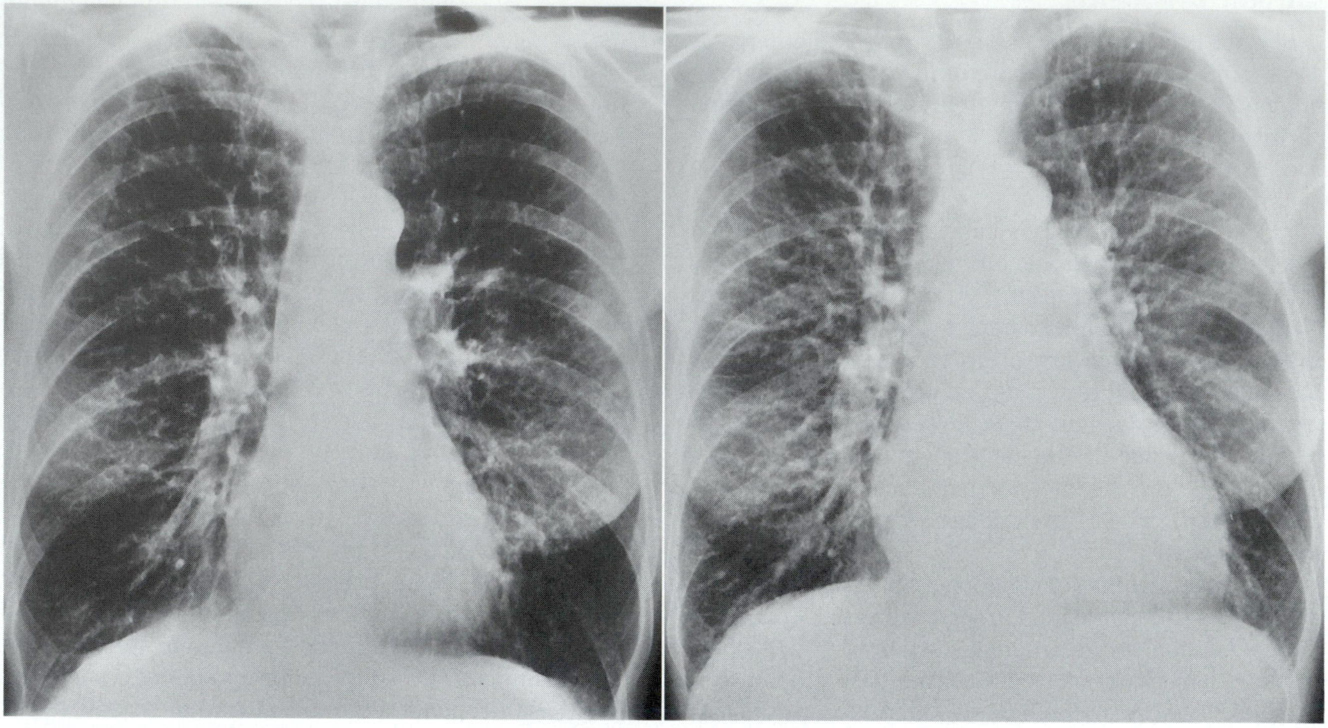

FIGURE 17-33
Cor pulmonale. **A,** Fifty-year-old man with chronic airflow obstruction. Lungs are large in volume, diaphragm is flat, and there is vascular attenuation at right apex. These features suggest emphysema, and this was supported by low carbon monoxide diffusion capacity. Lung markings are increased peripherally, particularly in left midzone. **B,** Patient became chronically hypoxic and, with respiratory infections, hypercapnic. One of these episodes was associated with cor pulmonale when patient became edematous, heart enlarged, and hilar and lung vessels enlarged. Emphysematous right upper zone shows less vascular engorgement and is relatively transradiant. Diaphragm is less depressed and more curved than before.

anterior or posterior segmental airways of the upper lobe. This is a normal finding, whereas visible side-on airways (tramline opacities) are always considered abnormal. Fraser and co-workers[141] assessed the frequency of detection of end-on airways and their wall thickness in approximately 150 control subjects and 150 patients with chronic bronchitis. They found end-on airways visible in about 80% of both groups and a slight increase in wall thickness in chronic bronchitis, which was of some value in distinguishing patients with chronic bronchitis from normal subjects, although the sign was subject to significant interobserver variation. The ratio of wall thickness to external diameter in end-on airways does not correlate with the degree of airflow obstruction.[65] Support for the finding of bronchial wall thickening in chronic bronchitis has come from an HRCT study in which proximal and distal bronchial wall thickening was present in 33% of smokers (compared with 18% of control subjects).[416] In this study the presence of cough and early morning sputum production was significantly correlated with the presence of bronchial wall thickening. Another sign described in the series of Bates and co-workers[30] was increased lung markings, detected in 18%. This feature again was rare in the British patients.[456,458] The sign

(Figure 17-33) consists of small, ill-defined linear opacities with or without accentuation of small vascular opacities.[147] It is a subjective sign that pathologic examination, in one study, showed to correlate with perivenous edema, inflammatory cell infiltration, and fibrosis.[127] It is considered by Fraser and associates[142] to be "useful evidence in support of a diagnosis of chronic bronchitis."

Bronchographic findings in chronic bronchitis are of historical interest only. They do, however, illustrate some pathologic features of the disease. Dilated mucous gland ducts in the proximal airways fill with contrast material in over 50% of patients.[174,458] However, Gamsu, Forbes, and Ovenfors[146] recorded this finding in a similar percentage of normal adults, and it cannot be regarded as specific for chronic bronchitis. It may be significant that these latter workers used powdered tantalum rather than a liquid contrast agent. Other bronchographic findings in chronic bronchitis include incomplete peripheral airway filling,[174] squared or truncated airway ends,[408,414,456] lack of proximal tapering,[458] and mild irregularity of outline.[174,458] Wall irregularity was also noted in some normal subjects.[146]

Cor pulmonale is a recognized complication of COPD and is seen almost exclusively in hypoxic patients at the chronic bronchitis end of the spectrum. With the onset of heart failure the heart and hilar and intermediate lung vessels become enlarged. Enlargement of vessels is present in all zones and affects particularly segmental vessels and a few divisions beyond, giving an appearance of plethora (Figure 17-33).[233] The changes of plethora probably reflect two processes: expansion of central blood volume and hypoxic vasoconstriction of small distal pulmonary arteries.

The size of central pulmonary arteries has been used to assess the level of pulmonary artery pressure. The most widely used measurement has been the width of the basal right pulmonary artery 1 cm beyond the right hilar Y point. In a study of 1085 normal adults (age range 18 to 72 years) the upper limit of normal range for the basal pulmonary artery diameter was 16 mm in men and 15 mm in women.[78] Two other studies of normal subjects give similar values: an upper range of 17 mm (men) and 15 mm (women)[492] and 17.4 mm for both sexes in a male-predominant series.[67] Other workers have looked at similar measurements in patients with COPD and tried to define criteria that might be used to separate subjects with and without pulmonary arterial hypertension.[79,252,320,492] These reports indicate that a reasonable threshold measurement with a low false-positive rate would be a diameter of 17 mm in women and 18 mm in men. Correlation coefficients in these studies have been low (r = 0.4 to 0.6), which means that while basal pulmonary artery diameter may be used to detect the presence or absence of pulmonary artery hypertension, it cannot be used to predict the exact level of pulmonary artery pressure. The main pulmonary artery segment, normally flat or slightly convex, becomes more prominent with pulmonary arterial hypertension. However, the presence or absence or the degree of prominence is not a reliable way of assessing pulmonary arterial hypertension, possibly because prominence is sensitive to patient rotation.[320] CT estimation of the size of the main pulmonary is not subject to the same limitations, and an upper limit of normal (mean + 2 SD) has been measured at 28.6 mm.[265] This value had a sensitivity of 100% in a series of patients with nonrespiratory pulmonary arterial hypertension.

Emphysema

Emphysema is a major cause of chronic airflow obstruction. It is a diagnosis that can be made only by using pathologic criteria. Thus emphysema is defined as "a condition of the lung characterized by abnormal, permanent enlargement of airspaces distal to the terminal bronchiole accompanied by the destruction of their (airspace) walls and without obvious fibrosis. The orderly appearance of the acinus and its contents are disturbed and may be lost."[465] This definition, unlike earlier ones,[81] makes destruction of airspace walls a necessary condition, thereby excluding, for example, compensatory "emphysema" and other conditions in which there is only airspace dilatation.

Pulmonary emphysema has a worldwide distribution but is more frequent in polluted and industrialized societies. It is very common, particularly in its milder forms; some degree of emphysema is recorded in 50% to 70% of autopsies from various centers around the world.[467] It has a peak prevalence at about 70 years of age and is two to three times more common in males.[467] The epidemiology of COPD has recently been reviewed.[447]

The pathogenesis is complex, but two mechanisms are particularly important. First is structural weakness caused by elastolysis, which itself may be secondary either to a constitutional disorder or to enhanced proteolysis. Second is airway obstruction caused either by loss of airway support or by inflammatory changes in the airway walls.

The most important etiologic factor by far is cigarette smoking, which exerts its effect in a variety of ways. Other inhaled pollutants have also been implicated, particularly cadmium chloride, nitrogen oxides, and phosgene. Various genetic disorders associated with emphysema are described, including alpha$_1$-antitrypsin deficiency, heritable diseases of connective tissue such as cutis laxa,[504] osteogenesis imperfecta, Marfan's syndrome,[51] and familial emphysema. A childhood onset with hemolytic anemia has been described.[18]

The pathologic classification of emphysema is based on the microscopic localization of disease within the acinus. With the use of such a system, it is not surprising that severe emphysema is often difficult to categorize. The principal types are decribed in the following paragraphs:

1. Panacinar emphysema. In this form the entire acinus is affected by dilatation and destruction. The features differentiating alveoli from alveolar ducts are lost, pores of Kohn enlarge, and fenestrations develop between alveoli. With progressive destruction, all that eventually remains are thin strands of tissue surrounding blood vessels. Panacinar emphysema is the most important type because it is the most widespread and severe and therefore the most likely to give rise to clinically significant disease. Pathologic changes are distributed throughout the lungs, but they are often basally predominant. Panacinar emphysema is the type occurring in alpha$_1$-antitrypsin deficiency, in Swyer-James (Macleod's) syndrome,[465] and in familial cases. Although generally considered the emphysema of nonsmokers, it also occurs in association with smoking-induced centriacinar emphysema.

2. Centriacinar emphysema. In this variety of emphysema, more commonly called centrilobular, there are selective dilatation and confluence of central elements in the acinus, particularly the respiratory bronchioles and their alveoli. The process tends to be most developed in the upper zones of the upper and lower lobes. It is strongly associated with smoking and chronic bronchitis, and it is much more common in men. Inflammatory changes in the small airways are a common association, with plugging, mural infiltration, and fibrosis leading to

stenosis, blockage, distortion, and destruction. Focal dust emphysema seen in coal workers may be considered a variety of centriacinar emphysema in which there is little airway inflammation and a more uniform distribution of disease throughout the lung.[465]

3. Periacinar emphysema. This variety of emphysema is commonly called paraseptal, emphasizing its main feature, selective expansion of alveoli adjacent to connective tissue septa and bronchovascular bundles, particularly at the margins of the acinus but also subpleurally and adjacent to bronchovascular bundles. It has a tendency to develop where lung margins are sharp. Airspaces in paraseptal emphysema often become confluent and develop into bullae, which may be large. Paraseptal emphysema is the basic lesion in bullous lung disease.[464] Airway obstruction and physiologic disturbance are often minor in paraseptal emphysema despite gross bulla formation.

4. Cicatricial emphysema. Scar emphysema is usually localized and of little clinical significance[464] except in the context of widespread scarring processes such as sarcoidosis or histiocytosis X.

5. Unclassified emphysema.[200]

The classification of emphysema depends on microscopic localization of the lesions. At a macroscopic level lesions may be focal, multifocal, or widespread and may show regional predilection, such as upper or lower zone.

Patients with small amounts of emphysema are frequently asymptomatic.[465] Widespread emphysema, however, causes nonproductive cough and progressive exertional dyspnea. With the exception of paraseptal emphysema, the degree of disability is related to the severity of the emphysema rather than to the type.[465] Emphysema tends to be associated with the "pink puffer" clinical picture,[102] characterized by early dyspnea, nonproductive cough, and relatively normal blood gases achieved at the expense of marked dyspnea.[422] There is, however, considerable overlap with the chronic bronchitis−associated "blue bloater" end of the spectrum. Patients with this latter syndrome have productive cough, episodes of deterioration associated with infection and bronchospasm, deranged blood gas levels (hypoxia and hypercapnia), and a tendency to develop pulmonary arterial hypertension and cor pulmonale.[422]

Respiratory function tests in emphysema reflect three major pathologic changes: (1) small airway obstruction caused loss of mural support and inflammatory wall change, (2) loss of lung recoil, and (3) loss of alveolar surface.[422] Airway obstruction reduces peak flow and FEV_1. Lung recoil is balanced by chest wall recoil; when the former is reduced, the chest wall moves out, and thus various static lung volumes increase (residual volume, functional residual capacity, and total lung capacity). Reduction in the alveolar gas exchange surface is reflected in a reduction in carbon monoxide diffusion. In addition, the work of breathing is increased, and eventually hypoxemia develops, initially during sleep or exer-

cise. Hypercapnia is not found, since responsiveness to arterial oxygen levels remains intact.

Airflow obstruction in emphysema is located at two sites: (1) peripherally in small airways and (2) in large central airways. The latter component of resistance is variable and present only in expiration, particularly at low lung volumes.[54,140,301] The behavior of large airways has been studied with bronchoscopy and cine bronchography.[128] The collapse of lobar and segmental airways in emphysematous subjects during forced expiration has been demonstrated,[70,140] and pressure measurements show these to be sites of high resistance.[301,303] Collapse of large airways is due principally to the large transmural pressures generated in emphysema during forced expiration. In addition, airway walls are probably less able to withstand such pressures because of mural atrophy[308] or altered cross-sectional geometry.[70,286]

A number of studies have tried to correlate chest radiographic findings and lung function tests in patients with nonspecific chronic airflow obstruction, many of whom have had emphysema. Reich, Weinshelbaum, and Yee[407] found that the length of the right lung and the height of the arc of the right hemidiaphragm correlated well with FEV_1 and the ratio FEV_1/VC.[407] In this study a right lung length of 30 cm or more identified 70% of the patients with airflow obstruction.[407] These workers found that if the absolute height of the right hemidiaphragm measured against the ribs was corrected for body surface area, this too correlated well with the degree of airflow obstruction. Other workers have not found such corrections to be necessary, and in one study of 189 patients all but 3% of those with the height of the right hemidiaphragm at or below the right seventh rib had airflow obstruction.[65] The sensitivity of this finding, however, was low, 30% to 40%. Similar findings have been reported by others[17,107] and emphasized in an editorial by Pratt[393] that concludes that chest radiographs reveal emphysema rather than airflow obstruction per se.

The chest radiographic findings in emphysema may be divided into four types: hyperinflation, vascular change, bullae, and increased markings. Hyperinflation and vascular change are usually the predominant findings, with hyperinflation reflecting a functional abnormality and vascular change reflecting the pathologic one of lung destruction.[397] In the early radiologic studies case selection of patients with emphysema lacked certainty because it was based on clinical features and respiratory function changes[459] and not on morphologic criteria. Between 1962 and 1976, however, a number of studies correlated radiologic and pathologic findings and attempted to assess the accuracy of various signs.* However, as Thurlbeck[495] points out, all these studies are flawed in that they have an excess of patients with chronic airflow obstruction, so that radiologic features of airflow obstruction are given "disproportionate value in recognizing

---

*References 248, 278, 369, 411, 482, 498, 499.

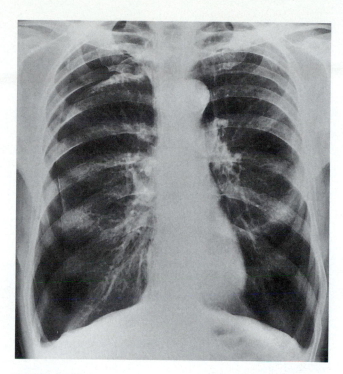

FIGURE 17-34
Emphysema. Posteroanterior chest radiograph demonstrates two of the most reliable signs of emphysema: (1) depression of right hemidiaphragm with its midpoint lying on upper border of seventh rib anteriorly and (2) flattening of both hemidiaphragms. Other, less reliable features include narrow heart with air density below it. There is right pneumothorax.

emphysema." In addition, in many of these studies sizable (20% to 30%) interobserver and intraobserver variation has occurred in the diagnosis of emphysema. Observer variation in the use of individual radiologic signs, particularly those based on vascular changes, has also been a problem.[248,369,482] Furthermore, it is difficult to give an overview of these studies because of the great variation in the severity of disease studied, the radiologic signs assessed, the pathologic methods used for quantifying emphysema, and the conclusions. Some of the studies have been critically reviewed recently.[393-395,434]

Hyperinflation is indicated by a number of signs:

1. The diaphragm is low (Figure 17-34). The right hemidiaphragm is usually assessed because it is not obscured by the heart. The right hemidiaphragm is considered to be low if its border, in the midclavicular line, is at or below the anterior end of the seventh rib.[282] Some workers have taken the sixth rib in pyknic individuals.[248] Occasionally normal individuals, particularly if young and fit, have a right hemidiaphragm lying at the level of the seventh rib.

2. The diaphragm is also flat (Figures 17-34 and 17-35). Flattening of a hemidiaphragm can be assessed subjectively, as well as objectively by drawing a line joining costophrenic and cardiophrenic angles and measuring the maximum perpendicular height from this line

to the diaphragm silhouette. A value of less than 1.5 cm indicates flattening. The combination of depression and flattening is specific for generalized emphysema, whereas depression on its own is seen with overinflation in nonemphysematous conditions such as acute asthma. Other signs are less reliable indicators of hyperinflation.

3. The retrosternal airspace may be increased (Figure 17-35). This measurement is taken on the lateral radiograph between the anterior aspect of the ascending aorta and the posterior surface of the sternum at a point 3 cm below the manubriosternal junction. Critical values indicating hyperinflation have ranged from 2.5 cm[369] to 4.5 cm.[459] The bigger values are more specific.

4. There may be an obtuse costophrenic angle on the posteroanterior or lateral chest radiograph (Figure 17-35).

5. A retrosternal airspace extending to within 3 cm of the diaphragm may be present (Figure 17-35).

6. The cardiac diameter may be less than 11.5 cm,[457] with a vertical heart and visible lung beneath the heart (Figure 17-34). Several studies have found that signs of overinflation are the best predictors of the presence and severity of emphysema.[248,369,482] Nicklaus and co-workers[369] found that a flat diaphragm on the posteroanterior chest radiograph was the best predictor, detecting 94% of patients with severe emphysema, 76% with moderate, and 21% with mild, with a false-positive rate of only 4%.

Several vascular signs have been ascribed to emphysema:

1. A region of transradiancy (Figures 17-36 and 17-37) may occur. Transradiancy may be a generalized change that makes reliable assessment difficult or may be localized, in which case it can be identified with reasonable certainty by comparison with "normal" areas.

2. The number and size of pulmonary vessels and their branches are reduced, particularly in the middle or outer aspect of the lung ("arterial deficiency"). Arterial deficiency may be localized or generalized (Figure 17-36).

3. Vessels are distorted and may be unduly straight or curved and have increased branching angles.

4. There may be transradiant, avascular areas with hairline curvilinear margins, at least in part, which represent bullae (Figure 17-37). Although bullae may be a feature of generalized emphysema, they can occur as a local manifestation of paraseptal emphysema in otherwise normal lungs. Several studies have found arterial deficiency a more reliable criterion of emphysema than hyperinflation.[278,498,499] Using arterial deficiency alone to detect emphysema, Thurlbeck and co-workers[498] found that its accuracy was similar to that described for hyperinflation criteria by Nicklaus and associates.[369] There were no false-positive results, and all patients with severe, 66% with moderate, and 35% with mild emphysema were identified.

Thurlbeck and co-workers[498] have described another vascular pattern in emphysema in which increased markings are present peripherally on the chest radio-

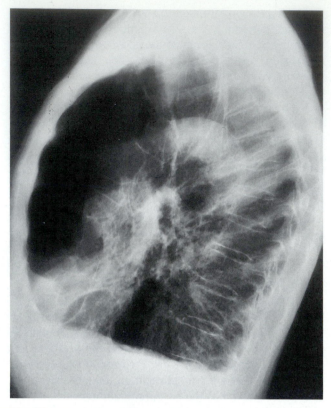

FIGURE 17-35
Emphysema. Lateral chest radiograph demonstrates characteristically large retrosternal transradiancy with increased separation of aorta and sternum measuring 4.6 cm, 3 cm below angle of Louis and extending to within 3 cm of diaphragm anteriorly. Both costophrenic angles are obtuse and both hemidiaphragms flat.

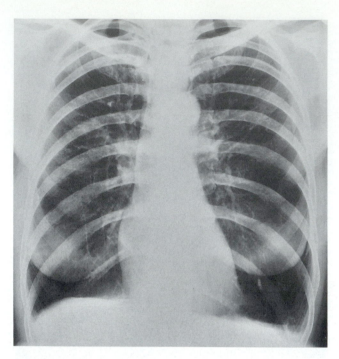

FIGURE 17-36
Panacinar emphysema with alpha₁-antitrypsin deficiency. Large-volume lungs with low flat diaphragms. Both lower zones are hypertransradiant, and vessels within these zones are reduced in size and number and are pruned. Distribution of these changes is typical of panacinar emphysema. Patient was 52-year-old woman. (Courtesy Dr. P. Gishen, London.)

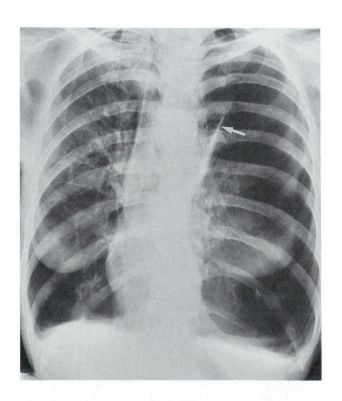

FIGURE 17-37
Emphysema with alpha₁-antitrypsin deficiency. In female patient, both diaphragms are low and flat. Mediastinum is displaced to right by large bulla, which occupies much of left hemithorax, compressing lung tissue medially and inferiorly. Part of wall of bulla can be identified *(arrow)*. Vasculature is reduced in right lower zone because of panacinar emphysema. Bulla formation is not a common feature of alpha₁-antitrypsin deficiency. (Courtesy Dr. P. Gishen, London.)

graph (Figure 17-33). These markings have been interpreted as caused by an increase in size and number of small vessels, although other factors such as edema, cellular infiltration, and scarring may play a part.[127] It is an appearance seen most commonly in the presence of pulmonary arterial hypertension, cor pulmonale, and centrilobular emphysema (Figure 17-33). Hyperinflation is commonly absent or mild.[498] Recognition of increased markings as a manifestation of emphysema allows cases to be detected radiologically that would otherwise be missed.[498] In one series of 73 patients with chronic airflow obstruction, 63% of those with severe emphysema had this pattern.[52]

The following conclusions may be drawn from radiologic and pathologic studies in generalized emphysema*: (1) The chest radiograph reliably detects severe emphysema and can be used to exclude severe disease. Mild disease is rarely detected, and moderate disease is detected in about 50% of patients. (2) The sensitivity of the chest radiograph is not good, ranging from about 50% to 80%[434]; in one study it was only 24%.[499] This exceptionally low figure was probably because most subjects had mild or moderate emphysema and only vascular radiologic signs were used. In contrast, specificity is good, between 95% and 100%, giving a low false-positive rate. Accuracy of the chest radiograph in diagnosing emphysema is in the order of 65% to 80%.[434] (3) There is a sizeable intraobserver and interobserver variation in relation to radiologic signs, for example, 12% intraobserver and 25% interobserver variation in the study by Nicklaus and co-workers.[369] Vascular signs, not surprisingly, are subject to more variation when being assessed than signs relating to hyperinflation.[434] (4) Most studies find that the best predictors of generalized emphysema are evidence of hyperinflation (particularly a low diaphragm) and flattening of the diaphragm.[248,369,411,482,498] Vascular criteria are generally less reliable, apart from two studies.[278,499]

When other chest conditions occur in emphysematous lungs, the radiologic appearances are modified. Thus with consolidation and centrilobular emphysema the emphysematous spaces produce rounded transradiancies in the airspace opacity (Figure 17-38). With heart failure, edema may spare emphysematous lung and the diaphragm tends to become more rounded and elevated as lung compliance falls (Figure 17-33).[333]

In contrast to the chest radiograph, CT has proved very sensitive and specific in assessing emphysema. CT has been used to detect and characterize emphysema and grade its severity since findings were first described in 1982.[161]

The signs of emphysema on CT have been reported.[38,39,138,161] There are areas of low attenuation with ill-defined margins (Figure 17-39). However, when areas become 1 to 2 cm in diameter, it is not unusual for part of their border to become well defined (Figure 17-40) because of marginating interlobular septa or vessels. In one study assessing various signs of centrilobular emphysema, nonperipheral, low-attenuation areas on in vivo CT correlated best with emphysema assessed post mortem.[138] Other signs of emphysema include bullae (focal air-containing cysts with well-defined, hairline walls), pruning and attenuation of vessels (Figure 17-40), and vascular distortion (Figure 17-41). Vessels may be stretched and swept, and branching angles are widened.

It may be possible, especially when HRCT is used in

*References 248, 278, 369, 411, 482, 498, 499.

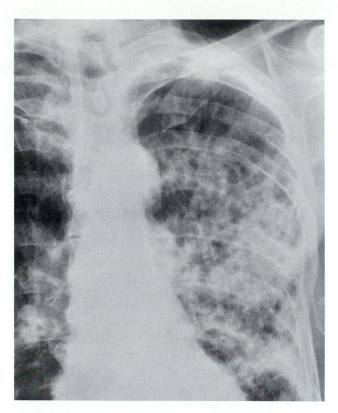

FIGURE 17-38
Emphysema. Localized posteroanterior radiograph of left upper zone shows infective consolidation superimposed on centrilobular emphysema. Emphysematous spaces create rounded transradiancies with pneumonia.

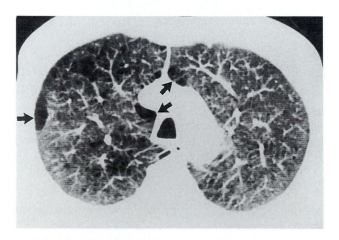

FIGURE 17-39
Centrilobular (and paraseptal) emphysema on conventional computed tomogram. There are numerous focal low-density areas. On left, lesions tend to be deep to pleura, small (2 to 5 mm), and poorly marginated. On right, changes are more advanced and small low-density areas have become confluent, forming lesions up to 2 cm in diameter. Larger lesions are often in part well marginated because of bordering septa or vessels. Subpleural low densities are due to paraseptal emphysema *(arrows)*.

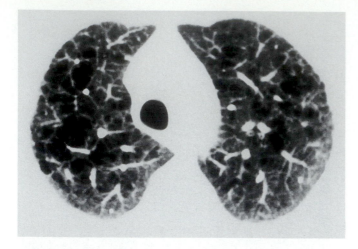

FIGURE 17-40
Centrilobular emphysema on conventional tomogram. Much of the lung is occupied by transradiant spaces, which are bigger than in Figure 17-39. Many of the low-density areas have well-defined margins formed by vessels and possibly septa.

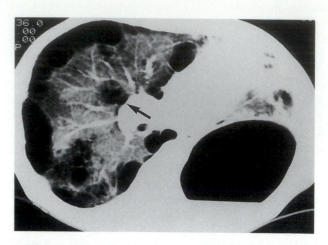

FIGURE 17-42
Advanced paraseptal emphysema on conventional computed tomogram. In this patient paraseptal emphysematous spaces are large, forming bullae. Characteristic peripheral (subpleural) distribution is present on right, with most lesions abutting chest wall and mediastinum. Lesions also commonly occur against bronchovascular structures *(arrow)*. On left side there is single large bulla with air-fluid level caused by adjacent infection.

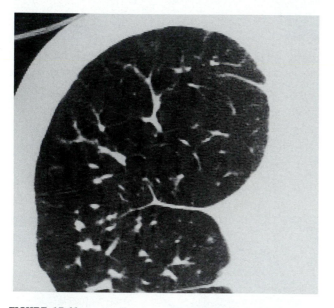

FIGURE 17-41
Panlobular emphysema on high-resolution computed tomogram. Low density is diffuse and not focal as in centrilobular emphysema. Vessels are attenuated, swept, and stretched.

patients with mild or mild to moderate disease, to distinguish among the various types of emphysema.[38,137] Centrilobular emphysema, particularly in early disease, has an upper zone predilection[138] and may be confined to this region. Low-density areas are typically focal, remote from the pleura (Figure 17-39),[138] and related to centrilobular arteries.[356] Lung immediately surrounding the low-density lesions appears normal. With progression of disease, centrilobular emphysematous lesions become confluent with obvious vascular abnormalities, and at this

stage the disease is morphologically indistinguishable from panlobular emphysema. In panlobular emphysema (Figure 17-41), lung destruction is much more uniform and gives rise to extensive low-density areas with vascular distortion and pruning. Small, focal, low-density areas as seen in centrilobular emphysema are not found. Mild panlobular emphysema is easily overlooked[332] because it is a diffuse process lacking the juxtaposed contrasting densities of normal lung and focal transradiancies as seen in centrilobular emphysema. Panlobular emphysema has a predilection for the lower zone. Paraseptal emphysema (Figure 17-39) is easily detected on CT[332] as well-marginated low-density areas with distinct hairline walls. Cysts occur peripherally in the secondary pulmonary lobule and are therefore commonly seen subpleurally (Figure 17-39) or in relation to bronchovascular bundles (Figure 17-42). Subpleural cysts are commonly found in the azygoesophageal recess, adjacent to the left ventricle, and in the anterior junctional region (Figure 17-42).[38] The intervening lung is normal.[137]

The distribution and severity of emphysema may be quantitated by CT. CT scans can be assessed visually or by density measurements. These techniques have been validated in a number of studies comparing in vitro and in vivo CT quantification with pathologic assessment in postmortem or surgical specimens. Pathologic evaluation in most studies has been of macroscopic emphysema assessed visually by counting lesions or panel matching. A few more recent studies have measured microscopic emphysema pathologically using an index: airspace wall surface area per unit volume.[164] Studies using various CT section thicknesses (between 1 and 10 mm) have shown

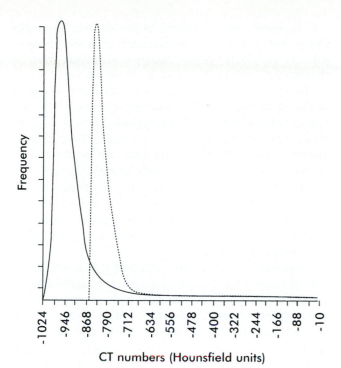

FIGURE 17-43
Graph of pixel density (computed tomogram [CT] numbers in Hounsfield units) derived from CT lung sections, plotted against pixel frequency for normal subject *(interrupted line)* and for patient with panacinar emphysema *(continuous line)*. Data for emphysematous patient were derived from study illustrated in Figures 17-41 and 17-44, *B.* Emphysematous changes in patient were gross, and there is little overlap with curve of normal subject.

good correlation between macroscopic pathology scores and visually assessed (HR)CT scores with r values ranging from about 0.6 to 0.8.[39,138,267,332] Intraobserver and interobserver variation in these studies has been low.[38,332,353] Emphysematous lesions are more conspicuous and reliably diagnosed on HRCT,[351,470] and CT-pathologic studies comparing sections 1.5 and 10 mm thick have shown improved correlations with pathologic scores: r = 0.85 (1.5 mm) versus r = 0.81 (10 mm) (mixed emphysema)[332] and r = 0.96 (1.5 mm) versus r = 0.90 (10 mm) (panacinar emphysema).[470] (HR)CT consistently underestimates the extent of centrilobular and panlobular emphysema,[470] since small lesions (less than 5 mm in diameter) are not reliably identified.[332] Thus in two CT-pathologic series there was an 18% (6:33)[332] and 33% (2:6)[138] false-negative rate for CT in patients with mild disease. The false-positive rate for (HR)CT is very low, about 2%,[434] which may be related at least in part to the misinterpretation of low-density movement artifacts.[490]

Emphysema can also be assessed by measuring lung density. CT lung density is related to the amount of air, tissue, interstitial fluid, and blood within a given voxel, and normal data have been reported.* In a recent study

*References 2, 143, 161, 199, 426, 518.

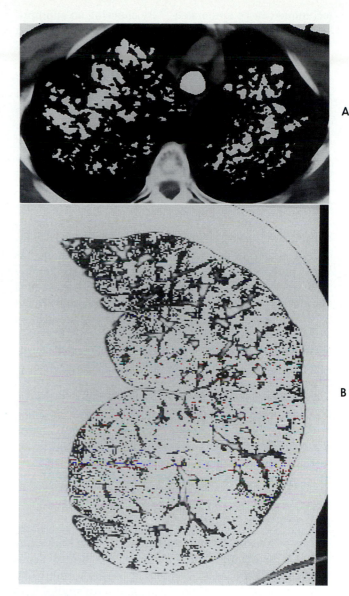

FIGURE 17-44
Pixel highlighting in emphysema. All pixels with computed tomogram number of −910 HU or less have been highlighted, identifying areas of probable emphysema. **A,** Centrilobular emphysema at level midway between aortic arch and carina. Highlighting emphasizes typically focal distribution of lesions, deep to pleura. **B,** Panlobular emphysema. Highlighted pixels are distributed in even, confluent pattern.

lung density values in normal subjects at full inspiration varied from −770 to −875 HU.[2] In addition, there is a gravitationally induced density gradient in the supine position; in one study posterior values were 20 to 70 HU greater than anterior ones.[329] The density of emphysematous lung is abnormally low. If a histogram plot is made of frequency against pixel density (HU), the emphysematous curve is shifted to the left compared with normal (Figure 17-43).[199] Pixels with values below a certain number can be highlighted on a CT image ("density masking") (Figure 17-44) and expressed as a percentage of the total pixels in a given section. This time-consuming technique can be automated.[19] By choosing an appropriate threshold level the operator can discriminate between "normal" lung and emphysematous lung. Muller and co-workers,[353] in a study comparing macroscopic emphysema as assessed by the "density mask" method and picture-graded pathology scores at the same level, found that a density of −910 (HU) gave the best discrimination between emphysematous and normal lung (r = 0.94). Caution is needed in uncritical extrapolation of the preceding findings to other machines because many technical factors can affect CT density measurements.[2] It has been recommended that threshold levels be established by experiment for any given scanner.[353] An alternative quantitative method to "density masking" is to calculate the percentage of pixels falling in the lowest fifth percentile of density values.[305] This percentage has been compared with the amount of microscopic emphysema as assessed by an index (airspace wall surface area per unit volume) and a moderately good correlation of r = 0.77 was found.[164] The use of a "density mask" method and both expiratory and inspiratory CT scans has been advocated as a means of distinguishing areas of simple hyperinflation without tissue destruction from areas of emphysema.[260]

A number of studies have compared the degree of CT-determined emphysema and respiratory function tests.[165,257,431,435] HRCT is capable of detecting emphysema in symptomatic patients with reduced diffusion capacity but no evidence of airflow limitation[259] and also in subjects with no defect of diffusion or airflow.[188]

Lung scintigraphy in chronic obstructive pulmonary disease

Both perfusion (Q) and ventilation (V) lung scintiscans are usually abnormal in COPD. In the United States xenon-133 is the agent commonly used for ventilation scans, whereas in the United Kingdom most studies have been performed with krypton-81m (^{81m}Kr). The longer half of life of ^{133}Xe (5.1 days) allows wash-in, equilibrium, and wash-out studies, which are precluded by the very short half-life of ^{81m}Kr (13 seconds). However, ^{81m}Kr gives a more accurate estimate of the true ventilation than does ^{133}Xe. The sensitivity of scintiscans is considered similar to that of spirometric tests in detecting COPD.[11]

The characteristic finding on a lung scintiscan in COPD is multiple, patchy, matched defects of both perfusion and ventilation (Figure 17-45), generally distributed throughout the lungs.[93] Emphysematous defects are due to areas of parenchymal destruction[126] and are therefore nonsegmental and fixed. They may or may not correspond to oligemic or bullous areas on the corresponding chest radiograph.[12] Scintiscans in emphysema using ^{133}Xe as the ventilation agent show in addition to the preceding findings a slow wash-in curve so that an equilibrium state may never be achieved.[11] Wash-out is also delayed and prolonged beyond the usual 3 minutes taken to achieve a background count level.[10]

Lung scintiscans of patients at the chronic bronchitis end of the COPD spectrum generally resemble those of patients with emphysema except that defects may be segmental,[126] although not all studies have found this.[93] Perfusion defects in chronic bronchitis are probably produced by hypoxic vasoconstriction secondary to hypoventilation caused by airway narrowing. Such a mechanism may explain why, in chronic bronchitis, perfusion defects are sometimes smaller than the corresponding ventilation defects.[126] Occasionally hypoxic vasoconstriction fails to occur,[468] and in this situation, typically seen at the lung bases in acute exacerbations of chronic bronchitis, ventilation defects are completely mismatched.[93] With resolution of the acute exacerbation such defects disappear.

A number of studies have assessed the usefulness of V/Q scintiscans for detecting pulmonary embolism in the presence of COPD.[9,284,473] In general these studies found that high-probability scintiscans for pulmonary embolism had a high positive predictive value and that low-probability and normal scintiscans had a predictive value similar to that in a control population without COPD. Compared with findings in a control population there was an excess of scintiscans of intermediate probability for pulmonary embolism.

Labeled aerosols may be used to study lung ventilation. In normal individuals gases and aerosols produce similar images.[76] In COPD, however, ventilation scintiscans produced by the two agents are strikingly different, with focal spots of high and low activity on the aerosol scintiscan.[198,288,436] Focal deposition tends to be central or mixed in emphysema and peripheral in chronic bronchitis.[198,226,288] Deposition of aerosol is thought to occur in airways at areas of fixed and dynamic narrowing by a variety of complex mechanisms.[198,226,489]

Positron emission tomography (PET) has had a limited use in studying the lung. Pulmonary applications of PET have recently been reviewed.[441] In a research context PET is capable of providing sophisticated physiologic information relating to COPD.[63]

Alpha$_1$-antitrypsin deficiency

The association between serum alpha$_1$-antitrypsin (A$_1$-AT) deficiency and COPD was first recognized in 1963,[277] and 6 years later an association with neonatal hepatitis and cirrhosis was recorded.[444]

A$_1$-AT is a serum protein that inhibits a number of lysosomal proteases released during inflammatory reactions, preventing the damaging effects of elastases released by macrophages and particularly neutrophils. Elastase has been shown to produce emphysema in lungs when administered into the airways,[398] and the elastase of neutrophils within the lung has the same potential.[224] It is not surprising therefore that some patients with reduced levels of A$_1$-AT are at risk for emphysema. This effect is augmented by smoking. Histologic study shows the emphysema to be of the panacinar type.[167,443,498]

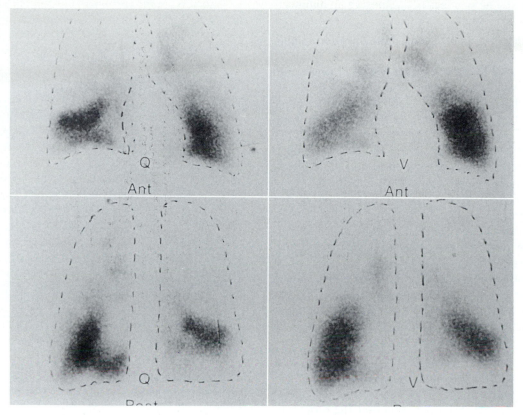

FIGURE 17-45
Ventilation-perfusion scintiscan in generalized emphysema (probably centrilobular). Upper images are anterior views and lower ones posterior, with perfusion scans on left and ventilation ones on right. There are multiple, matched defects of perfusion and ventilation distributed throughout lungs but most marked in middle and upper zones. In these zones, chest radiograph showed marked oligemic changes.

The serum level and type of A_1-AT depend on two codominant alleles that occupy one locus. Different alleles produce different types and amounts of A_1-AT. The type of A_1-AT may be recognized by electrophoresis, and the allele producing it is designated by Pi (protease inhibitor), followed by one of a number of capital letters. By far the most common allele is PiM, and when homozygous (PiMM) it is associated with normal A_1-AT levels. The frequency of the PiM allele in most studies from various countries has been on the order of 95% to 99%, but levels below 90% have been recorded in some populations.

Some alleles are associated with low serum levels of A_1-AT. Although there are a number of these, only a few are important clinically, particularly PiZ but also PiS and Pi-, the last having a silent allele. Homozygous PiZ individuals have about 10% to 15% of the expected serum A_1-AT levels, while heterozygotic PiMZ individuals have a level of about 60%.[121] Not only are A_1-AT levels depressed, but also they fail to rise in situations that stimulate an increase in acute-phase reactants. The PiZ allele has a frequency of about 1.2%, so that only one to

two individuals per 10,000 of the population are homozygotes.

A large study of 256 PiZZ patients showed that eventually emphysema developed in nearly every individual and life expectancy was lower.[276] The PiZZ type of emphysema is characterized by an early onset, between 35 and 50 years of age.[122,264,276] Symptoms develop about 10 years earlier in smokers than in nonsmokers,[264] and respiratory function impairment and radiologic change tend to be worse in smokers. Males outnumber females about 2:1.[158,264]

Opinion is divided over the relationship of the heterozygote state (PiMZ) and respiratory disease. The consensus is that no definite relationship exists between the two but that the heterozygote state may increase susceptibility to emphysema in the presence of other risk factors.[224]

Radiologic changes of emphysema can be seen in about 80% of patients who are homozygous and have COPD.[201] The striking feature of the emphysematous change is its lower zone predominance (Figure 17-36). In a study of 165 PiZ homozygotes, 98% had lower zone involvement,[158] and in 24% this was the only zone involved. In the same series only 3 of 140 patients with radiologic changes had isolated involvement of the upper or middle and upper zone.[158] Similarly, in a study of 52 PiZZ patients with COPD, 67% showed isolated lower zone emphysema, whereas this pattern was seen in only 8% of PiMM patients.[201] The lower zone predominance of emphysema in A_1-AT deficiency is also noted on lung scintiscans.[521] Bullae are not a major feature, but they do occur (Figure 17-37).[424] The pattern of emphysematous change in heterozygotes, such as PiMZ and PiMS genotypes, is like that in homozygous PiM individuals.

CT findings have been described is a series of 17 patients, all but one of whom had homozygous PiZ.[187] Emphysematous changes were seen in all zones but had a lower zone predominance, and 41% had bullae, although these were never a major feature. Bronchial wall thickening and/or dilatation was present in 41%. Other workers have reported an association between A_1-AT deficiency and bronchiectasis.[238] An association with bronchitis and asthma is also recognized.[287]

Bullae

A bulla is an emphysematous space within the lungs that has a diameter of more than 1 cm in the distended state and that causes a local protrusion from the surface of the removed lung.[81,410] Bullae may be single or multiple and may represent a localized abnormality (focal paraseptal emphysema) or, more commonly, be part of widespread panacinar emphysema. Occasionally they are familial.[156] Pathologists recognize three types of bullae, which differ in location, size of neck, and amount of contained residual lung tissue.[410]

Bullae communicate with the bronchial tree, but air enters and leaves slowly and generally bullae do not act as a clinically important dead space,[255] although exceptions have been noted.[28] During tidal breathing Po_2 in bullae is higher than arterial Po_2.[344] Bullae show "paper bag compliance," inflating more easily than lung up to a critical volume, after which they become stiff and much less compliant than lung.[500] The pressure in bullae is normally negative and the same as pleural pressure.[344]

On radiologic examination a bulla produces an avascular transradiant area, usually separated wholly or partly from the remaining lung by a thin curvilinear wall (Figures 17-37 and 17-46). Occasionally the wall is completely absent, and under these circumstances bullae can be difficult to detect. Plain radiographs markedly underestimate the number of bullae demonstrated at postmortem examination.[278] The wall is usually of hairline thickness. Sometimes segments of the wall are thicker when there are major contributions from redundant pleura or collapsed adjacent lung. Bullae caused by paraseptal emphysema are much more common in the upper zones,[53] but when they are associated with widespread panacinar emphysema, the distribution is much more even.[410] Bullae may be as small as 1 cm diameter or

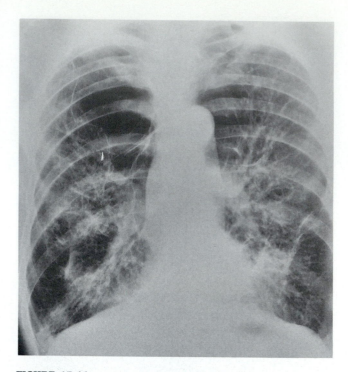

FIGURE 17-46
Bullae in patient with chronic airflow obstruction. In right upper zone there is large transradiant area associated with thin curvilinear opacities, representing walls of bullae. At right base, further transradiant zone is without curvilinear shadows.

may occupy the whole hemithorax, causing marked relaxation collapse of the adjacent lung (Figure 17-37). They may even extend across into the opposite hemithorax, particularly by way of the anterior junctional area.[133] CT is more sensitive than the chest radiograph in demonstrating bullae (Figure 17-47).[133,345,399] CT allows accurate assessment of the number, size, and position of bullae and is particularly useful when bullae are obscured by other lung abnormalities, such as diffuse interstitial fibrosis.[345] Computed tomograms taken on inspiration and expiration indicate the extent to which a bulla is ventilated, and the appearance of the rest of the lung helps in assessing the extent and degree of diffuse lung disease (Figure 17-47).[345] The foregoing capability of CT makes it extremely useful for identifying patients suitable for treatment with bullectomy.[343]

Bullae usually enlarge over months or years, but the rate is variable and a period of stability may be followed by a sudden expansion.[53] Bullae may also disappear either spontaneously[103] or following infection or hemorrhage.[53,322,478] The main complications of bullae are pneumothorax, infection, and hemorrhage, and an association with bronchial carcinoma has been described. When infected, bullae usually contain fluid and develop an air-fluid level (Figure 17-42).[307,322,478] The hairline wall often becomes thickened, and indeed this may be the only sign of infection. Infected bullae differ from an abscess in that the patient is less ill, the wall of the ring

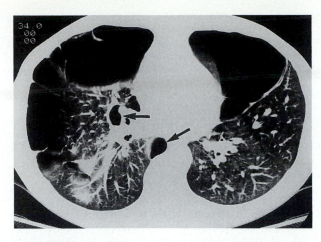

FIGURE 17-47
Bullous disease on high-resolution computed tomogram. Bullae are distributed in characteristic fashion. Several large bullae are situated anterolaterally. Smaller bullae *(arrows)* are present in azygoesophageal recess and against major vessels. Intervening lung, well seen paravertebrally, is reduced in volume but is otherwise normal with well-preserved vessels.

shadow is thinner and has a sharp inner margin, and there is less adjacent pneumonitis.[42] Following infection, bullae often disappear.[322] Hemorrhage into the bulla is a less common complication[42,231] that may be accompanied by hemoptysis and a decrease in hemoglobin level. As with infection, the bulla may disappear after bleeding occurs.[322] A few cases of carcinoma arising in or adjacent to bullae are described.[322] Suspicious signs in this context include a mural nodule, mural thickening, a change in diameter of the bulla, pneumothorax, and the accumulation of fluid within the bulla.[503] Evidence has not shown that a carcinoma arising in relation to a bulla is any more than a chance association, unlike the situation with a variety of lung cysts, most of which are probably congenital.[396]

Patients with isolated bullous disease are usually asymptomatic. Occasionally bullae produce breathlessness, which may be relieved by bullectomy.[28] The greatest benefit from surgery is seen in patients with a large bulla (occupying 50% or more of a hemithorax), a moderate reduction in FEV_1, a rapid onset of dyspnea, and no evidence of generalized emphysema.[144,255] The contribution of imaging to the assessment of patients before bullectomy has been reviewed.[144] CT has largely replaced many of the imaging studies performed in the past for bullous disease because it accurately shows the size, number, and site of bullae and permits evaluation of intervening lung for possible disease such as emphysema.

REFERENCES

1. Aaby GV, Blake HA: Tracheobronchiomegaly, *Ann Thorac Surg* 2:64-70, 1966.
2. Adams H, Bernard MS, McConnochie K: An appraisal of CT pulmonary density mapping in normal subjects, *Clin Radiol* 43:238-242, 1991.
3. Adenis L, Laurent JC, Charle J, et al: Tuberculose ganglionnaire mediastinale de l'adulte fistulisee dans l'oesophage, *Lille Med* 19:766-769, 1976.
4. Afzelius BA: A human syndrome caused by immotile cilia, *Science* 193:317-319, 1976.
5. Afzelius BA, Mossberg B: Immotile cilia (editorial), *Thorax* 35:401-404, 1980.
6. Aherne W, Bird T, Court SDM, et al: Pathological changes in virus infections of the lower respiratory tract in children, *J Clin Pathol* 23:7-18, 1970.
7. Akira M, Higashihara T, Sakatani M, et al: Diffuse panbronchiolitis: follow-up CT examination, *Radiology* 189:559-562, 1993.
8. Akira M, Kitatani F, Yong-Sik L, et al: Diffuse panbronchiolitis: evaluation with high-resolution CT, *Radiology* 168:433-438, 1988.
9. Alderson PO, Biello DR, Sacariah KG, et al: Scintigraphic detection of pulmonary embolism in patients with obstructive pulmonary disease, *Radiology* 138:661-666, 1981.
10. Alderson PO, Lee H, Summer WR, et al: Comparison of Xe-133 washout and single-breath imaging for the detection of ventilation abnormalities, *J Nucl Med* 20:917-922, 1979.
11. Alderson PO, Line BR: Scintigraphic evaluation of regional pulmonary ventilation, *Semin Nucl Med* 10:218-242, 1980.
12. Alderson PO, Secker-Walker RH, Forrest JV: Detection of obstructive pulmonary disease, *Radiology* 111:643-648, 1974.
13. Aliabadi P, Shafiepoor H: Bronchography in the recognition of congenital cystic bronchiectasis, *AJR* 131:255-257, 1978.
14. Al-Mallah Z, Quantock OP: Tracheobronchomegaly, *Thorax* 23:320-324, 1968.
15. Alroy GG, Lichtig C, Kaftori JK: Tracheobronchopathia osteoplastica: end stage of primary lung amyloidosis? *Chest* 61:465-468, 1972.
16. Amoury RA, Hrabovsky EE, Leoidas JC, et al: Tracheoesophageal fistula after lye ingestion, *J Pediatr Surg* 10:273-276, 1975.
17. Andersen PE, Andersen LH, Jest P: The chest radiograph in chronic obstructive lung disease compared with measurements of single-breath nitrogen washout and spirometry, *Clin Radiol* 33:51-55, 1982.
18. Anderson CE, Finklestein JZ, Nussbaum E, et al: Association of hemolytic anemia and early-onset pulmonary emphysema in three siblings, *J Pediatr* 105:247-251, 1984.
19. Archer DC, Coblentz CL, deKemp RA, et al: Automated in vivo quantification of emphysema, *Radiology* 188:835-838, 1993.
20. Arrigoni MG, Bernatz PE, Donoghue FE: Broncholithiasis, *J Thorac Cardiovasc Surg* 62:231-237, 1971.
21. Ashford NS, Buxton-Thomas MS, Flower CDR, et al: Aerosol lung scintigraphy in the detection of bronchiectasis, *Clin Radiol* 39:29-32, 1988.
22. Atwell SW: Major anomalies of the tracheobronchial tree with a list of the minor anomalies, *Dis Chest* 52:611-615, 1967.
23. Azizirad H, Polgar G, Borns PR, et al: Bronchiolitis obliterans, *Clin Pediatr* 14:572-584, 1975.
24. Bachman AL, Hewitt WR, Beekley HC: Bronchiectasis: a bronchographic study of 60 cases of pneumonia, *Arch Intern Med* 91:78-96, 1953.
25. Banner AS, Muthuswamy P, Shah RS, et al: Bronchiectasis following heroin-induced pulmonary edema, *Chest* 69:552-555, 1976.
26. Barbato A, Novello A, Zanolin D, et al: Diverticulosis of the main bronchi: a rare cause of recurrent bronchopneumonia in a child, *Thorax* 48:187-188, 1993.
27. Barker AF, Bardana EJ: Bronchiectasis: update of an orphan disease, *Am Rev Respir Dis* 137:969-978, 1988.
28. Bateman ED, Westerman DE, Hewitson RP, et al: Pneumonectomy for massive ventilated lung cysts, *Thorax* 36:554-556, 1981.

29. Bates DV: The fate of the chronic bronchitic: a report of the 10-year follow-up in the Canadian Department of Veterans Affairs co-ordinated study of chronic bronchitis, *Am Rev Respir Dis* 108:1043-1065, 1973.

30. Bates DV, Gordon CA, Paul GI, et al: Chronic bronchitis: report on the third and fourth stages of the co-ordinated study of chronic bronchitis in the Department of Veterans Affairs, Canada, *Med Serv J Can* 22:1-59, 1966.

31. Bateson EM, Woo-Ming M: Tracheobronchomegaly, *Clin Radiol* 24:354-358, 1973.

32. Batsakis JG, Fries GT, Goldman RT, et al: Upper respiratory tract plasmacytoma, *Arch Otolaryngol* 79:613-618, 1964.

33. Becker TS, Shum TK, Waller TS, et al: Radiological aspects of rhinoscleroma, *Radiology* 141:433-438, 1981.

34. Becklake MR, Goldman HI, Boxman AR, et al: The long-term effects of exposure to nitrous fumes, *Am Rev Tuberc* 76:398-409, 1957.

35. Becroft DMO: Bronchiolitis obliterans, bronchiectasis, and other sequelae of adenovirus type 21 infection in young children, *J Clin Pathol* 24:72-82, 1971.

36. Benjamin B, Pitkin J, Cohen D: Congenital tracheal stenosis, *Ann Otol Rhinol Laryngol* 90:364-371, 1981.

37. Berdon WE, Baker DH, Boyer J: Unusual benign and malignant sequelae to childhood radiation therapy, *AJR* 93:545-556, 1965.

38. Bergin C, Muller N, Miller RR: CT in the qualitative assessment of emphysema, *J Thorac Imag* 1:94-103, 1986.

39. Bergin C, Muller N, Nichols DM, et al: The diagnosis of emphysema: a computed tomographic–pathologic correlation, *Am Rev Respir Dis* 133:541-546, 1986.

40. Berkmen YM: The trachea: the blind spot in the chest, *Radiol Clin North Am* 22:539-562, 1984.

41. Berkmen YM, Auh YH: CT diagnosis of acquired tracheoesophageal fistula in adults, *J Comput Assist Tomogr* 9:302, 1985.

42. Bersack SR: Fluid collection in emphysematous bullae, *AJR* 83:283-292, 1960.

43. Bertelsen S, Struve-Christensen E, Aasted A, et al: Isolated middle lobe atelectasis: aetiology, pathogenesis, and treatment of the so-called middle lobe syndrome, *Thorax* 35:449-452, 1980.

44. Bhalla M, Grillo HC, McLoud TC, et al: Idiopathic larygotracheal stenosis: radiologic findings, *AJR* 161:515-517, 1993.

45. Bhargava DK, Verma A, Banti G, et al: Early observations on lung function studies in symptomatic "gas" exposed population of Bhopal, *Ind J Med Res* 86(suppl):1-10, 1987.

46. Bierman CW: Pneumomediastinum and pneumothorax complicating asthma in children, *Am J Dis Child* 114:42-50, 1967.

47. Black RJ: Congenital tracheo-oesophageal fistula in the adult, *Thorax* 37:61-63, 1982.

48. Blackie SP, Al-Majed S, Staples CA, et al: Changes in total lung capacity during acute spontaneous asthma, *Am Rev Respir Dis* 142:79-83, 1990.

49. Blades B, Dugan DJ: Pseudobronchiectasis, *J Thorac Surg* 13:40-48, 1944.

50. Blair DN, Coppage L, Shaw C: Medical imaging in asthma, *J Thorac Imag* 1:23-35, 1986.

51. Bolande RP, Tucker AS: Pulmonary emphysema and other cardiorespiratory lesions as part of the Marfan abiotrophy, *Pediatrics* 33:356-366, 1964.

52. Boushy SF, Aboumrad MH, North LP, et al: Lung recoil pressure, airway resistance, and forced flows related to morphologic emphysema, *Am Rev Respir Dis* 104:551-561, 1971.

53. Boushy SF, Kohen R, Billig DM, et al: Bullous emphysema: clinical, roentgenologic and physiologic study of 49 patients, *Dis Chest* 54:327-334, 1968.

54. Bowen JH, Woodard BH, Pratt PC: Bronchial collapse in obstructive lung disease, *Chest* 80:510-513, 1981.

55. Boyden EA: *Segmental anatomy of the lungs,* New York, 1955, McGraw-Hill.

56. Boyden EA: Developmental anomalies of the lungs, *Am J Surg* 89:79-89, 1955.

57. Brandstetter RD, Messina MS, Sprince NL, et al: Tracheal stenosis due to sarcoidosis, *Chest* 80:656, 1981.

58. Brashear RE, Meyer SC, Manion MW: Unilateral atelectasis in asthma, *Chest* 63:847-849, 1973.

59. Breatnach E, Abbott GC, Fraser RG: Dimensions of the normal human trachea, *AJR* 142:903-906, 1984.

60. Breatnach E, Kerr I: The radiology of cryptogenic obliterative bronchiolitis, *Clin Radiol* 33:657-661, 1982.

61. Brinkman GL, Block DL: The prognosis in chronic bronchitis, *JAMA* 197:1-7, 1966.

62. Brooks LJ, Cloutier MM, Afshani E: Significance of roentgenographic abnormalities in children hospitalized for asthma, *Chest* 82:315-318, 1982.

63. Brudin LH, Rhodes CG, Valind SO, et al: Regional structure-function correlations in chronic obstructive lung disease measured with positron emission tomography, *Thorax* 47:914-921, 1992.

64. Burke GJ: Pneumothorax complicating acute asthma, *S Afr Med J* 55:508-510, 1979.

65. Burki NK, Krumpelman JL: Correlation of pulmonary function with the chest roentgenogram in chronic airway obstruction, *Am Rev Respir Dis* 121:217-223, 1980.

66. Burrows B, Fletcher CM, Heard BE, et al: The emphysematous and bronchial types of chronic airways obstruction, *Lancet* 1:830-835, 1966.

67. Bush A, Gray H, Denison DM: Diagnosis of pulmonary hypertension from radiographic estimates of pulmonary arterial size, *Thorax* 43:127-131, 1988.

68. Butland RJA, Cole P, Citron KM, et al: Chronic bronchial suppuration and inflammatory bowel disease, *Q J Med* 50:63-75, 1981.

69. Caldarola VT, Harrison EG, Clagett OT, et al: Benign tumors and tumorlike conditions of the trachea and bronchi, *Ann Otol Rhinol Laryngol* 73:1042-1061, 1964.

70. Campbell AH, Young IF: Tracheobronchial collapse, a variant of obstructive respiratory disease, *Br J Dis Chest* 57:174-181, 1963.

71. Cantrell JR, Guild HG: Congenital stenosis of the trachea, *Am J Surg* 108:297-305, 1964.

72. Carasso R, Couropmitree C, Heredia R: Egg-shell silicotic calcification causing bronchoesophageal fistula, *Am Rev Respir Dis* 108:1384-1387, 1973.

73. Cardell BS: Pathological findings in deaths from asthma, *Int Arch Allergy Appl Immunol* 9:189-199, 1956.

74. Carilli AD, Kotzen LM, Fischer MJ: The chest roentgenogram in smoking females, *Am Rev Respir Dis* 107:133-136, 1973.

75. Carpenter BLM, Merten DF: Radiographic manifestations of congenital anomalies affecting the airway, *Radiol Clin North Am* 29:219-240, 1991.

76. Chamberlain MJ, Morgan WKC, Vinitski S: Factors influencing the regional deposition of inhaled particles in man, *Clin Sci* 64:69-78, 1983.

77. Chan CK, Hyland RH, Hutcheon MA, et al: Small-airways disease in recipients of allogenic bone marrow transplants: an analysis of 11 cases and a review of the literature, *Medicine* 66:327-340, 1987.

78. Chang CH: The normal roentgenographic measurement of the right descending pulmonary artery in 1085 cases, *AJR* 87:929-935, 1962.

79. Chetty KG, Brown SE, Light RW: Identification of pulmonary hypertension in chronic obstructive pulmonary disease from routine chest radiographs, *Am Rev Respir Dis* 126:338-341, 1982.

80. Choplin RH, Wehunt WD, Theros EG: Diffuse lesions of the trachea, *Semin Roentgenol* 18:38-50, 1983.

81. Ciba Guest Symposium: Terminology, definitions, and classification of chronic pulmonary emphysema and related conditions, *Thorax* 14:286-299, 1959.

82. Clark JG, Crawford SW, Madtes DK, et al: Obstructive lung disease after allogenic marrow transplantation: clinical presentation and course, *Ann Intern Med* 111:368-376, 1989.

83. Clark JG, Schwartz DA, Flournoy N, et al: Risk factors for airflow obstruction in recipients of bone marrow transplants, *Ann Intern Med* 107:648-656, 1987.

84. Clark NS: Bronchiectasis in childhood, *Br Med J* 1:80-88, 1963.

85. Clarke A, Skelton J, Fraser RS: Fungal tracheobronchitis: report of 9 cases and review of the literature, *Medicine* 70:1-14, 1991.

86. Colby TV, Myers JL: Clinical and histologic spectrum of bronchiolitis obliterans, including bronchiolitis obliterans organizing pneumonia, *Semin Respir Med* 13:119-133, 1992.

87. Conces DJ, Tarver RD, Vix VA: Broncholithiasis: CT features in 15 patients, *AJR* 157:249-253, 1991.

88. Cook AJ, Weinstein M, Powell RD: Diffuse amyloidosis of the tracheobronchial tree: bronchographic manifestations, *Radiology* 107:303-304, 1973.

89. Cooke JC, Currie DC, Morgan AD, et al: Role of computed tomography in diagnosis of bronchiectasis, *Thorax* 42:272-277, 1987.

90. Cooper G, Guerrant JL, Harden AG, et al: Some consequences of pulmonary irradiation, *AJR* 85:865-874, 1961.

91. Cornelius EA, Betlach EH: Silo-filler's disease, *Radiology* 74:232-238, 1960.

92. Crawford SW, Clark JG: Bronchiolitis associated with bone marrow transplantation, *Clin Chest Med* 14:741-749, 1993.

93. Cunningham DA, Lavender JP: Krypton 81m ventilation scanning in chronic obstructive airways disease, *Br J Radiol* 54:110-116, 1981.

94. Currie DC, Cooke JC, Morgan AD, et al: Interpretation of bronchograms and chest radiographs in patients with chronic sputum production, *Thorax* 42:278-284, 1987.

95. Currie DC, Needham S, Peters AM, et al: 111-Indium-labelled neutrophils migrate to the lungs in bronchiectasis, *Thorax* 41:256, 1986.

96. Currie DC, Saverymuttu SH, Peters AM, et al: Indium-111-labelled granulocyte accumulation in respiratory tract of patients with bronchiectasis, *Lancet* 1:1335-1339, 1987.

97. Curtin JJ, Webster ADB, Farrant J, et al: Bronchiectasis in hypogammaglobulinaemia — a computed tomography assessment, *Clin Radiol* 44:82-84, 1991.

98. Dallimore NS: Squamous bronchial carcinoma arising in a case of multiple juvenile papillomatosis, *Thorax* 40:797-798, 1985.

99. Davis EW, Katz S, Peabody JW: Broncholithiasis, a neglected cause of bronchoesophageal fistula, *JAMA* 160:555-557, 1956.

100. Dick JA, Morgan WKC, Muir DFC, et al: The significance of irregular opacities on the chest roentgenogram, *Chest* 102:251-260, 1992.

101. Dixon GF, Donnerberg RL, Schonfeld SA, et al: Advances in the diagnosis and treatment of broncholithiasis, *Am Rev Respir Dis* 129:1028-1030, 1984.

102. Dornhorst AC: Respiratory insufficiency, Frederick W. Price Memorial Lecture, *Lancet* 1:1185-1187, 1955.

103. Douglas AC, Grant IWB: Spontaneous closure of large pulmonary bullae: a report on three cases, *Br J Tuberc* 51:335-338, 1957.

104. Dowling EA, Johnson IM, Collier FCD, et al: Intratracheal goiter: a clinicopathologic review, *Ann Surg* 156:258-267, 1962.

105. Doyle AJ: Demonstration on computed tomography of tracheomalacia in tracheobronchomegaly (Mounier-Kuhn syndrome), *Br J Radiol* 62:176-177, 1989.

106. Dukes RJ, Rosenow EC, Hermans PE: Pulmonary manifestations of hypogammaglobulinaemia, *Thorax* 33:603-607, 1978.

107. Dull WL, Bohadana AB, Teculescu DB, et al: The standard chest roentgenogram for determining lung overinflation, *Lung* 160:311-314, 1982.

108. Dunne MG, Reiner B: CT features of tracheobronchomegaly, *J Comput Assist Tomogr* 12:388-391, 1988.

109. Dunnill MS: The pathology of asthma, with special reference to changes in the bronchial mucosa, *J Clin Pathol* 13:27-33, 1960.

110. Eber CD, Stark P, Bertozzi P: Bronchiolitis obliterans on high-resolution CT: a pattern of mosaic oligemia, *J Comput Assist Tomogr* 17:853-856, 1993.

111. Editorial: Chest radiographs in asthma, *Br Med J* 4:123-124, 1974.

112. Edmonds LC, Prakash UBS: Lymphoma, neutropenia, and wheezing in a 70-year-old man, *Chest* 103:585-587, 1993.

113. Effman EL, Fram EK, Vock P, et al: Tracheal cross-sectional area in children: CT determination, *Radiology* 149:137-140, 1983.

114. Eggleston PA, Ward BH, Pierson WE, et al: Radiographic abnormalities in acute asthma in children, *Pediatrics* 54:442-449, 1974.

115. Eliasson R, Mossberg B, Camner P, et al: The immotile-cilia syndrome: a congenital ciliary abnormality as an etiologic factor in chronic airway infections and male sterility, *N Engl J Med* 297:1-6, 1977.

116. Ell SR, Jolles H, Galvin JR: Cine CT demonstration of nonfixed upper airway obstruction, *AJR* 146:669-677, 1986.

117. Epler GR: Bronchiolitis obliterans and airways obstruction associated with graft-versus-host disease, *Clin Chest Med* 9:551-556, 1988.

118. Epler GR: Silo-filler's disease: a new perspective, *Mayo Clin Proc* 64:368-370, 1989.

119. Epler GR, Colby TV: The spectrum of bronchiolitis obliterans, *Chest* 83:161-162, 1983.

120. Epler GR, Snider GL, Gaensler EA, et al: Bronchiolitis and bronchitis in connective tissue disease: a possible relationship to the use of penicillamine, *JAMA* 242:528-532, 1979.

121. Eriksson S: Pulmonary emphysema and alpha$_1$-antitrypsin deficiency, *Acta Med Scand* 175:197-205, 1964.

122. Eriksson S: Studies in α_1-antitrypsin deficiency, *Acta Med Scand Suppl* 432:5-85, 1965.

123. Esterley JR, Heard BE: Multiple bronchiolar stenoses in a patient with generalized airway obstruction, *Thorax* 20:309-316, 1965.

124. Ettman IK, Keel DT: Tracheal diverticulosis, *Radiology* 78:187-191, 1962.

125. Fairfax AJ, Haslam PL, Pavia D, et al: Pulmonary disorders associated with Sjogrens syndrome, *Q J Med* 50:279-295, 1981.

126. Fazio F, Lavender JP, Steiner RE: 81mKr ventilation and 99mTc perfusion scans in chest disease: comparison with standard radiographs, *AJR* 130:421-428, 1978.

127. Feigin DS, Abraham JL: "Increased pulmonary markings" — a radiologic-pathologic correlation study (abstract), *Invest Radiol* 15:425, 1980.

128. Feist JH: Selective cinebronchography in obstructive and restrictive pulmonary disease, *AJR* 99:543-554, 1967.

129. Feist JH, Johnson TH, Wilson RJ: Acquired tracheomalacia: etiology and differential diagnosis, *Chest* 68:340-345, 1975.

130. Feldman F, Seaman WB, Baker DC: The roentgen manifestations of scleroma, *AJR* 101:807-813, 1967.

131. Felson B: Neoplasms of the trachea and main stem bronchi, *Semin Roentgenol* 18:23-37, 1983.

132. Findley LJ, Sahn SA: The value of chest roentgenograms in acute asthma in adults, *Chest* 80:535-536, 1981.

133. Fiore D, Biondetti PR, Sartori F, et al: The role of computed tomography in the evaluation of bullous lung disease, *J Comput Assist Tomogr* 6:105-108, 1982.

134. Fleischner FG: Reversible bronchiectasis, *AJR* 46:166-172, 1941.

135. Fletcher CM, Pride NB: Definitions of emphysema, chronic bronchitis, asthma, and airflow obstruction: twenty-five years on from the Ciba Symposium, *Thorax* 39:81-85, 1984.

136. Fortoul TI, Cano-Valle F, Oliva E, et al: Follicular bronchiolitis in association with connective tissue diseases, *Lung* 163:305-314, 1985.

137. Foster WL, Gimenez EI, Roubidoux MA, et al: The emphysemas: radiologic-pathologic correlations, *Radiographics* 13:311-328, 1993.

138. Foster WL, Pratt PC, Roggli VL, et al: Centrilobular emphysema: CT-pathologic correlation, *Radiology* 159:27-32, 1986.

139. Fox MA, Lynch DA, Make BJ: Thymoma with hypogammaglobulinemia (Good's syndrome): an unusual cause of bronchiectasis, *AJR* 158:1229-1230, 1992.

140. Fraser RG: The radiologist and obstructive airway disease, *AJR* 120:737-775, 1974.

141. Fraser RG, Fraser RS, Renner JW, et al: The roentgenologic diagnosis of chronic bronchitis: a reassessment with emphasis on parahilar bronchi seen end-on, *Radiology* 120:1-9, 1976.

142. Fraser RG, Pare JAP, Pare PD, et al: *Diagnosis of diseases of the chest,* vol 3, ed 3, Philadelphia, 1990, WB Saunders.

143. Fromson BH, Denison DM: Quantitative features in the computed tomography of healthy lungs, *Thorax* 43:120-126, 1988.

144. Gaensler EA, Jederlinic PJ, FitzGerald MX: Patient work-up for bullectomy, *J Thorac Imag* 1:75-93, 1986.

145. Gamsu G, Borson DB, Webb WR, et al: Structure and function in tracheal stenosis, *Am Rev Respir Dis* 121:519-531, 1980.

146. Gamsu G, Forbes AR, Ovenfors C-O: Bronchographic features of chronic bronchitis in normal men, *AJR* 136:317-322, 1981.

147. Gamsu G, Nadel JA: The roentgenologic manifestations of emphysema and chronic bronchitis, *Med Clin North Am* 57:719-733, 1973.

148. Gamsu G, Webb WR: Computed tomography of the trachea: normal and abnormal, *AJR* 139:321-326, 1982.

149. Gamsu G, Webb WR: Computed tomography of the trachea and mainstem bronchi, *Semin Roentgenol* 18:51-60, 1983.

150. Gans ROB, de Vries N, Donker AJM, et al: Circulating antineutrophil cytoplasmic autoantibodies in subglottic stenosis: a useful aid in diagnosing vasculitis in this condition? *Q J Med* 80:565-574, 1991.

151. Gardner S, Seilheimer D, Catlin F, et al: Subglottic coccidioidomycosis presenting with persistent stridor, *Pediatrics* 66:623-625, 1980.

152. Gay S, Dee P: Tracheobronchomegaly: the Mounier-Kuhn syndrome, *Br J Radiol* 57:640-644, 1984.

153. Geddes DM, Corrin B, Brewerton DA, et al: Progressive airway obliteration in adults and its association with rheumatoid disease, *Q J Med* 46:427-444, 1977.

154. Genereux GP: Radiology and pulmonary immunopathological disease. In Steiner RE, ed: *Recent advances in radiology and medical imaging,* vol 7, New York, 1983, Churchill Livingstone, pp 213-240.

155. Gibb WRG, Dhillon DP, Zilkha KJ, et al: Bronchiectasis with ulcerative colitis and myelopathy, *Thorax* 42:155-156, 1987.

156. Gibson GJ: Familial pneumothoraces and bullae, *Thorax* 32:88-90, 1977.

157. Gilles JD, Reed MH, Simons FER: Radiologic findings in acute childhood asthma, *J Can Assoc Radiol* 29:28-33, 1978.

158. Gishen P, Saunders AJS, Tobin MJ, et al: Alpha₁-antitrypsin deficiency: the radiological features of pulmonary emphysema in subjects of Pi type Z and Pi type SZ: a survey by the British Thoracic Association, *Clin Radiol* 33:371-377, 1982.

159. Glazer G, Webb WR: Laryngeal papillomatosis with pulmonary spread in a 69-year-old man, *AJR* 132:820-822, 1979.

160. Glynn AA, Michaels L: Bronchial biopsy in chronic bronchitis and asthma, *Thorax* 15:142-153, 1960.

161. Goddard PR, Nicholson EM, Laszlo G, et al: Computed tomography in pulmonary emphysema, *Clin Radiol* 33:379-387, 1982.

162. Gordon I, Helms P, Fazio F: Clinical applications of radionuclide lung scanning in infants and children, *Br J Radiol* 54:576-585, 1981.

163. Gosink BB, Friedman PJ, Liebow AA: Bronchiolitis obliterans: roentgenologic-pathologic correlation, *AJR* 117:816-832, 1973.

164. Gould GA, MacNee W, McLean A, et al: CT measurements of lung density in life can quantitate distal air space enlargement—an essential defining feature of human emphysema, *Am Rev Respir Dis* 137:380-392, 1988.

165. Gould GA, Redpath AT, Ryan M: Lung CT density correlates with measurements of airflow limitation and the diffusing capacity, *Eur Respir J* 4:141-146, 1991.

166. Greenberg SD, Boushy SF, Jenkins DE: Chronic bronchitis and emphysema: correlation of pathologic findings, *Am Rev Respir Dis* 96:918-928, 1967.

167. Greenberg SD, Jenkins DE, Stevens PM: The lungs in homozygous alpha₁-antitrypsin deficiency, *Am J Clin Pathol* 60:581-592, 1973.

168. Greene R: "Saber-sheath" trachea: relation to chronic obstructive pulmonary disease, *AJR* 130:441-445, 1978.

169. Greene R, Lechner GL: "Saber-sheath" trachea: a clinical and functional study of marked coronal narrowing of the intrathoracic trachea, *Radiology* 115:265-268, 1975.

170. Greenfield H, Herman PG: Papillomatosis of the trachea and bronchi, *AJR* 89:45-50, 1963.

171. Greenspan RH, Sagel S, McMahon J, et al: Timed expiratory chest films in detection of air-trapping, *Invest Radiol* 8:264-265, 1973.

172. Greenstone M, Rutman A, Dewar A, et al: Primary ciliary dyskinesia: cytological and clinical features, *Q J Med* 67:405-430, 1988.

173. Greenstone M, Rutman A, Pavia D, et al: Normal axonemal structure and function in Kartagener's syndrome: an explicable paradox, *Thorax* 40:956-957, 1985.

174. Gregg I, Trapnell DH: The bronchographic appearances of early chronic bronchitis, *Br J Radiol* 42:132-139, 1969.

175. Grenier P, Lenoir S, Brauner M: Computed tomographic assessment of bronchiectasis, *Semin Ultrasound CT MR* 11:430-441, 1990.

176. Grenier P, Maurice F, Musset D, et al: Bronchiectasis: assessment by thin-section CT, *Radiology* 161:95-99, 1986.

177. Grillo HC: Surgical treatment of postintubation tracheal injuries, *J Thorac Cardiovasc Surg* 78:860-875, 1979.

178. Griscom NT: Computed tomographic determination of tracheal dimensions in children and adolescents, *Radiology* 145:361-364, 1982.

179. Griscom NT: CT measurement of the tracheal lumen in children and adolescents, *AJR* 156:371-372, 1991.

180. Griscom NT, Vawter GF, Stigol LC: Radiologic and pathologic abnormalities of the trachea in older patients with cystic fibrosis, *AJR* 148:691-693, 1987.

181. Griscom NT, Wohl MEB: Tracheal size and shape: effects of change in intraluminal pressure, *Radiology* 149:27-30, 1983.

182. Griscom NT, Wohl MEB: Dimensions of the growing trachea related to age and gender, *AJR* 146:233-237, 1986.

183. Gronner AT, Trevino RJ: Tracheocoele, *Br J Radiol* 44:979-981, 1971.

184. Gross BH, Felson B, Birnberg FA: The respiratory tract in amyloidosis and the plasma cell dyscrasias, *Semin Roentgenol* 21:113-127, 1986.

185. Gudbjerg CE: Roentgenologic diagnosis of bronchiectasis, *Acta Radiol* 43:209-226, 1955.

186. Guerry-Force ML, Muller NL, Wright JL, et al: A comparison of bronchiolitis obliterans with organizing pneumonia, usual interstitial pneumonia and small airways disease, *Am Rev Respir Dis* 135:705-712, 1987.

187. Guest PJ, Hansell DM: High resolution computed tomography (HRCT) in emphysema associated with alpha-1-antitrypsin deficiency, *Clin Radiol* 45:260-266, 1992.

188. Gurney JW, Jones KK, Robbins RA, et al: Regional distribution of emphysema: correlation of high-resolution CT with pulmonary function tests in unselected smokers, *Radiology* 183:457-463, 1992.

189. Guynes WA, Dickinson WE, Sutherland RD, et al: Tracheoesophageal fistula following blunt chest trauma, *Texas Med* 75:52-53, 1979.

190. Haddad MC, Sharif HS, Jared MS, et al: Premature tracheobronchial, laryngeal and costochondral cartilage calcification in children, *Clin Radiol* 47:52-55, 1993.

191. Han BK, Dunbar JS, Striker TW: Membranous laryngotracheobronchitis (membranous coup), *AJR* 133:53-58, 1979.

192. Handelsman DJ, Conway AJ, Boylan LM, et al: Young's syndrome: obstructive azoospermia and chronic sinopulmonary infections, *N Engl J Med* 310:3-9, 1984.

193. Hansell DM, Strickland B: High-resolution computed tomography in pulmonary cystic fibrosis, *Br J Radiol* 62:1-5, 1989.

194. Hardy KA, Schidlow DV, Zaeri N: Obliterative bronchiolitis in children, *Chest* 93:460-466, 1988.

195. Haskin PH, Goodman LR: Normal tracheal bifurcation angle: a reassessment, *AJR* 139:879-882, 1982.

196. Hawley PC, Whitcomb ME: Bronchiolitis fibrosa obliterans in adults, *Arch Intern Med* 141:1324-1327, 1981.

197. Hayes JA: Distribution of bronchial gland measurements in a Jamaican population, *Thorax* 24:619-622, 1969.

198. Hayes M: Lung imaging with radioaerosols for the assessment of airway disease, *Semin Nucl Med* 10:243-251, 1980.

199. Hayhurst MD, MacNee W, Flenley DC, et al: Diagnosis of pulmonary emphysema by computerised tomography, *Lancet* 2:320-322, 1984.

200. Heard BE, Khatchatourov V, Otto H, et al: The morphology of emphysema, chronic bronchitis, and bronchiectasis: definition, nomenclature, and classification, *J Clin Pathol* 32:882-892, 1979.

201. Hepper NG, Mulm JR, Sheehan WC, et al: Roentgenographic study of chronic obstructive pulmonary disease by alpha-1-antitrypsin phenotype, *Mayo Clin Proc* 53:166-172, 1978.

202. Herzog CA, Miller RR, Hoidal JR: Bronchiolitis and rheumatoid arthritis, *Am Rev Respir Dis* 124:636-639, 1981.

203. Hill DJ, Landau LI, Phelan PD: Small airway disease in asymptomatic asthmatic adolescents, *Am Rev Respir Dis* 106:873-880, 1972.

204. Hines DW, Haber MH, Yaremko L, et al: Pseudomembranous tracheobronchitis caused by *Aspergillus*, *Am Rev Respir Dis* 143:1408-1411, 1991.

205. Hodson CJ, Trickey SE: Bronchial wall thickening in asthma, *Clin Radiol* 11:183-191, 1960.

206. Hodson ME, Simon G, Batten JC: Radiology of uncomplicated asthma, *Thorax* 29:296-303, 1974.

207. Hoeffler HB, Schweppe I, Greenberg SD: Bronchiectasis following pulmonary ammonia burn, *Arch Pathol Lab Med* 106:686-687, 1982.

208. Hogg JC: Bronchiolitis in asthma and chronic obstructive pulmonary disease, *Clin Chest Med* 14:733-740, 1993.

209. Hogg JC, Macklem PT, Thurlbeck WM: Site and nature of airway obstruction in chronic obstructive lung disease, *N Engl J Med* 278:1355-1360, 1968.

210. Holden WS, Ardran GM: Observations on the movements of the trachea and main bronchi in man, *J Faculty Radiol* 8:267-275, 1957.

211. Holinger PH, Gelman HK, Wolfe CK: Rhinoscleroma of the lower respiratory tract, *Laryngoscope* 87:1-9, 1977.

212. Holinger PH, Johnston KC, Basinger CE: Benign stenosis of the trachea, *Ann Otol Rhinol Laryngol* 59:837-859, 1950.

213. Holmes AH, Trotman-Dickenson B, Edwards A, et al: Bronchiectasis in HIV disease, *Q J Med* 85:875-882, 1992.

214. Holt RM, Schmidt RA, Goodwin JD, et al: High resolution CT in respiratory bronchiolitis−associated interstitial lung disease, *J Comput Assist Tomogr* 17:46-50, 1993.

215. Homma H, Yamanaka A, Tanimoto S, et al: Diffuse panbronchiolitis: a disease of the transitional zone of the lung, *Chest* 83:63-69, 1983.

216. Hopkirk JAC, Stark JE: Unilateral pulmonary collapse in asthmatics, *Thorax* 33:207-210, 1978.

217. Horvath ET, doPico GA, Barbee RA, et al: Nitrogen dioxide−induced pulmonary disease, *J Occup Med* 20:103-110, 1978.

218. Hosker HSR, Clague HW, Morritt GN: Ectopic right upper lobe bronchus as a cause of breathlessness, *Thorax* 42:473-474, 1987.

219. Hoskins MC, Evans RA, King SJ, et al: "Sabre sheath" trachea with mediastinal lipomatosis mimicking a mediastinal tumour, *Clin Radiol* 44:417-418, 1991.

220. Hossain S: Quantitative measurement of bronchial muscle in men with asthma, *Am Rev Respir Dis* 107:99-109, 1973.

221. Houk VN, Kent DC, Fosburg RG: Unilateral hyperlucent lung: a study in pathophysiology and etiology, *Am J Med Sci* 253:406-416, 1967.

222. Howland WJ, Good CA: The radiographic features of tracheopathia osteoplastica, *Radiology* 71:847-850, 1958.

223. Hunter TB, Kuhns LR, Roloff MA, et al: Tracheobronchiomegaly in an 18 month old child, *AJR* 123:687-690, 1975.

224. Idell S, Cohen AB: Alpha-1-antitrypsin deficiency, *Clin Chest Med* 4:359-375, 1983.

225. Imoto EM, Stein RM, Shellito JE, et al: Central airway obstruction due to cytomegalovirus-induced necrotizing tracheitis in a patient with AIDS, *Am Rev Respir Dis* 142:884-886, 1990.

226. Isawa T, Wasserman K, Taplin GV: Lung scintigraphy and pulmonary function studies in obstructive airway disease, *Am Rev Respir Dis* 102:161-172, 1970.

227. Jackson CL, Huber JF: Correlated applied anatomy of bronchial tree and lungs with system of nomenclature, *Dis Chest* 9:319-326, 1943.

228. Jackson GD, Littleton JT: Simultaneous occurrence of anomalous cardiac and tracheal bronchi: a case study, *J Thorac Imag* 3:59-60, 1988.

229. Jamal K, Cooney TP, Fleetham JA, et al: Chronic bronchitis: correlation of morphological findings to sputum production and flow rates, *Am Rev Respir Dis* 129:719-722, 1984.

230. Jardin M, Remy R: Segmental bronchovascular anatomy of the lower lobes: CT analysis, *AJR* 147:457-468, 1986.

231. Jay SJ, Johanson WG: Massive intrapulmonary hemorrhage: an uncommon complication of bullous emphysema, *Am Rev Respir Dis* 110:497-501, 1974.

232. Jazbi B, Goodwin C, Tackett D, et al: Idiopathic subglottic stenosis, *Ann Otol Rhinol Laryngol* 86:644-648, 1977.

233. Jefferson K, Rees S: *Clinical cardiac radiology*, ed 2, London, 1980, Butterworths.

234. Jesseph JE, Merendino KA: The dimensional interrelationships of the major components of the human tracheobronchial tree, *Surg Gynecol Obstet* 105:210-214, 1957.

235. Joharjy IA, Bashi SA, Abdullah AK: Value of medium-thickness CT in the diagnosis of bronchiectasis, *AJR* 149:1133-1137, 1987.

236. Johnson TH, Mikita JJ, Wilson RJ, et al: Acquired tracheomalacia, *Radiology* 109:577-580, 1973.

237. Johnston RF, Green RA: Tracheobronchiomegaly: report of five cases and demonstration of familial occurrence, *Am Rev Respir Dis* 91:35-50, 1965.

238. Jones DK, Godden D, Cavanagh P: Alpha-1-antitrypsin deficiency presenting as bronchiectasis, *Br J Dis Chest* 79:301-304, 1985.

239. Jones GR, Proudfoot AT, Hall JI: Pulmonary effects of acute exposure to nitrous fumes, *Thorax* 28:61-65, 1973.

240. Judd DR, Dubuque T: Acquired benign esophagotracheobronchial fistula, *Dis Chest* 54:237-240, 1968.

241. Kagan E, Soskolne CL, Zwi S, et al: Immunologic studies in patients with recurrent bronchopulmonary infections, *Am Rev Respir Dis* 111:441-451, 1975.

242. Kaneko K, Kudo S, Tashiro M, et al: Case report: computed tomography findings in Williams-Campbell syndrome, *J Thorac Imag* 6:11-13, 1991.

243. Kao SCS, Smith WL, Sato Y, et al: Ultrafast CT of laryngeal and tracheobronchial obstruction in symptomatic postoperative infants with esophageal atresia and tracheoesophageal fistula, *AJR* 154:345-350, 1990.

244. Karasick D, Karasick S, Lally JF: Mucoid pseudotumors of the tracheobronchial tree in two cases, *AJR* 132:459-460, 1979.

245. Karetzky MS: Asthma mortality: an analysis of 1 year's experience, review of the literature and assessment of current modes of therapy, *Medicine* 54:471-484, 1975.

246. Kartagener M: Zur pathogenese der Bronchiektasien: Bronchiektasien bei Situs viscerum inversus, *Beitr Klin Tuberk* 83:489-501, 1933.

247. Kass I, Zamel N, Dobry CA, et al: Bronchiectasis following ammonia burns of the respiratory tract: a review of two cases, *Chest* 62:282-285, 1972.

248. Katsura S, Martin CJ: The roentgenologic diagnosis of anatomic emphysema, *Am Rev Respir Dis* 96:700-706, 1967.

249. Katz I, LeVine M, Herman P: Tracheobronchiomegaly: the Mounier-Kuhn syndrome, *AJR* 88:1084-1094, 1962.

250. Katzenstein A-LA, Askin FB: *Surgical pathology of non-neoplastic lung disease*, Philadelphia, 1990, WB Saunders.

251. Kaufmann HJ, Mahboubi S, Spackman TJ, et al: Tracheal stenosis as a complication of chondrodysplasia punctata, *Ann Radiol* 191:203-209, 1976.

252. Keller CA, Shepard JW, Chun DS, et al: Pulmonary hypertension in chronic obstructive pulmonary disease, *Chest* 90:185-192, 1986.

253. Kindt GC, Weiland JE, Davis WB, et al: Bronchiolitis in adults: a reversible cause of airway obstruction associated with airway neutrophils and neutrophil products, *Am Rev Respir Dis* 140:483-492, 1989.

254. King TE: Respiratory bronchiolitis–associated interstitial lung disease, *Clin Chest Med* 14:693-698, 1993.

255. Kinnear WJM, Tattersfield AE: Emphysematous bullae: surgery is best for large bullae and moderately impaired lung function, *Br Med J* 300:208-209, 1990.

256. Kinney WW, Angelillo VA: Bronchiolitis in systemic lupus erythematosus, *Chest* 82:646-649, 1982.

257. Kinsella M, Muller NL, Abboud RT, et al: Quantitation of emphysema by computed tomography using a "density mask" program and correlation with pulmonary function tests, *Chest* 97:315-321, 1990.

258. Kinsella M, Muller NL, Staples C et al: Hyperinflation in asthma and emphysema: assessment by pulmonary function testing and computed tomography, *Chest* 94:286-289, 1988.

259. Klein JS, Gamsu G, Webb WR, et al: High resolution CT diagnosis of emphysema in symptomatic patients with normal chest radiographs and isolated low diffusing capacity, *Radiology* 182:817-821, 1992.

260. Knudson RJ, Standen JR, Kaltenborn WT, et al: Expiratory computed tomography for assessment of suspected pulmonary emphysema, *Chest* 99:1357-1366, 1991.

261. Kogutt MS, Swischuk LE, Goldblum R: Swyer-James syndrome (unilateral hyperlucent lung) in children, *Am J Dis Child* 125:614-618, 1973.

262. Kondoh Y, Taniguchi H, Yokoyama S, et al: Emphysematous change in chronic asthma in relation to cigarette smoking: assessment by computed tomography, *Chest* 97:845-849, 1990.

263. Kowal LE, Goodman LR, Zarro VJ, et al: CT diagnosis of broncholithiasis, *J Comput Assist Tomogr* 7:321-323, 1983.

264. Kueppers F, Black LF: α_1-Antitrypsin and its deficiency, *Am Rev Respir Dis* 110:176-194, 1974.

265. Kuriyama K, Gamsu G, Stern RG, et al: CT-determined pulmonary artery diameters in predicting pulmonary hypertension, *Invest Radiol* 19:16-22, 1984.

266. Kurklu EU, Williams MA, le Roux BT: Bronchiectasis consequent upon foreign body retention, *Thorax* 28:601-602, 1973.

267. Kuwano K, Matsuba K, Ikeda T, et al: The diagnosis of mild emphysema: correlation of computed tomography and pathology scores, *Am Rev Respir Dis* 141:169-178, 1990.

268. Kwong JS, Adler BD, Padley SPG, et al: Diagnosis of diseases of the trachea and main bronchi: chest radiography vs CT, *AJR* 161:519-522, 1993.

269. Kwong JS, Muller NL, Miller RR: Diseases of the trachea and main-stem bronchi: correlation of CT with pathologic findings, *Radiographics* 12:645-657, 1992.

270. Lahdensuo A, Mattila J, Vilppula A: Bronchiolitis in rheumatoid arthritis, *Chest* 85:705-708, 1984.

271. Lallemand D, Chagnon S, Buriot D, et al: Tracheomegaly and immune deficiency syndromes in childhood, *Ann Radiol* 24:67-72, 1981.

272. Landay MJ, Shaw C, Bordlee RP: Bilateral left lungs: unusual variation of hilar anatomy, *AJR* 138:1162-1164, 1982.

273. Landing BH, Dixon LG: Congenital malformations and genetic disorders of the respiratory tract (larynx, trachea, bronchi, and lungs), *Am Rev Respir Dis* 120:151-185, 1979.

274. Landing BH, Lawrence T-YK, Payne VC, et al: Bronchial anatomy in syndromes with abnormal visceral situs, abnormal spleen and congenital heart disease, *Am J Cardiol* 28:456-462, 1971.

275. Laraya-Cuasay LR, DeForest A, Huff D, et al: Chronic pulmonary complications of early influenza virus infection in children, *Am Rev Respir Dis* 116:617-625, 1977.

276. Larsson C: Natural history and life expectancy in severe alpha$_1$-antitrypsin deficiency, PiZ, *Acta Med Scand* 204:345-351, 1978.

277. Laurell CB, Ericksson S: The electrophoretic α_1 globulin pattern of serum in α_1-antitrypsin deficiency, *Scand J Clin Invest* 15:132-140, 1963.

278. Laws JW, Heard BE: Emphysema and the chest film: a retrospective radiological and pathological study, *Br J Radiol* 35:750-761, 1962.

279. Lee KS, Bae WK, Lee BH, et al: Bronchovascular anatomy of the upper lobes: evaluation with thin-section CT, *Radiology* 181:765-772, 1991.

280. Lee KS, Im J-G, Bae WK, et al: CT anatomy of the lingular segmental bronchi, *J Comput Assist Tomogr* 15:86-91, 1991.

281. Legge DA, Tiede JJ, Peters GA, et al: Death from tension pneumothorax and chlorpromazine cardio-respiratory collapse as separate complications of asthma, *Ann Allergy* 27:23-29, 1969.

282. Lennon EA, Simon G: The height of the diaphragm in the chest radiograph of normal adults, *Br J Radiol* 38:937-943, 1965.

283. Lentz D, Bergin CJ, Berry GJ, et al: Diagnosis of bronchiolitis obliterans in heart-lung transplantation patients: importance of bronchial dilatation on CT, *AJR* 159:463-467, 1992.

284. Lesser BA, Leeper KV, Stein PD, et al: The diagnosis of acute pulmonary embolism in patients with chronic obstructive pulmonary disease, *Chest* 102:17-22, 1992.

285. Libshitz HI, Shuman LS: Radiation-induced pulmonary change: CT finding, *J Comput Assist Tomogr* 8:15-19, 1984.

286. Liddelow AG, Campbell AH: Widening of the membranous wall and flattening of the trachea and main bronchi, *Br J Dis Chest* 58:56-60, 1964.

287. Lieberman J, Colp C: A role for intermediate heterozygous alpha$_1$-antitrypsin deficiency in obstructive lung disease, *Chest* 98:522-523, 1990.

288. Lin MS, Goodwin DA: Pulmonary distribution of an inhaled radioaerosol in obstructive pulmonary disease, *Radiology* 118:645-651, 1976.

289. Lincoln JCR, Deverall PB, Stark J, et al: Vascular anomalies compressing the oesophagus and trachea, *Thorax* 24:295-306, 1969.

290. Little AG, Ferguson MK, Demeester TR, et al: Esophageal carcinoma with respiratory tract fistula, *Cancer* 53:1322-1328, 1984.

291. Lloyd DC, Taylor PM: Calcification of the intrathoracic trachea demonstrated by computed tomography, *Br J Radiol* 63:31-32, 1990.

292. Lomasney L, Bergin CJ, Lomasney J, et al: CT appearance of lunate trachea, *J Comput Assist Tomogr* 13:520-522, 1989.

293. Longstreth GF, Weitzman SA, Browning RJ, et al: Bronchiectasis and homozygous alpha-1-antitrypsin deficiency, *Chest* 67:233-235, 1975.

294. Lowry T, Schuman LM: "Silo-filler's disease" — a syndrome caused by nitrogen dioxide, *JAMA* 162:153-160, 1956.

295. Lundgren R, Stjernberg NL: Tracheobronchopathia osteochondroplastica: a clinical bronchoscopic and spirometric study, *Chest* 80:706-709, 1981.

296. Lynch DA: Imaging of small airways diseases, *Clin Chest Med* 14:623-634, 1993.

297. Lynch DA, Brasch RC, Hardy KA, et al: Pediatric pulmonary disease: assessment with high-resolution ultrafast CT, *Radiology* 176:243-248, 1990.

298. Lynch DA, Newell JD, Tschomper BA, et al: Uncomplicated asthma in adults: comparison of CT appearance of the lungs in asthmatic and healthy subjects, *Radiology* 188:829-833, 1993.

299. MacFarlane JD, Dieppe PA, Rigden BG, et al: Pulmonary and pleural lesions in rheumatoid disease, *Br J Dis Chest* 72:288-300, 1978.

300. Macklem PT: The pathophysiology of chronic bronchitis and emphysema, *Med Clin North Am* 57:669-679, 1973.

301. Macklem PT, Fraser RG, Brown WG: Bronchial pressure measurements in emphysema and bronchitis, *J Clin Invest* 44:897-905, 1965.

302. Macklem PT, Thurlbeck WM, Fraser RG: Chronic obstructive disease of small airways, *Ann Intern Med* 74:167-177, 1971.

303. Macklem PT, Wilson NJ: Measurement of intrabronchial pressure in man, *J Appl Physiol* 20:653-663, 1965.

304. MacLeod WM: Abnormal transradiancy of one lung, *Thorax* 9:147-153, 1954.

305. MacNee W, Gould G, Lamb D: Quantifying emphysema by CT scanning: clinicopathologic correlates, *Ann NY Acad Sci* 624:179-194, 1991.

306. Macpherson RI, Cumming GR, Chernick V: Unilateral hyperlucent lung: a complication of viral pneumonia, *J Can Assoc Radiol* 20:225-231, 1969.

307. Mahler D, D'Esopo NO: Peri-emphysematous lung infection, *Clin Chest Med* 2:51-57, 1981.

308. Maisel JC, Silvers GW, George MS, et al: The significance of bronchial atrophy, *Am J Pathol* 67:371-383, 1972.

309. Mangiulea VG, Stinghe RV: The accessory cardiac bronchus: bronchologic aspect and review of the literature, *Dis Chest* 54:433-436, 1968.

310. Mannes GPM, van der Jagt EJ, Wouters B, et al: Dextrocardia? *Chest* 96:391-392, 1989.

311. Margolin HN, Rosenberg LS, Felson B, et al: Idiopathic unilateral hyperlucent lung: a roentgenologic syndrome, *AJR* 82:63-75, 1959.

312. Marmorstein BL, Cianciulli FD: Planimetric measurement of total lung capacity in asthma, *Chest* 66:378-381, 1974.

313. Marti-Bonmati L, Catala FJ, Perales FR: Computed tomography differentiation between cystic bronchiectasis and bullae, *J Thorac Imag* 7:83-85, 1991.

314. Marti-Bonmati L, Perales FR, Catala F, et al: CT findings in Swyer-James syndrome, *Radiology* 172:477-480, 1989.

315. Martin CJ: Tracheobronchopathia osteochondroplastica, *Arch Otolaryngol Head Neck Surg* 100:290-293, 1974.

316. Martin KW, McAlister WH: Intratracheal thymus: a rare cause of airway obstruction, *AJR* 149:1217-1218, 1987.

317. Martini N, Goodner JT, D'Angio GJ, et al: Tracheoesophageal fistula due to cancer, *J Thorac Cardiovasc Surg* 59:319-324, 1970.

318. Maruyama Y, Petter JR, Green CR: Acquired esophagotracheal fistula secondary to a foreign body in the esophagus, *N Engl J Med* 260:126-127, 1959.

319. Matsuba K, Thurlbeck WM: Disease of the small airways in chronic bronchitis, *Am Rev Respir Dis* 107:552-558, 1973.

320. Matthay RA, Schwartz MI, Ellis JH, et al: Pulmonary artery hypertension in chronic obstructive pulmonary disease: determination by chest radiography, *Invest Radiol* 16:95-100, 1981.

321. McCarthy D, Milic-Emili J: Closing volume in asymptomatic asthma, *Am Rev Respir Dis* 107:559-570, 1973.

322. McCluskie RA: Unusual fate of emphysematous bullae, *Thorax* 36:77, 1981.

323. McGuinness G, Naidich DP, Garay S, et al: AIDS associated bronchiectasis: CT features, *J Comput Assist Tomogr* 17:260-266, 1993.

324. McGuiness G, Naidich DP, Garay SM, et al: Accessory cardiac bronchus: CT features and clinical significance, *Radiology* 189:563-566, 1993.

325. McGuiness G, Naidich DP, Leitman BS, et al: Bronchiectasis: CT evaluation, *AJR* 160:253-259, 1993.

326. McLaughlin FJ, Strieder DJ, Harris GBC, et al: Tracheal bronchus: association with respiratory morbidity in childhood, *J Pediatr* 106:751-755, 1985.

327. McLoud TC, Epler GR, Colby TV, et al: Bronchiolitis obliterans, *Radiology* 159:1-8, 1986.

328. Meisner P, Hugh-Jones P: Pulmonary function in bronchial asthma, *Br Med J* 1:470-475, 1968.

329. Millar AB, Fromson B, Strickland BA, et al: Computed tomography based estimates of regional gas and tissue volume of the lung in supine subjects with chronic airflow limitation or fibrosing alveolitis, *Thorax* 41:932-939, 1986.

330. Miller AH: Scleroma of larynx, trachea and bronchi, *Laryngoscope* 59:506-514, 1949.

331. Miller RD, Divertie MB: Kartagener's syndrome, *Chest* 62:130-135, 1972.

332. Miller RR, Muller NL, Vedal S, et al: Limitations of computed tomography in the assessment of emphysema, *Am Rev Respir Dis* 139:980-983, 1989.

333. Milne EN, Bass H: Roentgenologic and functional analysis of combined chronic obstructive pulmonary disease and congestive cardiac failure, *Invest Radiol* 4:129-147, 1969.

334. Milne JE: Nitrogen dioxide inhalation and bronchiolitis obliterans: a review of the literature and report of case, *J Occup Med* 11:538-547, 1969.

335. Milner AD, Murray M: Acute bronchiolitis in infancy: treatment and prognosis, *Thorax* 44:1-5, 1989.

336. Mitchell RE, Bury RG: Congenital bronchiectasis due to deficiency of bronchial cartilage (Williams-Campbell syndrome), *J Pediatr* 87:230-234, 1975.

337. Mitchell RS, Ryan SF, Petty TL, et al: The significance of morphologic chronic hyperplastic bronchitis, *Am Rev Respir Dis* 93:720-729, 1966.

338. Moles KW, Varghese G, Hayes JR: Pulmonary involvement in ulcerative colitis, *Br J Dis Chest* 82:79-83, 1988.

339. Moncada RM, Venta LA, Venta ER, et al: Tracheal and bronchial cartilaginous rings: warfarin sodium − induced calcification, *Radiology* 184:437-439, 1992.

340. Mont JL, Botey A, Subias R, et al: Unilateral pulmonary hemorrhage in a patient with Goodpasture's and Swyer-James' syndrome, *Eur J Respir Dis* 67:145-147, 1985.

341. Moore ADA, Godwin JD, Dietrich PA, et al: Swyer-James syndrome: CT findings in eight patients, *AJR* 158:1211-1215, 1992.

342. Mootoosamy IM, Reznek RH, Osman J, et al: Assessment of bronchiectasis by computed tomography, *Thorax* 40:920-924, 1985.

343. Morgan MDL, Denison DM, Strickland B: Value of computed tomography for selecting patients with bullous lung disease for surgery, *Thorax* 41:855-862, 1986.

344. Morgan MDL, Edwards CW, Morris J, et al: Origin and behaviour of emphysematous bullae, *Thorax* 44:533-538, 1989.

345. Morgan MDL, Strickland B: Computed tomography in the assessment of bullous lung disease, *Br J Dis Chest* 78:10-25, 1984.

346. Morrish WF, Herman SJ, Weisbrod GL, et al: Bronchiolitis obliterans after lung transplantation: findings at chest radiography and high-resolution CT, *Radiology* 179:487-490, 1991.

347. Morrison SC: Case report: demonstration of a tracheal bronchus by computed tomography, *Clin Radiol* 39:208-209, 1988.

348. Morrissey WL, Gould IA, Carrington CB, et al: Silo-filler's disease, *Respiration* 32:81-92, 1975.

349. Mounier-Kuhn P: Dilatation de la trachee: constatations radiographiques et bronchoscopiques, *Lyon Med* 150:106-109, 1932.

350. Mueller RE, Keble DL, Plummer J, et al: The prevalence of chronic bronchitis, chronic airway obstruction and respiratory symptoms in a Colorado city, *Am Rev Respir Dis* 103:209-228, 1971.

351. Muller NL: CT diagnosis of emphysema: it may be accurate, but is it relevant? *Chest* 103:329-330, 1993.

352. Muller NL, Bergin CJ, Ostrow DN, et al: Role of computed tomography in the recognition of bronchiectasis, *AJR* 143:971-976, 1984.

353. Muller NL, Staples CA, Miller RR, et al: "Density mask": an objective method to quantitate emphysema using computed tomography, *Chest* 94:782-787, 1988.

354. Munro NC, Cooke JC, Currie DC, et al: Comparison of thin section computed tomography with bronchography for identifying bronchiectatic segments in patients with chronic sputum production, *Thorax* 45:135-139, 1990.

355. Murata K, Itoh H, Senda M, et al: Stratified impairment of pulmonary ventilation in "diffuse panbronchiolitis": PET and CT studies, *J Comput Assist Tomogr* 13:48-53, 1989.

356. Murata K, Itoh H, Todo G, et al: Centrilobular lesions of the lung: demonstration by high-resolution CT and pathologic correlation, *Radiology* 161:641-645, 1986.

357. Murphy KC, Atkins CJ, Offer RC, et al: Obliterative bronchiolitis in two rheumatoid arthritis patients treated with penicillamine, *Arthritis Rheum* 24:557-560, 1981.

358. Myers JL, Colby TV: Pathologic manifestations of bronchiolitis, constrictive bronchiolitis, cryptogenic organizing pneumonia, and diffuse panbronchiolitis, *Clin Chest Med* 14:611-622, 1993.

359. Myers JL, Veal CF, Shin MS, et al: Respiratory bronchiolitis causing interstitial lung disease: a clinico-pathologic study of six cases, *Am Rev Respir Dis* 135:880-884, 1987.

360. Nadel HR, Stringer DA, Levison H, et al: The immotile cilia syndrome: radiological manifestations, *Radiology* 154:651-655, 1985.

361. Naidich DP, Funt S, Ettenger NA, et al: Hemoptysis: CT-bronchoscopic correlations in 58 cases, *Radiology* 177:357-362, 1990.

362. Naidich DP, McCauley DI, Khouri NF, et al: Computed tomography of bronchiectasis, *J Comput Assist Tomogr* 6:437-444, 1982.

363. Naidich DP, Terry PB, Stitik FP, et al: Computed tomography of the bronchi: normal anatomy, *J Comput Assist Tomogr* 4:746-753, 1980.

364. Naidich DP, Zinn WL, Ettenger NA, et al: Basilar segmental bronchi: thin-section CT evaluation, *Radiology* 169:11-16, 1988.

365. Neeld DA, Goodman LR, Gurney JW, et al: Computerized tomography in the evaluation of allergic bronchopulmonary aspergillosis, *Am Rev Respir Dis* 142:1200-1205, 1990.

366. Nelson SW, Christoforidis A: Reversible bronchiectasis, *Radiology* 71:375-382, 1958.

367. Nelson SW, Christoforidis AJ: Bronchography in diseases of the adult chest, *Radiol Clin North Am* 11:125-152, 1973.

368. Neville E, Brewis RAL, Yeates WK, et al: Respiratory tract disease and obstructive azoospermia, *Thorax* 38:929-933, 1983.

369. Nicklaus TM, Stowell DW, Christiansen WR, et al: The accuracy of the roentgenologic diagnosis of chronic pulmonary emphysema, *Am Rev Respir Dis* 93:889-899, 1966.

370. Niederman MS, Gambino A, Lichter J: Tension ball valve mucus plug in asthma, *Am J Med* 79:131-134, 1985.

371. Niewoehner DE: New messages from morphometric studies of chronic obstructive pulmonary disease, *Semin Respir Med* 8:140-146, 1986.

372. Nishimura K, Kitaichi M, Izumi T, et al: Diffuse panbronchiolitis: correlation of high-resolution CT and pathologic findings, *Radiology* 184:779-785, 1992.

373. O'Dell CW, Taylor A, Higgins CB, et al: Ventilation-perfusion lung images of the Swyer-James syndrome, *Radiology* 121:423-426, 1976.

374. Okada K, Lee M-O, Hitomi S, et al: Sinus histiocytosis with massive lymphadenopathy and tracheobronchial lesions: CT and MR findings, *J Comput Assist Tomogr* 12:1039-1040, 1988.

375. Onitsuka H, Hirose N, Watanabe K, et al: Computed tomography of tracheopathia osteoplastica, *AJR* 140:268-270, 1983.

376. Osborne D, Vock P, Godwin JD, et al: CT identification of bronchopulmonary segments: 50 normal subjects, *AJR* 142:47-52, 1984.

377. Ostrow D, Buskard N, Hill RS, et al: Bronchiolitis obliterans complicating bone marrow transplantation, *Chest* 87:828-830, 1985.

378. Otsuji H, Hatakeyama M, Kitamura I, et al: Right upper lobe versus right middle lobe: differentiation with thin-section, high-resolution CT, *Radiology* 172:653-656, 1989.

379. Padley S, Varma N, Flower CDR: Case report: tracheobronchomegaly in association with ankylosing spondylitis, *Clin Radiol* 43:139-141, 1991.

380. Padley SPG, Adler BD, Hansell DM, et al: Bronchiolitis obliterans: high resolution CT findings and correlation with pulmonary function tests, *Clin Radiol* 47:236-240, 1993.

381. Paganin F, Trussard V, Seneterre E, et al: Chest radiography and high resolution computed tomography of the lungs in asthma, *Am Rev Respir Dis* 146:1084-1087, 1992.

382. Panitch HB, Callahan CW, Shidlow DV: Bronchiolitis in children, *Clin Chest Med* 14:715-731, 1993.

383. Paradis I, Yousem S, Griffith B: Airway obstruction and bronchiolitis obliterans after lung transplantation, *Clin Chest Med* 14:751-763, 1993.

384. Penn CC, Liu C: Bronchiolitis following infection in adults and children, *Clin Chest Med* 14:645-654, 1993.

385. Perez-Guerra F, Walsh RE, Sagel SS: Bronchiolitis obliterans and tracheal stenosis: late complications of inhalation burn, *JAMA* 218:1568-1570, 1971.

386. Peters ME, Arya S, Langer LO, et al: Narrow trachea in mucopolysaccharidoses, *Pediatr Radiol* 15:225-228, 1985.

387. Peters ME, Dickie HA, Crummy AB, et al: Swyer-James-MacLeod syndrome: a case with a baseline normal chest radiograph, *Pediatr Radiol* 12:211-213, 1982.

388. Petheram IS, Kerr IH, Collins JV: Value of chest radiographs in severe acute asthma, *Clin Radiol* 32:281-282, 1981.

389. Peto R, Speizer FE, Cochrane AL, et al: The relevance in adults of air-flow obstruction, but not of mucus hypersecretion, to mortality from chronic lung disease, *Am Rev Respir Dis* 128:491-500, 1983.

390. Pontius JR, Jacobs LG: The reversal of advanced bronchiectasis, *Radiology* 68:204-208, 1957.

391. Prabhu MB, Barber D, Cockroft DW: Bronchiolitis obliterans and *Mycoplasma* pneumonia, *Respir Med* 85:535-537, 1991.

392. Pradham DJ, Rabuzzi D, Meyer JA: Primary solitary lymphoma of the trachea, *J Thorac Cardiovasc Surg* 70:938-940, 1975.

393. Pratt PC: Conventional chest films can reveal emphysema, but not COPD, *Chest* 92:8, 1987.

394. Pratt PC: Radiographic appearance of the chest in emphysema, *Invest Radiol* 22:927-929, 1987.

395. Pratt PC: Role of conventional chest radiography in diagnosis and exclusion of emphysema, *Am J Med* 82:998-1006, 1987.

396. Prichard MG, Brown PJE, Sterrett GF: Bronchiolo-alveolar carcinoma arising in longstanding lung cysts, *Thorax* 39:545-549, 1984.

397. Pugatch RD: The radiology of emphysema, *Clin Chest Med* 4:433-442, 1983.

398. Pushpakom R, Hogg JC, Woolcock AJ, et al: Experimental papain-induced emphysema in dogs, *Am Rev Respir Dis* 102:778-789, 1970.

399. Putman CE, Godwin JD, Silverman PM, et al: CT of localized lucent lung lesions, *Semin Roentgenol* 19:173-188, 1984.

400. Rahbar M, Tabatabai D: Tracheobronchiomegaly, *Br J Dis Chest* 65:65-68, 1971.

401. Rakower J, Moran E: Unilateral hyperlucent lung (Swyer-James syndrome), *Am J Med* 33:864-872, 1962.

402. Ramirez-R J, Dowell AR: Silo-filler's disease: nitrogen dioxide-induced lung injury; long-term follow-up and review of the literature, *Ann Intern Med* 74:569-576, 1971.

403. Randolph J, Grunt JA, Vawter GF: The medical and surgical aspects of intratracheal goiter, *N Engl J Med* 268:457-461, 1963.

404. Ravin CE, Handel DB, Kariman K: Persistent endotracheal tube cuff overdistension: a sign of tracheomalacia, *AJR* 137:408-409, 1981.

405. Rebuck AS: Radiological aspects of severe asthma, *Aust Radiol* 14:264-268, 1970.

406. Reed WB, Lopez DA, Landing B: Clinical spectrum of anhidrotic ectodermal dysplasia, *Arch Dermatol* 102:134-143, 1970.

407. Reich SB, Weinshelbaum A, Yee J: Correlation of radiographic measurements and pulmonary function tests in chronic obstructive pulmonary disease, *AJR* 144:695-699, 1985.

408. Reid L: Chronic bronchitis and emphysema: a symposium. III. Pathological findings and radiological changes in chronic bronchitis and emphysema. A. Pathological finding in chronic bronchitis, *Br J Radiol* 32:291-292, 1959.

409. Reid L: Measurement of the bronchial mucous gland layer: a diagnostic yardstick in chronic bronchitis, *Thorax* 15:132-141, 1960.

410. Reid L: *The pathology of emphysema*, London, 1967, Lloyd-Luke Ltd.

411. Reid L, Millard FJC: Correlation between radiological diagnosis and structural lung changes in emphysema, *Clin Radiol* 15:307-311, 1964.

412. Reid L, Simon G: Unilateral lung transradiancy, *Thorax* 17:230-239, 1962.

413. Reid LM: Reduction in bronchial subdivision in bronchiectasis, *Thorax* 5:233-247, 1950.

414. Reid LM: Correlation of certain bronchographic abnormalities seen in chronic bronchitis with the pathological changes, *Thorax* 10:199-204, 1955.

415. Remy-Jardin M, Remy J: Comparison of vertical and oblique CT in evaluation of bronchial tree, *J Comput Assist Tomogr* 12:956-962, 1988.

416. Remy-Jardin M, Remy J, Boulenguez C, et al: Morphologic effects of cigarette smoking on airways and pulmonary parenchyma in healthy adult volunteers: CT evaluation and correlation with pulmonary function tests, *Radiology* 186:107-115, 1993.

417. Remy-Jardin M, Remy J, Gosselin B, et al: Lung parenchymal changes secondary to cigarette smoking: pathologic-CT correlations, *Radiology* 186:643-651, 1993.

418. Restrepo GL, Heard BE: Air trapping in chronic bronchitis and emphysema: measurements of the bronchial cartilage, *Am Rev Respir Dis* 90:395-400, 1964.

419. Rifkin MD, Pritzker HA: Tracheobronchial cartilage calcification in children: case reports and review of the literature, *Br J Radiol* 57:293-296, 1984.

420. Rindsberg S, Friedman AC, Fiel SB, et al: MRI of tracheobronchomegaly, *J Can Assoc Radiol* 38:126-128, 1987.

421. Ritsema GH: Ectopic right bronchus: indication for bronchography, *AJR* 140:671-674, 1983.

422. Robins AG: Pathophysiology of emphysema, *Clin Chest Med* 4:413-420, 1983.

423. Roca J, Granena A, Rodriquez-Roison R, et al: Fatal airway disease in an adult with chronic graft-versus-host disease, *Thorax* 37:77-78, 1982.

424. Rosen RA, Dalinka MK, Gralino BJ, et al: The roentgenographic findings in alpha-1-antitrypsin deficiency (AAD), *Radiology* 95:25-28, 1970.

425. Rosenbaum HD, Alavi SM, Bryant LR: Pulmonary parenchymal spread of juvenile laryngeal papillomatosis, *Radiology* 90:654-660, 1968.

426. Rosenblum LJ, Mauceri RA, Wellenstein DE, et al: Density patterns in the normal lung as determined by computed tomography, *Radiology* 137:409-416, 1980.

427. Rott HD: Kartagener's syndrome and the syndrome of immotile cilia, *Hum Genet* 46:249-261, 1979.

428. Royle H: X-ray appearances in asthma: a study of 200 cases, *Br Med J* 1:577-580, 1952.

429. Rubenstein J, Weisbrod G, Steinhardt MI: Atypical appearances of "saber-sheath" trachea, *Radiology* 127:41-42, 1978.

430. Rubin BK: Immotile cilia syndrome (primary ciliary dyskinesia) and inflammatory lung disease, *Clin Chest Med* 9:657-668, 1988.

431. Sakai F, Gamsu G, Im J-G, et al: Pulmonary function abnormalities in patients with CT-determined emphysema, *J Comput Assist Tomogr* 11:963-968, 1987.

432. Sakula A: Tracheobronchopathia osteoplastica: its relationship to primary tracheobronchial amyloidosis, *Thorax* 23:105-110, 1968.

433. Saleh M, Miles AI, Lasser RP: Unilateral pulmonary edema in Swyer-James syndrome, *Chest* 66:594-597, 1974.

434. Sanders C: The radiographic diagnosis of emphysema, *Radiol Clin North Am* 29:1019-1030, 1991.

435. Sanders C, Nath PH, Bailey WC: Detection of emphysema with computed tomography: correlation with pulmonary function tests and chest radiology, *Invest Radiol* 23:262-266, 1988.

436. Santolicandro A, Ruschi S, Fornai E, et al: Imaging of ventilation in chronic obstructive pulmonary disease, *J Thorac Imag* 1:36-53, 1986.

437. Sato A, Chida K, Iwata M, et al: Study of bronchus-associated lymphoid tissue in patients with diffuse panbronchiolitis, *Am Rev Respir Dis* 146:473-478, 1992.

438. Sato P, Madtes DK, Thorning D, et al: Bronchiolitis obliterans caused by *Legionella pneumophila*, *Chest* 87:840-842, 1985.

439. Scadding JG: The bronchi in allergic aspergillosis, *Scand J Respir Dis* 48:372-377, 1967.

440. Scadding JG: Definition of clinical categories of asthma. In Clark TJH, Godfrey S, eds: *Asthma*, London, 1977, Chapham & Hall, p 5.

441. Schuster DP: Positron emission tomography: theory and its application to the study of lung disease, *Am Rev Respir Dis* 139:818-840, 1989.

442. Selman-Lama M, Perez-Padilla R: Airflow obstruction and airway lesions in hypersensitivity pneumonitis, *Clin Chest Med* 14:699-714, 1993.

443. Semple PDA, Reid CB, Thompson WD: Widespread panacinar emphysema with alpha-1-antitrypsin deficiency, *Br J Dis Chest* 74:289-295, 1980.

444. Sharp HL, Bridges RA, Krivit W, et al: Cirrhosis associated with alpha-1-antitrypsin deficiency: a previously unrecognized inherited disorder, *J Lab Clin Med* 73:934-939, 1969.

445. Shepard JO, Grillo HC, McLoud TC, et al: Right-pneumonectomy syndrome: radiological findings and CT correlation, *Radiology* 161:661-664, 1986.

446. Sherman S, Skoney JA, Ravikrishnan KP: Routine chest radiographs in exacerbations of chronic obstructive pulmonary disease, *Arch Intern Med* 149:2493-2496, 1989.

447. Sherrill DL, Lebowitz MD, Burrows B: Epidemiology of chronic obstructive pulmonary disease, *Clin Chest Med* 11:375-387, 1990.

448. Shin MS, Berland LL, Myers JL, et al: CT demonstration of an ossifying bronchial carcinoid simulating broncholithiasis, *AJR* 153:51-52, 1989.

449. Shin MS, Ho KJ: Broncholithiasis: its detection by computed tomography in patients with recurrent hemoptysis of unknown etiology, *Comput Radiol* 7:189-193, 1983.

450. Shin MS, Jackson RM, Ho K-J: Tracheobronchomegaly (Mounier-Kuhn syndrome): CT diagnosis, *AJR* 150:777-779, 1988.

451. Shuttleworth JS, Self CL, Pershing HS: Tracheopathia osteoplastica, *Ann Intern Med* 52:234-242, 1960.

452. Siegel MJ, Shackelford GD, Francis RS, et al: Tracheal bronchus, *Radiology* 130:353-355, 1979.

453. Silverman G: Tuberculosis of the trachea and major bronchi, *Dis Chest* 11:3-17, 1945.

454. Silverman PM, Godwin JD: CT/bronchographic correlations in bronchiectasis, *J Comput Assist Tomogr* 11:52-56, 1987.

455. Silvers GW, Maisel JC, Petty TL, et al: Flow limitation during forced expiration in excised human lungs, *J Appl Physiol* 36:737-744, 1974.

456. Simon G: Chronic bronchitis and emphysema: a symposium. III. Pathological findings and radiological changes in chronic bronchitis and emphysema. B. Radiological changes in chronic bronchitis, *Br J Radiol* 32:292-294, 1959.

457. Simon G: Radiology and emphysema, *Clin Radiol* 15:293-306, 1964.

458. Simon G, Galbraith HJB: Radiology of chronic bronchitis, *Lancet* 2:850-852, 1953.

459. Simon G, Pride NB, Jones NL, et al: Relation between abnormalities in the chest radiograph and changes in pulmonary function in chronic bronchitis and emphysema, *Thorax* 28:15-23, 1973.

460. Singer DB, Greenberg SD, Harrison GM: Papillomatosis of the lung, *Am Rev Respir Dis* 94:777-781, 1966.

461. Singh AK, Kothawla LK, Karlson KE: Tracheo-esophageal and aortoesophageal fistulae complicating corrosive esophagitis, *Chest* 70:549-551, 1976.

462. Skeens JL, Fuhrman CR, Yousem SA: Bronchiolitis obliterans in heart-lung transplantation patients: radiologic findings in 11 patients, *AJR* 153:253-256, 1989.

463. Smith KR, Morris JF: Reversible bronchial dilatation: a report of a case, *Dis Chest* 42:652-656, 1962.

464. Snider GL: A perspective on emphysema, *Clin Chest Med* 4:329-336, 1983.

465. Snider GL, Kleinerman J, Thurlbeck WM, et al: The definition of emphysema: report of a National Heart, Lung, and Blood Institute, Division of Lung Diseases workshop, *Am Rev Respir Dis* 132:182-185, 1985.

466. Sobonya R: Fatal anhydrous ammonia inhalation, *Hum Pathol* 8:293-299, 1977.

467. Sobonya RE, Burrows B: The epidemiology of emphysema, *Clin Chest Med* 4:351-358, 1983.

468. Sostman HD, Neumann RD, Gottschalk A, et al: Perfusion of nonventilated lung: failure of hypoxic vasoconstriction? *AJR* 141:151-156, 1983.

469. Soto B, Pacifico AD, Souza AS, et al: Identification of thoracic isomerism from the plain chest radiograph, *AJR* 131:995-1002, 1978.

470. Spouge D, Mayo JR, Cardoso W, et al: Panacinar emphysema: CT and pathologic findings, *J Comput Assist Tomogr* 17:710-713, 1993.

471. Stanbridge RD: Tracheo-esophageal fistula and bilateral recurrent laryngeal nerve palsies after blunt chest trauma, *Thorax* 37:548-549, 1982.

472. Starshak RJ, Sty JR, Woods G, et al: Bridging bronchus: a rare airway anomaly, *Radiology* 140:95-96, 1981.

473. Stein PD, Coleman RE, Gottschalk A, et al: Diagnostic utility of ventilation-perfusion lung scans in acute pulmonary embolism is not diminished by preexisting cardiac or pulmonary disease, *Chest* 100:604-606, 1991.

474. Stephens RW, Lingeman RE, Lawson LJ: Congenital tracheoesophageal fistulas in adults, *Ann Otol Rhinol Laryngol* 85:613-617, 1976.

475. Stern EJ, Graham CM, Webb WR, et al: Normal trachea during forced expiration: dynamic CT measurements, *Radiology* 187:27-31, 1993.

476. St John RC, Dorinsky PM: Cryptogenic bronchiolitis, *Clin Chest Med* 14:667-675, 1993.

477. Stokes D, Sigler A, Khouri NF, et al: Unilateral hyperlucent lung (Swyer-James syndrome) after severe *Mycoplasma pneumoniae* infection, *Am Rev Respir Dis* 117:145-152, 1978.

478. Stone DJ, Schwartz A, Feltman JA: Bullous emphysema: a long-term study of the natural history and the effects of therapy, *Am Rev Respir Dis* 82:493-507, 1960.

479. Sugiyama Y: Diffuse panbronchiolitis, *Clin Chest Med* 14:765-772, 1993.

480. Suprenant EL, O'Loughlin BJ: Tracheal diverticula and tracheobronchomegaly, *Dis Chest* 49:345-351, 1966.

481. Sutherland JB, Palser RF, Pagtakhan RD, et al: Xenon-133 ventilation and perfusion studies in bronchiectasis, *J Can Assoc Radiol* 31:242-245, 1980.

482. Sutinen S, Christoforidis AJ, Klugh GA, et al: Roentgenologic criteria for the recognition of nonsymptomatic pulmonary emphysema, *Am Rev Respir Dis* 91:69-76, 1965.

483. Sweatman MC, Millar AB, Strickland B, et al: Computed tomography in adult obliterative bronchiolitis, *Clin Radiol* 41:116-119, 1990.

484. Swischuk LE, Hayden CK: The trachea in children, *Semin Roentgenol* 18:7-14, 1983.

485. Swyer PR, James GCW: A case of unilateral pulmonary emphysema, *Thorax* 8:133-136, 1953.

486. Tager IB, Speizer FE: Risk estimates for chronic bronchitis in smokers: a study of male-female differences, *Am Rev Respir Dis* 113:619-625, 1976.

487. Takasugi JE, Godwin JD: The airway, *Semin Roentgenol* 26:175-190, 1991.

488. Tandon MK, Campbell AH: Bronchial cartilage in chronic bronchitis, *Thorax* 24:607-612, 1969.

489. Taplin GV, Poe ND, Greenberg A: Lung scanning following radioaerosol inhalation, *J Nucl Med* 7:77-87, 1966.

490. Tarver RD, Conces DJ, Godwin JD: Motion artifacts on CT simulate bronchiectasis, *AJR* 151:1117-1119, 1988.

491. Taybi H, Capitanio MA: Tracheobronchial calcification: an observation in three children after mitral valve replacement and warfarin sodium therapy, *Radiology* 176:728-730, 1990.

492. Teichmann V, Jezek V, Herles F: Relevance of width of right descending branch of pulmonary artery as a radiological sign of pulmonary hypertension, *Thorax* 25:91-96, 1970.

493. Theodore J, Starnes VA, Lewiston NJ: Obliterative bronchiolitis, *Clin Chest Med* 11:309-321, 1990.

494. Thompson JW, Ahmed AR, Dudley JP: Epidermolysis bullosa dystrophica of the larynx and trachea: acute airway obstruction, *Ann Otol Rhinol Laryngol* 89:428-429, 1980.

495. Thurlbeck WM: Chronic airflow obstruction in lung disease. In Bennington JL, ed: *Major problems in pathology*, vol 5, Philadelphia, 1976, WB Saunders.

496. Thurlbeck WM: Pathophysiology of chronic obstructive pulmonary disease, *Clin Chest Med* 11:389-403, 1990.

497. Thurlbeck WM, Angus GE: A distribution curve for chronic bronchitis, *Thorax* 19:436-442, 1964.

498. Thurlbeck WM, Henderson JA, Fraser RG, et al: Chronic obstructive lung disease: a comparison between clinical, roentgenologic, functional and morphologic criteria in chronic bronchitis, emphysema, asthma and bronchiectasis, *Medicine* 49:82-145, 1970.

499. Thurlbeck WM, Simon G: Radiographic appearance of the chest in emphysema, *AJR* 130:429-440, 1978.

500. Ting EY, Klopstock R, Lyons HA: Mechanical properties of pulmonary cysts and bullae, *Am Rev Respir Dis* 87:538-544, 1963.

501. Toledo TM, Moore WL, Nash DA, et al: Spontaneous pneumopericardium in acute asthma: case report and review of the literature, *Chest* 62:118-120, 1972.

502. Tsuji H, Takazakura E, Terada Y, et al: CT demonstration of spinal epidural emphysema complicating bronchial asthma and violent coughing, *J Comput Assist Tomogr* 13:38-39, 1989.

503. Tsutsui M, Araki Y, Shirakusa T, et al: Characteristic radiographic features of pulmonary carcinoma associated with large bulla, *Ann Thorac Surg* 46:679-683, 1988.

504. Turner-Stokes L, Turton C, Pope FM, et al: Emphysema and cutis laxa, *Thorax* 38:790-792, 1983.

505. Turton CW, Williams G, Green M: Cryptogenic obliterative bronchiolitis in adults, *Thorax* 36:805-810, 1981.

506. Vandevivere J, Spehl M, Dab I, et al: Bronchiectasis in childhood, *Pediatr Radiol* 9:193-198, 1980.

507. Vix VA: Radiographic manifestations of broncholithiasis, *Radiology* 128:295-299, 1978.

508. Vock P, Spiegel T, Fram EK, et al: CT assessment of the adult intrathoracic cross section of the trachea, *J Comput Assist Tomogr* 8:1076-1082, 1984.

509. Wanderer AA, Ellis EF, Goltz RW, et al: Tracheobronchiomegaly and acquired cutis laxa in a child: physiologic and immunologic studies, *Pediatrics* 44:709-715, 1969.

510. Watanabe Y, Nishiyama Y, Kanayama H, et al: Congenital bronchiectasis due to cartilage deficiency: CT demonstration, *J Comput Assist Tomogr* 11:701-703, 1987.

511. Way SPB: Tracheopathia osteoplastica, *J Clin Pathol* 20:814-820, 1967.

512. Wayne KS, Taussig LM: Probable familial congenital bronchiectasis due to cartilage deficiency (Williams-Campbell syndrome), *Am Rev Respir Dis* 114:15-22, 1976.

513. Webb WR, Glazer G, Gamsu G: Computed tomography of the normal pulmonary hilum, *J Comput Assist Tomogr* 5:476-484, 1981.

514. Weber AL, Grillo HC: Tracheal stenosis: an analysis of 151 cases, *Radiol Clin North Am* 16:291-308, 1978.

515. Weber AL, Grillo HC: Tracheal tumors: a radiological, clinical and pathological evaluation of 84 cases, *Radiol Clin North Am* 16:227-246, 1978.

516. Weed LA, Andersen HA: Etiology of broncholithiasis, *Dis Chest* 37:270-277, 1960.

517. Weg JG, Krumholz RA, Hackelroad LE: Unilateral hyperlucent lung: a physiologic syndrome, *Ann Intern Med* 62:675-684, 1965.

518. Wegener OH, Koeppe P, Oeser H: Measurement of lung density by computed tomography, *J Comput Assist Tomogr* 2:1251-1256, 1978.

519. Weiss W: Cigarette smoke, asbestos, and small irregular opacities, *Am Rev Respir Dis* 130:293-301, 1984.

520. Weiss W: Cigarette smoking and small irregular opacities, *Br J Ind Med* 48:841-844, 1991.

521. Welch MH, Richardson RH, Whitcomb WH, et al: The lung scan in alpha-1-antitrypsin deficiency, *J Nucl Med* 10:687-690, 1969.

522. Wells AU, du Bois RM: Bronchiolitis in association with connective tissue disorders, *Clin Chest Med* 14:655-666, 1993.

523. Westcott JL, Cole SR: Traction bronchiectasis in end-stage pulmonary fibrosis, *Radiology* 161:665-669, 1986.

524. White CS, Cole RP, Lubetsky HW, et al: Acute asthma: admission chest radiography in hospitalized adult patients, *Chest* 100:14-16, 1991.

525. White RI, James AE, Wagner HN: The significance of unilateral absence of pulmonary artery perfusion by lung scanning, *AJR* 111:501-509, 1971.

526. Whitehouse G: Tracheopathia osteoplastica, *Br J Radiol* 41:701-703, 1968.

527. Whitelaw A, Evans A, Corrin B: Immotile cilia syndrome: a new cause of neonatal respiratory distress, *Arch Dis Child* 56:432-435, 1981.

528. Whitwell F: A study of pathology and pathogenesis of bronchiectasis, *Thorax* 7:213-239, 1952.

529. Whyte KF, Williams GR: Bronchiectasis after *Mycoplasma* pneumonia, *Thorax* 39:390-391, 1984.

530. Wieder S, Rabinowitz JG: Fibrous mediastinitis: a late manifestation of mediastinal histoplasmosis, *Radiology* 125:305-312, 1977.

531. Wiggins J, Strickland B, Chung KF: Detection of bronchiectasis by high-resolution computed tomography in the yellow nail syndrome, *Clin Radiol* 43:377-379, 1991.

532. Wilcox P, Miller R, Miller G, et al: Airway involvement in ulcerative colitis, *Chest* 92:18-22, 1987.

533. Wilks S: Ossific deposits on the larynx, trachea and bronchi, *Trans Pathol Soc Lond* 8:88, 1857.

534. Williams H, Campbell P: Generalized bronchiectasis associated with deficiency of cartilage in the bronchial tree, *Arch Dis Child* 35:182-191, 1960.

535. Williams JL, Markowitz RI, Capitanio MA, et al: Immune deficiency syndromes, *Semin Roentgenol* 10:83-89, 1975.

536. Winterbauer RH, Bedon GA, Ball WC: Recurrent pneumonia, *Ann Intern Med* 70:689-700, 1969.

537. Wiot JF: Tracheobronchial trauma, *Semin Roentgenol* 18:15-22, 1983.

538. Wohl MEB, Chernick V: Bronchiolitis, *Am Rev Respir Dis* 118:759-781, 1978.

539. Wolfe F, Schurle DR, Lin JJ, et al: Upper and lower airway disease in penicillamine treated patients with rheumatoid arthritis, *J Rheumatol* 10:406-410, 1983.

540. Woodford DM, Coutu RE, Gaensler EA: Obstructive lung disease from acute sulfur dioxide exposure, *Respiration* 38:238-245, 1979.

541. Woodring JH, Barrett PA, Rehm SR, et al: Acquired tracheomegaly in adults as a complication of diffuse pulmonary fibrosis, *AJR* 152:743-747, 1989.

542. Woodring JH, Howard RS, Rehm SR: Congenital tracheobronchomegaly (Mounier-Kuhn syndrome): a report of 10 cases and review of the literature, *J Thorac Imag* 6:1-10, 1991.

543. Woolcock AJ, Read J: Lung volumes in exacerbations of asthma, *Am J Med* 41:259-273, 1966.

544. Woolcock AJ, Rebuck AS, Cade JF, et al: Lung volume changes in asthma measured concurrently by two methods, *Am Rev Respir Dis* 104:703-709, 1971.

545. Wright JL: Inhalational lung injury causing bronchiolitis, *Clin Chest Med* 14:635-644, 1993.

546. Wright JL, Cagle P, Churg A, et al: Diseases of the small airways, *Am Rev Respir Dis* 146:240-262, 1992.

547. Wychulis AR, Ellis FH, Anderson HA: Acquired nonmalignant esophagotracheo-bronchial fistula: report of 36 cases, *JAMA* 196:117-122, 1966.

548. Yamashita H: *Roentgenologic anatomy of the lung,* Stuttgart, 1978, Georg Thieme.
549. Young K, Aspestrand F, Kolbenstvedt A: High resolution CT and bronchography in the assessment of bronchiectasis, *Acta Radiol* 32:439-441, 1991.
550. Young RH, Sandstrom RE, Mark GJ: Tracheopathia osteoplastica: clinical, radiologic and pathological correlations, *J Thorac Cardiovasc Surg* 79:537-541, 1980.
551. Yousem SA, Colby TV, Carrington CB: Follicular bronchitis/bronchiolitis, *Hum Pathol* 16:700-706, 1985.
552. Yousem SA, Colby TV, Carrington CB: Lung biopsy in rheumatoid arthritis, *Am Rev Respir Dis* 131:770-777, 1985.
553. Yousem SA, Colby TV, Gaensler EA: Respiratory bronchiolitis–associated interstitial lung disease and its relationship to desquamative interstitial pneumonia, *Mayo Clin Proc* 64:1373-1380, 1989.
554. Zieverink SE, Harper AP, Holden RW, et al: Emergency room radiography of asthma: an efficacy study, *Radiology* 145:27-29, 1982.

18 Chest Trauma

PAUL DEE

SKELETAL TRAUMA

Rib fractures are commonly encountered in clinical practice, and the majority are of limited clinical significance. Certain fractures assume a greater significance by virtue of specific features.

The presence of certain rib fractures indicates a severe trauma or an increased likelihood of damage to certain organs. For example, because the first, second, and third ribs are well protected by the shoulder girdles and the associated musculature, a considerable force is necessary to fracture these ribs. The possibility of damage to important structures such as the aorta and the great vessels is therefore greater.[6] However, patients with significant damage to intrathoracic vascular structures have additional clinical and radiographic evidence of vascular damage. Thus the finding of fractures of the first three ribs in the absence of such additional evidence is not felt to be an indication for angiography.[28,78,110] On the other hand, the presence of fractures of the tenth, eleventh, or twelfth ribs should suggest the possibility of rupture of the liver, kidneys, or spleen.

Fractured rib ends may lacerate the pleura or lung with resultant bleeding or pneumothorax. This possibility constitutes perhaps the main reason to perform radiography in the average patient.

Fractures of a large number of ribs on one side may result in a flail chest with inspiratory chest retraction on that side and potentially serious clinical consequences. The definition of flail chest varies, but the fracturing of four or more contiguous ribs makes flailing a distinct clinical possibility.

Pathologic fractures are clearly of the utmost clinical significance. The diagnosis hinges on identifying a fracture through a destructive process, and obtaining detailed views or tomography may be necessary to confirm the suspicion of focal bone destruction. The majority of such fractures relate to metastatic neoplasm or myeloma, but on occasion they relate to a benign process such as eosinophilic granuloma.

Rib fractures are commonly seen in children subjected to physical abuse.[50] Indeed the finding of occult rib fractures may be a critical clue to the fact that the child has been abused. Rib fractures are uncommon in infants and young children, and when present they can ordinarily be attributed to a known episode of significant trauma. Underlying conditions that may predispose to rib fractures such as rickets or osteogenesis imperfecta must be excluded. Rib fractures in abused children are often bilateral and at varying stages of healing. Callus formation may be prominent, a feature making the fractures more readily visible.

As previously indicated, rib fractures are often clinically inconsequential. Also, a major degree of internal thoracic trauma can occur in the absence of rib fractures, particularly in younger individuals. The thoroughness with which the physician strives to determine the presence or absence of rib fractures depends on the particular circumstances of the case and medicolegal considerations. Inevitably, significant amounts of time, money, and resources are expended in many patients with suspected rib fractures, with little practical result in most cases. A thorough examination of the chest with supplementary rib detail films probably requires a minimum of five films and at least 5 to 10 minutes of room time, when in practice a single frontal upright chest radiograph should suffice. Danher, Eyes, and Kumar[18] studied the radiographs from over 1100 cases of chest trauma and found that only 17 patients were admitted to the hospital for reasons related exclusively to rib trauma. In only two of these cases did oblique views give additional information, and even this information was clinically inconsequential. Other authors[20,98] have supported these findings.

Certain fractures have distinct or noteworthy features:

1. Stress fractures. Fractures of the first or second ribs may be stress fractures as a result of activity, such as backpacking. The bony reaction and callus formation may give a spurious appearance of an apical pulmonary parenchymal process. Apical lordotic and rib detail views plus the clinical circumstances should resolve the diagnosis.

2. Cough fractures. These may also be stress fractures but occur in older patients in the posterolateral aspects of the lower ribs. The patient may experience localized rib pain. The condition is usually of some standing, and callus formation around the fractures may be conspicuous.

3. Excessive callus formation in cushingoid patients. Patients with Cushing's syndrome or receiving intensive steroid therapy are frequently osteoporotic and have an increased tendency to fractures. An interesting and characteristic feature in these patients is the exuberant callus formation that occurs in relation to the fractures.[82] This exuberant callus may simulate a pulmonary parenchymal process.

4. Multiple rib fractures in alcoholics. Hard-core alcoholic patients frequently have multiple bilateral rib fractures in varying stages of healing.[51] Such fractures may be an indicator of other medical consequences of alcohol abuse.

5. Pseudarthroses of ribs. On occasion, rib fractures evolve into pseudarthroses, since ribs are difficult to immobilize. As with stress fractures or excessive callus formation, an unwary or unobservant physician may diagnose a parenchymal lesion.

Other skeletal injuries or their secondary effects may be encountered. The presence of a sternal fracture usually indicates significant chest trauma, and the physician should be alert to the possibility of a deceleration injury to the aorta, the great vessels, or the myocardium.[8,41] As many as 8% of patients admitted with blunt chest trauma have sternal fractures.[41] These fractures cannot be visualized on frontal chest radiographs and may be relatively inconspicuous on lateral chest radiographs. In the appropriate circumstances, careful attention should be paid to the sternal contours on the lateral view. Sternal fractures as such do not generally cause problems either in healing or by direct damage to adjacent structures. Costochondral separation may occur in younger individuals, and this usually also indicates significant trauma. The diagnosis of costochondral separation, however, is essentially based on clinical findings.

Dislocation of the sternoclavicular joint with posterior displacement of the inner end of the clavicle may cause compression of the trachea and the adjacent great vessels with significant clinical consequences.[30] Dislocation of a sternoclavicular joint may be difficult or impossible to detect, particularly in a patient with major trauma in whom the radiographic examination is restricted. However, tracheal deviation may be noted and paratracheal soft tissue thickening may be apparent. The diagnosis of dislocation of the sternoclavicular joint is readily made with computed tomography (CT).[10] Clinical awareness of the possibility of such an injury is the key factor in its recognition, with radiographs often helping to confirm the diagnosis.

Major trauma to the root of the neck, on occasion, may damage the phrenic nerve with resultant diaphragmatic paresis or paralysis. In a severely traumatized patient the development of lower zone or lower lobe atelectasis is fairly common. The atelectasis might be responsible for the diaphragmatic elevation rather than the reverse. Once suspected, the diagnosis can be confirmed by fluoroscopy or ultrasound examination.

Fractures of the thoracic spine are not usually of much direct consequence to the respiratory system. The paravertebral soft tissue thickening adjacent to these fractures, however, may be conspicuous on the chest radiographs, and due allowance should be made when diagnosing lower lobe collapse or aortic injury.[23,111]

PULMONARY PARENCHYMAL TRAUMA

Contusion of the lung parenchyma is common in major trauma and may be seen underlying the point of injury or as a contrecoup lesion. The radiographic appearances are those of a diffuse ill-defined alveolar process with patchy, often confluent shadowing in the lungs (Figure 18-1). Presumably the bleeding into the lung parenchyma must continue for a period of time following the injury, and therefore the changes should wax during that time. However, it is unusual to be able to radiograph a severely injured patient within 1 hour of the trauma with all the inevitable problems, such as transport and resuscitation. In the majority of cases the findings are manifest at the time of the initial examination and show little tendency to increase in severity with subsequent examinations. Radiographic clearing of pulmonary contusion may be relatively rapid, and the signs of contusion have often resolved within 48 hours.

Pulmonary contusion is distributed according to the spread of a shock wave and does not localize in a lobar or segmental pattern. The interlobar fissures do not dampen the spread of the shock wave, and contusion may be seen on either side of the fissures. CT examinations are now performed with greater frequency in patients with trauma and demonstrate lung contusion with great clarity (Figure 18-2). Schild and others[89] imaged experimentally induced pulmonary contusions with computed tomography (CT) and plain radiographs. CT detected 100% of contusions immediately after the trauma, whereas the plain films failed to detect 20% of contusions even after

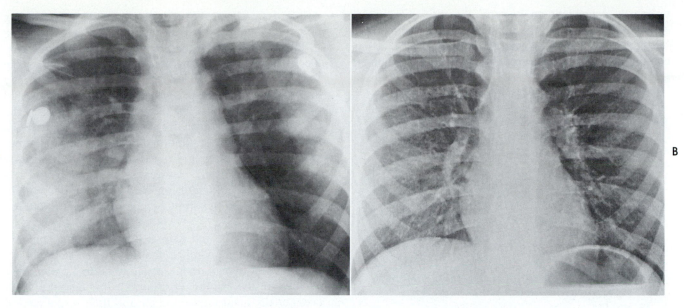

FIGURE 18-1
A, Radiograph of a young man within 2 hours of a motor vehicle accident. B, Same patient 72 hours later. All evidence of pulmonary contusion has disappeared.

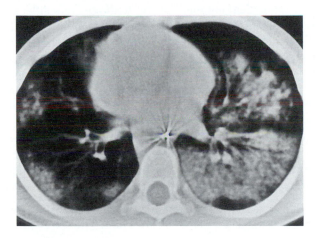

FIGURE 18-2
Computed tomography scan of the patient in Figure 18-1 showing widespread patchy alveolar densities representing contused lung.

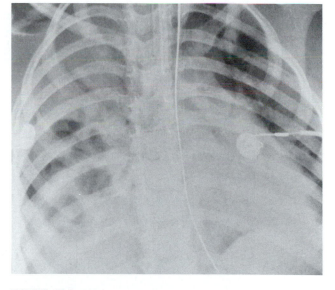

FIGURE 18-3
Radiograph of a child involved in an automobile accident, showing severely contused lung and several pneumatoceles.

sequential examination. Lung contusion in itself is not an indication for CT examination.

Pneumatoceles may be encountered in association with pulmonary contusion. Shock waves cause shearing of a portion of the lung parenchyma with escape of air into the resultant fissure. This localized internal leak of air plus the retraction of lung caused by its inherent elasticity results in a localized rounded airspace in the lung parenchyma (Figure 18-3). The resultant pneumatocele may contain a variable quantity of fluid, presumably blood. Indeed, if the entire space fills with blood, the result is a pulmonary hematoma. Pneumatoceles and hematomas may be multiple but are more commonly isolated lesions. On occasion they are extremely large, up to 14 cm in diameter, but most are 2 to 5 cm in diameter. Pneumatoceles or hematomas are usually first seen several hours after the injury. Possible explanations for this slight delay include obscurity of the lesions because the initial lung contusion may be severe, or enlargement of the parenchymal space because of an air leak or continued oozing of blood. A pneumatocele usually does not have a well-defined wall, at least in the early stages following injury. The visibility of a pneumatocele is ordinarily dependent on its size, the fluid it contains, and the surrounding pulmonary contusion. Distinguishing between a pneumatocele and a hematoma that has communicated with the bronchial tree may be difficult (Figures 18-4 and 18-5). A hematoma becomes more visible as a circumscribed density as the surrounding pulmonary parenchymal contusion clears (Figure 18-6).

Both pneumatoceles and hematomas resolve, pneumatoceles faster than hematomas. Hematomas may take some months to resolve and for a considerable period may be the only visible sequela of a previous trauma. Since by this stage a hematoma is a circumscribed lung mass, the lesion may be mistaken for a neoplasm (Figure 18-7). During the phase of resolution a hematoma may communicate with the bronchial tree and appear as a cavitary process (Figure 18-8). Awareness of these features is important to avoid confusion with more serious pulmonary processes. Cavitating hematomas resolve without treatment.

Pneumothoraces and pleural effusions are a common accompaniment of parenchymal injury and may require prompt chest tube drainage. Severely injured patients are usually in the supine position for radiography. This occasionally makes detecting air and fluid in the pleural space difficult, unless it is localized to the minor fissure, the subpulmonic spaces, or the mediastinal pleural space. In the supine position a patient tends to collect air anteriorly and to layer fluid posteriorly. Anterior pneumothoraces can be detected on frontal projections taken with the patient supine, but the findings are subtle and easily disregarded. The mediastinal contours on the affected side may be seen with unusual clarity, and the anterior portion of the diaphragm may be depressed, revealing more of the base of the heart on that side.[35] Pleural effusions may cause a diffuse haze over the lung field resulting from the filtering effect of the posteriorly positioned fluid layer. If the effusion is large enough, it may extend around the lung and produce a band of density along the lateral chest wall and over the apex. Cross-table lateral views can be helpful for both pneumothoraces and pleural effusions. CT is highly accurate

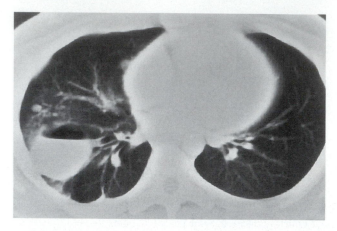

FIGURE 18-4
Computed tomography scan showing a pneumatocele containing fluid and air with some surrounding lung contusion.

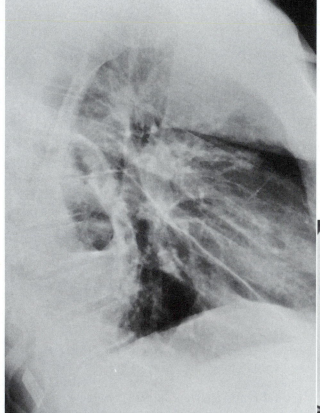

A

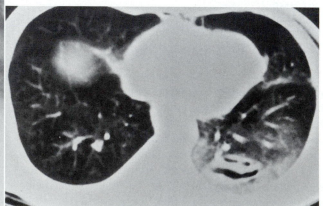

B

FIGURE 18-5
A, Lateral chest radiograph and, B, computed tomography scan showing a left lower lobe airspace containing fluid 1 week following major thoracic trauma. Airspace appears to have thickened wall, but clinical evidence did not suggest evacuation of a hematoma. Airspace was present on the initial examination immediately after the accident and therefore was regarded as a pneumatocele.

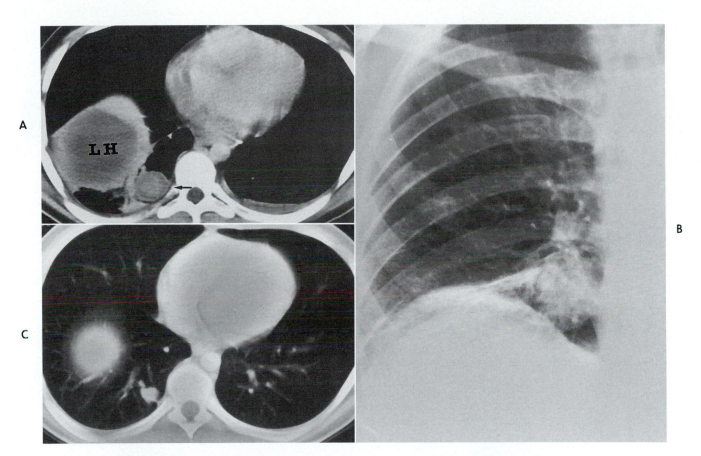

FIGURE 18-6
A, Computed tomography scan of a young man involved in a motor vehicle accident. Note the large hematoma in liver *(LH)*. Pulmonary hematoma *(arrow)* is partially obscured by right lower lobe consolidation and atelectasis. **B,** Hematoma becomes visible on chest radiograph 1 week later. **C,** Follow-up scan 6 weeks later shows a smaller well-circumscribed resolving hematoma.

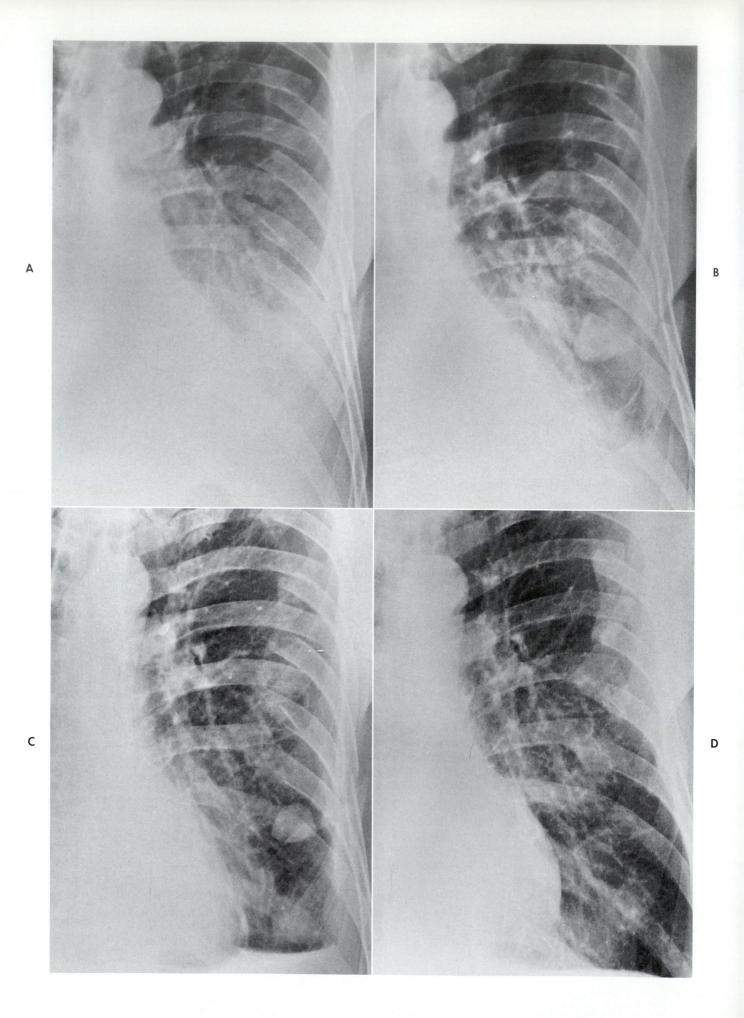

FIGURE 18-7
A, Admission film following major trauma to the patient's left chest. Note multiple rib fractures, left pleural effusion, and left basal pulmonary parenchymal opacification. **B,** Two days later, a pulmonary hematoma is visible. **C,** Two weeks later, the hematoma is the only residual parenchymal lesion. **D,** Six months later, the hematoma has resolved.

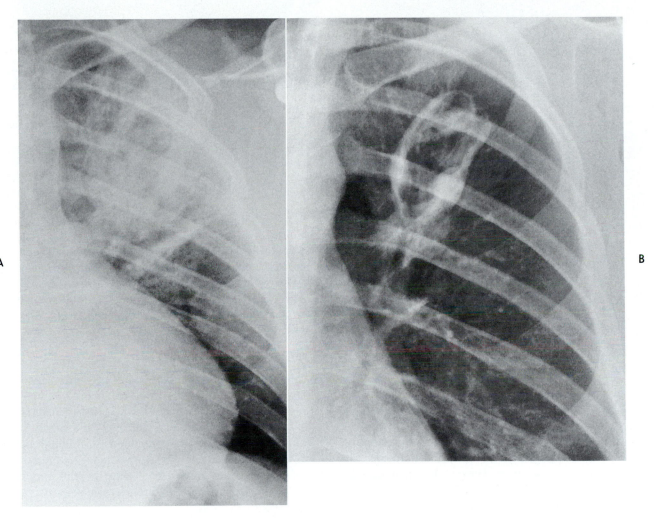

A

B

FIGURE 18-8
A, Left upper lobe pulmonary contusion following a motor vehicle accident. **B,** Four weeks later a well-circumscribed cavitary lesion represents the hematoma that has communicated with the bronchial tree and evacuated. Resolution was eventually complete.

for both, and the lung bases should always be covered during the abdominal CT examination for visceral injury (Figure 18-9).[104] McGonigal and others[60] showed that CT detected 100% of pneumothoraces, whereas supine frontal chest radiographs detected only 40%. This is in accordance with Tocino and associates' finding[100] that only 50% of pneumothoraces in trauma patients are detected by supine chest radiographs.

GUNSHOT, BLAST, AND STAB WOUNDS

Most gunshot wounds to the lungs in civilian practice are the result of low-velocity missiles. Although the missiles may fragment, the devastating fragmentation of a high-velocity missile is not seen. In addition, the shock waves of low-velocity missiles are not nearly so severe or extensive in their effects. The lung is a low-density structure of high elasticity, and the degree of damage is

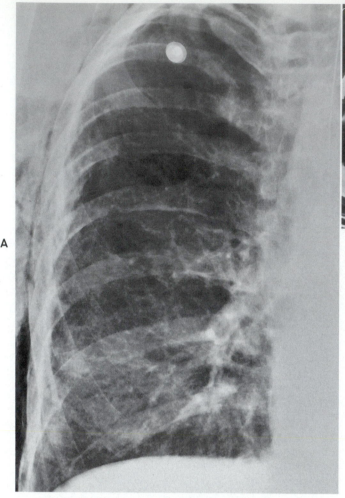

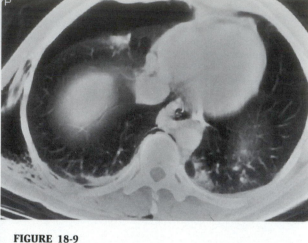

FIGURE 18-9
A, Supine radiograph on admission following an automobile accident. Air is seen in the chest wall, but no pneumothorax is identified. **B,** Computed tomography scan shows an anteriorly positioned pneumothorax.

much less than in high-density, low-elasticity structures such as liver or brain.[47] A low-velocity missile traversing the lung forms a distinct track that may be air filled or occupied by hematoma (Figure 18-10).[32] Surrounding this track is a variable zone of lung contusion. On occasion the track itself is visible, and gauging the thickness and extent of the surrounding contusion may be possible. This observation applies particularly to cases with an air-filled track radiographed in the axis of the track. Shotgun injuries are generally severe because of the intermediate muzzle velocity of these weapons and the large mass of the shot (Figure 18-11). Shotgun injuries to the chest are stated to be nearly 10 times more lethal than wounds from other weapons.[91] The pleura is inevitably involved in pulmonary damage from gunshots, and hemothorax or pneumothorax is common. The chest radiograph is a critical factor in determining whether or not the pleural space should be drained. In damage confined to the lungs and pleura, drainage may be the only direct intervention required.

Stab wounds do not generate shock waves, and the resultant contusion of lung parenchyma is less. As with gunshot wounds the significance of stab wounds relates to the extent and severity of damage to major vascular structures and the pleura or pericardium. The actual trauma to pulmonary parenchyma is less significant.

Blast injuries are relatively uncommon. In described cases the changes are typically bilateral and centered on the major airways, with perihilar edema and contusion.[57,107]

TORSION OF THE LUNG

Torsion of a lung or a lobe of lung is an extremely rare but serious condition that may result from compressive trauma to the chest.[26] The victim is almost invariably a child and has usually been run over by a car. In adults lung torsion may occur spontaneously, although usually an inciting lesion, such as a lung tumor, is present.[36,71] Torsion of lung may also occur in the immediate postoperative period following thoracic surgery, usually after lobar resection.[72]

Diagnosis of lung torsion is extraordinarily difficult. A key factor is awareness of the existence of this condition and the circumstances under which it occurs. The radiographic findings may be subdivided:

1. Results of torquing of the airways and the lung vessels. Airway torquing may result in an abrupt cutoff in the airway at the hilum with the development of atelectasis. Torquing of the hilar vessels also may result in hemorrhagic infarction of lung. Thus a range of findings in the lung parenchyma from normal aeration through varying degrees of lobar or whole lung atelectasis to expansile consolidation of lung is possible.

2. Anatomic malpositioning. By identifying anatomic malposition, the physician can make a definitive diagnosis of lung torsion before exploration. The hilar vessels or the interlobar fissures may be observed to be rotated away

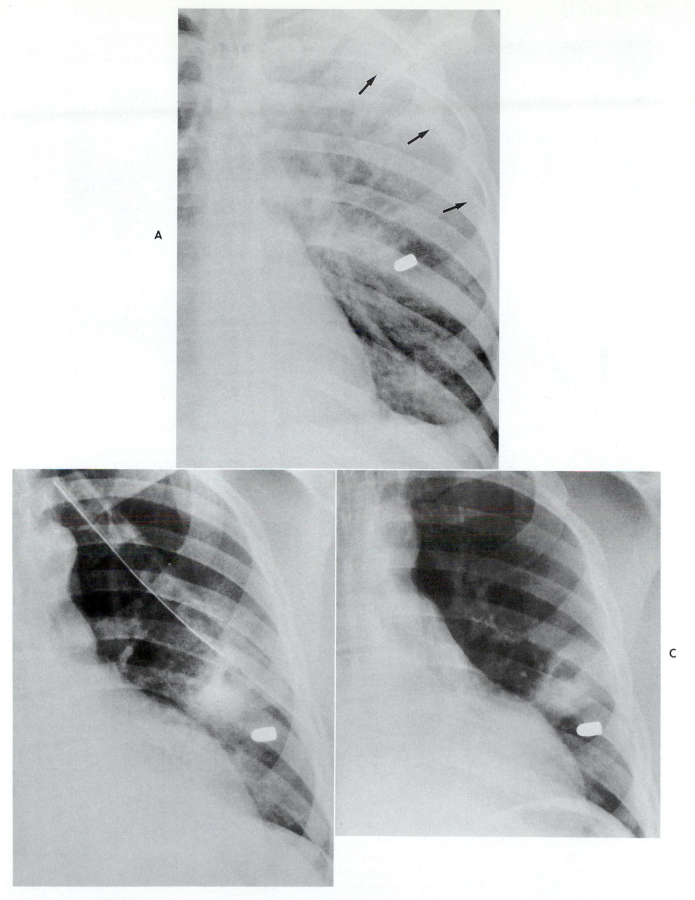

FIGURE 18-10

A, Supine chest radiograph on admission after the patient suffered a gunshot wound from a handgun. Hemothorax is layering posteriorly and extending around lung laterally and over apex *(arrows).* **B,** Day 2 following chest tube drainage of hemothorax. Note the rounded, ill-defined zone of contusion around the bullet track. **C,** Day 4. Zone of contusion has become more defined, and a distinct air-filled bullet track is evident.

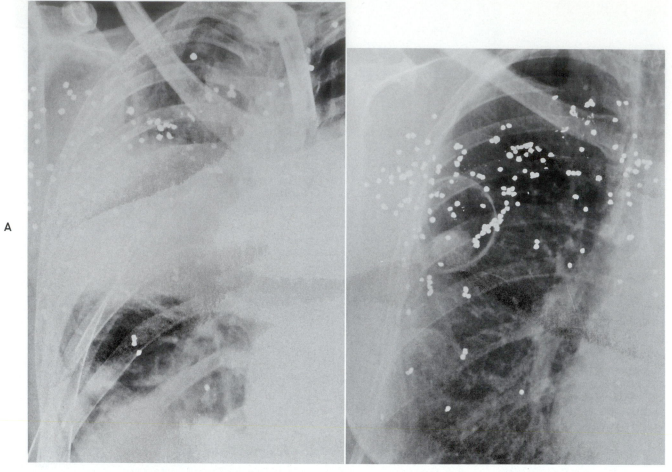

FIGURE 18-11
A, Massive pulmonary contusion following a shotgun wound to chest. Hemothorax had been drained by a chest tube. **B,** Radiograph 5 years later shows that the cavity has persisted following the shotgun wound and now contains a mycetoma.

from their normal position. Alternatively, if previous films are available, an identifiable structure such as a lung nodule may have shifted position in an inexplicable fashion.

TRACHEAL OR BRONCHIAL RUPTURE

Tracheal or bronchial rupture may result from penetrating injuries or intubation.[86] Blunt trauma must be severe to cause airway rupture, and significant damage to other structures such as the thoracic cage, lungs, and aorta is likely. Indeed, tracheobronchial rupture is associated with a 30% overall mortality rate, chiefly from associated injuries.[37] High-speed traffic accidents are the usual cause of tracheal or bronchial rupture. Diagnosis is by no means easy, and a significant proportion of cases go undiagnosed until complications develop either at the site of rupture, such as bronchial stenosis, or in the lung distal to the rupture, such as septic complications or persistent atelectasis (Figure 18-12).[43,52,54] The findings of airway rupture are sometimes subtle and may be overshadowed by the other injuries. Alternatively, more obvious signs of

rupture may be wrongly attributed to damage to other structures.

There are two main radiographic manifestations of tracheal or bronchial rupture: evidence of air leakage at the site of rupture and disturbed ventilation of the lung distal to the rupture. Evidence of air leakage is the more critical, and absence of air leakage makes the diagnosis of a breach in a major airway difficult, if not impossible. The most common finding is a pneumothorax, found in 60% to 100% of cases (Figure 18-13).[48,97] Another indication of an airway leak is the presence of a pneumomediastinum (Figure 18-14).[97,102] The coexistence of a pneumothorax and a pneumomediastinum is the strongest indication of a bronchial rupture. On the other hand, if the outer adventitial sleeve of the bronchus remains intact, no air leak may exist — a situation that occurs in approximately 10% of cases of tracheobronchial fracture.[14] Pneumomediastinum may be the only visible sign of an air leak in ruptures of the trachea or the intramediastinal portions of the bronchi.

The pneumothorax is frequently large and under

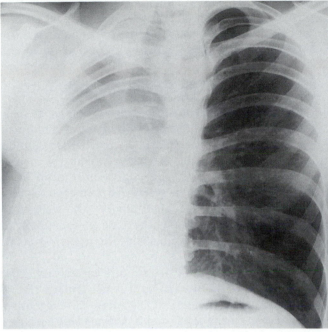

A

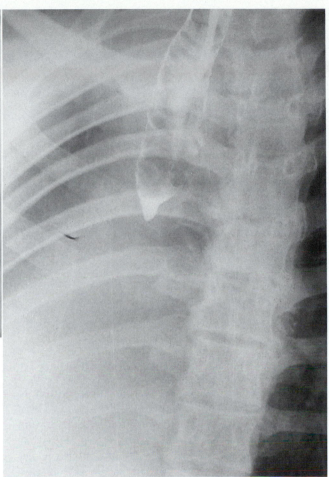

B

FIGURE 18-12
A, Chest radiograph of an 18-year-old man showing the total right lung collapse. **B,** Bronchogram shows total occlusion of the right bronchus thought to result from a major accident when the patient was 9 years of age.

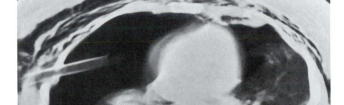

FIGURE 18-13
Computed tomography scan of a patient severely injured in an automobile accident. In spite of a well-placed chest tube, a large pneumothorax and considerable chest wall emphysema develop. Severe air leak is the result of bronchial transection. (Courtesy Dr. Mark Shogry, Greensboro, N.C.)

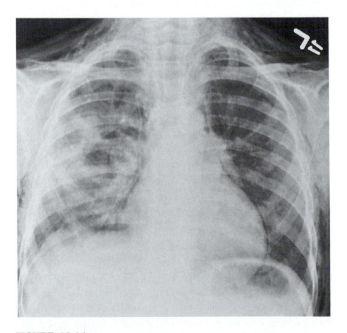

FIGURE 18-14
Radiograph of a young man involved in a motor vehicle accident. Right lung contusion with pneumatocele formation is evident. Pneumomediastinum tracking to the neck indicates tracheobronchial rupture.

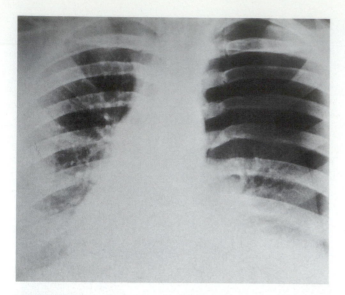

FIGURE 18-15
Complete bronchial transection showing a large left pneumothorax and a sagging left lung. (Courtesy Dr. Nicholas Badin, Petersburg, Va.)

tension; an air leak may be persistent after insertion of pleural tubes. In these circumstances the lung fails to reexpand. One unusual but characteristic feature that may be encountered in patients with bronchial disruption and a large pneumothorax is that bronchial fracture may allow the lung to sag away from the hilum inferiorly and laterally, giving rise to the "fallen lung" sign (Figure 18-15). Normally with a pneumothorax the lung recoils inward toward the hilum. The vascular pedicle remains intact, and the lung remains perfused although underventilated.[73] The consequent ventilation-perfusion mismatch may result in hypoxia and cyanosis.

The presence of a pneumomediastinum is a critical finding in patients with chest trauma. A pneumothorax is not an infrequent accompaniment to rib fractures, and its potential significance may be overlooked. A pneumomediastinum following trauma is a more specific sign of a breach of airway integrity. Air in the mediastinum is seen as streaky lucencies in the carinal region extending superiorly as the air dissects in the tissue planes around the trachea, aorta, and great vessels. On the margins of the mediastinum the air dissects and elevates the mediastinal parietal pleura from the aorta and the heart. On lateral films a pneumomediastinum is best appreciated in the retrosternal space.

The second major effect of a major airway rupture is to disturb the ventilation of the affected lung.[42] Loss of bronchial continuity combined with hemorrhage and edema results in atelectasis. The diagnostic problems in these cases are numerous. In severely traumatized patients, atelectasis may develop for reasons other than bronchial rupture or significant associated pulmonary abnormalities such as lung contusion or aspiration changes may be present. Collapse of a lung is expected in

the presence of a pneumothorax, particularly if the pneumothorax is large and under tension. Atelectasis in bronchial rupture is usually persistent and unresponsive to normal therapeutic endeavors. Bronchial stenosis or occlusion at the site of rupture is a frequent consequence in the untreated case. Septic complications may be encountered in the affected lung.

In a small number of cases the diagnosis of major airway injury has been made by observing an abnormally positioned endotracheal tube or an unusual configuration of the air-filled cuff of the tube. Particularly in cases associated with a traumatic intubation, the tip of the endotracheal tube may be seen to be positioned too far to the right of the tracheal air column.[87] The walls of the trachea ordinarily confine the cuff of the tube. The air-filled cuff may be overdistended to a rounder configuration.[64]

The diagnosis of bronchial rupture depends on awareness of this possibility in cases of severe thoracic trauma. In a significant number of instances the diagnosis is missed in the acute phase and is detected only because of persistent lung or lobar atelectasis. Bronchoscopy should be performed in any case in which the features described previously provide at least some suspicion of an airway rupture.

INJURY TO THE AORTA AND GREAT VESSELS

Deceleration forces can cause marked shearing stresses, particularly in zones where a structure changes from being relatively fixed to being relatively unsupported. Such a zone occurs in the aortic isthmus in the region of attachment of the ligamentum arteriosum. Below this point the descending aorta is tethered by the intercostal arteries, whereas the aortic arch is capable of movement in rapid deceleration. Transection of the aorta at this point is a major cause of death in motor vehicle or aircraft crashes. An alternative mechanism for injuries to the aortic isthmus has been proposed by Crass and Cohen.[15,16] These authors hypothesize that compression of the anterior chest causes the manubrium to arc posteriorly and inferiorly, the axis of rotation being the spinal attachments of the first rib. The aortic isthmus is then "pinched" between the manubrium and the spine.

Ninety-five percent of aortic ruptures encountered clinically occur in the region of the isthmus, and the other 5% occur in the ascending aorta, presumably from posterior shearing of the aortic arch.[53] Approximately 1% of partial ruptures occur in the descending aorta well beyond the isthmus (Figure 18-16).[79] In survivors of aortic injury the degree of damage falls just short of complete transection and immediate exsanguination. In these cases the adventitial layer may just maintain the continuity of the aorta, at least for a time. However, the risk of ultimate rupture is high: more than 50% rupture within the first 24 hours and most of the remainder within the next few weeks. Only 2% survive indefinitely

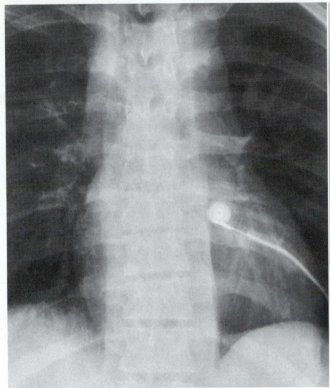
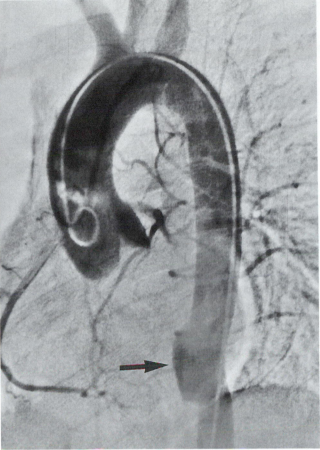

FIGURE 18-16
A, Radiograph showing lower thoracic paravertebral soft tissue thickening in a young victim of an automobile accident. No fracture is seen. B, Aortogram shows aortic disruption immediately above the diaphragm *(arrow).*

with a chronic pseudoaneurysm.[38] Immediate diagnosis is therefore vital, and the chest radiograph is crucial in this regard.

In the great majority of medical centers angiography is used to definitively diagnose damage to the aorta and the great vessels. Few if any surgeons would operate without an angiogram. CT can diagnose the presence of aortic damage,[11,45] but the use of CT as a primary method of investigation in these circumstances is unlikely. Magnetic resonance imaging (MRI) elegantly demonstrates the aorta in multiple planes but is in general poorly suited to the investigation of severely injured patients requiring continuous monitoring. Transesophageal echocardiography is well suited to examining the aortic isthmus region and has the advantage of being rapid and safe when performed by experienced clinicians. Partial ruptures have been observed with transesophageal echocardiography,[12,19,34,92,95] but its role has not yet been fully evaluated. While transesophageal echocardiography shows promise of being of some utility, the same cannot be said of intravascular ultrasound at this time.[106] The method appears to be too invasive and too time consuming to be of value.

The diagnosis of damage to the aorta and the great vessels depends largely on the nature and severity of the trauma and the findings on the chest radiograph. In most cases there are no findings on clinical examination to indicate such damage.[83] The chest radiograph is used to determine the need for angiography. A completely normal chest radiograph has been stated to have a 98% negative predictive value for aortic rupture.[65] Nevertheless, in a review of the literature Woodring[108] noted that over 7% of patients with traumatic rupture of the aorta had an initially normal chest radiograph. On the other hand an abnormal chest radiograph is a poor predictor of aortic rupture. Only 10 % to 20% of angiograms are positive in patients with suspected aortic rupture,[96] and therefore an additional noninvasive screening test would be useful. CT is now readily available and widely employed in patients with head, skeletal, and abdominal trauma; indeed many patients with possible aortic rupture require CT for other injuries. The changes on the plain radiograph in acute aortic rupture are largely the result of mediastinal bleeding. Study of aortograms in cases of aortic rupture does not suggest that aneurysmal dilatation is a significant cause of the plain radiographic changes.[108] Contrast-enhanced CT examinations readily detect periaortic soft tissue thickening with a far greater sensitivity than plain films. Thus a normal CT examination should have a better negative predictive value than a normal chest radiograph.

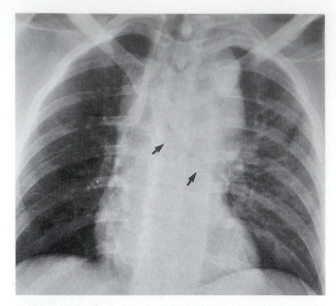

FIGURE 18-17
Traumatic aortic rupture resulting from an automobile accident. Note diffuse mediastinal widening with loss of aortic contours. Left main bronchus is depressed and elongated *(arrows)*. Note the left apical pleural cap and soft tissue thickening in the left paravertebral region.

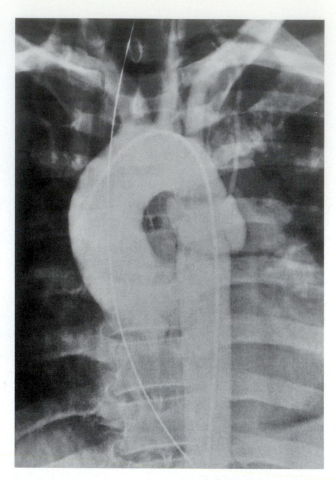

FIGURE 18-18
Aortogram showing a traumatic false aneurysm at the aortic isthmus. Note the wide deviation of the nasogastric tube from the aorta.

In two series comprising a total of over 480 trauma cases examined with CT, no false-negative examinations were noted.[70,81] In the combined series 155 patients had abnormal chest radiographs, and in this group 110 had normal CT scans seemingly obviating the need for aortography. On the other hand, some series have demonstrated the limitations of CT in identifying cases of transected aorta and major aortic branch injuries without CT evidence of mediastinal hemorrhage.[62,63] Experience with CT and chest radiography indicates that CT is more likely to detect mediastinal abnormalities. CT scanning could be used for screening cases with a low-to-moderate risk of aortic rupture, particularly in cases with equivocal chest radiographs or as an adjunct to CT examination of head, spinal, or abdominal injuries.[67,84] A disadvantage of CT is that intravenous contrast media are usually used, increasing the contrast load if recourse to aortography is necessary. However, modern fast scanners give excellent enhancement with lower contrast volumes, and aortography may be performed with digital subtraction techniques, limiting the total dose of contrast media.[68]

Plain film findings have been comprehensively reviewed by Woodring and others and are as follows (Figure 18-17)[109]:

1. Diffuse widening of the mediastinum with obscuring of the aortic contours and obliteration of the aortopulmonary window. These changes result from perivascular hematoma formation. Unfortunately, in many instances the chest radiographs must be obtained in the supine position with a short focus-film distance. Moreover, the patient may be incapable of full inspiration. The problems are compounded if the patient is short, thickset, and obese. In these circumstances a normal mediastinum can easily appear unusually wide. If possible, an upright chest film with a 6-foot film-focus distance should be obtained. Establishing reliable measurement criteria for mediastinal widening is difficult given the variations in patient positioning, body build, and age. Proposed criteria include a mediastinal width exceeding 8 cm just above the aortic knob[56] or a ratio of the width of the mediastinum to the width of the chest exceeding 0.25 at the level of the aortic knob.[90] However, although Gundry and others[39] found mediastinal widening to be the single most reliable sign of traumatic rupture of the aorta, they found basing the evaluation of the mediastinum on absolute figures impractical. Furthermore, rupture of the aorta or the great vessels may be observed with mediastinal measurements less than those quoted previously.[27] Care must be taken not to confuse paraspinal hematomas associated with

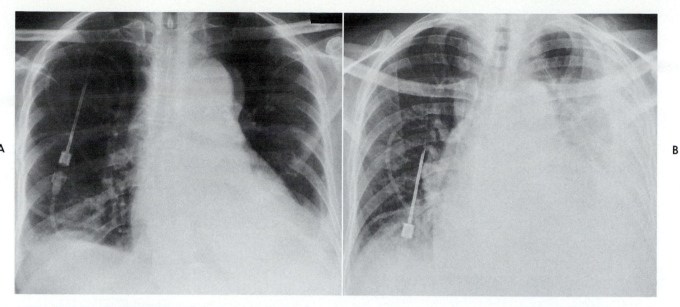

FIGURE 18-19
A, Mediastinal hematoma following thoracic trauma. B, Three hours later, a large hemothorax has developed on the left side.

spine fractures with mediastinal hematomas caused by aortic rupture.[23]

2. Evidence of hematoma displacing normal structures. Hematoma formation around the isthmus of the aorta commonly displaces the left main bronchus downward and the trachea and esophagus to the right. Depression of the left bronchus to below 40 degrees from the horizontal has been stated to be a significant indication of aortic rupture.[55] Tracheal deviation may be more difficult to assess because the trachea normally deviates to the right at the level of the aortic knob, and small degrees of patient rotation can be critical. Deviation of the esophagus as indicated by the position of a nasogastric tube is a good indication of hematoma formation. Normally the esophagus is closely related anatomically to the isthmus and the descending aorta (Figure 18-18).[33,99]

3. Evidence of extension of bleeding into anatomically continuous regions. Extension of bleeding in a posterior direction may cause widening of the paravertebral lines (Figure 18-17).[77] Leakage of blood into a pleural cavity, most often the left pleural cavity, may result in the development of a hemothorax (Figure 18-19). The finding of a hemothorax in an injured patient should immediately raise the possibility of an aortic injury. Hematomas may also track out of the mediastinum over the lung apices, forming apical "caps" (Figure 18-17).[93] These are particularly significant when there are no fractures of the upper ribs to account for extrapleural thickening.

The diagnosis of aortic rupture is so critical that a large number of negative angiographic examinations have to be accepted. Mediastinal hematoma formation may indeed be present even in the absence of angiographic evidence of damage to the aorta or great vessels. In these cases the bleeding is presumably the result of small artery or venous hemorrhage.

INJURY TO THE ESOPHAGUS AND THORACIC DUCT

Rupture of the esophagus by blunt external trauma is rare, comprising only 10% of all cases.[9] Traumatic rupture of the esophagus usually results from a penetrating injury, particularly by instrumentation, or as a complication of dilatation of an esophageal stricture. The radiographic features include pneumomediastinum; pneumothorax or pleural effusion, most commonly on the left side; and evidence of mediastinitis, including abscess formation.

Penetrating injury or surgical damage during thoracic exploration is the usual cause of injury to the thoracic duct (Figure 18-20).[103] Thoracic duct damage from blunt external trauma is rare, with only 20 cases reported in the literature in the years up to 1988.[24] Fluid accumulation is characteristically slow, and several days may pass before significant quantities of fluid accumulate. The anatomic course of the thoracic duct may determine the side on which the fluid accumulates. The duct enters the thorax through the aortic opening in the diaphragm and ascends on the right anterolateral aspect of the spine. In the midthoracic region it trends to the left to ascend on the left anterolateral aspect of the spine. Finally it arches forward to enter the venous system in the region of the left jugular and subclavian vein junction. The definitive diagnosis rests on determining that an effusion is chylous in appropriate clinical circumstances.

Lymphography has been used successfully to determine the site of leakage before surgical intervention.

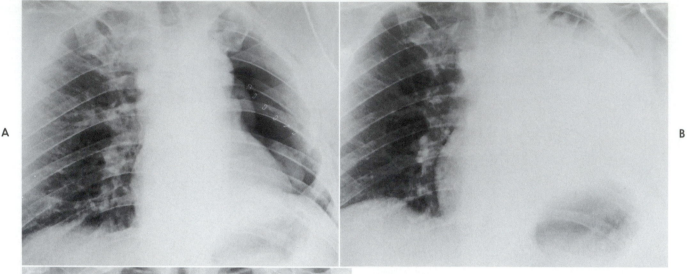

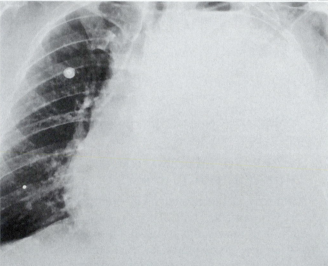

FIGURE 18-20
A, Postoperative film immediately following a pneumonectomy on the left side. B, Three days after surgery. Pleural effusion is collecting on the left side. C, One week after surgery. Left-sided effusion is massive and is displacing the mediastinum to the right. Thoracentesis reveals a chylous effusion.

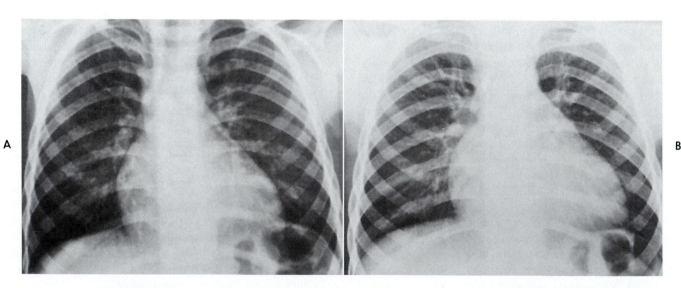

FIGURE 18-21
Chest radiographs of a 3-year-old boy who was run over by a reversing car. A, On admission the chest radiograph was normal in appearance. B, Two weeks later the heart has enlarged. Patient has pulmonary venous congestion.

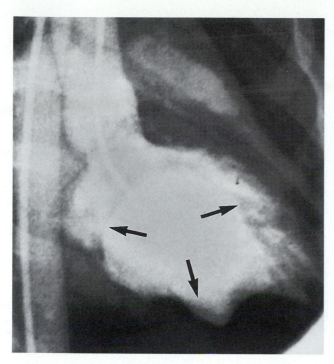

FIGURE 18-22
Frame from a left ventricular cineangiogram performed on the patient in Figure 18-21. Note the left ventricular aneurysm (arrows).

Sachs and others[88] studied 12 patients with chylous ascites or chylothorax following surgery and found abnormal lymphangiograms in seven, which facilitated diagnosis. Of five patients with normal lymphangiograms, four were successfully treated conservatively and one was found at surgery to have a leak from a gastroplasty anastomosis. These authors did not find that CT gave useful additional information.

INJURY TO THE HEART AND PERICARDIUM

The heart and pericardium appear to be well protected from nonpenetrating injury, and clearly documented traumatic lesions are uncommon. Penetrating trauma, on the other hand, is usually the result of a felonious assault, and the mortality is high. The following abnormalities may be encountered following chest trauma:

1. Myocardial contusion or infarction
2. Myocardial laceration leading to hemopericardium and tamponade
3. Septal defects and true and false myocardial aneurysms
4. Coronary artery damage with hemopericardium, false aneurysm formation, and infarction
5. Chordal rupture with valve insufficiency
6. Pneumopericardium
7. Postpericardiectomy syndrome and constrictive pericarditis as possible late sequelae
8. Dislocation of the heart through a pericardial tear (exceedingly rare)[29,49]
9. Bullet embolization

The majority of these conditions have radiologic features that are similar to their nontraumatic equivalents. A graphic example of cardiac injury following nonpenetrating trauma is illustrated in Figures 18-21 and 18-22.

DIAPHRAGMATIC RUPTURE

Acute rupture of the diaphragm results from either a penetrating injury or major abdominal trauma. It may result in herniation of abdominal contents into the chest either in the acute phase or in a delayed fashion. Major herniation can cause severe cardiopulmonary compressive effects. Herniated bowel may also strangulate, sometimes years after the initial injury.[4] Penetrating injuries of the diaphragm are caused by knives or bullets: abdominal injuries requiring laparotomy occur in at least 75% of patients, and diaphragmatic injuries are often detected by direct inspection.[21] Demetriades and others[21] encountered herniation in 15% of a series of 150 cases of penetrating injury of the diaphragm. Fourteen cases were diagnosed during the acute phase, but 10 cases were diagnosed during a subsequent admission. Major abdominal trauma causing diaphragmatic rupture is usually the result of a high-speed motor vehicle accident or a fall from a considerable height. A high incidence of associated injury is reflected in reported mortality rates of up to 25%.[69,86]

Diaphragmatic rupture resulting from abdominal trauma is more common on the left side, presumably because the liver acts as a buffer on the right. Rodriguez-Morales, Rodriguez, and Shatney[86] in an analysis of 60 cases found that 70% of diaphragmatic ruptures occurred on the left. Similarly, Gelman, Mirvis, and Gens[31] encountered rupture of the left diaphragm in 88% of a series of 50 cases. Rupture of the right diaphragm actually may be more common than these series suggest because right diaphragmatic hernias are more likely to be clinically inapparent. Despite the presence of a rupture in the diaphragm, herniation of abdominal contents is by no means invariable, particularly if positive-pressure ventilation is used.[3] Thus a significant number of diaphragmatic ruptures are discovered incidentally during abdominal exploration in the acute phase.[69] In a number of cases the rupture remains undiscovered during the patient's initial hospital stay only to be diagnosed by follow-up chest radiography or when complications of visceral herniation ensue, sometimes months or years later.[4,61] Delayed diagnosis is particularly likely to occur when the rupture is in the right hemidiaphragm.[5,31] In series that have analyzed all cases of diaphragmatic rupture with or without visceral herniation, only 40% to 50% of cases have been identified radiographically before surgical intervention.[3,69,86] Clearly radiographic examination must have been limited in some of these cases because of the need for urgent surgical intervention. In other cases the absence of visceral herniation rendered a radiographic diagnosis impossible. Diagnosis of diaphragmatic rupture has many pitfalls, particularly in cases in which addi-

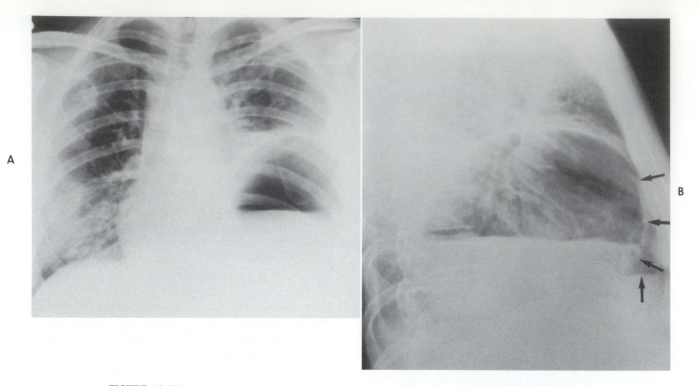

FIGURE 18-23
A, Posteroanterior and, B, lateral radiograph of a posttraumatic diaphragmatic hernia. Margin of stomach wall simulates the curve of the diaphragm. However, the anterior margin of the stomach curves down to the actual level of the diaphragm *(arrows)*.

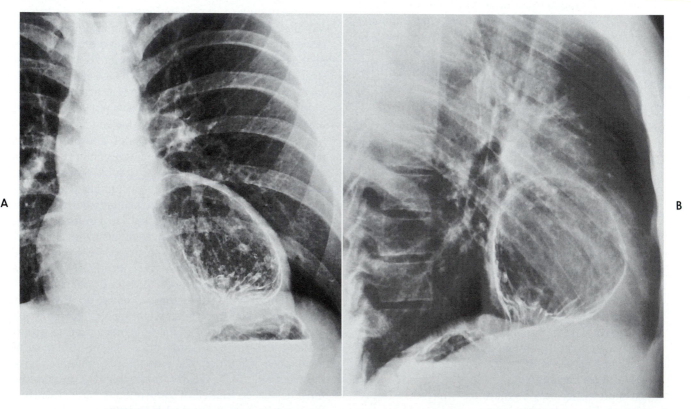

FIGURE 18-24
Chest radiographs taken after a barium study demonstrate a diaphragmatic hernia. Herniation is believed to result from an episode of trauma that occurred months previously.

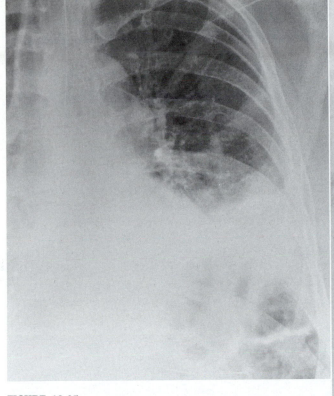

A

B

FIGURE 18-25
A, Radiograph of a young male patient soon after a stab wound to the left side of chest. Diaphragm is obscured by pleural fluid and consolidated or collapsed lung. Gas-filled bowel loops may be under an elevated diaphragm. **B,** At 2-month follow-up examination a knuckle of colon is seen to be herniating through a lateral diaphragmatic defect.

tional major injury makes the radiographic examination more difficult and extended.

The diagnosis of diaphragmatic rupture can be made or suspected only with demonstrable herniation of visceral contents through the rent in the diaphragm or evidence of transit of fluid or air between the abdominal and pleural cavities. Herniation of hollow viscera may be readily recognized by the characteristic gas pattern of the herniated stomach and bowel (Figure 18-23). Continuity of these loops of bowel with infradiaphragmatic bowel may be apparent, possibly with some constriction or gathering of loops at the site of the rupture. The normal diaphragmatic contours are obscured, although problems may arise if the herniated stomach forms an arclike contour simulating a paralyzed or eventrated diaphragm (Figure 18-23). The passage of a nasogastric tube may be helpful with herniations of the stomach into the left chest; the nasogastric tube either is held up at the esophageal hiatus or turns upward beyond the hiatus into the left chest. Contrast studies of the gastrointestinal tract are rarely necessary or even appropriate in the acute phase following the trauma. Barium studies of the stomach or the colon may be useful for patients presenting in a delayed

fashion (Figure 18-24). Herniation of solid viscera or omentum results in diagnostic problems and accounts in large part for the difficulties in diagnosing rupture of the right hemidiaphragm.[94] If only a small knuckle of bowel herniates, it may be obscured by pleural fluid and contused or collapsed lung (Figure 18-25). Diaphragmatic herniation may be simulated by posttraumatic diaphragmatic paralysis or by posttraumatic pneumatoceles. Abnormal communication between the abdominal or pleural cavities can only be inferred from the seemingly inappropriate passage of air or fluid across this barrier. For example, peritoneal lavage fluid may be detected in the pleural cavity at a subsequent CT examination, or an inexplicable association of a pneumothorax with a pneumoperitoneum may be seen.

Several other imaging procedures may help in the diagnosis of diaphragmatic rupture. CT performed for general abdominal or chest trauma may strongly suggest a localized herniation of bowel or omentum through the diaphragm.[22,44,101] However, CT simply indicates focal visceral herniation and usually cannot identify the actual defect in the diaphragm in the absence of herniation (Figure 18-26).[2] CT has, on occasion, identified disrup-

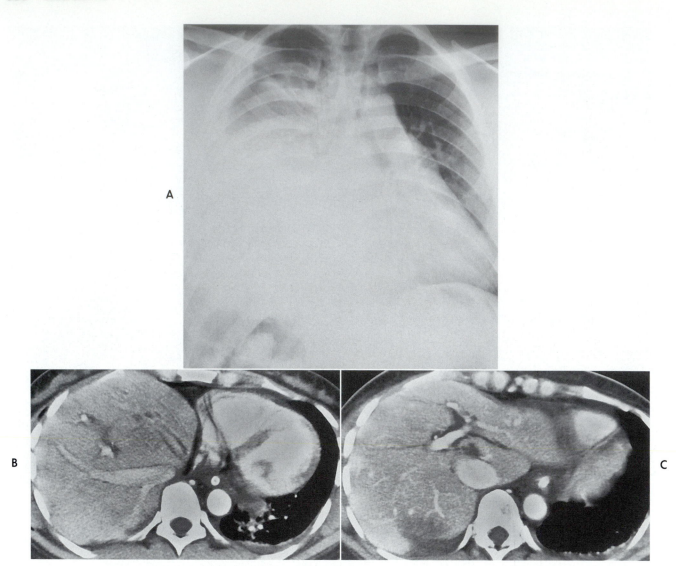

FIGURE 18-26

A, Chest radiograph of a victim of an automobile accident. Right side of diaphragm is elevated (gas in the bowel marks the approximate position of the lower liver edge). Heart is displaced to left. **B,** Computed tomography (CT) scan at midthoracic level. Note engorgement of hepatic veins and perivascular edema in liver. **C,** CT scan at xiphoid level. Note dilatation of inferior vena cava and defect in diaphragm and liver posteriorly. At surgery, liver was herniating through a large sagittal tear in diaphragm.

tion of the diaphragm in the absence of herniation, but only portions of the diaphragm can be sufficiently delineated to allow such a diagnosis to be made.[46]

MRI has been used to diagnose diaphragmatic rupture with some success, but only in a few cases (Figure 18-27).[31,66] MRI is capable of imaging in multiple planes with excellent tissue discrimination and would probably be used more were it not for the difficulty of monitoring patients during the examination.

Real-time ultrasound may also succeed in identifying visceral herniation.[94] The diaphragm is a readily identifiable structure on real-time ultrasound studies; bowel is also identifiable by its peristaltic movement. The difficulty with ultrasound, however, is in obtaining an adequate

window into the chest, particularly on the left side.

Diagnostic pneumoperitoneography has been used in the past to demonstrate communication between the abdomen and the chest but has fallen out of favor because of a high incidence of false-negative results.[76] Similarly, radionuclide peritoneography with technetium-99m-labeled macroaggregated albumin can be used,[40,80] but its value has yet to be determined. Isotope liver and spleen scanning can be used to diagnose herniation of the liver into the right side of the chest.[5] Herniation is distinguished from upward displacement of the liver associated with an elevated right hemidiaphragm by a variable degree of liver constriction at the site of the rent in the diaphragm.

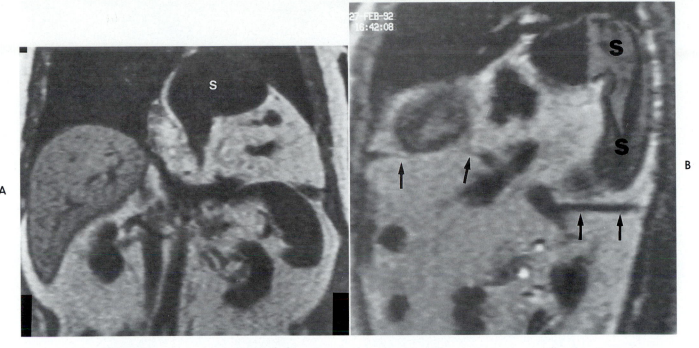

FIGURE 18-27
A, Coronal and, B, sagittal magnetic resonance images of a patient with traumatic rupture of left side of diaphragm. Stomach *(S)* has herniated into the chest together with some small bowel loops. Diaphragm is indicated *(arrows)*.

INDIRECT EFFECTS OF TRAUMA ON THE LUNGS

Severe trauma can have indirect effects on the lungs that may severely complicate the clinical and radiographic diagnosis. Three main processes require consideration: fat embolism, adult respiratory distress syndrome, and neurogenic pulmonary edema. Only fat embolism is described here; the other two conditions are discussed in Chapter 9.

Fat embolism

Skeletal trauma, particularly trauma involving the pelvis and the major long bones, may cause neutral fat droplets to enter the bloodstream. These fat droplets are 20 to 40 μm in diameter and cause occlusions in the vascular bed of the lungs and other organs. Autopsy and special clinical studies indicate that subclinical fat embolization is much more common than is generally realized.[13,59,74] The term "fat embolism syndrome" is often reserved for cases that have overt clinical findings attributable to the effects of fat embolization on the lungs and other organs such as the brain, kidneys, and skin. Fat embolization may be detected by examination of the blood and urine in as many as 90% of cases following major trauma, whereas the incidence of fat embolism syndrome in this patient group is approximately 3%.[25]

In the mechanical theory of fat embolization, fat is disrupted in the soft tissues and the bone marrow. The liberated fat enters the lacerated ends of veins in the traumatized area, possibly aided by a rise in the intramedullary pressure in bone or by movement of bony fragments. Fat embolization is stated to be less common in compound or open fractures in which a rise in intramedullary pressure is less likely. Rapid immobilization of fractures, particularly early operative fixation, decreases the incidence of fat embolization.[85]

Trauma is the major cause of fat embolism syndrome. However, fat embolization may occur in the absence of trauma in a diverse series of conditions, including diabetes mellitus, acute decompression sickness, chronic pancreatitis, alcoholism, burns, severe infections, sickle cell disease, inhalational anesthesia, and renal infarction.[7] A biochemical theory of fat embolization proposed to account for these nontraumatic cases states that the embolic fat is derived from circulating blood lipids and from fat mobilized from fat depots. Neutral fat in the blood is normally emulsified in the form of chylomicrons, which are less than 1 μm in diameter. During the metabolic response to stress, chylomicrons may coalesce to form fat globules of up to 40 μm in diameter, and these globules are capable of causing capillary occlusion.

However, the deleterious effects of fat embolization are not simply the result of vascular occlusion by neutral fat.[1,7] Hydrolysis of neutral fat by tissue lipase forms free fatty acids that have a toxic effect on the vascular endothelium and lung parenchyma. The result is endothelial damage leading to increased capillary permeability and damage to the alveolar lining cells, and thus to loss of

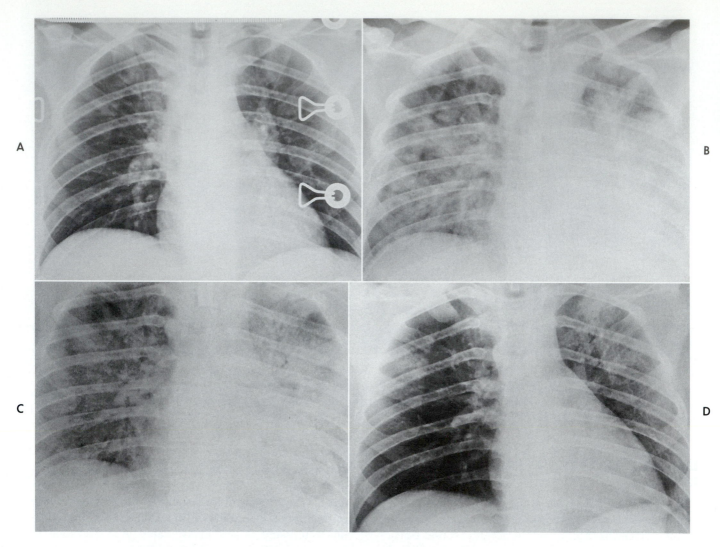

FIGURE 18-28
A, Admission radiograph on a young male with severe pelvic and lower extremity fractures. B, Seventy-two hours later, the patient had severe respiratory distress with clinical evidence of fat embolism syndrome. C, At 96 hours. D, Eleven days after admission the pulmonary changes have largely regressed.

surfactant activity and the formation of hyaline membranes. Furthermore, platelets adhere to neutral fat and intravascular coagulation may supervene. Excessive breakdown of platelets releases vasoactive amines such as serotonin and 5-hydroxytryptamine that, together with histamine released from damaged lung parenchyma and vasoactive amines released from the injury site, cause vasospasm and pulmonary capillary congestion. The biochemical and hematologic interactions therefore are complex but are almost certainly crucial to the development of the fat embolism syndrome. In rare cases acute cor pulmonale occurs within hours of an injury, attributable to a major degree of occlusion of the pulmonary vascular bed by neutral fat.[58] A latent period of 12 to 48 hours before fat embolism syndrome supervenes is almost invariable. This latent period can be readily explained by

the time required to hydrolyze neutral fat and for the secondary vasculitis and pneumonitis to develop.

The chief clinical manifestations of fat embolism syndrome involve the lungs, central nervous system, and skin. The pulmonary manifestations are generally the first to appear: within 72 hours of the trauma, dyspnea, tachypnea, and cyanosis develop. The arterial oxygen tension decreases to 50 mm Hg or less. At the same time generalized cerebral symptoms may develop, ranging from headache and irritability to delirium, stupor, seizures, and coma. Focal neurologic signs are generally absent. Funduscopic examination may reveal petechial hemorrhages. A petechial rash appears in many, but not all, cases after 2 to 3 days. The rash is distributed over the neck and trunk.

A chest radiograph broadly reflects the severity of the

syndrome; it may remain normal in mild cases of the fat embolization syndrome. Otherwise, radiographic abnormalities develop after a 12- to 72-hour latent period. The classic response is the development of either multiple focal alveolar densities or a diffuse interstitial or alveolar pulmonary edema pattern. Pleural effusions are not a feature of fat embolization syndrome. On occasion the degree of shadowing becomes remarkably severe, yet clearing generally occurs in 7 to 14 days (Figure 18-28). On the other hand, adult respiratory distress syndrome (ARDS) may develop with prolongation of the clinical course and a significantly increased mortality. Curtis and others[17] in a study of 30 patients with fat embolization syndrome identified 10 patients with complicating ARDS. Six of these patients died, as compared with two of 18 patients with fat embolization syndrome in an uncomplicated form. Two other patients in the series died of the effects of acute paradoxic fat embolization. All 10 patients with complicating ARDS had evidence of intravascular coagulopathy, a feature not detected in the other patients. The radiographic features of ARDS are discussed further on pp. 411 to 414.

The development of hypoxia, particularly in a patient with a normal chest radiograph, may indicate ventilation-perfusion scintigraphy. Ventilation is normal in fat embolism syndrome, but a perfusion scan may show multiple peripheral subsegmental defects that give the scan a diffusely mottled appearance.[75,105] This is quite unlike the larger and more focal defects commonly associated with multiple thromboembolism.

The diagnosis of fat embolism syndrome is based on the correlation of the clinical features, the chest radiographic appearances, and the laboratory findings, especially the results of blood gas analysis. The radiographic findings are not specific and may be found in other conditions in which trauma plays a part, including pulmonary contusion, massive aspiration of gastric contents, thermal damage, toxic gas inhalation, transfusion reactions, neurogenic and other causes of pulmonary edema, and gram-negative sepsis. The latent period before the radiographic and clinical findings of fat embolism syndrome develop has great diagnostic importance. In many of the conditions mentioned previously the chest radiograph is abnormal from the outset. ARDS may supervene in any severely traumatized individual, and fat embolization as a precipitating cause may go unrecognized.

REFERENCES

1. Alho A: Fat embolism syndrome: etiology, pathogenesis and treatment, *Acta Chir Scand Suppl* 499:75-85, 1980.
2. Ammann A, Brewer W, Maull K, et al: Traumatic rupture of the diaphragm: real time sonographic diagnosis, *AJR* 140:915-916, 1983.
3. Arendrup HC, Skov Jensen B: Traumatic rupture of the diaphragm, *Surg Gynecol Obstet* 154:526-530, 1982.
4. Aronchick JM, Epstein DM, Gefter WB, et al: Chronic traumatic diaphragmatic hernia: the significance of pleural effusion, *Radiology* 168:675-678, 1988.
5. Ball T, McCrory R, Smith JO, et al: Traumatic diaphragmatic hernia: errors in diagnosis, *AJR* 138:633-637, 1982.
6. Barcia TC, Livoni JP: Indications for angiography in blunt thoracic trauma, *Radiology* 147:15-19, 1983.
7. Batra P: The fat embolism syndrome, *J Thorac Imag* 2(3):12-17, 1987.
8. Ben-Menachem Y: Avulsion of the innominate artery associated with fracture of the sternum, *AJR* 150:621-622, 1988.
9. Bladergroen MR, Lowe JE, Postlethwait RW: Diagnosis and management of esophageal perforation and rupture, *Ann Thorac Surg* 42:235-239, 1986.
10. Brooks S, Cmolik B, Young J, et al: Transesophageal echocardiographic examination of a patient with traumatic aortic transection from blunt chest trauma: a case report, *J Trauma* 31:841-845, 1991.
11. Brooks AP, Olson LK: Computed tomography of the chest in the trauma patient, *Clin Radiol* 40:127-132, 1989.
12. Brooks AP, Olson LK, Shackford SR: Computed tomography in the diagnosis of traumatic rupture of the thoracic aorta, *Clin Radiol* 40:133-138, 1989.
13. Chan KM, Tham KT, ChuI HS, et al: Post traumatic fat embolism — its clinical and subclinical presentations, *J Trauma* 24:45-49, 1984.
14. Chesterman JT, Satsangi PN: Rupture of the trachea and bronchi by closed injury, *Thorax* 21:21-27, 1966.
15. Cohen AM, Crass JR, Thomas HA, et al: CT evidence for the "osseous pinch" mechanism of traumatic aortic injury, *AJR* 159:271-274, 1992.
16. Crass JR, Cohen AM, Motta AO, et al: A proposed new mechanism of traumatic aortic rupture: the osseous pinch, *Radiology* 176:645-649, 1990.
17. Curtis AMcB, Knowles GD, Putman CE, et al: The three syndromes of fat embolism: pulmonary manifestations, *Yale J Biol Med* 52:149-157, 1979.
18. Danher J, Eyes BE, Kumar K: Oblique rib views after blunt chest trauma: an unnecessary routine? *Br Med J* 289:1271, 1984.
19. Davis GA, Sauerisen S, Chandrasekaran K, et al: Subclinical traumatic aortic injury diagnosed by transesophageal echocardiography, *Am Heart J* 123:534-536, 1992.
20. Deluca SA, Rhea JT, O'Malley TO: Radiographic evaluation of rib fractures, *AJR* 138:91-92, 1982.
21. Demetriades D, Kakoyiannis S, Parekh D, et al: Penetrating injuries of the diaphragm, *Br J Surg* 75:824-826, 1988.
22. Demos TC, Solomon C, Posniak HV, et al: Computed tomography in traumatic defects of the diaphragm, *Clin Imag* 13:62-67, 1989.
23. Dennis LN, Rogers LF: Superior mediastinal widening from spine fractures mimicking aortic rupture on chest radiographs, *AJR* 152:27-30, 1989.
24. Dulchavsky SA, Ledgerwood AM, Lucas CE: Management of chylothorax after blunt chest trauma. *J Trauma* 28:1400-1401, 1988.
25. Feldman F, Ellis K, Gren WM: The fat embolism syndrome, *Radiology* 114:535-542, 1975.
26. Felson B: Lung torsion: radiographic findings in nine cases, *Radiology* 162:631-638, 1987.
27. Fisher RG, Hadlock F, Ben-Menachem Y: Laceration of the thoracic aorta and brachiocephalic arteries by blunt trauma: report of 54 cases and review of the literature, *Radiol Clin North Am* 19:91-110, 1981.
28. Fisher RG, Ward RE, Ben-Menachem Y, et al: Arteriography and the fractured first rib: too much for too little? *AJR* 138:1059-1062, 1982.
29. Fulda G, Brathwaite CEM, Rodriquez A, et al: Blunt traumatic rupture of the heart and pericardium: a ten-year experience (1979-1989), *J Trauma* 31:167-173, 1991.
30. Gazak S, Davidson SJ: Posterior sternoclavicular dislocations: two case reports, *J Trauma* 24:80-82, 1984.

31. Gelman R, Mirvis SE, Gens D: Diaphragmatic rupture due to blunt trauma: sensitivity of plain chest radiographs, *AJR* 156:51-57, 1991.

32. George PY, Goodman P: Radiographic appearance of bullet tracks in the lung, *AJR* 159:967-970, 1992.

33. Gerlock AJ, Muhletaler CA, Coulam CM, et al: Traumatic aortic aneurysm: validity of esophageal tube displacement sign, *AJR* 135:713-718, 1980.

34. Goarin JP, LeBret F, Riou B, et al: Early diagnosis of traumatic thoracic rupture by transesophageal echocardiography, *Chest* 103:618-619, 1993.

35. Gordon R: The deep sulcus sign, *Radiology* 136:25-27, 1980.

36. Graham RJ, Heyd RL, Raval VA, et al: Lung torsion after percutaneous needle biopsy of lung, *AJR* 159:35-37, 1992.

37. Guest JL, Anderson JN: Major airway injury in closed chest trauma, *Chest* 72:63-66, 1977.

38. Gundry SR, Burney RE, MacKenzie JR: Traumatic pseudoaneurysms of the thoracic aorta, *Arch Surg* 119:1055-1060, 1984.

39. Gundry SR, Williams S, Burney RE, et al: Indications for aortography: radiography after blunt chest trauma; a reassessment of the radiographic findings associated with traumatic rupture of the aorta, *Invest Radiol* 18:230-237, 1983.

40. Haldorsson A, Esser MJ, Rappaport W, et al: A new method of diagnosing diaphragmatic injury using intraperitoneal technetium: case report, *J Trauma* 33:140-142, 1992.

41. Harley DP, Mena I: Cardiac and vascular sequelae of sternal fractures, *J Trauma* 26:553-555, 1986.

42. Hartley C, Morritt GN: Bronchial rupture secondary to blunt chest trauma, *Thorax* 48:183-184, 1993.

43. Harvey-Smith W, Bush W, Northrop C: Traumatic bronchial rupture, *AJR* 134:1189-1193, 1980.

44. Heiberg E, Wolverson MK, Hard RN, et al: CT recognition of traumatic rupture of the diaphragm, *AJR* 125:369-372, 1980.

45. Heiberg E, Wolverson MK, Sundaram M, et al: CT in aortic trauma, *AJR* 140:1119-1124, 1983.

46. Holland DG, Quint LE: Traumatic rupture of the diaphragm without visceral herniation: CT diagnosis, *AJR* 157:17-18, 1991.

47. Hollerman JJ, Fackler ML, Coldwell DM, et al: Gunshot wounds: bullets, ballistics and mechanisms of injury, *AJR* 155:685-690, 1990.

48. Hood RM, Sloan HE: Injuries of the trachea and major bronchi, *J Thorac Cardiovasc Surg* 38:458-480, 1959.

49. Kermond AJ: The dislocated heart: an unusual complication of major chest injury, *Radiology* 119:59-60, 1976.

50. Kleinman PK: Bony thoracic trauma. In Kleinman PK, editor: *Diagnostic imaging of child abuse,* Baltimore, 1987, Williams & Wilkins.

51. Lindsell DRM, Wilson AG, Maxwell JD: Fractures on the chest radiograph in detection of alcoholic liver disease. *Br Med J* 285:597-599, 1982.

52. Lotz PR, Martel W, Rohwedder JL, et al: Significance of pneumomediastinum in blunt trauma to the thorax, *AJR* 132:817-819, 1979.

53. Lundell CJ, Quinn M, Rinck E: Traumatic laceration of the ascending aorta: angiographic assessment, *AJR* 145:715-719, 1985.

54. Mahboubi S, O'Hara AE: Bronchial rupture in children following blunt chest trauma, *Pediatr Radiol* 10:133-138, 1981.

55. Marnocha KE, Maglinte DDT: Plain-film criteria for excluding aortic rupture in blunt chest trauma, *AJR* 144:19-21, 1985.

56. Marsh DG, Sturm JT: Traumatic aortic rupture: roentgenographic indications for angiography, *Ann Thorac Surg* 21:337-340, 1976.

57. Martin N, Bollaert PE, Bauer P, et al: Two case reports of pulmonary blast injury, *Cah Anesthiol* 35(2):133-137, 1987.

58. Mayron R, Ruiz E, Meslitz ST, et al: Tissue-fat pulmonary embolism occurring in a patient with a severe pelvic fracture, *J Emerg Med* 2:251-256, 1985.

59. McCarthy B, Mammen E, Leblanc LP, et al: Subclinical fat embolism: a prospective study of 50 patients with extremity fractures, *J Trauma* 13:9-16, 1973.

60. McGonigal MD, Schwab CW, Kauder DR, et al: Supplemented emergent chest computed tomography in the management of blunt torso trauma, *J Trauma* 30:1431-1435, 1990.

61. McHugh K, Ogilvie BC, Brunton FJ: Delayed presentation of traumatic diaphragmatic hernia, *Clin Radiol* 43:246-250, 1991.

62. McLean T, Olinger G, Thorsen M. Computed tomography in the evaluation of the aorta in patients sustaining blunt chest trauma, *J Trauma* 31:254-256, 1991.

63. Miller FB, Richardson JD, Thomas HA, et al: Role of CT in diagnosis of major arterial injury after blunt thoracic trauma, *Surgery* 106:596-603, 1989.

64. Millham FH, Raji-Khorasani A, Birkett DF, et al: Carinal injury: diagnosis and treatment — case report, *J Trauma* 31:1420-1422, 1991.

65. Mirvis S, Bidwell J, Buddemeyer E, et al: Value of chest radiography in excluding traumatic aortic rupture, *Radiology* 163:487-493, 1987.

66. Mirvis S, Keramati B, Buchman R, et al: MR imaging of traumatic diaphragmatic rupture, *J Comput Assist Tomogr* 12:147-149, 1988.

67. Mirvis SE, Kostrubiak I, Whitley NO, et al: Role of CT in excluding major arterial injury after blunt thoracic trauma, *AJR* 149:601-605, 1987.

68. Mirvis SE, Pais SO, Gens DR: Thoracic aortic rupture: advantages of intra-arterial digital subtraction angiography, *AJR* 146:987-991, 1986.

69. Morgan AS, Flanchbaum L, Esposito T, et al: Blunt trauma to the diaphragm: an analysis of 44 patients, *J Trauma* 26:565-567, 1986.

70. Morgan PW, Goodman LR, Aprahamian C, et al: Evaluation of traumatic aortic injury: does dynamic contrast-enhanced CT play a role? *Radiology* 182:661-666, 1992.

71. Moser ES, Proto AV: Lung torsion: case report and literature review, *Radiology* 162:639-642, 1987.

72. Munk PL, Vellet AD, Zwirewich C: Torsion of the upper lobe of the lung after surgery: findings on pulmonary angiography, *AJR* 157:471-472, 1991.

73. Oh KS, Fleischner FG, Wyman SM: Characteristic pulmonary finding in traumatic complete transection of a main stem bronchus, *Radiology* 92:371-372, 1969.

74. Palmovic V, McCarroll JR: Fat embolism in trauma, *Arch Pathol* 80:630-635, 1965.

75. Park HM, Ducret RP, Brindley DC: Pulmonary imaging in fat embolism syndrome, *Clin Nucl Med* 11:521-522, 1986.

76. Payne J, Yellin A: Traumatic diaphragmatic hernia, *Arch Surg* 117:18-24, 1982.

77. Peters DR, Gamsu G: Displacement of the right paraspinous interface: a radiographic sign of acute traumatic rupture of the thoracic aorta, *Radiology* 134:599-603, 1980.

78. Poole GU: Fracture of the upper ribs and injury to the great vessels, *Surg Gynecol Obstet* 169:275-282, 1989.

79. Rabinsky I, Sidhu GS, Wagner RB: Mid-descending aortic traumatic aneurysms, *Ann Thorac Surg* 50:155-160, 1990.

80. Ramirez JS, Moreno AJ, Otero C, et al: Detection of diaphragmatic disruptions by peritoneoscintigraphy using technetium-99m diethylene-triamine pentacetic acid, *J Trauma* 28:818-882, 1988.

81. Raptopoulos V, Sherman RG, Phillips DA, et al: Traumatic aortic tear: screening with chest CT, *Radiology* 182:667-673, 1992.

82. Resnick D: Disorders of other endocrine glands and of pregnancy. In Resnick D, Niwayama G, eds: *Diagnosis of bone and joint disorders,* ed 2, Philadelphia, 1988, WB Saunders.

83. Rich NM, Spencer FC: *Vascular trauma,* Philadelphia, 1978, WB Saunders.

84. Richardson P, Mirvis SE, Scorpio R, et al: Value of CT in determining the need for angiography when the findings of mediastinal hemorrhage on chest radiographs are equivocal, *AJR* 156:273-279, 1991.

85. Riska EB, Myllynen P: Fat embolism in patients with multiple injuries, *J Trauma* 22:891-894, 1982.

86. Rodriguez-Morales G, Rodriguez A, Shatney CH: Acute rupture of the diaphragm in blunt trauma: analysis of 60 patients, *J Trauma* 26:438-444, 1986.

87. Rollins RJ, Tocino I: Early radiographic signs of tracheal rupture, *AJR* 148:695-698, 1987.

88. Sachs PB, Zelch MG, Rice TW, et al: Diagnosis and localization of laceration of the thoracic duct: usefulness of lymphangiography and CT, *AJR* 157:703-705, 1991.

89. Schild HH, Strunk H, Weber W, et al: Pulmonary contusion: CT vs plain radiograms, *J Comput Assist Tomogr* 13:417-420, 1989.

90. Seltzer SE, D'Orsi C, Kirshner R, et al: Traumatic aortic rupture: plain radiographic findings, *AJR* 137:1011-1014, 1981.

91. Shafer N, Wilkenfeld M, Shafer R: Gunshot wounds. In Wecht C, ed: *Legal medicine*, Philadelphia, 1982, WB Saunders.

92. Shapiro M, Yanofsky S, Trapp J: Cardiovascular evaluation in blunt thoracic trauma using transesophageal echocardiography (TEE), *J Trauma* 31:835-840, 1991.

93. Simeone JF, Deren MM, Cagle F: The value of the left apical cap in the diagnosis of aortic rupture, *Radiology* 139:35-37, 1981.

94. Somers JM, Gleeson FV, Flower CDR: Rupture of the right hemidiaphragm following blunt trauma: the use of ultrasound in diagnosis, *Clin Radiol* 42:97-101, 1990.

95. Sparks MB, Burchard KW, Marrin CA, et al: Transesophageal echocardiography: preliminary results in patients with traumatic thoracic rupture, *Arch Surg* 126:711-714, 1991.

96. Sturm JT, Hankins DG, Young G: Thoracic aortography following blunt chest trauma, *Am J Emerg Med* 8:92-96, 1990.

97. Taskinen SO, Salo JA, Halttumen PEA, et al: Tracheobronchial rupture due to blunt chest trauma: a follow-up study, *Ann Thorac Surg* 48:846-849, 1989.

98. Thompson BM, Finger W, Tonsfeldt D, et al: Rib radiographs for trauma: useful or wasteful? *Ann Emerg Med* 15:261-265, 1986.

99. Tisnado J, Tsai FY, Alo A, Roach JF: A new radiographic sign of acute traumatic rupture of the thoracic aorta: displacement of the nasogastric tube to the right, *Radiology* 125:603-608, 1977.

100. Tocino IM, Miller MH, Frederick PR, et al: CT detection of occult pneumothorax in head trauma, *AJR* 143:987-990, 1984.

101. Toombs BD, Sandler CM, Lester RG: Computed tomography of chest trauma, *Radiology* 140:733-738, 1981.

102. Unger JM, Schuchmann GG, Grossman JE, et al: Tears of the trachea and main bronchi caused by blunt trauma: radiologic findings, *AJR* 153:1175-1180, 1989.

103. Vallieres E, Shamji FM, Todd TR: Post pneumonectomy chylothorax, *Ann Thorac Surg* 55:1006-1008, 1993.

104. Wall SD, Federle MP, Jeffrey RB, et al: CT diagnosis of unsuspected pneumothorax after blunt abdominal trauma, *AJR* 141:919-921, 1983.

105. Williams AG, Mettler FA, Christie JH, et al: Fat embolism syndrome, *Clin Nucl Med* 7:495-497, 1986.

106. Williams DM, Simon HJ, Marx MV, et al: Acute traumatic aortic rupture: intravascular US findings, *Radiology* 182:247-249, 1992.

107. Williams JR, Stembridge VA: Pulmonary contusion secondary to nonpenetrating chest trauma, *AJR* 91:284-290, 1964.

108. Woodring JH: The normal mediastinum in blunt traumatic rupture of the thoracic aorta and bronchiocephalic arteries, *J Emerg Med* 8:467-476, 1990.

109. Woodring JH, Dillon ML: Radiographic manifestations of mediastinal hemorrhage from blunt chest trauma, *Ann Thorac Surg* 37:171-178, 1984.

110. Woodring JH, Fried AM, Hatfield DR, et al: Fractures of first and second ribs: predictive value for arterial and bronchial injury, *AJR* 138:211-215, 1982.

111. Woodring JH, Lee C, Jenkins K: Spinal fractures in blunt chest, *J Trauma* 28:789-793, 1988.

19 Interventional Techniques

DAVID M. HANSELL

Virtually all of the imaging-guided interventional techniques used in other parts of the body have been adapted for diagnostic and therapeutic purposes in the chest. Many of these procedures have come to be recognized as the diagnostic method or treatment of choice in difficult thoracic problems. Each of these interventional procedures is discussed in terms of indications, technique, complications, and efficacy compared with other techniques.

PERCUTANEOUS NEEDLE BIOPSY OF THE LUNG

Several techniques are available for obtaining a sample of lung tissue for histologic, cytologic, or bacteriologic examination. The most common methods include an open lung or thoracoscopic biopsy (both of which require a general anesthetic), a transbronchial bronchoscopic biopsy, and a percutaneous needle biopsy. Selecting the most appropriate technique depends on the site, size, and likely nature of the pulmonary lesion. Percutaneous needle biopsy is not new. In 1883 Leyden made a diagnosis of pneumonia by needle aspiration,[78] and 3 years later Menetier used it to diagnose lung cancer.[25] The technique did not gain widespread acceptance for many years because use of relatively large-bore needles (3 mm diameter or more) carried a significant complication rate, particularly hemorrhage and pneumothorax.[56] A further handicap was the lack of any means of guidance for the precise placement of the needle. It was not until the 1960s that percutaneous needle biopsy became more widely performed, with the development of fine-bore aspiration needles, improved cytologic diagnosis, and the widespread availability of image intensification.[72] The indications and limitations of the technique are now widely recognized.[4,116,171,181]

Indications

The frequency with which percutaneous needle biopsy of lung lesions is performed in any institution is governed by local circumstances, particularly the availability of thoracic surgery and cytopathologic examination. Whether another biopsy technique is more appropriate for a given patient should always be considered.

Percutaneous needle biopsy is usually performed to confirm a suspected pulmonary malignancy (primary or secondary),[82] to prove the benign nature of a pulmonary lesion, to obtain microorganisms from an area of consolidation or lung abscess,[21,135] or to diagnose a mediastinal mass.[53]

The value of percutaneous needle biopsy is unquestioned in patients with a suspected pulmonary malignancy who are inoperable on the basis of metastatic disease, an invasive tumor, poor lung function, or general debility. Apart from confirming the clinical diagnosis, management decisions will be based on the histologic type of tumor. The utility of percutaneous needle biopsy is less clear cut in patients with suspected lung cancer who are otherwise operable.[11] A certain benign diagnosis (that would obviate the need for surgery) is infrequently made from a percutaneous needle biopsy, and when malignancy is not definitively confirmed by needle biopsy, a subsequent thoracotomy may be necessary to establish the diagnosis. Such patients' management is not influenced by percutaneous needle biopsy.[16]

Contraindications

Although there are no absolute contraindications to percutaneous needle biopsy, a number of factors significantly increase the risk of complications. The most important relative contraindications are an uncooperative patient, severe chronic obstructive pulmonary disease, pulmonary arterial hypertension, a contralateral pneumonectomy, and a significant coagulopathy.

The need for a considered decision in undertaking a percutaneous needle biopsy in a high-risk patient is paramount. Full discussion with the referring physician about the risks to the patient and the likelihood of success and a readiness to deal with acute complications that may be catastrophic in such a patient are obviously necessary.[22] The type of needle (aspiration versus cutting) and the number of passes by the operator are factors that can be modified for high-risk patients. Careful selection of the route traversed by the biopsy needle may lessen the chance of a pneumothorax. For example, centrally placed masses that abut the mediastinum or vertebral column may allow the biopsy to be performed without the needle traversing aerated lung.

While the risk of serious hemorrhage from the inadvertent puncture of a pulmonary artery in patients with pulmonary arterial hypertension would be expected to be higher than in the normal population, pulmonary arterial hypertension is not universally regarded as an absolute contraindication.[181] Nevertheless, if percutaneous needle biopsy is deemed necessary in a patient with raised pulmonary arterial pressure, a fine-caliber (22-gauge) aspiration needle rather than a larger bore or cutting needle would seem prudent.

Patients with a pulmonary mass that is thought to be a hydatid (echinococcal) cyst or an arteriovenous malformation should not be subjected to percutaneous lung biopsy because of the theoretical risks of an anaphylactic reaction and hemorrhage, respectively. However, in the case of hydatid disease three patients have been reported to have undergone needle aspiration without any complication.[85]

In summary, there are no absolute contraindications to percutaneous needle biopsy, although some patients clearly are at high risk from the procedure. These patients need a careful explanation of the need for the procedure and close attention during and after the biopsy.

Technique of percutaneous needle biopsy

TYPES OF NEEDLE. Percutaneous biopsy needles can be broadly categorized into those that are used to aspirate material for cytologic examination and those that have a cutting action and so provide a core of tissue for histologic examination. Some needles are a compromise between these two types and yield small fragments of tissue as well as a cellular aspirate.[47] The trend over the last few years has been to use smaller diameter needles (19 gauge or smaller), mainly because of the higher incidence of significant bleeding associated with the use of larger bore needles.[52,107,131,190] An ideal needle should be of narrow enough gauge to be used safely in any part of the thorax, retain enough rigidity to prevent deviation as it passes through different tissues, have a sufficiently large luminal diameter to enable the recovery of material for both histologic and cytologic examination, and finally be sharp enough to transfix and enter small fibrous or calcified lesions. No single needle satisfies all of these requirements, and the radiologist performing needle biopsies will usually become familiar with two or three different needles to deal with different eventualities. The smallest diameter needles that are widely available are the spinal or Chiba aspiration needles (22 to 25 gauge)[146]; at diameters of less than 22 gauge the great flexibility of the needle becomes a problem, often preventing precise placement of the needle. An adequate cytopathologic service is a prerequisite for the use of this type of needle, since fragments of tissue suitable for histopathologic examination are not reliably obtained with such fine-bore aspiration needles.

Many types of needle have been designed to improve the yield of solid fragments of tissue by modifying the cutting edge.[34,46,76,172] One of the most popular of these is the 22-gauge Westcott needle,[177] which has a central stylet, obtuse beveled tip, and small slot adjacent to the tip into which a fragment of tissue can be aspirated.

Other modifications include two- and three-component coaxial needles with cutting edges; a coaxial system requires a larger outer needle but has the advantage that multiple samples can be obtained by one needle pass.[46,163] Some authorities advocate the use of a screw-type needle.[102,106] However, there is no evidence that any single needle is superior in terms of diagnostic yield or low complication rate compared with another.

Certain histopathologic diagnoses can be made only when the lung architecture is intact. In these conditions aspirated cellular material or minute fragments of disorganized lung will prove nondiagnostic. Such diseases are often characterized by areas of focal or multifocal consolidation. In these cases a powered Tru-Cut type of needle that will obtain a large core of tissue with the minimum of disruption to the specimen is recommended. Recently, 20-gauge powered cutting needles have been developed (Biopty, Bard Inc., Billerica, Mass., and Temno, Becton Dickinson, Rutherford, N.J.). The action of cutting a core of tissue, powered by a spring-activated handle, results in the tip of the needle traveling between 0.5 and 2 cm. Spring-powered needles are therefore unsuitable for the biopsy of small lesions (less than 2.5 cm diameter) and should probably not be used for the biopsy of masses immediately adjacent to the major cardiovascular structures. A number of benign and malignant histologic diagnoses can be made with confidence from intact tissue specimens provided by these needles, including bronchioloalveolar cell carcinoma, lymphoproliferative disorders, Wegener's granulomatosis, and cryptogenic organizing pneumonia. Furthermore, 18- to 14-gauge powered cutting needles can reliably obtain diagnostic material from pleural, chest wall, and mediastinal masses.[15,40,98,133,185]

IMAGING GUIDANCE. Of the imaging techniques used for the guidance of percutaneous needle biopsy, fluoroscopy is the most commonly used method. It is generally quicker and easier than computed tomography (CT) or ultrasonography for smaller intrapulmonary lesions.[66,67] Probably because of the speed with which fluoroscopically guided biopsies can be performed, the rate of pneumothorax is less than with CT-guided biopsies.[32,161]

Giving definitive guidelines about which imaging technique is most appropriate in any given situation is impossible. The size, nature, and site of the lesion (particularly relation to its cardiovascular structures) and the preference of the operator have a bearing on which technique provides the optimal guidance. In some instances two techniques are desirable; for example, when fluoroscopy is used, CT may provide additional information about the safest route to the lesion (Figure 19-1).[42] The yield from fluoroscopically guided biopsy is extremely high with a sensitivity for the detection of malignancy of up to 95%.[88,129,177]

In contrast, the yield from CT-guided biopsies does not, overall, equal that of fluoroscopic-guided biopsies. This discrepancy is probably due to differences in case selection, since CT is often reserved for lesions in more difficult sites.[37,161] Nevertheless, there is no doubt that CT guidance is less satisfactory for small intrapulmonary lesions, particularly those in the lower zones that have great mobility because of normal respiratory excursion. Another factor that may reduce the accuracy of CT guidance is the partial volume effect that may affect the apparent position of the needle tip; theoretical methods of overcoming this error — which is significant only in the biopsy of very small lesions and when an angled approach is required — include scanning with narrow collimation, minimizing the distance to be traversed within the patient, and using long needles.[187] CT-guided biopsy is the unequivocal method of choice in a few instances: lesions not clearly seen on fluoroscopy (for example, masses in the costophrenic recess, at the extreme lung apex, or overlying the hilum) and lesions abutting the major cardiovascular structures.* CT may also be useful in the few instances in which a transosseous approach is required.[41]

Ultrasonographic guidance is a particularly useful technique for peripheral pulmonary consolidation or masses when they abut the chest wall and so allow sonographic access.† Many reports have confirmed the use of ultrasonography for guiding the percutaneous biopsy of anterior mediastinal masses.[133,152,188]

PRACTICAL ASPECTS OF PERCUTANEOUS NEEDLE BIOPSY. The techniques for fluoroscopic and ultrasound-guided biopsies are similar and differ from CT-guided biopsies in that the latter requires repeated rescanning and is not performed in real time.

Before a fluoroscopic-guided biopsy is performed, the lesion must be accurately localized using posteroanterior and lateral radiographs. If the lesion is not visible on a lateral radiograph (and therefore unlikely to be seen on the lateral projection of biplane fluoroscopy), CT is used to gauge the precise depth of the lesion. Tests to exclude a coagulation defect are desirable but not essential. Premedication is rarely necessary if the procedure has been carefully explained to the patient. Discussing the risks of the procedure with the patient is essential and includes the chance of pneumothorax with the possible necessity of a chest drain and the possibility of hemoptysis. Warning the patient before starting the procedure that several needle passes may be necessary is also useful.

The most appropriate approach can usually be determined before positioning the patient on the fluoroscopy table. Once the lesion has been identified, the patient is asked to suspend respiration, usually on inspiration, to identify where the lesion lies in relation to the overlying intercostal spaces. A marker is then placed on the skin (a small lead shot is useful for this purpose). Once an unimpeded approach has been chosen, the lead shot can be pressed onto the skin to make a visible mark. The skin is cleaned with disinfectant, and the potential track is infiltrated with local anesthetic down to, and through, the pleura while the patient suspends respiration. In choosing the exact site of needle entry in the intercostal space, having the needle close to a superior, rather than inferior, rib surface is preferable to prevent damage to the intercostal neurovascular bundle.

Before insertion the needle is marked so that its tip will lie within the lesion. Measurements are taken from either the lateral radiograph, which must include an allowance for magnification, or CT. The needle should be advanced smoothly along the line of the central x-ray beam with breath held at the predetermined phase of respiration judged to bring the lesion into line with the intercostal space. Depending on the consistency of the lesion, the needle tip is usually felt entering the lesion. The patient is then asked to breathe quietly. The position of the needle within the lesion can be confirmed by fluoroscopy (Figure 19-2). On single-plane fluoroscopy a satisfactory position is suggested when the lesion is seen to move synchronously and with the same excursion as the tip of the needle. The method of obtaining fragments of material depends largely on the design of the needle. Most needles have a central stylet that is removed while the patient suspends respiration; as soon as this is done, a finger should be placed over the hub of the needle to reduce the possibility of air embolism. For straightforward aspiration a syringe is attached and the plunger pulled back while a

---

*References 19, 32, 37, 98, 138, 161.
†References 15, 18, 58, 62, 185, 186, 189.

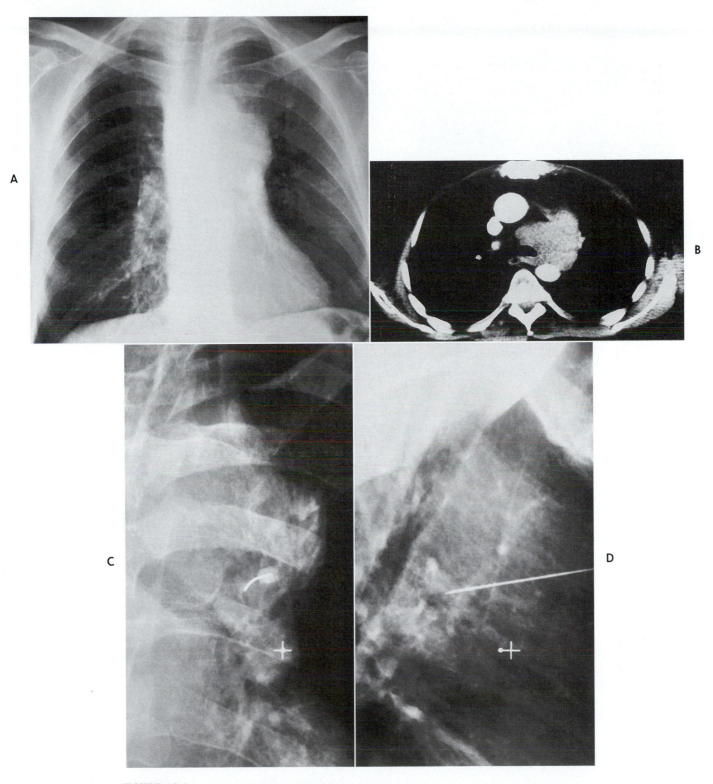

FIGURE 19-1
A, Posteroanterior radiograph of a 55-year-old smoker showing a large mass in the aortopulmonary window. B, Computed tomography confirms the location of the mass and its relationship to great vessels. C, Anteroposterior and, D, lateral fluoroscopic spot films showing the tip of the needle within the mass that proved to be undifferentiated adenocarcinoma.

FIGURE 19-2
A, Anteroposterior fluoroscopic film of a 22-gauge needle in the lateral aspect of a 1 cm nodule *(arrowheads)*. **B,** Lateral fluoroscopic film confirms the position of the needle tip within the lesion *(arrowheads)*. Cytologic examination showed a well-differentiated adenocarcinoma.

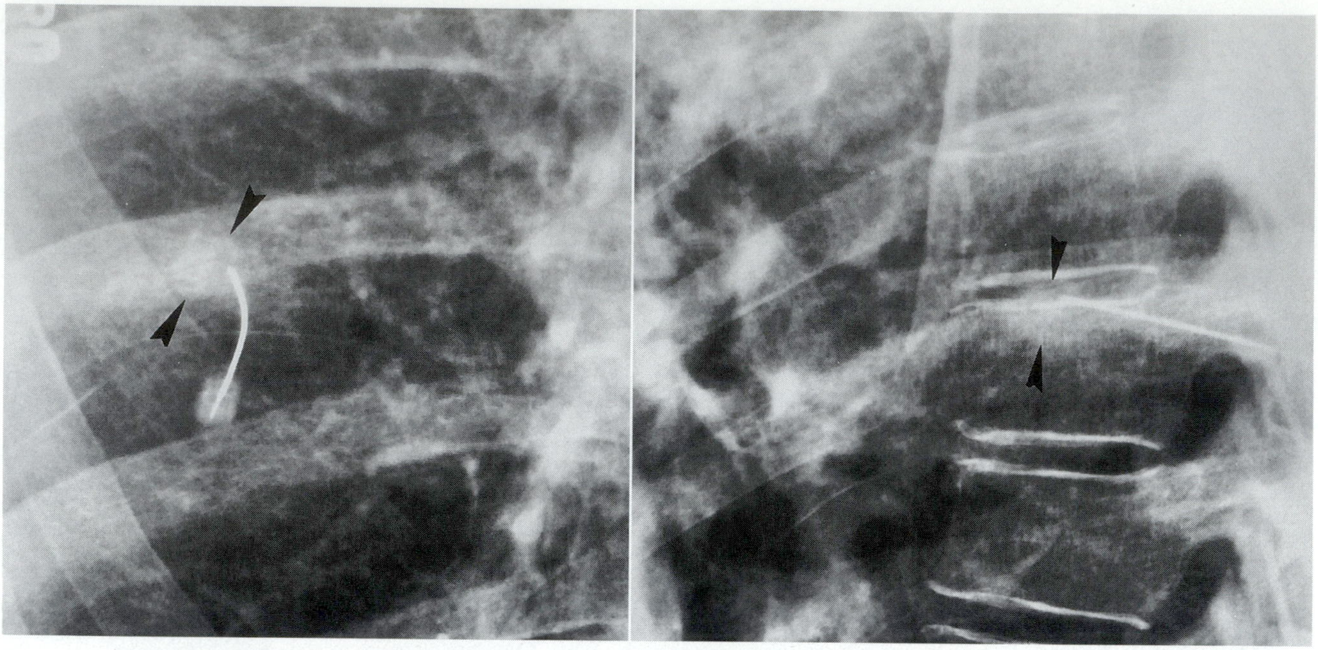

slight jiggling motion is used to free material into the needle lumen.[68,69] Releasing negative pressure before the needle is withdrawn from the patient is usually recommended. Processing the aspirated material depends on whether a cytopathologist is present at the procedure. In general the aspirate should be fixed in 95% alcohol for cytology, although sometimes air-dried specimens are required. Fragments large enough for histopathologic examination, usually greater than 3 mm across, should be placed in a formalin-saline solution. The possibility of an infective cause should not be overlooked, and material for microscopy and culture should be placed in sterile saline solution or the specific medium recommended by the microbiologists. The number of passes performed depends on the adequacy of the biopsy specimen. The only guarantee that a positive sample has been obtained comes from the cytopathologist, who can assess sufficient material for a diagnosis. Without this facility, up to three passes suffices in the majority of cases. Injection of a coagulant in the needle track as the needle is withdrawn may reduce the rate of pneumothorax.[10,84,167] However, there is no clear evidence that this procedure has much effect on the overall rate of significant pneumothoraces, and in most centers "patch" techniques are not routinely done.

An expiratory chest radiograph is usually obtained within the first 3 hours after the procedure. However, if the mass is large and obviously involves the chest wall so that no normal lung is traversed,[50] the need for a chest radiograph in the absence of any symptoms of respiratory distress is questionable. If no pneumothorax has developed at 4 hours and the patient is asymptomatic, many centers allow outpatients to leave the hospital,[118] since the subsequent development of a pneumothorax becomes increasingly unlikely.[114,148]

Complications of percutaneous needle biopsy

The complication rate of percutaneous needle biopsy has decreased over the years, probably because the combination of smaller caliber needles and improved imaging guidance allows safer and faster placement of needles. Patient selection is an important factor in the complication rate; for example, a young fit patient is at far less risk than an elderly smoker with advanced emphysema.

The most common complications of percutaneous needle biopsy are pneumothorax and minor hemoptysis. Rarer complications include air embolism, major hemoptysis, hemothorax with or without empyema formation, cardiac tamponade, bronchopleural fistula, lung torsion, implantation of tumor in the needle track, and tumor embolism.* The frequency of biopsy-associated pneumothorax is difficult to gauge; most series suggest a frequency of between 10% and 35% for fluoroscopic-guided biopsies. However, lower and much higher frequencies of 8% and 61% have been reported.[181] Factors that substantially increase the likelihood of a pneumothorax include preexisting lung disease (particularly chronic obstructive pulmonary disease), an increased

*References 1, 6, 45, 70, 71, 87, 88, 90, 99, 137, 141, 154.

number of passes,[95] traversing more than one visceral pleural surface,[46] deep lesions, and advanced age. Of these, chronic obstructive pulmonary disease is the most important.[33,89] Contrary to expectation, the caliber of the biopsy needle does not seem to be a major factor in determining the rate of pneumothorax.[141]

Several modifications to the technique of percutaneous needle biopsy have been suggested to reduce the rate of significant pneumothorax: maintaining complete suspension of respiration while traversing the visceral pleura,[46] placing the patient in a lateral decubitus position after the procedure with the biopsy side dependent,[14,94,95] administering 100% oxygen to the patient during the procedure,[119] and instilling a coagulant or placing foam plugs into the needle track during withdrawal of the needle.[28,84,143,150,167] Whether any of these techniques makes a significant contribution to reducing the occurrence of pneumothorax is not clear; probably the single most important factor is the experience of the operator.

Percutaneous needle biopsy should not be performed unless the operator is prepared to treat an iatrogenic pneumothorax instantly. The number of patients requiring a chest drain following percutaneous needle biopsy is small and in most operators' experience is well under 10%. Small, asymptomatic stable pneumothoraces detected on chest radiography do not need to be treated. However, if symptoms develop or if the pneumothorax exceeds 50% of the volume of the hemithorax, a chest drain should be inserted. Any patient who shows acute respiratory distress, even when the classic signs of a tension pneumothorax are absent, should have a drain inserted immediately. A small-bore drain (6F to 9F) is almost invariably successful for the treatment of an iatrogenic pneumothorax, and this can conveniently be connected to a one-way valve until the air leak seals. A Heimlich valve (Becton Dickinson, Rutherford, N.J.) and other types of flutter valves have been specifically designed for the emergency treatment of pneumothoraces.[92,130] Most leaks heal within 2 days, but occasionally an air leak persists. In these cases active suction may be necessary.[13,115]

Bleeding is potentially the most dangerous complication of percutaneous needle biopsy. Trivial hemoptysis is often briefly preceded by a cough and occurs in about 10% of cases. Massive fatal hemoptyses fortunately are rare and usually follow biopsy with larger caliber (greater than 18-gauge) cutting needles.[8,52,107,110] This dread complication is extremely rare with needles of 20 gauge or smaller.[181]

Clinically apparent air embolism is an even rarer complication of percutaneous needle biopsy. It occurs when the needle lies within a pulmonary vein and allows the ingress of air either from the surrounding lung or via the needle lumen. In the documented cases,[1,154,176] coughing at the time of needle placement is common to every case, and for this reason, as well as the increased chance of tearing the visceral pleura, removing the needle

swiftly is probably advisable in the event of a bout of coughing. The occurrence of malignancy seeding along the needle track is much less common than is generally supposed. It is most likely to occur with larger caliber needles[141] and when the tumor, particularly a mesothelioma, is already invading the chest wall.[142]

Accuracy of percutaneous needle biopsy

In most centers the positive yield from patients with lung carcinoma is 85% to 95% with the widest spectrum of reported positive yields in lung cancer ranging from 78%[153] to 99%.[129] Factors influencing the rate of true-positive diagnosis include the needle size, number of passes, type of imaging guidance, nature of the lesion (particularly the size and site[8]), and experience of both the radiologist and the pathologist. The false-positive rate for pulmonary malignancy is extremely low, probably less than 2%.[16]

The cytologic or histopathologic statement "negative for malignant disease" may be deceptive because it encompasses two quite different situations: (1) nodules from which no malignant cells are identified but for which no specific diagnosis is offered by the pathologist (the majority)[11] and (2) nodules in which a specific benign diagnosis can be reached (for example, pulmonary infarct or hamartoma). In the latter case the diagnosis may be accepted as such unless the clinical or radiographic suspicion of malignancy is high, in which case a repeat biopsy or even surgical resection will have to be considered. However, a definitive benign biopsy by percutaneous needle biopsy is rare, ranging from 5%[16] to 16%[183]; the likelihood of obtaining benign diagnosis will depend heavily on the prevalence of lung cancer in the population under study. Percutaneous needle biopsy specimens that are reported as containing "inflammatory" or necrotic material should be considered nonspecific and should never be taken as excluding malignancy. The frequency of a cancer-positive result on further biopsy following an initial negative result may be as high as 35% to 45%.[111,131,177] Causes for a failure to obtain a positive malignant diagnosis include extensive necrosis of the tumor, a desmoplastic reaction to the tumor causing intense fibrosis, or, most frequently, missing a small lesion altogether.

The true-positive diagnostic rate for malignant mediastinal and hilar masses ranges from 85% to 95%.* The rate with which specific benign diagnoses is made is higher than that for pulmonary lesions and is approximately 30%.[147] Fine needle biopsy does not achieve the same high diagnostic accuracy for lymphomas as for other neoplasms.† The more undifferentiated the lymphoma, the easier a purely cytologic diagnosis. However, in well-differentiated lymphoma, the lymph node architecture is important for typing the lymphoma, and larger

---

*References 2, 42, 91, 127, 173, 178, 180.
†References 2, 91, 98, 170, 173, 178.

intact cores of tissue are needed. Furthermore, in nodular sclerosing Hodgkin's lymphoma, obtaining sufficient cellular material to make a definitive diagnosis by aspiration alone is often impossible.[2,91,127] In cases in which lymphoma is suspected, larger cutting needles significantly improve the specificity of histologic diagnoses.[49,91,98,188] In patients with known lymphoma in whom intrathoracic recurrence is suspected, aspiration of material for cytology is often sufficient to confirm the diagnosis of recurrence, and in these instances larger fragments of tissue are not always needed.[66,67] A coaxial technique may be useful to allow multiple samples to be taken from a questionable area of mediastinal recurrence.[184]

The need for classifying the cell type of lung cancer from fragments obtained from percutaneous needle biopsy is clinically important. The agreement between the results of cytologic examination of needle aspirate and the final histopathologic findings ranges from approximately 60% to 90%.[88,112,191] Interestingly, most discordance occurs among large cell carcinoma, squamous carcinoma, and adenocarcinoma.[47] Since the crucial distinction is between small cell and non–small cell carcinomas, this disagreement usually does not affect management of patients. Depending on the exact technique and type of needle used, percutaneous needle biopsy may provide both cytologic material and small tissue fragments suitable for histopathologic examination. Even with a 22-gauge needle, fragments of tissue can be obtained in up to 92% of cases, and these subsequently provided a histopathologic diagnosis in 72% of cases.[47] The value of obtaining material suitable for histopathologic examination in patients with a low probability of lung cancer should not be overlooked. Some conditions can be diagnosed with certainty only from the histopathologic material, for example, focal organizing pneumonia (in which identification of delicate intraalveolar granulation tissue is needed) and Wegener's granulomatosis (in which inclusion of a vessel showing granulomatous vasculitis is needed).

PERCUTANEOUS DRAINAGE OF INTRATHORACIC FLUID COLLECTIONS

The application of percutaneous drainage techniques of fluid collection within the thorax has increased with improved image guidance, particularly ultrasonography[81,96] and CT.[159] A further advantage of cross-sectional imaging is the ability to identify distant loculations and, in the case of ultrasonography, septations within the pleural collection (Figure 19-3) that may alter the management strategy. Supplementary techniques include the instillation of fibrinolytic agents for the treatment of loculated empyemas (Figure 9-3)[75] and sclerotherapy for malignant effusions.[97]

Indications

The indications for the percutaneous drainage of an intrathoracic fluid collection include relief of symptoms caused by the mass effect of a large effusion; drainage of an empyema or infected bulla; drainage of a mediastinal pus collection[43] (most often post sternotomy), and drainage of a sterile chronic pleural collection, for example, a malignant effusion. The indications and technique for the drainage of intrapulmonary abscesses are in most respects similar to those of pleural collections. These two clinical problems are considered together. While the indications for drainage of a subacute pleural effusion depend largely on its size, chronicity, and etiology, opinions on the timing and method of drainage are highly variable and usually reflect whether the patient is being managed by a physician or a surgeon. In common with other treatment options, patient selection is probably the most important factor in determining the success of percutaneous drainage of a pleural collection. In patients in whom medical treatment of a parapneumonic pleural effusion or lung abscess fails, the decision of whether to proceed to surgical resection or percutaneous drainage has to be made. In general, these decisions are not usually the result of faultless clinical logic. There are some overriding factors that determine how the patient is managed; for example, young children usually cannot tolerate an indwelling chest drainage tube, and conversely elderly patients may be better served by percutaneous drainage than by a surgical procedure.

Contraindications

There are no absolute contraindications to the percutaneous drainage of intrathoracic fluid collections apart from a patient who is unable to cooperate. Impaired hemostasis is a relative contraindication to the procedure, usually when the platelet count is less than 50,000 or partial prothrombin time is greater than 1.4 times the control. A problem, but not strictly a contraindication, is inaccessibility of the collection, although with careful analysis of the CT examination a direct route for the drainage catheter can usually be found (Figure 19-4).

Technique of percutaneous drainage

TYPES OF CATHETER. Although there are many different types of chest drainage catheters, each with its own advocates, the most commonly used is a polyethylene nephrostomy-type pigtail catheter (8F to 12F). The two design features of a drainage catheter that are most likely to influence successful drainage of a collection are its internal luminal diameter and number of side holes. A larger bore (14F to 24F) drainage catheter is obviously less likely to clog when the collection contains fibrinous material, blood clots, or necrotic debris. For this reason having two or three catheters of varying caliber readily available is useful so that the type of catheter can be decided at the time of the procedure when fluid is first aspirated. Smaller bore tubes are better tolerated by patients, especially children, and drainage catheters as small as 8F are satisfactory for nonviscous fluid collections.

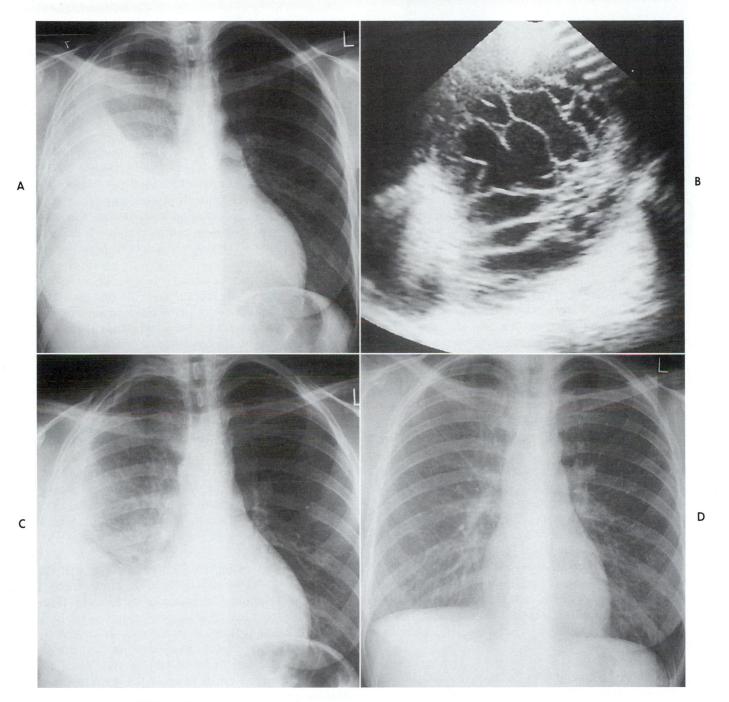

FIGURE 19-3
A, Large right parapneumonic pleural effusion in a 23-year-old patient. **B,** Ultrasonography shows numerous septations within the effusion. **C,** Incomplete drainage of the effusion after insertion of a pigtail catheter. **D,** Minimal residual pleural thickening in the right hemithorax 2 months after successful treatment by infusion of streptokinase into the loculated effusion. (Courtesy Dr. M.B. Rubens, London.)

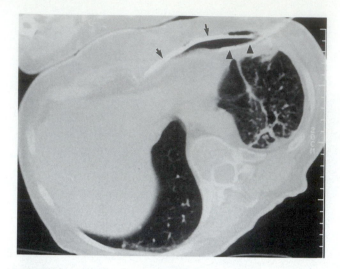

FIGURE 19-4
Computed tomography scan used for the precise guidance of narrow-bore drainage catheter *(arrowheads)* into an infected collection located beneath a left chest wall prosthesis *(arrows)*.

IMAGING GUIDANCE. The choice of imaging guidance lies among fluoroscopy, ultrasonography, or CT (Figure 19-5) and is determined by the site and size of the collection, as well as the operator's preference.

Establishing from the preliminary imaging of the patient whether the fluid collection lies within the pleural space or lung is not always easy. In patients with severe bullous emphysema this may be impossible, even with CT. Furthermore, fluid collections in abdominal viscera may sometimes mimic collections in the lower part of the chest.[23,104,164] Fluoroscopy can be used to guide the positioning of catheters in large collections. However, with an air-fluid level within the space, positioning the catheter in the most dependent part of the cavity will be possible only if the patient is in the erect position. In these instances CT guidance allows more precision in placing the catheter. Ultrasonography is a quick and efficient technique for identifying pleural collections,[81] provided that no subcutaneous air or calcification is in the pleural rind to prevent sonographic access. Ultrasonography can also be used for localizing intrapulmonary abscesses as long as no aerated lung is between the abscess and chest wall.

TECHNIQUE OF DRAIN PLACEMENT. Once the route of access (ideally a straight line) has been chosen, the skin is cleaned and the proposed entry site is infiltrated with local anesthetic. A 22-gauge needle may then be inserted directly into the cavity to confirm that there is no bony obstacle and also to aspirate fluid for laboratory analysis. The type and bore of the drainage catheter to be used are influenced by the nature of the fluid aspirated. At this stage, if CT is being used to guide placement, a further scan is obtained to confirm the location and path of the needle. With large collections this stage may be omitted. The needle can then be exchanged for either a needle with

a bore sufficient to accept a standard J-tip guidewire or, bypassing the guidewire step, the assembled narrow-bore catheter and central needle can be inserted directly. The use of a guidewire is necessary when positioning of the catheter is likely to be difficult, and a guidewire can also be used to position the catheter in the most dependent part of the cavity. Track dilatation is necessary if a guidewire is used and has the added advantage of obviating snagging of the catheter end, which is a frequent problem with single-step types of pigtail catheters. Snagging can be minimized by using a scalpel with an appropriately designed long, near parallel-edged blade.

While coiling some of the drainage catheter within the cavity is ideal, the side holes should be below the fluid level in the dependent part of the cavity when the patient is erect or semierect. Once air in the cavity can reach the side holes, the effects of applied suction are lost. Maintaining negative or at least neutral pressure is important so that contents of the catheter cannot be aspirated back into the cavity; this is most effectively obtained with a water seal. Suction at a pressure of approximately 20 cm water is needed to aspirate pus through small-bore catheters. Although irrigation has been recommended, no controlled studies have shown whether it gives any therapeutic benefit; it is probably of no value if the fluid collection is draining freely but is obviously useful if the catheter becomes blocked by viscid fluid. The efficacy of fibrinolytic agents in the treatment of multiloculated empyemas has been reported in one series[75]: in a prospective study of ten patients with loculated infective empyemas, nine patients were successfully treated by instillation of 100,000 units of urokinase daily until radiographic resolution of the collection was achieved. Whether the benefits of this costly treatment outweigh surgical treatment of drainage by rib resection or pleural decortication is uncertain, but this technique clearly provides a useful nonsurgical alternative in selected patients.

Patients with malignant pleural effusions that have been drained with small-bore drainage catheters may be treated by instilling sclerosing agents into the pleural space to prevent reaccumulation of the effusion. In one series 15 of 21 patients were successfully treated with either bleomycin or tetracycline (no longer available for pleurodesis in the United States) in this way.[97] The common factor in patients in whom the procedure fails is that the effusions drain at a rate of more than 100 ml/day before the sclerotherapy.

Establishing the success rate of image-guided drainage of pleural and intrapulmonary collections is difficult because of the wide variations in patient selection, technique, and aftercare. This last factor is particularly important and often overlooked by radiologists. In one series 59% of patients with chest or abdominal catheters placed by radiologists were found to have catheter-related problems that were discovered on daily rounds following

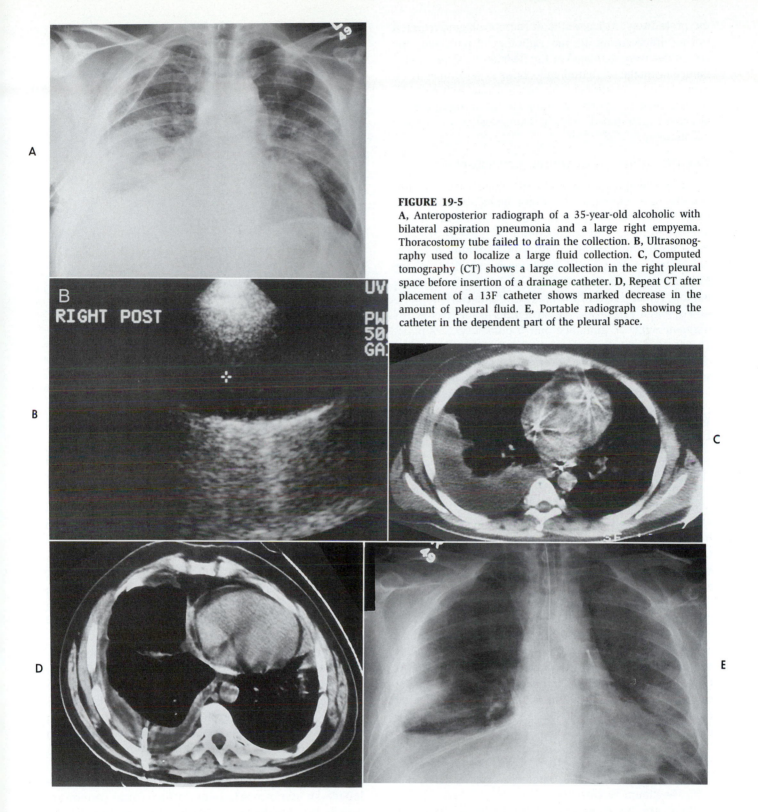

FIGURE 19-5
A, Anteroposterior radiograph of a 35-year-old alcoholic with bilateral aspiration pneumonia and a large right empyema. Thoracostomy tube failed to drain the collection. **B,** Ultrasonography used to localize a large fluid collection. **C,** Computed tomography (CT) shows a large collection in the right pleural space before insertion of a drainage catheter. **D,** Repeat CT after placement of a 13F catheter shows marked decrease in the amount of pleural fluid. **E,** Portable radiograph showing the catheter in the dependent part of the pleural space.

the procedures. At least 30% of these problems required further intervention in the radiology department; the remainder were managed at the bedside.[44] When image-guided drainage of pleural collections is performed by an experienced practitioner, the success rate is high.* Although fewer, reports of drainage of intrapulmonary abscesses after failed medical management are equally encouraging.[5,109,160,162,174]

Complications of drainage procedures

Serious complications of percutaneous catheter drainage are rare, the most important being severe hemorrhage.† Pain at the site of catheter insertion can be minimized by careful consideration of the least troublesome site for the patient (ideally anterolaterally, avoiding the posterior chest wall). Kinking and blockage of the catheter occur frequently but can often be rectified without replacement of the catheter.[44] Inadvertent puncture of major cardiovascular structures or the liver is less frequent with CT guidance and a guidewire technique. The creation of a bronchopleural fistula is a theoretical possibility when a lung abscess is drained. In the two small series reported to date, this does not appear to be a frequent problem.[160,162]

BRONCHIAL ARTERIOGRAPHY AND EMBOLIZATION

The indications for bronchial arteriography have changed over the years, and it is now most often performed as a precursor to embolization to stop a massive hemoptysis in patients unsuitable for surgical management.‡ Surgical resection is still regarded as the treatment of choice in patients with massive hemoptysis (defined as more than 600 ml in 24 hours). Without surgical intervention the mortality in such patients is more than 50%.[36]

The most common causes of bronchial artery hypertrophy and consequent intrapulmonary hemorrhage are suppurative lung diseases (particularly the bronchiectasis of cystic fibrosis[20,151,155]) and posttuberculous cavities containing mycetomas. Less common causes of hemorrhage from the bronchial circulation include bronchial carcinoma, chronic pulmonary abscess,[117] congenital malformations (Figure 19-6), and cyanotic heart disease.[79] In some hemorrhagic pulmonary lesions the vascular supply is complex with contributions from the pulmonary circulation, systemic bronchial arteries, and sometimes the nonbronchial systemic arteries that transgress the pleura (Figure 19-7).[63]

There are no contraindications to bronchial artery embolization, although the patient should be hemodynamically stable and able to lie flat for the duration of the

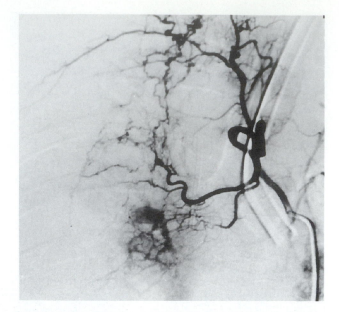

FIGURE 19-6
Digital subtraction bronchial arteriogram performed during active hemorrhage with a patient under general anesthetic (note selective intubation of the left lung). Contrast medium can be seen pooling in the right midzone, probably in a lobar bronchus. No predisposing cause for the abnormally hypertrophied bronchial circulation was identified in this patient.

procedure. If a spinal artery arising from a bronchial artery is identified, special care should be taken if embolization of that bronchial artery is contemplated.[24] However, spinal arteries may become visible only following embolization when there is preferential flow into the small spinal artery. Fast-flowing blood in the hypertrophied bronchial artery will theoretically direct embolic material to the abnormal intrapulmonary circulation rather than to the spinal artery.[20] The frequency with which the spinal artery is identified is variable[123,182]; in one series the spinal artery was identified in 55% of patients.[20]

The number and origins of the bronchial arteries are highly variable. Up to 20% of bronchial arteries arise from vessels other than the descending aorta.[9] The most common arrangement is one main right bronchial artery from a common intercostobronchial trunk arising from the thoracic aorta at approximately the level of T5 and two left bronchial arteries arising more inferiorly.[120] In the studies reported to date the number of left bronchial arteries always exceeds the number on the right.[9] The bronchial arteries conforming to the typical pattern are usually found within a 2 cm radius of the center of the left main bronchus. The wide variation in both the numbers and the origins of the bronchial arteries needs to be remembered when comprehensive bronchial arteriography is contemplated. Up to 35% of patients have either multiple vessels or unusual origins.[20,86] Bronchial arteries may arise from the thyrocervical trunk, the internal mammary artery, the costocervical trunk, the subclavian

---

*References 57, 65, 81, 139, 165, 179.
†References 5, 57, 65, 139, 165, 179.
‡References 20, 30, 31, 55, 83, 122, 123, 125, 149, 151, 157, 158, 182.

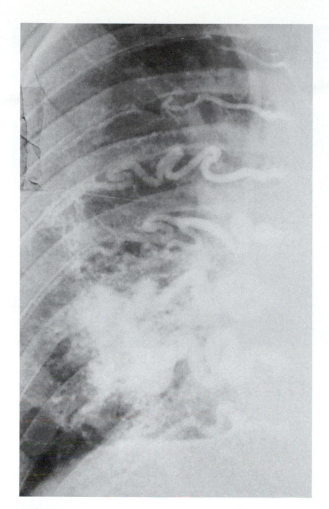

FIGURE 19-7
Aortogram showing hypertrophied intercostal arteries penetrating the pleura and supplying the underlying right lung. Trauma sustained in a road traffic accident was thought to be responsible; the patient had a hemoptysis 4 years after the incident.

artery, a lower intercostal artery, the inferior phrenic artery, or even the abdominal aorta.[9,20,63]

Many different catheter shapes have been recommended for the selective catherization of bronchial arteries arising from the thoracic aorta. The ideal catheter design depends on whether the right or left bronchial artery is to be catheterized. The right intercostal bronchial trunk takes off from the aorta at an acute upward angle, whereas the left bronchial arteries leave the aorta more or less at right angles. Despite this difference, most bronchial arteries can be selectively catheterized with a cobra, shepherd's crook, or Mikahelson catheter, provided that the tip tapers to 5F or smaller. Coaxial catheter systems may be useful for the superselective catheterization of the bronchial circulation, allowing precise delivery of embolic material and so preventing spillover into the aorta or inadvertent embolization of the spinal artery. There is the theoretical danger of wedging the catheter in the bronchial artery, which could result in spinal cord ischemia.

Use of small volumes (less than 10 ml boluses) of low-osmolar contrast media is thought to reduce the risk of spinal cord damage.[24,158]

Fiberoptic bronchoscopy is sometimes advocated before bronchial artery embolization to establish the site of hemorrhage. However, a large hemoptysis almost invariably results in vigorous coughing and spreads blood throughout the bronchial tree, making localization at a lobar level (or indeed, the side) impossible.[151] Few criteria exist to determine which angiographically demonstrated bronchial arteries should be embolized. Guidelines are particularly relevant when several bronchial arteries have been identified and the site of hemorrhage is not obvious from the prior thoracic imaging. Embolization obviously should be directed at the vessels considered most likely to be the source of hemorrhage. Bronchial arteries with a diameter greater than 3 mm can be considered to be pathologically enlarged. Patients may be surprisingly reliable at localizing the origin of the hemoptysis, for example, a gurgling or curious sensation in one part of one lung. In patients with diffuse suppurative lung disease, most commonly cystic fibrosis, an attempt should be made to embolize all significantly enlarged bronchial arteries bilaterally.[20,149,151] If no abnormal bronchial arteries are identified, a systematic search should be made for aberrant bronchial arteries. When a patient continues to have hemoptyses after embolization of all suspicious systemic arteries, investigating the pulmonary circulation for a source of hemorrhage may be necessary.[31] Such an approach is demanding for both patient and operator. An appreciation of the anatomy and pathophysiology of these complex disorders will reduce the incidence of complications.[124]

A variety of embolic materials have been used for the embolization of bronchial arteries ranging from particles of polyvinyl alcohol foam (Ivalon, Pacific Medical Industries, Calif.); pledgets of absorbable gelatin; and sometimes combinations, for example, particles of Spongostan and Mersilene threads.[35] For grossly hypertrophied bronchial arteries, Gianturco metal coils can be used. Coils lodged proximally in the bronchial artery have the disadvantage of preventing recatheterization, which may be necessary at a later date. The use of agents capable of obliterating the microcirculation (particularly ethyl alcohol) is inappropriate because of the theoretical risk of such a material being diverted to the spinal artery and causing spinal cord damage.[101]

Following bronchial artery embolization (Figure 19-8) most patients experience a transient fever and chest pain.[30] After 48 hours some patients cough up small amounts of altered blood, possibly because of limited bronchial infarction. Serious complications after bronchial artery embolization are rare. Most of the reported cases of transverse myelitis have been caused by contrast toxicity rather than inadvertent embolization[24,64,105] and predate the introduction of low-osmolar contrast media. Necrosis of the mainstem bronchi is an exceedingly rare

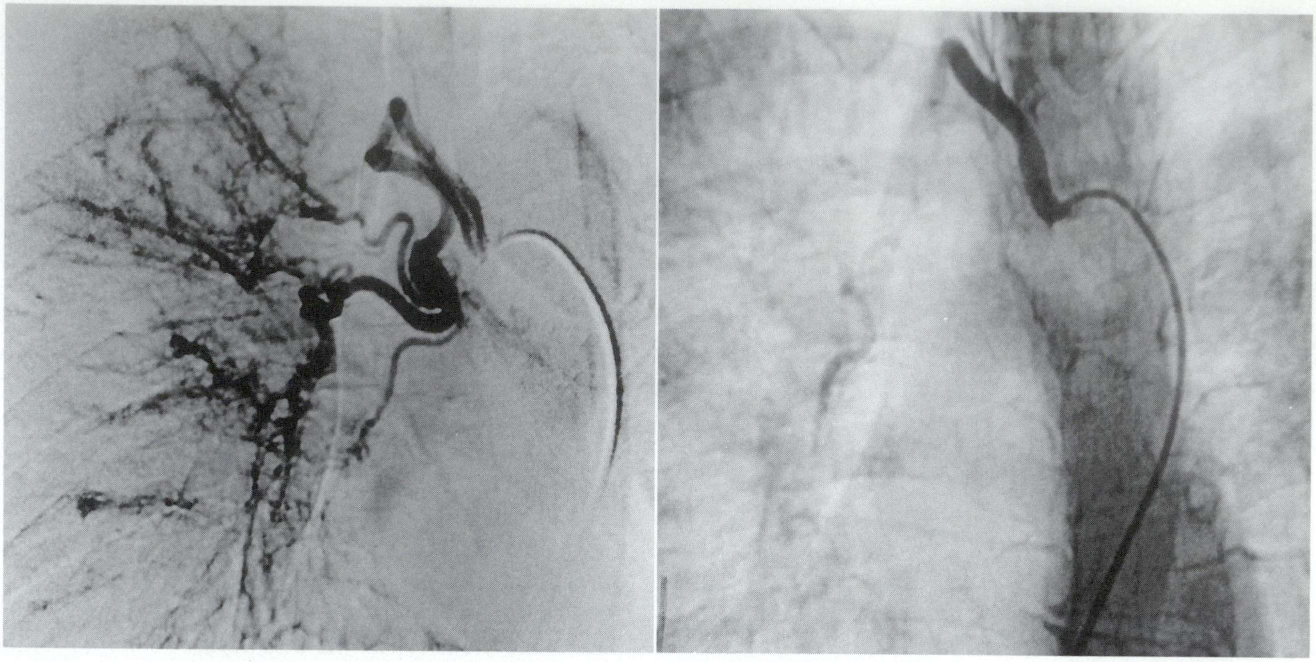

FIGURE 19-8
A, Selective right bronchial arteriogram in a patient with cystic fibrosis who presented with a hemoptysis. B, Following embolization, only the stump of the bronchial artery is opacified.

complication and has been reported only twice.[61,123] A later development of a bronchoesophageal fistula has been reported in one patient.[100] Spillover of embolization material into the thoracic aorta may cause distant ischemia or infarction in the legs or abdominal organs; a single case of fatal ischemic colitis has been reported.[77]

The aim of bronchial artery embolization, which is the immediate control of life-threatening hemoptysis, is achieved in 75% to 90% of patients.[51,122,123,151,158] Failures are caused by an inability to complete the procedure, failure to identify significant (possibly aberrant) bronchial arteries, and an inability to maintain the catheter position and proceed to embolization. Up to 20% of patients rebleed within 6 months following an initially successful bronchial artery embolization.[64,123] The reasons cited for recurrent hemorrhage are recanalization of previously embolized vessels,[29] incomplete initial embolization, and hypertrophy of small bronchial arteries not initially embolized.[122] Bronchial artery embolization usually can be successfully repeated in patients who rebleed.

TRACHEOBRONCHIAL STENTS

Occlusion or stenosis of a main airway by bronchial carcinoma is a significant and distressing cause of morbidity. Major airway obstruction can cause breathlessness, recurrent infections, and in extreme cases asphyxiation. Nonmalignant causes of tracheal or bronchial stenoses are numerous and include iatrogenic interference (notably following lung transplantation[134]),

relapsing polychondritis, tracheomalacia, and granulomatous diseases.

The palliative treatments of malignant obstruction of the major airways include internal or external radiotherapy[73,144] and repeated resection of recurrent endobronchial tumor by diathermy[74] or laser.[54] The rapid recurrence of bronchial carcinoma is not satisfactorily dealt with by any of these techniques. Stenoses of benign origin may be dilated by bougienage,[7] but long-term success is not universal.

Stenting is indicated in patients with major airway obstruction in whom other treatments have failed to provide long-term palliation. The first stents were made of silicon and had various configurations, including an inverted Y that rested on the carina. Stents were subsequently developed that were less likely to migrate.[93,175] Short-length strictures in the main bronchi have been successfully treated with straight silicon stents that have a collar at each end to prevent displacement.[59] Such stents are railroaded into position over a guidewire using a ridged bronchoscope.

The use of metallic stents in tracheal and bronchial strictures has undergone a revival since the first modern description of a stainless steel wire coil used for the treatment of an anastomotic stenosis of the trachea.[108] The most widely available expanding metallic stents currently available are the Gianturco* and the Wall-

*References 26, 38, 103, 132, 140, 166, 168.

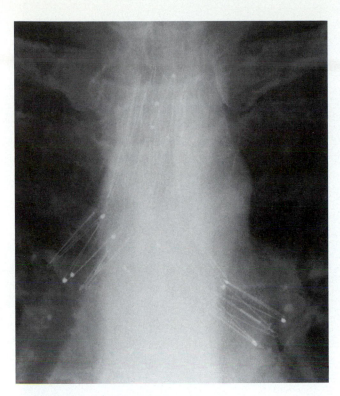

FIGURE 19-9
Multiple Gianturco stents holding open the lower trachea and main bronchi in a patient with fibrosing mediastinitis.

stent.[59,128,156] Both of these stents are positioned through an introducing sheath. Unlike the stents made of silicon tubing, the metallic stents are collapsed and preloaded in a cartridge (of approximately 10F) and are easier to position. Metallic stents can also cross the orifice of an adjacent bronchus without obstructing that airway. Although placement can be performed under either fluoroscopic or bronchoscopic control alone, in practice the procedure is best performed by a combination of the two techniques. Without fluoroscopy seeing the lower end of the stricture bronchoscopically may be impossible when the introducing sheath is in position.

These metallic mesh stents rapidly become covered by epithelium, and this process is usually complete within 1 month.[59] These stents are most effective when the stenosis is caused by extrinsic compression of the airways by a tumor or in holding open a floppy malacic segment. Multiple stents can be placed for long stenoses (Figure 19-9). The Gianturco stent is theoretically more effective because of its greater expansile radial force, compared with the Wallstent, and the former may show progressive dilatation of a tough fibrous stricture over a period of weeks on sequential radiographs. However, in one of the largest series reported to date, in which 35 and 39 patients were treated with Gianturco and Wallstent prostheses, respectively, there was a much higher complication rate with the Gianturco stent. In 30% of patients the Gianturco stent either migrated or ruptured.[128] Recent

design modification of the Gianturco stent by the manufacturers has attempted to overcome these problems. Endobronchial tumors or inflammatory strictures, in which there is rapid neoplastic growth or exuberant granulation tissue, ultimately obstruct open-mesh stents because of the ingrowth of tissue. An approach to the problem of tumor ingress through the mesh is to cover the stent with material such as silicon.[39]

SUPERIOR VENA CAVA STENTS

Superior vena cava obstruction (SVCO) is a distressing condition characterized by marked facial and upper limb swelling, intractable headache, and shortness of breath. SVCO is usually caused by advanced mediastinal malignancy, and conventional palliative treatment relies on radiation therapy, chemotherapy, and sometimes surgery.[48,80,113] Although radiation therapy often produces an initial improvement, recurrence of symptoms is the rule. Balloon angioplasty of both benign and malignant causes of SVCO has been attempted,[3,136] but not surprisingly symptoms are liable to recur rapidly after angioplasty alone.

The percutaneous placement of metallic stents for the treatment of SVCO has practical attractions. With increasing experience, reliable and successful palliation of SVCO has been reported with the Gianturco stent,[12,17,60,121,126] Palmaz stent,[27,145] and Wallstent.[169] A superior vena cavagram (Figure 19-10, *A*) is mandatory to identify the length of the stenosis and its site (in relation to the confluence of the brachiocephalic veins and to the right atrium) and to exclude intraluminal thrombus or tumor (an absolute contraindication to the procedure). If the stenosis is close to the point of entry of the superior vena cava into the right atrium, a stent might be placed with one end lying free within the cavity of the right atrium. In the case of the Wallstent, each end of the stent has to be anchored in the vascular endothelium because a free end within the right atrium renders the stent unstable.

Following balloon dilatation (Figure 19-10, *B*), the stent is positioned across the stricture to a diameter of at least 12 mm (Figure 19-10, *C*), and a postplacement cavagram is performed to confirm patency and free flow of blood into the right atrium (Figure 19-10, *D*). Patients are usually anticoagulated with intravenous heparin for at least 72 hours. After angioplasty and stent placement, relief of SVCO symptoms is usually rapid and dramatic. In two of six patients symptoms recurred: in one case this was due to venous thrombosis and in the other to tumor progression distal to the stent.[145] In another series of five patients there was no recurrence of SVCO symptoms before death.[169]

Although there is the risk of superior vena cava rupture at time of angioplasty, this complication has not been reported to date, possibly because most patients have received radiation therapy, which results in an envelope of fibrosis around the superior vena cava. The only complication of the procedure reported so far has been a

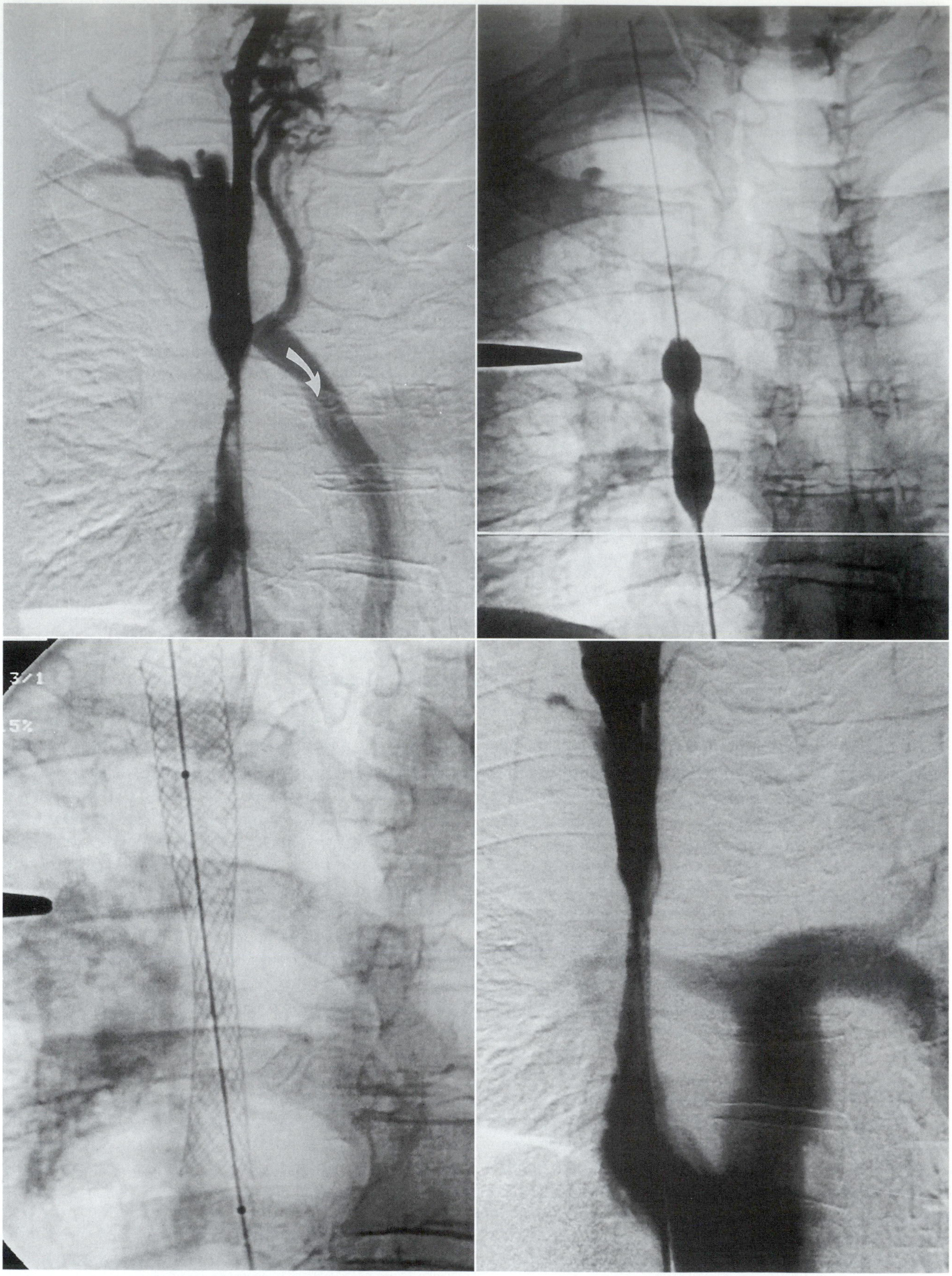

FIGURE 19-10
A, Digital subtraction superior vena cavagram showing stenosis of the lower superior vena cava caused by surrounding tumor and radiation fibrosis. There are collaterals at the thoracic inlet and retrograde flow down the azygos vein *(arrow)*. B, Balloon angioplasty of the stenosis before stent placement. C, Magnified view of the Wallstent traversing the site of the dilated stenosis. D, Cavagram after placement of the Wallstent showing free flow of contrast into the right atrium and pulmonary circulation. After the procedure the patient experienced immediate relief of his symptoms.

transient phrenic nerve palsy, postulated to be caused by compression of the nerve against the surrounding tumor and radiation fibrosis.[60]

The role of intravascular stents in nonmalignant SVCO has not been defined. Patients with SVCO from fibrosing mediastinitis have been successfully treated,[60,169] although the likelihood of late recurrence of the stenosis either from progression of the mediastinal fibrosis or from endothelial proliferation within the superior vena cava is not known.[192]

REFERENCES

1. Aberle DR, Gamsu G, Golden JA: Fatal systemic arterial air embolism following lung needle aspiration, *Radiology* 165:351-353, 1987.
2. Adler OB, Rosenberger A, Peleg H: Fine needle aspiration of mediastinal masses: evaluation of 136 experiences, *AJR* 140:893-896, 1983.
3. Ali MK, Ewer MS, Balakrishnan PV, et al: Balloon angioplasty for superior vena cava obstruction, *Ann Intern Med* 107:856-857, 1987.
4. American Thoracic Society: Guidelines for percutaneous transthoracic needle biopsy, *Am Rev Respir Dis* 140:255-256, 1989.
5. Aronberg DJ, Sagel SS, Jost RG, et al: Percutaneous drainage of lung abscess, *AJR* 132:282-283, 1979.
6. Baker BK, Awwad EE: Computed tomography of fatal cerebral air embolism following percutaneous aspiration biopsy of the lung, *J Comput Assist Tomogr* 12:1082-1083, 1988.
7. Ball JB, Delaney JC, Evans CC, et al: Endoscopic bougie and balloon dilatation of multiple bronchial stenoses: 10 year follow up, *Thorax* 46:933-935, 1991.
8. Berquist TH, Bailey PB, Cortese DA, Miller WE: Transthoracic needle biopsy: accuracy and complications in relation to location and type of lesion, *Mayo Clin Proc* 55:475-481, 1980.
9. Botenga ASJ: *Selective bronchial and intercostal arteriography,* Baltimore, 1970, Williams & Wilkins.
10. Bourgouin PM, Shepard JO, McLoud TC, et al: Transthoracic needle aspiration biopsy: evaluation of the blood patch technique, *Radiology* 166:93-95, 1988.
11. Calhoun P, Feldman PS, Armstrong P, et al: The clinical outcome of needle aspirations of the lung when cancer is not diagnosed, *Ann Thorac Surg* 41:592-596, 1986.
12. Carrasco CH, Charnsangavej C, Wright KC, et al: Use of the Gianturco self-expanding stent in stenoses of the superior and inferior venae cavae, *J Vasc Intervent Radiol* 3:409-419, 1992.
13. Casola G, vanSonnenberg E, Keightley A, et al: Pneumothorax: radiologic treatment with small catheters, *Radiology* 166:89-91, 1988.
14. Cassel DM, Birnberg FA: Preventing pneumothorax after lung biopsy: the roll-over technique, *Radiology* 174:282, 1990.
15. Chang DB, Yang PC, Luh KT, et al: Ultrasound-guided pleural biopsy with Tru-Cut needle, *Chest* 100:1328-1333, 1991.
16. Charig MJ, Stutley JE, Padley SPG, Hansell DM: The value of negative needle biopsy in suspected operable lung cancer, *Clin Radiol* 44:147-149, 1991.
17. Charnsangavej C, Carrasco CH, Wallace S, et al: Stenosis of the vena cava: preliminary assessment of treatment with expandable metallic stents, *Radiology* 161:295-298, 1986.
18. Cinti D, Hawkins HB: Aspiration biopsy of peripheral pulmonary masses using real-time sonographic guidance, *AJR* 142:1115-1116, 1984.
19. Cohan RH, Newman GE, Braun SD, Dunnick NR: Fluoroscopically guided transthoracic needle aspiration biopsy, *J Comput Assist Tomogr* 8:1093-1098, 1984.
20. Cohen AM, Doershuk CF, Stern RC: Bronchial artery embolization to control hemoptysis in cystic fibrosis, *Radiology* 175:401-405, 1990.
21. Conces DJ, Clark SA, Tarver RD, Schwenk GR: Transthoracic aspiration needle biopsy: value in the diagnosis of pulmonary infections, *AJR* 152:31-34, 1989.
22. Conces DJ, Jr, Schwenk GRJ, Jr, Doering PR, Glant MD: Thoracic needle biopsy: improved results utilizing the team approach, *Chest* 91:813-816, 1987.
23. Dawson SL, Neff CC, Mueller PR, et al: Fatal hemorrhage after inadvertent transpleural biliary drainage, *AJR* 141:33-34, 1983.
24. Di Chiro G: Unintentional spinal cord arteriography: a warning, *Radiology* 112:231-233, 1974.
25. Dick R, Heard BE, Hinson KFW, et al: Aspiration needle biopsy of thoracic lesions: an assessment of 227 biopsies, *Br J Chest* 68141:8633-8694, 1974.
26. Egan AM, Flower CDR: Expandable metal stents for tracheobronchial obstruction, *Clin Radiol* 49:162-165, 1994.
27. Elson JD, Becker GJ, Wholey MH, Ehrman KO: Vena caval and central venous stenoses: management with Palmaz balloon-expandable intraluminal stents, *J Vasc Intervent Radiol* 2:215-223, 1991.
28. Engeler CE, Hunter DW, Castaneda-Zuniga W, et al: Pneumothorax after lung biopsy: prevention with transpleural placement of compressed collagen foam plugs, *Radiology* 184:787-789, 1992.
29. Fairfax AJ, Ball J, Batten JC, Heard BE: Pathological study following bronchial artery embolization for haemoptysis in cystic fibrosis, *Br J Dis Chest* 74:345-352, 1980.
30. Fellows KE, Khaw KT, Schuster S, Shawchman H: Bronchial artery embolization in cystic fibrosis: technique and long-term results, *J Pediatr* 95:959-963, 1979.
31. Ferris EJ: Pulmonary hemorrhage: vascular evaluation and interventional therapy, *Chest* 80:710-714, 1981.
32. Fink I, Gamsu G, Harter LP: CT guided aspiration biopsy of the thorax, *J Comput Assist Tomogr* 6:958-962, 1982.
33. Fish GD, Stanley JH, Miller KS, et al: Post-biopsy pneumothorax: estimating the risk by chest radiography and pulmonary function tests, *AJR* 150:71-74, 1988.
34. Franseen CC: Aspiration biopsy with a description of a new type of needle, *N Engl J Med* 224:1054-1058, 1941.
35. Garcarek J, Marciniak R: Application of Spongostan and Mersilene for embolization of bronchial arteries, *Eur Radiol* 2-4:287-291, 1992.
36. Garzon AA, Gourin A: Surgical management of massive haemoptysis, *Ann Thorac Surg* 187:267-271, 1978.
37. Gatenby RA, Mulhern JR, Broder GJ, Moldofsky PJ: Computed tomographic guided biopsy of small apical and peripheral upper lobe lung masses, *Radiology* 150:591-592, 1984.
38. George PJM, Irving JD, Khagani A, Dick R: Role of the Gianturco expandable metal stent in the management of tracheobronchial obstruction, *Cardiovasc Intervent Radiol* 15:375-381, 1992.
39. George PJM, Irving JD, Mantell BS, Rudd RM: Covered expandable metal stents for recurrent tracheal obstruction, *Lancet* 335:581-582, 1990.
40. Gleeson F, Lomas DJ, Flower CDR, et al: Powered cutting needle biopsy of the pleura and chest wall, *Clin Radiol* 41:199-201, 1990.
41. Glynn TP: Transosseous approach for thoracic needle biopsy, *Radiology* 177:278-279, 1990.
42. Gobien RP, Skucas J, Panis S: CT assisted fluoroscopically guided aspiration biopsy of central hilar and mediastinal masses, *Radiology* 141:443-447, 1981.
43. Gobien RP, Stanley JH, Gobien BS, et al: Percutaneous catheter aspiration and drainage of suspected mediastinal abscesses, *Radiology* 151:69-71, 1984.
44. Goldberg MA, Mueller PR, Saini S, et al: Importance of daily rounds by the radiologist after interventional procedures of the abdomen and chest, *Radiology* 180:767-770, 1991.
45. Graham RJ, Heyd RL, Raval VA, Barrett TF: Lung torsion after percutaneous needle biopsy of lung, *AJR* 159:35-37, 1992.

46. Greene R: Transthoracic needle aspiration biopsy. In Athanasoulis CA et al, eds: *Interventional radiology*, Philadelphia, 1982, WB Saunders.

47. Greene R, Szyfelbein WM, Isler RJ, et al: Supplementary tissue-core histology from fine-needle transthoracic aspiration biopsy, *AJR* 144:787-792, 1985.

48. Gutowicz MA, Quinones-Baldrich WJ, Lieber CP, et al: Operative treatment of refractory superior vena caval syndrome, *Ann Surg* 50:399-401, 1984.

49. Haaga JR, LiPuma, JP, Bryan PJ, et al: Clinical comparison of small and large-caliber cutting needles for biopsy, *Radiology* 146:665-667, 1983.

50. Haramati LB, Austin JHM: Complications after CT-guided needle biopsy through aerated versus nonaerated lung, *Radiology* 181:778, 1991.

51. Hayakawa K, Tanaka F, Torizuka T, et al: Bronchial artery embolization for hemoptysis: immediate and long-term results, *Cardiovasc Intervent Radiol* 15:154-159, 1992.

52. Herman PG, Hessel SJ: The diagnostic accuracy and complications of closed lung biopsies, *Radiology* 125:11-14, 1977.

53. Herman SJ, Holub RV, Weisbrod GL, Chamberlain DW: Anterior mediastinal masses: utility of transthoracic needle biopsy, *Radiology* 180:167-170, 1991.

54. Hetzel MR, Millar MO, Ayesh R, et al: Laser treatment for carcinoma of the bronchus, *Br Med J* 286:12-16, 1983.

55. Hickey NM, Peterson RA, Leech JA, et al: Percutaneous embolotherapy in life threatening hemoptysis, *Cardiovasc Intervent Radiol* 11:270-273, 1988.

56. House AJS: Biopsy techniques in the investigation of diseases of the lung, mediastinum, and chest wall, *Radiol Clin North Am* 17:393-412, 1979.

57. Hunnam GR, Flower CDR: Radiologically guided percutaneous catheter drainage of empyemas, *Clin Radiol* 39:121-126, 1988.

58. Ikezoe J, Sone S, Higashihara T, et al: Sonographically guided needle biopsy for diagnosis of thoracic lesions, *AJR* 143:229-234, 1984.

59. Irving JD, Goldstraw P: Tracheobronchial stents, *Semin Intervent Radiol* 8:295-304, 1991.

60. Irving JD, Kurdziel JC, Reidy JF, et al: Gianturco self expanding stents: clinical experience in the vena cava and large veins, *Cardiovasc Intervent Radiol* 15:328-333, 1992.

61. Ivanick MJ, Thorwarth W, Donohue J, et al: Infarction of the left mainstem bronchus: a complication of bronchial artery embolization, *AJR* 141:535-537, 1983.

62. Izumi S, Tamaki S, Natori H, et al: Ultrasonically guided aspiration needle biopsy in disease of the chest, *Am Rev Respir Dis* 125:460-464, 1982.

63. Jardin M, Remy J: Control of hemoptysis: systemic angiography and anastomoses of the internal mammary artery, *Radiology* 168:377-383, 1988.

64. Kardjiev V, Symeonov A, Charkov I: Etiology, pathogenesis and prevention of spinal cord lesions in selective angiography of the bronchial and intercostal arteries, *Radiology* 112:81-83, 1974.

65. Keller FS, Rosch J, Barker AF, et al: Percutaneous interventional catheter therapy for lesions of the chest and lungs, *Chest* 81:407-412, 1982.

66. Khouri NF, Meziane MA: Transthoracic needle aspiration biopsy — optimizing the yield, *J Thorac Imag* 2:18-26, 1987.

67. Khouri NF, Stitik FP, Erozan YZ, et al: Transthoracic needle aspiration biopsy of benign and malignant lung lesions, *AJR* 144:281-288, 1985.

68. Kreula J: Effect on sampling technique on specimen size in fine needle aspiration biopsy, *Invest Radiol* 25:1294-1299, 1990.

69. Kreula J, Virkunnen P, Bondestam S: Effect of suction on specimen size in fine needle aspiration biopsy, *Invest Radiol* 25:1175-1181, 1990.

70. Kucharczyk W, Weisbrod GL, Cooper JD, et al: Cardiac tamponade as a complication of thin needle aspiration lung biopsy, *Chest* 82:120, 1982.

71. Lalli AF, McCormack LJ, Zelch M, et al: Aspiration biopsies of chest lesions, *Radiology* 127:35-40, 1978.

72. Lalli AF, Naylor B, Whitehouse WM: Aspiration biopsy of thoracic lesions, *Thorax* 22:404, 1967.

73. Law MR, Henk JM, Goldstraw P, Hodson ME: Bronchoscopic implantation of radioactive gold grains into endobronchial carcinoma, *Br J Chest* 79:147-151, 1985.

74. Ledingham SJM, Goldstraw P: Diathermy resection and radioactive gold grains for palliation of obstruction due to recurrence of bronchial carcinoma after external irradiation, *Thorax* 44:48-51, 1989.

75. Lee KS, Im JG, Kim YH, et al: Treatment of thoracic multiloculated empyemas with intracavitary urokinase: a prospective study, *Radiology* 179:771-775, 1991.

76. Lee LH: A new biopsy needle and its clinical use, *AJR* 121:854-859, 1974.

77. Lemoigne F, Rampal P, Petersen R: Fatal ischemic colitis after bronchial artery embolization, *Nouv Presse Med* 12:2056-2057, 1983.

78. Leyden T: Uber infektiose pneumonie, *Dtsch Med Wochenschr* 9:52-54, 1883.

79. Lois JF, Gomes AS, Smith DC, Laks H: Systemic-to-pulmonary collateral vessels and shunts: treatment with embolization, *Radiology* 169:671-676, 1980.

80. Lokich JJ, Goodman R: Superior vena caval syndrome: clinical management, *JAMA* 231:58-61, 1975.

81. Lomas DJ, Padley SG, Flower CDR: The sonographic appearances of pleural fluid, *Br J Radiol* 66:619-624, 1993.

82. Mathisen DJ: A surgeon's view of interventional radiology in general thoracic surgery patients, *Semin Intervent Radiol* 8:85-87, 1991.

83. Mauro MA, Jaques PF, Morris S: Bronchial artery embolization for control of hemoptysis, *Semin Intervent Radiol* 9:45-51, 1992.

84. McCartney R, Tait D, Stilson M, Seidel GF: A technique for the prevention of pneumothorax in pulmonary aspiration biopsy, *AJR* 120:872-875, 1974.

85. McCorkell SJ: Unintended aspiration of pulmonary echinococcal cysts, *AJR* 143:123, 1984.

86. McPherson S, Routh WD, Nath H, Keller FS: Anomalous origin of bronchial arteries: potential pitfall of embolotherapy for hemoptysis, *J Vasc Intervent Radiol* 1:86-88, 1990.

87. Meyer JE, Ferrucci JT, Janower ML: Fatal complications of percutaneous lung biopsy, *Radiology* 96:47-48, 1970.

88. Meyer JE, Gandbhir LH, Milner LB, et al: Percutaneous needle biopsy of nodular lung lesions, *J Thorac Cardiovasc Surg* 73:787-791, 1977.

89. Miller KS, Fish GB, Stanley JH, Schabel SI: Prediction of pneumothorax rate in percutaneous needle aspiration of the lung, *Chest* 93:872-875, 1988.

90. Milner LB, Ryan K, Gullo J: Fatal intrathoracic haemorrhage after percutaneous lung biopsy, *AJR* 132:280-281, 1979.

91. Moinuddin SM, Lee LH, Montgomery JH: Mediastinal needle biopsy, *AJR* 143:531-532, 1984.

92. Molina PL, Solomon SL, Glazer HS, et al: A one-piece unit for treatment of pneumothorax complicating needle biopsy: evaluation in 10 patients, *AJR* 155:31-33, 1990.

93. Montgomery WW: T-tube tracheal stent, *Arch Otolaryngol* 82:320-321, 1965.

94. Moore EH, LeBlanc J, Montesi SA, et al: Effects of patient positioning after needle aspiration lung biopsy, *Radiology* 181:385-387, 1991.

95. Moore EH, Shepard JO, McLoud TC, et al: Positional precautions in needle aspiration lung biopsy, *Radiology* 175:733-735, 1990.

96. Moore PO, Mueller PR, Simeone JF, et al: Sonographic guidance in diagnostic and therapeutic interventions in the pleural space, *AJR* 149:1-5, 1987.

97. Morrison MC, Mueller PR, Lee MJ, et al: Sclerotherapy of malignant pleural effusions through sonographically placed small-bore catheters, *AJR* 158:41-43, 1992.

98. Morrissey B, Adams H, Gibbs AR, Crane MD: Percutaneous needle biopsy of the mediastinum: review of 94 procedures, *Thorax* 48:632-637, 1993.

99. Müller NL, Bergin CJ, Miller RR, Ostrow DN: Seeding of malignant cells into the needle tract after lung and pleural biopsy, *J Can Assoc Radiol* 37:192-194, 1986.

100. Munk PL, Morris DC, Nelems B: Left main bronchial-esophageal fistula: a complication of bronchial artery embolization, *Cardiovasc Intervent Radiol* 13:95-97, 1990.

101. Naar CA, Soong J, Clore F, Hawkins IF Jr: Control of massive hemoptysis by bronchial artery embolization with absolute alcohol, *AJR* 140:271-272, 1983.

102. Nahman BJ, Van Aman ME, McLemore WE, O'Toole RV: Use of the Rotex needle in percutaneous biopsy of nodular lung lesions, *AJR* 145:97-99, 1985.

103. Nashef SA, Dromer C, Velly JF, et al: Expanding wire stents in benign tracheobronchial disease: indications and complications, *Ann Thorac Surg* 54:937-940, 1992.

104. Neff CC, Mueller PR, Ferrucci JT, et al: Serious complications following transgression of the pleural space in drainage procedures, *Radiology* 152:335-341, 1984.

105. Newton TH, Preger L: Selective bronchial arteriography, *Radiology* 84:1043-1051, 1965.

106. Nordenstrom B: New instruments for biopsy, *Radiology* 117:474, 1975.

107. Norenberg R, Claxton CP, Takaro T: Percutaneous needle biopsy of the lung: report of two fatal complications, *Chest* 66:216-218, 1974.

108. Pagliero KM, Shepherd MP: Use of stainless steel wire coil in treatment of anastomotic dehiscence after cervical tracheal resection, *J Thorac Cardiovasc Surg* 67:932-935, 1974.

109. Parker LA, Melton JW, Delany DJ, Yankaskas BC: Percutaneous small bore catheter drainage in the management of lung abscesses, *Chest* 92:213-218, 1987.

110. Pearce JG, Patt NL: Fatal pulmonary hemorrhage after percutaneous aspiration lung biopsy, *Am Rev Respir Dis* 110:346-349, 1974.

111. Pedersen OM, Aasen TB, Gulsvik A: Fine needle aspiration biopsy of mediastinal and peripheral pulmonary masses guided by real-time sonography, *Chest* 89:504-508, 1986.

112. Penketh ARL, Robinson AA, Barker V, Flower CDR: Use of percutaneous needle biopsy in the investigation of solitary pulmonary nodules, *Thorax* 42:967-971, 1987.

113. Perez CA, Presant CA, van Amburg IL: Management of superior vena caval obstruction, *Semin Oncol* 5:123-134, 1978.

114. Perlmutt LM, Braun SD, Newman GE, et al: Timing of chest film follow-up after transthoracic needle aspiration, *AJR* 146:1049-1050, 1986.

115. Perlmutt LM, Braun SD, Newman GE, et al: Transthoracic needle aspiration: use of a small chest tube to treat pneumothorax, *AJR* 148:849-851, 1987.

116. Perlmutt LM, Johnston WW, Dunnick NR: Percutaneous transthoracic needle aspiration: a review, *AJR* 152:451-455, 1989.

117. Philpott NJ, Woodhead MA, Wilson AG, Millard FJC: Lung abscess: a neglected cause of life threatening haemoptysis, *Thorax* 48:674-675, 1993.

118. Poe RH, Kallay MC: Transthoracic needle biopsy of lung in non-hospitalized patients, *Chest* 92:676-678, 1987.

119. Poe RH, Kallay MC, Wicks CM, Odoroff CH: Predicting risk of pneumothorax in needle biopsy of the lung, *Chest* 85:232-235, 1984.

120. Pump KK: Distribution of bronchial arteries in the human lung, *Chest* 62:447-451, 1972.

121. Putnam JS, Uchida BT, Antonivic R, Rosch J: Superior vena cava syndrome associated with massive thrombosis: treatment with expandable stents, *Radiology* 167:727-728, 1988.

122. Rabkin JE, Astafjev VI, Gothman LN, Grigorjev YG: Transcatheter embolization in the management of pulmonary hemorrhage, *Radiology* 163:361-365, 1987.

123. Remy J, Arnaud A, Fardou H, et al: Treatment of hemoptysis by embolization of bronchial arteries, *Radiology* 122:33-37, 1977.

124. Remy-Jardin M, Wattinne L, Remy J: Transcatheter occlusion of pulmonary arterial circulation and collateral supply: failures, incidents and complications, *Radiology* 180:699-705, 1991.

125. Roberts AC: Bronchial artery embolization therapy, *J Thorac Imag* 5:60-72, 1990.

126. Rosch J, Bedell JS, Putnam J, et al: Gianturco expandable wire stents in the treatment of superior vena cava syndrome recurring after maximum tolerance radiation, *Cancer* 60:1243-1246, 1987.

127. Rosenberger A, Adler O: Fine needle aspiration biopsy in the diagnosis of mediastinal lesions, *AJR* 131:239-242, 1978.

128. Rousseau H, Dahan M, Lauque D, et al: Self-expandable prostheses in the tracheobronchial tree, *Radiology* 188:199-203, 1993.

129. Sagel SS, Ferguson TB, Forrest JR, et al: Percutaneous transthoracic aspiration needle biopsy, *Ann Thorac Surg* 26:399-405, 1978.

130. Samelson SL, Goldberg EM, Ferguson MK: The thoracic vent, clinical experience with a new device for treating simple pneumothorax, *Chest* 100:880-882, 1991.

131. Sargent EN, Turner AF, Gordonson J, et al: Percutaneous pulmonary needle biopsy: report on 350 patients, *AJR* 122:758-768, 1974.

132. Sawada S, Tanigawa N, Kobayashi M, et al: Malignant tracheobronchial obstructive lesions: treatment with Gianturco expandable metallic stents, *Radiology* 188:205-208, 1993.

133. Sawhney S, Jain R, Berry M: Tru-Cut biopsy of mediastinal masses guided by real-time ultrasound, *Clin Radiol* 44:16-19, 1991.

134. Schafers H, Haydock DA, Cooper JD: The prevalence and management of bronchial anastomotic complications in lung transplantation, *J Thorac Cardiovasc Surg* 101:1044-1052, 1991.

135. Scott WW, Kuhlman JE: Focal pulmonary lesions in patients with AIDS: percutaneous transthoracic needle biopsy, *Radiology* 180:419-421, 1991.

136. Sherry CS, Diamond NG, Meyers TP, Martin RL: Successful treatment of superior vena cava syndrome by venous angioplasty, *AJR* 147:834-835, 1986.

137. Shevland JE: Right ventricular perforation: a rare complication of percentaneous lung biopsy, *J Thorac Imag* 6:85-86, 1991.

138. Sider L, Davis TM: Hilar masses: evaluation with CT guided biopsy after negative bronchoscopic examination, *Radiology* 164:107-109, 1987.

139. Silverman SG, Mueller PR, Saini S, et al: Thoracic empyema: management with image guided catheter drainage, *Radiology* 169:5-9, 1988.

140. Simmonds AK, Irving JD, Clark SW, Dick R: Use of expandable metal stents in the treatment of bronchial obstruction, *Thorax* 44:680-681, 1989.

141. Sinner WN: Complications of percutaneous transthoracic needle aspiration biopsy, *Acta Radiol* 17:813-828, 1976.

142. Sinner WN, Zajicek J: Implantation metastasis after percutaneous transthoracic needle aspiration biopsy, *Acta Radiol* 17:473-480, 1976.

143. Skupin A, Gomez F, Husain M, et al: Complications of transthoracic needle biopsy decreased with isobutyl 2-cyanoacrylate: a pilot study, *Ann Thorac Surg* 43:406-408, 1987.

144. Slawson RG, Scott RM: Radiation therapy for bronchogenic carcinoma, *Radiology* 132:175-176, 1979.

145. Solomon N, Holey MH, Jarmolowski CR: Intravascular stents in the management of superior vena cava syndrome, *Cathet Cardiovasc Diagn* 23:245-252, 1991.

146. Stanley JH, Fish GD, Andriole JG, et al: Lung lesions: cytologic diagnosis by fine needle biopsy, *Radiology* 162:389-391, 1987.

147. Sterrett G, Whitaker D, Shilkin KB, et al: The fine needle aspiration cytology of mediastinal lesions, *Cancer* 51:127-135, 1983.

148. Stevens GM, Jackman RJ: Outpatient needle biopsy of the lung; its safety and utility, *Radiology* 151:301-304, 1984.

149. Stoll JF, Bettmann MA: Bronchial artery embolization to control hemoptysis: a review, *Cardiovasc Intervent Radiol* 11:263-269, 1988.

150. Surprenant EL: Transthoracic needle aspiration biopsy: evaluation of the blood patch technique, *Radiology* 168:285, 1988.

151. Sweezey NB, Fellows KF: Bronchial artery embolization for severe hemoptysis in cystic fibrosis, *Chest* 97:1322-1326, 1990.

152. Tikkakoski T, Lohela P, Leppanen M, et al: Ultrasound-guided aspiration biopsy of anterior mediastinal masses, *J Clin Ultrasound* 19:209-214, 1991.

153. Todd TRJ, Weisbrod G, Tao LC, et al: Aspiration needle biopsy of thoracic lesions, *Ann Thorac Surg* 32:154-161, 1981.

154. Tolly TL, Feldmeier JE, Czarnecki D: Air embolism complicating percutaneous lung biopsy, *AJR* 150:555-556, 1988.

155. Tonkin ILD, Hanissian AS, Boulden TF, et al: Bronchial arteriography and embolotherapy for hemoptysis in patients with cystic fibrosis, *Cardiovasc Intervent Radiol* 14:241-246, 1991.

156. Tsang V, Williams AM, Goldstraw P: Sequential Silastic and expandable metal stenting for tracheobronchial strictures, *Ann Thorac Surg* 53:856-860, 1992.

157. Uflacker R, Kaemmerer A, Neves C, Picon PD: Management of massive hemoptysis by bronchial artery embolization, *Radiology* 146:627-634, 1983.

158. Uflacker R, Kaemmerer A, Picon PD, et al: Bronchial artery embolization in the management of hemoptysis: technical aspects and long term results, *Radiology* 157:637-644, 1985.

159. Ulmer JL, Choplin RH, Reed JC: Image-guided catheter drainage of the infected pleural space, *J Thorac Imag* 6:65-73, 1991.

160. van Moore A Jr, Zuger JH, Kelley MJ: Lung abscess: an interventional radiology perspective, *Semin Intervent Radiol* 8:36-43, 1991.

161. vanSonnenberg E, Casola G, Ho M, et al: Difficult thoracic lesions: CT guided biopsy experience in 150 cases, *Radiology* 167:457-461, 1988.

162. vanSonnenberg E, D'Agostino HB, Casola G, et al: Lung abscess: CT-guided drainage, *Radiology* 178:347-351, 1991.

163. vanSonnenberg E, Lin AS, Deutsch AL, et al: Percutaneous biopsy of difficult mediastinal, hilar and pulmonary lesions by computed tomographic guidance and a modified coaxial technique, *Radiology* 148:300, 1983.

164. vanSonnenberg E, Mueller PR, Ferrucci JTJ: Percutaneous drainage of 250 abdominal abscesses and fluid collections. Part 1. Results, failures and complications, *Radiology* 151:337-341, 1984.

165. vanSonnenberg E, Nakamoto SK, Mueller PR, et al: CT and ultrasound guided catheter drainage of empyemas after chest-tube failure, *Radiology* 151:349-353, 1984.

166. Varela A, Maynar M, Irving JD, et al: Use of Gianturco self-expandable stents in the tracheobronchial tree, *Ann Thorac Surg* 49:806-809, 1990.

167. Vine HS, Kasdon EJ, Simon M: Percutaneous lung biopsy using the Lee needle and a track-obliterating technique, *Radiology* 144:921-922, 1982.

168. Wallace MJ, Charnsangavej C, Ogawa K, et al: Tracheobronchial tree: expandable metallic stents used in experimental and clinical applications, *Radiology* 158:309-312, 1985.

169. Watkinson AF, Hansell DM: Expandable Wallstent for the treatment of superior vena cava obstruction, *Thorax* 49:915-920, 1993.

170. Weisbrod GL: Percutaneous fine needle aspiration biopsy of the mediastinum, *Clin Chest Med* 8:27-41, 1987.

171. Weisbrod GL: Transthoracic percutaneous fine-needle aspiration biopsy in the chest and mediastinum, *Semin Intervent Radiol* 8:1-14, 1991.

172. Weisbrod GL, Herman SJ, Liang-Che T: Preliminary experience with a dual cutting edge needle in thoracic percutaneous fine needle biopsy, *Radiology* 163:300-302, 1987.

173. Weisbrod GL, Lyons DJ, Tao LC, Chamberlain DW: Percutaneous fine needle aspiration biopsy of mediastinal lesions, *AJR* 143:525-529, 1984.

174. Weissberg D: Percutaneous drainage of lung abscess, *J Thorac Cardiovasc Surg* 87:308-312, 1984.

175. Westaby S, Jackson JW, Pearson FG: A bifurcated silicone rubber stent for relief of tracheobronchial obstruction, *J Thorac Cardiovasc Surg* 83:414-417, 1982.

176. Westcott JL: Air embolism complicating percutaneous needle biopsy of the lung, *Chest* 63:108-110, 1973.

177. Westcott JL: Direct percutaneous needle aspiration of localized pulmonary lesions: results in 422 patients, *Radiology* 137:31-35, 1980.

178. Westcott JL: Percutaneous needle biopsy of hilar and mediastinal masses, *Radiology* 141:323-328, 1981.

179. Westcott JL: Percutaneous catheter drainage of pleural effusion and empyema, *AJR* 144:1189-1193, 1985.

180. Westcott JL: Transthoracic needle biopsy of the hilum and mediastinum, *J Thorac Imag* 2:41-48, 1987.

181. Westcott JL: Percutaneous transthoracic needle biopsy, *Radiology* 169:593-601, 1988.

182. Wholey MH, Chamorro HA, Rao G, et al: Bronchial artery embolization for massive hemoptysis, *JAMA* 236:2501-2504, 1976.

183. Winning AJ, McIvor J, Seed WA, et al: Interpretation of negative results in fine needle aspiration of discrete pulmonary lesions, *Thorax* 41:875-879, 1986.

184. Wittich GR, Nowels KW, Korn RL, et al: Coaxial transthoracic fine-needle biopsy in patients with a history of malignant lymphoma, *Radiology* 183:175-178, 1992.

185. Yang PC, Chang DB, Yu CJ, et al: Ultrasound-guided core biopsy of thoracic tumors, *Am Rev Respir Dis* 146:763-767, 1992.

186. Yang PC, Luh KT, Sheu JC, et al: Peripheral pulmonary lesions: ultrasonography and ultrasonically guided aspiration biopsy, *Radiology* 155:451-456, 1985.

187. Yankelevitz DF, Henschke CI, Davis SD: Percutaneous CT biopsy of chest lesions: an in vitro analysis of the effect of partial volume averaging on needle positioning, *AJR* 161:273-278, 1993.

188. Yu CJ, Yang BC, Chang DB, et al: Evaluation of ultrasonically guided biopsies of mediastinal masses, *Chest* 100:399-405, 1991.

189. Yuan A, Yang PC, Chang DB: Ultrasound-guided aspiration biopsy of small peripheral pulmonary nodules, *Chest* 101:926-930, 1992.

190. Zavala DC, Bedell GN: Percutaneous lung biopsy with a cutting needle: an analysis of 40 cases and comparison with other biopsy techniques, *Am Rev Respir Dis* 106:186-193, 1972.

191. Zavala DC, Schoell JE: Ultrathin needle aspiration of the lung in infectious and malignant disease, *Am Rev Respir Dis* 123:125-131, 1981.

192. Zollikofer C, Largiader I, Bruhlmann WF, et al: Endovascular stenting of veins and grafts: preliminary clinical experience, *Radiology* 167:707-712, 1988.

Index

A

Abdominal mass, hypoplasia of lung associated with, 620
Abdominal pain
  helminthic infection indicated by, 255
  pleural effusion caused by hepatic abscess indicated by, 673
ABMA; *see* Anti–basement membrane antibody disease
ABPA; *see* Allergic bronchopulmonary aspergillosis
Abscess
  amebic liver, 216
  brain
    computed tomographic scan of, 627f
    Legionnaire's disease and, 159
  central nervous system, bacterial infection as cause of, 238
  cutaneous cold, Job's syndrome and, 541
  hepatic, pleural effusion caused by, 673
  lung; *see* Lung abscess
  mediastinal, 883
  paraspinal, paraspinal mass caused by, 805
  pleural effusion caused by, 655, 672-673
  pulmonary, matched defects in ventilation scanning caused by, 379-380
  subcutaneous, blastomycosis indicated by, 204
Abscess cavity, pneumonia associated with, 153
Acanthosis nigricans, lung carcinoma associated with, 273
Accessory diaphragm, 635
ACE; *see* Angiotensin-converting enzyme
Acebutolol, pleural changes associated with, 679
Acetylsalicylic acid, pulmonary edema caused by, 465
Achondroplasia, hypoplasia of lung associated with, 620
Achromic patches, tuberous sclerosis associated with, 591
Acidemia, pulmonary hypertension associated with, 402
Acinar shadow
  asthma associated with, 844
  bleomycin adverse effects indicated by, 471
  cardiogenic alveolar edema associated with, 410
  definition of, 66
  description of, 113-114
  diffuse pulmonary hemorrhage indicated by, 523
  examples of, 68f
  helminthic infection indicated by, 255
  high-resolution computed tomography and, 133
  pulmonary alveolar proteinosis indicated by, 597
  sarcoidosis associated with, 578
Acinetobacter, pneumonia caused by, 157
Acinus, description of, 21
Acquired immunodeficiency syndrome, 229-271
  bacterial infections associated with, 238-240
  Castleman's disease and, 756
  cryptococcosis associated with, 200
  disseminated histoplasmosis and, 239
  herpes simplex pneumonia and, 215
  lymphocytic interstitial pneumonitis associated with, 333

Acquired immunodeficiency syndrome — cont'd
  malignancies in, 240-244
  mediastinal and hilar node enlargement caused by, 747
  Mycobacterium tuberculosis associated with, 230-232
  Nocardia infection associated with, 190
  nontuberculous mycobacterial infection and, 232-233
  pneumothorax caused by, 691
  pulmonary infections in, 229-240
  pulmonary tuberculosis associated with, 176
  reactivation tuberculosis associated with, 172
Acromegaly, lung carcinoma associated with, 273
ACTH; *see* Adrenocorticotropic hormone
Actinomycetes, extrinsic allergic alveolitis and, 541
Actinomycin D, radiation effects heightened by, 478
Actinomycosis
  broncholithiasis associated with, 836
  description of, 192
  radiograph of, 193f
  tracheoesophageal fistula caused by, 825
Acute chest syndrome, description of, 406
Acute inhalational injury, description of, 450-452
Acute respiratory distress syndrome, inhalational injury and, 451
Addison's disease, thymic hyperplasia associated with, 730
Adenocarcinoma
  bronchial, 272, 274
    calcification in solitary pulmonary nodule and, 99f
    computed tomographic scan of, 279f
    pleural effusion caused by, 297t
  central tumor, lymph node involvement and, 288
  computed tomographic scan of, 102, 278f
  cryptogenic fibrosing alveolitis associated with, 492
  peripheral nodule associated with, 298
  pleural effusion in, 297
  rate of growth of, 277
  scarred lung associated with, 273
  systemic sclerosis associated with, 516
  tracheal tumor and, 312
Adenoma
  multiple endocrine, thymic carcinoid and, 728
  parathyroid, 723
    computed tomography for detection of, 9
    needle aspiration of, 723
Adenoma sebaceum
  tuberous sclerosis associated with, 591-592
Adenopathy; *see also* Lymph node; Lymphadenopathy
  focal, tuberculosis identified by, 176
  histoplasmosis and, 195
  Hodgkin's disease and, 318
  lymphoma in acquired immunodeficiency syndrome and, 243
  mediastinal; *see* Mediastinal adenopathy
  Mycobacterium avium-intracellulare infection indicated by, 233
  retroperitoneal, Hodgkin's disease and, 318
  sarcoidosis and, 571-573

---

f indicates a figure; *t* indicates a table.